CLINICAL NURSING SKILLS

BASIC TO ADVANCED SKILLS

Fourth Edition

CLINICAL NURSING SKILLS

BASIC TO ADVANCED SKILLS

Fourth Edition

Sandra F. Smith, RN, MS, ABD
President, National Nursing Review
Los Altos, California

Donna J. Duell, RN, MS, ABD
Director of Nursing
Cabrillo College
Aptos, California

with

Barbara C. Martin, RN, MS, CS
Professor, School of Nursing
The University of Tulsa
Tulsa, Oklahoma

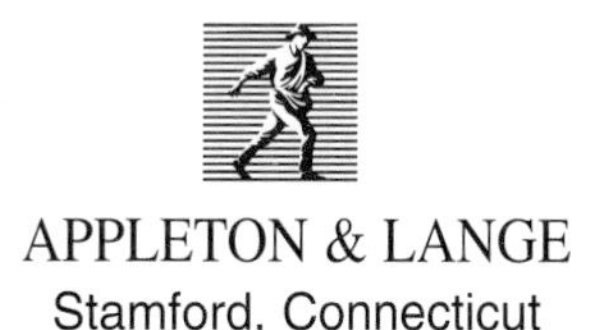

APPLETON & LANGE
Stamford, Connecticut

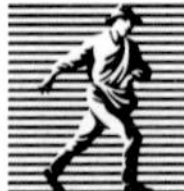

96 97 98 99 / 10 9 8 7 6 5 4 3 2

Prentice Hall International (UK) Limited, *London*
Prentice Hall of Australia Pty. Limited, *Sydney*
Prentice Hall Canada, Inc., *Toronto*
Prentice Hall Hispanoamericana, S.A., *Mexico*
Prentice Hall of India Private Limited, *New Delhi*
Prentice Hall of Japan, Inc., *Tokyo*
Simon and Schuster Asia Pte. Ltd., *Singapore*
Editora Prentice Hall do Brasil Ltda., *Rio de Janeiro*
Prentice Hall, *Upper Saddle River, New Jersey*

Library of Congress Cataloging-in-Publication Data

Smith, Sandra Fucci.
Clinical nursing skills : basic to advanced skills / Sandra F. Smith, Donna J. Duell; with Barbara C. Martin. —4th ed.
p. cm.
Includes bibliographical references and index.
ISBN 0-8385-1389-1 (pbk. : alk. paper)
1. Nursing. I. Duell, Donna. II. Martin, Barbara, M.S. III. Title.
[DNLM: 1. Nursing Process. WY 100 S659c 1996]
RT41.S5826 1996
610.73—dc20
DNLM/DLC 95-31491
for Library of Congress CIP

Acquisitions Editor: David P. Carroll
Editor-in-Chief: Sally J. Barhydt
Production Editor: Sondra Greenfield
Designer: Mary Skudlarek

PRINTED IN THE UNITED STATES OF AMERICA

Contributors

Joan N. Althaus, RN, MSN, CCRN
Doctoral Candidate
Medical Electronics Clinical Specialist
Hewlett-Packard
Dallas, Texas

Abby S. Bloch, MS, RD
Clinical Nutrition Specialist
Memorial Sloan Kettering Cancer Center
New York, New York

Christine Bolwell, RN, MSN, CCRN
Publisher
Nurse Educator's Microworld
Saratoga, California

Randy Caine, RN, MS, EdD
Associate Professor of Nursing
California State University
Long Beach, California

Janet W. Cook, RN, MS
formerly
Assistant Professor
University of North Carolina
Greensboro, North Carolina

Jacqueline Dowling, RN, MS
Director, Nursing Laboratory
University of Massachusetts
Lowell, Massachusetts

Lou Ann Emerson, RN, MSN
Assistant Professor
University of Cincinnati
Cincinnati, Ohio

Rita Fahrner, RN, MS
Clincial Nurse Specialist, AIDS
San Francisco, California

Joan Frommhagen, RN, MS, MA, CET
Assistant Director of Nursing
Cabrillo College
Aptos, California

Nancy Meyer Holloway, RN, MSN, CCRN, CEN
Clinical Specialist and Consultant
Orinda, California

Jill D. Holmes, RN, MS
Legal Nurse Consultant
Gray, Carey, Ames & Frye
San Diego, California

Kathleen Kaplan, RN, MSN, CNM
formerly
Associate in Nursing
Columbia University
New York, New York

Terry W. Miller, RN, MSN, PhD
Associate Professor
San Jose State University
San Jose, California

Susan D. North, RN, MS, ScD
Consultant
Johns Hopkins Program for International Education
Baltimore, Maryland

Sally Talley, RN, ET
Specialist in Enterostomal Therapy
San Jose, California

Jean O. Trotter, RN, C, MS
Assistant Professor
University of Maryland
Baltimore, Maryland

Katherine H. West, RN, BSN
Infection Control Consultant
Springfield, Virginia

Judith A. Yanda, RN, MS
Inservice Education
Santa Teresa Hospital
San Jose, California

Mary G. Yarbrough, RN, MS, MPH
President & CEO
Mercy Healthcare Arizona
Phoenix, Arizona

Contents

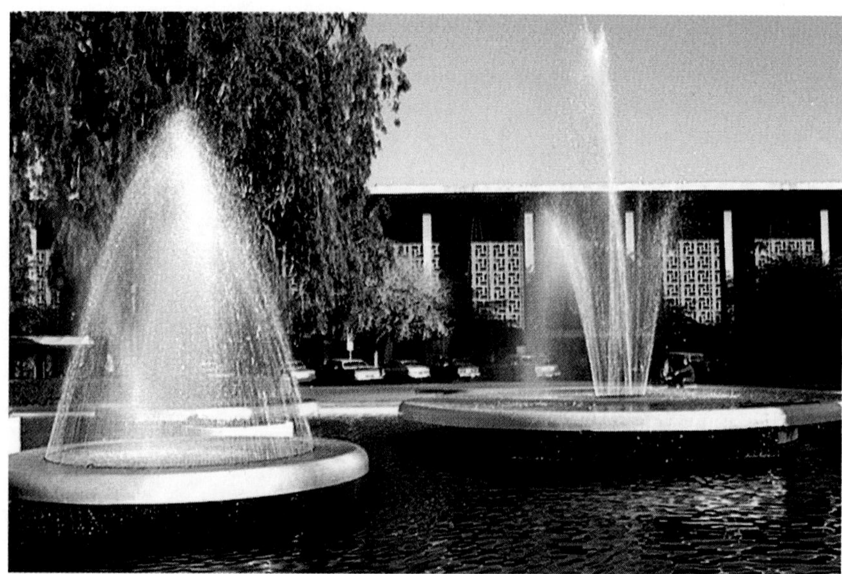

Stanford University Hospital

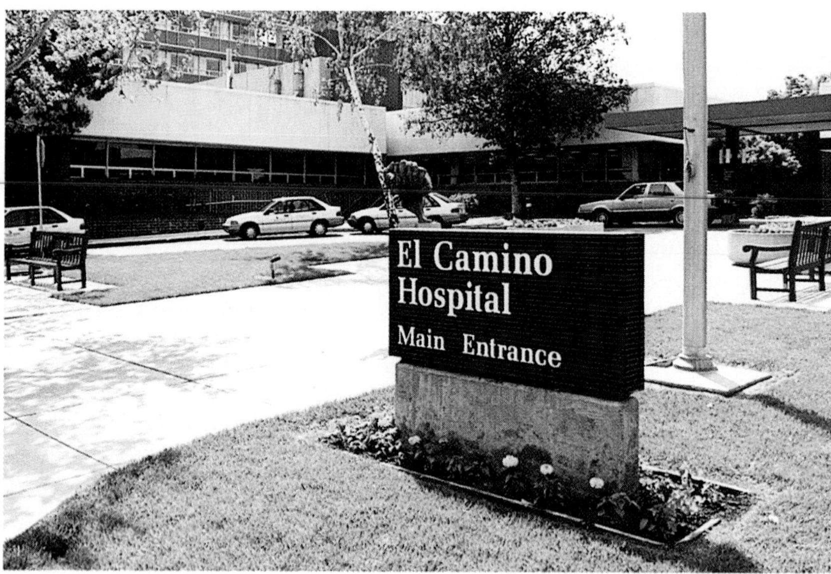

El Camino Hospital

Preface

The authors' goal for the fourth edition of *Clinical Nursing Skills* is to continue the quality presentation of nursing skills that characterized the first three editions of this text. This text is presented in a format adaptable to any curriculum. It is designed for all levels of nursing students—baccalaureate, associate degree, and diploma—who are attempting to master nursing procedures in the clinical setting as a component of their nursing education.

An effective nursing skills text must be current, innovative, and relevant as well as comprehensive so that it will be used by students from basic to intermediate to the advanced level of skills. Thus, this text is appropriate for beginning students learning nursing fundamentals to senior students mastering advanced medical–surgical nursing and finally to nurses working in home care settings. The text first describes basic concepts and then applies them to clinical situations in a nursing process framework.

To use this book in the most effective way, it is important that the reader understand that the material is organized from the most basic level of mastery to the more complex skills. This approach enables the student to perform a specific skill, including how to assess the client, formulate nursing diagnoses, perform the procedure, evaluate the results, and document. Each procedure includes equipment, preparation and the step-by-step performance necessary to master the skill. The nurse can easily access the material for immediate reference in the clinical area. Extensive illustrations and photographs within each unit visually relate to the concepts presented.

Although the nursing process provides the organizing framework for this textbook, additional learning aids have been included to help the student assimilate the immense amount of nursing content. The *critical thinking application* following each unit encourages the student to consider potential problems that may arise while performing skills and offer critical thinking options for problem resolution. *Rationale* for specific nursing actions assists the student to understand why certain actions are performed. *Clinical alerts* call attention to safety issues, critical information, or actions. *Boxed information* emphasizes specific aspects of client care and the additional knowledge necessary for mastery of a particular skill. *Client teaching principles* are included as appropriate. Finally, *geriatric considerations,* a new section following each chapter, present specific concepts underlying nursing care of the elderly.

Special features and benefits that distinguish this book from other similar texts include:

- Comprehensive coverage of over 550 basic and intermediate to advanced skills in the nursing process framework.
- Over 625 new full-color photographs of step-by-step procedures. These clear, specific, and up-to-date illustrations show new equipment, new procedures, and nursing actions.
- The skill format is clear and concise, with step-by-step presentation of individual skills and content that includes rationale, clinical alerts, and adjunct information in boxes.
- Pedagogic features include learning objectives, terminology, nursing diagnoses, references, and bibliographies that focus attention on critical elements and content.
- Rationale for specific nursing actions increases learning but does not overload the student by being presented for every minor step in each skill.

- Critical thinking applications are included for every unit to assist the student in applying the process of critical thinking to clinical situations. If the student encounters an unexpected outcome or event, critical thinking options provide a basis for corrective intervention.
- This edition includes additional higher level medical–surgical skills as well as critical care procedures such as a new chapter on venous access devices.
- Every chapter includes *geriatric considerations.* Due to expanded clinical experience in long-term or subacute care settings and the increased age of hospitalized clients, students are caring for more elderly clients than ever before. This section helps students understand concepts underlying nursing care of the elderly and adjust the skills accordingly.
- A new chapter (Chapter 6), *Stress, Holistic Health, and Alternative Treatment Methods,* focuses on changes in attitudes about health care. This chapter addresses current trends toward alternative medicine, presents material that will assist the student to incorporate new concepts of stress and adaptation, and includes holistic methods for teaching the client how to alleviate stress.
- A second new chapter, *Vascular Access Devices* (Chapter 28), presents the latest methods of administering long-term IV therapy via central lines, cannulas, infusion ports, and peripheral intravenous central catheters (PICC).
- A totally revised chapter on infection control (Chapter 15) incorporates the latest CDC guidelines for nursing care of clients.
- Identification of safety issues and considerations provides critical information essential for student learning. Because the licensing examination focuses on safe clinical judgment, it is important for students to know how to perform skills in a safe and competent manner in order to pass the NCLEX.

For faculty who adopt *Clinical Nursing Skills* a valuable *Instructor's Manual* is available. Each chapter of the manual includes teaching/learning strategies, critical thinking exercises, content examinations, answers to critical thinking exercises and content exams. The last section of the manual consists of the skills checklists in printed form for duplication by the instructor. The checklists are also available on computer disk, packaged with the book for the convenience of the instructor.

The authors are confident that students and faculty will find this new edition of *Clinical Nursing Skills* relevant, useful, and adaptable to their learning needs. Furthermore, the authors hope that faculty will find this textbook a valuable teaching tool and reference for clinical practice.

Sandra F. Smith
Donna J. Duell

Acknowledgments

The authors express their appreciation to the many people who assisted with the fourth edition of *Clinical Nursing Skills*. Through the assistance and generosity of Stanford University Hospital, El Camino Hospital, Watsonville Community Hospital, and Dominican Santa Cruz Hospital, we were able to complete extensive photography in the appropriate clinical environment. We extend our thanks to the administrators and staff, and particularly to the staff development group at these hospitals. We especially express our gratitude to the coordinator of photography, Karen Hoxeng, and our photographer, Ron May; the professional consultants for photography, Sally Miller, Constance Troulinos, Debra Solerno, Karen Isilker, and Sally Talley; and the models for photography, Fiore Solerno, Tarah Smith, Samantha Menna, Audrey Henry Griffiths, Megan Hoxeng, Ellen Duell, Pat Emmons, and Joan Frommhagen. We also wish to extend our thanks to the many unnamed clients who consented to be in the photographs. Last, but by no means least, we wish to thank our friends and families for their encouragement and support during this project.

1

Professional Nursing

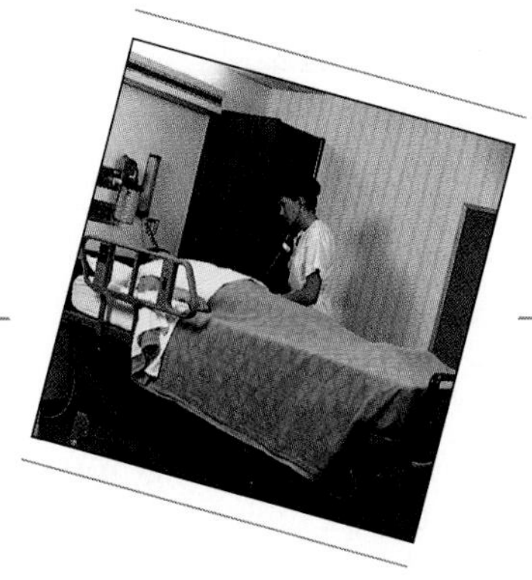

LEARNING OBJECTIVES

- Discuss what is meant by the concept "professional role of the nurse."
- Define the term "accountable."
- List three ways you can assist the client to assume and adapt to the client role.
- Identify the guidelines that will assist you to convey nursing competence to your clients.
- Describe the nursing practice act.
- Define the term nurse licensure.
- State four functions that the Board of Registered Nursing performs.
- Discuss four grounds for licensure revocation for professional misconduct.
- Explain the legal issues of drug administration.
- Describe what is meant by "clients' rights."
- List four actions or guidelines that you need to complete to prepare for daily client care.
- Describe the steps of planning for client care.
- State what is meant by advanced directives.

PROFESSIONAL ROLE

As you enter the profession of nursing, you will experience some of the most frustrating and some of the most rewarding situations of your life. To decrease the frustrations and increase the positive experiences, this chapter introduces you to the role of the nurse. Emphasis is placed on those procedures that will assist you to become a functioning member of the health team, even with limited experience.

The information in this chapter will help you through the first few critical days of your clinical experience. In addition, legal aspects of the nursing profession are discussed to make you aware of the far-reaching consequences of nursing actions. Clients' rights and the Nurse Practice Act are also presented for your information.

As a nurse you will be held accountable and responsible for your actions. What does all this mean? To be accountable means that you are answerable for all your activities surrounding client care. Accountability can be observed and measured by a variety of factors. Nursing actions are evaluated against a set of standards, frequently referred to as standards of performance. In this evaluation the nurse is judged according to predetermined factors in which all nurses should be competent.

Responsibility means that the nurse is conscientious and honest in all professional activities. A good example of responsibility deals with not betraying confidential information concerning clients in the hospital. In addition, a responsible nurse respects clients' rights and abides by the Patient's Bill of Rights.

Nurses must function within the nurses' code of ethics. The code of ethics is a set of formal guidelines for governing professional action. It assists the nurse to problem solve where judgment is required. More emphasis is now being placed on the professional organizations to uphold the code of ethics and to admonish those nurses who violate the code.

American Nurses Association Code for Nurses

1. The nurse provides services with respect for human dignity and the uniqueness of the client, unrestricted by considerations of social or economic status, personal attributes, or the nature of the health problems.
2. The nurse safeguards the client's right to privacy by judiciously protecting information of a confidential nature.
3. The nurse acts to safeguard the client and the public when health care and safety are affected by the incompetent, unethical, or illegal practice of any person.
4. The nurse assumes responsibility and accountability for individual nursing judgments and actions.
5. The nurse maintains competence in nursing.
6. The nurse exercises informed judgment and uses individual competence and qualifications as criteria in seeking consultation, accepting responsibilities, and delegating nursing activities to others.
7. The nurse participates in activities that contribute to the ongoing development of the profession's body of knowledge.
8. The nurse participates in the profession's efforts to implement and improve standards of nursing.
9. The nurse participates in the profession's efforts to establish and maintain conditions of employment conducive to high-quality nursing care.
10. The nurse participates in the profession's effort to protect the public from misinforma-

tion and misrepresentation and to maintain the integrity of nursing.

11. The nurse collaborates with members of the health professions and other citizens in promoting community and national efforts to meet the health needs of the public.

Assuming the Client Role

Assisting the client to adapt to hospitalization is one of the primary functions of the nurse. The less resistive the client is to receiving treatment during hospitalization, the more open he or she is to curative methods. The nurse can assist in adaptation by understanding that all clients have individual needs, concerns, and perceptions that require discussion and planning as they take on the role of client in the health care setting. You must accept the client's perceptions of his or her new surroundings. Be aware that anxiety is a natural reaction to an unfamiliar setting, to new procedures, and to new people. If, for example, a client is extremely fatigued or overwhelmed by traveling to the hospital and the admission procedure, you can help him or her adapt to the surroundings, regain a sense of control and identity, and accept the changed circumstances.

Another way to assist the client to retain his or her identity and uniqueness is to communicate with the client as an individual. Ask questions and observe verbal responses as well as nonverbal cues. Provide ways to care for a client's personal possessions, clothing, and physical comfort so that the client adapts more easily to the change in environment and feels more secure and in control.

Be aware that the medical condition is only one part of the client's life and that the changes that have led up to admission affect other areas of his or her well-being. Clients may have concerns about new routines, financial matters, their families, or their future. By responding to clients' total needs at the time of admission, you can help them establish a positive attitude toward their total care.

Acknowledge and accept any statements or behavior the client uses to adapt to his or her new surroundings. Even though various cultures and groups differ in their response to illness and some responses may differ from your personal beliefs, acknowledge the client's individuality. Support the client's beliefs and behavior as long as they do not increase the risk of injury or illness. Be sensitive to any past health care experiences that may influence the client's feelings at the time of admission. A prior experience in the hospital may determine how a client responds to the current environment.

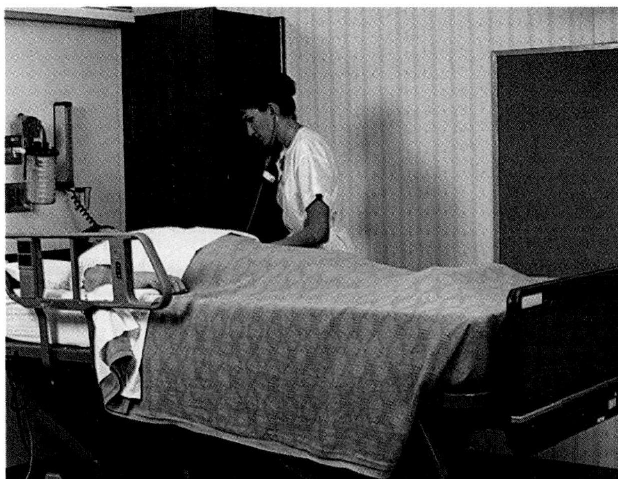

Relate to clients as worthwhile individuals who deserve respect and consideration.

Assuming the Nursing Role

Your actions, both verbal and nonverbal, influence the client's feelings and ideas regarding your level of competence, the role of nursing in administering care, and the client's overall adaptation to hospitalization. Assuming a professional role means that you behave as a professional person. Following the guidelines below will assist you to convey nursing competence, not only to clients but also to your peers and other nursing staff.

- Always dress neatly in appropriate, clean attire, and follow the dress code of your school or facility.
- Speak in correct English without slang or inappropriate language.
- Relate to the clients as worthwhile individuals who deserve respect and consideration. Call the client by his or her surname, and use the appropriate honorific (Mr., Ms., Miss, Mrs.). Do not use nicknames or first names.
- Do not "talk down" to or patronize the client. Remember that the client knows more about his or her own body, symptoms, feelings, and responses than anyone else. Listen and pay attention to what the client says about himself or herself.
- Remain in a professional role at all times. Do not socialize with the clients. They need to view you as a knowledgeable professional who brings healing, caring, and teaching roles to the relationship.
- Use yourself as a therapeutic tool to convey caring and healing. Use body language to reinforce

honest and direct verbalization, not to contradict it.

- Be accountable and answerable for your behavior and nursing actions and the nursing care you are expected to provide. If you do not understand what is expected, seek assistance from a staff member. Your responsibility is to remain reliable, honest, and trustworthy in administering nursing care.

LEGAL ASPECTS

Legal issues and regulations play a dominant role in nursing practice today. The law provides a framework for establishing nursing actions in the care of clients. Laws determine and set boundaries and maintain a standard of nursing practice.

The Nurse Practice Act defines professional nursing and recommends those actions that the nurse can practice independently and those actions that require a physician's order before completion.

Each state has the authority to regulate and they *administrate* health care professionals. Although the provisions of Nurse Practice Acts are quite similar from state to state, it is imperative that the nurse know the licensing requirements and the grounds for license revocation defined by the state in which he or she works.

Legal and ethical standards for nurses are complicated by a myriad of federal and state statutes and the continually changing interpretation of them by the courts of law. Nurses are faced today with the threat of legal action based on negligence, malpractice, invasion of privacy, and other grounds. This chapter covers the basic legal issues and topics, from clients' rights and nurses' liability in the administration of drugs and grounds for proceedings to address professional misconduct.

The Nurse Practice Act

The Nurse Practice Act is a series of statutes enacted by a state to regulate the practice of nursing in that state. Subjects covered by Nurse Practice Acts include definition of the scope of practice, education, licensure, and grounds for disciplinary actions. Nurse Practice Acts are quite similar throughout the United States, but the professional nurse is held legally responsible for the specific requirements for licensure and regulations of practice as defined by the state in which she or he works.

The responsibilities of the professional nurse involve a level of performance for a defined range of health care services. These services include assessment, implementation, and evaluation of nursing action, as well as teaching and related services, such as counseling. A summary of the skills and functions that professional nurses perform in daily practice follows.

- Provide direct and indirect client care services
- Perform and deliver basic health care services
- Implement testing and prevention procedures
- Observe signs and symptoms of illness
- Administer treatments per physician's order
- Observe treatment reactions and responses
- Administer medications per physician's order
- Observe medication responses and any side effects
- Observe general physical and mental conditions of individual clients
- Document nursing care
- Supervise allied nursing personnel
- Coordinate members of the health care team

Nurse Licensure

The authorization to practice nursing is defined legally as the right to practice nursing by an individual who holds an active license issued by the state in which she or he intends to work. The licensing process is administered by the state board of registration, frequently called the BRN. This board may also grant endorsement or reciprocity to an applicant who holds a current license in another state. The applicant for RN licensure must have attended an accredited school of nursing, be a qualified nursing professional or paraprofessional, or have met specific prerequisites if licensed in a foreign country.

Board of Registered Nursing Functions

- Establishes and oversees educational standards
- Establishes professional standards
- Monitors examinations for licensure (NCLEX)
- Registers and renews licenses
- Conducts investigations of violations of the statutes and regulations
- Issues citations
- Holds disciplinary hearings for possible suspension or revocation of the license
- Imposes penalties following disciplinary hearings

Standards of Nursing Practice

These standards were first published in 1973 by the American Nurses Association and implemented by nursing service departments throughout the country. The standards describe the specific function and activities of nurses and provide criteria for evaluating the quality and effectiveness of nursing care. Six defined standards encompass the use of the nursing process in the delivery of client care. The standards are authoritative descriptions of the responsibility and accountability of the professional nurse.

The standards of nursing practice are divided into two sections: The first section, standards of care, describes the six standards of care using the nursing process. The second section, standards of professional performance, includes standards referring to quality of care, performance appraisals, ethics, and so on.

American Nurses' Association Standards of Nursing Practice

1. The collection of data about the health status of the client/patient is systematic and continuous. The data are accessible, communicated, and recorded.
2. Nursing diagnoses are derived from health status data.
3. The plan of nursing care includes goals derived from the nursing diagnoses.
4. The plan of nursing care includes priorities and the prescribed nursing approaches or measures to achieve the goals derived from the nursing diagnoses.
5. Nursing actions provide for client/patient participation in health promotion, maintenance, and restoration.
6. The nursing actions assist the client/patient to maximize his [or her] health capabilities.
7. The client/patient's progress or lack of progress toward goal achievements is determined by the client/patient and the nurse.
8. The client/patient's progress or lack of progress toward goal achievement directs reassessment, reordering of priorities, new goal setting, and revision of the plan of nursing care.

Liability and Legal Issues

Each state defines and regulates the grounds for professional misconduct. Even though many states have similar standards the practicing nurse must know how her state defines professional misconduct. Any one of the following actions would be considered professional misconduct.

- Obtaining an RN license through fraudulent methods
- Practicing in an incompetent or negligent manner
- Practicing when ability to practice is severely impaired
- Being habitually drunk or dependent on drugs
- Being convicted of or committing an act constituting a crime under federal or state law
- Refusing to provide health care services on the grounds of race, color, creed, or national origin
- Permitting or aiding an unlicensed person to perform activities requiring a license
- Practicing nursing while license is suspended
- Practicing medicine without a license

The penalties for professional misconduct include probation, censure and reprimand, suspension of the license, or revocation of the license. The state's Board of Registered Nursing has the authority to impose any of the above penalties for professional misconduct.

Drugs and the Nurse

In their daily work, most nurses handle a wide variety of drugs. Failure to give the correct medication or improper handling of drugs may result in serious problems for the nurse due to strict federal and state statutes relating to drugs. The Comprehensive Drug Abuse Prevention Act of 1970 provides the fundamental federal regulations for compounding, selling, and dispensing narcotics, stimulants, depressants, and other controlled items. Each state has a similar set of regulations for the same purpose.

LEGAL ISSUES IN DRUG ADMINISTRATION

- Nurses must not administer a specific drug unless allowed to do so by the particular state's Nurse Practice Act.
- Nurses are to take every safety precaution in whatever they are doing.
- Nurses are to be certain that employer's policy allows them to administer a specific drug.
- A drug may not lawfully be administered unless all the above items are in effect.
- General rules for drug dispensing:
  - Never leave tray with prepared medicines unattended.
  - Always report errors immediately.
  - Send labeled bottles that are unintelligible back to pharmacist for relabeling.
  - Store internal and external medicines separately if possible.

Noncompliance with federal or state drug regulations can result in liability. Violation of the state drug regulations or licensing laws are grounds for the board of nurse registration to initiate disciplinary action.

Negligence/Malpractice

The doctrine of negligence rests on the duty of every person to exercise due care in his/her conduct toward others from which injury may result. To find liability there must be a duty of care on the part of the nurse and a causal relationship between damage or harm to the client as well as an act or an omission to act by the nurse.

Gross negligence is the intentional failure to perform a duty in reckless disregard of the consequences affecting the client. It is viewed as a gross lack of care to such a level as to be considered willful and wanton.

Criminal negligence also consists of a duty on the part of the nurse and an act that is the proximate cause of the injury or death of a client. This type of negligence is usually defined by statute and as such is punishable as a crime. The act being punished would be a flagrant and reckless disregard of the safety of others and/or a willfull disregard to the injury liable to follow so as to convert the act into a crime when it results in personal injury or death. One is not "negligent" unless he/she fails to exercise the degree of reasonable care that would be exercised by a person of ordinary prudence under all the existing circumstances in view of probable danger of injury.

Malpractice is any professional misconduct that is an unreasonable lack of skill or fidelity in professional duties. In a more specific sense it means bad, wrong, or injurious treatment of a client resulting in injury, unnecessary suffering, or death to a client proceeding from ignorance, carelessness, lack of professional skill, disregard of established rules, protocols, principles or procedures, neglect, or a malicious or criminal intent.

CIVIL LAW	**CRIMINAL LAW**
Contract	Assault
Unintentional tort	Battery
Intentional Tort	Murder
Negligence	Manslaughter

Legal doctrine holds that an employer may also be liable for negligent acts of employees in the course and scope of employment. Physicians, hospitals, clinics, and other employers may be held liable for negligent acts of their employees. This doctrine does not support acts of gross negligence or acts that are outside the scope of employment.

CLASSIFICATIONS OF LAW RELATED TO NURSING

Classification	*Example*
Constitutional	Clients' rights to equal treatment
Administrative	Licensure and the state BRN
Labor relations	Union negotiations
Contract	Relationship with employer
Criminal	Handling of narcotics
Tort	
Medical malpractice	Reasonable and prudent client care
Product liability	Warranty on medical equipment

CLIENTS' RIGHTS

In the United States all but 10 states have some provision for the rights of clients. A right of the claim may be moral or legal or both; a legal right can be enforced in a court of law. It is important to remember that within a health care system all clients retain their basic constitutional rights, such as freedom of expression, due process of law, freedom from cruel and inhumane punishment, equal protection, and so forth.

Because clients' rights may conflict with the nursing function, you should be familiar with the key elements of these rights. Rights include consent, confidentiality, and involuntary commitment. In considering these rights, however, remember that they may be modified by the client's mental or physical condition.

Consent to Receive Health Services

Consent is the client's approval to have his or her body touched by specific individuals, such as doctors, nurses, and laboratory technicians. Informed consent refers to the process of informing the client prior to granting a consent regarding treatment, such as tests and surgery, and must be understood by the client in terms of the intended outcome and the potential harmful results. The client may rescind a prior consent verbally or in writing.

The authority to sign a consent must be given by a mentally competent adult. Court-authorized persons may give consent for mentally incompetent adults. In emergency situations, if the client is in immediate danger of serious harm or death, action may be taken to preserve life without the client's consent.

The nurse's liability in terms of consent is to ensure that the client is fully informed before being asked to sign a consent form. The physician, nurse, or other health personnel must inform the client of any potentially harmful effects of the treatment. If this is not done, it may result in the nurse's being held personally liable. The nurse must respect the right of a mentally competent adult client to refuse health care; however, a life-threatening situation may alter the client's right to refuse treatment.

Clients' Rights

Clients are protected by law (invasion of privacy) against unauthorized release of personal clinical data, such as symptoms, diagnoses, and treatments. Nurses, as well as other health care personnel, may be held personally liable for invasion of privacy, should litigation arise from the unauthorized release of client data. Confidential information, however, may be released with the client's consent. Information release is mandatory when ordered by a court or when state statutes require reporting child abuse, communicable diseases, or other incidents. Nurses have a legal and ethical responsibility to become familiar with their employer's policies and procedures regarding protection of clients' information.

Medical records are the key written account of such client information as signs and symptoms, diagnosis, treatment, and responses to treatment. Not only do these records document care given to clients, but they also provide effective means of communication among health care personnel. These records contain important data for insurance and other expense claims and are used in court in the event of litigation.

Health professionals are becoming more aware of the implications of clients' rights as society in general becomes more aware of every human being's basic rights. Although there are still gaps in the legal process, many states are beginning to grapple with the status of laws applicable to clients who are hospitalized. It is essential that nurses be aware of the particular state's laws and statutes affecting clients and themselves. Nurses as well as physicians are accountable for their actions, and the threat of civil and criminal prosecution is becoming more prevalent.

The Client's Bill of Rights

1. The client has the right to considerate and respectful care.
2. The client has the right to obtain from his or her physician complete current information concerning diagnosis, treatment, and prognosis in terms the client can be reasonably expected to understand.
3. The client has the right to receive from the physician information necessary to give informed consent prior to the start of any procedure or treatment. . . . Where medically significant alternatives for care or treatment exist, or when the client requests information concerning medical alternatives, the client has the right to such information [and] to know the name of the person responsible for the procedures or treatment.
4. The client has the right to refuse treatment to the extent permitted by law and to be informed of the medical consequences of his or her action.
5. The client has the right to every consideration of privacy concerning his or her own medical care program.
6. The client has the right to expect that all communications and records pertaining to his or her care should be treated as confidential.
7. The client has the right to expect that within its capacity a hospital must make reasonable response to the request of a client for services.
8. The client has the right to obtain information as to any relationship of the hospital to other health care and educational institutions insofar as his or her care is concerned [and] any professional relationships among individuals, by name, who are treating him or her.
9. The client has the right to be advised if the hospital proposes to engage in or perform human experimentation affecting his or her care or treatment [and] has the right to refuse to participate.
10. The client has the right to expect reasonable continuity of care.
11. The client has the right to examine and receive an explanation of his or her bill regardless of source of payment.
12. The client has the right to know what hospital rules and regulations apply to his or her conduct as a client.

Advanced Directives

An advanced directive is a document that allows clients to make legal decisions about how they wish to receive future medical treatment. It is written and signed before any such care becomes necessary. Within this document, the client may indicate the person or persons he or she wishes to make medical decisions in situations in which the client is unable to do so. The document needs to be signed and witnessed, and copies should be kept on file in the physician's office and the hospital. The witness to this document should not be a hospital employee, relative, or heir to the estate. Advanced directives vary among states and therefore the nurse must be knowledgeable about the use and type of directives in the state in which he or she practices.

ADVANCED DIRECTIVES

The Omnibus Budget Reconciliation Act (OBRA) of 1990 requires states to provide advanced directives as options for clients. This document should be completed and signed before treatment is necessary. The nurse should check with the client's physician to determine that advanced directives are on file.
Documents include

- Client's choice in continuing medical care when the client is unable to speak or make decisions
- Living will, power of attorney for health care, or a notarized handwritten document
- Documents available in client's medical record
- Documents witnessed by persons other than medical personnel or relatives of the client or heirs to the client's estate

Living Will. A living will is a type of advanced directive, indicating the client's wishes regarding prolonging life using life support measures, refusing or stopping medical interventions, or making decisions about his or her medical care. Living wills are executed while the client is competent and able to make sound decisions. As conditions change, a living will needs to be evaluated for relevance. (States differ in their acceptance of living wills as legal documents.)

Durable Power of Attorney for Health Care. This legal document gives power to make health care decisions to a designated individual in the event the client is unable to make competent decisions for him or herself. The designated person is obligated to follow the directives outlined in the document. Decisions regarding withdrawing or using life support, organ donation, or consent to treatment or procedures are included in the directives.

CLINICAL PRACTICE

Before your first clinical experience, you should review the most essential components of client care to enable you to practice safe and efficient nursing care. Guidelines for clinical practice, the parts of a client chart, communication techniques, principles of medical asepsis, a basic nursing assessment, and protocols for nursing care procedures are presented to give you confidence and background information in providing nursing care.

Guidelines for Clinical Practice

Before attempting to provide client care, you need to familiarize yourself with all aspects of the care the client requires. The following guidelines will assist you in this preparation. Usually the preparation is completed the night before you go to the clinical setting. If this is not possible, you need to identify those aspects of preparation that will render you a safe practitioner.

- Obtain the clinical assignment in sufficient time to be able to prepare for safe practice.
- Read the client's chart and obtain all the data necessary to assist you in client care. This usually encompasses the following items: history and physical, physician's progress notes, graphic sheet, medication record, laboratory findings, nurses' notes or flow sheets or both, admissions data base, client care plan, Kardex card, and physician's orders. Each of these documents is illustrated later in this chapter.
- Review all procedures that you will provide for the client. Use your skills and fundamentals books for your review.
- Research the diagnosis so that you are more aware of signs and symptoms the client may exhibit. Identify alterations from normal such as altered laboratory values, vital signs, and so forth.
- Research all medications you will administer to the client. Many instructors require medication cards be completed on all medications to be administered.
- Plan your day's schedule by developing a time plan to help keep you organized and to enable you to complete client care in a timely manner.
- Practice charting the procedures you will be administering so that you can identify appropriate vocabulary and include necessary information. Pertinent charting information is included with each procedure described in this text.

Providing Client Care

You have prepared for this clinical practice before coming to the nursing unit. Now you receive an update on the client's condition, and a team leader goes over nursing procedures you will be completing. This is accomplished during a report period. Each hospital has a method for presenting the report. Some facilities tape a report from the off-going shift that is listened to by the on-coming staff. Other nursing units give a verbal report in which they review the information obtained by the previous shift. Facilities where primary nursing is practiced have a one-to-one report between the on-coming nurse and the off-going nurse for a specific group of clients. At this time a work sheet is completed that lists times for treatments and medications. Following the report, the team leader or your preceptor nurse goes over all aspects of the care you will deliver for the client. This is the time to ask any questions you may have regarding policy or procedure for the nursing unit or the client. Your medication cards or unit-dose sheet is checked at this time to ensure that you have all necessary medications and equipment to prepare and administer the drugs.

The following outline of client care will assist you in planning your nursing care for the day.

1. Wash your hands.
2. Gather equipment, such as a stethoscope, sphygmomanometer, thermometer, and linen.
3. Check the client's identaband. Introduce yourself to the client and explain the nursing care you will be giving.
4. Check if the client has any preference for the order in which the care is to be given.
5. Complete a nursing assessment. You may use the basic nursing assessment outlined in this chapter as a guide if your instructor does not have one she or he prefers you to use.
6. Document your findings as you are completing the physical assessment, and enter it in the nurses' notes section of the chart.
7. Take vital signs if it is the policy of the unit.
8. Complete all nursing interventions, and document the findings immediately after completion.
9. Administer all medications. Document medication administration in the appropriate place, and observe for signs of side effects or unusual findings.
10. During your nursing care, practice good communication techniques.
11. Complete all charting.
12. Terminate the relationship with the client.
13. Report off to the appropriate person.
14. Wash your hands before leaving the nursing unit.

Client's Records

The following documents are those you will be using most often in clinical practice. Become familiar with each form, its placement in the chart, and the information that it contains. Examples of these forms are included at the end of the chapter.

Kardex. The Kardex card represents the "hub" for all client activities. Physician's orders are transcribed on the card. Laboratory tests, medications, and activity levels are just a few items documented in designated areas of the Kardex.

Care Plan. The care plan identifies the client's usual or potential problems, expected outcomes, and nursing actions. Discharge criteria is also an integral part of the care plan.

Client's Chart

The chart itself contains several forms that are important to your preparation and administration of nursing care.

Nurses' Notes. Nurses' notes do not necessarily have a particular or specific format as do graphic records or physician's orders. One type of narrative nurses' notes is illustrated on page 15. Clinical observations and nursing interventions are documented in nurses' notes. Flow sheets are frequently used for documenting activities of daily living and nursing interventions.

Medication Records. Medication records are usually similar to the one illustrated on page 14. All medications should be documented on a medication record. Some facilities chart routine medications on one medication sheet and prn and one-time only medications on another sheet. Check the institution's policy for each record's use.

Graphic Records. Temperature, pulse, and respirations are graphed on the graphic sheet. Blood pressure readings, intake and output records, and dietary intake are also recorded on this form.

Physician's Orders. Physician's orders are written on forms with carbon copies attached. This form allows copies of the orders to be sent to the pharmacy or CSR for supplies. Each facility dictates where each sheet is sent.

Physician's Progress Notes. Physician's progress notes contain daily observations and thoughts regarding treatments, signs, and symptoms experienced by the client, operative risks explained to the client, and the client's responses to therapy.

History and Physical. The physician's report of his assessment is written on a special form. Most hospitals type the history and physical from dictated notes by the physician. When this occurs, it may be several days before this information is available.

Laboratory Forms. Laboratory results are sent back to the unit on the original laboratory order form. The information from each form may be transcribed to a laboratory data flow sheet. This sheet provides a valuable overview of all laboratory results.

Communicating with the Client

The foundation of the person's perception of him or herself and the world is the result of communicated messages received from significant others. Communication is a basic human need, and since we live in a social society, everyone has a need to in some way communicate with others in the world. A basic proposition of communication is that a person cannot *not* communicate. Everything you observe in another person is a form of communication: the way one stands and moves, the gestures, total body position, and all the nuances of speech, like tone, pace, and choice of words. The communication process includes both verbal and nonverbal expressions. It is affected by the individual's experience, his or her relationship, and the context in which the communication takes place. It is also affected by the purpose of the sender in sending the message, the content of the message, the manner in which the message is sent, and, finally, the effect on the receiver. As you can see, the communication process can be very complex. As a beginning practitioner, however, the most important factor to remember is that *what* you say and *how* you say it has a very great influence on your client.

One of the most important skills you must master is to be able to talk therapeutically to clients and to be able to listen to them. Nurse–client communication is an intimate process of providing nursing care. In fact, the initial step in the nursing process—assessment—comprises observation, interview, and examination. The interview involves talking and listening to the client. Initially it may be difficult for you to concentrate on both talking and listening, since you have not yet mastered the basic skills, such as a bedbath or backrub. As you gain experience, however, these skills will become more familiar and you can focus on the communication-interaction process with the client.

Learning to talk with clients and listening to them is the beginning of a nurse–client relationship. Some of you come to nursing with many of these basic communication skills already mastered. Others experience shyness, hesitancy, and awkwardness in relating to clients. Try to keep in mind that you are being educated to be a professional person—a nurse—and as such you have a great deal to give to your clients. They will learn to respect your skill, value your presence, and depend on you when they are ill. One of the most rewarding aspects to nursing is experiencing a communication between you and your client. If you do feel shy or hesitant, remember that communication skills can be learned. Begin by practicing or role playing with your classmates until you feel comfortable in the initial phases of a relationship.

In establishing nurse–client communication, some basic guidelines should be remembered.

- Accept the client as a valued and worthwhile individual, for this acceptance is a prerequisite for a nurse–client relationship.
- Be aware of the total client, not just his or her physical needs. The client's social, emotional, and spiritual needs are also important.
- Understand your own needs, feelings, and reactions so that they do not interfere with the therapeutic process with the client.
- Be prepared to feel some degree of emotional involvement with your client, evidencing caring and concern for his or her welfare. At the same time, however, it is necessary to maintain objectivity.
- Remember that the nurse–client interaction is a professional one. As such, you as the nurse possess the skills, abilities, and resources to relieve the other person's pain and discomfort and your client seeks comfort and assistance for alleviation of some existing problem.
- A nurse–client relationship does not require a long-term agreement or formal meetings between nurse and client to be effective. You may still meet the objectives of such a relationship in a short clinical experience.

Basic Nursing Assessment

Each nurse develops her or his own routine for completing a basic nursing assessment. There is no right or wrong way, although it should be consistent and complete. The following outline for basic assessment is a simple approach to the assessment and one you may wish to adopt until you have established a good system for yourself.

The basic assessment is completed at the beginning and end of each shift. The assessment should take no longer than 5 to 10 minutes to complete. You should concentrate on the specific physiologic system that correlates with the client's diagnosis. For a more in-depth discussion of each system in the assessment, see the chapter on physical assessment.

The following outline will assist you in completing a basic physical assessment.

1. Vital signs
    a. Temperature (method dictated by condition)
    b. Radial pulse: rate, volume, and rhythm
    c. Respirations: rate, depth, and rhythm
    d. Blood pressure: Korotkoff's sounds
2. State of comfort: location and intensity of pain; response to medications if given
3. Emotional responses: client behavior, reactions, and demeanor; general mood (crying, depression)
4. Skin: presence or absence of abrasions, contusions, erythema, decubitus ulcers, incision line, color, turgor, temperature
5. Musculoskeletal: activity level, general mobility, gait, range of motion
6. Neurological: pupils (size, response, equality); hand grips; strength and sensation of all extremities; ability to follow commands; level of consciousness
7. Respiratory: breath sounds; sputum color and consistency; cough (productive or nonproductive)
8. Cardiovascular: heart sounds; presence of pulses; edema; presence of hair on extremities
9. Gastrointestinal: bowel pattern and sounds; presence of nausea or vomiting; abdominal distention; consumption of diet
10. Genitourinary: voiding; color, odor, and consistency of urine; dysuria; vaginal drainage or discomfort; penile discharge

If any unusual findings are assessed, complete a more in-depth assessment of the particular system affected. Throughout the day, continue to assess changes in the client's condition by paying particular attention to the alterations from normal that you identified in the initial assessment. At the end of the shift, make a notation of any changes in the client's condition.

MEDICAL ASEPSIS PRINCIPLES

Microorganisms are found everywhere in nature. Pathogenic microorganisms, or pathogens, cause disease; nonpathogenic microorganisms, or nonpathogens, do not cause disease. Some microorganisms are nonpathogens in their normal body environment. An example of this is *Escherichia coli*, which is normally present in the intestinal tract and does not cause a problem until it inhabits another environment such as the urinary tract.

The spread of microorganisms is prevented by the use of two forms of asepsis: medical asepsis and surgical asepsis. Medical asepsis occurs when there is an absence of pathogens. Surgical asepsis occurs when there is an absence of all organisms. Medical asepsis is often referred to as "clean technique," whereas surgical asepsis is termed "sterile technique." A discussion of surgical asepsis can be found later in this book. This chapter discusses medical asepsis as it affects nursing care.

Principles of medical asepsis are used in all aspects of client care. In fact, the use of medical asepsis begins before you report to the nursing unit. To ensure protection for the client, you begin practicing medical asepsis by limiting jewelry to only a wedding band and perhaps small earrings for pierced ears when administering client care. Fingernails are short and in good repair. Your hair is off your collar and under control to prevent contaminating sterile fields and falling into client's food or wounds.

While providing client care, the following principles should be kept in mind.

- Linen rooms or carts are considered clean; therefore linen not used for client care cannot be returned.
- Utility rooms are designated as areas for clean and dirty supplies. Cross-contamination must be avoided by not placing articles in the wrong area.
- Linen and articles are carried away from your uniform and are not held close to your body.
- Articles dropped on the floor are considered contaminated and must be discarded appropriately. If linen is accidentally dropped on the floor, it is placed in a soiled linen hamper. Clients are to wear slippers or shoes when out of bed.
- Each client has his or her own supplies and equipment, which are not used by other clients. Sterilization or disinfection is carried out between use.
- If you are not feeling well, you should not report for clinical experience. If you are running a temperature or have a cold and a runny nose, call the appropriate person and report that you are ill.
- Paper tissue is used for removing client's secretions. Discard the tissue in the trash basket.

- Equipment is cleaned and rinsed with cold water to remove secretions or substances before being returned to the central supply area. Heat coagulates the substances and makes it more difficult to remove.
- Soap and water are considered the best cleansers because they help break down soil so it can be more readily removed. Detergents may be more effective in hard or cold water; however, tissue damage can result from their use. Germicides may be added to soap or detergent and increase the effectiveness of the cleansing agent.
- Friction is used to facilitate soil removal. A brush, sponge, or cloth may be used to produce the friction.
- When aseptic technique is used, cleaning is conducted from the cleanest to the least clean area. For example, always clean the incision area from the center of the incision to the periphery of the skin.

Handwashing

The single most effective medical aseptic practice is handwashing. When you first arrive at the nursing unit and before beginning nursing practice, you should complete a medical handwashing procedure. The important concept to remember is that you soap and rinse your hands twice before providing any nursing care to the client. Hands are washed before all procedures and in between clients. The specific step-by-step handwashing procedure is covered in Chapter 9, *Bathing and Bedmaking*.

Unsterile gloves may be used with unsterile procedures, such as enemas or cleaning excreta, to prevent contamination of the nurse's hands. The use of gloves decreases cross-contamination between clients. Clients frequently feel "unclean" when gloves are used in client care; therefore gloves should be used only when necessary. When gloves are no longer needed, dispose of them in the utility room, not in the client unit.

PROTOCOL FOR PROCEDURES

Each procedure in this textbook follows a basic protocol. To save space and prevent repetition, all steps in the protocol are frequently not outlined in detail for each procedure. Remember, however, that these steps are important and must be followed if complete and responsible nursing care is to be delivered to the patient.

- Check physician's orders.
- Check client care plan or Kardex.
- Identify client.
- Introduce yourself to the client.
- Explain procedure to be done.
- Wash your hands.
- Gather equipment and fill out charge slips.
- Take all of the required equipment to the room.
- Provide privacy for the client by drawing curtain or screen around bed.
- Raise bed to HIGH position.
- Lower side rail nearest you.
- Drape client (if appropriate).
- Perform procedure according to protocol.
- Clean client as necessary.
- Remove drape and position client for comfort.
- Raise side rail to UP position.
- Lower bed.
- Replace call bell.
- Pull back curtain or remove screen.
- Remove equipment and clean, dispose, and disperse used equipment.
- Document or chart findings.

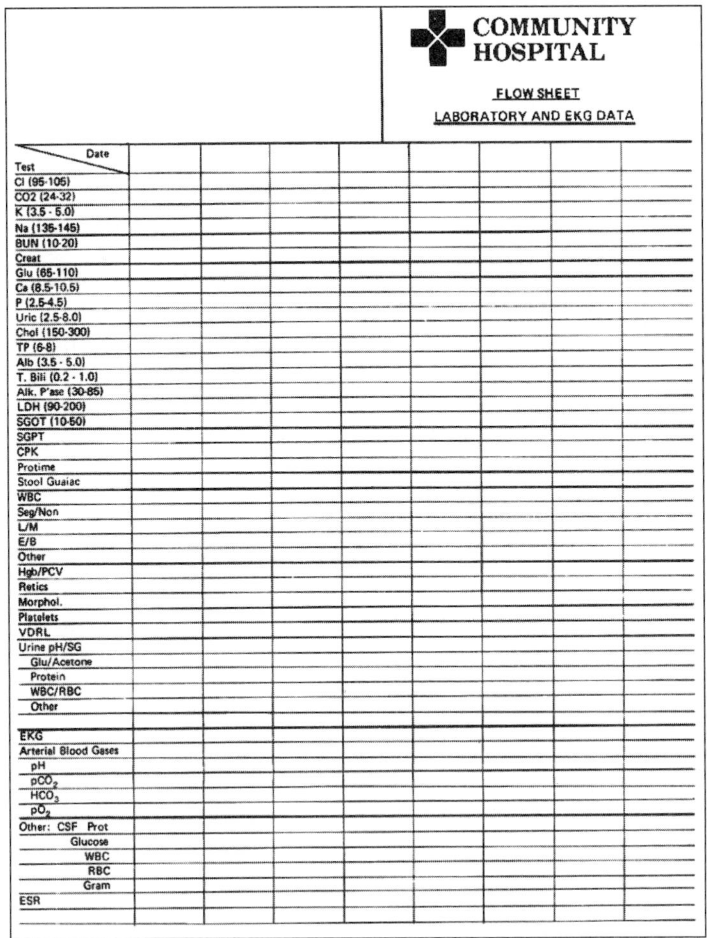

COMMUNITY HOSPITAL

FLOW SHEET

LABORATORY AND EKG DATA

Test / Date								
Cl (95-105)								
CO2 (24-32)								
K (3.5 - 5.0)								
Na (135-145)								
BUN (10-20)								
Creat								
Glu (65-110)								
Ca (8.5-10.5)								
P (2.5-4.5)								
Uric (2.5-8.0)								
Chol (150-300)								
TP (6-8)								
Alb (3.5 - 5.0)								
T. Bili (0.2 - 1.0)								
Alk. P'ase (30-85)								
LDH (90-200)								
SGOT (10-50)								
SGPT								
CPK								
Protime								
Stool Guaiac								
WBC								
Seg/Non								
L/M								
E/B								
Other								
Hgb/PCV								
Retics								
Morphol.								
Platelets								
VDRL								
Urine pH/SG								
Glu/Acetone								
Protein								
WBC/RBC								
Other								
EKG								
Arterial Blood Gases								
pH								
pCO_2								
HCO_3								
pO_2								
Other: CSF Prot								
Glucose								
WBC								
RBC								
Gram								
ESR								

Laboratory results flow sheet.

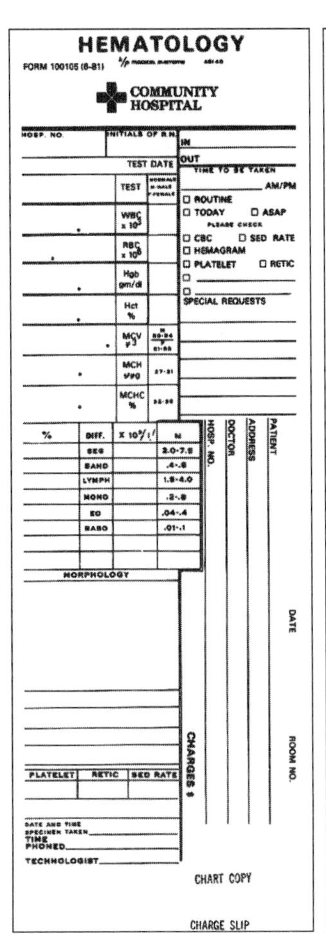

HEMATOLOGY

FORM 100105 (6-81)

COMMUNITY HOSPITAL

HOSP. NO. | INITIALS OF R.N. | IN | OUT

TEST DATE | TIME TO BE TAKEN | AM/PM

TEST | NORMALS MALE / FEMALE

WBC x 10³ | RBC x 10⁶ | Hgb gm/dl | Hct % | MCV μ³ | MCH μμg | MCHC %

☐ ROUTINE ☐ TODAY ☐ ASAP (PLEASE CHECK)

☐ CBC ☐ SED RATE ☐ HEMAGRAM ☐ PLATELET ☐ RETIC ☐ ☐

SPECIAL REQUESTS

%	DIFF.	x 10⁹/l	N
	SEG		2.0-7.5
	BAND		.4-.8
	LYMPH		1.5-4.0
	MONO		.2-.8
	EO		.04-.4
	BASO		.01-.1

MORPHOLOGY

PLATELET | RETIC | SED RATE

DATE AND TIME SPECIMEN TAKEN ____

TIME PHONED ____

TECHNOLOGIST ____

HOSP. NO. | DOCTOR | ADDRESS | PATIENT | DATE | ROOM NO. | CHARGES $

CHART COPY

CHARGE SLIP

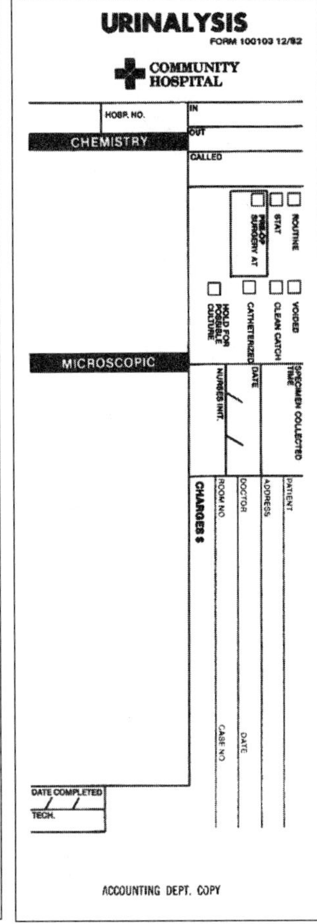

URINALYSIS

FORM 100103 12/82

COMMUNITY HOSPITAL

HOSP. NO. | IN | OUT | CALLED

CHEMISTRY

☐ PRE-OP SURGERY AT ☐ STAT ☐ ROUTINE

☐ HOLD FOR POSSIBLE CULTURE ☐ CATHETERIZED ☐ CLEAN CATCH ☐ VOIDED

MICROSCOPIC

NURSES INIT. | DATE | SPECIMEN COLLECTED TIME

CHARGES $ | ROOM NO. | DOCTOR | ADDRESS | PATIENT | CASE NO. | DATE

DATE COMPLETED / /

TECH.

ACCOUNTING DEPT. COPY

Laboratory order forms.

COMMUNITY HOSPITAL

ACTIVITIES	HYGIENE	DIET		BLADDER/BOWEL	DATE ORDERED	TO BE DONE	LABORATORY	DATE SENT
Complete Bedrest; BR c Commode; BR c BRP; Amb c help; Amb ad lib; Up in chair; Other	Complete bed bath; Partial bath; Shower Tub; Oral Care; Dentures	NPO; Clear Liq.; Full Liq.; Soft; Regular; Nourishments; Assist Feed; Tube Feeding	Restrict Fluids; 24 ___; days ___; pms ___; nocs ___; Push Fluids ___; Special ___	Peri-Care; date last BM; Ostomy Care			ADMIT CBC - VDRL - UA	
Vital Signs	THERAPY: PT; OT	SAFETY: Restraints; Wrist; Rails up; Rails down; Side rail release	INTAKE AND OUTPUT	RESPIRATORY: IPPB; Incentive Spirometer; O_2 cannula ___ mask ___				
Neuro Signs; S & A; WEIGHT	Isolation			STROKE PROGRAM				

TREATMENTS

DATE	

X-RAY/OTHER

ADMIT CHEST

ALLERGIES | SURGICAL PROCEDURE | OLD CHART REQUESTED ____ RECEIVED ____

ROOM | NAME | ADM. DATE | AGE | DIAGNOSIS | PHYSICIAN

Kardex card—Activities of daily living (ADL) information.

FROM UNIVERSITY MEDICAL CENTER

TO MEDICATION ADMINISTRATION RECORD

INTRAMUSCULAR/SUBCUTANEOUS SITE CODES		PAIN SCALE	SEDATION SCALE
A-Right Arm	F-Right Thigh	0-No Pain	1-Wide Awake
B-Left Arm	F-Left Thigh	1-Mild Pain	2-Drowsy
C-Right Hip	G-Right Abdomen	2-Discomforting	3-Dozing Intermittently
D-Left Hip	H-Left Abdomen	3-Distressing	4-Mostly Sleeping
		4-Horrible	5-Awakens Only When Aroused
		5-Excruciating	

	MEDICATIONS AND DIRECTIONS	RT	2301-0700	0701-1500	1501-2300
03/11	Dilantin 2 caps PO Every Morning (Phenytoin Sodium Cap 100 Mg)				
03/11	Phenobarbital 1 Tab PO Bedtime (Phenobarbital Tab 30 Mg)				
03/11	Folvite Generic 1 Tab PO Once Daily (Folic Acid Tab 1 Mg)				
03/11	A-Methylpred 40 Mg IV Every 12 HR from 9 AM (Methylprednisolone Sod Sul)				
03/11	Prilosec 1 Cap PO Every 24 Hours (Omperazole Cap 20 Mg)				
03/11	Xylocaine Viscous 5-10 mL PO Every 4 Hours-PRN (Lidocaine Viscous Soln 3%)				
	To wash mouth				

MESSAGE — MAR CHECKED

Time	
Pain Rating	
Sedation Level	
Respiration Rate	

NURSE INITIALS AND SIGNATURE	NURSE INITIALS AND SIGNATURE	NURSE INITIALS AND SIGNATURE

CONFIDENTIAL INFORMATION

Rm & Bed # Name CHART COPY Med Rec # Page___ of___

Medical administration record (MAR).

KARDEX / RAND CLIENT CARE PLAN

CLIENT EDUCATION PROGRAM	DATE Start	DATE Finish	DISCHARGE CRITERIA	DISCHARGE PLAN	Addressograph
Diabetic____			PLAN: Stroke Rehab Eval ____	Discharge Coordinator	
Coronary____			Cardiac Rehab Eval ____	Date Involved ____	
Other____			SOCIAL SERVICE	Home ____	
____			Date Involved ____	ECF____	
			Comment:	OTHER____	

Date	Client Problem	Deadline Date	Expected Outcome	Health Team Action

Discharge and teaching plan.

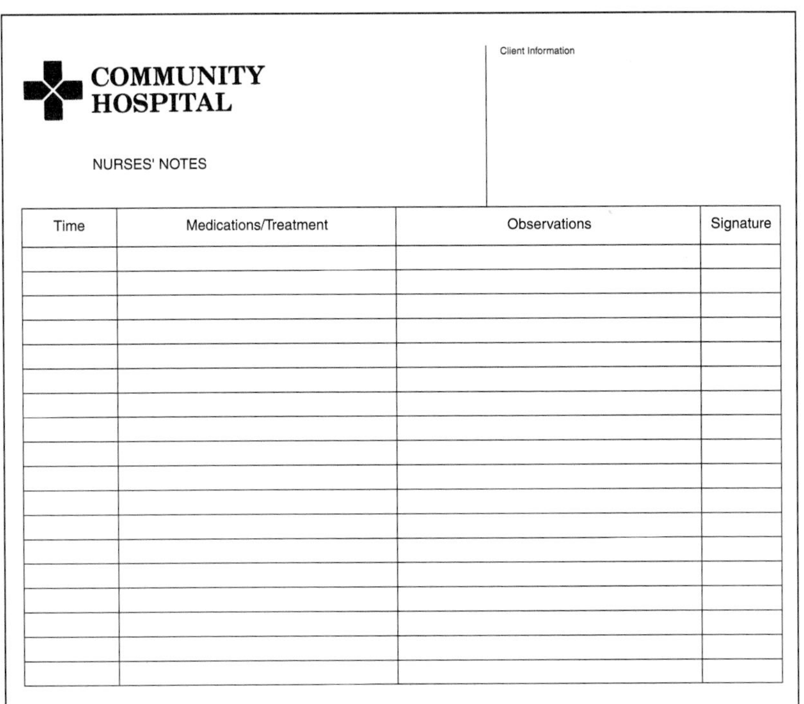

COMMUNITY HOSPITAL

NURSES' NOTES

Client Information

Time	Medications/Treatment	Observations	Signature

Nurses' notes.

COMMUNITY HOSPITAL

ROUTINE

PRESS HARD

MEDICATION DOSAGE ROUTE	SHIFT	/ /19	/ /19	/ /19	/ /19
	2300-0700				
	0700-1500				
	1500-2300				
	2300-0700				
	0700-1500				
	1500-2300				
	2300-0700				
	0700-1500				
	1500-2300				
	2300-0700				
	0700-1500				
	1500-2300				
	2300-0700				
	0700-1500				
	1500-2300				
	2300-0700				
	0700-1500				
	1500-2300				
	2300-0700				
	0700-1500				
	1500-2300				
	2300-0700				
	0700-1500				
	1500-2300				
	2300-0700				
	0700-1500				
	1500-2300				
	2300-0700				
	0700-1500				
	1500-2300				
SITE CODE: - RUOQ, - LUOQ, - R THIGH, - L THIGH, - R LOWER ABD, - L LOWER ABD, - R DELTOID, - L DELTOID	2300-0700				
	0700-1500				
	1500-2300				

CHART COPY

Medication record.

COMMUNITY HOSPITAL

CLINICAL RECORD

DATE																		
HOSP DAY/POSTOP DAY																		
TIME	0200	0600	1000	1400	1800	2200	0200	0600	1000	1400	1800	2200	0200	0600	1000	1400	1800	2200

KEY	PULSE	TEMP. C	TEMP. F
BLACK – PULSE & RESPIRATIONS RED – TEMPERATURE	140	40.6	105
	130	40.0	104
	120	39.4	103
	110	38.8	102
	100	38.3	101
	80	37.7	100
	90	37.2	99
	70	36.6	98
	60	36.1	97
	50	35.5	96
	RESPIRATIONS		
	BLOOD PRESSURE		

HEIGHT	WEIGHT			WEIGHT			WEIGHT		
	BREAKFAST	LUNCH	DINNER	BREAKFAST	LUNCH	DINNER	BREAKFAST	LUNCH	DINNER
DIET – TYPE									
% CONSUMED									
INTAKE & OUTPUT HOURS	0600-1400	1400-2200	2200-0600	0600-1400	1400-2200	2200-0600	0600-1400	1400-2200	2200-0600
INTAKE									
Oral									
IV									
Blood - Plasma									
Other									
8 Hr. Total									
Output									
Urine									
Emesis									
Stools									
GI Suction									
8 Hr. Total									
24 Hr. Intake									
24 Hr. Output									
SIGNATURE									

DATE:

CLINICAL RECORD

Graphic record.

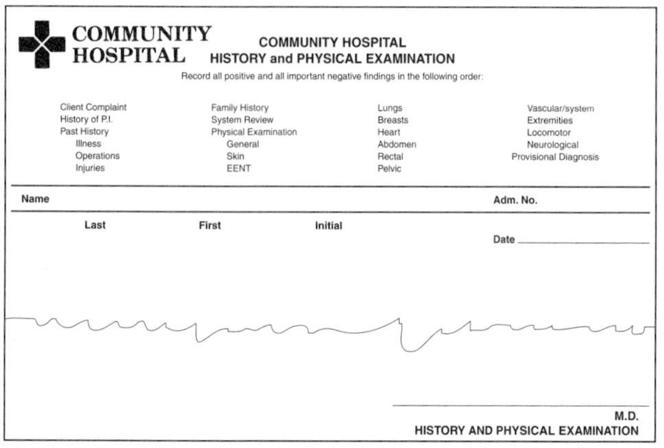

COMMUNITY HOSPITAL

COMMUNITY HOSPITAL
HISTORY and PHYSICAL EXAMINATION

Record all positive and all important negative findings in the following order:

Client Complaint	Family History	Lungs	Vascular/system
History of P.I.	System Review	Breasts	Extremities
Past History	Physical Examination	Heart	Locomotor
Illness	General	Abdomen	Neurological
Operations	Skin	Rectal	Provisional Diagnosis
Injuries	EENT	Pelvic	

Name — Adm. No.

Last — First — Initial — Date ______

M.D.
HISTORY AND PHYSICAL EXAMINATION

Physician's history and physical record.

COMMUNITY HOSPITAL

Client Information

PROGRESS NOTES

Date	Note progress of case, complications, change in diagnosis, condition on discharge

Physician's progress notes.

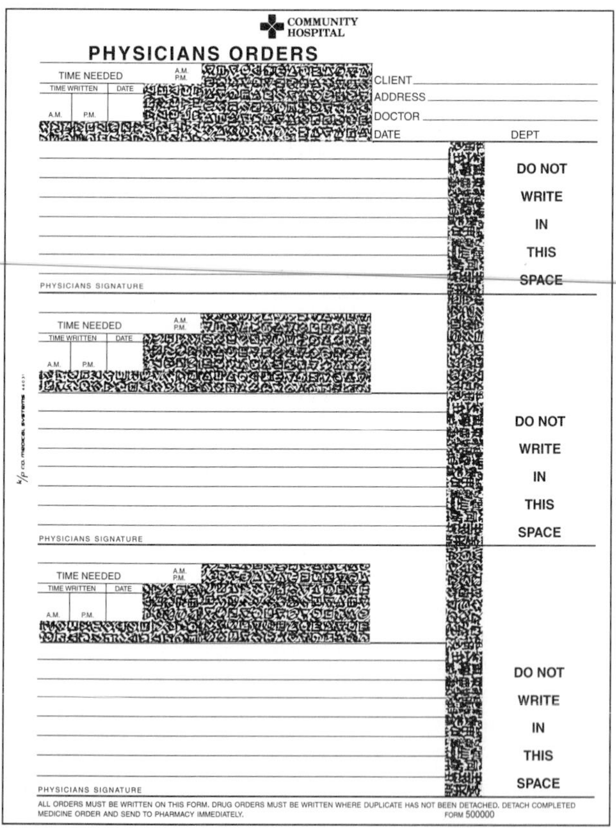

COMMUNITY HOSPITAL

PHYSICIANS ORDERS

TIME NEEDED A.M. P.M. — CLIENT ______
TIME WRITTEN — DATE — ADDRESS ______
A.M. — P.M. — DOCTOR ______
DATE — DEPT

DO NOT WRITE IN THIS SPACE

PHYSICIANS SIGNATURE

TIME NEEDED A.M. P.M.
TIME WRITTEN — DATE
A.M. — P.M.

DO NOT WRITE IN THIS SPACE

PHYSICIANS SIGNATURE

TIME NEEDED A.M. P.M.
TIME WRITTEN — DATE
A.M. — P.M.

DO NOT WRITE IN THIS SPACE

PHYSICIANS SIGNATURE

ALL ORDERS MUST BE WRITTEN ON THIS FORM. DRUG ORDERS MUST BE WRITTEN WHERE DUPLICATE HAS NOT BEEN DETACHED. DETACH COMPLETED MEDICINE ORDER AND SEND TO PHARMACY IMMEDIATELY. FORM 500000

Physician's order sheet.

2

Nursing Process

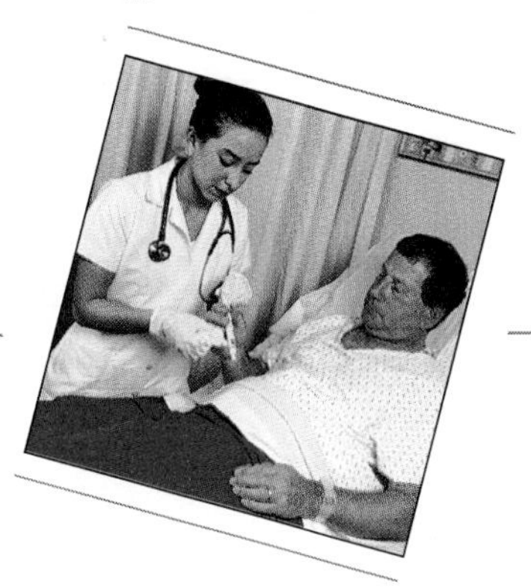

LEARNING OBJECTIVES

- Define the term "nursing process."
- Describe how the nursing process relates to nursing.
- Discuss the term "assessment," and describe how it influences the nursing process.
- List the components of the assessment step.
- Describe the primary purpose of the analysis phase of the nursing process.
- Define planning and give an example of this step in the nursing process.
- Define what is meant by the implementation phase of the nursing process.
- Explain evaluation and include your understanding of why it is an important step in the nursing process.
- Explain how critical thinking is used in each step of the nursing process.
- Define the term "nursing diagnosis."
- Differentiate nursing diagnosis from medical diagnosis.
- State two examples of nursing diagnoses.
- Describe how etiology and defining characteristics relate to a nursing diagnosis.

NURSING PROCESS

Nursing process is a familiar term in nursing and is used as a way of organizing nursing actions in health care delivery. By definition, the term *process* refers to a series of actions that lead toward a particular result. When attached to nursing, the term *nursing process* becomes a general description of a nursing care plan: assessment, analysis/nursing diagnosis, planning, implementation, and evaluation. Although the five steps can be described separately and in logical order, in practice the steps overlap and events may not always occur in the order listed here. For purposes of understanding this process, however, it is appropriate to work through each phase in logical progression.

The five steps of the nursing process are presented, defined, and illustrated to assist you in understanding the importance of integrating this framework in your beginning mastery of nursing content. A model of each step will enable you to visualize how the individual components can be translated into direct nursing actions or behaviors.

Assessment

Assessment, the first step in the nursing process, refers to the establishment of a data base for a specific client. Assessment requires skilled observation, reasoning, and a theoretical knowledge base to gather and differentiate, verify and organize data, and document the findings. The nurse gathers information relevant to the client from a variety of sources and then assigns meaning to this data. Assessment is a critical phase because all the other steps in the process depend on the accuracy and reliability of the assessment.

Assessment is based on concepts of physiology, pathophysiology, psychology, and social adjustment.

Assessment

Gather data
  Objective data
  Subjective data
Verify data
Confirm observations
Organize data
Communicate data

Observe—Interview—Examine

Identify client needs
Be aware of staff reactions to client
Assess sources of data
  Client history
  Data from family
  Client status—physical/emotional
  Signs and symptoms
  Test results and findings
Recall stored knowledge

Nursing Diagnosis

Nursing diagnosis is an integral component of the nursing process. Following the assessment step of the nursing process, the formulation of a nursing diagnosis is made. Nursing diagnosis is the statement of a client problem derived from the systematic collection of data and its analysis. It is a clinical judgment about a designated client, family, or community that provides the basis for completion of the nursing process. Nursing diagnosis includes the etiology, when known, and relates directly to the defining characteristics. Nursing diagnosis provides the foundation for each individual client's therapeutic plan of care, and once it is established, the nurse is accountable for actions that occur within the scope of this nursing diagnosis framework.

A nursing diagnosis is a judgment about a client in response to actual or potential health problems. It provides the basis for selecting nursing interventions that assist the client to achieve stated expected outcomes.

Nursing Diagnosis

Analyze collected data
Examine defining characteristics, both major and minor
Determine clusters of clues
Identify related factors
Identify potential nursing diagnoses
Develop nursing diagnosis appropriate to client problem

Planning

The planning phase refers to the identification of nursing actions that are strategies for achieving the goals or the desired outcome of nursing care. This planning phase should be directly related to solving or alleviating the problems identified in the nursing diagnosis. It includes a plan, goals, strategies for goal outcome, and nursing measures for the delivery of care.

Planning

Develop a plan based on goals, including a teaching plan
Anticipate needs of client and family based on priorities
Select nursing behaviors needed to accomplish goals
Specify deadlines for completion of plan
Coordinate care and community resources
Consider contingencies for modifying plan
Record relevant information

Clients should be involved in the planning phase to ensure that the client's and the health team members' goals are congruent. If they are not, goal achievement can be impaired. Planning focuses on the development of a plan of care individualized for a specific client.

Planning is based on client's health care needs, selected goals, and strategies directed toward goal achievement. It is a plan of care in which the appropriate nursing actions and client's desires are considered and chosen to achieve a goal.

Implementation

The fourth phase in the nursing process is the implementation, or intervention, phase. This phase refers to the priority nursing actions or interventions performed to accomplish a specified goal. It explicitly describes the action component of the nursing process. This phase involves initiating and completing those nursing actions necessary to accomplish the identified client goals. Nursing actions must be appropriate, individualized for the client, and based on safe nursing practice; they should be formulated on scientific principles and derived from the problem-solving process. Finally, the interventions must be congruent with the total medical as well as nursing treatment plan. Implementation of the plan involves giving direct care to the client to accomplish the specified goal.

Implementation

Implement client care plan by giving direct care based on goals
Perform actions and procedures in accordance with client needs
Counsel and teach client or family or both
Use preventive, palliative, or emergency measures for client's welfare
Encourage independence and self-care
Motivate and maintain optimum wellness
Communicate to client's family and allied staff
Supervise work of staff for whom nurse is respon sible
Record data
Continue assessment process

Implementation is based on accurate and complete assessment, interpretation of data, identified client needs, goals, nursing diagnosis, and strategies to achieve goals.

Evaluation

The final phase of the nursing process is evaluation. Evaluation is the examination of the outcome of nursing actions or the extent to which the expected outcomes or goals were achieved. Was the goal achieved? What parts of the goal were not achieved? Was client behavior modified? Evaluation is a necessary phase to complete the nursing process. It allows the nurse to continue to identify goals in the overall treatment plan and to alter the current plan to the client's needs.

> ***Evaluation***
>
> Determine effects of nursing actions
> Determine extent to which goals were achieved
> Examine appropriateness of nursing actions
> Investigate effect and degree of compliance for client and family
> Reassess care plan—judge if goal modification is necessary
> Consider alternative nursing actions
> Record client responses

Evaluation is based on the previous phases of the nursing process (assessment, analysis, planning, and implementation). The evaluation phase completes the process and examines the outcome.

The nursing process has provided the framework for the immense amount of nursing content that is contained in this textbook. The rationale for choosing this framework is that it provides a way to organize and present nursing knowledge as well as being an essential component of providing quality client care.

CRITICAL THINKING

Nurses are required to be problem solvers and decision makers, to acquire nursing judgment skills, and to think critically in order to practice in today's nursing climate. Decision-making and problem-solving skills are necessary for managing and delivering client care. Both of these skills require critical thinking.

Critical thinking has been defined by many authors; however, the most relevant to nursing is the definition by Watson and Glaser.* They describe critical thinking as a process that defines a problem, selects pertinent information for a solution, recognizes stated and unstated assumptions, formulates and selects relevant hypotheses, draws conclusions, and judges the validity of inferences. The outcome of critical thinking is forming a conclusion and stating the justification for that conclusion. This is what differentiates critical thinking from usual thinking.

Nurses who are considered critical thinkers are those who use logic, creativity, and good communication, and are flexible and competent in delivery of client care. Nurses use critical thinking skills as they relate theory to practice, apply the nursing process in client care, and make critical clinical decisions. The ability to use critical thinking skills assists the nurse to recognize and analyze problems and to solve them using a systematic approach.

To acquire critical thinking skills, the nurse must first develop a sound theoretical knowledge base. This means studying the concepts appropriate to each clinical discipline (i.e., disease state and client problem in each area of nursing practice) and transferring that knowledge to provide safe client care and make independent judgments.

Critical thinking is a process as well as a cognitive skill that is used to identify and define problems, assess clients, and evaluate their responses to treatment and care. Nurses select and classify data and organize it into clusters or patterns to support nursing diagnoses. Critical thinking is used when alternative nursing actions are evaluated and the most appropriate action is selected for each client problem. After the client intervention is carried out, the effectiveness of the intervention and client outcome is evaluated using critical thinking. It is easy to see from this statement that critical thinking is used throughout the steps of the nursing process.

The following examples demonstrate how critical thinking is used throughout the steps of the nursing process.

Assessment

Identifying essential assessment data and where the data can be found requires critical thinking. Obtaining, classifying, and organizing data is a principal function of critical thinking.

Nursing Diagnosis

Before a nursing diagnosis is made, the nurse critically analyzes, clusters, and interprets all the collected data to ensure an accurate nursing diagnosis.

Planning

Client's long- and short-term goals are formulated after deliberating with the client, family, and other health team members. Defining realistic goals that are acceptable to the client requires critical thinking. A prioritized plan of care is developed during this phase of the nursing process that includes client outcomes.

Implementation

Nursing interventions are specific strategies developed to achieve positive client outcomes. These interventions are determined by using the critical thinking skills of generalizing, explaining, and predicting outcomes. After consideration of all possible actions, nursing interventions are implemented.

Evaluation

During the final phase of the nursing process, the nurse critically analyzes each of the client outcomes. If the client need was not satisfied, the plan would be revised.

In addition to using critical thinking skills when providing client care, nurse managers use these skills in assigning client care and delegating activities, an example of which is the assignment of client care to a nursing assistant. The nurse manager must determine the skill level of the nursing assistant and the critical nature of the client, as well as other staffing assignments before the assignment is completed.

NURSING DIAGNOSIS

An important implication of nursing diagnosis is that it refers to a health problem or condition that nurses are legally licensed to treat. The establishment and acceptance of this diagnostic category demonstrates recognition and legal sanction of nursing as a profession with its own body of knowledge, education, and experience.

The term *nursing diagnosis* is not comparable to or the same as medical diagnosis. Nursing diagnosis is derived from the assessment phase of the nursing process and is based on both subjective and objective data. As the data base evolves, patterns of health problems emerge, and alterations from normal health states are identified. A nursing diagnosis is a statement of an actual health problem or a potential one within the

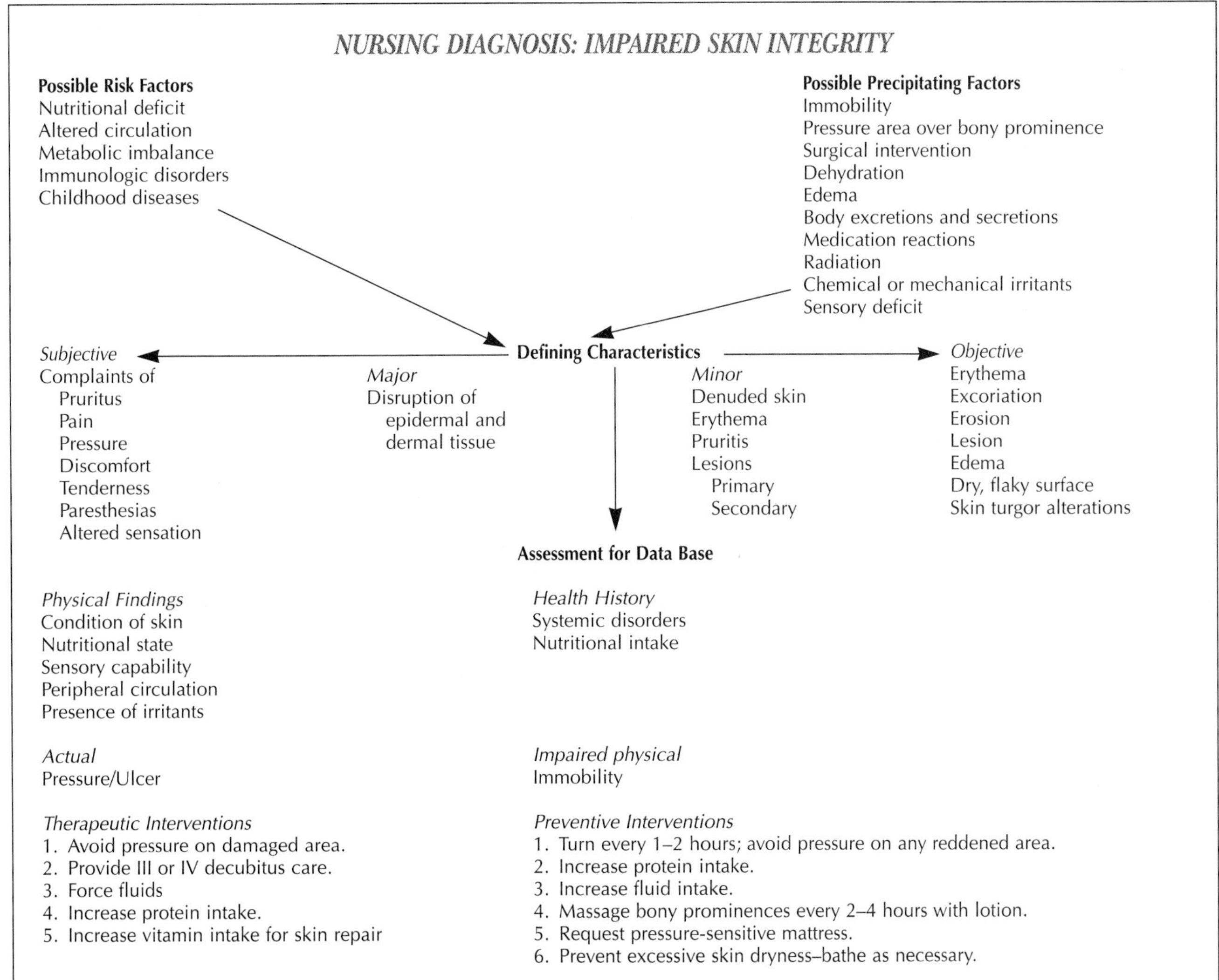

client's biologic, social, or personal system. The specific problem identified implies that the nurse is qualified and prepared to intervene and treat that condition. The nurse is not legally able to intervene and treat a medical diagnosis without specific physician's orders. Thus, the nurse is not able to intervene if the client has a diagnosis of *potential atelectasis* or *pneumonia.* This is a medical diagnosis, whereas *ineffective breathing pattern* is a nursing diagnosis and nursing interventions can be instituted to assist the client.

Components of the nursing diagnosis are divided into three major categories: the diagnosis of a client's condition as potential or actual, the etiology to which the condition is related, and the defining characteristics that support the etiology. Thus, in practice, the client's nursing diagnosis could be stated, for example, Impaired Skin Integrity. This statement is followed by the related factors, if known, and the defining characteristics.

The rationale for specifying whether a diagnosis is actual or potential is that this judgment gives direction to the nursing interventions and enables the nurse to evaluate them on a realistic basis. Since many causes of a condition are possible, the term *related factors* identifies possible etiologies. And since there are also various interventions possible for different etiologies, the statement needs to be specific to individualize client care. Finally, the third component of nursing diagnosis includes the defining characteristics or the observable signs and symptoms that directly relate to the etiology and, in turn, to the actual or potential nursing diagnosis.

Since the steps of the nursing process are based on formulating a nursing diagnosis, it is a critical component of providing high-level professional nursing care. To ensure that the nursing terms used in diagnosis are standardized throughout the nursing profession, the National Conference Group Classification of Nursing Diagnosis established a list of accepted nursing diagnoses. This list standardized diagnostic terms to clearly communicate a client's problems and needs. The accepted nursing diagnoses are listed at the end of this chapter.

The standardized list assists nurses to define and classify the scope of nursing practice. This classification system will assist the profession to expand its body of knowledge based on a firm scientific foundation.

A nursing diagnosis describes a client's response that can be altered through independent nursing practice interventions. An actual nursing diagnosis is determined after validating clinical data (major defining characteristics). A nursing diagnosis comprises four components:

Label, or *nursing, diagnosis*: A descriptor of the client's condition determined through a subjective and objective assessment. The conditions can be identified as actual or potential.

Definition: A clear statement that accurately defines the nursing diagnosis. Most established definitions have been developed by the North American Nursing Diagnosis Association (NANDA).

Defining characteristics: Clinical behaviors, signs and symptoms, either observed or verbalized by the client or family. Both subjective and objective signs and symptoms determine the nursing diagnosis. Defining characteristics are separated into major and minor designations. Major characteristics are critical indicators present 80–100% of the time. Minor characteristics are present 50–79% of the time.

Related factors: Etiologies or contributing factors that influence the client's condition. These factors can be grouped into physiological, psychological, situational, maturational, or treatment-related categories.

Diagnostic Statements

Two common types of diagnostic statements, or nursing diagnoses, are generally used. A two-part statement includes the label and related factors that contributed to the client's condition. Impaired Skin Integrity "related to" prolonged immobility is an example of such a statement. A three-part statement includes the label, related factors, and the signs and symptoms related to the diagnosis: for example, Impaired Skin Integrity "related to" prolonged immobility as evidenced by a 2×2-cm lesion on coccyx.

The "related to" phrase indicates a relationship between the nursing diagnosis and the related factors. It does not imply a cause-and-effect relationship. The more specific the related factors are stated, the more relevant and accurate the nursing actions or interventions can be determined.

The PES framework is a commonly used approach or organizing framework developed by Marjory Gordon that uses the three-part diagnostic statement.

P refers to the *problem,* or state of health, of the individual, family, or community. This problem is expressed as clearly as possible, for example, Impaired Skin Integrity.

E describes the *etiology*, or probable cause, of the health problem. This may refer to many factors that include client behaviors, environmental components, or the interaction of both. The etiology is combined with the problem statement by using the words "related to," for example, prolonged bedrest.

S signifies the relevant *signs and symptoms*—usually a summary of the objective assessment findings (signs) and subjective data reported by the client (symptoms). The phrase that connects this part of the statement is "manifested by," for example, Impaired Skin Integrity, "related to" prolonged bedrest, *manifested* by open lesion, 2 × 2 cm on coccyx.

Although there are several approaches to formulating a statement of nursing diagnosis, the PES system is used by many schools of nursing throughout the United States.

NANDA APPROVED NURSING DIAGNOSES FOR CLINICAL USE AND TESTING (1994).

Pattern 1: Exchanging

Altered Nutrition: More than Body Requirements
Altered Nutrition: Less than Body Requirements
Altered Nutrition: Potential for More Than Body Requirements
* Risk for Infection
* Risk for Altered Body Temperature
Hypothermia
Hyperthermia
Ineffective Thermoregulation
Dysreflexia
Constipation
Perceived Constipation
Colonic Constipation
Diarrhea
Bowel Incontinence
Altered Urinary Elimination
Stress Incontinence
Reflex Incontinence
Urge Incontinence
Functional Incontinence
Total Incontinence
Urinary Retention
Altered (Specify Type) Tissue Perfusion (Renal, cerebral, cardiopulmonary, gastrointestinal, peripheral)
Fluid Volume Excess
Fluid Volume Deficit
* Risk for Fluid Volume Deficit
Decreased Cardiac Output
Impaired Gas Exchange
Ineffective Airway Clearance
Ineffective Breathing Pattern
Inability to Sustain Spontaneous Ventilation
Dysfunctional Ventilatory Weaning Response (DVWR)
* Risk for Injury
Risk for Suffocation
* Risk for Poisoning
* Risk for Trauma
* Risk for Aspiration
* Risk for Disuse Syndrome
Altered Protection
Impaired Tissue Integrity
Altered Oral Mucous Membrane
Impaired Skin Integrity
* Risk for Impaired Skin Integrity
# Decreased Adaptive Capacity: Intracranial
# Energy Field Disturbance

Pattern 2: Communicating

Impaired Verbal Communication

Pattern 3: Relating

Impaired Social Interaction
Social Isolation
Risk for Loneliness
Altered Role Performance
Altered Parenting
* Risk for Altered Parenting
# Risk for Altered Parent/Infant/Child Attachment
Sexual Dysfunction

Altered Family Processes
Caregiver Role Strain
* Risk for Caregiver Role Strain
# Altered Family Process: Alcoholism
Parental Role Conflict
Altered Sexuality Patterns

Pattern 4: Valuing

Spiritual Distress (Distress of the Human Spirit)
Potential for Enhanced Spiritual Well-Being

Pattern 5: Choosing

Ineffective Individual Coping
Impaired Adjustment
Defensive Coping
Ineffective Denial
Ineffective Family Coping: Disabling
Ineffective Family Coping: Compromised
Family Coping: Potential for Growth
Potential for Enhanced Community Coping
Ineffective Community Coping
Ineffective Management of Therapeutic Regimen (Individuals)
Noncompliance (Specify)
Ineffective Management of Therapeutic Regimen: Families
Ineffective Management of Therapeutic Regimen: Community
Ineffective Management of Therapeutic Regimen: Individual
Decisional Conflict (Specify)
Health Seeking Behaviors (Specify)

Pattern 6: Moving

Impaired Physical Mobility
* Risk for Peripheral Neurovascular Dysfunction
# Risk for Perioperative Positioning Injury
Activity Intolerance
Fatigue
* Risk for Activity Intolerance
Sleep Pattern Disturbance
Diversional Activity Deficit
Impaired Home Maintenance Management
Altered Health Maintenance
Feeding Self Care Deficit
Impaired Swallowing
Ineffective Breastfeeding
Interrupted Breastfeeding
Effective Breastfeeding
Ineffective Infant Feeding Pattern
Bathing/Hygiene Self Care Deficit
Dressing/Grooming Self Care Deficit
Toileting Self Care Deficit
Altered Growth and Development
Relocation Stress Syndrome
Risk for Disorganized Infant Behavior
Disorganized Infant Behavior
Potential for Enhanced Organized Infant Behavior

Pattern 7: Perceiving

Body Image Disturbance
Self Esteem Disturbance
Chronic Low Self Esteem
Situational Low Self Esteem
Personal Identity Disturbance
Sensory/Perceptual Alterations (Specify) (Visual, Auditory, Kinesthetic, Gustatory, Tactile, Olfactory)
Unilateral Neglect
Hopelessness
Powerlessness

Pattern 8: Knowing

Knowledge Deficit (Specify)
Impaired Environmental Interpretation Syndrome
Acute Confusion
Chronic Confusion
Altered Thought Processes
Impaired Memory

Pattern 9: Feeling

Pain
Chronic Pain
Dysfunctional Grieving
Anticipatory Grieving
* Risk for Violence: Self-Directed or Directed at Others
* Risk for Self-Mutilation
Post-Trauma Response
Rape-Trauma Syndrome
Rape-Trauma Syndrome: Compound Reaction
Rape-Trauma Syndrome: Silent Reaction
Anxiety
Fear

#New diagnoses added in 1994 classified at level 1.4 using new Criteria for Staging (see reference later in this book).
*Diagnoses with modified label terminology in 1994. (This change was recommended by the NANDA Taxonomy Committee and adopted to remain consistent with the ICD.)

3

Client Care Management

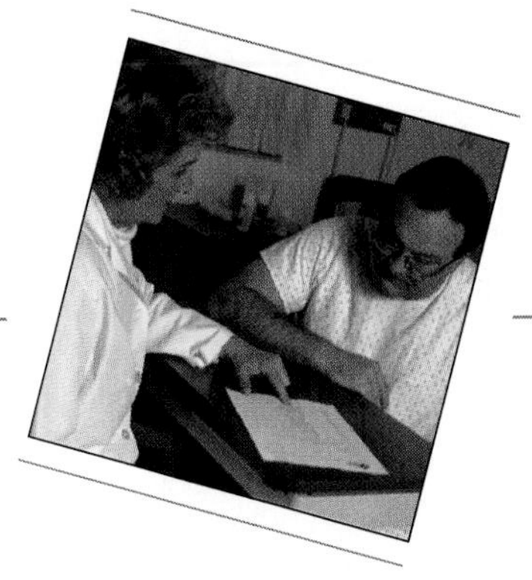

LEARNING OBJECTIVES

- Describe the components of the client care plan.
- State the two types of client care plan.
- Explain the method for individualizing the care plan when a standard care plan is used.
- Compare and contrast the initiation of a standard and individualized care plan.
- Define the term client problem or need.
- State the most important reason for using nursing diagnosis in care planning.
- Describe the relationship between expected outcomes or goals and client care.
- Define the use of deadlines and checkpoints in the client care plan.
- Describe the relationship between long-term goals and discharge criteria.
- State how the client care plan and nurses' notes relate to each other.
- Discuss the RN's role in delegating client care.
- Complete a data collection tool based on a clinical situation.
- Develop a time-management work sheet for client care.

CARE PLANS

Client care plans are an integral part of providing nursing care. Without them, quality and consistency of client care may not be obtained. Client care plans provide a means of communication among nurses and other health care providers. The plan should serve as a focal point for client care assignments and reporting.

Regardless of the type of care plan used, the following information should be included: client's needs or problems both actual and potential, stated as nursing diagnoses, expected outcomes or short-term goals, nursing interventions or actions, and discharge criteria or long-term goals.

Once the goals of client care are established, they are formulated in a care plan. Each step in meeting these goals is detailed, including specific observations and how often the observations are made. Step-by-step directions are included for difficult problems, such as lengthy and involved dressing changes. Individualized client teaching programs are described on the care plan. As is evident, all of this information is essential in providing continuity of client care.

Format

Client care plans are available in several formats. The client's plan of care may be outlined on the Kardex, or on a specific hospital form and placed in the client's chart.

Types

Client care plans consist of two types: an individualized care plan completely written by the nurse for each specific client and a standard client care plan. Because of the large amount of time necessary to write individualized care plans, hospital nursing departments are developing preprinted standard care plans based on the most frequent hospital admission diagnoses for the hospital. The standard care plan outlines the usual problems or needs that occur with a specific diagnosis. It contains a list of usual nursing actions or interventions and the standard expected outcomes for each problem.

Individualizing Care Plans

All clients must have an individualized plan of care even though the standard care plan is used. To individualize the care plan, space is generally provided at the end of the preprinted form to allow the nurse to identify unusual problems or needs. Standard care plans can also be individualized by activating only those problems that pertain to a particular client. For example, the figure illustrates a standard care plan that has been individualized. Items 1 and 3 have been activated by circling, dating, and initialing the item number. The nurse may add another problem to the bottom of the form to further individualize the care plan.

Initiating the Plan

The client care plan is formulated after the assessment phase of the nursing process. The nurse, after completing the nursing history and assessment, determines if a standard care plan is available for the client's medical diagnosis or if an individualized care plan must be written. If a standard care plan is available, the nurse need only circle, date, and initial the needs that are relevant for that client. When an individualized care plan is being written, the nurse translates the client's needs or problems into nursing diagnoses and writes them on the care plan. Nursing diagnoses are the acceptable terminology for use on client care plans throughout the country. The terminology was established by the

KARDEX / RAND CLIENT CARE PLAN

CLIENT EDUCATION PROGRAM			DISCHARGE CRITERIA	DISCHARGE PLAN	Addressograph
	DATE		PLAN:		
Diabetic______	Start	Finish	Stroke Rehab Eval ______	Discharge Coordinator	
Coronary______			Cardiac Rehab Eval ______	Date Involved ______	
Other______			SOCIAL SERVICE	Home ______	
______			Date Involved ______	ECF______	
			Comment:	OTHER______	

Date	Client Problem	Deadline Date	Expected Outcome	Health Team Action

Kardex card form is not retained as a permanent part of the medical record.

COMMUNITY HOSPITAL

CLIENT CARE PLAN
Individualized

Client Information

Discharge Criteria
1) *Verbalizes understanding of discharge meds*
2) *States available resource agencies*
3)
4)

Admitting Diagnosis
Relevant Info:

Date	Problem/Need	Expected Outcome/Goal	CP	DL	Nursing Interventions	Update / DC	Initial
3/22/96	*1. Knowledge*	*Verbalizes*	*q̄ shift*	*Prior to disch.*	*1. a) Instruct in actions of and times for*		
	Deficit R/t	*understanding*			*administration of each drug.*		
	discharge meds.	*of discharge meds.*			*b) Ask client to recite s/s of side effects*		
		States s/s of side			*of meds.*		
		effects.					
	2. Ineffective	*Able to*	*q̄ shift*	*Prior to disch.*	*2. a) Determine level of understanding*		
	Individual	*demonstrate*			*of diagnosis and prognosis.*		
	Coping	*effective coping.*					

Individualized client care plan is a permanent part of the medical record.

National Conference on Classification of Nursing Diagnosis, published for the first time in 1973.

Client Problems or Needs

A client problem or need is a condition that requires assistance or intervention from a health team member to return the client to a healthy state. The client problem is identified as any unmet need. It can be as basic as the need for adequate comfort or nourishment to the more complex psychosocial needs.

On many care plans, problems are identified as either actual or potential. An actual problem is one that exists at that time. Interventions are planned to resolve or alter the problem. A potential problem describes a condition that frequently occurs with the client's diagnosis or health problem. An actual problem, for example, is a reddened coccyx related to urinary incontinence. Interventions are developed to treat the reddened area to prevent further breakdown or decubitus ulcer formation. A potential problem, such as "Ineffective Breathing Patterns *related to* acute pain" following gallbladder surgery, could affect any client with

COMMUNITY HOSPITAL

CLIENT CARE PLAN

Client Information

Discharge Criteria
1) Lungs clear to auscultation.
2) Voiding qs and continent of urine.
3) Verbalizes an understanding of discharge instructions and medications.
4)

Admitting Diagnosis

Relevant Info:

Date	Problem/Need	Expected Outcome/Goal	CP	DL	Nursing Interventions	Update / DC	Initial
1/18/96	(1.) Ineffective Breathing Pattern related to pain.	Absence of respiratory complications.	q2h x24h then q4h x48h then q8h q3-4 h	POD 3 1/21 3 pm	1a. Encourage turning, coughing and deep breathing exercises (TCDB) q2h. b. Teach client to splint incision when coughing. c. Instruct in use of breathing device, if ordered. d. Place in semi-Fowler's position. e. Assess need for pain med. f. Medicate for pain 1/2hr. before TCDB. g. Auscultate breath sounds.		
	2. Altered Urinary Elimination related to incontinence.	Continent of urine. Absence of urinary tract infection (UTI).	q4h	cath. out	2a. Check urinary output for signs and symptoms of UTI, i.e. color, odor, consistency. b. Provide catheter care according to protocol. c. Force fluids to 2500mL. d. Give cranberry juice, 240mL q shift.		
1/18/96	(3.) Knowledge Deficit related to administration of discharge meds.	Verbalizes understanding of discharge meds, including listing signs and symptoms of side effects.	q24h	prior to disch	3a. Instruct in action of Maxaquin b. Review side effects with client and/or family. c. Have client state signs and symptoms of side effects prior to discharge. d. Provide Take Home Medication pamphlet.		
	4. Impaired Skin Integrity related to prolonged immobility.	Skin clean and intact.	q4h q2h	prior to disch	4a. Provide skin care. Use alcohol in a.m., lotion thereafter. b. Turn side to side. c. Keep linens dry and wrinkle free.		

*You may use approved abbreviations from the facility when writing care plans.

Preprinted standardized client care plan using Nursing Diagnosis format.

that condition. Interventions are planned to prevent the problem. Some potential problems are identified to assess more carefully for them. For example, a debilitated client with poor nutrition is assessed for possible wound infection.

Nursing Diagnosis

Using a nursing diagnosis to state the client's real or potential problems takes the problem out of the realm of a medical diagnosis. The nursing diagnosis does not focus on a problem or disease state but rather on a physical, psychological, or behavioral response. Nursing diagnosis can change frequently as the client's health status changes and potential health problems become actual health problems. The nursing diagnosis approach, unlike the medical model or systems approach to care planning, allows for this flexibility in focus.

The use of nursing diagnosis in care planning is a universal method of communication to all health team members. When the diagnosis "Impaired Skin Integrity" is written, the entire health team knows that the client has a broken area on the skin with destruction of skin layers. The relationship of skin impairment to cause is usually stated as "Impaired Skin Integrity, *related to* prolonged immobility."

Expected Outcomes or Goals

After the problems have been identified, the nurse sets goals or expected outcomes for client care that are congruent with the goals of the client or significant other. Client-centered goals should be clear, concise, realistic, and should identify specific observable and measurable behaviors. Expected outcomes or goals should indicate what is to be expected when the goal is achieved, by whom, when, to what degree of accuracy, and should be

COMMUNITY HOSPITAL

CLIENT CARE PLAN

Client Information

Discharge Criteria
1) Lungs clear to auscultation.
2) Voiding qs and continent of urine.
3) Verbalizes an understanding of discharge instructions and medications.
4)

Admitting Diagnosis
Relevant Info:

Date	Problem/Need	Expected Outcome/Goal	CP	DL	Nursing Interventions	Update / DC	Initial
1/18/96	(1.) Ineffective Breathing Pattern related to pain.	Absence of respiratory complications.	q2h x24h then q4h x48h then q8h	POD 3 1/21 3 pm	(1)a. Encourage turning, coughing and deep breathing exercises (TCDB) q2h. b. Teach client to splint incision when coughing. c. Instruct in use of breathing device, if ordered. d. Place in semi-Fowler's position.		
			q3-4 h		e. Assess need for pain med. f. Medicate for pain 1/2hr. before TCDB. g. Auscultate breath sounds.		
	2. Altered Urinary Elimination related to incontinence.	Continent of urine. Absence of urinary tract infection (UTI).	q4h	cath. out	2a. Check urinary output for signs and symptoms of UTI, i.e. color, odor, consistency. b. Provide catheter care according to protocol. c. Force fluids to 2500mL. d. Give client cranberry juice, 240mL q shift.		
1/18/96	(3.) Knowledge Deficit related to administration of discharge meds.	Verbalizes understanding of discharge meds, including listing signs and symptoms of side effects.	q24h	prior to disch	(3)a. Instruct in action of Maxaquin b. Review side effects with client and/or family. c. Have client state signs and symptoms of side effects prior to discharge. d. Provide Take Home Medication pamphlet.		
	4. Impaired Skin Integrity related to prolonged immobility.	Skin clean and intact.	q4h q2h	prior to disch	4a. Provide skin care. Use alcohol in a.m., lotion thereafter. b. Turn side to side. c. Keep linens dry and wrinkle free.		

*You may use approved abbreviations from the facility when writing care plans.

Expected outcomes and nursing interventions.

time-limited. The figure shows several examples of a client-centered goal and the nursing interventions necessary to attain each goal.

Interventions

After problems and expected outcomes are written on the care plan, the nurse determines appropriate nursing interventions that meet the goals of care. Interventions, if written properly, specify the exact nursing actions to be carried out or provide explicit instructions on how care is to be delivered. Time and frequency of the intervention should also be provided.

Checkpoints and Deadlines

The standard care plan illustrated in this text includes checkpoint (CP) and deadline (DL) columns. The checkpoint indicates how often the action or intervention should be checked, observed, or carried out and therefore how often it should be charted. The deadline column indicates the time when the goal should be met or the action is no longer necessary. It is important to document the exact time and date when the nursing action should be completed to communicate this information to the entire nursing staff. In the example, notice that item 1—breathing patterns ineffective—should be alleviated by the third postoperative day, in this case, January 21 at 3:00 PM. The checkpoints are listed in sequence to meet the goal. For the first 24 hours the nursing interventions (1a through 1d) should be completed every 2 hours and then advanced to every 4 hours for the next 48 hours.

Short- and Long-Term Goals

Client care plans must include both short- and long-term goals. Long-term goals are frequently stated as discharge criteria and as such should be met prior to dis-

COMMUNITY HOSPITAL

CLIENT CARE PLAN

Client Information

Discharge Criteria

1) Lungs clear to auscultation.
2) Voiding qs and continent of urine.
3) Verbalizes an understanding of discharge instructions and medications.
4)

Admitting Diagnosis

Relevant Info:

Date	Problem/Need	Expected Outcome/Goal	CP	DL	Nursing Interventions	Update / DC	Initial
1/18/96	(1.) Ineffective Breathing Pattern related to pain.	Absence of respiratory complications.	q2h x24h then q4h x48h then q8h q3-4 h	POD 3 1/21 3 pm	(1)a. Encourage turning, coughing and deep breathing exercises (TCDB) q2h. b. Teach client to splint incision when coughing. c. Instruct in use of breathing device, if ordered. d. Place in semi-Fowler's position. e. Assess need for pain med. f. Medicate for pain 1/2hr. before TCDB. g. Auscultate breath sounds.		
	2. Altered Urinary Elimination related to incontinence.	Continent of urine. Absence of urinary tract infection (UTI).	q4h	cath. out	2a. Check urinary output for signs and symptoms of UTI, i.e. color, odor, consistency. b. Provide catheter care according to protocol. c. Force fluids to 2500mL. d. Give cranberry juice, 240mL q shift.		
1/18/96	(3.) Knowledge Deficit related to administration of discharge meds.	Verbalizes understanding of discharge meds, including listing signs and symptoms of side effects.	q24h	prior to disch	(3)a. Instruct in action of Maxaquin b. Review side effects with client and/or family. c. Have client state signs and symptoms of side effects prior to discharge. d. Provide Take Home Medication pamphlet.		
	4. Impaired Skin Integrity related to prolonged immobility.	Skin clean and intact.	q4h q2h	prior to disch	4a. Provide skin care. Use alcohol in a.m., lotion thereafter. b. Turn side to side. c. Keep linens dry and wrinkle free.		

*You may use approved abbreviations from the facility when writing care plans.

Checkpoints, deadlines, and discharge criteria.

charge, if possible. Short-term goals usually appear in the form of expected outcomes for each problem. They are designed as stepping stones to assist the client to meet discharge criteria or long-term goals. Some hospitals, particularly rehabilitation facilities, use short-term goals differently. They frequently set weekly steps or phases in the rehabilitative process that clients meet before the final expected outcome is achieved. For example, to meet the long-term goal of ambulation without use of devices, a short-term goal is to ambulate with a walker without assistance. These types of goals are prioritized and updated regularly.

Updating Care Plans

To ensure that client care plans are current and relevant, they should be reviewed on a daily basis and updated at least every 24 to 48 hours. There are several ways to update a care plan. Some facilities have spaces designated on the nursing Kardex or nurses' notes. In the figure, the update column is used when the original deadline is reached but the problem persists. A new deadline must then be established. If the ineffective breathing pattern exists beyond the third postoperative day, a new time frame for goal achievement is determined and documented in the update column. As the example shows, the fourth postoperative day is determined to be the new time frame. The update would then read 1/22 @ 3PM.

Activating Care Plans

When standard care plans are used, a systematic approach to activation and deactivation must be understood by all nursing personnel. As already stated, a common approach is to circle, date, and initial problems

COMMUNITY HOSPITAL

CLIENT CARE PLAN

Client Information

Discharge Criteria
1) Lungs clear to auscultation.
2) Voiding qs and continent of urine.
3) Verbalizes an understanding of discharge instructions and medications.
4)

Admitting Diagnosis

Relevant Info:

Date	Problem/Need	Expected Outcome/Goal	CP	DL	Nursing Interventions	Update / DC	Initial
1/18/96	(1.) Ineffective Breathing Pattern related to pain.	Absence of respiratory complications.	q2h x24h then q4h x48h then q8h q3-4 h	POD 3 1/21 3 pm	(1)a. Encourage turning, coughing and deep breathing exercises (TCDB) q2h. b. Teach client to splint incision when coughing. c. Instruct in use of breathing device, if ordered. d. Place in semi-Fowler's position. e. Assess need for pain med. f. Medicate for pain 1/2hr. before TCDB. g. Auscultate breath sounds.	Cont, 1/22 @ 3 pm	DD
	2. Altered Urinary Elimination related to incontinence.	Continent of urine. Absence of urinary tract infection (UTI).	q4h	cath. out	2a. ~~Check urinary output for signs and symptoms of UTI, ie. color, odor, consistency.~~ b. ~~Provide catheter care according to protocol.~~ c. Force fluids to 2500mL. d. Give cranberry juice, 240mL q shift.	1/21 1/21	DD DD
1/18/96	(3.) Knowledge Deficit related to administration of discharge meds.	Verbalizes understanding of discharge meds, including listing signs and symptoms of side effects.	q24h	prior to disch	(3)a. ~~Instruct in action of Maxaquin~~ b. ~~Review~~ side effects with client and/or family. c. Have client state signs and symptoms of side effects prior to discharge.	1/21	DD

Updating and inactivating of care plan.

that are relevant for the individual client. Any problem that is not circled remains inactivated and should not be assessed, treated, or documented. From the example, you can see that the client has two of the problems listed, a potential ineffective breathing pattern and a knowledge deficit regarding discharge medication. Items 1 and 3 are circled. In the date column, date, time, and initials of the nurse activating the problem are entered. The second problem is not activated; therefore a circle is not placed around the number.

Inactivating Care Plans

To inactivate the problem, a single line through the problem or intervention with a black pen can be made. In the update/DC column the date, time, and nurse's initials should be placed next to the crossed out, inactivated information. If only one of the interventions is not necessary, a line is drawn through that intervention and initials placed next to it in the initial column. The other interventions are left current and active.

COMMUNICATION

Documentation

Documentation of findings in the nurses' notes should closely parallel the intervention column for all activated problems. When a problem is assessed every 2 hours, it should be documented appropriately in the client's chart every 2 hours. If breath sounds are auscultated every 4 hours, they are documented on a flow sheet or in the nurses' notes every 4 hours. If a chart audit is done on the client's chart, the quality assurance auditor should be able to find each activated problem identified in the chart with appropriate interventions documented.

Care Plans

Client care needs are identified and appropriate interventions determined to meet these needs. This data is written on the care plan as a means of communicating the client's needs to all health care workers.

Clinical Pathway for Total Hip Replacemen

	1	2	3
Underscore at care event needs initials or time.	Admit/Operation Date or Time ______	Postoperative day (POD) 1 Date/Time ______	POD 2 Date/Time ______
ASSESSMENT A	q 8° ✓:general assessment, CMS, Drsg, I&O, B/S, Abd dist, flatus, SaO2 q 4 hr. ✓: V.S, Hemovac(HV)	q 8° ✓:gen assessment CMS, Drsg, HV, I&O, IV q 4° ✓: VS BID: Homan sign SaO2>90 DC O2	q 8° ✓:gen asses CMS, Drsg, I&O, VS, IV site HV dcd BM passed
PHYSICAL ACTIVITY P	Bedrest, move in bed with assist	OOB chair,transf & gait training	1 gait training Amb BID if able
TREATMENT T	I.S., TCDB, TED/SCD, Hip Precautions	TED/SCD, I.S., TCDB, Hip Precautions	Hip Prec., TED/SC I.S.,DC Foley
MEDICATIONS IV,PO,IM,SQ,ETC M	Ancef 8hr x 24hr, Antiemetic PRN, Anticoagulant	Stool softener, Iron supp. if HBG <10 & Anticoagulant	Stool softener, I supp, Anticoagular cathartic if no B
IV FLUIDS/ BLOOD PRODUCTS I	Transfuse/reinfuse PRN, IV at 75/100 cc till tol P.O.	IV at TKO	IV TKO or hep. LOK
NUTRITION N	Advance diet as tolerated	DAT	DAT
COMFORT/PAIN C	PCA/Epidural or other pain medication	PCA/Epidural or other pain medication	PCA/Epidural tape give PO pain meds
EDUCATION E	Pre & Postop., clinical pathway,TED/SCD, Analgesia method	Reinforce Postop. & clinical pathway, TED/SCD, Analgesia	Analgesia method

Sample of Clinical Pathway.

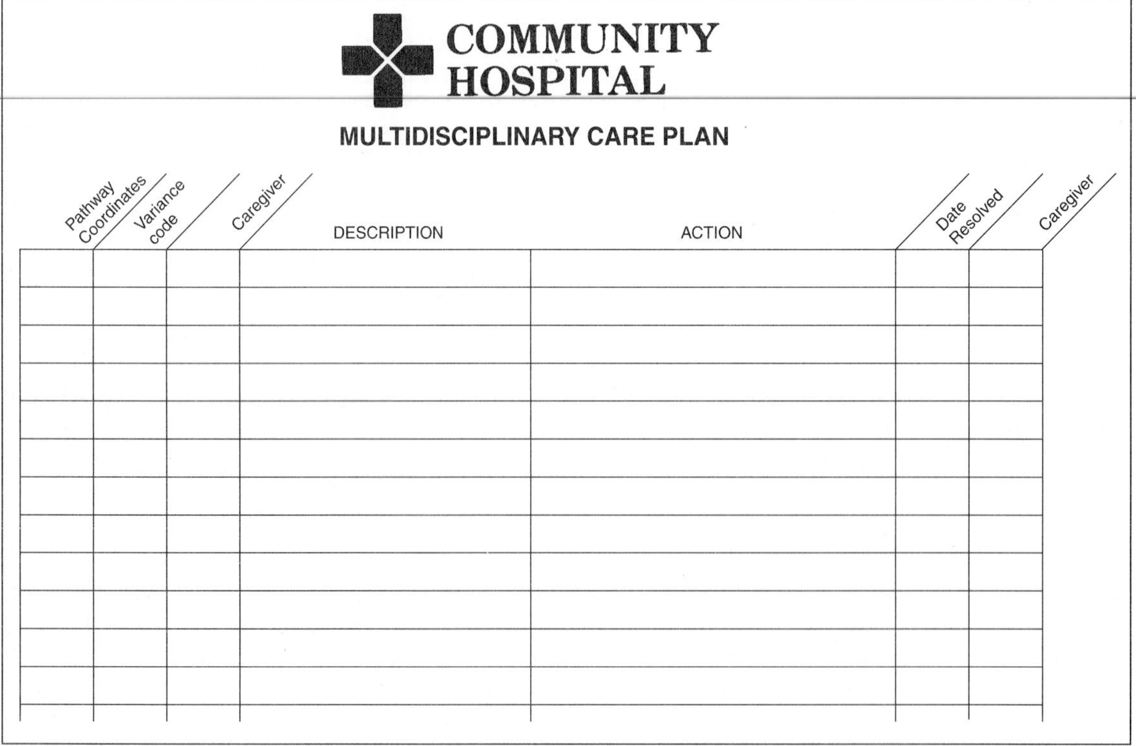

COMMUNITY HOSPITAL

MULTIDISCIPLINARY CARE PLAN

Pathway Coordinates	Variance code	Caregiver	DESCRIPTION	ACTION	Date Resolved	Caregiver

Multidisciplinary Care Plan.

Careplan Formats

As computers are being used more commonly to document nursing care and workplace redesign is transforming how we deliver nursing care, the type and method of using the nursing care plan is changing. The Joint Commission on the Accreditation of Healthcare Organization's requirements are becoming more flexible and are allowing new ways to document client care. Critical paths, protocols, and standardized nursing care plans are used with or are replacing the more traditional care plans.

Computerized Client Care Plans. The format used in computer software packages individualizes client care plans according to each health care facility's specifications. This type of format is very popular now that computerized documentation systems have been implemented in many facilities. Preparation time for writing individualized care plans is decreased and standardized plans are developed and written by clinical experts. One disadvantage of this software is that nurses must carefully determine the relevance and appropriateness of the care plan for each individual client. The care plan for each client is generated by the computer each shift. Changes must be entered into the computer frequently to ensure the accuracy of the plan.

Critical Paths or Clinical Pathways. This type of documentation is used primarily with managed care delivery systems. In this system, traditional nursing care plans do not exist. A critical path or clinical pathway is a standardized multidisciplinary plan of care developed for clients with common or prevalent conditions. It is a tool developed collaboratively by all health team members to facilitate achievement of client outcomes in a predictable and established time frame. The plan indicates the actions and interventions achieved at designated times in order to meet the criteria for reimbursable length of stay. For example, a client with a total hip replacement has a critical path that states time frames for out of bed, gait training, and ambulation listed under the physical activity section of the form. On the first postoperative day the client should move from bed to chair and participate in gait training. Nursing diagnoses are not always incorporated in the critical path. If the client does not achieve the expected outcome in the specified time a "variance" occurs, and an individual plan of care is developed that may then incorporate nursing diagnosis. For example, if a client is unable to ambulate by day three a nursing diagnosis can be used to individualize the client's variance from the critical path expectations. An individualized care plan is initiated, and charting continues on the variance until it is resolved. The individualized section of the care path is usually found on the back of the form. All other documentation continues on the care path. Documentation of nursing activities completed in response to the critical path varies according to facility policies and guidelines. Some facilities initial each day's completed tasks on the critical path document, whereas others use flow charts and narrative charting.

Protocols. There are several uses for protocols within the various health care settings. Protocols can be used when specific equipment, such as a Roto Bed, is used in client care. They are also useful for specific nursing interventions such as administration of IV antifibrinolytic agents. In both of these situations, specific actions must be taken to ensure accurate and safe care of clients requiring these treatments. Using protocols in these situations promotes safety.

Protocols can be used in conjunction with standard care plans, standardized care plans, and critical paths. The use of protocols decreases the amount of documentation required on the care plan as actions and interventions are described in detail on the protocol.

In some areas of the hospital, protocols are used in place of care plans. This is particularly true in emergency departments, outpatient surgery, labor and delivery, postanesthesia departments, and operating rooms. Protocols for client care in each of these areas are practical because clients have common needs. For example, clients in the postanesthesia area must have their respiratory status monitored, fluid balance maintained, and level of consciousness assessed. These clients must also meet certain criteria for discharge from the unit. There is no real requirement for an individualized plan of care for the clients in these settings. The time spent in these specialty areas is usually very limited and the service very specific.

Report

A shift-to-shift report should be given not only from the Kardex but from the client care plan. There is no need to review particular procedures for such activities as dressing changes when they are outlined on the care plan. A simple statement to the effect that the procedure is listed on the care plan is all that is necessary. This decreases both time and repetition of information.

To avoid confusion from shift to shift, specific times for treatments and for activities of daily living (ADLs) are indicated. For example, it is noted on the care plan that the client prefers his bath before 8 AM to avoid having to ask him every day when he wants his bath. This consistency promotes a feeling of confidence in the nursing staff and alleviates fear.

Care Conferences

Client care conferences and care plans play an integral role in planning and delivering health care for difficult or unusual problems. The client care conference can focus on developing the care plan or on identifying difficult problems. A conference can then be scheduled to plan appropriate interventions and to inform all health team members of the goals for that client's care.

Delegating Client Care

Client care assignments should be based on careful analysis of each client's needs and goals of care. The care plan can be consulted for an effective use of health team members to their best advantage as well as for the client's welfare. A client requiring extensive sterile dressing changes, frequent assessments, and IV medications is more appropriately assigned to a professional nurse. A client who is convalescing following a stroke and requires mainly bathing and ambulation assistance can usually be assigned to another member of the health team such as a nursing assistant.

In most health care facilities, delegating client care to health care workers is under the jurisdiction of the registered nurse (RN). To delegate appropriate tasks, the nurse must be familiar with the Nurse Practice Act for RNs and Licensed Vocational Nurses (LVNs) in their state and with the hospital's job descriptions for each level of health care worker. The hospital cannot expand the duties of health care workers beyond those legally allowed by the state. The hospital may, however, decrease their task levels and require certification or credentials for some tasks.

General Principles of Delegation

Safe, effective management of client care is an important nursing responsibility. The following principles present guidelines for care.

- RNs are legally responsible for assigned client care.
- RNs are responsible for (1) delegation of care to all levels; (2) evaluation of care given; and (3) teaching and support.
- LVNs work with RNs to initiate care plans.
- LVNs do not initiate client teaching with the exception of a standard care plan.
- IV parameters vary by state; for example, some states do not allow LVNs to do IV push or to add medications to the IV bag.

Client Acuity Systems

State law, such as Title 22 of the California Code of Regulation, provides information on how staffing is determined in hospitals within that state. Title 22 states the following regulations regarding staffing.

> There shall be a method for determining staffing requirements based on assessment of client needs. This assessment shall take into consideration at least the following:
>
> 1. The ability of the client to do self-care
> 2. Degree of illness
> 3. Requirements for special nursing activities
> 4. Skill level of personnel required in delivery care
> 5. Placement of the client in the nursing unit
>
> There shall be documentation of the methodology used in making staffing determinations. Such documentation shall be part of the records of the nursing service and be available for review.

Various systems to determine staffing patterns have been used for many years. With the advent of diagnosis-related groups (DRGs), acuity systems for planning staffing needs are being used in many hospitals. This system forms the basis for client care delivery. Categories of nursing care are identified, and a numerical value is assigned to each category. These categories of care include areas such as ADLs, ambulation, client teaching, and medication administration. The numerical values assigned to each category are based on a point scale. For example, using a scale of 1 to 5, a score of 1 indicates the client can function independently in certain tasks; a score of 5 indicates complete dependency on a caregiver for that category.

The scores from all categories are totaled; this score is divided by the number of categories in the acuity system. The final score is designated as the client's acuity level, which is determined for each 8-hour shift. Every nursing unit has a predetermined number of client care hours assigned for each acuity level. For example, a client acuity level of 4.0 on the day shift is allotted 2.8 hours of nursing care for that shift.

After all clients in the nursing unit are assigned an acuity level, the total client care acuity number is used to determine the number of nursing staff required for the next shift. Then, the acuity level of individual clients is used to plan care assignments for the staff. A nurse may be able to safely care for a total acuity of 16. This method seems equitable, since each staff member is assigned to clients based on acuity. Thus, instead of assigning the nursing staff to clients based on room location or number of clients, the acuity level is used to allocate staff resources. Staffing patterns based on the acuity system have been found to be the most practical, equitable, and manageable.

Evaluation

The evaluation of how well the client care plan was individualized to meet the needs of the client is tested at discharge. If the care plan was appropriate, the discharge criteria is met. The nursing interventions and problems are then inactivated or discontinued. Frequently there are clients who, on discharge, have not met the discharge criteria for various reasons. The documentation in the chart should reflect those problems that still exist, the extent to which the problem is being resolved, and additional information to indicate which plans were formulated for goal achievement.

STUDENT CLINICAL PLANNING

Preclinical Planning

To assist students with client care planning prior to clinical experience, many nursing programs have developed a Student Clinical Prep Form. This form helps focus the student's attention on the information neces-

STUDENT CLINICAL PREP FORM

IDENTIFYING DATA

Client Initials ______ Room # ________ Age ______ M ____ F ____ Date of Admission __________ Allergies ________________

Cultural/Ethnic Background __________________ Primary Language Spoken ________________ Religious Preference ________________

Occupation ______________________________ Retired ________ Family/Living Arrangements ______________________________

Admitting Diagnosis ______________________________ Diagnostic Procedures (dates): ______________________________

Brief History of Present Illness ______________________ Surgical Procedures (dates): ______________________________

______________________________ Pertinent Lab Data: ______________________________

PHYSICAL Assessment Findings ______________________

PATHOPHYSIOLOGY of Primary & Secondary Diagnoses

Medications (Routine & PRNs currently taking)

Drug	Dosage	Route	Classification	Expected Effects	Usual Side Effects	Critical Assessment Data

IV Solutions	Additives	Drip rate	Site Assess.

Special Equipment/Considerations

Interventions	Time	Outcome	

Drains/Tubes

Student clinical prep form.

sary to ensure safe nursing practice. Most forms of this type, such as the example provided, include information related to the client's biographical data, history and physical assessment findings, medical diagnosis, nursing diagnosis, medications including IVs, and nursing interventions.

Time Management

Implementing time management techniques during your student clinical experience will assist you not only in organizing client care management but also in completing your assignment efficiently. Some techniques you may find helpful are listed below.

- Design a time management work sheet you can follow.
- Collect the appropriate information you will require to identify client care tasks (e.g., RN report, care plan, Kardex, medication record).
- Identify specific tasks of client care and the time frame needed for completion.
- Prioritize tasks included in the client care plan.
- Make an initial visit to assess your client's status.
- Revise priorities based on your assessment.
- Plan nursing interventions in sequence.
- Group client care activities for accomplishment in the same time frame in sequence. Allocate time to complete client assignment.
- Consider client's wishes for completing nonpriority tasks, such as bathing and grooming.
- Identify tasks for which you will require assistance.
- Notify the appropriate colleague to assist you (e.g., ambulating your client).
- Identify and collect necessary equipment for task completion.
- Complete client care, implementing the prioritized plan of action (POA) using your time management worksheet.
- Allocate appropriate time to interact with your client.
- Mark off tasks on the time management sheet as you complete them, leaving a record for giving verbal report to the nurse when leaving the unit.
- Document client care as soon as feasible, or at least every 2 hours, on the appropriate records.

Client #1 ________	7 AM 8	9 10	11 12	1 2	3	Assessment Data
Room number ____			VS BP TPR Meds	I&O I O		Neuro ________
Med Diag: ________						Resp ________
________						GU ________
________						GI ________
Nsg Diag: ________						M/S ________
________						Psy/Soc ________
Diet ________						
Activity level ______						
________						
IV Solution ______						
IV# ______						
Credit ______						
Rate ______						
IV to follow ______						
IV# ______	Lab: ________					
Rate ______	X-ray: ________					
	Special Procedures: ________					

Time management work sheet.

4

Documentation

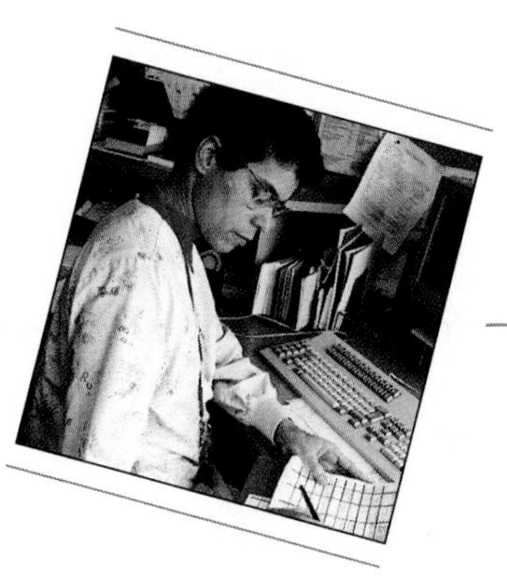

LEARNING OBJECTIVES

- Define the term "charting."
- Explain at least three purposes of charting.
- Describe at least three major components of accurate charting.
- Differentiate between the advantages and disadvantages of the three charting systems: source-oriented, problem-oriented, and computer-assisted charting.
- Explain the importance of relating the nursing process to charting.
- Complete a charting exercise in all three charting systems using a simulated situation.
- Describe the rationale for using flow sheets.
- List the four items that should be charted for every client.
- Discuss the relationship between the nursing assessment data base, nursing problem list, and problem-oriented medical records.
- Define the terms "subjective" and "objective data," "assessment," and "plan" when referring to SOAP notes.
- Discuss the major difference between focus and SOAP charting.
- Explain the information contained in a discharge summary when using POMR charting.
- Describe the legal ramifications for completing unusual occurrence reports.
- Discuss specific client activities requiring consent forms.
- Discuss the legal risks of computer charting.

TERMINOLOGY

Care Plan, Client: a plan of care, usually written, that meets the special needs of each client.

Charting: process of recording information about a client concerning the progress of his or her disease and treatment.

Computer-assisted charting: client information is entered into the computer for storage and retrieval at a later time.

Flow sheets: client data are recorded or graphed to show patterns or alterations in findings.

Incident report: recording of an unusual happening or event that could affect client or staff safety also commonly referred to as unusual occurrences.

Kardex: a convenient and readily accessible file of cards containing current client information.

Nursing process: a set of actions that includes assessment, planning, intervention, and evaluation.

Problem-oriented medical record (POMR): a client record that is organized according to the person's specific health problems.

Report: to give an account of something that has been seen, heard, done, or considered.

SOAP notes: nursing notes organized consistently by what the client feels "subjectively"; what the nurse observes "objectively"; how the nurse "assesses" the situation; and what the nurse "plans."

SOAPIE: nursing notes similar to SOAP with additional data; implementation (i) and evaluation (e).

Source-oriented charting: information in the chart is organized according to its source, for example, physician's progress notes, nurses' notes.

Systems charting: charting or documentation relative to the assessment data obtained during the physical assessment of the client.

CHARTING

Next to direct client care, charting is one of the nurse's most important functions. Charting, the process of recording vital information, serves many important purposes:

- Charting communicates information, such as facts, figures, and observations, to other members of the client's health care team.
- Charting assists supervisory personnel to evaluate the staff's performance on a day-by-day basis for specific clients.
- Charting provides a permanent record for future reference that may become a legal document in the event of litigation or prosecution.

Charting—A Method of Communication

In communicating your observations and actions, charting helps to ensure both quality and continuity of health care for your clients. Information recorded by you becomes a valuable data base for nurses on subsequent shifts. Then, when you reassume responsibility

COMMUNITY HOSPITAL

Client Information

NURSES' NOTES

Time	Medications/Treatment	Observations	Signature
1/6/96 8:30 A		Grimacing and not moving in bed. States pain is 8 on	
		pain scale.	D. Jones RN
9 A	Roxanol SR 30 mg P.O.	For pain	D. Jones RN
9:30A		Pain now 2 on pain scale. Able to turn and cough.	D. Jones RN

Nurses notes.

for the client, you can determine what events occurred during prior time periods. In addition to the client's attending physician, other personnel interested in the chart may include the infection control nurse, discharge coordinator, utilization review personnel, or other hospital staff specialists who are checking on the client's progress or lack of positive reaction to treatment.

The client, as an individual, should receive individualized attention that focuses on his or her specific needs. As these needs are identified by each member of the health care team, they can be communicated to the others. Since nurses have the greatest amount of direct client contact, it is appropriate for the nurse to coordinate the important function of charting.

Charting provides one means for assessing the quality and effectiveness of nursing care. Nurse managers, team leaders, and supervisors use nurses' notes as a basis for staff evaluations. Because charts are documented descriptions of nursing actions, the quality of nursing care may be evaluated on the basis of the quality of charting notes.

Complete and accurate charting is essential to protect both the client and the nurse. Since charting describes nursing interventions and their outcomes, other health care personnel can determine if subsequent treatment should be changed. Frequently a client's reaction time is nearly as important as the reaction itself; therefore accuracy of time observations becomes an integral part of the charting process.

A client's record includes all charting and becomes part of a legal document. Should a client's hospital record be introduced in court, the notes become a legal record of the care provided by each health care provider. Legally, care that is not recorded is considered to be care that was not provided. It is necessary therefore to chart all care that you *do* provide, as well as any care that you *do not* provide.

The legal requirement for charting is found in state laws and professional requirements. For example, Title 22 of the California Code of Regulation states

> Nurses' notes which shall include but not be limited to the following: concise and accurate record of nursing care administered; record of pertinent observations including psychosocial and physical manifestations as

> well as incidents and unusual occurrences, and relevant nursing interpretation of such observations; name, dosage and time of administration of medications and treatment. Route of administration and site of injection shall be recorded if other than by oral administration; record of type of restraint and time of application and removal. The time of application and removal shall not be required for soft tie restraints used for support and protection of the patient.

In addition to the nurses' notes Title 22 requires that a written client care plan must be a permanent part of the medical record.

> There shall be a written patient care plan developed for each patient in coordination with the total health team. This plan shall include goals, problems/needs, and approach and shall be available to all members of the health terms.

The Joint Commission on Accreditation of Healthcare Organizations (JCAHO) also states their requirements for documentation in their nursing care standards. Examples of the documentation standards include: an admission assessment performed and documented by a registered nurse that includes consideration of biophysical, psychosocial, environmental, self-care, educational, and discharge planning; nursing care based on identified nursing diagnoses or client care needs and client care standards; needs that are consistent with the therapies of other disciplines; interventions identified to meet the client's needs; the actual client care provided while hospitalized; educational information provided; and the ability of the client or family to manage the continuing care on discharge.

The Charting Process

The format of the chart varies from hospital to hospital. Most important is the content of the notes. First, your notes should describe the assessment that you completed at the beginning of your shift. This information provides a baseline for changes that may occur later in the client's condition. If there are no such changes, this fact should be entered as the final note. Some hospitals require that all parts of the assessment be documented; others require that only abnormalities be documented.

As your shift progresses, you should always include certain items in your notes, including changes in the client's medical, mental, or emotional condition. Nurses are well attuned to medical changes, such as shock, hemorrhage, or a change in level of consciousness; however, the nurse may overlook subtle emotional changes. Anger, depression, or joy should also be documented because these emotions often are indications of the client's response to the illness. Recording these changes is absolutely necessary if other nurses are to act appropriately during subsequent shifts. You should also chart if *no* changes occurred in the client's condition so that treatments can be modified as necessary. Normal aspects of the client's condition should be noted also.

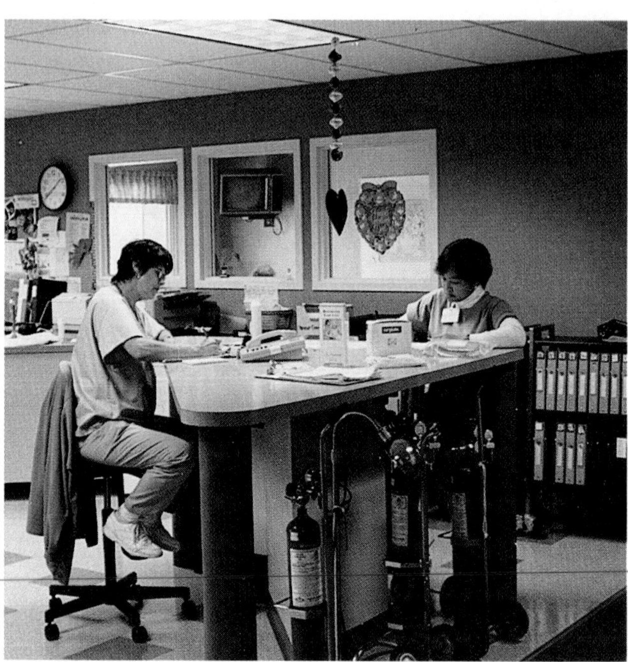

Charting is completed during the day immediately following client care.

Reactions to any unscheduled or prn medications must be recorded. Because each medication is given to meet a specified need, the client's response or lack of response must be recorded to document whether the need was met. To complete this part of the entry, note the time the medication was given, the problem for which the medication was given, and the expected solution. For example: "7 AM c/o moderate ROQ abdominal incisional pain, "7" on pain scale. Roxanol, 30 mg, PO for pain." When the effects of the medication are known, write another note: "8 AM States pain relieved."

Finally, it is important to record the client's response to teaching. These notes may describe return demonstrations, verbalization of learning, or resistance to instruction. Because most teaching takes place over a period of days, record both what you taught and how the client responded. Then other nurses will know whether to repeat the previous instructions, reinforce them, or start a new topic.

Frequently, repetitive aspects of nursing care, such as vital signs and intake and output, are recorded on flow sheets. If flow sheets are used, you need not repeat the same information in your notes. An exception is an abnormal measurement that is a part of a larger assessment. For example: "c/o sharp abd. pain. BP 78/50. P 136. Skin cold & diaphoretic. NG tube draining bright red bloody fluid c̄ small clots. Reported to Dr. Jones."

Charting for Potential Legal Problems

- Use facts. If you chart "physician notified," include time called, facts you gave, and his or her response.
- Do not use pat phrases. Be specific and use individual assessment parameters. Do not chart global assessments such as IV running.
- Be professional when you chart. Do not make interpretations; state what happened, for instance, "suggested to physician that client requires heart monitor" and physician responded "case does not warrant a monitor." If this client were later to be involved in a lawsuit, these notes indicate that the nurse was observant, alert, and aware that the client might be in danger.
- Chart potentially serious situations; include observations, reports to the physician and supervisor, and whether any action was taken. Be precise; add quotes or specific communication. This is the only kind of charting that holds up in court.
- Use correct language and medical terms. Do not use slang or abbreviations that are not generally accepted. Your charting, for legal reasons, must be specific, clear, and precise.
- Report problems to appropriate authorities such as suspected child abuse to social services.
- Provide the best care you are capable of giving; then precisely chart your observations, interventions, and communications; this is the best deterrent to later legal problems.

Charting and the Nursing Process

The nursing process provides the framework for decision making throughout all phases of nursing care. The components of the nursing process are assessment, planning, implementation (or intervention), and evaluation. This cycle is applied by the nurse both to routine situations and critical care emergencies.

It is important to relate the nursing process to charting because for experienced nurses, the process may become only a mental exercise. The nurse "thinks through" the situation, makes decisions, takes action, and then observes the results. Unless the entire process is recorded on the client care plan and documented in the chart, the next nurse who encounters a similar situation with the same client is deprived of important and potentially valuable background data. The second nurse, without knowing the full background, may repeat the entire process, resulting in a loss of valuable time and an increase in client discomfort. When similar nursing interventions completed by different nurses have the same positive results, the client experiences a feeling of reassurance that may not be achieved if each nurse attempts a totally different set of interventions to reach the same objective.

The client, in a strange environment with unknown people doing unfamiliar and often uncomfortable things, often tries to find reassurance in any type of routine. The client soon expects a certain procedure to be done by the same person in the same way and at a predictable hour. Changes in the procedure are often upsetting to the client. It is imperative that the steps of any procedure, especially those that are complicated or personalized to the client, be documented in detail on the client care plan so that each nurse does it the same way. The detailed description of how to perform a dressing change, however, is written in the client's care plan, not in the nurses' notes.

The nurses' notes describe the amount, color, consistency, and odor of the drainage. In addition, the amount and type of irrigating solution and type of abdominal dressing are noted. It is important to add a statement as to the client's tolerance of the procedure.

Charting Systems

The three main charting systems are source-oriented, problem-oriented, and computer-assisted charting. The most common system is the source-oriented chart, so named because the information is organized and presented according to its source. For example, there are separate sections for doctors' progress notes, nurses' notes, and respiratory therapy notes. To obtain a complete "picture" of the client, one must read through all sections and piece together the separate bits of data. This may be a time-consuming process, and the result may not produce an accurate or complete assessment of the client. Narrative charting is found within this charting system.

A second system for chart organization is the problem-oriented medical record. In this system the chart is based on the problem list—all problems, present or potential, identified with that client. Using the problems as reference points, each person giving care charts progress notes on the same sheets. In this way assessment of a specific incident by everyone concerned (e.g., physician, RN, dietitian, enterostomal therapist) is in the same location, and the client's overall picture can be easily seen.

The third type of organizing data is computer-assisted charting. This type of charting constantly updates information from many sources. For example,

COMMUNITY HOSPITAL

CLIENT CARE PLAN

Client Information

Discharge Criteria
1) Lungs clear to auscultation.
2) Voiding qs and continent of urine.
3) Verbalizes an understanding of discharge instructions and medications.
4)

Admitting Diagnosis
Relevant Info:

Date	Problem/Need	Expected Outcome/Goal	CP	DL	Nursing Interventions	Update / DC	Initial
3/22/96	(1.) Ineffective Breathing Pattern related to pain.	Absence of respiratory complications.	q2h x24h then q4h x48h then q8h q3-4 h	POD 3 3/25 3 pm	1a. Encourage turning, coughing and deep breathing exercises (TCDB) q2h. b. Teach client to splint incision when coughing. c. Instruct in use of breathing device, if ordered. d. Place in semi-Fowler's position. e. Assess need for pain med. f. Medicate for pain 1/2hr. before TCDB. g. Auscultate breath sounds.		
	2. Altered Urinary Elimination related to incontinence.	Continent of urine. Absence of urinary tract infection (UTI).	q4h	cath. out	2a. Check urinary output for signs and symptoms of UTI, ie. color, odor, consistency. b. Provide catheter care according to protocol. c. Force fluids to 2500mL. d. Give cranberry juice, 240mL q shift.		
3/22/96	(3.) Knowledge Deficit related to administration of discharge meds.	Verbalizes understanding of discharge meds, including listing signs and symptoms of side effects.	q24h	prior to disch	3a. Instruct in action of Maxaquin b. Review side effects with client and/or family. c. Have client state signs and symptoms of side effects prior to discharge. d. Provide Take Home Medication pamphlet.		

COMMUNITY HOSPITAL

CLIENT CARE PLAN
Individualized

Client Information

Discharge Criteria
1) *Wound healing progressing satisfactorily*
2) *Verbalizes ability to care for wound at home*
3) *Verbalizes understanding of discharge instructions*
4)

Admitting Diagnosis
Relevant Info:

Date	Problem/Need	Expected Outcome/Goal	CP	DL	Nursing Interventions	Update / DC	Initial
3/22/96	*Impaired skin integrity related to prolonged immobility*	*Wound healing s̄ complications*	*q̄ 4th*	*Prior to discharge*	*4a. Place on Lt. side c̄ chux under hips & abd. Gently move into this position. Do not rush c̄ move.* *b. Note drainage, location, quantity, color & odor.* *c. Irrig. wound c̄ 50 mL. saline solution. Use asepto syringe. Catch solution in emesis basin.* *c. Cover wound with ABD dressings. Use Montgomery straps.*		

Individualized client care plan.

physiologic measurements are recorded and updated on the computer terminal at least hourly.

The information is easily retrievable by the nursing personnel as questions arise. Reference material for common nursing problems ensures quick reference and easily retrieved information to provide safe nursing care.

Two charting systems, focus charting and charting by exception, are currently gaining more acceptance. Focus charting is similar to SOAP (subjective, objective, assessment, plan) charting except it uses the term "focus" in place of "problem," which eliminates the negative connotation of the word "problem." The focus is not necessarily written as a nursing diagnosis. It can encompass terms such as "signs and symptoms" (increased temperature), a significant client event or a change in client status (need for surgical intervention), or an acute change in status (vital signs or excessive bleeding). The progress notes are organized using the DAR format: data, action, and response. Data includes the information that supports the focus; action is the nursing intervention used to treat the problem and response is how the client responds to the intervention and the outcome. The following is an example of focus charting:

D: Client found grimacing, hands clenched, and body rigid. Verbalized pain at 9 on pain scale.
A: Administered 15 mg MS IV push. Called physician to request PCA for client.
R: Pain moderately relieved after 35 minutes. Able to understand instruction in use of PCA.

Charting by exception uses flow sheets, protocols and standards of practice, nursing diagnosis, care plans, SOAP progress notes, and a nursing data base. A nursing and physician order flow sheet is used to document physical assessments and implementation of physician and nursing orders as well as completion of nursing and physician orders. The form also contains the teaching record and discharge notes.

Some legal or reimbursement issues, such as admissability in court, may be related to charting by exception. At this time the rule "if it wasn't charted, it wasn't done" is still the prevailing attitude in legal issues.

Source-Oriented Systems Charting. Systems charting is a common and efficient way of organizing client information in source-oriented nurses' notes. An outline of the systems to be reviewed, and sometimes specific subheadings for each, is established. Medical units may use one type of systems nurses' notes, and critical care may use another.

At the beginning of the shift the nurse performs a physical assessment on each client to determine that client's current status. This information becomes the initial systems charting. When changes occur, they are noted with the time under the appropriate system. If no changes occur during the shift, no other charting of this type may be necessary.

To record all pertinent client information, several flow sheets are commonly used in conjunction with the systems form. One flow sheet is the vital signs sheet, which contains information, such as temperature, pulse, blood pressure, respiration, urine output, hemodynamic monitoring values, infusion rates of vasoactive drugs, and daily weights. Other flow sheets may include a medication and an intake and output record. Special sheets, such as neurologic monitoring sheets and diabetic sheets, are used as necessary. Flow sheets eliminate the need to write excessive notes and avoid duplication of information. Flow sheets do not negate the need for narrative descriptions.

Refer back to the client care plan to ensure that all problems have been assessed and documentation completed. It is a good idea to check the care plan several times a day.

Source-Oriented Narrative Charting. Narrative charting is based on chronology rather than systems. Information is charted in chronologic order regardless of the subject of the note. For example, the nurses' notes for a client could appear as follows:

0730 Blood glucose 240 mg/dL
0745 5 units Reg. Insulin administered Rt. Abd.
0815 Assessment completed.

Hospitals usually have maximum time requirements for this type of note, with common parameters being every 2 or 3 hours. Although there may be a requirement for frequency of charting, there usually is not one for charting content. This leads to the primary deficiency of narrative charting; it is very easy to chart without specifying why the client is in the hospital or what the client's overall condition is. Note the example illustrated in the figure. Why is the client in the hospital? What is the client's general condition? How is the client progressing?

When using narrative charting, an assessment should be performed at the beginning of the shift and as needed thereafter. When assessment is the initial entry in narrative charting, subsequent entries are more relevant and understandable. This combination

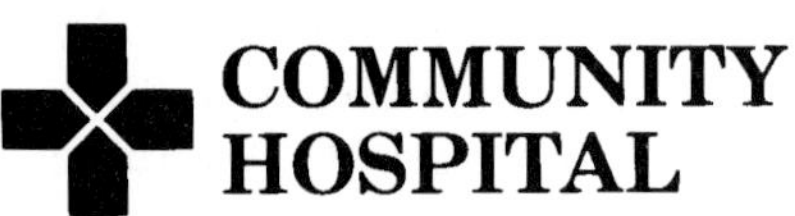

COMMUNITY HOSPITAL

NURSES' NOTES

Client Information

Time	Medications/Treatment	Observations	Signature
1/23/96			
7:30 A		Blood glucose 240 mg/dl.	D. Jones RN
7:45 A	5 units Reg. Insulin	Administered Rt. Abd.	D. Jones RN
8:15 A		Assessment completed.	
		Neuro: Alert and oriented, PERL reflexes WNL	
		Cardio: p. 102, irregular c̄ pericardial friction rub	
		present.	
		Resp: Rales present bilaterally in bases. Non-produc-	
		tive cough.	
		GI: Bowel sounds present, Abd. soft and non-tender.	
		GU: Voiding lge. amts. light straw-colored urine s̄	
		sediment.	
		M/S: No c/o pain or limitation of movement.	
		Skin: clean and moist, no reddened areas or	
		breakdown noted.	D. Jones RN

Source-oriented narrative charting using systems charting format.

of assessment and narrative charting is the best technique to ensure that adequate information about the client is recorded for all personnel who use nurses' notes.

Because the client's chart is considered a legal document, it is important that nurses chart relevant, accurate, and appropriate information in a timely manner. The following rules for charting narrative notes will assist you in maintaining an acceptable chart.

1. Use black ink, not felt pen or pencil. Black ink microfilms best.
2. Correct errors by drawing a single line through the error, write the word mistaken entry (ME) above it, and then initial the error. The error must be readable. Ink eradication, erasures, or use of occlusive materials is not acceptable. The word "error" is not longer advised because juries tend to associate the word "error" with an actual nursing care mistake.
3. Sign each entry with your first initial, last name, and status, for example, SN for student nurse, LVN for licensed vocational nurse, or RN for registered nurse. Script, not printing, is used for the signature. Each signature should appear at the right hand margin of the nurses' notes.
4. Notes should appear on each succeeding line.

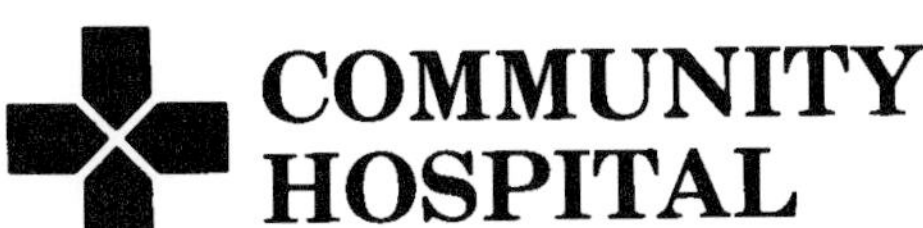

ICU NEURO/SPINAL FLOW CHART

Date: 3/22/96		Time:	8 AM		
Pupils	Right:	size	4 MM		
		Reaction	S		
	Left:	Size	4 MM		
		Reaction	S		
		Visual Acuity	C		
Mental Status					
COMA SCALE	Eyes Open	Spontaneously			
		To Speech			
		To Pain	+		
		Never			
	Verbal Response	Clear			
		Confused			
		Inappropriate	+		
		Incomprehensible			
		None			
MOVEMENT	Arms	Normal Power			
		Weakness	+		
		Flexion			
		Extension			
		No Response			
	Legs	Normal Power			
		Weakness	+		
		Flexion			
		Extension			
		No Response			
Reflexes		Gag/Cough	0		
		Corneal	+		
		Babinski R/L	+/+		
		Oculocephalic	0		
Respiratory		Pattern	Reg.		
		Rate	28		
Seizures		Type	0		
		Duration			
Fluid Drainage from Ears or			0		
Nose			0		

Signature D. Jones RN

Neurologic flow sheet.

Lines should not be omitted in the nurses' notes. A horizontal line is drawn to "fill up" a partial line. Continuous charting is done for each entry unless a time change occurs. You do not need a new line for each new idea or statement.

5. Entries should be concise. Complete sentences are not required. Start each entry with a capital letter, and end the entry with a period even if the entry is a single word or phrase.
6. The date is entered in the data column on the first line of every page of nurses' notes and whenever the date changes.
7. Time is entered in the time column whenever a new time entry occurs. Do not put time changes in the text of the nurses' notes. If only one time is entered for block charting, enter the last time you were with the client.
8. Chart objective facts, not your interpretations. For example, chart "ate 100%," not "good appetite." If the client complains, place the complaint in quotation marks to indicate that it is his or her statement. For example, "c/o chest pain radiating down left arm."
9. Objective data is to be charted as well. In addition to the statement offered by the client, the nurse should chart his or her observations: "Skin cold and clammy. Diaphoretic. Vital signs stable."
10. Refusal of medications and treatments must be documented. A circle is placed around the time the medication or treatment is to be given in the appropriate area of the chart. An explanation as to the reason medication was not given is entered in the nurses' notes.
11. Sign each entry before it is replaced in the chart rack. An entry is not to be left unsigned. If all the charting is completed for the shift at one time, a single signature is placed at the end of the charting.
12. Accuracy is important. Describe behaviors rather than feelings. This allows other health team members to determine the client's actual problems.
13. Chart only those abbreviations and symbols approved by the facility. Information can be misinterpreted or misleading when unfamiliar abbreviations are used. (See the listing at the end of the chapter for examples of commonly used abbreviations.)
14. Spell correctly, using proper terminology and grammar.

COMMUNITY HOSPITAL

DIABETIC RECORD

DIRECTION: Test second voiding whenever possible.

DATE		3/22/96	3/22/96	3/22/96									
TIME	1st void / 2nd void	6 am / 6^{15}am	11 am / 11^{30}am	4^{15}pm / 4^{30}pm									
VOLUME	1st void / 2nd void	200cc / 60cc	150cc / 45cc	350cc / 25cc									
SUGAR		1+	Neg	2+									
ACETONE		Neg	Neg	Neg									
INSULIN	TYPE	Reg	-0-	Reg									
	DOSE	5 u		10 u									
	TIME	6^{30}am		4^{49}pm									
	ROUTE	SQ		SQ									
	SITE	RU arm		LU arm									
SIGNATURE		D. Jones RN		D. Jones RN									

Diabetic flow sheet.

15. Write legibly. If your writing is not legible, then print.
16. Only chart what you personally have done or observed. An exception to this rule is when you are responsible for charting for nonprofessional personnel.
17. Do not use the word "client" in the chart. The chart belongs to that client.
18. Do not double the chart. If something appears on a flow sheet, it does not need to appear on the nurses' narrative record unless there is an alteration from normal.
19. Do not squeeze information into a space because you forgot to chart it earlier. Add the information on the first available line. Write in the time the event occurred, not the time you entered the information.
20. The following information should be charted.
    a. Physician's visits.
    b. Times the client leaves and returns to the

NARRATIVE CHARTING

Advantages

- Can be used in conjunction with flow sheets and other documentation systems
- Quick method of charting chronologic data
- Familiar method of charting
- Easy to use
- Used in all types of clinical settings

Disadvantages

- Lack of systematic structure leading to difficulty in determining data relationships
- Time-consuming
- Frequently lacks information on client care outcomes
- Difficult to monitor data for quality assurance
- Relevant information found in several areas in chart

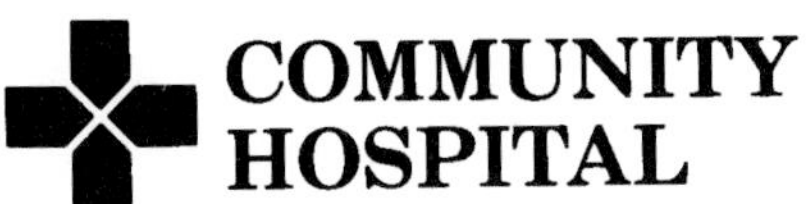

NURSES' NOTES

Client Information

Time	Medications/Treatment	Observations	Signature
3/22/96 7:35 AM		c/o moderate pain in RLQ incisional area, 7 on pain	
		scale.	D. Jones RN
7:45 AM	Roxanol 30 mg. P.O.	For incisional pain.	D. Jones RN
8:20 AM		States pain relieved.	
8:45 AM	Dressing change	Inc. area clean s̄ edema or erythema. Scant serous	
		drainage on dressing.	
9:30 AM		Amb. in hall c̄ assistance.	D. Jones RN
12:15 AM		Dr. Peter visited.	D. Jones RN

Nurses' notes.

unit, mode of transportation, and destination.

c. Medications (chart immediately after given). Include dosage, route of administration (if parenteral, where given), whether pain was relieved (if pain medication), and side effects.

d. Treatments (chart immediately after given).

Problem-Oriented Medical Records

The second major type of charting is the problem-oriented medical records, or POMR. This system differs from source-oriented narrative charting, not only in format but in philosophy. Problem-oriented medical records focus on the client's status rather than on the source of the information, such as department or member of the health care team who is originating the information. Narrative charting typically consists of doctors' progress notes, physical therapy progress notes, nurses' notes, and respiratory therapy progress notes. With POMR, only one set of progress notes is used, and all personnel caring for the client record their data on this set.

The PIE charting format, which stands for problem-identification, intervention, and evaluation, is a newer, condensed version of the problem-oriented charting system. This type of charting uses the nursing process and nursing diagnosis while incorporating the plan of care into the nurses' progress notes. The PIE charting system does not use the traditional nursing care plan. Client problems, teaching needs, and discharge planning needs are identified during the initial client assessment, the P of the PIE format. Based on the assessment, nursing diagnoses are identified and numbered on a problem list. Interventions that are carried out are documented for each specific nursing diagnosis (I). Each shift evaluates the outcome of the interventions in resolving the client's problem (E). The following is an example of PIE documentation:

P#1 Pain r/t postoperative incisional drainage tube placement.

P. Instruct in use of PCA and positioning for comfort.

I. Instruction given on how to use PCA pump. Positioned on unoperative side with pillows to back and between knees.

E. Using PCA appropriately, pain tolerable, identified as 3 on pain scale. Positioning has assisted in decreasing pain and allowed client to rest comfortably for longer periods of time.

In its purest form, a POMR consists of five distinct parts: the data base (initial assessment), problem list, initial plan, progress notes, and discharge summary. The data base is made up of information from and about the client that is used to develop the problem list. Because the POMR system is systematic and well defined, the data base consists of specific types of data, including the chief complaint (why the client came to the hospital), personal and family medical history, allergies and reactions, medications taken at home, physical assessment, mental and emotional assessment, and lifestyle.

Development of a complete data base requires skill and practice. Basic features of client interviewing and physical assessment are covered in other sections of this text, but a few tips and reminders may help to sharpen your skills. First, select a time mutually acceptable to you and the client. Know how much time you have for the interview and whether the client has scheduled appointments or tests. Be aware of the client's physical and emotional comfort, the physical environment of the interview location, and pending meal times. Second, consider how your questions might affect the client. Phrase questions that require the client to explain and answer—a "yes" or "no" is not sufficiently informative. Do not make the client defensive by being judgmental about his or her actions. Clients who believe you do not approve of their actions often withhold potentially important information. Third, avoid leading statements. Many clients try to respond in an agreeable manner. For example, "You don't . . ." statements may be answered by "No, of course not." Also, avoid using medical jargon unfamiliar to the client. Some words you use daily may be unknown to your client. The client answers what he or she *thinks* you asked to avoid showing ignorance. This situation may result in an invalid data base because the data is incorrect.

After completing the data base, the nurse next defines the client problems for the problem list. A "problem" is any difficulty that the client cannot handle alone—the client needs assistance from someone on the health care team. The difficulty may be a physical symptom, such as pain or infection; an emotional problem caused by fear of impending surgery or worry about a family member; or a social problem, such as loss of job and income or inability to live independently at home. Problems are usually defined as active (acute or chronic) or inactive (resolved). Active problems may also be potential—not yet present but likely to occur. Examine the following list of problems and see if you can determine how to categorize them.

Upper GI bleeding, 3 days' duration	Active
Children, 2 and 5 years old, at home with father	Active
Possible skin breakdown	Active—Potential
Appendectomy 1954	Resolved
Asthma since childhood	Active—Chronic

Medical diagnoses are included on the problem list if they are definite. If they are only tentative, the client's symptoms should be put on the list until the actual diagnosis is made. Of course, many of the symptoms may qualify as part of the nursing diagnosis, since they can be defined as interfering with the client's sense of well-being. For example, anxiety related to one's medical diagnosis is a nursing diagnosis.

The categories of the POMR closely approximate the steps in the nursing process. The data base and problem list equate to assessment; the initial plan equates to planning; the progress notes discuss intervention; and the discharge summary is an evaluation.

After you complete the data base and start the problem list, you then formulate the client care plan (CCP). For each major problem or group of problems, the CCP should include the following information: date, problem, expected outcome, check point, deadline, and nursing actions.

In the POMR system, one set of progress notes is

COMMUNITY HOSPITAL

NURSING ASSESSMENT DATA BASE

Date	Time	Room #	Admit by:
3/22/96	4 P.M.	110 A	ambulatory ___ guerney ___ W/C ✓ ambulance ___

T.P.R.	B/P RT	B/P LT	Height	Weight
998-110-24	160/90	164/94	5'6"	200 #

Instructed in use of:

Yes	No	
✓		Telephone
✓		Bed-Controls
✓		Lights
✓		Nurse call System
✓		Visiting hours

Articles at bedside (describe item)

✓	Ring	Yellow Metal
	Watch	
✓	Money (amt.)	$10.50
✓	Eyeglasses	
	Hearing Aid	

	Contact Lenses	
	Dentures: Upper	✓
	Lower	✓
	Other	

Reason for No: ___ Other ___

Tests completed on admission

	Lab Work	✓	X-ray	Chest
✓	UA		Other	

Above information obtained by: KMead, RN

Previous illness	Meds taken @ home on routine basis	Meds taken today state time	Meds brought to hospital
Diabetes	Lasix 40 mg P.O.		None
✓ Hypertension	Digoxin 0.25 mg P.O.		
✓ Heart Disease			
Lung Disease			
Other			

Disposition of Meds: ☐ Home ☐ Pharmacy

Allergies:

✓ FOOD Shellfish, Citrus fruits

✓ DRUGS ASA, Codeine

☐ None Known

Data base record.

COMMUNITY HOSPITAL

NURSING PROBLEM LIST

Date Problem Began	Prob. #	Problem	Date Resolved	Date Recurred
3/22/96	1	Altered Urinary Elimination R/t incontinence.		
3/22/96	2	Unilateral Neglect R/t right-sided weakness.		
3/22/96	3	Altered Nutrition: Less than Body Requirement R/t aversion to eating and difficulty swallowing.		
3/22/96	4	Impaired Skin Integrity R/t emaciation.		

Problem list.

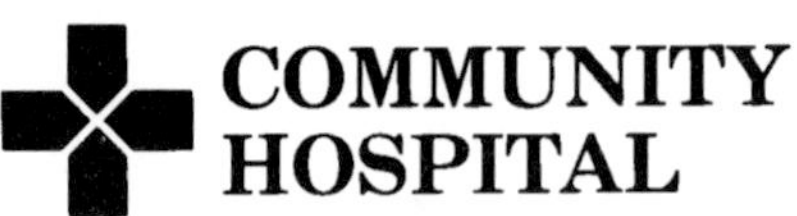

COMMUNITY HOSPITAL

Client Information

PROGRESS NOTES

Date	Note progress of case, complications, change in diagnosis, condition on discharge
3/22/96	Problem #3
	S Refuses to eat. States "I'm afraid to swallow because I choke sometimes and I don't like the food."
	O Has difficulty swallowing fluids. Chokes if not sitting upright.
	A Swallowing difficulty — probably related to CVA.
	P Contact dietitian to see client re: food preferences.
	Place in high-Fowler's position when feeding.
	Feed slowly and reassure client often. D. Jones RN

Progress notes using SOAP charting.

used by everyone. This means that all members of the health care team write their observations on the same part of the chart. The entries on the problem list are always numbered, so when the nurse, physician, and the respiratory therapist all refer to problem 3 in their progress notes, everyone knows that they are referring to "Ineffective airway clearance, *related* to pain."

Within the well-organized POMR system, progress notes have a specific format, usually called SOAP or SOAPIE. These acronyms translate as:

Subjective: Client's symptoms and own description of problem

Objective: Clinical findings; include observations and factual data, for instance, intake and output, vital signs, drainage, presence of rash.

Assessment: Your conclusions about the problem based on subjective and objective data. Nursing diagnoses may be written here.

Plan: What you decide to do about the problem.

Implementation: Your nursing interventions.

Evaluation: How the implementation worked.

When writing progress notes, remember that a separate SOAP or SOAPIE note is needed for each problem. You should not combine problems. It is not always necessary to include the I, E, portions of the note; however, always include the S, O, A, and P parts, even if the client does not supply subjective statements.

The discharge summary, the final step in the POMR system as well as all forms of charting, includes both a summary of the client's hospitalization and documentation of client teaching. SOAPIE notes are again used as the charting format, and a summary should be written for each problem on the problem list. If the problem is fully resolved during hospitalization, that fact and the date it occurred (from the progress notes) are all that is necessary. The discharge summary is not a day-by-day account of the client's stay but a short review. It is beneficial to include specific highlights such as the highest serum glucose level or the highest temperature, but all the values need not be included. Remember, a separate SOAPIE note should be written for each problem that is not fully resolved at the time of the discharge.

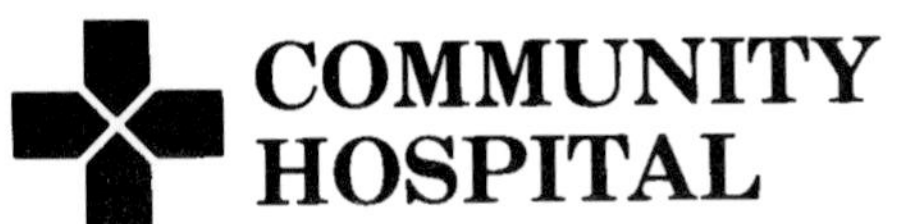

Client Information

PROGRESS NOTES

Date	Note progress of case, complications, change in diagnosis, condition on discharge
4/17/96	Mr. Rappaport was admitted to the restorative care unit on 3/15/96 with right-sided weakness, difficulty swallowing,
	inability to perform ADL's, 10# weight loss, and coccyx area reddened with Stage 1 pressure ulcer. Laboratory values WNL
	except for a urinary tract infection 1 week prior to admission which has been resolved with P.O. Gantrisin (Problem #1)
	Continues to exhibit right-sided weakness. Unable to perform ADL's-right handed (Problem #2) O.T. working on alternative
	ways to become independent in ADL's. Instructions given to client to swallow on left side. Weight loss has stabilized, dietitian
	working with client to determine food preferences. Hi-protein, hi-calorie liquids between meals started 4/10/96. (Problem #3)
	Skin care with transparent dressings continues. Area remains unchanged (Problem #4) Plan is to begin preparation for
	discharge. Instructions on dietary needs and skin care given to wife and daughter. O.T. will continue at home to work on
	ADL's.
	D. Jones RN

Discharge summary.

All invasive procedures, surgical interventions, and major diagnostic tests should be listed and the results outlined. Braces, equipment, and supplies (e.g., for dressing changes, catheterizations) should be included in the summary. If the equipment or braces are difficult to use or apply, it is helpful if pictures or diagrams are included. Completed client teaching, discharge medications, and specific teaching regarding the medications should also be documented.

Referrals to other health care services should be identified with the name of the agency and the contact person listed on the chart. If clients are being discharged to other health care facilities or to a visiting nurse, it is helpful if they receive not only a copy of the discharge summary but a copy of the last client care plan. This provides for a smooth transition of care from one health care setting to another.

Because of the many changes necessary when implementing POMR, hospitals often use only part of it or are changing to it in stages; therefore it is common to find situations in which parts of several systems are in use. For example, SOAP nursing notes may be used and the remainder of the chart is source-oriented, or doctors may use the problem list and SOAP progress notes and nurses use systems charting for nurses' notes. Although progress is rather slow, it appears that many more hospitals are adopting the POMR system not only for its format and ease of use but also for its completeness on documenting client care.

SOAP AND SOAPIE CHARTING

Problem #1: Fluid Volume, Excess, *related to* poor compliance to medication administration.

- S "My rings are tight and my shoes don't fit."
- O Fingers are edematous. 3+ pitting edema of both ankles.
- A Due to fluid overload as a result of refusing diuretics.
- P Elevate feet. Explain necessity for diuretics. Administer drug, obtain order for IM med if nec. Observe dietary intake of Na^+ to determine if compliant to diet.
- I Client education completed regarding use of LASIX.
- E Could state signs and symptoms of low potassium.

Problem #2: Ineffective Airway Clearance, *related to* pain.

- S "I'm having difficulty bringing up mucus."
- O Lungs sound congested, rales present bilaterally in lower bases.
- A Unable to deep breathe and cough due to high abdominal incision.
- P Elevate HOB 45 degrees. Enc. coughing and deep breathing. Medicate for pain q3h. Splint inc. when coughing.
- I Expectorating large amounts of clear mucus.
- E Lung sounds continue to reflect rales.

PROBLEM-ORIENTED CHARTING

Advantages

- Focuses on client problem
- Implements problem-solving approach
- Ease in retrieving information about each problem
- Problem resolution is clearly documented
- Problem list assists in identifying priority needs of client
- May be used effectively in acute or long-term care settings
- Consistency in documentation format
- Effectively uses nursing process in documentation
- Readily used in conjunction with standard nursing care plan
- Integrated documentation system promotes collaboration among all health care providers
- PIE charting uses flow sheet, which decreases documentation time and redundancy

Disadvantages

- Difficult to obtain agreement on what should be included in record
- Physician's vary in their acceptance of all disciplines using same list
- Duplication of information necessary on several forms
- Need for constant updating of problem list and determining whose responsibility it is to do so
- Format is frequently not used in pure form, making it difficult to use effectively
- Not efficient because each problem requires a separate PROM entry
- PIE charting incorporates use of care planning which is responsibility of RN, therefore it is difficult to use LVNs in documentation system

Computer-Assisted Charting

Computers have become a valuable tool in documenting client care. One common system focuses on the client's physiologic information. With input from various monitoring devices, such as an arterial line and a Swan–Ganz catheter, the computer can automatically determine and frequently update many pieces of data, including hematology and chemistry tests, ABGs (arterial blood gases), cardiac output, vital signs, and central venous pressures, to name only a few. These results can be viewed on a VMT (video matrix terminal similar to a television screen) or printed out on paper. The VS (vital sign) and hemodynamic data are continually updated, and many of the laboratory tests can be updated at least every hour.

Another type of computer system records, stores, and retrieves many pieces of data about the client that must be communicated throughout the hospital for the client to receive optimal care. For example, when a client is admitted and the physician enters orders into the computer, many things automatically happen. The dietary department is notified of the diet needs, pharmacy is notified of medications and IVs that are ordered, CSR is notified of special equipment needs, and the laboratory is notified of required tests. It is no longer necessary for the nurse to make out and deliver requests to all these departments and then arrange for delivery or pick up of the desired items. This has been a basic and broad overview of some of the functions of the Technicon Medical Information System (MIS), which is used in many hospitals throughout the country.

Each nursing station in a hospital using this system has several computer terminals. The VMT shows a matrix-like television picture, from which the nurse can select specific categories. These matrices are grouped together in a logical order so that general categories of information can be recorded. The nurse records the information by either pointing the light pen at the proper word or phrase or entering the data into the computer via the keyboard. The nurse can record "Client admitted ambulatory from the emergency room." If the client speaks only Spanish, the nurse types in "Spanish." All the pertinent information obtained while admitting the client and doing the initial physical assessment can easily and quickly be recorded using only the light pen and typing in data such as how the client feels about hospitalization. The admitting sheets the nurse takes to the bedside correlate to the information on the matrices, so that the data are easy to transfer and nothing is omitted.

Hospitals usually have programs that contain special matrices such as "the nursing master guide." This is an example of a matrix that only lists other matrices

```
MATRIX NO. 1347          HOSP. NO. 01          01/05/96
DYNAMIC MATRIX

          GENERAL ADMIT NOTES

*CLIENT ADM:         /GURNEY
AMB        /WC     /AMBULANCE    FROM EMERG RM
           FROM--
                                         **
(PRIMARY LANGUAGE OTHER THAN ENGLISH)
CLIENT SPEAKS--                          **
(CLIENT HAS:) (LOCATED AT :) (HOME) (HOSP)
  GLASSES                         **      **
  CONT LENSES                     **      **
  HEARING AID                     **      **
  CANE                            **      **
  CRUTCHES                        **      **
  WALKER                          **      **
  DENTURES                        **      **
  PROSTHESIS                      **      **
  --                   (HOME) UPPER    U&L
  --                   (HOSP) LOWER    PARTIAL
                           ADMIT VITAL SIGNS
```

General admission notes matrix.

```
MATRIX NO. 1347          HOSP. NO. 01          01/05/96
DYNAMIC MATRIX

      NSG MASTER GUIDE - GENERAL                          01
                                                          02
RN/LVN--------------------------
*VS-RESULTS, OBSV         *GEN REPORTING                  03
*VS-OBSV ONLY             *GEN RPTG-SURG                  04
*DIET, FLD BAL                                            05
*UNIT TESTS/EXAMS         *IMMED POST-OP:                 06
*HYG, ACTIV, SAFETY       *ADMIT NOTES                    07
*PROCEDURES                                               08
                          *MISC DATA                      09
*BASIC CARE NEEDS                                         10
*PHYSICAL ASSESS          *SPECIAL OBSV                   11
*TEACH/DISCH PLANS                                        12
                          *READY FOR THE OR               13
*UNSCHED, MISC MED        *TO THE OR                      14
*MED FOLLOW-UP                                            15
                          *NSG DISCH SUMMARY              16
*IV, BLD BEGIN            *NSG TRANS SUMMARY              17
*IV, BLD END              *EXC CHARTING                   18
*IV, BLD GEN OBSV                                         19
*IV, NO.0---              *CHANGE SPECIALTY               20
```

General nursing master guide.

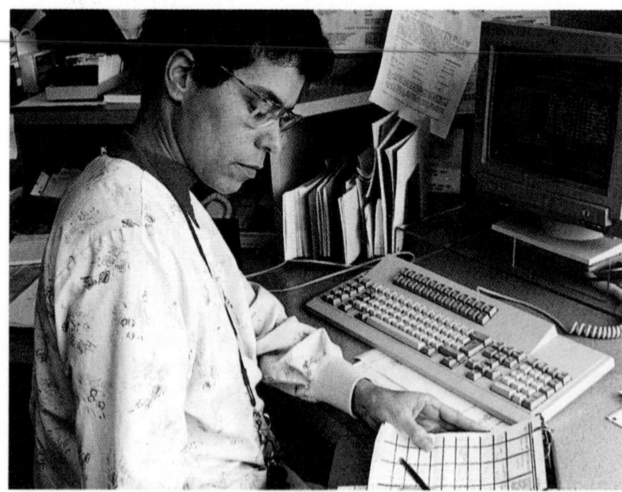

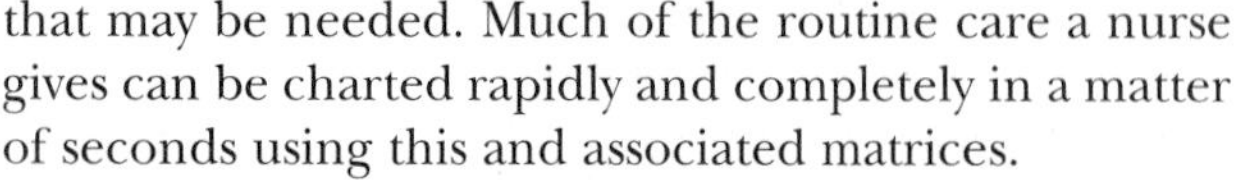

Entry data becomes part of permanent record.

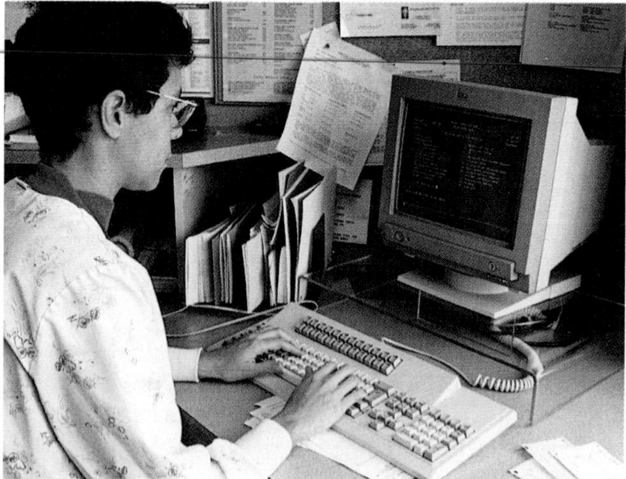

Client data is entered into computer at nurse's station.

that may be needed. Much of the routine care a nurse gives can be charted rapidly and completely in a matter of seconds using this and associated matrices.

When the nurse has completed the charting, the VMT automatically displays all the data. At this time the nurse can make corrections, additions, or deletions. If the data displayed are correct, the nurse enters the data and it becomes a permanent part of the computer record for that client, and a hard copy is printed out to be put in the chart. There are also ways of retrieving and changing mistakes. Also it is easy to see the logical progression of the charting process. The matrix titles act as gentle reminders of what needs to be charted.

When the client is to be discharged, the nursing discharge summary is completed. This shows not only the client's physical condition but also the status of client teaching and follow-up plans. Again, it is simply punched or tapped on the terminal and the data are

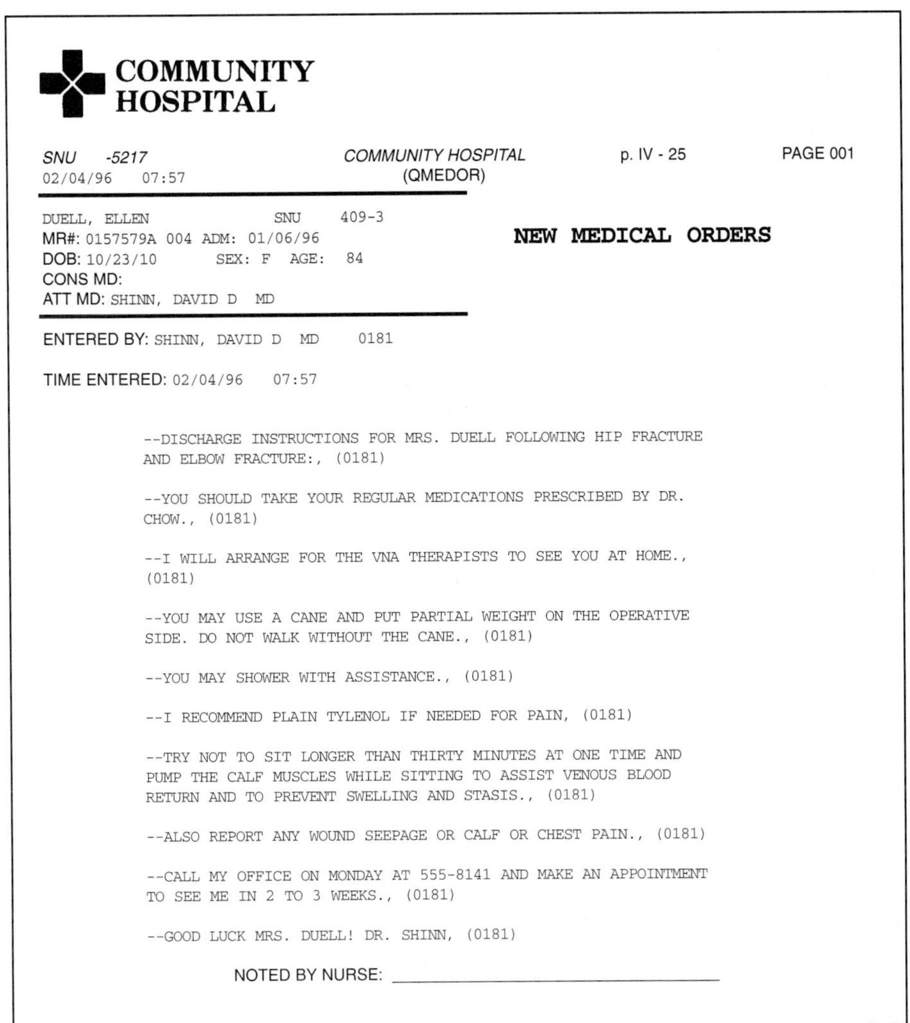

COMMUNITY HOSPITAL

SNU -5217 COMMUNITY HOSPITAL p. IV - 25 PAGE 001
02/04/96 07:57 (QMEDOR)

DUELL, ELLEN SNU 409-3
MR#: 0157579A 004 ADM: 01/06/96
DOB: 10/23/10 SEX: F AGE: 84
CONS MD:
ATT MD: SHINN, DAVID D MD

NEW MEDICAL ORDERS

ENTERED BY: SHINN, DAVID D MD 0181

TIME ENTERED: 02/04/96 07:57

--DISCHARGE INSTRUCTIONS FOR MRS. DUELL FOLLOWING HIP FRACTURE AND ELBOW FRACTURE:, (0181)

--YOU SHOULD TAKE YOUR REGULAR MEDICATIONS PRESCRIBED BY DR. CHOW., (0181)

--I WILL ARRANGE FOR THE VNA THERAPISTS TO SEE YOU AT HOME., (0181)

--YOU MAY USE A CANE AND PUT PARTIAL WEIGHT ON THE OPERATIVE SIDE. DO NOT WALK WITHOUT THE CANE., (0181)

--YOU MAY SHOWER WITH ASSISTANCE., (0181)

--I RECOMMEND PLAIN TYLENOL IF NEEDED FOR PAIN, (0181)

--TRY NOT TO SIT LONGER THAN THIRTY MINUTES AT ONE TIME AND PUMP THE CALF MUSCLES WHILE SITTING TO ASSIST VENOUS BLOOD RETURN AND TO PREVENT SWELLING AND STASIS., (0181)

--ALSO REPORT ANY WOUND SEEPAGE OR CALF OR CHEST PAIN., (0181)

--CALL MY OFFICE ON MONDAY AT 555-8141 AND MAKE AN APPOINTMENT TO SEE ME IN 2 TO 3 WEEKS., (0181)

--GOOD LUCK MRS. DUELL! DR. SHINN, (0181)

NOTED BY NURSE: ______________________

Computerized medical orders.

displayed. This information and the client instruction sheet generated by the computer is sent home with the client.

In addition to making the charting of client care and the communication between departments much simpler and less time-consuming, the computer provides reference material for common nursing problems. For example, a matrix may show the signs and symptoms associated with diabetes mellitus. If the nurse is unsure of the signs and symptoms of the different forms of this disease, he or she can easily find them in the computer, and, if needed, this information can be printed out and put in the chart. In this way the nurse can be quickly updated about the client's condition and thereby provide optimal care.

As in many professions, use of the computer in nursing and medicine has become more common and its possible uses are rapidly expanding. If learning the skills of computer use is viewed as a challenge and the reward is more efficient nursing care and less time spent on paperwork, the learning time will have been well spent.

Minimizing Legal Risks of Computer Charting

The American Nurses' Association, the American Medical Record Association, and the Canadian Nurses' Association offer guidelines and strategies for computer safety in charting.

- Your personal password or computer signature should not be given to anyone: neither another nurse on the unit, a float nurse, nor a physician. The hospital issues a short-term password with access to certain records for infrequent users.
- Do not leave a computer terminal unattended after you have logged on. Some computers have a timing device that shuts down a terminal when it has not been used for a certain time.

COMPUTER-ASSISTED CHARTING

Advantages

- Computers store large volumes of information
- Quick communication between departments
- Quick access to information
- Confidentiality is maintained with records
- Bedside computers increase accuracy and speed of documentation
- Nursing information systems improve documentation and meet JACHO standards
- They track client outcomes
- They increase speed and completeness of reimbursement through accurate documentation
- Information is legible

Disadvantages

- Computer system is expensive to purchase and update
- "Downtime" can create problems of not receiving information or it is not charted on time
- Computer may increase charting time if numbers of terminals there are insufficient
- Nurses rely on computers and don't question information when it may be wrong

- Computer entries are part of the client's permanent record and, as such, cannot be deleted. It is possible, however, to correct an error before the material has been stored. If the entry has already been moved to storage, handle the error by marking the entry "mistaken entry," add correct information, date and initial the entry. If you record information in the wrong chart, write "mistaken entry," add "wrong chart," and sign off.
- Once information about a client is stored, it is difficult to delete accidentally. Do check that stored records have back-up files. This is an important safety check. If you inadvertently delete a part of the permanent record (this is difficult to do, since the computer always asks if you are sure), type an explanation into the computer file with date, time, and your initials. Submit an explanation in writing to your supervisor.
- Do not leave computer information about a client displayed on a monitor where others have access to it. Also, do not leave printed files unattended. Keep a log that accounts for every copy of a computerized file that you have generated from the system.
- A positive diagnosis of human immunodeficiency virus (HIV) or hepatitis (HBV) is part of the client's confidential record. Disclosure of this information to unauthorized people may have legal implications. If the diagnosis is entered as any other diagnosis, take steps to follow your hospital's confidentiality procedures. Check your state's special protocols for treatment of a client's HBV or HIV status.

REPORTING

Intrashift Reports

Reporting your observations and interventions to other health team members is as essential as documenting them on the client's chart. Intrashift reports are usually verbal reports relayed to team members, team leaders, or charge nurses to keep them informed of changes in the client's conditions. Examples of findings that need to be communicated to other health team members include significant changes in vital signs, unusual responses to treatments, medications, or changes in the client's physical or emotional condition.

Intershift Reports

Intershift reports disseminate client information between shifts. It may be accomplished through a verbal report or by tape recording the information. The intershift report should include the following data: client's name, room number, physician's name, diagnosis, and date of surgery when appropriate. In addition, report unusual findings based on the nursing assessment, response to treatments or medications, unusual occurrences, laboratory results, laboratory studies, tests to be completed on the next shift, and any physical or psychosocial problems that exist.

Physician Notification

Physicians should be notified whenever treatment or nursing care parameters are exceeded, significant alterations occur in physical assessment findings, or abnormal laboratory findings and test results are obtained.

Before calling the physician, have all data available to allow you to answer questions: current vital signs, laboratory results, when medications were given last, and so on. It is a good idea to have the entire chart with you.

When calling the physician, identify yourself by name, your status (RN or SN), nursing unit, and the client's name. State the exact reason you are calling. Give pertinent and succinct information.

Nurse Manager

Written or verbal reports are given to nurse managers, nursing supervisors, or clinical coordinators during each shift. The report includes information on all critically ill clients, those with unusual occurrences or complications, and clients with conditions that are difficult to manage. It is also a good idea to alert the supervisor to problems with families, physicians, or other health disciplines so she or he can assist you in the problem solving.

DOCUMENTATION

Unusual Occurrence, or Incident Report

Unusual occurrence, also called incident report (IR), serves three main purposes: to help document quality of care, to identify areas where in-service education is needed, and to record the details of an incident for possible legal reference.

With some staff nurses, IRs have a poor reputation and, perhaps, with some justification. When something goes wrong and a nurse is told to "make out an IR," it is interpreted as a form of punishment.

Although IRs should be completed regularly with any unusual occurrence and may, on occasion, be used as a form of reprimand, they are no more nor less than what their title suggests: a report of an incident.

As a tool for documenting quality of care, IRs inform the quality assurance coordinator and the head nurse of areas of practice on the unit that need improvement. For example, there may be an increase in the number of clients who fell out of bed. Further research may show that because the census is up, the staff is very busy and is forgetting to reposition clients' overbed tables. In their attempts to get water or tissues, for example, more clients are falling out of bed. The solution to the problem may be to speak with the staff regarding the consequences of this action, and as a group find a mutually acceptable way of preventing this type of incident from recurring.

IRs also suggest and document the need for in-service education. For example, when an unusual number of IRs are written regarding a new piece of equipment, the head nurse may conclude that the staff, especially those on evening and night shifts, needs instruction on operating this equipment properly and effectively. Another example is an increase in IRs regarding IVs that are behind or ahead of schedule. This might indicate that the nurses do not know how to apply and regulate the IV pump correctly. A solution to this problem is to conduct a series of classes for all shifts in which the operation of the IV pump is discussed and hands-on practice is given. Such classes could be given by someone in the hospital's in-service education department or by a representative of the manufacturer of the IV pumps.

Incident reports may also record the details of an occurrence for possible legal use. In some hospitals incident reports are called unusual occurrences and cover any situation that prevented the client from having a normal recovery. These incidents could include nonnursing actions such as returning to surgery for control of bleeding or having chest tubes inserted for a pneumothorax. In most situations, though, IRs pertain to nurse–patient activities.

When completing an IR with possible legal implications, it is doubly important to record all details of the incident. It is not easy to recall details of the care you gave a client 1 or 2 months ago. Frequently lawsuits are not filed for months or even years after an incident, so it is essential that you record important details promptly.

Information to record on the IR includes general details of the incident, the client's response, your action or reaction to the incident, and a list of other personnel who were aware of the details of the incident. Often there is space on the IR in which to record the physician's report of the client's condition following the incident. To fill in the section regarding the physician's report, the nurse later copies the doctor's progress notes from the chart onto the IR. At no time is the incident report given to the physician. This is a written document between the hospital and its insurance carrier, not the physician.

On completion, IRs are forwarded to the unit head nurse and then to nursing administration. Information from the report of interest to in-service education or quality assurance departments can be obtained at this time. Ultimately the IR is passed along to the hospital's legal department to be retained indefinitely in the event that legal action is later initiated on behalf of the client.

Consent Forms

When an individual enters a hospital, some of his or her basic legal rights are affected. So that these rights are not violated, the client must give permission (consent) for all treatment. If consent is not obtained, the hospital, physician, or nurse may be charged with committing "battery" against the client. Battery, as defined by

UNUSUAL OCCURRENCE

COMPLETE IMMEDIATELY FOR EVERY INCIDENT AND SEND TO ADMINISTRATOR

________________________ HOSPITAL NAME

ADMINISTRATOR:
Please forward to
Hospital Attorney

________________________ CITY

________________________ FOR ADDRESSOGRAPH PLATE

CONFIDENTIAL REPORT OF INCIDENT (NOT A PART OF MEDICAL RECORD)

CLIENT ________ (LAST NAME) ________ (FIRST NAME) AGE ____ SEX ____ (M OR F) ROOM ________

ADMITTING DIAGNOSIS ________ DATE OF ADMISSION ________

ATTENDING PHYSICIAN ________ DATE OF INCIDENT ________ TIME ____ M

WERE BED RAILS UP? ________ WAS SAFETY BELT IN USE? ________

WAS CLIENT RATIONAL? ________ HI LO BED POSITION ________

SEDATIVES ________ DOSE ________ TIME ________

NARCOTICS ________ DOSE ________ TIME ________

{ GIVEN WITHIN 12 HOURS PREVIOUS TO INCIDENT

TIME DOCTOR WAS CALLED ______ A.M. ______ P.M. TIME RESPONDED ______ A.M. ______ P.M.

(I.E., HOUSE PHYSICIAN-RESIDENT-INTERN-ETC.)

I NOTIFIED DR. ________ TIME ____ M BY ________

NURSE'S ACCOUNT OF THE INCIDENT (INCLUDE EXACT LOCATION)

____
____
____
____

LIST PERSONS FAMILIAR WITH DETAILS OF INCIDENT - AND OTHER CLIENTS IN THE SAME ROOM

NAME ________ ADDRESS ________

NAME ________ ADDRESS ________

NAME ________ ADDRESS ________

HISTORY OF INCIDENT AS RELATED BY CLIENT ________
____
____
____

DATE OF REPORT ________ ________________________ SIGNATURE OF NURSE OR SUPERVISOR REPORTING

____

DOCTOR'S REPORT OF CLIENT'S CONDITION (FROM PROGRESS REPORT) ________
____
____
____

ORIGINAL TO HOSPITAL ATTORNEY

Unusual occurrence, or incident, report.

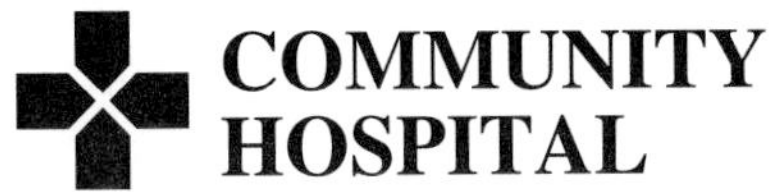

Client Information

AUTHORIZATION FOR AND CONSENT TO SURGERY, ADMINISTRATION OF ANESTHETICS, SPECIAL DIAGNOSTIC OR THERAPEUTIC PROCEDURES

Date ______________ Time ______________

Your admitting physician is ____, M.D.

Your surgeon is ____, M.D.

1. The hospital staff and facilities assist your physicians and surgeons in the performance of various surgical operations and other diagnostic and therapeutic procedures. These surgical operations and special diagnostic or therapeutic procedures all may involve calculated risks of complications, injury or even death, from both known and unknown causes and no warranty or guarantee has been made as to result or cure. Except in a case of emergency or exceptional circumstances, these operations and procedures are not performed upon clients unless and until the client has had an opportunity to discuss them with his/her physician. Each client has the right to consent to or to refuse any proposed operation or special procedure (based upon the description or explanation received).
2. Your physicians and surgeons have determined that the operations or special procedures listed below may be beneficial in the diagnosis or treatment of your condition. Upon your authorization and consent, the operations or special procedures will be performed by your physicians and surgeons and their staff. The persons in attendance for the purpose of administering anesthesia or performing other specialized professional services, such as radiology, pathology and the like, are not the agents, servants or employees of the hospital or your physician or surgeon, but are independent contractors performing specialized services on your behalf and, as such, are your agents, servants, or employees. Any tissue or member severed in any operation will be disposed of in the discretion of the pathologist, except ______________________________ and those body parts specified as donor organs.
3. Your signature opposite the operations or special procedures listed below constitutes your acknowledgement (a) that you have read and agreed to the foregoing, (b) that the operations or special procedures have been adequately explained to you by your attending physicians or surgeons and that you have all of the information that you desire, and (c) that you authorize and consent to the performance of the operations or special procedures.

Operation or Procedure

____

____

Signature ______________________________ Signature ______________________________
Client Witness

(If client is a minor or unable to sign, complete the following): Client is a minor, is unable to sign because

____

____
Father Guardian

____
Mother Other person and relationship

Consent form.

law, is an "offensive touching" of the client. This could include injection or any breaking of the skin's surface, use of x-rays, or insertion of tubes, for example.

Before you panic and attempt to get a consent signed for such a routine procedure as taking the client's next blood pressure, you should know that routine nursing care is "consented to" when the client signs the "conditions of admissions" form. Also, certain procedures, such as injections, intubations, and dressings are treatments ordered by the physician and agreed to by the client. If the client has listened to the explanation of a specific procedure and has agreed to allow the procedure to be carried out, he or she is giving implied consent; however, the client has the right to refuse any treatment, including changing his or her mind about a procedure previously agreed to. In that case the physician must be contacted regarding alternative actions.

When discussing the formal written or explicit consents, the two key activities are obtaining and witnessing consent. Obtaining consent is not a nursing function because it includes the explanation of what is to be done, the risks of the procedure to that client, alternative procedures, and probable outcomes. This information should be given by the doctor.

The nurse's role is to witness the signing of the consent. When the consent form is presented to the client, it should be explained, and the client should be encouraged to read it thoroughly before signing. Occasionally a nurse is asked to explain or expand the physician's presentation. Acceptable practice is for the nurse to clarify, define a medical term, or add more details to the physician's initial information. If the nurse feels that the client does not really understand what is going to occur, it is the nurse's responsibility to notify the doctor to give further explanation before the client signs the consent. An easy way to determine what the client understands is to ask him or her to repeat the physician's explanation. Under ordinary circumstances, only one witness to signing the consent is necessary. The witness does not have to be an RN, just someone over the age of 18 years.

There are many rules and regulations governing consents. If you have questions about them, consult the consent manual for your hospital, or a supervisory person. There are several important situations in which more information may be needed. One relates to the client's mental competency. Generally the client must sign personally, and spouses are unable to sign for the client. Permanent incompetence usually involves legal action to assign someone else as conservator. Temporary incompetence may be the result of hospital treatments, such as drugs or anesthetics. When a narcotic or sedative has been given, at least 4 hours lapsed time is recommended before the client is considered competent to sign a consent. A second situation concerns the client who is a minor. The age of consent varies by state and also according to specific situations, such as emancipation (being away from the family and self supporting) and the type of medical problem (reportable diseases or pregnancy). An associated problem may arise when deciding who can legally sign for a minor.

WORD ROOTS, PREFIXES, AND SUFFIXES

a, an: without, not
ab: away from
abd: abdominal
a.c.: before meals
acro: extreme, top, extremity
acu: sharp
ad, al: to, toward
adeno: gland
adip: fat
ad lib.: freely, as desired
-aemia: blood
aero: air, gas
-aesthesia: sensation
-al: action, process
alg: pain
-algesia, algia: suffering pain
amb.: ambulatory, walking
amput: cut away, cut off
amt.: amount
ante: before
anti: against, opposed to
ap, apo: away from
arteri: artery
arthro: joint
-ase: enzyme
aur: ear
auto: self
bacill: rod
bacter: rod
bi: double, two
bid: twice each day
bile: bile
bio: life
blephar: eyelid
BM: bowel movement
brachi: arm
brady: slow
BRP: bathroom privileges
bucc: check
c̄: with
cale: stone
capit: head
cardi, cardio: heart
cathart: cleansing
caud: tail
cav: hollow
cec: blind
cent: hundred
-chem, -chemo: chemical
chole: bile
chron: time

cid: kill
-cide: causing death
cili: eyelid
circum: ring, circle
C/O: complains of
cogni: know
colo: colon
com, con: with, together
crani: skull
cry: cold
cut: skin
cyan: blue
cyst: bladder
cyt: cell
-cyte: cell
DC: discontinue
demi: half
dent: tooth
derm: skin
di, dis: double, separation, reversal
dors: back
dur: hard
dy: two
-dynia: pain
dys: abnormal, different
e, ec: out from
-ectomy: cutting out
em, en: in, within
embol: inserted a wedge
-emesis: vomiting
-emia: blood
emulsi: milk out, exhaust
endo: within
entero: intestinal
epi: upon
erythro: red
eso: inside
-esthesia: sensation
et: and
eu: normal
ex: out of
exo: the outside, beyond
fore: before, in front of
gastro: stomach
genito: genital
-gens, -gent: clan, tribe
glosso: relating to the tongue
glyco: sugar
-gram: tracing, a mark
-graphy: a writing, a record
grav: heavy
gyn: woman
H_2O: water
hemi: half
hemo: blood
hepar, hepatio: liver
hisc: open
homeo: same, similar
homo: same, similar
HS: bedtime
hydro: related to water
hyper: above, beyond
hypo: under, below
I&O: intake and output
-iasis: condition, pathologic state
ile, ilo: intestine
in: not, within, into
in.: inch
incont: incontinent
infra: below
inter: between
intra: inside
is: equal
isch, ischo: hold, suppress
-ism: condition, theory
itis: inflammation
juxta: next to
latero: side
lb or #: pound
leuko: white
lip: fat
lith: stone
ly: loose, dissolve
-lysis: dissolving, decomposition
macro: large, big
mal: bad, poor
mamm: breast
man: hand
mani: mental alterations
megaly: large
meta: beyond
metra, metro: uterus
micro: small
ne: young, new
nebul: cloud, mist
necr, necro: dead
neo: new
neuro: nerve
noct: night
-nos, -noso: disease
npo: nothing by mouth
nucleo: nucleus
nutri: nourish
ob: against
oc: occlude
olig: few, small
oob: out of bed
opisth: backward
-opsy: examination
opthalm: eye
-orrhaphy: repair of
ortho: straight, normal
-osis: process, condition
oss, ost: bone
-ostomy: creation of an opening
-otomy: opening into
palp: touch, feel
pan: all, entire
para: beside, beyond
paten, patent: spreading open
path: disease, sickness
pc: after meals
ped, pedi, pedo: foot
ped, pedo: child
pen: lack of
per: by, through
peri: around
pet: tend toward
pha: speak
phag: eat
phleb: vein
phon: sound
phot: light
phthi: waste away
-phylaxis: protection
-plasm: to mold
-plasty: formed or repaired by plastic surgery
platy: broad, flat
-plegia: paralysis
pleur: rib
plur: more
pne: breathing
-pnea: respiration, respiratory condition
pneumo: air, gas, lung
post: after, behind
pre: before
prn: whenever necessary
pro: before
pruri: itch
pseud, pseudo: false
psych: the soul, mind
-ptosis: a lowered position of an organ
pulmo: lung
pur: pus
pyo: pus
pyro: fire
qd: every day

qh: every hour
qid: four times each day
qs: as much as required
q2h: every 2 hours
q3h: every 3 hours
q4h: every 4 hours
ren: kidneys
retro: backwards
-rhage, -rhagia: hemorrhage, excessive flow or discharge
s̄: without
-sclerosis: dryness, hardness
-scopy: to see
sedat: soothed, calm
semi: half
sens: sense
sept: wall off
socio: social
som: sleep
spiro: breathe
stasis: stoppage, slowing
stat: immediately
steat: fat
sub, sup: under, below
super: over, above, higher
syn: with, together
tach: fast
therm: heat
therapeu: serve, treatment
thromb: clot
tid: three times each day
-tomy: cut
top: place
toxic: poisonous
troch: wheel
trop: turn, change
-trophy: nutrition, nourishment
ultra: beyond, excessively
un: one
-uria: a specific condition of, or related to urine
vaso: vessel
veno: vein
ventro: abdomen
°: degree

5

Communication and the Nurse–Client Relationship

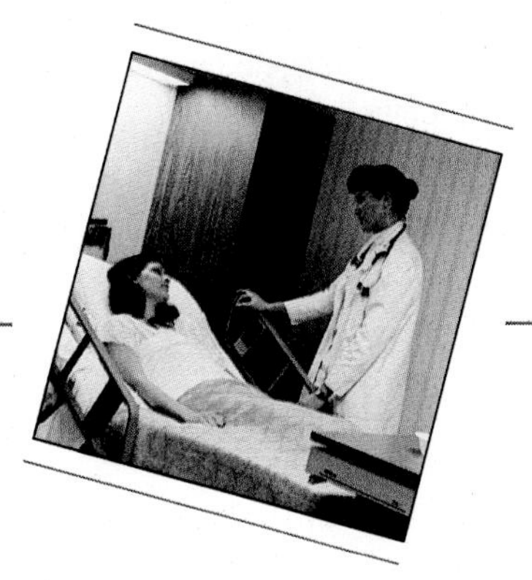

LEARNING OBJECTIVES

- Define the term "communication."
- Explain why communication is such an important concept in nursing.
- Describe what is meant by the communication process.
- Discuss four factors that affect communication.
- List five examples of therapeutic communication.
- List five examples of blocks to communication.
- Demonstrate the steps for beginning a client interaction.
- Explain why it is therapeutic to encourage the client to express feelings and thoughts.
- State two nursing diagnoses that relate to communication with clients.
- Describe the phases of a nurse–client relationship.
- List three components for maintaining a nurse–client relationship.
- Describe the rationale for discussing termination at the beginning of the relationship.

TERMINOLOGY

Acceptance: favorable reception; basic acknowledgment.

Agitation: excessive restlessness and increased mental and especially physical activity.

Anxiety: a state of uneasiness and distress; diffuse apprehension.

Apprehension: a fearful or uneasy anticipation of the future; dread.

Assistance: aiding, helping, or giving support.

Attitude: a state of mind or feeling with regard to some matter; disposition.

Behavior: the actions or reactions of persons under specified circumstances.

Clarify: to make clear or easier to understand.

Cliché: stereotyped response; a trite or overused expression or idea.

Cognition: the mental process or faculty by which knowledge is acquired.

Communication: the exchange of thoughts, information, or messages.

Confusion: disorder; jumble; distraction; bewilderment.

Congruence: agreement; conformity.

Consent: to agree; to be of the same mind.

Convey: to communicate or make known; to impart.

Coping mechanism: a means by which to adjust or adapt to disequilibrium; defense mechanism against anxiety.

Counseling: to give support or to provide guidance.

Depression: a mental state characterized by dejection, lack of hope, and absence of cheerfulness.

Emotion: any strong feeling, as of joy, hate, sorrow, love.

Empathy: ability to readily comprehend the feelings, thoughts, and motives of another person.

Esteem: to consider as of a certain value; regard; respect.

Evaluate: to examine and judge; appraise.

Expression: to manifest or communicate; make known.

Feedback: the return of information to the place of origin.

Helping relationship: an interaction of individuals that sets the climate for movement of the participants toward common goals.

Maladaptive: inability to, or faulty adjustment or adaptation.

Noncompliance: failure or refusal to comply or go along with something.

Overdependence: the state of needing or relying on someone or something too much.

Perception: the process of receiving and interrupting sensory impressions.

Rapport: a feeling of mutual trust experienced by persons in a satisfactory relationship.

Refer: to send or direct someone for action or help.

Relationship: an interaction of individuals over a period of time.

Self-esteem: a sense of pride in oneself; self-love.

Social: involvement with communities and other persons.

Support: to lend strength or give assistance to.

Termination: the end of something; a limit or boundary; conclusion or cessation.

Therapeutic: having medicinal or healing properties; a healing agent.

Touch: a tactile sense.

Understanding: to perceive and comprehend the nature and significance of; to know.

Unique: being the only one of its kind.

Validate: to substantiate or verify.

COMMUNICATION

Communication is the process of sending and receiving messages by means of symbols, words, signs, gestures, or other actions. It is a multilevel process consisting of the content, or information, part of the message and the part that defines the meaning of the message. Messages sent and received define the relationship between people. From the point of view of a learned skill, communication is intended to accomplish a defined goal. It is the transmission of facts, feelings, and meaning through the communication process.

The communication process forms one of the primary bases for administering all skills. Without clear communication the nurse cannot assess, administer, or evaluate his or her actions in performing the skill. The principles of therapeutic communication also form a basis for interviewing and counseling skills.

Communication is a vital element in nursing. Everything that occurs within the nurse–client interaction involves some form or mode of communication, whether it includes listening to an upset family member, assisting a client in health teaching, or performing a nursing procedure. Without communication the nurse could not give nursing care.

The communication process includes both verbal and nonverbal expressions and is affected by the intrapersonal framework of the person, the relationship between the participants, and the purpose of the sender. The content of the message and the context also influence the communication process. The manner in which the message is sent and the effect on the receiver also play a role in the eventual outcome of the communication process.

Guidelines That Influence Effective Communication

- A person cannot *not* communicate. This idea is basic to communication. We have an inherent need to communicate, whether it be verbal or nonverbal. Even silence is a form of communication.
- There is a content, or informational, value to messages sent and received that explains what the message is about and expresses how the sender regards the receiver.
- The message sent is not necessarily the message received.
- Messages contain overt and covert meanings. The sender is aware of the overt, or direct, message and may or may not be aware of the hidden, or covert, meaning.
- Communication becomes dysfunctional when a person does not assume responsibility for his or her communication. Dysfunctional communications result from failing to learn to communicate properly and leaving the responsibility for communicating to others.

All communication between nurse and client should be therapeutic, whether it involves obtaining information for an assessment, interacting with the client during a bed bath, or doing client teaching. The difference between therapeutic communication and a therapeutic relationship is that a relationship has a beginning, middle, and end with specified goals for each phase. Therapeutic communication techniques should be used in all forms of communication.

Guidelines for Communicating with Clients

- Take an active role and guide the conversation if the client is overly hesitant. For example, "I'm here to listen to any concerns you might have, Mr. Smith. You were mentioning having trouble understanding. . . ."
- Give broad opening statements and ask open-ended questions to help the client describe what is happening to him or her. Pick up cues and follow through with the subject that the client introduces to provide continuity.
- Use body language to convey empathy, interest, and encouragement to facilitate communication.
- Use silence as a therapeutic tool, as it allows the client to pace and direct his or her own communications. Long periods of silence, however, may increase the client's anxiety level, so use this technique wisely.

THERAPEUTIC COMMUNICATION TECHNIQUES

Communication includes the totality of the human person and reflects what is happening within and outside of us. Body sensations, thoughts, feelings, emotions, ideas, perceptions, judgments, previous experiences, and memories are all part of how and what we communicate. Effective, functional communication only occurs when what is happening within is congruent with what we share with the outside. It is important to be a therapeutic as well as a functional communicator and not to disturb the communication process by using nontherapeutic techniques or blocks to communication.

Therapeutic communication techniques assist the flow of communication and always focus on the client. Nontherapeutic communication techniques block or hinder communication and generally focus on the nurse and meet the nurse's needs. The major therapeutic and nontherapeutic techniques are listed below.

Acknowledgment

Acknowledging the client without inserting your own values or judgments. Acknowledgment may be simple and with or without understanding, verbal or nonverbal.

Example:
In the response "I hear what you're saying," the nurse acknowledges a statement without agreeing with it.

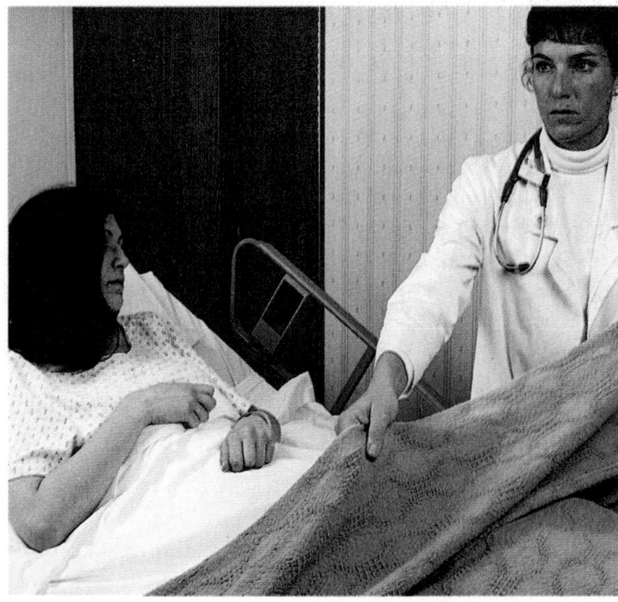

Therapeutic communication implies the nurse is focusing on the client. Here we see an example of nontherapeutic communication.

Example:
"Yes, go on." "Uh huh."

Clarification

Clarifying the client's message. Check out or make clear either the intent or hidden meaning of the message, or determine if the message sent was the message received.

Example:
"I don't understand. Can you say it in a different way."
Example:
"Are you saying . . . "(Repeat meaning of client's message)

Feedback

Using feedback to relay to the client the effect of his or her words. This method helps keep the client on course or alters the course. It involves acknowledging, validating, clarifying, extending, and altering.

Example:
"You did that well."
Example:
"When you say that, it makes me feel uncomfortable." (If the client is making personal comments about the nurse.)

Focus

Focusing or refocusing on the client's statement. Pick up on central topics or "cues" given by the client.

Example:
"You were telling me how hard it was to talk to your mother."
Example:
"You said the test tomorrow is frightening."

Incomplete Sentences

Encouraging the client to continue.

Example:
"Then your life is . . ."

Listening

Consciously receiving the client's message.

Example:
Listening eagerly, actively, responsively, and seriously.

Minimum Verbal Activity

Keeping your own verbalization minimal and letting the client lead the conversation.

Example:
"You feel . . . ?"
"Go on."

Mutual Fit or Congruence

Creating harmony of verbal and nonverbal messages.

Example:
A client is crying, and the nurse says, "I'll sit with you awhile," and puts his or her hand on the client's shoulder.
Example:
A client tells the nurse he or she feels fine but the client's body language indicates that he or she feels depressed and not fine. "You say you feel fine, but you don't look like you feel fine."

Nonverbal Encouragement
Using body language to communicate interest, attention, understanding, support, caring, and listening to promote data gathering.

Example:
The nurse nods appropriately as the client talks.
Example:
The nurse leans forward.

Open-ended Questions
Asking questions that cannot be answered with a simple "yes" or "no" or "maybe." Generally ask questions requiring an answer of several words to broaden conversational opportunities and to help the client communicate.

Example:
"How did your weekend pass go?" rather than "Did you have a good weekend?"

Paraphrase
Rewording or summarizing what has been said.

Example:
"You are saying you're unhappy."
Example:
After the client gives a long description of his or her family, the nurse asks the client, "You feel uncomfortable with your family?"

Reflection
Identifying and sending back a message acknowledging the feeling or repeating the last few words the client said. (Conveys acceptance and great understanding.)

Example:
". . . distrust your doctor?"

Restatement
Repeating the client's statement as encouragement for him or her to continue.

Example:
"You said that you hear voices."

Validation
Verifying the accuracy of the sender's message.

Example:
"Yes, it is confusing with so many people around."

BLOCKS TO COMMUNICATION

Changing the Subject
Introducing new topics inappropriately, a pattern that may indicate anxiety.

Example:
The client is crying and discussing his or her fear of surgery when the nurse asks, "How many children do you have?"

False Reassurance
Using cliches, pat answers, "cheery" words, advice, and "comforting" statements in an attempt to reassure the client. Most of what is called "reassurance" is really false reassurance.

Example:
"It's going to be all right."
Example:
"Don't worry. This pain medication always works."

Giving Advice
Telling the client what to do. Giving your opinion or making decisions for the client implies he or she cannot handle his or her own life decisions and that you are accepting responsibility for him or her.

Example:
"If I were you. . . ."
Example:
"You should change doctors if you are unhappy."

Incongruence
Sending verbal and nonverbal messages that contradict one another; two or more messages, sent via different levels, seriously contradicting one another. The contradiction may be between the content, verbal, nonverbal, or content (time, space).

Example:
"I'd like to talk to you." (But I'm just too busy) said while nurse is turning away from the client.

Assumptions
Making an assumption about the meaning of someone else's behavior that is not validated by the other person.

Example:
The nurse finds the suicidal patient smiling and tells the staff he's in a cheerful mood and much better.

Invalidation
Ignoring or denying another person's presence, thoughts, or feelings.

Example:
Client: "Hi, how are you?" Nurse: "I can't talk now, I'm on my way to lunch."

Overloading
Talking rapidly, changing subjects, and giving more information than can be absorbed at one time.

Example:
"What's your name? I see you're 48 years old and that you like sports. Where do you come from?"

Social Response
Responding in a way that focuses attention on the nurse instead of the client.

Example:
"This sunshine is good for my roses. I have a beautiful rose garden."

Underloading
Remaining silent and unresponsive, not picking up cues, and failing to give feedback.

Example:
Nurse asking, "What's your name?" as he or she smiles and walks away.

Value Judgments
Giving one's own opinion, moralizing or implying one's own values by using words, such as "nice," "good," "bad," "right," "wrong," "should," and "ought."

Example:
"I think he's a very good doctor."
Example:
"I think it's good that you changed your dress."

RELATIONSHIP THERAPY

Nurses are given the unique opportunity to share part of who they are with others who have asked directly or indirectly for assistance. It is within this interpersonal framework that the nurse–client relationship begins to develop and take on its individual characteristics.

Both individuals bring into the relationship their thoughts, feelings, sense of self or self-worth, behavior patterns, abilities to adapt and cope, belief systems, and points of view about life and how they interact with it.

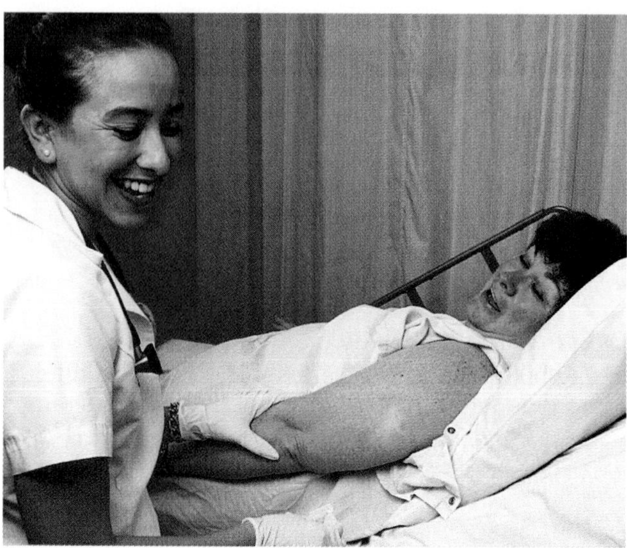

Within the interpersonal framework, nurses share part of who they are with the client.

Within all these complex variables, there is a commonly shared point at which the nurse–client relationship begins.

This relationship may be defined as the interaction between the nurse and a client with shared therapeutic goals and objectives. Characteristics of the relationship include acceptance, honesty, understanding, and empathy of the nurse toward the client who is willingly or unwillingly seeking help. Generally it is important for the nurse to view the client as a unique individual who is responsible for his or her own feelings, actions, and behaviors and who is an active participant in a health care program. The relationship is more effective if the client shows a willingness to accept responsibility and actively participates in the therapeutic relationship. In psychiatry, however, this is not always possible, and the nurse must begin the relationship by accepting the level at which the client is able to participate. This, at times, is a difficult and frustrating process. The goal of relationship therapy is to assist the client to identify and meet his or her own needs. The nurse may assist the client in reaching the goals by demonstrating acceptance so that the client can experience the feeling of being accepted as an individual; by developing mutual trust through consistent, congruent nursing behaviors; by providing corrective emotional experiences to increase self-esteem; and finally by creating a safe, supportive environment. Some degree of emotional involvement and honest, open communication is essential throughout the relationship. The nurse must encourage the client to express his or her feelings within safe limits.

Relationship Principles

Principles underlying a helping relationship include:

- Awareness of the total client, including physical needs
- Some degree of emotional involvement while maintaining objectivity
- The setting of appropriate limits and consistency
- Empathetic understanding focusing on the client
- Open, honest, clear communication
- Encouragement of the expression of feelings
- Focus on "here and now"

Dangers to the relationship include overemotional involvement and judgmental attitudes on the part of the nurse and the staff.

Phases in Nurse–Client Relationship Therapy

Initiation, or Orientation, Phase

- Establish boundaries of the relationship.
- Identify problems.
- Assess your own anxiety levels and those of the client.
- Identify expectations.

Continuation, or Active Working, Phase

- Promote an attitude of acceptance.
- Use specific therapeutic and problem-solving techniques to develop a working relationship.
- Continually assess and evaluate problems.
- Focus on increasing the client's independence and decreasing his or her reliance on the nurse.
- Maintain the goal of client's confronting and working through identified problems.

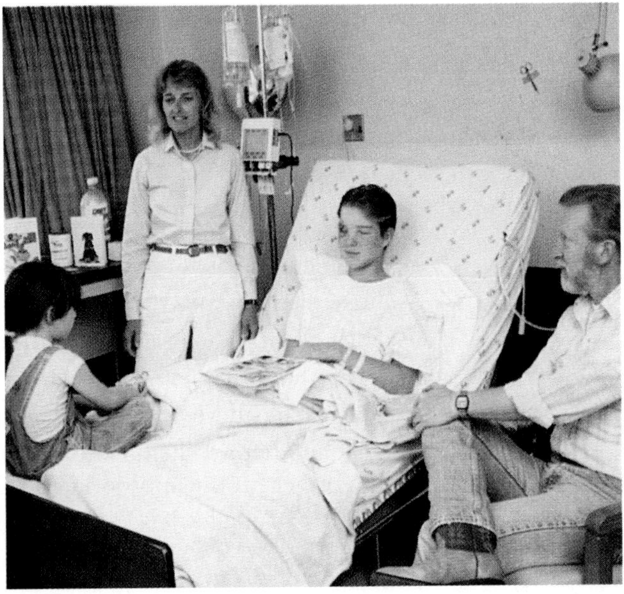

Relationship therapy includes bringing the family together to discuss client care needs.

Termination Phase

- Plan for termination early in the development of the relationship.
- Maintain initially defined boundaries.
- Anticipate problems of termination: Client may become too dependent on the nurse; encourage client to become independent. Termination may recall client's previous separation experiences, causing feelings of abandonment, rejection, and depression. Discuss client's previous experiences.
- Discuss client's feelings about termination of the relationship.

NURSING DIAGNOSES

The following nursing diagnoses may be appropriate to include in a client care plan when the components are related to establishing and maintaining a nurse–patient relationship.

NURSING DIAGNOSIS	RELATED FACTORS
Communication, Impaired Verbal	Psychologic barrier, inability to speak dominant language, impaired cognitive function, lack of privacy
Powerlessness	Perceived lack of control resulting in dissatisfaction
Social Interactions, Impaired	Lack of motivation, anxiety, depression, lack of self-esteem, disorganized thinking, delusions, hallucinations
Social Isolation	Hospitalization, terminal illness
Thought Processes, Altered	Depression, anxiety, fear of unknown, emotional trauma, unclear communication, negative response from others

unit 1

THERAPEUTIC COMMUNICATION

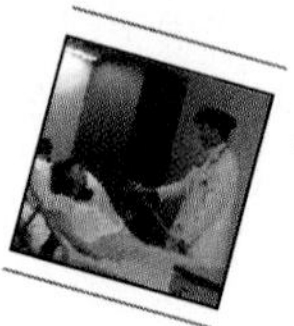

NURSING PROCESS DATA

ASSESSMENT Data Base

Determine individual's ability to process information at the cognitive level.

Evaluate mental status data to establish baseline for intervention.

Evaluate client's ability to communicate on a verbal level.

Observe what is happening with the client here and now.

Identify client's developmental level so interaction expectations will be realistic.

Determine whether client exhibits primarily verbal or nonverbal behavior so you can relate to him or her on the appropriate level.

Assess client's anxiety level because anxiety interferes with communication.

PLANNING Objectives

To assist client to meet his or her own needs

To assist client to experience the feeling of being accepted

To increase client's self-esteem

To provide a supportive environment for change

To institute therapeutic rather than casual or nongoal-oriented communication

To affect or influence the client's physical, emotional, and social environment

IMPLEMENTATION Procedures

Introducing Yourself to a Client

Beginning a Client Interaction

Assisting a Client to Describe Personal Experiences

Encouraging a Client to Express Needs, Feelings, and Thoughts

Using Communication to Increase a Client's Sense of Self-Worth

EVALUATION Expected Outcomes

Client develops the ability to assess and meet his or her own needs.

Communication becomes clearer, more explicit, and centered on problem areas.

A supportive environment is created so that the client can reduce the level of anxiety and experience change.

INTRODUCING YOURSELF TO A CLIENT

Procedure

1. Obtain client assignment.
2. Read chart and review physician's orders.
3. Check client care plan.
4. Clarify any questions about client assignment.
5. Proceed to client's room and check room number.
6. Introduce yourself to the client. (Example: "Good morning, Mr. Jones. My name is Miss Barnes. I am a student nurse from the Bellington School of Nursing, and I will be caring for you today.")
7. If the client is blind, introduce yourself as you come into the door: tell exactly what you are doing and when you are leaving. **Rationale:** Blind clients become anxious when they hear someone enter the room who does not speak.
8. Begin to establish a nurse–client relationship using clear, open communication.

BEGINNING A CLIENT INTERACTION

Procedure

1. Following introduction (at which time you call the client by name and tell the client your name), relate purpose of interaction.
2. Tell client specifically what you will be doing in terms of his or her care.
3. Ask if the client understands or has any questions.
4. Encourage client to describe how he or she is feeling at the time.
5. Encourage client to participate in his or her care—both verbally and nonverbally.
6. Pay attention to communication as well as the procedure you are administering. **Rationale:** Often, your best data base is drawn from observation.
7. Complete communication by asking client for feedback.
8. Complete interaction by telling client when you will return.
9. Follow through on agreed on meeting time to build client trust.

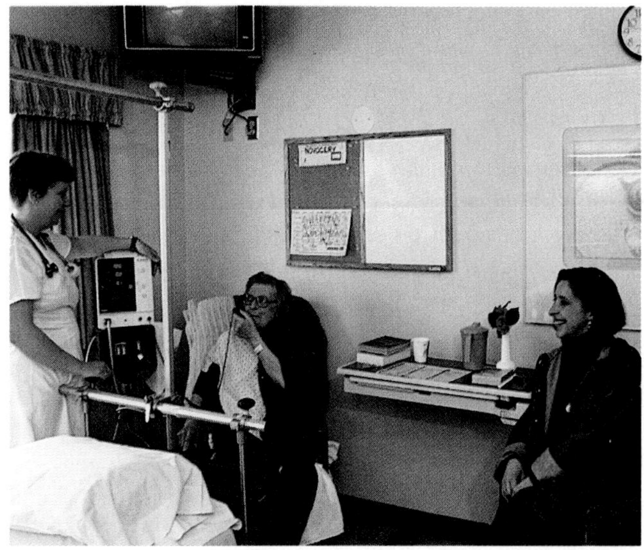

When interacting with a client, the nurse includes friends as an important element in client's support system.

ASSISTING A CLIENT TO DESCRIBE PERSONAL EXPERIENCES

Procedure

1. Encourage client to describe his or her perceptions and feelings.
2. Focus on communication as well as body reactions.
3. Don't dominate the conversation. **Rationale:** The less you say, the more you encourage spontaneity and verbalization from the client.
4. Assist client to clarify feelings.
5. Maintain an accepting, nonjudgmental attitude. **Rationale:** Making value judgments, even nonverbal ones, negatively affects the nurse–client relationship.
6. Give broad opening statements, and ask open-ended questions. **Rationale:** This open approach enables the client to describe what is happening.

ENCOURAGING A CLIENT TO EXPRESS NEEDS, FEELINGS, AND THOUGHTS

Procedure

1. Focus on feelings rather than superficial topics during interactions.
2. Assist client to identify thoughts and feelings.
3. Pick up on verbal cues, leads, and signals from the client.
4. Convey attitude of acceptance and empathy toward the client. **Rationale:** Being aware of your own feelings and attitudes and separating them from the client's contributes to acceptance.
5. Note what is said as well as what is not said.
6. Assist the client to become aware of differences between behavior, feelings, and thoughts.
7. Give honest, nonjudgmental feedback to the client.

USING COMMUNICATION TO INCREASE THE CLIENT'S SENSE OF SELF-WORTH

Procedure

1. Use body language as well as verbal communication to convey empathy. **Rationale:** Sitting down at the client's bedside or not acting as if you are in a hurry encourages communication.
2. Respect the client's need for emotional privacy, but be available to client.
3. Encourage the client to apply the problem-solving approach to different situations.
4. Be nonjudgmental (see example of making judgmental responses.)
5. Mutually identify goals to meet the client's individual needs.
6. Keep all agreements with the client.
7. Become the client's advocate.
8. Give client positive feedback when appropriate.

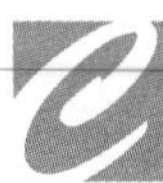

CHARTING for Therapeutic Communication

- Identification of client needs
- Explicit goals of interaction
- Communication patterns of client
- Emotional state of client
- Expressed feelings and thoughts if relevant

CRITICAL THINKING APPLICATION

CLINICAL PROBLEMS	CRITICAL THINKING OPTIONS
Therapeutic communication is not achieved.	• Eliminate blocks to communication from interaction style. If a block does occur, recognize it. Move to correct communication by using therapeutic modes of communication. • Evaluate your own process of communication during and after interaction. • If client needs to verbalize and you cannot help him or her do so, contact another nurse or the social worker.
Client's demanding behavior interferes with the therapeutic communication process.	• Do not ignore demands; they will only increase in intensity. • Attempt to determine causal factors of behavior, such as high anxiety level. • Set limits to response patterns when client is demanding. Control own feelings of anger and irritation. • Teach alternative means to getting needs met.

unit 2 NURSE–CLIENT RELATIONSHIP

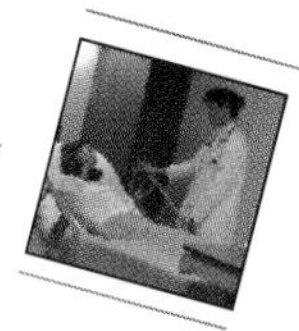

NURSING PROCESS DATA

ASSESSMENT Data Base

Determine the purpose of establishing a nurse–client relationship.

Consider the overall condition of client to determine if he or she can benefit from a nurse–client relationship.

A specific relationship could feed into secondary gains of anxiety.

An individual with chronic organic brain disorder cannot benefit from a relationship per se.

Identify client expectations of a therapeutic relationship to determine if you can meet these needs.

Examine your own feelings and expectations to evaluate potential effect on such a relationship.

PLANNING Objectives

To provide an environment in which client can feel secure enough to alter behavior patterns

To allow a client to experience a positive, satisfying relationship

To enable client to test more adaptive ways to handle anxiety

To provide a climate conducive to raising the client's self-esteem

To allocate enough time to complete planned process of interaction

To terminate relationship successfully

IMPLEMENTATION Procedures

Initiating a Nurse–Client Relationship

Facilitating a Nurse–Client Relationship

Terminating a Nurse–Client Relationship

EVALUATION Expected Outcomes

Principles of therapeutic communication are used.

Boundaries of professional relationship are maintained.

The appropriate environment for interaction is established.

Termination of the relationship is completed successfully.

INITIATING A NURSE–CLIENT RELATIONSHIP

Procedure

1. Assess client's symptoms and problems, and communicate a willingness to help alleviate these discomforts.
2. Assess client's need for and ability to handle trust, and then approach client accordingly. **Rationale:** Open, honest, congruent communication and consistent behavior help lay the groundwork for trust.
3. Establish mutual goals as a basis for the relationship. **Rationale:** Goals mutually set and agreed on

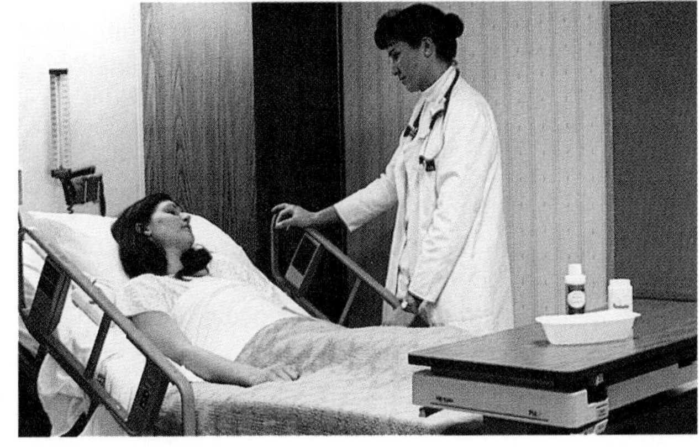

Initiating a relationship is an important component of client care.

are more easily accepted by both parties in the relationship.

4. Demonstrate to client that the nurse can be trusted. Do what you say you will do, and only make promises you are willing to keep. **Rationale:** The most important element of the initiating phase is the beginning of trust. Without trust the nurse–client relationship is ineffective.
5. Encourage client's participation in his or her care. **Rationale:** This focus enhances compliance to treatment.
6. Set limits on the client's behavior. **Rationale:** Limits protect the client from him or herself and show that the nurse cares enough to intervene when behavior is inappropriate.
7. Approach client in a warm, accepting manner. **Rationale:** The client may interpret a cool, aloof manner as lack of interest.

FACILITATING A NURSE–CLIENT RELATIONSHIP

Procedure

1. Assume the role of facilitator in the relationship.
2. Accept client as having value and worth as an individual. **Rationale:** Basic acceptance is a fundamental prerequisite of a relationship.
3. Provide a safe environment conducive to client's willingness to share.
4. Maintain the relationship on a professional level. **Rationale:** Responding on a professional rather than a social level defines the relationship.
5. Keep interaction reality-oriented, that is, in the here and now. **Rationale:** Discussion of past or future experiences does not contribute to a change in behavior now.
6. Listen actively; that is, responding to the client's cues.
7. Use nonverbal communication to support and encourage client.
   a. Recognize meaning and purpose of nonverbal communication.
   b. Keep verbal and nonverbal communication congruent.
8. Focus content and direction of conversation on client's cues.
9. Interact on client's intellectual, developmental, and emotional level.
10. Focus on "how," what," "when," "where," and "who" rather than "why." **Rationale:** Asking "why" places the client on the defensive because it requires justification of behavior.
11. Teach client problem solving to correct maladaptive patterns.
12. Assist client to identify, express, and cope with feelings.
13. Help client develop alternative coping mechanisms that are more adaptive.
14. Recognize a high level of anxiety, and assist client to deal with it.

TERMINATING A NURSE–CLIENT RELATIONSHIP

Procedure

1. Work closely with the client in planning the termination of the relationship from its beginning. **Rationale:** This approach promotes the client's independence and increases his or her sense of self-esteem.
2. Remember that expression of feelings by both the nurse and the client is a necessary component of this phase. **Rationale:** Verbalization can, in itself, be a growth-producing experience by providing time for the nurse and client to share their feelings of caring for each other.
3. Anticipate problems of termination and plan for their resolution. **Rationale:** Saying goodbye is often uncomfortable and difficult for both the client and the nurse.
4. Be aware that the client's behavior may reflect overdependence, depression, and withdrawal. **Rationale:** Allowing this behavior to be expressed helps the client to work it through.
5. Do not terminate the relationship too abruptly or allow it to persist beyond the client's needs.
6. Complete a satisfactory termination of the relationship. **Rationale:** This enables the client to move on to other relationships with positive feelings.

CHARTING for Nurse–Client Relationship

- Primary goals of nurse–client relationship and identified client needs
- Ongoing process of relationship therapy, including client's expressed feelings, thoughts, and so forth.
- Client's behavior and changes in behavior, both positive and negative
- Cues to other team members on how best to relate to this particular client

CRITICAL THINKING APPLICATION

CLINICAL PROBLEMS	CRITICAL THINKING OPTIONS
Client refuses to participate in a nurse–client relationship.	• Comply with client's request, and do not force or impose relationship therapy. • Continue to offer relationship therapy at intervals. • Suggest that another team member attempt to establish a relationship.
Nurse–client relationship frequently degenerates into a social conversation.	• Reevaluate the goals for the relationship, and remind client of terms originally established. • Set firm limits, and continually reexamine progress.
Termination of the nurse–client relationship is not successful.	• Reexamine the process of termination (termination should begin at the beginning of the relationship). • Devote more interaction time to this aspect of the relationship. • Attempt to elicit feelings about termination from the client as well as examining your own feelings. • Allow the client's behavior to be expressed without making value judgments, and assist the client to discuss his or her feelings.

GERIATRIC CONSIDERATIONS

Physical changes that affect communication

- Hearing changes (e.g., presbycusis, tympanic membrane atrophy, and distorted sounds) may make communication difficult. The nurse must speak clearly, loudly, and in view of the client. Use simple sentences, request feedback to validate understanding.
- Visual changes, such as presbyopia, pupil, cornea, and lens impairment, diminish visualization. The nurse should be aware of eye changes and check that client sees clearly enough to perform required activities.

Psychosocial changes that affect communication

- Relationships change with age. There is a loss of nurturing functions within the family. The nurse may need to perform this function with the elderly.
- Role changes within and outside the family occur—loss of spouse and loss of support systems. Elderly may require more support from caregivers.
- Elderly have fears of physical dependency, chronic illness, and loneliness. Caregiver may need to address these fears and work with client through communication and relationship to reduce them.

6

Stress, Holistic Health, and Alternative Treatment Methods

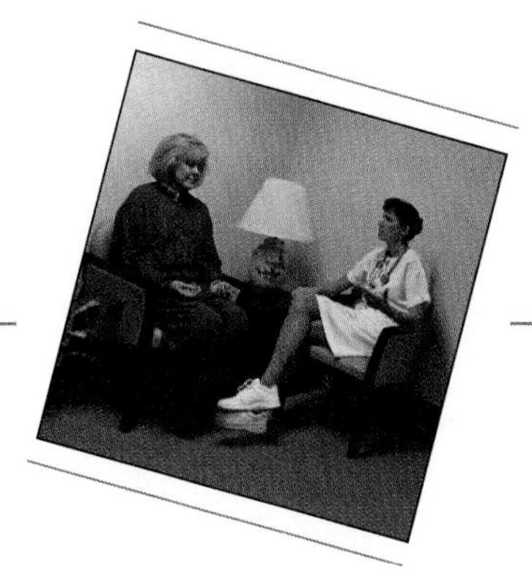

LEARNING OBJECTIVES

- Define the term "stress" according to Dr. Selye.
- Discuss the psychologic effect of stress on the body.
- Describe the body's physiologic response to stress, and include at least two body systems.
- Explain Selye's general adaptation syndrome, and differentiate between the three stages.
- List at least three different categories of stressors.
- Identify at least five danger signals of stress.
- Outline factors identified as causes of stress.
- Discuss a specific method the client can use to control stress.

TERMINOLOGY

Adaptive reaction: a response by which the person attempts to improve or alter his or her condition in relation to the environment.

Alleviate: to make more bearable; reduce (pain, grief, or suffering).

Anxiety: a state of uneasiness and distress; diffuse apprehension.

Apathy: indifference; insensibility; without emotion; sluggish.

Apprehension: a fearful or uneasy anticipation of the future; dread.

Ataraxia: the absence of all anxiety.

Autonomic nervous system: the part of the nervous system that regulates the functioning of internal organs and glands; it controls such functions as digestion, respiration, and cardiovascular activity.

Cerebral cortex: the extensive outer layer of grey tissue of the cerebral hemispheres (brain), responsible for higher nervous functions.

Coping mechanisms: means by which an individual adjusts or adapts to a threat or a challenge; actions that assist in maintaining homeostasis.

Defense mechanism: conscious or unconscious processes used to protect oneself from threats or to alleviate anxiety.

Delusion: a fixed, false belief.

Dynamics of homeostasis: danger or its symbols, whether internal or external, resulting in the activation of the sympathetic nervous system and the adrenal medulla. The organism prepares for fight or flight.

Emotional: affected by strong feelings, as of joy and sorrow.

Fight or flight: one's immediate response to stress that is, although archaic and often inappropriate, part of our central nervous system biologic heritage.

General adaptation syndrome: a general theory of stress response formulated by Dr. Hans Selye; describes the action of stress response in three stages: the alarm reaction, the stage of resistance, and the stage of exhaustion.

-Genic: suffix indicating generation or production.

Hallucination: false perception having no relation to reality and not accounted for by external stimuli.

Health: the state of physical, psychologic, and sociologic well-being.

Holistic: a way of looking at individuals and organisms as a whole rather than a sum of the parts.

Homeostasis: the maintenance of a constant state in the internal environment through self-regulatory techniques that preserve an organism's ability to adapt to stress.

Hypertension: a condition in which the client has a higher blood pressure than judged to be normal.

Illness: a state characterized by the malfunction of the biopsychosocial organism.

Impulsive: act of driving onward with sudden force.

Insomnia: inability to sleep.

Lifestyle: the manner in which one is accustomed to living.

Meditation: the act of reflecting on or pondering; contemplation.

Musculo: pertaining to the muscles.

Musculoskeletal: pertaining to the muscles and the skeleton.

Neuro: prefix pertaining to nerves.

Pain: a sensation in which a person experiences discomfort, distress, or suffering.

Parasympathetic nervous system: a division of the autonomic nervous system that regulates acetylcholine and conserves energy expenditure; it slows down the system.

Perspective: subjective evaluation of relative significance; a view.

Pressure: the act of bearing down; exerting force.

Psychogenic: of mental origin.

Relaxation: a lessening of tension or activity in a part.

Stamina: constitutional energy; strength; endurance.

Stress: a nonspecific response of the body to any internal or external event or change that impinges on a person's system and creates a demand.

Stressor: a specific demand that gives rise to a coping response.

Sympathetic nervous system: a division of the autonomic nervous system that controls energy expenditure and mobilizes for action when confronted with a threat.

Tachycardia: abnormally rapid heart action; above 100 beats per minute.

Tranquilizer: a drug that acts to reduce tension and anxiety without interfering with normal mental activity.

Wellness: a state of physical, psychologic, and sociologic well-being of a whole person. Synonym for health.

STRESS

Stress is a universal phenomenon; all human beings in all cultures experience it as a part of their everyday existence. Although stress is a natural component of life, it can sap energy and contribute to the presence of disease. The concept of stress has been with us since the beginning of time, but it was not until William Osler and Walter Cannon began their investigations in the early 1900s that stress was actually linked to illness. By 1950, Dr. Hans Selye, a Canadian endocrinologist and biologist, scientifically demonstrated that stress plays a major role in certain diseases, such as gastric ulcers and high blood pressure. Since Dr. Selye's early research, authorities from medicine as well as all areas of science have studied and written thousands of articles on this subject. With the undeniable fact that stress affects an individual's total life, nurses should have a basic understanding of this phenomenon, its effect on humans, how humans cope and adapt to stress, and how the nurse can deal with his or her own stress and help clients deal with theirs. To examine stress and its influence on human beings in this culture, we have to examine the total scope of life experience. The stress of life is life itself according to Dr. Barbara Brown, a nurse–author.

Western medicine is entering an era of transformation. The whole context of the medical profession is changing. Client and professionals alike are examining alternatives to traditional patterns of treatment and are devising new modes of health care delivery. These changes are occurring at a time when the health care system in this country, and indeed the world, desperately needs a new structure to deal with health and illness.

Perhaps the greatest impetus for these changes has developed in response to new knowledge about the role of stress in our lives. Dr. Selye, the acknowledged expert on stress, believed that efforts to manage and find cures for diseases would be ineffective as an approach to wellness. He and other prominent scientists think that the only viable answer is to examine our ability to cope and adapt to stress. At the second international conference on stress held in Monte Carlo, the eminent physician, Dr. Arnold Fox, stated that stress is either the main cause or a strong contributing factor in all diseases of humankind. In fact, most scientists now attribute 70–80% of all diseases to stress and lifestyle.

The view that disease is caused by invading microorganisms, or that ill people are merely victims, or even that all disease can be cured by modern science is misleading and limiting. New definitions of existing problems necessitate finding new solutions. The current emphasis on stress is relevant to our times, and we, as nurses, need to recognize and understand stress and its influence on us as individuals, on our profession, and, most particularly, on our clients.

Stress is a difficult term to define precisely, for it does not have a single specific source or one definite response. Dr. Selye stated that stress may be viewed as the common denominator of all the body's adaptive reactions. Stress may be grief as well as joy, pleasure as well as unhappiness, cold as well as heat, fear as well as elation. In fact, stress covers the total range of mental, emotional, and physical demands on the body, and responds with predictable biochemical and general adaptation changes. If the body is in a state of balance and the whole organism functions in harmony, the body is healthy. Stress can be defined as a state of arousal or agitation that throws the body out of balance. Although a certain amount of stress is necessary for survival, when it becomes prolonged and intense, our adaptive responses weary, and the negative aspects begin to take their toll on our bodies and our minds. When this occurs, it can be said that disease or dis-ease has overtaken the body and an unhealthy state exists.

The Effect of Stress

Physiologically, stress may be viewed as the experience an individual has when the demands placed on the body exceed the ability to cope, and the body is thrown out of balance. Chemically, stress initiates certain bodily processes, such as the "fight-or-flight" mechanism, which result in a threat to homeostasis. Early in the 1900s Dr. Cannon, a Harvard physiologist, coined the term "homeostasis." As a result of his work, certain adjustment mechanisms of the body, such as blood sugar level, temperature, and hydration, were identified. According to Dr. Cannon, the stress response resulted in these mechanisms being activated, which in turn threw the body out of balance.

Rather than a specific response, Dr. Selye focused on a general adaptation process as a response to stress. This process is the body's attempt to adapt and maintain homeostasis. Dr. Selye further defined stress as the rate of wear and tear on the body and stated that the only freedom from stress is death.

Dr. Selye's general adaptation syndrome occurs in three stages. The first stage, the *alarm stage,* occurs when the generalized response throughout the body responds to stressors, such as trauma, infection, pain, cold, heat, and fear. The purpose of the alarm reaction is to mobilize the body's defenses to meet the stressor. Biochemically, during the alarm stage, the adrenal cortex produces the antiinflammatory hormones, the adrenocorticotropin hormones (cortisone and cortisol), and the proinflammatory hormones (aldosterone and desoxycorticosterone). The shock phase is when the autonomic nervous system comes into full play. The second stage, the *resistance stage,* occurs when the body's defenses are mobilized to produce hormones to cope with the alarm stage. The body chemistry either repels or adapts to the stressor. During this phase the organ-

Selye's Stress Adaptation Syndrome

Stage	General Function	Interpersonal	Behavioral	Affective	Cognitive	Physiological
1 Alarm reaction	Mobilization of body defenses	Interpersonal communication effectiveness decreases	Task oriented Increases restlessness Apathy, regression Crying	Feelings of anger, suspiciousness, helplessness Anxiety level increases	Alert Thinking becomes narrow and concrete Symptoms of thought blocking, forgetfulness, and decreased productivity	Muscle tension Increase in epinephrine and cortisone Stimulation of adrenal cortex and lymph glands Increase in blood pressure, heart rate, blood glucose
2 Stage of resistance	Adaptation to stresses Resistance increases	Interpersonal communication self-oriented Uses interpersonal relationships to meet own needs	Automatic behaviors Self-oriented behaviors Fight or flight behavior apparent	Increased use of defense mechanisms Emotional responses may be automatic or exaggerated	Thought processes more habitual than problem-solving oriented	Hormonal levels return to prealarm stage All physiological responses return to normal or are channeled into psychosomatic symptoms
3 Stage of exhaustion	Depletion or exhaustion of organs and resources Loss of ability to resist stress	Disintegration of personal interactions Communication skills ineffective and disorganized Self-oriented	Restless, withdrawn, agitated; may become violent or self-destructive Diminished productivity	Depressed, flat or inappropriate affect Exaggerated or inappropriate use of defense mechanisms Decreased ability to cope	Thought disorganization, hallucinations, preoccupation Reduced intellectual processes	Exhaustion, with increase demands on organism Adrenal cortex hormone depletion Death, if stress is continuous and excessive

ism is successful in adapting to the stressor, and the biochemical changes resulting from the alarm phase return to the prealarm stage. Any life change causes alarm and resistance, and the stress accrued through life reduces the body's adaptive abilities at a much greater rate than normal stress levels. The *final stage* occurs when the stress is prolonged and the body can no longer cope effectively. The result is exhaustion and the body may become ill with disease. The organism's adaptive abilities are depleted, and the organism loses its ability to deal with the stress. The organism goes into shock, and, if the stress is not alleviated, the result may be death of the organism. The general adaptation syndrome varies widely in intensity. Reaction to positive stimuli, such as getting married or a job promotion, also activates a stress response. The response may, however, result in less damage than a negative stressor, even though it does temporarily throw the body out of balance. Furthermore, a person does not respond with the same intensity to all negative stressors. For example, one doesn't respond with the same degree of intensity to jumping in a cold pool as to turning a corner and seeing a man with a gun.

The local adaptive syndrome is the manifestation of stress in a limited part of the body. The body responds locally to the stressor, such as a burn or cut to a finger. The local response may also trigger a general response if the ability of the body to respond to the specific area is greatly affected by the condition of the whole organism. An upper respiratory infection causes a much different response within a healthy child than in a child with cystic fibrosis. The better the organism as a whole adapts to stress, the more effective the local adaptive response.

SIGNALS OF STRESS

Physiologic

Fatigue, lethargy
Muscle tension—neck, back, legs, and so forth
Frequent headaches—tension, migraine
Shaking, trembling, spasms
Cold extremities, poor circulation
Digestion disturbances—acid, nausea, ulcers, gas cramps
Eating disorders—compulsive eating, loss of appetite
Elimination disorders—diarrhea, constipation
Sleep problems—insomnia, nightmares, excessive sleep, early awakenings
Pain—backache, teeth grinding
Excessive sweating
Heart problems—palpitations, racing, variable heartbeat, chest pain
Breathing complications—hyperventilation
High blood pressure
Skin eruptions—rash, hives, itching, eczema, acne
Sexual difficulties—impotence, low libido (desire), nonorgasmic, vaginitis
Amenorrhea (absence of menstrual period)

Psychologic

Anxiety
Panic disorder
Depression
Pessimism
Melancholy
Impatience
Anger
Irritability
Boredom
Confusion
Helplessness
Apathy
Alienation
Isolation
Numbness
Self-consciousness
Purposeless

Behavioral Indicators

Restlessness
Loss of memory, poor concentration
Nervous mannerisms—tics, grimaces, finger tapping, hair twisting
Speech difficulties—stuttering, stammering
Hyperactivity
Disorganization
Passivity
Aggressiveness
Indecisivenes
Tardiness
Inflexibility
Nonproductivity
Poor problem solving
Alcohol and drug abuse
Phobic responses
Overeating

Individual Responses to Stress

Responses to stress, then, can be categorized into several different patterns: the *physiologic response*, in which there is loss or gain in weight over time, hormone levels increase, blood pressure increases, or possibly a somatoform (psychosomatic) symptom appears; the *psychologic response*, which may also result in a psychosomatic illness or psychiatric manifestations, such as depression, mania, withdrawal from reality, or anxiety; and, the *behavioral response,* in which one hits out, becomes aggressive (fights), or withdraws; one may also become immobilized, or turn inward (physical or emotional flight). The *interpersonal mode* can reflect stress when communication effectiveness decreases, relationships deteriorate, trust in others diminishes, and the ability to form and maintain close, intimate, loving ties with another person decreases. Finally, the affective response may be present when one's emotions are affected so that anxiety is high and emotions are unstable, labile, unpredictable, and inappropriate to the situation. All of the above-mentioned modes of response relate to the negative elements of response patterns. Of course, these modes can be used in a positive way so that stress becomes nondetrimental. There is no way to eliminate stress completely, but individuals can learn to minimize the harmful effects and use their response modes in a positive way.

DANGER SIGNALS OF STRESS

Depression, lack of interest in life
Uncontrolled hyperactive behavior
Lack of concentration, inability to focus
Feelings of unreality
Loss of control, emotional instability
Pervasive high anxiety level
Physical manifestations
- Irregular heartbeats
- Tremors, tics
- Gastrointestinal disturbance
- Skin disturbance
- Changes in respiratory patterns

Insomnia
Disease
Increased dependence on alcohol, drugs

Stressors may be chemical, physical, developmental, and emotional. Graduating from nursing school, being promoted, failing to be promoted, having arguments, and playing a tough game of racquetball are all stressful events and require adaptation and change at some level. By understanding stress, we can more easily identify stress factors and their effects on clients who need or seek health care. Whether a client is having a baby, undergoing open heart surgery, or seeking counseling for emotional problems, each of these individuals is experiencing stress in his or her own particular manner. How the individual adapts or fails to adapt depends on several factors: personality and emotional makeup and past experiences in dealing with stress (response repertoire).

People are able to create many different forms of disease as well as emotional and spiritual scars. And the more we use up our reserves of adaptation energy, the more likely we are to age and hasten our death. In fact, Dr. Selye warned that there is no evidence that the basic reserves of energy for adaptation can be restored. These may be genetically programmed. The more reserves we use handling everyday stress, the less we have for major crises or for growing older. The latest research indicates that there is a direct relationship between the amount of stress encountered in everyday life and aging.

Stress and Disease

Stress and an individual's method of handling it have been associated with the risk of developing heart disease, cancer, and other illnesses. Although stress is an inevitable part of life, excessive amounts of it can contribute to poor health. When one goes through a very stressful period, it is important to work through that stress, rather than ignore it.

The mechanisms by which stress leads to disease may differ for heart disease and cancer. Perceived stress leads to a release of adrenaline, cortisol, and other hormones within the body. These substances, in turn, increase the heart rate, blood pressure, cholesterol level, and platelet stickiness. When stress becomes chronic, these physiologic changes can accelerate atherosclerosis, the process that causes coronary heart disease.

Individuals with Type A behavior are known to be at increased risk of heart disease. Type A behavior is defined as having a constant sense of time urgency and a feeling of free-floating anger at the world in general. These behavior patterns can be seen as a maladaptive way of dealing with chronic stress. The famous 20-year study of the causative factors in heart disease, the Framingham study, examined many aspects of heart disease. Results revealed that males who were classified as Type A developed chest pains three times as often as their more peaceful Type B counterparts. Another fascinating conclusion was that those who remained calm and serene (Type B personalities) rarely developed high cholesterol levels regardless of their diet.

The immune system may be the stress, cancer the connection. Chronic stress causes changes in the immune system that can interfere with its ability to recognize and destroy cancerous cells. Several researchers have shown that cancer clients have a characteristic personality pattern years before the cancers are diagnosed. Part of this personality pattern involves difficulty dealing with stress and turning conflict inward instead of confronting it directly.

It is important to remember that the stress syn-

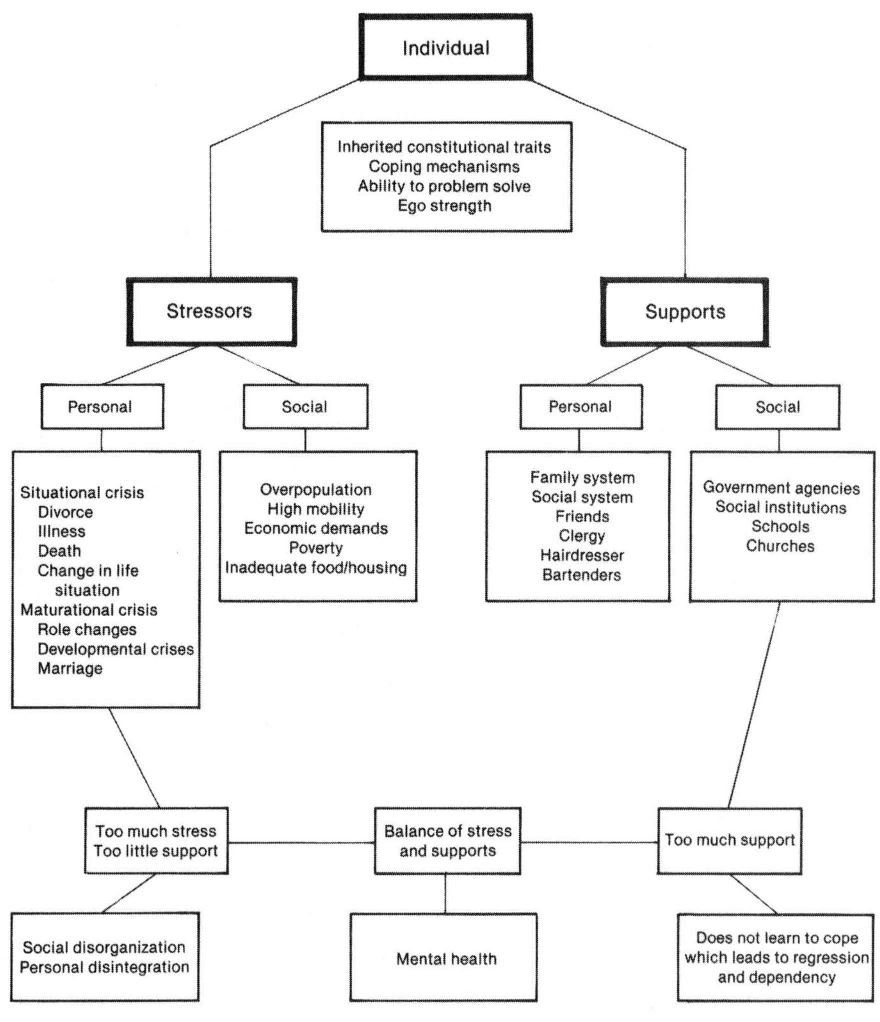

Stress Model

drome can be both positive and negative. Any change or alteration in the balance of life can create stress. The Holme and Rahe stress scale is an excellent example of the varying conditions in life that result in stress. We are all unique individuals, and we respond differently to various stressors. Thus, it does not matter whether the stress is positive or negative, light or severe. What matters is how we develop adaptive mechanisms to cope with these stressors. The ability to cope or solve a problem can be translated as the ability to withstand stress and create life experiences that do not work against us. The implications of stress theory—that by being able to withstand stress, by coping with it, diluting it when it occurs, or eliminating it we can actually affect our life—are tremendously exciting. It means that we are not doomed to inevitable illness later in life, nor are we preprogrammed for premature aging. In fact every individual controls his or her own health. To quote the *Journal of American Medical Association*, "Nature did not intend us to grow old and ill; we were designed to die young in old age but free of disease." In other words, even when we are old we should feel "young" (healthy) and be free of disease.

Along with coping with one's own stress, it is the responsibility of the nurse to be aware that clients suffer from stress phenomena and that part of the nurse's role is to assist clients to adapt and cope with stress.

Guidelines for Implementing Stress Objectives in Nursing

The nurse must have an understanding of the role of stress.

- Understand and accept the theory of stress—what it is and what effect it has on the body.

- Be cognizant of the manifestations of stress: tiredness, apathy, frequent illness, lack of interest or liveliness, unwillingness to seek out new challenges, inability to cope with change, and many other symptoms.
- Elicit the factors that alter resistance to stress (illness, hospitalization, pain, medication, family pressures, etc.).
- Assist in making a plan and implementing it, designing specific actions to reduce stress, such as relaxation methods.
- Educate the individual about how to control his or her own stressors.

The nurse may carry out specific behaviors in the hospital setting to reduce stress.

- Assist in reducing the negative aspects of stress.
- Counsel the client and family on the theory of stress; together, examine how the client's particular stressors affect his or her lifestyle.
- Reinforce the client's adaptive process by meeting his or her needs, listening to concerns, administering care, and providing emotional support.
- Assist the client to alter adaptive behaviors to cope more effectively with stress.

A NEW PARADIGM FOR HEALTH

The way the western world views health is undergoing a change. Even the terms we use to describe health are changing; new terms, like *holistic health* and *alternative, unconventional,* or *complementary medicine* are being heard more frequently in both medical and nonmedical circles. In the past, good health meant the absence of disease. The new definition of holistic health goes beyond physical health to encompass the health of the whole person, including mental, emotional, and spiritual health. The World Health Organization (WHO) formulated a new definition of health in 1970 that has significantly influenced the medical model of health care. WHO described health as "a state of complete physical, mental, and social well-being, not merely the absence of disease or infirmity." What made this definition innovative is that it took into account the mind as well as the body. In fact, this new interpretation of health almost enters the spiritual dimension. Though critics have pointed out that by this definition no one is truly healthy, it is the beginning of a view of health as an open system in a holistic framework. A holistic redefinition of health emphasizes high-level wellness or going beyond the absence of disease toward one's maximum health potential. This section focuses on the connection among mind, body, spirit, and environment and discusses how one can use this connection to reach the possible highest level of health and wellness.

A Holistic Approach to Health

The 1990s are witnessing a significant growth in a new dimension of health—the holistic approach. As shown in a recent Gallup survey completed for *American Health Magazine,* many people in our society now include a very broad range of issues in their concept of personal health. Certainly their top health concern is still oriented toward personal health—"staying free of disease." Their third-highest priority, however—"living in an environment with clean air and water"—expresses a much more global health perspective. Many of their top concerns show that they regard not only physical status but also mental and emotional status as important components of personal health. Today's significant health goals may even include having a positive outlook on life and sharing love with friends and family. Wellness can be thought of as a state of being; holistic health is the means of achieving it.

The term "holistic" implies wholeness; a harmonious individual that integrates mind, body, and spirit into a functioning unit. A holistic stress model implies modifying all parts of one's life so that stress is both encountered and alleviated from an integrated perspective.

In recent decades, a new view of health has developed in Western thought. In 1926, South African Jan Smuts coined the word *holism.* He used this term to refer to the tendency in nature to synthesize and organize toward greater wholes. He wrote that the meaning of the whole organism is greater than the sum of the parts. His theory suggests that we think of the human organism not as separate parts, but rather as the sum of all its parts—physical, psychologic, social, and spiritual; in this way, the whole person becomes the focus of health. Holistic medicine postulates a constant interchange between mind and body, psyche and soul.

In the modern era, Carl Jung was one of the first physicians and therapists to discuss the prevention of illness in terms of using one's inner resources. He discussed the inner self and themes of self-renewal in relation to growth, spirituality, and health. As our body of research knowledge grows, more and more physicians are employing spiritual growth techniques as a health tool. For example, Dr. Carl Simonton has been using meditation and imagery as adjunct therapy for clients with cancer and has shown that clients recover faster and have less pain when guided imagery was used. He has also demonstrated that cancer clients showed a heightened immune response. Dr. Joan Broysenko at the Harvard Mind-Body Clinic is also using meditation as a medical tool; Dr. Norman Shealy, founder of the American Holistic Medical Association and the Shealy Institute for Comprehensive Pain and Health Care, has used alternative methods of health care for many years. The current literature, much of it authored by prominent physicians, exemplifies today's trend toward the holistic, or alternative, model.

The holistic paradigm suggests that the body, psyche, and environment are one and interact as an open system. This idea can assist us to view our client's health as well as our personal health from a new dimension. In the holistic view, health care includes three types of actions: disease and injury prevention, treatment, and health promotion.

Alternative treatments may include treatments that require involvement on the client's part, such as changes in eating patterns and other lifestyle behaviors; or physical treatments, such as acupuncture or vitamin therapy. The client is counseled to take the initiative and assume responsibility for his or her own health, and the role of the nurse and physician is to guide clients to various health care options. Truly holistic treatment involves an integrated assessment of all aspects of health.

ALTERNATIVE MEDICINE

Alternative, or unconventional, medicine is not nearly as unknown, untried, or unaccepted as traditional physicians believed. In 1993, the *New England Journal of Medicine* found that Americans made 425 million visits to these alternative providers in 1990, compared with 388 million visits to all other mainstream primary care physicians. Furthermore, Americans spent $13.7 billion on alternative medicine in 1990, three-quarters of this total not reimbursed by insurance. This figure is more than the amount Americans paid for nonreimbursed hospital care. Many physicians, on learning the results of this survey, were stunned because they had no idea Americans were seeking alternative therapies in such numbers. Another startling find was that 72% of those using alternative therapies did not tell their primary care physician.

The National Institutes of Health, a conservative, scientifically based organization, has made its first foray into the field of alternative medicine by dispensing $2 million (a fraction of its $10.3 billion annual budget) to a new Office of Alternative Medicine. This office was founded because of congressional pressure to investigate new approaches to the degenerative diseases killing Americans.

Alternative Treatment Methods

Following is a short sampling of alternative treatment methods that may be used alone or in tandem with the more conventional medical treatments. Alternative methods may be classified as lifestyle (holistic medicine; ayurvedic medicine), botanical (homeopathy, herbal, aromatherapy), manipulative (chiropractic, acupressure and acupuncture, reflexology, massage), and mind-over-matter (meditation, guided imagery, biofeedback, color healing, and hypnotherapy).

Acupuncture. An ancient Chinese method of relieving pain and treating disease, acupuncture is based on the belief that energy, or *qi*, flows along 12 lines, or meridians, in the body creating a balance between two principles of nature called yin and yang. Each meridian is connected to a particular organ or system. It is believed that lack of energy flow or blocked energy along the meridians leads to illness or disease. Acupuncture treatment involves inserting sharp needles under the skin along the meridian lines, thereby unblocking energy, stimulating flow, and restoring balance and health of internal organs. Since the 1960s in the United States, Chinese doctors, as well as some U.S. physicians, have performed major surgery with acupuncture as the only anesthetic.

Applied Kinesiology. Applied kinesiology is a form of treatment based on the theory that the condition of a person's muscles reflect certain internal disorders or problems. Body imbalances or disorders are identified when certain muscle groups are tested and appear weak. Certain foods, medications, or herbs are held in a person's hand or placed next to their skin. If the substance is not appropriate for the body, the muscles respond to testing by appearing weak. When the substance is removed, the muscles regain their strength. Based on identifying weak muscles, various treatments, such as diet therapy, acupressure, or chiropractic, are suggested.

Ayurveda. A form of medicine that originated in India, ayurveda, meaning the science of life, has been practiced in India for over 5000 years and has just recently become known in the West. This system is based on the concept of three metabolic body types: slim, athletic, and heavy. Each body type utilizes food and herbs in a different way, thus treatment includes dietary changes, herbs, and exercise, as well as specific practices, such as yoga, meditation, massage with herbal remedies, and medicated inhalations. This form of medicine has recently gained popularity in the West after several Indian physicians opened clinics based on this system of treatment. Notable among them is Dr. Deepak Chopra, an endocrinologist, who has written several popular books on the subject.

Biofeedback. This technique employs an instrument to monitor physiologic processes of the body and to "feed back" measurements to the individual being monitored. A scale, thermometer, and pulse monitor are common feedback devices, as are more technically sophisticated machines having electronic sensors and digital readouts. Recent research has confirmed that many people can influence or control their autonomic processes (heart rate, temperature, digestive functions, etc.). As the client becomes more adept at controlling body responses, the need to use monitoring devices decreases—and the mental skills can be used independently.

Chiropractic. Originating in ancient Greece and literally meaning "done by the hands," chiropractic suggests that one cause of disease and dysfunction in the body is a misalignment of the spinal column that interferes with proper nerve function. These conditions cause or contribute to some diseases and lower the body's resistance to others. Spinal adjustments and manipulation restore structural integrity, thus enabling the body to heal itself. Studies have shown that chiropractic can relieve pain and structural disorders in the joints and muscles. The focus of treatment is general and includes correction of such disorders as headaches; allergies; pain in the back, hip, or spinal column; or gastrointestinal problems.

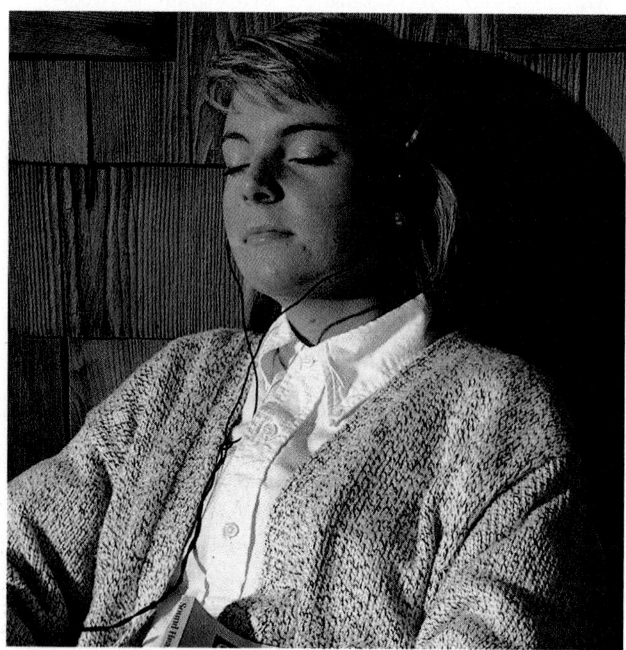

Sound and visualization are alternative treatment methods.

Energy Medicine. This contemporary view of health views the human body as comprised of electronic vibrations. It suggests that 21st century care will be based on principles of energy in which interventions involving the mind and body will interface with environmental, spiritual, and vibrational aspects of healing. Special high and low frequencies of sound and light are already being used for healing. For example, sound therapy is used to speed healing through a cast; full-spectrum light frequencies are being used to affect moods such as seasonal affective disorder (SAD); and documented studies have shown that certain individuals have the ability to transmit healing energy to others. A special photographic process called Kirlian photography has shown the energy moving from the healer to a client.

Homeopathy. Based on the work of the German physician Dr. Samuel Hahnemann in the early 1800s, homeopathy is a system of treatment that rests on the theory that extremely small doses of certain substances, usually herbal or chemical, cause a response in a person that mimics a particular disease. These substances, or homeopathic remedies, are administered to a person with a disease exhibiting a similar symptom pattern, stimulating the body's natural healing response. This is called "treatment by similars, or like cures like." The practice of homeopathy is becoming more popular; there is even a software package designed to assist physicians in the homeopathic diagnosis and treatment of disease.

Naturopathy. According to this school of thought, diseases are the body's attempt to heal itself through release of impurities. Treatments are designed to increase the client's "vital force" by eliminating toxins, thus allowing the body to heal. The methods used include anything except drugs, such as nutrition, herbs, massage, and exercise.

Nutrition. The holistic approach dictates that an individual pay close attention to nutritional status as a critical component of wellness. Research strongly points to diet as a major contributor to health or disease. This is especially so when a person has a diet of high fat, refined sugars, red meat, additives, preservatives, or junk food. Nutrition can also play a major role in prevention of disease; more and more emphasis is currently being placed on the role of antioxidants (vitamins C, E, beta-carotene, pycnogenol, etc.) in preventing such diseases as cancer and heart disease. Many alternative practitioners focus on incorporating all aspects of life (including nutrition) into a treatment plan.

Reflexology. Also called "zone therapy," reflexology is a method of treatment that proposes that diseases and organ dysfunction can be both diagnosed and treated by pressing on certain areas of the hands or feet. Each area of the body is represented by a corresponding area on the feet or hands; pressing on specific points is said to stimulate blood, nutrient, and energy flow to the diseased area of the body.

Relaxation and Visualization. Stress experts have carefully studied the effects of deep relaxation on the mind and body. They found that individuals who regularly practice relaxation exercises experience less stress than people who don't. The relaxation response is actually the physiologic opposite of the stress response. People adept at invoking the relaxation response use their minds to control their autonomic nervous system—oxygen consumption, respiratory rate, heart rate, blood pressure, and muscle tension. Their alpha brain waves, the waves associated with feelings of well-being, increase. Effective body relaxation techniques have existed for centuries. Several have gained significant popularity in recent years. The following short descriptions should familiarize you with the leading techniques.

1. *Deep Breathing*: Emphasized by virtually all relaxation exercises, deep breathing is a key to reducing stress. When you are tense, your breathing becomes rapid, irregular, and shallow. Healthy deep breathing increases the amount of oxygen in your blood, cleanses your system of carbon dioxide and other waste chemicals, relaxes your muscles, and encourages your heart rate to return to normal. Learning to take deep, slow, full breaths and exhale completely, effects mastery of this key relaxation technique. B. K. S. Iyengar, a world-class yoga teacher, suggests a breathing technique for stress reduction. Try it and instruct your clients in this technique.

   - Inhale as you normally do.
   - Exhale as you normally do.
   - Pause as long as comfortable.
   - Repeat the first three steps.

   Simple? Yes. Effective: Yes. This technique allows your lungs to empty more completely, continuing the normal exhalation process. Why is this simple exercise effective? Because the completed exhalation enables the mind to quiet—a rest from the jumble of one thought upon another. Iyengar says that if you learn this "secret," you can control stress. It also provides the foundation for meditation.
2. *Autogenic Training*: In this form of relaxation warmth and heaviness are visualized: two physical sensations associated with the relaxed state. The warmth represents increased blood flow throughout the body, and heaviness is perceived as relaxation of the skeletal muscles. During progressive relaxation, specific muscles or groups of muscles are tensed and released throughout the body. This technique is especially effective for clients who are fearful and stressed.
3. *Meditation*: Originating thousands of years ago, meditation is based on Eastern cultures and religions. The effects of meditation are similar to those associated with deep relaxation. Meditation is the process of bringing the mind to stillness. It sounds easy, but if you have tried meditation, you know from experience how difficult and frustrating this process can be. There are many methods of meditation, from the traditional transcendental meditation (TM) and Zen meditation to the repetition of a word such as "one," advocated by Dr. Herbert Benson of Harvard University. TM is a structured form of meditation popularized in the United States in the 1960s by Maharishi Mahesh Yogi. In TM, a mantra is selected (a word or sound) that is repeated mentally while seated quietly in a tranquil place.

   Perhaps the easiest meditation technique is to sit in a comfortable position with the spine straight (the lotus position is perfect if the legs can stand it), eyes closed, and to relax. While meditating, one concentrates on relaxing the muscles and organs throughout the body, then focuses on breathing. One is to inhale fully, then exhale, watching the breath come out "in one's mind's eye." If a thought comes in, it should be made to slip away and one should continue inhaling and exhaling. No thoughts should be allowed to rush in to break the concentration.
4. *Visualization*. Visualization is a proven technique for healing, stress management, and positive

goal attainment. When a mental picture is created, the body responds as if it were a real experience. Visualization can assist a client to feel more confident in circumstances filled with uncertainties. It can also assist with reducing pain. Teach the client to first relax (through one of the techniques mentioned in this chapter), then deep breathe, and finally to see the pain in the mind's eye becoming less and less severe.

5. *T'ai Chi Ch'uan*: This slow, graceful Chinese technique for relaxation is actually a system to both stimulate and balance subtle life energies. Thirty minutes a day devoted to the gentle, flowing movements of t'ai chi is relaxing, centering, and invigorating—a great way to relax and an interesting alternative to energetic Western exercise.
6. *Yoga*: Yoga is an ancient Indian discipline that begins with postures, or asanas, that stretch and strengthen muscles. It progresses to meditative relaxation or breathing techniques. Yoga is not sport or exercise as such; nor does it have to be a religion. The system is devised completely for health and well-being. The best way to begin yoga is to find an experienced teacher who can correct postures and guide the individual through the breathing and relaxation exercises.

NURSING DIAGNOSES

The following nursing diagnoses may be appropriate to include in a client care plan when the components are related to decreasing stress and promoting adaptation.

NURSING DIAGNOSIS	RELATED FACTORS
Anxiety	Increased stress, for instance, illness, trauma, loss
Ineffective Individual Coping	High stress on person, for example, individual inability to adapt, length and duration of stressor
Defensive Coping	Denial of problem, rationalization of failure, such as increased demands on individual
Altered Health Maintenance	High stress level, from illness, abuse, or psychologic factors
Social Isolation	Maladaptive coping to stressor, such as long-term or high level of stress
Post-trauma Response	Reexperiencing a traumatic event, exhibiting altered lifestyle, psychic numbness

unit 1

STRESS AND ADAPTATION

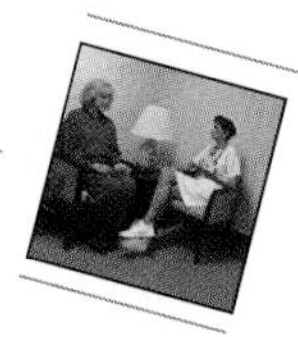

NURSING PROCESS DATA

ASSESSMENT Data Base

Identify the client who demonstrates stressed behavior.

Evaluate, with the client, the past and present stressors that the client has experienced.

Evaluate the stressors' effect on the client's body and signs of distress in the body.

Examples of stress effects are

- *Cardiovascular system*: increased pulse and blood pressure, evidence of angina, arrhythmias, migraine headaches, disturbance of heat and cold mechanisms
- *Gastrointestinal system*: ulcers, ulcerative colitis, constipation or diarrhea, imbalance in sugar absorption
- *Musculoskeletal system*: backache, tension headaches, arthritis, proneness to accidents
- *Autoimmune system*: infections, flu, allergies, rheumatoid arthritis, cancer

Assess client's level of energy and the degree to which it is depleted.

Evaluate client's awareness of thoughts, attitudes, values, and beliefs that influence stress response and adaptation.

Assess present level of distress in the client's body.

Assess possible causes of stress that are affecting client:

- *Environmental stressors*: input overload, such as sights, sounds, smells; actions and demands of others in the environment; or monotony
- *Physical stressors*: hunger, heat or cold, dangerous environment, injury, or pain
- *Emotional stressors*: loss of something of value, frustrations of needs and drives, threats to self-concept
- *Psychosocial stressors*: Conflicting cultural values (i.e., the American values of competition and assertiveness vs. the need to be dependent).
- *Future shock*: physiologic and psychologic stress resulting from an overload of the organism's adaptive systems and decision-making processes brought about by too rapidly changing values and technology
- *Cultural shock*: stress developing in response to the transition from a familiar environment to unfamiliar one; involves unfamiliarity with communication, technology, customs, attitudes and beliefs (i.e., immigrating, being confined in a hospital or prison); crowding, and urban life
- *Job choice and the work environment* (About 80% of the workers in our country are estimated to be unhappy in their jobs.)

Assess the factors that influence how the client responds to stress.

- *Characteristics of the stressful event*: magnitude, intensity, duration
- *Client's biologic and psychologic inclinations*
- *Appropriateness of support system*

PLANNING Objectives

To identify presence of stress in client

To identify how stress affects the body

To identify the current sources that result in stressed behavior

To determine the client's response to stress

To evaluate stress interventions that have a positive effect on stressed client

IMPLEMENTATION Procedures

Determining the Effect of Stress

Determining Response Patterns

Managing Stress

Manipulating the Environment to Reduce Stress

Teaching Coping Strategies
Managing Stress Using a Holistic Model
Alleviating Stress Using Controlled Breathing
Alleviating Stress Using Body Relaxation
Alleviating Stress Using Meditation

EVALUATION **Expected Outcomes**

Client is able to evaluate the general stressors and identify sources of stress in his or her life.
Client is aware of response patterns to stress and is able to alter patterns appropriately.
Client is aware of body–mind stress and its influence on his or her body.
Client is able to reduce environmental stressors.
Client is able to identify and alleviate stress caused by mental concerns.

DETERMINING THE EFFECT OF STRESS

Procedure

1. Identify client's stress tolerance level.
   a. Recognize the body's alarm signals (see major signals in assessment).
   b. Assess signal correctly as signifying high level of stress.
2. Discuss the concept of stress to elicit understanding of the effect on client's body.
   a. Stress may be physical, chemical, or emotional and may cause bodily or mental tension that may be a factor in disease causation.
   b. Stress tends to alter existing equilibrium.

DR. SELYE'S DEFINITION OF STRESS

- Stress is a specific syndrome that consists of all nonspecifically induced changes within the biologic system.
- The body is the common denominator of all adaptive responses.
- Stress is manifested by measurable changes in the body.
- Stress causes a multiplicity of changes in the body.

3. Encourage client to feel free to discuss life patterns that relate to stress.
4. Discuss the effect of stress. **Rationale:** Directing the conversation to the emotional, mental, and social sources of stress assist the client in examining its total effect.
5. Assist the client in formulating a plan to reduce or eliminate at least some sources of stress.

DETERMINING RESPONSE PATTERNS

Procedure

1. Evaluate adaptation factors that influence stress management.
   a. *Age*: adaptation is greatest in youth and young middle life and least at the extremes of life.
   b. *Environment*: does environment support managing stress?
   c. *Time*: the client can more easily adapt to stress over a period of time than suddenly.
   d. *Flexibility*: degree of flexibility of the individual influences survival.
   e. *Expenditure of energy*: the individual usually uses the adaptation mechanism that is most economic in terms of energy.
   f. *Presence of illness*: disease decreases the person's capacity to adapt to stress.
2. Assess the effects of stress on the client.
   a. Increased anxiety, anger, helplessness, hopelessness, guilt, shame, disgust, fear, frustration, or depression
   b. Behaviors resulting from stress:
      (1) Apathy, regression, withdrawal
      (2) Crying, demanding
      (3) Physical illness
      (4) Hostility, manipulation
      (5) Senseless violence, lashing out

MANAGING STRESS

Procedure

1. Discuss the client's body response to stress.
   a. The body's response to stress is a self-preservation mechanism that automatically and immediately becomes activated in times of danger.
   b. Assist client to understand response patterns.
2. Teach client to be aware of stress sensations in his or her body—recognize physical symptoms.
3. Suggest that client frequently monitor thought patterns to identify those thoughts that cause automatic tensing responses (tight muscles, increase in heartbeat, butterflies in stomach.)
4. Assist client to decide whether these thoughts are essential to survival or if they can be changed, eliminated, or replaced.
5. Assist client in planning to set aside periods each day for self-stress evaluation.
6. Provide problem-solving assistance so the client can examine new, more appropriate response patterns.
7. Refer client to resources (therapy classes, books, relaxation tapes) that will assist in developing new responses.

MANIPULATING THE ENVIRONMENT TO REDUCE STRESS

Procedure

1. Modify client's external environment so that adaptation responses are within his or her capacity.
2. Support the efforts of the client to adapt or to respond.
3. Provide client with the materials required to maintain constancy of his or her environment.
4. Understand the body's mechanisms for accommodating stress.
5. Prevent additional stress.
6. Reduce external stimuli and input through senses.
7. Reduce or increase physical activity depending on the cause of and response to stress.

TEACHING COPING STRATEGIES

Procedure

1. Analyze client's stress status.
   a. Estimate total amount of stress client is experiencing—too high a level of stress indicates need for intervention.
   b. Recognize where in body or mind the stress is manifesting.
2. Discuss various options for reducing stress—which alternatives fit with client.
3. Suggest client use diversion methods of coping.
   a. *Physical diversion*: jogging, swimming, cooking, cleaning
   b. *Mental diversion*: reading, painting, going to a movie, or simply thinking about a pleasant memory
4. Plan with client how to use rest as a way to cope with stress.
   a. Vacation, leave of absence from job, frequent naps
   b. Eliminate major stressors so result is rest from stress input.
   c. Plan with client how to manage time so that input can be reduced and goals limited.
5. Teach client how to use concentration, body relaxation, breathing, or meditation techniques to relieve mind stress.
6. Remind client that laughter is a great tranquilizer and healer as well as a stress reducer, and assist client to plan how to use this concept.

SUGGESTIONS FOR COPING

- Rank tasks to be completed, and identify activities that need to be accomplished.
- Forget unimportant details; do not try to remember too many things. Concentrate on the essential issues and details.

- Eliminate past unpleasant events from the mind and focus on the present.
- Do not cling to unpleasant experiences and emotions that impair emotional ability to respond to here and now.
- Discard habit of anticipating negative outcomes, which is often worse than the actual event.
- Do not yearn for things relating to the past or the future; focus attention on present desires.

MANAGING STRESS USING A HOLISTIC MODEL

Procedure

1. Manage stress through exercise.
   a. Poor physical condition becomes a stressor—this state contributes to lethargy, a constant fatigue level, low resistance for illness, and lessens adaptive responses.
   b. Good physical condition results in stamina, reserves necessary to withstand stress, and protection against unpredictable stress periods.
   c. Exercise prepares the body physically for stress caused by environmental conditions.
   d. Consistent exercise prepares body to handle stress emotionally.
2. Manage stress through diet.
   a. Certain foods and drug substances (caffeine, alcohol, sugar, junk foods, preservatives, tobacco) are potent stressors to our bodies.
   b. Consuming high-stress foods results in negative body changes, such as hypertension, high cholesterol, labile blood sugar levels, and a rapid, bounding pulse rate.
   c. Consuming a low-stress diet results in more energy and stamina to cope with stress.
   d. Teach client that a low-stress diet includes saturated fat and protein intake to equal 10–15% of consumed calories. Remainder of intake should be raw or barely cooked vegetables, fruits, whole grains, nuts, low-fat dairy products, and plenty of liquids. Eliminate sodas, caffeine products, and most alcohol. Exclude refined sugars and carbohydrates and convenience or processed foods.
   e. Encourage the use of vitamin supplements: vitamin C, B-complex, mineral supplements. Assist client to examine diet and experiment with different vitamin-mineral supplements.
3. Manage stress by altering lifestyle patterns.
   a. Counsel clients to eliminate unnecessary stressors in their life—change parts of life that are particularly stressful.
   b. Assist client to develop personal methods for coping with stress: walking in the woods, painting, listening to music, reading, or practicing yoga.
   c. Encourage client to assess lifestyle periodically and alter habits as necessary to reduce stress.

ALLEVIATING STRESS USING CONTROLLED BREATHING

Procedure

1. Instruct client to sit so that his or her back is well supported, with spine straight but not rigid.
2. Have client place feet flat on floor and place hands on legs.
3. If client is lying down, have him or her place hands at side.
4. Suggest client find a comfortable position, close eyes, and take a deep, slow breath through nostrils.
5. Continue giving the client the following instructions.
   a. Extend your abdominal muscles.

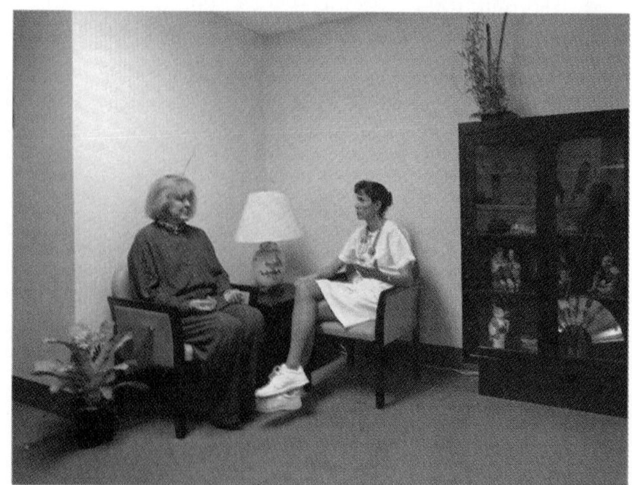

Find a quiet room to teach relaxation process.

b. Hold your breath for the count of four. Then very slowly release the air through slightly parted lips, making a whoosh sound.
c. When you think that all the air is out, hold your stomach in to push out even more air.
d. Repeat this breathing pattern several times so that your body relaxes.
e. Breathe in through your nostrils to the count of four—1-2-3-4. Hold it—1-2-3-4—and expel the breath all the way out slowly, slowly releasing the air through your mouth.
f. As the air goes out, feel all of the tension drain out with it.
g. Now double the count, and breathe in slowly, filling your lungs all the way to the top to the count of eight. 1-2-3-4-5-6-7-8. Hold it—1-2-3-4—and now slowly release the breath—5-6-7-8.
h. Again breathe in slowly to the count of 10 and count for the client—1-2-3-4-5-6-7-8-9-10. Hold it to the count of eight—1-2-3-4-5-6-7-8—and slowly release the air through your mouth to the count of 10—1-2-3-4-5-6-7-8-9-10. Pause.
i. Continue with your regular breathing pattern, letting the air breathe for you.

6. Stop the process by having the client open his or her eyes.

ALLEVIATING STRESS USING BODY RELAXATION

Procedure

1. Place client in a comfortable position.
   a. Have client sit so that back is well supported and spine is straight. Have client put both feet on the floor and hold hands comfortably in lap.
   b. If sitting is uncomfortable, have client lie on a bed and support areas of the body so that he or she is comfortable.
2. Instruct client to concentrate on each key muscle of the body, tensing and relaxing each muscle until it is totally relaxed.
3. Ask client to tense and release the muscles in the left toes, left foot, left calf, left thigh, and left leg.
4. Now have the client continue the process on the right leg, trunk, upper torso, arms, shoulders, neck, and face. Then have the client check to see that every muscle is relaxed.
5. Ask the client to check for tight areas, any tension, any uncomfortable areas or sensations and then to let it all go. Ask the client if he or she is willing to let all of the tension go.
6. Ask client to practice being totally relaxed.

ALLEVIATING STRESS USING MEDITATION

Procedure

1. Meditation is the process of relaxing the body and focusing and quieting the mind. The essence of this method depends on the ability to concentrate on an object, a word, or nothing at all.
2. The process of meditation begins with slow, quiet breathing and deep muscle relaxation. (See Alleviating Stress Using Controlled Breathing and Body Relaxation.)
3. Instruct the client in meditation techniques—suggest books or tapes that focus on meditation.
4. Encourage the client to begin meditation—suggest positive outcomes.
   a. During meditation, there is a decrease in oxygen consumption, blood pressure, pulse rate, respiration, brain wave activity, and blood lactate level (high in anxious people).
   b. Research indicates that meditation has a measurable effect on stress-related conditions.

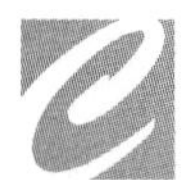

CHARTING for Stress

- Identification of stressed behavior observed in client
- Separation of physical from emotional and environmental stressors
- How client is responding to stress
- Pertinent verbalizations of client related to stress
- Nursing interventions related to stress reduction

CRITICAL THINKING APPLICATION

CLINICAL PROBLEMS	CRITICAL THINKING OPTIONS
Client moves into the stage of exhaustion, and stress becomes dangerous to health.	• Immediately take measures to remove stressors through medication, complete rest, and so forth. • Implement specific stress-reducing measures, such as relaxation processes, visualization, and biofeedback.
Client refuses to acknowledge that stress is affecting his or her life.	• Attempt to elicit feelings of client before giving information about the role of stress and effect on one's body. • Refer client to resources, articles, and knowledgeable persons who can discuss the effect of stress and the importance of eliminating stressors.

GERIATRIC CONSIDERATIONS

The influence of stress on aging is significant and affects response and coping ability.

- Elderly have less resistance to stressors: mental, emotional, environmental, and physical.
- Homeostatic imbalance is more common in the elderly and causes additional stress on the body.
- Adaptation to stress lessens with age (depends in part on genetic makeup and personal learning to deal with life crises).
- Nursing care should focus on adaptive responses to stress—assist client to develop mechanisms to deal with the stress of illness and hospitalization.

7

Admission and Discharge

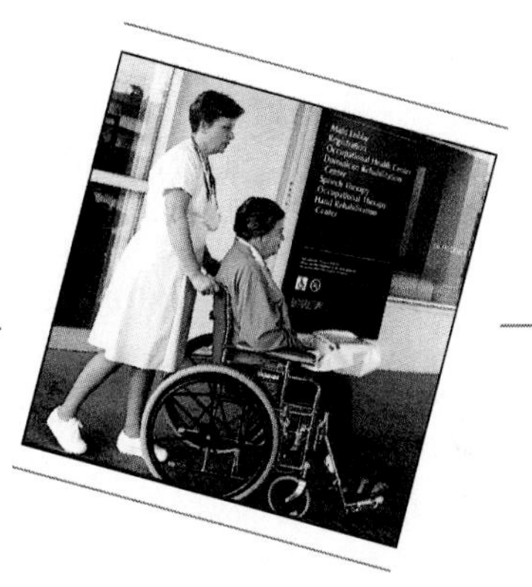

LEARNING OBJECTIVES

- Explain the steps of admitting a client to a health care unit.
- Describe the client assessment that is completed at the time of admission.
- List the data that are included in charting when admitting a client to the health care environment.
- Describe the disposition process for client's valuables when hospitalized.
- Outline the steps in transferring a client within the hospital environment.
- Describe two suggested solutions for clients who are unable to adapt to the hospital environment.
- Discuss the discharge procedures when a client leaves the health care unit.
- Identify three suggested solutions for a client leaving the hospital against medical advice.
- Describe the expected outcomes for clients being discharged from the hospital.
- Complete discharge charting on a client record using specific criteria.

TERMINOLOGY

Adaptation: ability to adjust to a change in environment.

Admit: the process of getting a client signed into the hospital.

Ambulatory: able to walk, or not confined to bed.

Antiembolic: a preventative measure, such as elastic hosiery, to avoid emboli.

Aseptic: sterile; free from bacteria and infection.

Assessment: critical evaluation of information; the first step in the nursing process.

Behavior: a person's total activity—actions or reactions; especially, conduct that can be observed.

Blood count: enumeration of the red corpuscles and leukocytes per milliliter. A blood count indicates the total number of cells.

Cardio: prefix pertinent to the heart

Client Care Plan: a plan for care of a specific client or one designed especially for one client.

Comfort: to ease physically; relieve, as of pain.

Communication: to convey or transmit knowledge, information, or messages to another person.

Comprehensive health care: a total system of health care that takes the whole person into account.

Criteria: a standard, rule, or test on which a judgment or decision can be based.

Diagnostic test: a test used to determine a diagnosis or to determine the cause and nature of a pathological condition.

Disability: a disabled state or condition; incapacity; a handicap.

Discharge: to let go, as in discharging a client from the hospital; the flowing away of a secretion or excretion of pus, feces, urine.

Home care assistance: nursing care given in the client's home.

Homeostasis: state of equilibrium of the internal environment.

Hygiene: the study of health and observance of health rules.

Hypoallergenic: a substance deemed to cause very little, if any, allergic response.

Hypotension: decrease of systolic and diastolic blood pressure below normal.

Identaband: a band, usually worn on a client's wrist, with the client's name and medical record number.

Kardex: a system of cards that contains pertinent medical information about clients.

Limitation: the state of being limited or restricted

Maladaptation: inability to adjust to a change in environment.

Potential: possible but not yet realized.

Procedure: a particular way of accomplishing a desired result.

Radiology: the branch of medicine concerned with radioactive substances.

Regression: a turning back or return to a former state.

Serology: the scientific study of serum.

Serum: any serous fluid, especially the fluid that moistens the surfaces of serous membranes; the watery portion of blood after coagulation.

Specimen: a part of a thing intended to show kind and quality of the whole, as a specimen of urine.

Stress: a state of agitation that throws the body out of balance.

Supervise: to direct or inspect performance; to oversee.

Termination: the spatial or temporal end of something; a limit or boundary.

Therapeutic: having healing or curative powers.

Transfer: to convey or shift from one person or place to another.

Transition: the process or an instance of changing from one form, state, activity, or place to another.

Verbalize: to express in words.

Void: to urinate or evacuate the bowels.

Volunteer: a person who performs or gives his or her services of his or her own free will.

ADMISSION, TRANSFER, AND DISCHARGE

The admission procedure for clients can be a negative experience if it is impersonal, mechanized, or impolite. It can be a positive step in health care if handled with attention and care. The impressions formed by the clients during the admission process strongly affects their attitude toward their total care. Because the admission procedure can be the initial introduction into the health care system, the nurses should consider this process a key step in client care.

Admission to the Hospital

The process of admitting a client to a health care facility varies in institutions, such as nursing homes, clinics, and hospitals. Regardless of the size or type of facility, the admission process is vitally important to provide safe, adequate care. Because the nurse–patient relationship begins with admission, the nurse should have a thorough understanding of the standard admission process.

If a client enters the hospital in an emergency situation, he or she may feel insecure or fearful because he or she has had little time to make plans concerning family, travel, finances, or employment. When a client enters the hospital for elective treatment or surgery, the nurse has time to orient and prepare the client for a hospital stay.

When the client arrives at the hospital, the first contact is usually with the admitting receptionist, who assigns a hospital number and interviews the client. If preadmission material was mailed to the client, it is verified by the receptionist at this time; otherwise, the client must answer questions about age, address, financial or insurance status, next of kin, religion, employment, and consent for treatment. If the client cannot answer these questions due to age or condition, a relative usually gives the information. A parent or guardian must do this for a child.

During admission, clients should be requested to place valuables in the hospital safe or to send them home with their family. Valuables include jewelry, money, credit cards, and blank checks. Clients also receive identification bracelets or identabands at this time.

Unless laboratory procedures are carried out in the client's room, the client is directed or escorted to the clinical laboratory for baseline values on hemoglobin, hematocrit, complete blood count, differential, and serologic screening for syphilis. Depending on the policy of the facility, the client may then proceed to the electrocardiographic laboratory and to radiology to obtain a chest x-ray.

These procedures sometimes take several hours. Delays often result in physical and emotional strain for the client. When an alternative is offered, such as having laboratory procedures performed the day before admission, the client should be encouraged to use these options to decrease emotional and physical fatigue. More time can then be allowed on the actual admission day for adapting to the hospital environment.

ADMISSION PROTOCOL

Advanced directives are made available to clients.

The client's bill of rights is presented to each client.

The admission assessment is completed by a registered nurse within a specified time after admission.

All clients must be clearly identified by a legible identification band.

When consent forms are required (for surgical procedures), they must be signed by an adult or guardian who is mentally and physically competent. The adult must give voluntary consent, understand the risks and benefits of the treatment, and have the opportunity to ask questions.

Admission to the Nursing Unit

When admission to the hospital is complete, the client is either directed to the nursing unit or escorted by a volunteer. The client may be met by a staff nurse assigned to admissions for that day or by the nurse who will be working with the client during the client's stay in the hospital. It is at this time that the nurse must begin

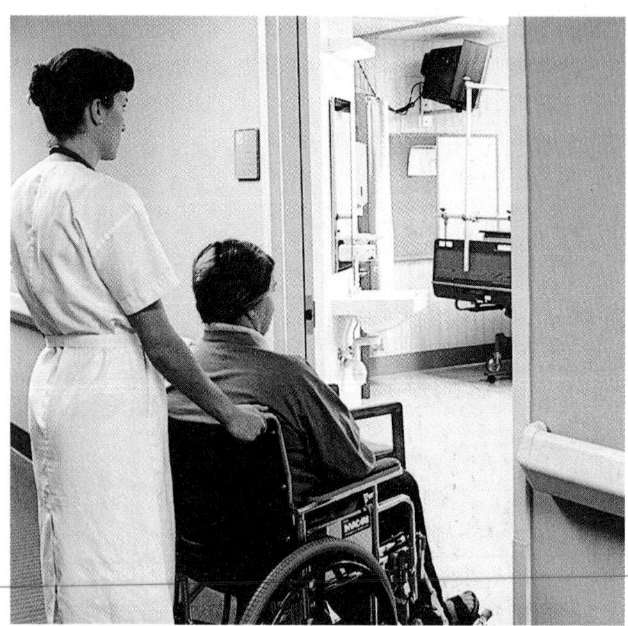

Client may be admitted to the hospital in a wheelchair.

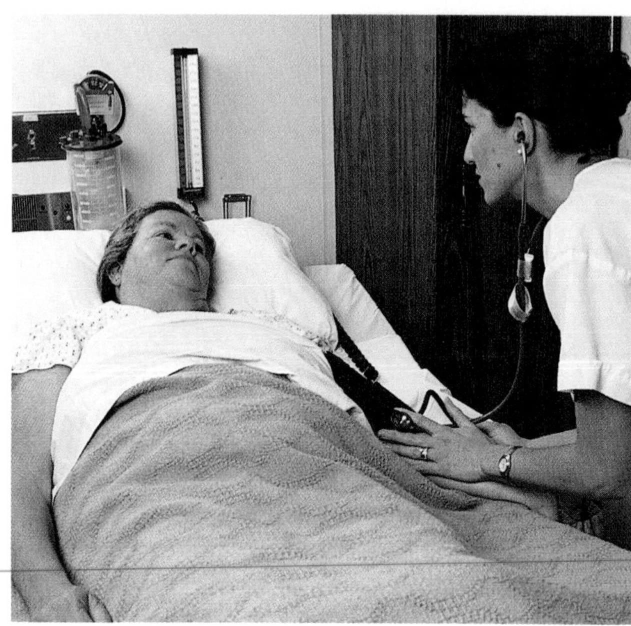

Vital signs are obtained during the admission procedure.

to assess the client's needs and to plan care. The nurse is required to prioritize the client's needs and to initiate the nursing care plan.

In 1992, the Joint Commission on Accreditation of Healthcare Organizations (JCAHO) required every person admitted to the hospital to have an admission assessment completed or directed by a registered nurse within a specified time frame.

When you meet a client, introduce yourself and any other personnel who will provide care, including the ward clerk. Explain your role and functions to the client. Your initial contact leaves a lasting impression, so try to present information in an uninterrupted, organized, and friendly manner. If other clients are in the room, introduce them to the new client.

Tell the client about mealtimes, visiting hours, telephone use, requests for clergy, recreational and lounge use, physicians' visits, and other schedules. Drugs may *not* be kept at the bedside without a physician's order. Some hospitals have printed booklets describing this information. The more information your client receives, the more control he or she has over the environment.

Help the client become familiar with his or her immediate physical space by showing the location and the operation of the intercom system or call bell, the location of the bathroom, and the operation of the call system inside the bathroom. If electric beds are used, show the client how to operate bed controls. You may also want to show the client how to operate the television and the radio set. Explain the cost and availability if not included with the room charges.

Because clients may not be sure of their role while in the hospital, many hospitals have adopted versions of the American Hospital Association's *Patient's Bill of Rights.* This bill includes the following rights: to obtain information about the client's illness or injury, to refuse medication or treatment, to participate in his or her own care, to know the rationale and risks of the treatment, and to receive courteous care. Make sure your clients understand their rights. Clear, uncomplicated explanations help them adapt to their new environment.

Once you have completed introductions and the environmental orientation, you may begin the nursing history and assessment to establish baseline data about the client's general condition (see Chapter 14, Basic Physical Assessment).

Transfer from Unit to Unit

Clients are frequently transferred from one unit to another as their condition fluctuates. When a client is moved, all of the records, charts, drugs, belongings, and personal hygiene and special equipment are transferred with him or her. After accompanying the client to a new unit, introduce him or her to new roommates,

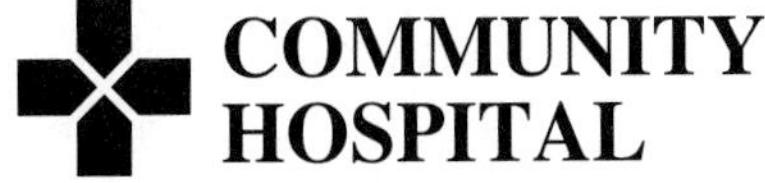

LIST OF PATIENT RIGHTS IN CALIFORNIA

In accordance with section 70707 of the California Administrative Code, the hospital and medical staff have adopted the following list of patient rights. Each patient has the right to:

1. Exercise these rights without regard to sex or cultural, economic, educational, or religious background or the source of payment for his care.
2. Considerate and respectful care.
3. Knowledge of the name of the physician who has primary responsibility for coordinating his care and the names and professional relationships of other physicians who will see him.
4. Receive information from his physician about his illness, his course of treatment, and his prospects for recovery in terms that he can understand.
5. Receive as much information about any proposed treatment or procedure as he may need in order to give informed consent or to refuse this course of treatment. Except in emergencies, this information shall include a description of the procedure or treatment, the medically significant risks involved in this treatment, alternate course of treatment or nontreatment and the risks involved in each, and to know the name of the person who will carry out the procedure or treatment.
6. Participate actively in decisions regarding his medical care. To the extent permitted by law, this includes the right to refuse treatment.
7. Full consideration of privacy concerning his medical care program. Case discussion, consultation, examination, and treatment are confidential and should be conducted discreetly. The patient has the right to be advised as to the reason for the presence of any individual.
8. Confidential treatment of all communications and records pertaining to his care and his stay in the hospital. His written permission shall be obtained before his medical records can be made available to anyone not directly concerned with his care.
9. Reasonable responses to any reasonable requests he may make for service.
10. Leave the hospital even against the advice of his physicians.
11. Reasonable continuity of care and to know in advance the time and iocation of appointment as well as the physician providing the care.
12. Be advised if hospital/personal physician proposes to engage in or perform human experimentation affecting his care or treatment. The patient has the right to refuse to participate in such research projects.
13. Be informed by his physician or a delegate of his physician of his continuing health care requirements following his discharge from the hospital.
14. Examine and receive an explanation of his bill regardless of source of payment.
15. Know which hospital rules and policies apply to his conduct as a patient.
16. Have all patients' rights apply to the person who may have legal responsibility to make decisions regarding medical care on behalf of the patient.

The American Hospital Association adopted a Patients' Bill of Rights in 1973 and revised it in 1992. Note example of a states' Bill of Rights above.

the charge nurse, and the nurse who will be responsible for his or her care. Assist him or her to get settled in the new room. Make a complete report to the nursing staff using the client care plan.

Discharge from a Unit

When a client is discharged from a health care unit, preparations must be made to help the client transfer from a dependent role to a more independent role. Discharge from the hospital can be a welcome relief for the client, but it can also be a time of anxiety and fear. During this transition, the nursing staff can facilitate the process by being aware of individual client needs.

During the discharge process, you must take into consideration the physical, emotional, and psychosocial needs of the client and family. Your responsibilities for the discharge process include assessing the client's posthospitalization needs and planning with the client and family to meet discharge needs. It is also important to communicate with appropriate health team members and community agencies. The final responsibilities of the discharge process are to terminate the nurse–client relationship and evaluate the discharge process.

See Chapters 31 (Client Education and Discharge Planning) and 34 (Home Care Management) for further information on discharging clients to home or another health care facility.

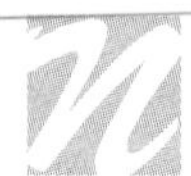

NURSING DIAGNOSES

The following nursing diagnoses are appropriate to use on client care plans when the components are related to admission, transfer, and discharge of a client.

NURSING DIAGNOSIS	RELATED FACTORS
Impaired Adjustment	Unavailable or inadequate support systems, loss of limb or bodily function
Anxiety	Actual or perceived threat to self-concept, threat to biologic integrity, unfamiliar environment and treatments, change in socioeconomic status
Anticipatory Grieving	Loss of function, change in lifestyle, lack of social support system, change in social role
Altered Health Maintenance	System impairment, surgery, musculoskeletal impairment, visual disorders, external devices
Social Isolation	Hospitalization, chemical dependency, altered appearance

unit 1

ADMISSION AND TRANSFER

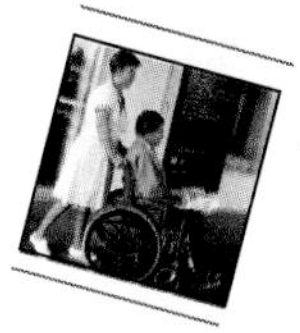

NURSING PROCESS DATA

ASSESSMENT Data Base

Observe and record client's physical, emotional, and intellectual status.

Observe and record client's ability to adapt to the environment of a hospital unit. Observe for disabilities or limitations.

Identify medications client is currently taking.

Assess the client's level of comfort or discomfort.

Determine client's understanding of his or her disease and its limitations.

Assess condition prior to transfer.

PLANNING Objectives

To assist client to adapt to hospital environment with minimal distress

To encourage the client to participate in his or her own plan of care

To provide a comfortable and aesthetically pleasing environment for the client

To provide the client with some control over his or her immediate environment

To provide the client with an opportunity to verbalize his or her feelings about hospitalization

To facilitate transfer if required

IMPLEMENTATION Procedures

Admitting a Client

Transferring a Client

EVALUATION Expected Outcomes

Client adapts to hospital environment.

Client participates in his or her own plan of care.

Client exercises some degree of control over his or her environment.

Client accepts transfer to new unit.

ADMITTING A CLIENT

Equipment

Admission kit for personal hygiene
Thermometer
Blood pressure cuff and stethoscope
Urine container
Kardex card and client care plan
Client's chart

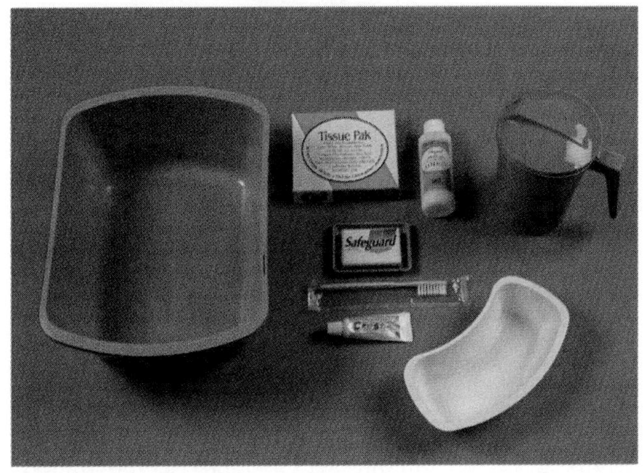

The admissions kit usually contains necessary personal hygiene items including lotion and mouth wash.

Procedure

1. Introduce yourself to the client and family and begin to establish a therapeutic nurse–patient relationship.

COMMUNITY HOSPITAL

Admission questionnaire

Addressograph Plate

Please answer the following questions so that we may plan your nursing care more efficiently and your discharge when it occurs. If you do not understand a question, please ask for help.

1. What health problem was responsible for admission to the Hospital at this time? __________
2. How long have you had this problem? __________
3. Briefly state what your understanding is of your present problem? __________
4: If known, what are your doctor's plans for you? __________
5: How long do you expect to be in the Hospital? __________
6: List any other health problems you are aware of besides the one other than hospitalized for: __________
7. List any major health problems, illnesses, surgeries, or hospitalizations you have had in the past, including the date of each: __________
   (Date) __________
   (Date)
8. Do you have any food allergies or restrictions? ❑ YES ❑ NO
   If yes, explain __________

2. Introduce the client and family to staff and to roommate if present. **Rationale:** Reduces anxiety about hospital stay.
3. Explain equipment and hospital routines.
4. Complete a general nursing assessment.
5. Check physician's orders for treatments to be instituted immediately. **Rationale:** This prevents delay of treatments that could affect client's condition.
6. Obtain client's health history. **Rationale:** Complete history provides total picture of client's condition and problems.
7. Obtain the patient's weight and height.
8. Obtain urine specimen and vital signs.
9. Inform laboratory that client is available for chest x-ray and routine blood work if not obtained earlier.
10. Identify client's problem areas and needs.
11. Notify physician that the client has been admitted, and obtain orders if policy permits.

OBTAINING A NURSING HISTORY

Past medical history or health problems, including those for which client was not hospitalized
Signs and symptoms according to client's perceptions
Assessment of health status (include lifestyle, habits)
Diet and nutrition, hydration status, elimination, exercise, habits (i.e., smoking, drinking), sleep patterns, cognitive function
Relationships and social support systems
Values, beliefs, religious or spiritual practices
History of allergies, especially drugs and foods, and restrictions
Medication history—use and allergies
Risk factors for health—weight, smoking habit, age, general health, and so on
Client's knowledge of illness (understanding of present illness) and expectations of care
Risk analysis for discharge (ability to manage self-care at home)
Special data base for elderly client: level of independence, ability to complete activities of daily living (ADLs), toxic reactions or side effects of medications, history of recent loss of loved one, management of chronic conditions (arthritis, incontinence, etc.)

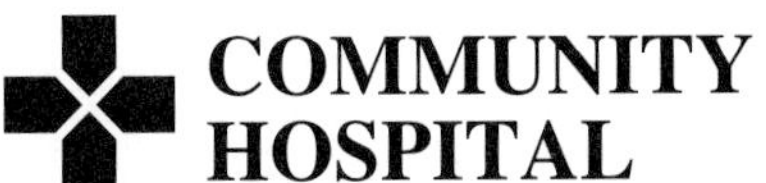

Belongings List

Patient's Naxme ______________________________ Date ____________

Male ☐ Female ☐

Admitting Unit ______________________________

☐ Discharged

☐ Decreased

☐ Transferred

Unit and Rm # From ______________________

Unit and Rm # To ______________________

CLOTHING LIST				MISCELLANEOUS	
PLEASE DESCRIBE	NUMBER	PLEASE DESCRIBE	NUMBER	PLEASE DESCRIBE	NUMBER
Bathrobe		Shoes		Cane	
Belt		Slacks/Shorts		Crutches	
Blouse		Slippers		Dentures ☐ Upper ☐ Lower ☐ Partial	
Coat		Skirts			
Dress		Sweater		Flowers or Plants	
Gloves		Tie		Glasses or Contact Lens	
Gown		Underclothes		Jewelry Remaining with Pt.	
Hat					
Helmet					
Hose/Socks/Pantihose				Luggage	
Jacket				Radio	
Pajamas				Wallet/Purse	
Shirt				Watch	
				Wig	

Signature of Person Listing ________________________________

Signature of Personnel Handling Belongings ________________________________

Signature of Receiving Personnel or Relative ________________________________

If Relative: Address ______________________________ Phone ____________

TABLE 7–1. Religious Guidelines for Client Care

Religious Group	Baptism	Death Rituals	Health Crisis	Diet
Adventist	Opposed to infant baptism	No last rites	Communion or baptism may be desirable	No alcohol, coffee, tea, or any narcotic
Baptist	Opposed to infant baptism	Clergy supports and counsels	Some believe in healing and laying on of hands Some sects resist medical help	Condemn alcohol Some do not allow coffee and tea
Black Muslim	No baptism	Prescribed procedures for washing body and shrouding after death	No faith healing	Prohibit alcohol and port
Buddhist	Rites are given after child is mature	Send for Buddhist priest Last rite chanting	Family should request priest to be notified	Usually no restrictions although some are vegetarian
Christian Scientist	No baptism	No last rites No autopsy	Deny the existence of health crises Many refuse all medical help, blood transfusions, or drugs	Alcohol, coffee, and tobacco viewed as drugs and not allowed
Episcopalian	Infant baptism mandatory	Last rites not essential for all members	Medical treatment acceptable	Some do not eat meat on Fridays
Jehovah's Witness	No infant baptism	No last rites	Opposed to blood transfusions	Do not eat anything to which blood has been added
Judaism	No baptism but ritual circumcision on eighth day after birth	Ritual washing of body after death	All ill people seek medical care	Orthodox observe kosher dietary laws, which prohibit pork, shellfish, and the eating of meat and milk products at the same time
Methodist	Baptism encouraged	No last rites	Medical treatment acceptable	No restrictions
Mormon	Baptism eight years or older	Baptism for the dead can be done by proxy	Do not prohibit medical treatment, although they believe in divine healing	Do not allow alcohol, caffeine, tobacco, tea, and coffee
Roman Catholic	Infant baptism mandatory	Last rites required	Sacrament of the sick	Most ill people are exempt from fasting

Note: There may exist circumstances that require a court order to supervene religious practices (e.g., a blood transfusion to save the life of a child).

12. Reassess client's level of comfort and ability to adapt to hospitalization (see Table 7–1 on religious guidelines).
13. Complete client teaching for all unfamiliar procedures or interventions.
14. Fill out Kardex card and client care plan.
15. Document information on appropriate forms in chart.

NURSING ASSESSMENT DATA BASE

COMMUNITY HOSPITAL

Date	Time	Room #	Admit by:	ambulatory—— W/C——	guerney —— ambulance ——

T.P.R.	B/P AT	B/P LT	Height	Weight

Instructed in use of:

Yes	No	
☐	☐	Telephone
☐	☐	Bed-Controls
☐	☐	Lights
☐	☐	Nurse call System
☐	☐	Visiting hours

Reason for No: ______

Above information obtained by: ______

Articles at bedside (describe item)

☐ Ring ______
☐ Watch ______
☐ Money (amt.) ______
☐ Eyeglasses ______
☐ Hearing Aid ______
Other ______

☐ Contact Lenses ______
☐ Dentures: Upper ______
☐ Lower ______
☐ Other ______

Tests completed on admission
☐ Lab Work ☐ X-ray ______
☐ UA ☐ Other ______

Previous illness	Meds taken @ home on routine basis	Meds taken today state time	Meds brought to hospital	Allergies:
☐ Diabetes				☐ FOOD ______
☐ Hypertension				
☐ Heart Disease				
☐ Lung Disease				
☐ Other				☐ DRUGS ______
			Disposition of Meds ☐ Home ☐ Pharmacy	☐ None Known

See Chapter 31 for sample discharge plan.

TRANSFERRING A CLIENT

Equipment

Wheelchair or guerney
Warm covering for guerney
Client's records, chart, and client care plan
Medications and medication cards
Personal hygiene equipment
Special equipment (e.g., sheepskin)
Personal belongings
Valuables receipt

Procedure

1. Obtain physician's order if needed. **Rationale:** Physicians order client transfers from and to critical care unit. They do not always order transfers within departments.
2. Contact admitting office to arrange for transfer.
3. Communicate with transfer unit to determine the best time for moving the client.
4. Inform and talk to client of impending transfer. **Rationale:** Discussing the rationale for transfer and eliciting the client's feelings facilitate adjustment to the transfer unit.
5. Gather equipment, belongings, and records.
6. Wash hands. **Rationale:** This prevents transfer of microorganisms to new unit.
7. Obtain necessary staff assistance for smooth transfer.

8. Transfer client to wheelchair or guerney unless client is remaining in bed for the transfer.
9. Cover client to provide warmth and to avoid exposure during transfer.
10. Notify head nurse when you arrive on the new unit.
11. Introduce and acquaint client with new roommates.
12. Introduce client to new staff, especially the nurse who will be caring for the client that day.
13. Give a complete report to staff, using the client care plan and Kardex. Give information concerning individualized care needs, client problems, progress, when next medications or treatments are due. **Rationale:** Complete communication maintains continuity of care after transfer.
14. Notify physician when client's transfer is completed.
15. Notify the switchboard and admitting office when transfer is completed. A written transfer slip must be sent to the appropriate departments.
16. Notify dietary department, x-ray, and the laboratory if tests were scheduled or results pending.

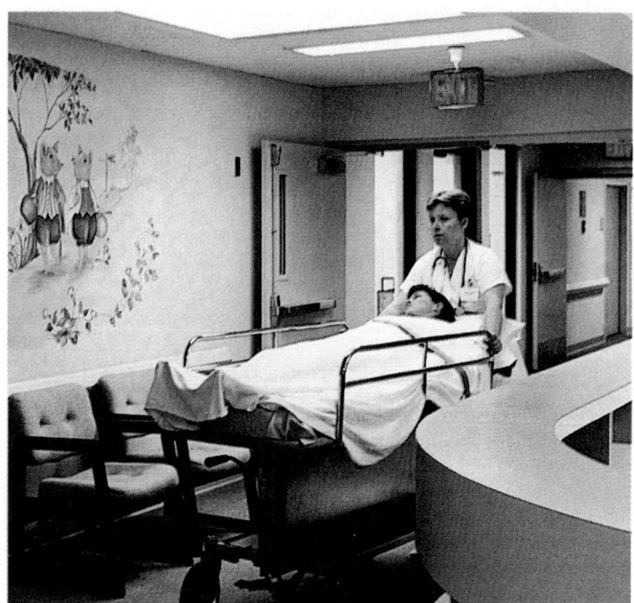

Clients are often admitted or transferred on a guerney.

17. Determine that valuables receipt is either with client or on chart.

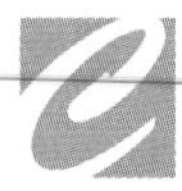

CHARTING for Admitting and Transferring

- Admission procedures
- Adaptation to hospitalization
- Admission assessment data: height, weight, vital signs, physical assessment findings
- Laboratory specimens obtained and sent
- Types of x-rays
- Transfer, time of arrival to new unit, method of transfer, and condition of the client

CRITICAL THINKING APPLICATION

CLINICAL PROBLEMS	CRITICAL THINKING OPTIONS
■ Client is unable to adapt to hospital environment.	• Assess physiologic and emotional basis for maladaptation. Request consultation with nurse manager, client advocate, physician.
■ Client resists transfer.	• Allow client an opportunity to ventilate feelings. • If possible, allow some choice (room, bed, number of roommates) in new unit.
■ Following transfer, client's personal belongings are lost.	• Return to previous unit and check with staff. • Ascertain that belongings were in fact at the hospital. • Check the clothing list for actual articles brought to hospital.

unit 2

HEIGHT AND WEIGHT

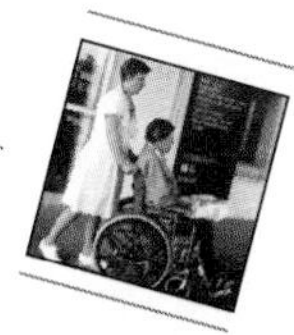

NURSING PROCESS DATA

ASSESSMENT Data Base

Check the need for daily or weekly body weight measurements.

Determine appropriate method for obtaining client's weight (bedside scale, bed scale).

Determine ability to stand for height measurement.

PLANNING Objectives

To establish baseline data to check against total body fluid balance

To identify excess or deficits of fluid balance

To establish baseline data for diagnostic tests that involve dye and radioactive material injections

To determine drug dosage

IMPLEMENTATION Procedure

Obtaining Height and Weight

EVALUATION Expected Outcomes

Client's weight, depending on status, disease state, and therapy, shows expected losses, gains, or stabilization.

Weight is obtained and recorded as ordered by the physician.

Height is obtained and recorded in admission form.

OBTAINING HEIGHT AND WEIGHT

Equipment

Balance beam scale (for clients who are able to stand without assistance)

Bed scale (for clients who are confined to bed or who are unable to stand)

Bed scale that is built into the bed

Floor scale (for clients in wheelchairs) with height bar

Preparation

1. Ask client to void before weighing.
2. Weigh client in the morning before breakfast.
3. Use the same scale each time you weigh the client. **Rationale:** For consistency in weight from day to day, keep as many variables the same as possible.
4. Make sure the client wears the same type of clothing (e.g., gown or robe) for each weighing.
5. If the client is bedridden, weigh linens used for covering the client each time the client is weighed.
6. Change wet gowns or heavily saturated dressings before weighing the client.

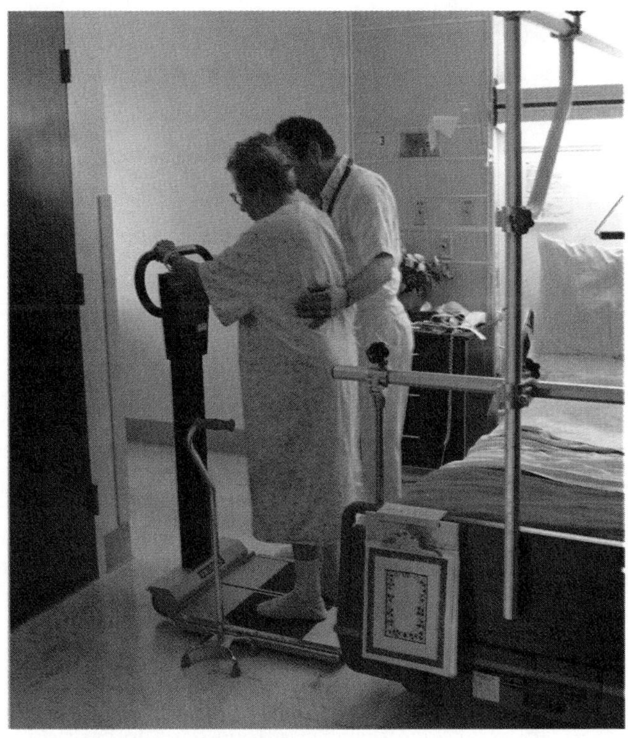

Weigh client in the morning using the same scale each time.

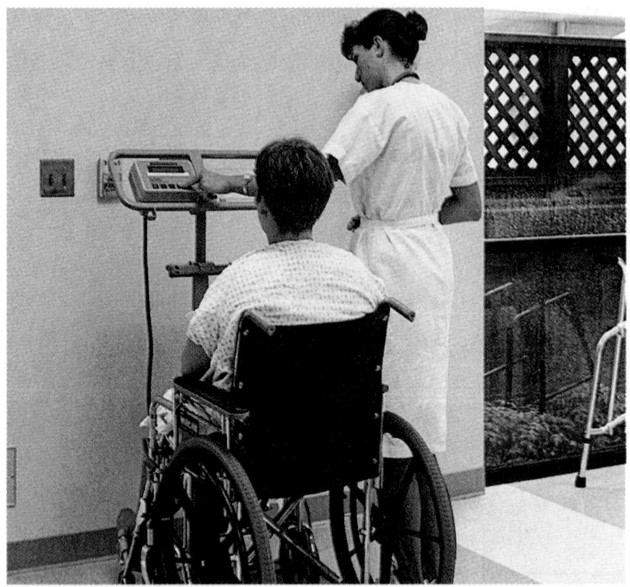

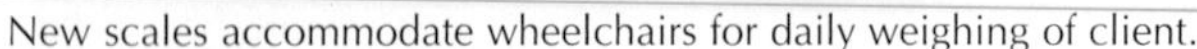

New scales accommodate wheelchairs for daily weighing of client.

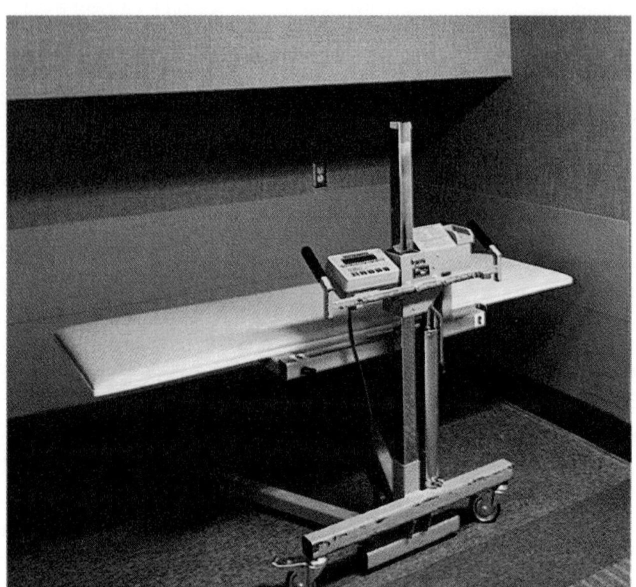

Bed scale is used to weigh clients who are on total bed rest.

TABLE 7.2. Weight Chart
Desirable Weights in Pounds, According to Frame (in Indoor Clothing)

Height Men *Feet*	*Inches*	Small Frame	Medium Frame	Large Frame	Height Women *Feet*	*Inches*	Small Frame	Medium Frame	Large Frame
5	2	112–120	118–129	126–141	4	8	92–98	96–107	104–119
5	3	115–123	121–133	129–144	4	9	94–101	98–110	106–122
5	4	118–126	124–136	132–148	4	10	96–104	101–113	109–125
5	5	121–129	127–139	135–152	4	11	99–107	104–116	112–128
5	6	124–133	130–143	138–156	5	0	102–110	107–119	115–131
5	7	128–137	134–147	142–161	5	1	105–113	110–122	118–134
5	8	132–141	138–152	147–166	5	2	108–116	113–126	121–138
5	9	136–145	142–156	151–170	5	3	111–119	116–130	125–142
5	10	140–150	146–160	155–174	5	4	114–123	120–135	129–146
5	11	144–154	150–165	159–179	5	5	118–127	124–139	133–150
6	0	148–158	154–170	164–184	5	6	122–131	128–143	137–154
6	1	152–162	158–175	168–189	5	7	126–135	132–147	141–158
6	2	156–167	162–180	173–194	5	8	130–140	136–151	145–163
6	3	160–171	167–185	178–199	5	9	134–144	140–155	149–168
6	4	164–175	172–190	182–204	5	10	138–148	144–159	153–173
					5	11	142–152	148–163	157–177
					6	0	146–156	152–167	161–181
					6	1	150–160	156–171	165–185
					6	2	154–164	160–175	169–189

This table was prepared in 1959 by the Metropolitan Life Insurance Company. Many health practitioners recommend using this version instead of the revised 1979 version, which gives higher weight ranges and may lead many individuals to greater complacency about their weight. Studies reported in 1995 indicate that lower weight parameters reduce the risk of cardiovascular disease, especially for women.
Source: Metropolitan Life Insurance Company.

Procedure

1. Transport client to scale or bring scale to bedside.
2. Balance scale so that weight is accurate. (See Table 7–2 for desirable weights.)
3. Place a clean paper towel on scale and ask client to remove shoes.
4. Assist client to stand with back toward balancing bar.

5. Move weights until the weight bar is level or balanced.
6. Record weight on appropriate record.
7. Place height bar level on top of the client's head.
8. Read client's height as measured.
9. Record height on appropriate record.
10. Throw away paper towel on scale and assist client back to room.

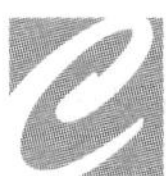

CHARTING for Height and Weight

- Client's weight and height recorded in weight book or on graphic sheet
- Type of scale used for weighing
- Bed linens, gowns, and equipment weighed (record on care plan or on Kardex)

CRITICAL THINKING APPLICATION

CLINICAL PROBLEMS	CRITICAL THINKING OPTIONS
Weight varies excessively from one day to the next.	• Check if same scale was used for both weighings. • Check what clothing or linen was on the client when he or she was weighed on both days. • Check that scale was balanced appropriately. • Reweigh the client to determine if an error was made in the weight.
Client is too critically ill to be weighed accurately because of mechanical devices used to sustain life.	• Estimate weight loss and gain by assessing other factors, such as skin turgor, output, presence of edema. • Weigh the client on a bed scale and note equipment used.

unit 3

DISCHARGE

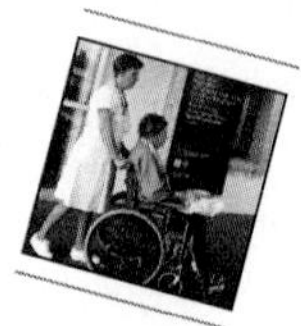

NURSING PROCESS DATA

ASSESSMENT Data Base

Identify physical, emotional, and psychosocial information concerning client's discharge.

Assess client's health care needs for discharge.

Identify disabilities and limitations that will extend after discharge.

Observe client's strengths.

Assess need for health care assistance in the home.

PLANNING Objectives

To prepare the client for discharge and complete discharge planning.

To assist in the transfer of a client whose condition necessitates care at another facility

To allow the client to verbalize his or her feelings about discharge and to identify the client's strengths and weaknesses

To help the client become aware of potential changes in environment and lifestyle due to his or her disability or limitation

IMPLEMENTATION Procedures

Discharging a Client

Discharging a Client against Medical Advice (AMA)

EVALUATION Expected Outcomes

Client verbalizes his or her feelings about being discharged and identifies strengths and weaknesses.

Client is aware of potential changes in environment and lifestyle due to his or her disability or limitations.

Client and family discuss how they can work together to help the client maximize his or her potential.

Client knowledgeably discusses all points included in the nurse–client teaching, including medication and self-care.

Home care assistance is arranged when needed.

DISCHARGING A CLIENT

Equipment

Educational pamphlets

Telephone numbers and information regarding clinic appointments or special groups

Specific equipment, such as wheelchair or commode, needed on discharge

Medications

Materials for dressing changes (if indicated) or antiembolic stockings

Preparation

1. Determine that physician's discharge orders have been written.
2. Notify family or significant other to arrange transportation. If unavailable, notify discharge coordinator for arrangements.
3. Notify all hospital departments: admitting, cashier, dietary.
4. Ensure that all laboratory work, x-rays, treatments, and procedures are completed prior to discharge.

5. Provide opportunities for client to discuss impending discharge.
6. Complete client teaching if applicable. (See Chapter 31, Client Education and Discharge Planning.)

Procedure

1. Review details of discharge with client (See discharge planning unit in Chapter 31).
2. Assist client with hygiene, dressing, packing. Check closets and drawers for client's belongings. Account for all valuables.
3. Review instructions and answer questions about medications, physical care, and supplies.
4. Terminate relationship with the client. Remember that each individual handles termination in his or her own way. **Rationale:** Providing an opportunity for the client to express his or her feelings and impressions contributes to a positive termination.
5. Follow hospital's prescribed procedure for client discharge, including discharge time and method of leaving hospital unit. **Rationale:** Many hospitals insist that clients be transported by wheelchair to prevent falls and injury.
6. Document the client's discharge on the chart.
7. Document discharge planning information given to client.

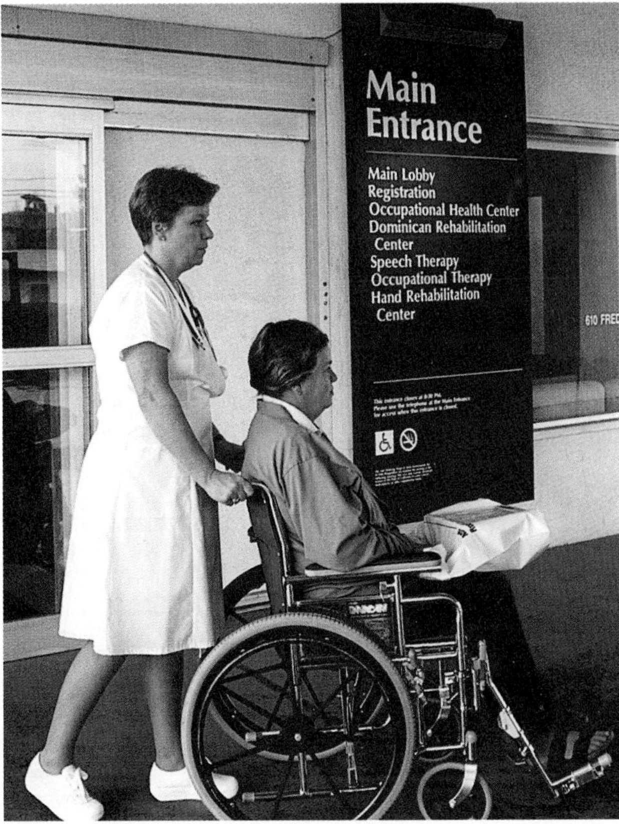

Clients are discharged in a wheelchair for their safety.

DISCHARGING A CLIENT AGAINST MEDICAL ADVICE (AMA)

Equipment

Form for discharge against medical advice
Pen

Procedure

1. If client insists on leaving the hospital, notify the physician.
2. Ascertain from the client exactly why he or she wants to leave the hospital.
3. Explain and validate the physician's reasons that continued hospital care is necessary.
4. If client still insists on leaving, offer him or her the appropriate form and request him or her to sign it. **Rationale:** This form states that the hospital is relieved from responsibility for the client's condition.
5. If client refuses to sign the form, note this fact on the form and have it witnessed. **Rationale:** This fulfills legal requirements if the client insists on discharge AMA without signing form.
6. Put the copy of the form on the client's chart.
7. Notify the appropriate people—the physician, nursing supervisor, administration—when the client leaves.
8. Escort the client to the door as you would any discharged client. **Rationale:** The hospital is still responsible for the client while he or she is on hospital property.

COMMUNITY HOSPITAL

RELEASE FROM RESPONSIBILITY - I

TREATMENT OF MISCARRIAGE OR PARTIAL ABORTION
(Other Than Therapeutic) Date ______ Time ______

I, the undersigned, a patient at the above named hospital, am advised by my doctor that I may be in a condition of abortion. I hereby declare that neither the physician nor any person employed by or connected with the said hospital has performed any act which may have contributed to the interruption of my pregnancy and do hereby absolve the said hospital and treating physician from any responsibility for my condition. My condition has been caused by the following facts occurring prior to the time of my admission to the hospital and treatment by my physician.

____

Witness ______________________ Signature ______________________
PATIENT

This form to be completed in the case of patients who are or MAY BE in a condition of abortion. Patient should state facts of her case in her own handwriting whenever possible.

LEAVING HOSPITAL AGAINST ADVICE Date ______ Time ______

This is to certify that ______________________

a patient in the above named hospital, is leaving the hospital against the advice of the attending physician and the hospital administration. I acknowledge that I have been informed of the risk involved and hereby release the attending physician, and the hospital, from all responsibility and any ill effects which may result from this action.

Witness ______________________ Signature ______________________
PATIENT

TEMPORARY ABSENCE RELEASE Date ______ Time ______

Having received permission from the attending physician to be absent from the above named hospital for my convenience from ______ m to ______ m, date ______________ I assume all responsibility for myself or ______________ patient, who is my ______________ (specify relationshiip), during this temporary absence and hereby release the above named hospital, its employees and the attending physicians from all responsibility during this absence and for my or patient's condition as result thereof.

I understand that I am remaining an inpatient at the above named hospital. My accommodation is being held for me, and I am responsible for all the usual hospital charges that would be payable by me if I remained in the hospital.

Witness ______________________ Signature ______________________
(PATIENT, PARENT OR LEGAL GUARDIAN)

CONSENT TO PHOTOGRAPH Date ______ Time ______

The undersigned do hereby authorize the above named hospital, and the attending physician to photograph or permit other persons to photograph ______________________

while under the care of the above institution, and agree that they may use or permit other persons to use the negatives or prints prepared therefrom for such purposes and in such manner as may be deemed necessary.

Witness ______________________ Signature ______________________
(PATIENT, PARENT OR LEGAL GUARDIAN)

RELEASE OF SIDE RAILS Date ______ Time ______

Having been informed by the above named hospital that protective side rails should be placed on my bed and raised for my personal protection, I hereby instruct the hospital and its employees not to place or raise protective side rails on my bed and hereby assume all risks in connection therewith and fully release the said hospital, its employees and my physician from any and all liability for any injury or damage to me by reason of its failure to place or raise protective side rails on my bed.

Witness ______________________ Signature ______________________

FORM 000060 (7-83)

CHARTING for Discharging a Client

- Day-to-day preparatory activities, such as teaching, return demonstrations, discussion with dietician
- If specific discharge forms or client teaching sheets are used, record data using these forms
- Discharge data, such as time, how discharged (ambulatory, wheelchair, ambulance), if accompanied by relative or nurse, and client's physical and psychosocial condition
- Discharge medications, special equipment, and materials taken home by client
- Discharge criteria that was not met and reason criteria was not met as identified on client care plan

CRITICAL THINKING APPLICATION

CLINICAL PROBLEMS	CRITICAL THINKING OPTIONS
■ Client is discharged to an extended care facility (ECF).	• Reinforce physician's explanation as to why client needs to go to an ECF. • Provide time for client and family to deal with the loss of the client's independence and his or her previous role in the home setting.
■ Client does not understand the discharge process.	• Repeat information as needed to help clarify unfamiliar terms or statements. • Explain to the client's relative the necessary care that will be required on discharge.
■ Client wants to leave the hospital AMA.	• Attempt to identify client's reasons for wanting to leave AMA. • Provide alternatives to leaving the hospital. • Do not force the adult client to remain in the hospital, but do encourage discussion about the situation. • Notify the charge nurse or supervisor that he or she should contact the client advocate, a social worker, or the clergy to discuss the situation with the client. • If possible, consult your hospital's policies and procedures regarding AMA before releasing client. • Have client sign AMA form, if possible. • If client will not sign AMA form, have another nurse witness refusal, and chart details of discharge.

GERIATRIC CONSIDERATIONS

U.S. demographics affect hospital admissions.

- By the year 2000, more than 28 million persons (13% of the U.S. population) are predicted to be over age 65.
- Average life expectancy has increased to 75 years.
- Health care services are used more by the aged than any other group.
- The older the age of the person, the longer stay in the hospital.
- Three out of four elderly people die of heart disease, cancer, or stroke.

Elderly clients admitted to the hospital require special consideration.

- Level of fatigue and pain may be pronounced; thus admission procedure may need to be altered to meet client's needs.
- May require special, repeated orientation due to confusion, impairment in hearing, visualization, mobilization, and so forth.
- Special attention may need to be oriented to family of the elderly client.
- Special problems associated with age need to be anticipated and nursing care planned to intervene appropriately.
- Discharge planning needs to take into account client's age and handicaps.

8

Safe Client Environment

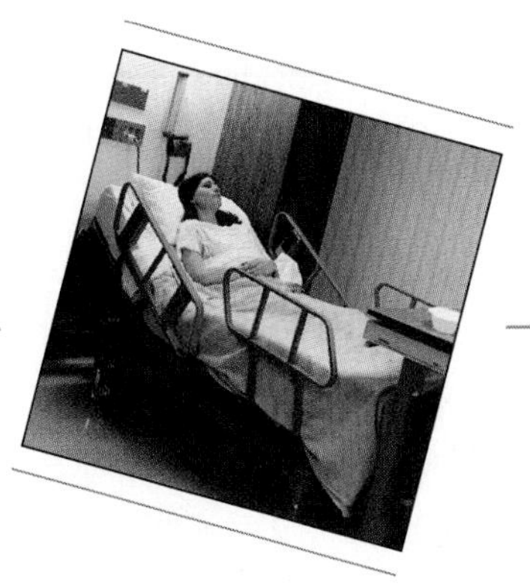

Unit One: A Safe Environment

Unit Two: Restraints

LEARNING OBJECTIVES

- Define the term "adaptation."
- Describe three characteristics that influence adaptation.
- Outline four sociocultural dimensions of environmental adaptation.
- State two nursing diagnoses that can be used to maintain a safe environment.
- Outline the objectives for providing a safe environment.
- List and briefly describe at least four guidelines for using restraints to prevent mechanical injuries.
- Explain four methods of preventing drug injuries.
- List the guidelines for providing safety when clients are receiving radioactive materials.
- Demonstrate two methods of client evacuation when a fire occurs in a nursing unit.
- Demonstrate the application of wrist restraints.
- Demonstrate the application of a posey restraint.
- Identify at least five actions that maintain a safe environment for infants.
- List the components that should be included when charting for application of restraints.

TERMINOLOGY

Adaptation: ability of an organism to adjust to a change in environment.

Ambiance: the pervading atmosphere of the surrounding environment.

Ambulation: to move from place to place by walking.

Aseptic: sterile; a condition free from bacteria and infection.

Assessment: critical evaluation of information; the first step in the nursing process.

Behavior: a person's total activity—actions or reactions; especially conduct that can be observed.

Comprehensive health care: a total system of health care that takes the whole person into account.

Contaminated waste: radioactive waste, which, if improperly disposed of, may be harmful or cause a radiation hazard.

Decibel: a unit for measuring difference in acoustic signals; a unit of intensity and volume of sound.

Ecosystem: the biologic and physical dimensions of the environment that refers to all living and nonliving elements.

Epidemiologist: one who studies the causes, distribution, and frequency of disease outbreaks in a human community.

Homeostasis: a state of equilibrium of the internal environment.

Hygiene: pertinent to a state of health and its preservation.

Limitation: the state of being limited or restricted.

Maladaptation: inability of an organism to adjust to a change in environment.

Nosocomial: infection or disease originating in a hospital.

Physiologic: in accord with or characteristic of the normal functioning of a living organism.

Psycho: prefix referring to the mind or mental processes of an individual.

Psychosocial: a term that refers both to psychologic and social factors.

Restraint: containment of a person in a chair or bed to provide safety.

Sociocultural: a term that refers both to society and culture.

Stress: pressure, strain, or force sufficient to throw an individual out of balance.

Supervise: to direct or inspect performance; to oversee.

Therapeutic: having healing or curative powers.

Thermal: pertaining to using, producing, or caused by heat.

ORIENTATION TO THE CLIENT ENVIRONMENT

Maintaining Homeostasis

As a nurse, one of your primary responsibilities is to make sure your clients have a safe and comfortable health care environment. It is your responsibility to help clients adapt to this environment as well as to their health care in general.

From a holistic view, the term "environment" can generally be explained as the total of all the conditions and influences, both external and internal, that affect the life and development of an organism. As human beings we are constantly exposed to changing physical, biologic, and social conditions. To survive, we continually assess our relationship to our changing surroundings. We also learn how to make adjustments that help us control and improve our environment. This complex process is called "adaptation."

Adaptation includes adjustments in all conscious and unconscious forms. People in most situations are able to control or adapt to their immediate surroundings. Usually the individual knows best how to adapt to the conditions that are specifically affecting him or her. Although no two people respond to the environment in exactly the same way, common principles related to adaptation can be found in all human beings:

- All adaptations are attempts to maintain optimum physical and chemical states, or homeostasis.
- Individuals retain their own identity and uniqueness regardless of the degree of adaptation required.
- Adaptation affects all aspects of human existence.
- Human beings have limits in the process and degree of their adaptation.
- Adaptation is measured in relationship to time.
- Adaptive responses to the environment may or may not be adequate or appropriate.
- Adaptive attempts may be stressful.
- The degree and process of adaptation varies from individual to individual.
- Adaptation is an ongoing process about which the individual may be consciously or unconsciously aware.

Each of us adjusts to our immediate environment in a way that is unique to us. When this environment changes suddenly, for instance when we are hospitalized, we may not be able to adapt independently to our immediate surroundings safely and comfortably. It is at this point that assistance must be provided.

CHARACTERISTICS THAT INFLUENCE ADAPTATION

The characteristics that make all people unique also provide information about the process of adaptation to the environment. These factors must be considered when assessing clients' needs and abilities to safely adjust to their immediate surroundings.

Age

A client's age is a critical factor in the assessment process. Because terms such as "elderly" and "young" can be interpreted in many different ways, the nurse may need to look at the client's developmental stage (physical and mental growth) rather than at the client's chronologic age.

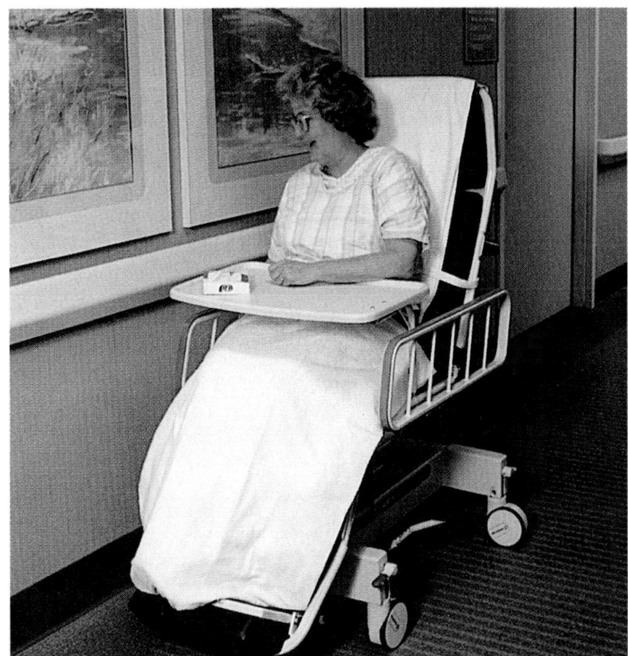

Ensure client safety when sitting in a chair.

As people develop, sensory receptors help process day-to-day events. Human beings learn how to protect themselves and how to adjust to changing needs through experiencing these events. During the learning process, young children may require entirely different protection than teenagers. A 30-year-old man who has learned through experience how to protect himself in a routine environment may not have adequate skills in an unfamiliar atmosphere.

The older adult often requires special assistance. Sensory impairments, such as slowness of movement, poor vision or hearing, loss of balance, and even diminished acuity for taste and touch, are not uncommon. When impairments occur, interpretation of sensory messages is altered. This can result in a decreased ability to sense harmful environmental stimuli. The older person may not see or hear an approaching car, detect the taste of spoiling food, or move quickly enough to avoid falling.

Level of Consciousness

The ability to perceive and react to environmental stimuli is closely related to level of consciousness. Adapting to a new or different environment requires learning through experience and possessing an awareness of the immediate surroundings. Making adjustments to the environment requires stimuli to travel over the sensory pathways of nerves to the central nervous system. To respond to stimuli, such as avoiding a burn from a hot object, motor neurons carry impulses to muscles to cause an involuntary reflex action, such as withdrawing the hand from hot water. Sensory impulses traveling to the cerebral cortex of the brain inform the person that this stimulus is potentially harmful. Voluntary movement then provides additional adaptation.

Consciousness is the state in which individuals are aware of themselves and their relationship to their surroundings. Unconsciousness indicates a lack of response or awareness of the environment. Levels of consciousness range from fully conscious to comatose. Difficulty in adapting to the immediate environment due to varying levels of consciousness can manifest itself in a variety of ways:

- Disoriented clients often view their environment in a fearful, distorted way. This condition can lead to extreme behavioral changes, self-injury, or combativeness.
- Neurologically injured clients may have decreased perceptions of stimuli such as heat, cold, pain, or friction. In extreme cases, they may have no perception of stimuli at all.
- Partial or total paralysis inhibits movement and is accompanied by a loss of position sense (dangling limbs or poor body alignment).
- Alterations in communication, sight, or hearing because of altered consciousness are barriers to sharing fears or concerns with others.
- Fluctuating levels of consciousness create difficulty in promoting self-care and self-image because of an inability to follow directions.

Continuous assessment of changes in the client's level of consciousness is essential. Degree of awareness influences the type and amount of assistance the client needs while in less than familiar surroundings.

States of Illness

Illness or injury causes a person to focus more intensely on him or herself. The very nature of disease or trauma requires the individual to use physical and mental energy to adapt to the situation and to become more egocentric. A client often cannot perform even the simplest daily activity. Fatigue or pain may render clients helpless. Assistance with activities, such as bathing, eating, skin care, and elimination, may be necessary.

Some medications produce such side effects as drowsiness, which prevent the individual from adequately assessing the environment. Perceptions may be distorted, and the client is more vulnerable to hazards.

Emotional stress and anxiety can occur in mild to acute degrees. Although mild anxiety very often increases perceptual awareness, acute anxiety reduces perceptual awareness.

Because an individual is able to focus only on a specific amount of stimuli at one time, additional stimuli that may be equally important are not perceived. Potential environmental dangers are not processed. The client whose energy is focused on pain may not even hear instructions from the nurse. Depressed clients also require assistance. Depression often results in slower than normal responses to stimuli. Alcohol, a central nervous system depressant, also causes dull, slow reactions to stimuli.

When pain, anxiety, illness, injury, weakness, medications, or even lack of sleep cause a decrease in sensory acuity, awareness of potential hazards is altered. The client may not be able to make the necessary biologic, physical, or emotional adjustments to adapt to the immediate environment. Any of these conditions necessitates immediate assessment and action.

PHYSICAL AND BIOLOGICAL DIMENSIONS

The influences that make up an environment include the basic categories of biological and physical conditions. The biological dimensions of our environment covered in this section include all living things, such as plants, animals, and microorganisms. Water, oxygen, sunlight, organic compounds, and other components in which living things exist and develop make up the physical dimensions of an environment.

As you become more aware of the factors that affect environmental adaptation, providing a safe and comfortable atmosphere for your clients becomes a greater challenge. As you assess your clients and help them adapt to the environment of a health care facility, you should consider the following essential elements: space, lighting, humidity, temperature, ventilation, sound levels, surfaces and equipment, safety, food and water, and waste disposal.

Adequate Space

Everyone needs space in which to grow and develop. This space may consist of a room or an area as small as a shelf or corner. No matter what form space takes, individuals need to feel they have control over it—that they can arrange it or decorate it to their liking.

Providing space for clients encourages stimulation and experimentation. Toddlers need the space of an area like a recreation room for discovery and motor skills, since playtime is their primary source of development. Adults often enjoy the social activities of a lounge but may also require well-defined personal areas even if these areas are as simple as a bedside table or a bulletin board.

Natural and Artificial Light

Light, like space, is necessary for growth and development. The production of vitamin D, a critical component of bone metabolism, occurs from ultraviolet radiation on the skin. Natural light also helps wounds heal. In a hospital setting, natural light can be used to decrease feelings of isolation and to encourage clients to continue their normal routine.

Whether natural or artificial, adequate light is essential for the preservation of sight, for safety, and for accurate assessments and nursing care. Because eye strain, as well as nervousness and fatigue can result from improper lighting, care should be taken to avoid glare, sharp contrast, and flickering lights. Night lights promote safety and orientation for the elderly.

Humidity and Temperature

The ability to adapt to changes in humidity or temperature is directly related to comfort. Most people in this country are comfortable at a room temperature of between 18.3° and 25°C (65°–77°F) with the humidity at 30–60%. People in other cultures function equally well at lower or higher readings.

Conditions that may inhibit a person's ability to adjust to high temperatures include excessive physical work, dehydration, extremes in age (the very young and very old), decreased physical fitness, and inappropriate clothing. An individual who has difficulty adapting to high temperatures may experience a rapid rise in pulse rate, cramps, nausea, and vomiting. Severe inability to adapt to heat can result in heat stroke and death.

An individual who has difficulty adapting to lower temperatures may experience a change in behavior, depressed vital signs, and eventual unconsciousness. Hypothermia, or abnormally low body temperature, occurs when there is an imbalance between heat loss and heat production.

Extreme heat or extreme cold increases the incidence of infection and adds to discomfort. Temperatures in health care institutions can be regulated with air conditioners and dehumidifiers, although care should be taken to avoid drafts and excessive dryness.

Ventilation

Particular attention should be given to assessing the movement or air within a client's immediate environment. An adequately ventilated room should contain a comfortable amount of moisture; be free of irritating pollutants, odors, or noxious fumes; and be at a tolerable temperature.

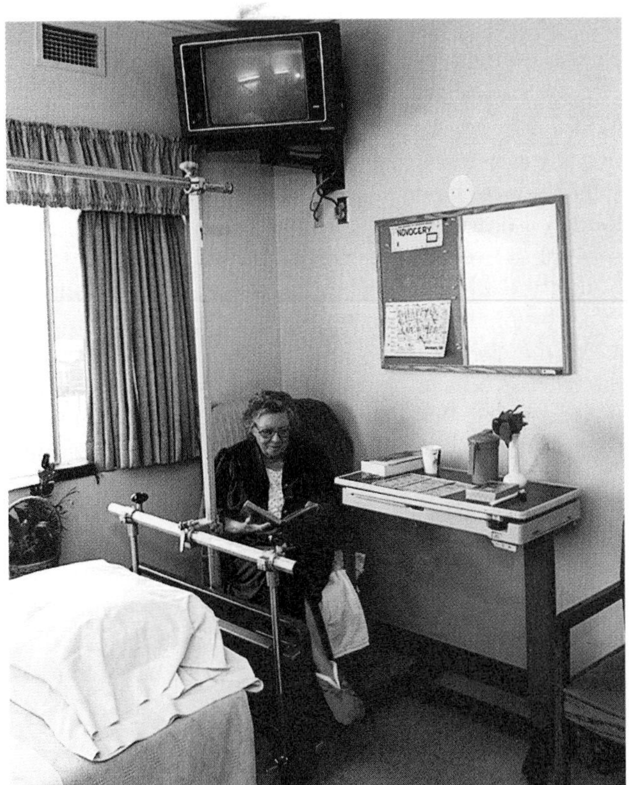

Provide a safe and comfortable environment with space for personal effects.

Adequate ventilation is especially important when more than one client is in a room. Other areas requiring optimum ventilation are operating rooms, delivery rooms, nurseries, isolation rooms, and sterile supply rooms.

A properly functioning ventilation system reduces airborne contaminants by regulating the amount of air movement within an enclosed area. When ventilation cannot be maintained by using doors and windows, mechanical devices, such as fans or air conditioners, may be used.

Comfortable Sound Levels

Noise can be defined as any undesirable sound. The intensity and kind of noise that is comfortable is highly individual and related to past experiences. A businessman who lives on a busy street in a city may not adjust well to the absolute quiet he may experience at night in a hospital room. On the other hand, a farmer from a rural community may be disturbed by the slightest sound. Infants often sleep peacefully in an atmosphere of loud noise and activity.

Decibel is the unit for measuring the intensity of noise. At close range noise produced from heavy traffic, for example, has a decibel measure of 90, whereas a whisper at 3 feet has an intensity of 20 decibels.

At certain levels noise is considered hazardous. Temporary or permanent hearing loss or damage can occur when noise is present for a prolonged time at intensities over 90 decibels. Other effects of sustained loud noise are muscle tension, increased blood pressure, blood vessel constriction, pallor, increased secretion of the adrenal hormone, and nervous tension.

The pitch, quality, and duration of noise may also affect the client's environment. Unwanted sounds produced by sirens, traffic, and aircraft are often beyond the control of the nurse. But noise within a hospital setting, such as television, call systems, careless handling of dishes and other equipment, visitors, excessive conversation at the nurses' station, and some care-related sounds (e.g., beeping monitors) can be controlled.

Nursing personnel should always be aware of the noise level and its effects on the clients' well-being. Very ill individuals are often more sensitive to excessive or meaningless stimuli. Certain sounds can be reassuring because they represent activity or assistance to the client.

Furniture and Clean Surfaces

Today, most health care facilities are designed to be attractive, orderly, efficient, and clean. Since a person's outlook is strongly influenced by the surroundings, careful attention to appearance and cleanliness can assist with adjustment to the health care environment. Although it is essential to assess the routines and standards of cleanliness of each client, the nurse may also have to teach the client how to organize and clean up. In some cases, instruction to the client may be critical to maintaining or improving a health care condition.

The standards and routine cleaning procedures of the hospital are generally not a nursing function now because hospital housekeeping has become a specialized occupation. Maintaining an organized, clean environment, however, requires coordination by all health care providers.

Furnishings should be arranged to be physically safe, comfortable, aesthetically appealing for the client, and easily cleaned. Adequate cleaning of the room should be done at a time of day that is coordinated with the client's needs so that the resulting sense of security adds to the client's ability to adapt adequately to the surroundings. The ambiance of the room and a sense of order contribute to the client's sense of well-being.

Hospital beds are usually adjustable in height from the floor; when the bed is in LOW position the client can more easily and safely get in or out of it; when it is in HIGH position, the nursing staff can more efficiently render care. A step stool may be necessary to enable some clients to get in and out of bed safely. The head and sometimes, the knee areas of the bed can be elevated; this is accomplished by electric controls or by hand cranks. The cranks, if used, are at the foot of the

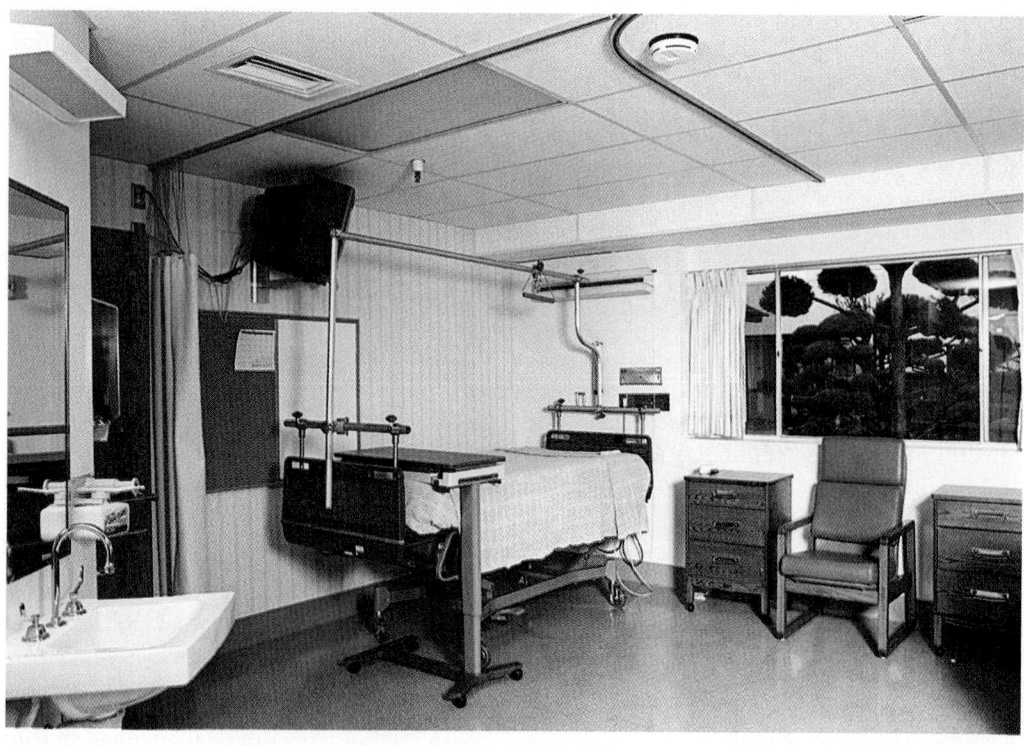

A pleasant environment promotes a sense of well being.

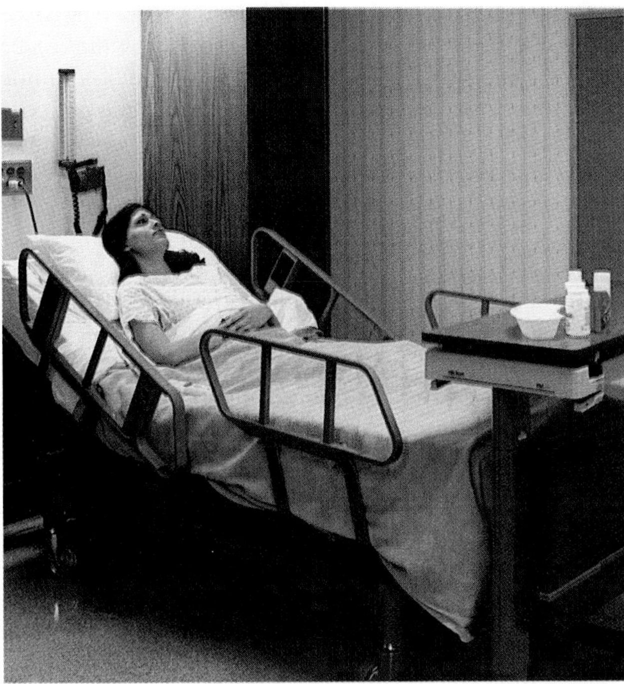
A neat, clean environment helps the client to adjust to the healthcare environment.

bed, with the "head" crank on the left and the "knee" crank on the right. Remember to replace the cranks under the bed when not in use. This placement prevents the hospital staff from running into them. The electric controls are found on the foot, the side of the bed, or on the side rails. When placed at the side, the client can more easily control bed positions. Bed wheels should be equipped with locks. Adjustable full or half side rails are placed on both sides of the client's bed for safety and a sense of security. Hospital policy dictates the use of side rails. One-half or three-fourths rails are normally preferred so clients can get in and out of bed without having to climb over the rails. Always replace them in position when you have completed client care. Most agencies require a signed release by clients who do not want side rails used.

The overbed table is adjustable in height and slides over the bed to provide space for self-care activities or additional working surface for the nurse. The overbed table may also be used when the client sits in a chair. Small bed trays are sometimes convenient when the overbed table cannot be used.

The bedside table, similar to a nightstand, holds the client's personal possessions in drawers. A cabinet section in the table can be used to store bathing or toiletry equipment, and the top provides space for the client's familiar items, such as pictures or books.

A chair with firm back and arm supports should always be a part of the client's furnishing. Chairs should be made of durable, easily cleanable materials, such as plastic or naugahyde. The client should be instructed to avoid contact between skin surfaces and the chair when sitting in a chair. A small towel or blanket can be placed under the client for this purpose.

A signaling system is also essential for the client to call for assistance. A signaling system may be an intercom, buzzer, electric light, or handbell. Whatever device is available must be within the client's reach and ability to use.

Food and Water

Fresh, nourishing food and clean water, are vital to recovering and maintaining health and must be planned for and ensured in appropriate amounts in health care facilities. A client's well-being can be positively affected by the ingestion of the correct number of calories, fat, proteins, carbohydrates, minerals, vitamins, and water, but it is well known that many people have nutritional habits that can negatively affect their well-being. A careful nutritional assessment is a critical step in helping the client adjust to the environment.

Waste Disposal

All waste products, whether contaminated equipment, human body wastes, garbage, soiled dressings, or refuse, must be disposed of in a way that prevents the

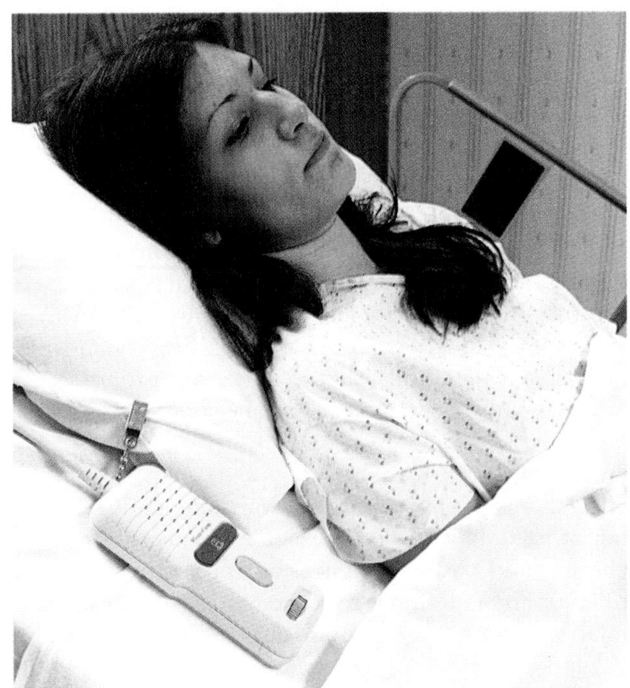
Ensure that call light is within easy reach of client to provide access to nursing staff.

spread of microorganisms. Hospital wastes can be hazardous and highly infective. If wastes cannot be properly removed, the client is at a risk and may not be able to adjust safely and comfortably to the surroundings.

Nurses must be aware of potential dangers to themselves as well as to their clients when disposing of waste materials. Most health care agencies have specific guidelines regarding the removal of various types of contaminated or hazardous materials. Many of these guidelines have been established by experts (epidemiologists) knowledgeable in the detection and spread of disease. The U.S. Public Health Service Centers for Disease Control, the American Hospital Association, and state departments of health are some of the agencies that prepare guidelines for the disposal of dangerous products.

In some health care facilities, a position of infection control nurse has been created to gather data on the type and frequency of various infections found in the hospital. Data about infections help the infection control nurse locate the source of the problem, predict its spread, and identify the best method of preventing its recurrence. Many of the nosocomial (hospital-originated) disease states can be traced to inappropriate or careless disposal of wastes. Each nurse plays a significant role in establishing a safe environment for the client by carrying out the recommended methods of waste disposal.

SOCIOCULTURAL DIMENSIONS

The first two dimensions of the environment, the biologic and physical, or ecosystem, refer to all living and nonliving elements. The third dimension of an environment is sociocultural, which includes both past and present influences from the people and the culture surrounding the individual. Customs, religious and legal systems, and economic and political beliefs are all part of this environment. This dimension also involves responses and adjustments to the ideals, concepts, beliefs, activities, and pressure of various groups, such as social clubs, peer groups, or colleagues.

Organization of Time

How clients perceive and deal with time and the passing of time depend on their age, immediate situation, culture, and past experiences as well as their present physical and emotional condition. To a mother waiting for her child to return from surgery, hours seem like days. Small children generally do not have a well-developed sense of time. A 3-year-old may act out feelings of abandonment when separated from a parent for just a few minutes. In an intensive care unit, time can be severely disrupted, since health care activities continue around the clock. The ability to organize time is a critical element in adaptation. Helping clients assess and plan their time is one of the most important ways you can help them cope with their new surroundings.

Privacy

Many people who enter a health care facility fear exposure and loss of identity. Providing privacy for a client is more than a luxury or a mere courtesy. It is necessary and vitally important to the individual's attitude toward health care.

Clients should be given as much privacy as possible. Most individuals give clues to the nurse about the degree of privacy they need. The client's culture, past experience, values, and age should all be considered when planning for privacy.

Hospital routines should be planned to promote privacy. If an embarrassing or upsetting situation occurs, the feelings of the client must be protected. People require time and space to think, organize, and reflect. Privacy is necessary for human development even at home. In the hospital, privacy is critical to the client's attitude and well-being.

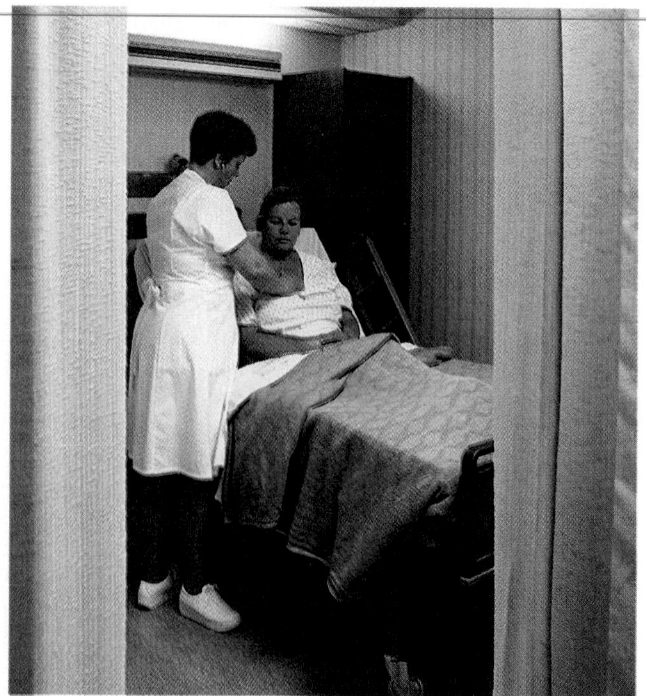

Clients should be given as much privacy as possible by drawing curtains or using screens.

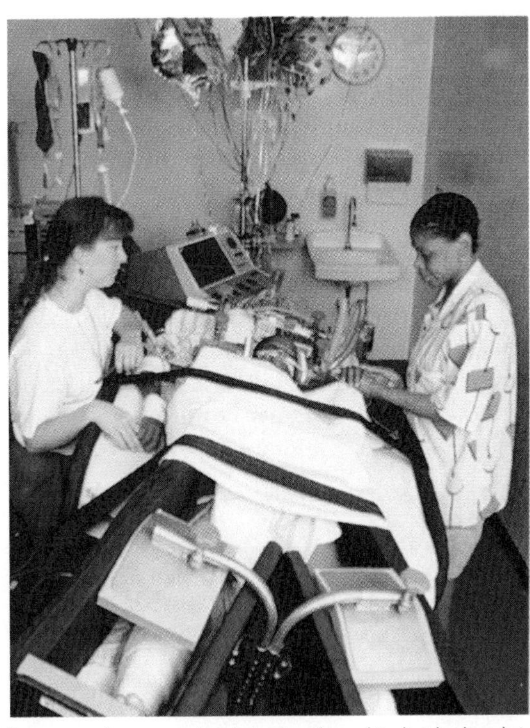

Providing an environment that is both safe and individualized, is a challenging task for the nursing staff.

Privacy can be promoted by drawing curtains or screens. Doors and window shades may also be used. Signs stating "Do Not Enter without checking at desk," posted on room entrances give the client a sense of security from disturbances. This is especially important during physical examinations, personal care, or emotional upset. Knocking or asking for permission to enter the client's room or area promotes mutual respect and enhances a sense of emotional space.

Privacy also extends beyond the physical need of the individual. Health status, conversation, and records are privileged information. A more trusting, therapeutic relationship evolves if the client understands that confidences shared with nurses are used appropriately.

Individualized Care

Providing an environment that is comfortable, safe, and individualized to meet the specific needs of a client is a challenging task. The client's ability to adapt to the immediate environment can either improve or interfere with his or her well-being. To assist the client in adjusting to the environment, a careful assessment of the situation should always include the person's usual routines, self-care abilities, cultural beliefs, and past experiences. To promote the best adaptation to a different environment, encourage as much independence as possible with each client. You may be required to use your resourcefulness, imagination, and ingenuity to assist the client through difficult periods. Open communication from client to staff is essential if positive adaptation is to occur.

Hospitalized clients also need emotional space. This form of space is that psychologic area where the person can experience a sense of self. This is particularly difficult to achieve in a hospital setting when caretakers exercise control over many of the activities of daily living. It is important that the staff be aware of this psychologic need so that they can provide adequate privacy, quiet, and freedom of choice over all of the areas that the client can control. The staff must also be aware that the client rarely needs to relinquish total responsibility for his or her care.

Information and Teaching

The amount of information the client has about the environment and immediate situation directly affects his or her ability to adjust safely and comfortably. When the individual is given information and explanation about strange equipment, diagnostic procedures, or unfamiliar health care personnel, fears and feelings of helplessness can be reduced and a shared sense of responsibility enhanced. The client becomes more

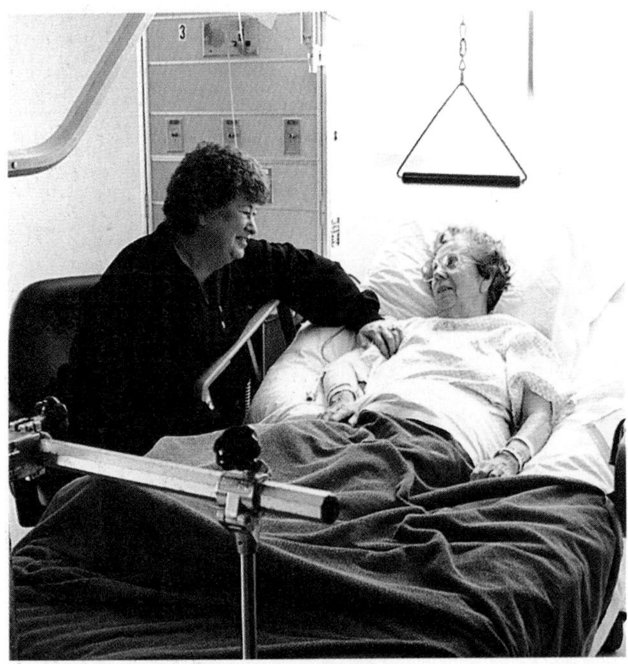

Providing a safe environment involves instructing the client and visitors in safety measures.

capable of asking questions and expressing concerns if prepared for unfamiliar occurrences.

Providing the client and his or her family, if appropriate, with information about the client's environment is the responsibility of the nurse. As more people assume the role of consumers of health care, there is more demand for knowledge about aspects of health care. Including the client in planning and caring for himself or herself promotes a sense of responsibility, independence, and self-respect.

Teaching the client about various aspects of health care is one method of information sharing. Over the years, the focus has changed from the professional staff doing everything for the client to helping the client be more independent. This change enables the client to adapt to the environment with guided assistance from nurses. As the client learns about his or her own health care and becomes involved in meeting his or her particular needs, a sense of trust, responsibility, and usefulness develops.

A SAFE ENVIRONMENT

Providing a safe environment involves a number of people, including the client, visitors, and health care providers. Providing protection from hazardous situations and education about safety precautions is one of your most important responsibilities as a nurse.

Clients who are moved from their usual environment into one that is unfamiliar and often frightening may act in ways that are very different from their usual behavior. A threatening situation can interfere with the individual's adaptation to the immediate surroundings.

The design and decor of the client's room must satisfy two needs: comfort and safety. Tasteful, unobtrusive colors help to normalize the hospital room. Interesting color combinations and patterns generally appeal more to the senses than do the traditional white or green choices. Pictures, flowers, cards, colorful linens, and curtains can add variety and familiarity to a room.

Safety Precautions

The client's age influences the specific safety precautions that need to be taken to provide a safe environment. For example, infants require constant supervision, since they may attempt to put anything in their mouths or noses.

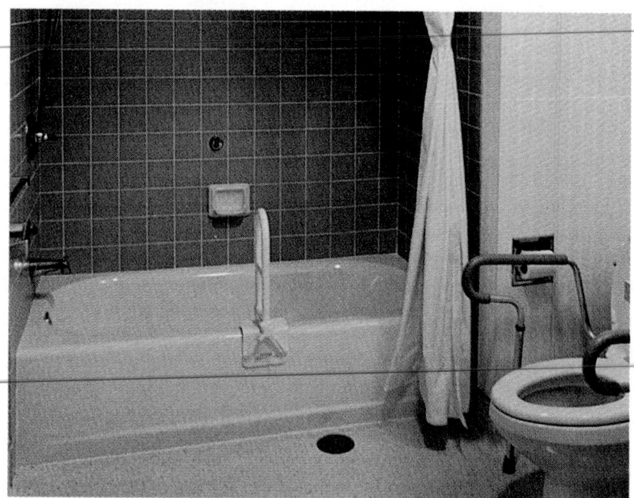

Safety features such as handrails in tub prevent client falls.

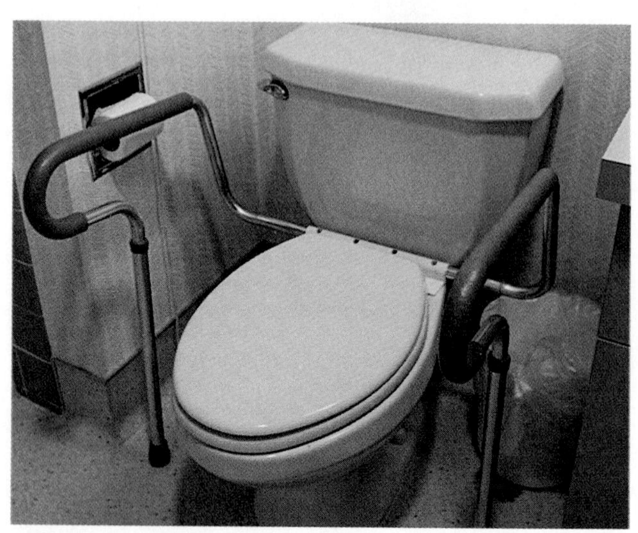

Rails next to the toilet prevent client falls.

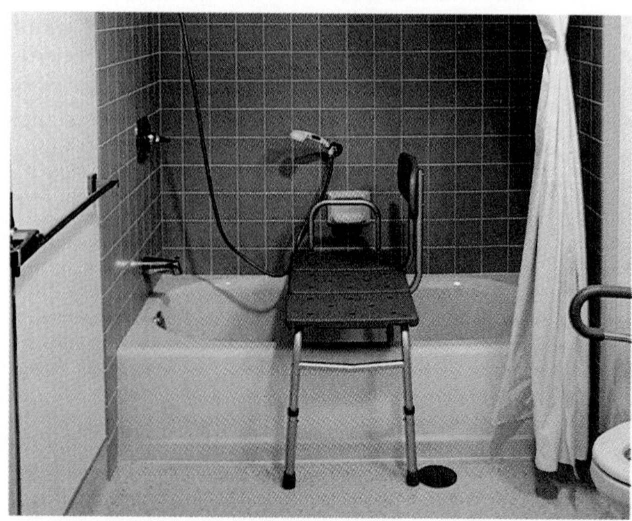

Shower chairs provide for client safety.

Preschool-aged children can be taught more detailed aspects of safety. Fire precautions and guidelines for bathing should be stressed.

Elementary school-aged children can usually protect themselves from hazards. They do, however, require instruction on how to operate mechanical equipment as well as information about fires and emergency exits.

All hospitals in the United States are required to be smoke-free facilities. Teenagers, adolescents, and adults should be given instruction about nonsmoking, the use of special equipment, and emergency exits. In addition, general information regarding their safety during hospitalization should be explained.

SMOKING POLICIES

Joint Commission for Accreditation of Health Care Organizations (JCAHO) standards require hospital smoking policies be disseminated and enforced throughout hospital buildings.

- Directives on smoking policy should be conveyed to each client on admission.
- Smoking is prohibited throughout the hospital.
- A physician may write orders for an exception to this policy for an individual client.
- A designated smoking area may be made available for family or visitors.

Elderly adults are especially susceptible to injury from falls. Poor vision, decreased balance and stability, disorientation, or chronic physical problems such as arthritis contribute to the high incidence of falls among the elderly. Specialized safety equipment, such as toilets and bathtubs with railings or modified seats, are often used in geriatric units to prevent injuries during bathroom use.

It is sometimes difficult to balance the need for client safety with that for autonomy. Use of surveillance by personnel or alarm systems or special monitoring devices provide creative alternatives to the use of restraints in promoting client safety.

Guidelines for the Use of Restraints

Although studies show that the use of restraints does not prevent falls or injury and may be a violation of the client's human rights, they are still deemed appropriate for some clients. The clients for whom restraints may be necessary include: the wandering mentally impaired; the unconscious; the unsafely mobile; those who are so active that essential care measures cannot be implemented; and the physically aggressive. Restraint use must be based on documented client behavior and should be applied only as a result of collaborative decision making among health team members.

Restraints should be a last resort and are legal only if necessary to protect the client or others from foreseeable harm. Clients may refuse their use or a nurse may be charged with assault if restraints are used when not needed. A nurse may also be charged with negligence when not using restraints when they have been medically ordered.

A physician's order must be specific regarding the purpose, type of restraint, and length of time to be used. Restraints are not to be ordered as prn. In an emergency, however, a nurse can legally restrain a client without an order. The use of restraints increases nursing responsibility.

The decision to use restraints should trigger further assessment and planning to correct the problem leading to the need for restraints.

If restraints are necessary, these guidelines should be followed.

- Review hospital policy for the use of restraints.
- Use restraints for the client's protection, not for the nurse's convenience.
- Use the least amount of restraint possible.
- Allow clients as much freedom of movement as possible. Use slip knots for quick release. Do not use square knots.
- Always explain the purpose of the restraint to the client and family.
- Remember that restraints can cause emotional, mental, and physical deterioration and increase the risk of injury if falls occur.
- Remember that circulation and skin integrity can be affected by restraints.
- Special precautions should be taken for adult females in restraints to protect breast tissue.
- Release restraints every 2 hours to inspect areas and provide joint range of motion to prevent circulatory impairment or broken skin. When a client is combative, release only one restraint at a time.
- Pad bony prominences, such as wrist and ankles, beneath a restraint.
- Attempt to make restraints as inconspicuous as possible for the sake of the client's relatives and friends, who may be upset by seeing restraints.
- Clearly document rationale and precautions taken for client safety.
- Assess client's fluid and elimination needs every 2 hours.

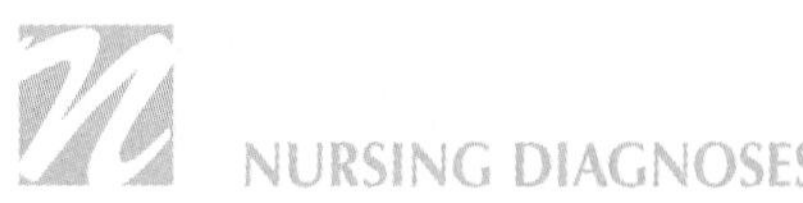

NURSING DIAGNOSES

The following nursing diagnoses may be appropriate to include in a client care plan when the components are related to maintaining a safe environment.

NURSING DIAGNOSIS	RELATED FACTORS/RISK FACTORS
Risk for Injury	Motor, sensory, or cognitive alterations; incontinence; bleeding tendency; physiologic instability due to medications or illness; environmental hazards; fire hazards.
Sensory-Perceptual Alteration	Substance abuse, altered sensory function, altered environmental conditions
Impaired Tissue Integrity	Restraints, chemical irritants or thermal factors, mechanical factors, trauma
Risk for Trauma	Altered cerebral function, mobility, impaired sensory function

unit 1

A SAFE ENVIRONMENT

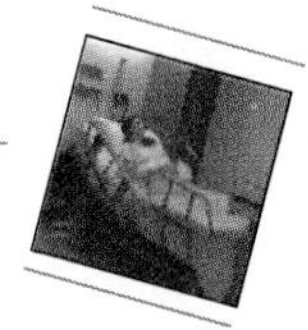

NURSING PROCESS DATA

ASSESSMENT Data Base

Identify client's age, previous or chronic sensory impairments, previous level of mobility, ambulatory aids used, and general health history.

Observe and record client's present level of consciousness, orientation, mobility, and restrictions.

Identify any impending loss of sensory or motor abilities due to illness or injury.

Evaluate client's ability to comprehend instruction about how to use potentially dangerous equipment.

Assess need for specific devices to promote a safe environment.

Assess type of fire extinguisher needed for specific types of fires or use ABC extinguisher.

Assess the need for protection while administering care to clients with radioactive implant.

Evaluate client's ability to make judgments.

Assess the client's reliability as an accurate health historian.

PLANNING Objectives

To assist client to interpret environmental stimuli relevant to his or her safety

To provide protection when states of illness decrease the individual's ability to receive and interpret environmental stimuli

To enhance degrees of mobility in a safe environment

To determine that all electrical equipment is intact and operated safely

To place all personal articles and call light within easy reach of client

To determine safety equipment necessary to promote a safe environment

To determine the protective devices needed when caring for clients receiving radioactive material

IMPLEMENTATION Procedures

Preventing Mechanical Injuries

Preventing Thermal Injuries

Providing Safety for Clients during a Fire

Providing Safety for Clients Receiving Radioactive Materials

EVALUATION Expected Outcomes

Client receives information regarding mechanical, chemical, and thermal safety precautions appropriate to his or her needs.

Client's immediate environment is safe from potential mechanical, chemical, and thermal hazards.

All electrical equipment is intact and operated safely.

If oxygen is used, appropriate safety measures are in effect.

All personal articles and call light are within easy reach of the client.

Personnel are protected from radioactive material.

PREVENTING MECHANICAL INJURIES

Equipment

Side rails

Restraints

Locks for movable equipment, such as wheelchairs and guerneys

Procedure

1. Orient new clients to their surroundings. Include use of call light and emergency signal in bathroom.
2. Put bed in low position when you are not providing direct client care.
3. Tell clients who are weak, sedated, in pain, or who have had surgery to ask for assistance before getting out of bed.
4. Make sure floors are free of debris that might cause clients to slip and fall. Spilled liquids should be wiped up immediately. Encourage housekeepers to use signs for slippery areas.
5. Check to see that client's unit and hallway are neat and free of hazardous obstacles, such as foot stools, electrical cords, or shoes.
6. Place articles, such as call light and cups, within the client's reach.
7. Remind client and hospital personnel to lock wheelchairs and guerneys and to release the lock only after client is secure for transport.
8. Keep full side rails up for all confused, sedated, elderly, seizure, and surgical clients.
9. Keep top side rails up for all clients.
10. Secure physician's specific orders if restraints are deemed necessary.
11. Use two staff to transport client on guerney or wheelchair when nonattached equipment, such as chest-tube system or IV poles must accompany client in transport.
12. Instruct ambulatory client in use of toilet and shower controls and emergency signals in bathroom.

PREVENTING THERMAL INJURIES

Equipment

Fire extinguishers

Covers for heat and cold application devices

Procedure

1. Make sure that all electrical appliances are routinely checked and maintained.
2. Have all electrical appliances brought to the hospital by client (radios, electric razors, etc.) checked by hospital maintenance staff. It is best to discourage use of nonhospital equipment.
3. Make sure water in the tub or shower is not more than 110°F.
4. When heating pads, sitz bath, or hot compresses are used, check the client frequently for redness. Maximum temperature should not exceed 105°F.
5. Hospitals do not allow smoking in the facility. There may be designated smoking areas outside the building. Inform clients and visitors about the hospital's smoking regulations. Do not allow confused, sedated, or severely incapacitated clients to smoke without direct supervision.
6. Store all combustible materials securely to prevent spontaneous combustion.
7. Make sure that all staff and employees participate in and understand fire safety measures, such as extinguishing fires and evacuating clients.

CLINICAL ALERT

The elderly, diabetic, or comatose client is especially vulnerable to thermal injuries.

PROVIDING SAFETY FOR CLIENTS DURING A FIRE

Equipment

Appropriate extinguisher for fire:
- Water type
- Soda-acid type
- Foam type
- Dry chemical type
- Carbon dioxide type
- ABC extinguisher

Procedure

1. Follow hospital policy and procedure for type of fire safety program and for ringing the fire alarm to summon help.
2. Secure the burning area by closing all doors and windows.
3. Shut off all possible oxygen sources and electrical appliances in the fire area.
4. Remove all clients from the immediate area to a safe place. Be familiar with fire exits.
5. To remove a client safely from the fire, use carrying method that is most comfortable for you and safe for client.
   a. Place blanket (or bedspread) on floor. Lower client onto blanket. Lift up head end of blanket and drag client out of danger.
   b. Use two-person swing method. Place client in sitting position. Form a seat by having two people clasp forearms or shoulders. Lift client into "seat" and carry out of danger.
   c. Carry client using "back-strap" carry method. Step in front of client. Place client's arms around your neck. Grasp client's wrists and hold tight against your chest. Pull client onto your back and carry to safety.
6. If possible, employ the appropriate extinguishing method without endangering yourself. Fire extinguisher should not be used directly on a person.
7. Be familiar with the different types of fire extinguishers and their location.

Class A
   a. Water-under-pressure type or soda-acid type
   b. Use on cloth, wood, paper, plastic, rubber, leather.
   c. Never use on electrical or chemical fires due to danger of shock.

Class B
   a. Foam, dry chemical, carbon dioxide types
   b. Use on fires such as gasoline, alcohol, acetone, oil, grease, or paint thinner and remover.
   c. Class A extinguisher is never used on class B fires.

Class C
   a. Dry chemical or carbon dioxide types
   b. Use on electrical wiring, electrical equipment, or motors.
   c. Class A or class B extinguishers are never used on a class C fires.

Class ABC combination
   a. Contains graphite
   b. Use on any type of fire.
   c. Most common extinguisher in use

8. Keep fire exits clear at all times.

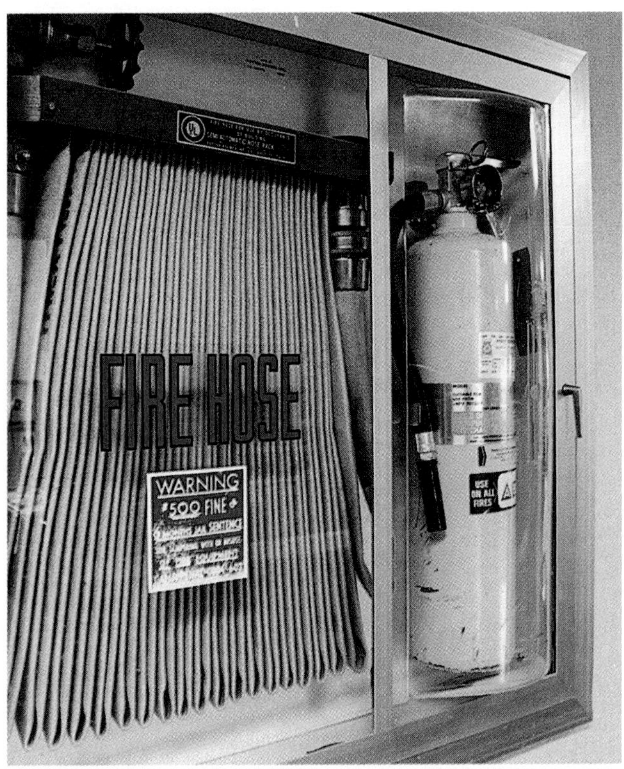

Become familiar with the use of fire extinguisher in the hospital.

PROVIDING SAFETY FOR CLIENTS RECEIVING RADIOACTIVE MATERIALS

Equipment

Protective shields for x-ray
Lead-shielded container if required
Film badge if required
Sign for client's door: "Caution, Radioactive Material"

> **■ CLINICAL ALERT**
>
> Pregnant nurses should check hospital policy regarding working with clients receiving radioactive materials.

Procedure

1. Review these guidelines
   a. Determine the type and amount of radiation used and its side effects and hazards.
   b. Increased time in the presence of a radioactive source increases exposure to radiation. Rotate care providers.
   c. Shields, such as lead walls or lead aprons, are used as protection from radioactive source.
   d. Exposure is greater the closer the person is to the radioactive source.
   e. When not in use, radioactive material must be stored in lead-shielded containers.
2. If nurse or family member is assisting with a radioactive procedure, they must put on a shield.
3. If a radioactive implant is used in a client, all nurses and visitors must be protected with a shield. Limit exposure with the client.
4. Keep track of how much time is spent in the presence of radioactive material. Request film badge if in area where ionizing radiation is used frequently.
5. Constantly assess and support clients who are undergoing radiation therapy. Bedrest, isolation, and unpleasant side effects are sometimes common.
6. Follow guidelines for working with clients with unsealed sources of Iodine-131.
   a. Wear rubber gloves at all times when providing care.
   b. Wash gloves before removing, and place in designated waste container.
   c. Wash hands with soap and water after removing gloves.
   d. Dispose of all bed linen in contaminated linen bag.
   e. Wrap all nondisposable items that have come in contact with client's blood, saliva, or gastric juices in plastic bag. Send to appropriate hospital department for decontamination (usually nuclear medicine department).
   f. Notify radiation safety officer (usually in radiology department) if clothes or shoes have been contaminated.

GENERAL GUIDELINES FOR RADIATION PRECAUTIONS*

Radioactive Implant

Private room: client should not leave room.
Care time not to exceed 15 minutes per employee per day.
No pregnant woman or anyone under age 18 should enter room.
No special handling of excreta other than universal precautions.
Bath usually omitted, client movement restricted.
Visitors limited to 1 hour/day, keeping distance from client.
All linens, gloves, trash, dressings, and so on kept in room until cleared by radiation safety officer.

Systemic Radioactive Material

No lab specimens to be taken without consent of radiation safety officer.
Use disposable dietary tray.
Handle all excreta and secretions with gloves.
Have client use toilet—flushing twice.
Shielding not needed.
No visitors without special instructions.
Keep gloves, dressings, linens, trash in contaminated container.

* Note: See Institutional Policy for Specifics.

CHARTING for Providing a Safe Environment

- Assessment notes
- Actual incidents involving mechanical, chemical, or thermal trauma
- Client education given
- Safety devices used

CRITICAL THINKING APPLICATION

CLINICAL PROBLEMS	CRITICAL THINKING OPTIONS
The client, nurse, or visitor experiences an accident or injury related to mechanical, chemical, or thermal trauma.	• Provide immediate first aid or care. • Assess vital signs, and notify physician. • Report the incident according to hospital procedure. Unusual occurrence forms are used to protect the injured individual as well as the nurse and the hospital. • Review safety procedures to ensure a safe environment. • Report all malfunctioning equipment immediately to the proper department.
Unfamiliarity with hospital fire and disaster protocol results in poor performance.	• Review protocols frequently to update knowledge base. • Participate in fire and disaster drills to become familiar with protocols.
Radium implant becomes dislodged and falls out.	• Put on lead gloves and pick up radium with forceps and place in lead-shielded container in client's room. • Notify physician and hospital radiation safety officer immediately. • Never touch radioactive source directly.
Spillage of excreta from client with systemic radioactive therapy.	• Cover spillage with absorbent material and notify radiation safety officer. • Wash with soap and water if skin contaminated. Notify radiation safety officer.

unit 2 RESTRAINTS

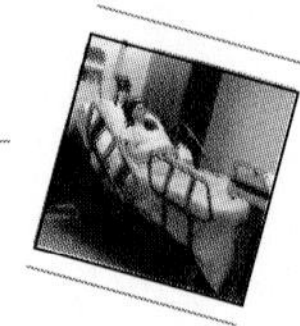

NURSING PROCESS DATA

ASSESSMENT Data Base

Assess need for restraints.
Identify appropriate type of restraint needed.
Assess area under and surrounding a restraint to ensure it is not restrictive.
Evaluate the affected extremity for circulation, sensation, and movement.

PLANNING Objectives

To identify clients who are at risk for injury
To obtain physician's order for restraints if deemed necessary
To prevent a client from injuring himself (herself) or others
To apply restraints safely and effectively
To restrain a child's elbow to prevent the child from reaching an incision
To promote client safety when ambulating or sitting in a chair

IMPLEMENTATION Procedures

Using Wrist Restraints
Using Mitt Restraints
Using Elbow Restraints
Applying a Safety Belt
Applying a Chest Restraint
Applying Mummy Restraints

EVALUATION Expected Outcomes

Restraints are applied appropriately.
Injuries to surrounding tissue are avoided when restraints are applied.
Client is prevented from injuring himself (herself) or others.
Child is prevented from reaching the incision site.

USING WRIST RESTRAINTS

Equipment

Kerlix gauze
Cloth restraints with flannel padding
Ace bandages of appropriate size for area to be immobilized
Call bell for communication

Procedure

1. Check physician's order for soft restraints if required.
2. Obtain Kerlix gauze or cloth restraint with flannel padding.

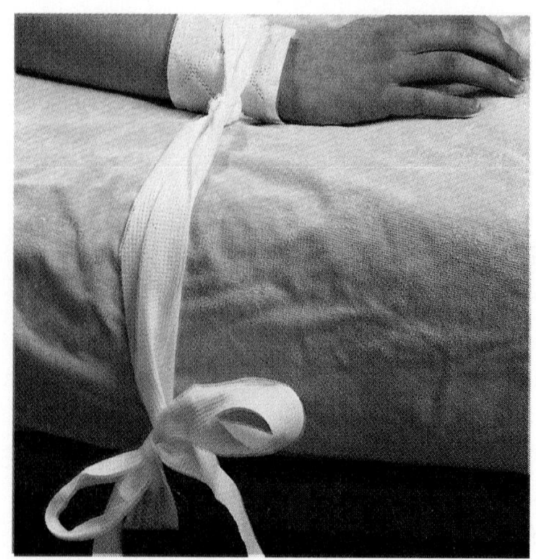

Tie soft wrist restraints firmly on bed frame.

3. When using Kerlix gauze, make a clove hitch to place over wrist or ankle, and secure under bed.
4. When using cloth restraint, place padded section over the wrist or ankle, wrap restraint around the wrist, and slide the strap through the slit in the wrist area. Tighten the strap securely, but maintain adequate circulation. Fasten strap under the bed frame.
5. Check limbs every 2 hours for circulation and skin condition.
6. Change client's position every 2 hours.
7. Release restraints every 2 hours, and administer skin care.
8. Put extremities through range of motion every 2 hours.
9. Document use of wrist restraints in nurses' notes.

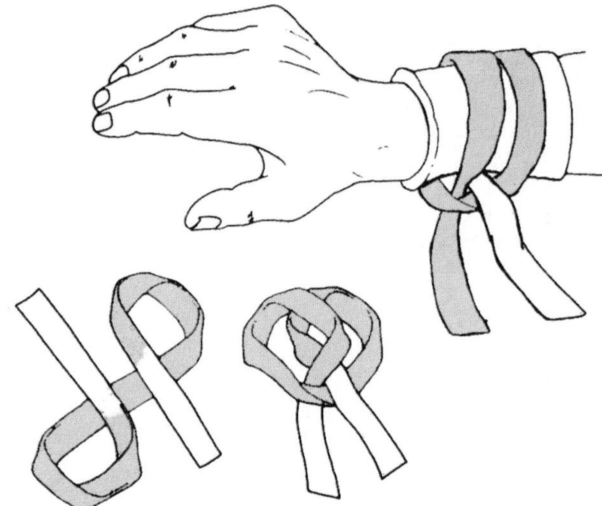

Clove hitch restraint.

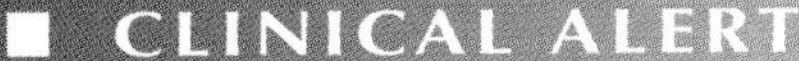

■ CLINICAL ALERT

If using leather restraints as wrist restraints, keep the key in client's room taped to the wall or top of bed. It must be in sight and easily accessible in case of emergency.

USING MITT RESTRAINTS

Equipment

Mitt restraint
Gauze padding
Call bell for communication

Procedure

1. Check physician's order or unit policy for use of soft restraint.

■ CLINICAL ALERT

Restraints are never used as a substitute for surveillance.

2. Check nursing care plan or Kardex for specifics.
3. Wash hands.
4. Obtain mitt restraint and gauze padding, if needed.
5. Identify the client by checking identaband.
6. Explain steps and purpose of procedure to client (to gain his or her cooperation) if client is able to understand.
7. Raise bed to high position.
8. Lower side rail.
9. Check condition of skin and circulation in involved extremity.
10. Wrap fingers with gauze to absorb moisture and prevent abrasion, if necessary.
11. Apply mitt; secure wrist ties snugly, but maintain circulation.
12. For hand control, tie restraints to immovable part of bed frame, not to side rail.
13. Place call light within easy reach for client, and monitor client frequently for safety.
14. Remove mitt every 2 hours to check adequacy of circulation, and skin condition, and provide range of motion.
15. Put extremity through range of motion.
16. Reposition client for comfort, and reapply mitt.

17. Raise bedrail and lower bed.
18. Wash hands.
19. Chart on nurses' notes: client behavior necessitating restraint; condition of skin and adequacy of circulation of involved extremity; time and site of mitt application; time of release and reaction of client.

USING ELBOW RESTRAINTS

Equipment

Elbow restraint
Soft padding

Procedure

1. Check physician's order and client care plan for elbow restraints.
2. Obtain elbow restraints (many types are available).
3. Explain necessity of restraints to child's parents.
4. Place restraints over elbow of both arms. You may need to insert tongue blades into pockets of restraint.
5. Wrap restraints snugly around the arm. Secure by tying the restraints at the top. Many restraints have ties long enough to cross under the child's back and tie under the opposite arm.
6. For small infants and children, tie or pin restraints to their shirts.
7. Release the restraints every 2 hours to allow joint mobility.
8. Assess position of restraints, circulation, skin condition, and sensation every hour.
9. Provide diversionary activity for small child.
10. Encourage parents or hospital personnel to hold child to promote a feeling of security.
11. Document use of restraints in nurses' notes.

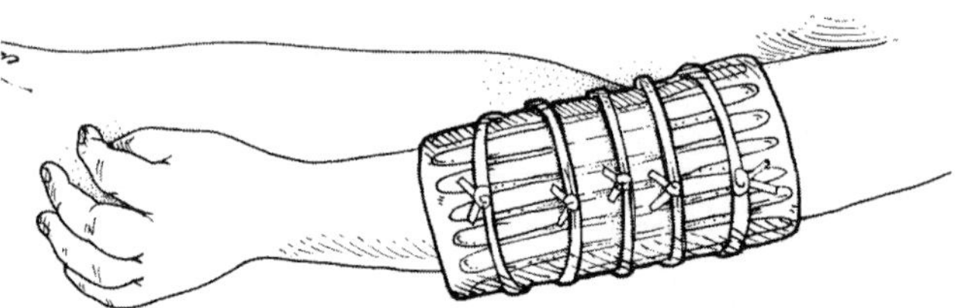

Elbow restraints prevent children from reaching equipment.

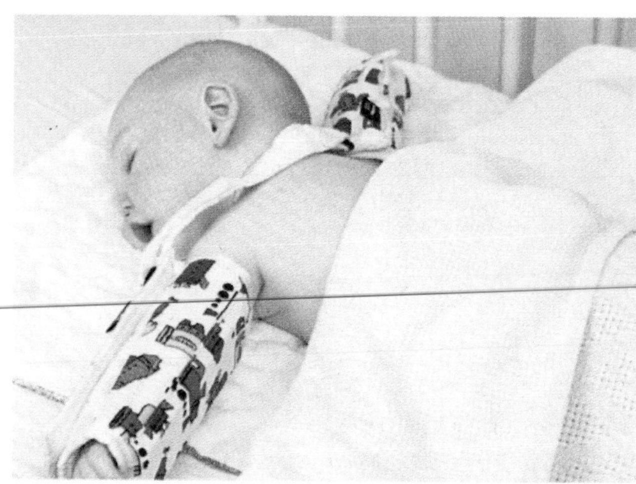

Elbow restraints may be used to prevent child from reaching his or her face or head.

APPLYING A SAFETY BELT

Equipment

Safety belt

Procedure

1. Check physician's order and client care plan for safety belt restraint.
2. Obtain safety belt. (Belts usually have a buckle to prevent slipping and to provide a snug fit.)
3. Explain necessity for safety belt to client.
4. Apply safety belt as follows:
   a. If client is ambulating, place belt around client's waist.
   b. If client is on a guerney, CircOlectric bed, or Stryker frame, fasten belt around client's abdomen.
   c. If client is in a wheelchair, place belt around client's abdomen and under arm rests, and secure in back.
5. If strap does not have a buckle, tie the belt in a slip knot to allow for quick removal in an emergency.
6. Document use of safety belt in nurses' notes.

APPLYING A CHEST RESTRAINT

Equipment

Safety vest
Call bell for communication

Procedure

1. Check physician's order and client care plan.
2. Explain necessity for jacket restraint to client and family.
3. Place jacket restraint over gown.
4. If using a safety vest rather than a jacket restraint, place safety vest on client so that closed side of vest is in back and front side of vest crosses over chest. **Rationale:** This prevents choking if client slumps forward.
5. Bring strap through slit in front of the vest. **Rationale:** Criss-crossing vest in the back may cause serious injury.
6. Tie straps to nonmovable part of spring frame, wheelchair kickspur, or geriatric chair frame. **Rationale:** This position minimizes risk of inadvertent release, which may cause subsequent injury.
7. Observe client frequently to ensure proper fit of jacket.
8. Document use of restraints in nurses' notes.

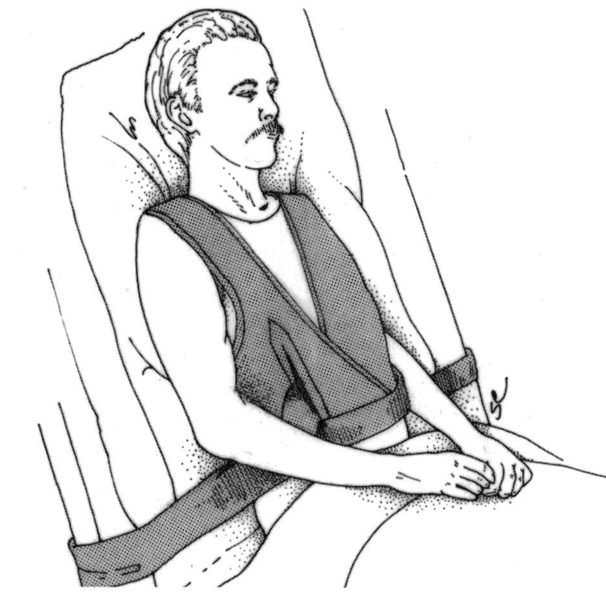

Restraints are most often used for the safety of the client.

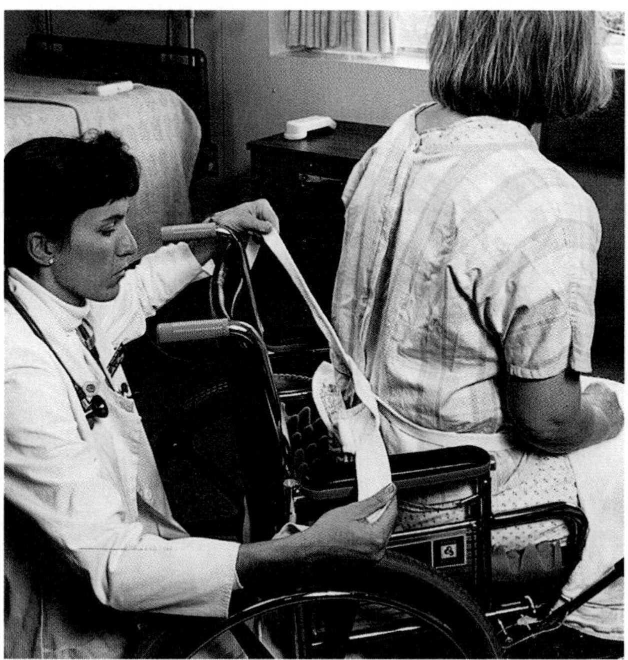

Place closed side of jacket restraint in back of client.

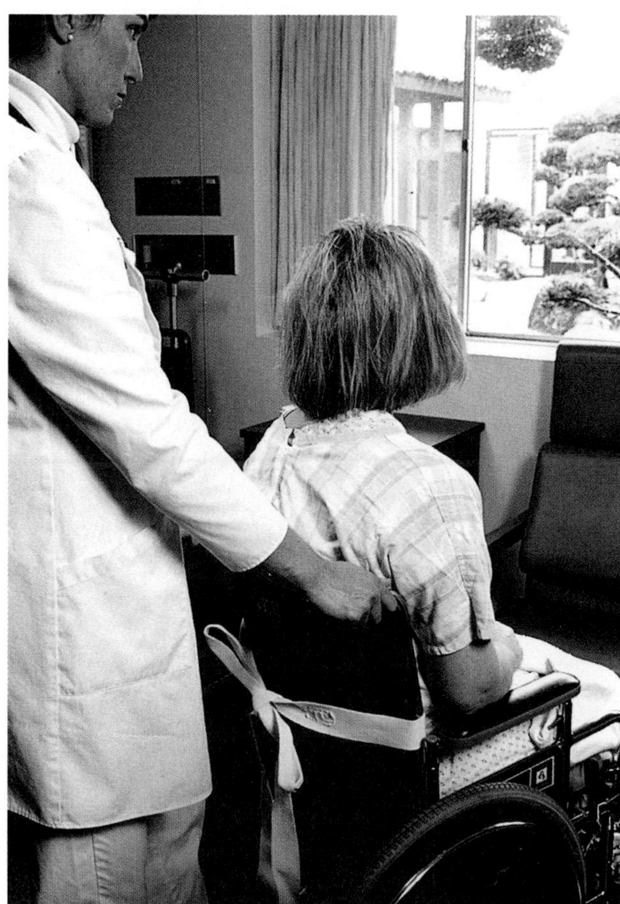

Tie jacket restraint securely at back of wheelchair.

APPLYING MUMMY RESTRAINTS

Equipment

Blanket large enough to fit child

Procedure

1. Place the blanket on a secure surface.
2. Fold down one corner of the blanket until the tip reaches the middle of the blanket.
3. Place the baby in a diagonal position with the head halfway off the folded edge of the blanket.
4. Bring one side of the blanket over the infant's arm and trunk, and tuck it under the other arm and around the back.
5. Tuck the bottom part of the blanket up onto the infant's abdomen.
6. Fold the second side over the infant, and tuck it snugly around the body.

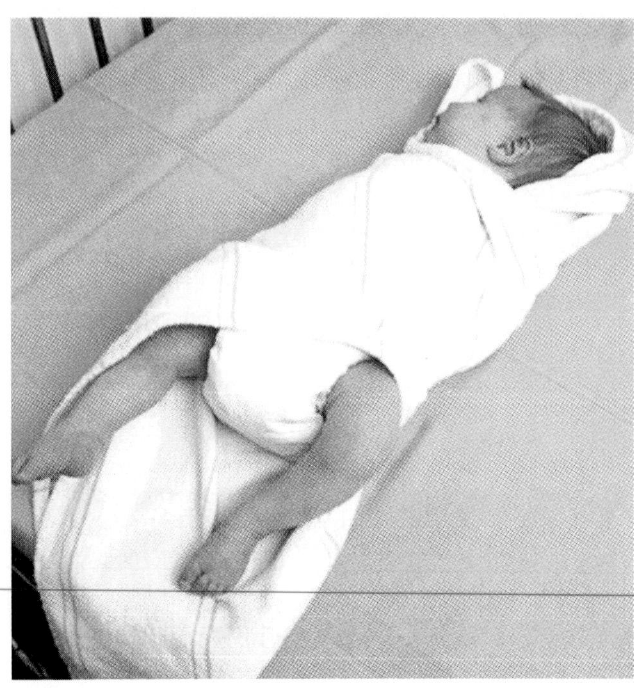

A mummy restraint is used when necessary for safety of the infant.

> Mummy boards with Velcro straps are used more often in the hospital setting. A diaper or Chux is placed on the board, the infant is placed on the board and secured with the Velcro straps.

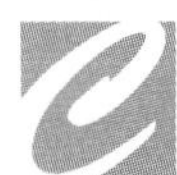

CHARTING for Applying Restraints

- Time and type of restraint applied
- Rationale for applying restraints
- Condition of extremity following application: skin color and temperature
- Time of removal and reapplication of restraint
- Effectiveness of restraint
- Client's tolerance of restraint

9

Bathing and Bedmaking

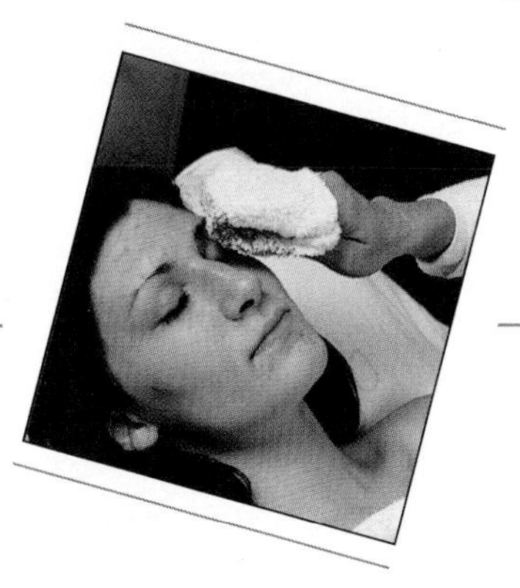

LEARNING OBJECTIVES

- Compare and contrast the steps in making an occupied, unoccupied, and surgical bed.
- Demonstrate the skill of folding a mitered corner.
- Outline the steps in bathing a bedridden adult client.
- Differentiate between bathing a bedridden client and a critically ill client.
- Compare and contrast the differences in bathing an infant and an adult client.
- Describe the assessment modalities completed while bathing a client.
- Outline the steps in providing morning care.
- Describe briefly the components of evening care.
- Define the three back care strokes and their use in back care.
- Complete client charting for evening care on nurses' notes.
- Write three nursing diagnoses appropriate for providing basic hygienic care to clients.

TERMINOLOGY

Bedmaking

Anesthesia (surgical, recovery) bed: a bed made in a specific manner for the client who is returning to the bed after having anesthesia or surgery.

Closed bed: a bed not being used by a client; the linens are left to cover the bed.

Occupied bed: the client remains in the bed while it is being made.

Open bed: a bed being used by a client; the linens are folded down.

Unoccupied bed: the client is out of the bed while it is being made.

Equipment Used with Beds

Aside from the standard types of equipment used on the basic hospital bed, specialized equipment can be added to meet the client's health care needs.

Balkan (overbed) frame: an overhead bed bar(s) used to support a trapeze, or a series of pulleys and weights used for traction equipment.

Bed cradle: a device attached to the lower end of the bed to prevent the bed linens from resting on the client's legs or feet. It is often used when a client has burns, ulcers, a wet cast, or specific circulatory diseases.

Footboard: usually a solid support placed on the bed where the soles of the feet touch. It is secured to the mattress or bed frame. Footboards are used to prevent permanent plantar flexion (footdrop) and to exercise leg muscles. The footboard may also have side supports to help maintain proper alignment of feet.

Sheets for Bedmaking

Contour sheets: sheets that have elastic at each corner; fitted sheets.

Drawsheets: sheets made of fabric, plastic, or rubber that are placed across the shoulder-to-knee area of the bed and tucked in on the sides.

Full sheets: regular full-length flat sheets that can be used as the top and bottom sheet.

Incontinent pads: large, disposable pads that can be placed under the buttocks area, head, drains, or any place where excess moisture or fluid may collect on the bed.

Pull sheets: sheets placed across the shoulder-to-knee area of the bed. The sides are not tucked under the mattress. The sheet is kept wrinkle-free and folded under the client. Pull sheets are used to lift the client in the bed.

Levels of Personal Care

Complete care: the client requires total assistance from the nurse because he or she is able to do little or nothing for him or herself. Complete bathing, skin care, oral care, nail and hair care, care of the feet, eyes, ears, and nose, and a total bed linen change are usually provided.

Early morning care: this type of care may or may not be a routine in some hospitals. If early morning care is provided, it is usually given by the night shift nurses. It may include bathing the hands and face, use of the bedpan or urinal, oral care, and other preparations before breakfast.

Evening care (H.S. care, hour of sleep care): evening care is usually provided to prepare the client for a relaxing, uninterrupted period of sleep. Activities include oral care, partial bathing, skin care and a soothing back massage, straightening or changing the bed linen, and offering the bedpan or urinal. The client should also be assessed for the need of food, drink, or medication before sleep.

O.R. care: clients who will be undergoing surgery or diagnostic tests may be required to bathe the evening before. Partial bathing is sometimes allowed in the morning if time permits. If the client is not allowed to have anything by mouth, care must be taken not to allow swallowing of water or dentifrice while providing oral care. The client is usually given a clean gown. All dentures, hairpins, make-up, nail polish, contact lenses, and jewelry are removed. Valuables are locked up. The client is encouraged to void before leaving for the operating room.

Partial care: the client performs as much of his or her own care as possible. The nurse completes the remaining care.

Skin Care

Acne: skin condition due to irritation and infection of the sebaceous glands.

Bedsore: a synonym for decubitus or pressure ulcer—area of cellular necrosis due to decreased circulation.

Blanching: a whitish hue to an area of the skin.

Ecchymosis: collection of blood underneath skin surface; bruise.

Emollient: soothing, softening agent applied to body surfaces.

Epidermis: superficial, or top, layer of skin.

Erythema: redness of skin associated with rashes, infections, and allergic responses.

Hyperemia: influx of blood into an area causing redness to the skin.

Ischemia: decreased, insufficient blood supply to body area.

Lesion: an area of broken skin.

Necrosis: cellular death.

Pediculosis: infestation of lice.

Pediculus capitis: head lice.

Pediculus corporis: body lice.

Pediculus pubis: crab lice.

Petechiae: pinpoint reddish spots.

Pressure ulcer: a synonym for bedsore or pressure sore area of cellular necrosis due to decreased circulation.

Purpura: reddish purple area.

Shearing force: layers of skin moving on each other.

Turgor: the degree of elasticity of the skin.

Back Care

Effleurage: long stroking motions of the hands up and down the back. Hands do not leave the skin surface. Pressure is light.

Petrissage: pinching of the skin, subcutaneous tissue, and muscle as you move up and down the client's back.

Tapotement: alternate striking of fleshy part of hands on client's back as you move up and down the back.

GENERAL TERMINOLOGY

Assessment: critical evaluation of information; the first step in the nursing process.

Complete bath: all areas of the body are bathed. This bath can be done completely by the nurse or by the client.

Cyanosis: blueness of the skin.

Erythema: a redness of the skin due to congestion of the capillaries.

Excreta: waste matter; materials cast out by the body.

Fissure: a groove, slit, or natural division; ulcer or crack-like sore.

Flush: a redness of the face and neck.

Hypoallergenic: against allergy, as hypoallergenic tape.

Incurvate: curved, especially inward.

Inflammation: swelling, pain, heat, and redness of tissue.

Intervention: the act of coming between, so as to hinder or modify.

Jaundice: yellowish appearance caused by deposition of bile pigment in the skin.

Mucosa: mucous membrane lining passages and cavities communicating with the air.

Pallor: paleness; absence of skin coloration.

Partial bath: certain parts of the body are bathed such as the face, hands, under arms, back and perineal area. Another definition of a partial bath is a bath that occurs when the nurse bathes areas which the client cannot reach and the client washes all other areas.

Pigment: any normal or abnormal coloring of the skin.

Plaque: a patch on the skin or on a mucous surface; a blood platelet.

Pressure point: area for exerting pressure to control bleeding; an area of skin that can become irritated with pressure, especially over bony prominences.

Sensory deprivation: enforced absence of usual and accustomed sensory stimuli.

Sensory overload: too much stimuli for the senses to adjust to at once.

Ulcer: an open sore or lesion of the skin or mucous membrane of the body.

BASIC HEALTH CARE

Clients enter the hospital environment because of an accident or acute illness requiring immediate care, or because the physician has recommended diagnostic procedures or surgery. The latter is commonly referred to as an "elective admission." Whatever the reason, the client must rapidly alter everyday routines and activities of daily living. The client may be concerned about his or her health and well-being and may experience varying degrees of anxiety as a reaction to unfamiliar procedures, hospital personnel, and the hospital environment.

After the client has been admitted to the health care unit, many independent actions, such as bathing, personal hygiene, and general care, may be curtailed by the nature of the illness and confinement. The client may require assistance with even the simplest of actions. Without therapeutic intervention, the total adaptation process may be put in jeopardy as additional physical problems occur.

Knowing when and how to intervene and performing such skills as bedmaking, bathing, and personal hygiene facilitate the client's process of adapting to the health care.

When the client is confined to bed even for a short time, comfort is essential in order to promote rest and sleep. Beds must be kept clean, free of debris and wrinkles, to prevent skin irritation and breakdown. The bed needs to be straightened frequently during the day to accomplish this. If the client is to remain in bed for an extended time, all care and daily routines are directed from bed. It becomes the center of activity.

There are many different types of beds and related equipment available to meet the special health care needs of individual clients.

Types of Beds

The hospital bed is a standard twin size bed in a frame that allows for different positions to facilitate care and comfort for the client. The height, head, and foot positions in most beds are electrically operated to assist both the client and the nursing staff. The nurse instructs the client in the proper use of bed controls and in bed positions that could be dangerous for the client.

The Stryker or Foster frame bed is generally used for individuals who are unable to move, such as those with spinal cord injuries, and for clients who must be placed in the prone position, such as those with decubitus ulcers. Canvas pieces are attached to a frame, which is placed over the client. It is then secured to the lower section of the frame so the client can be flipped over to the reverse position. The upper frame is then removed.

Another type of bed is the circular frame, an electrically operated bed that is attached to a circular frame. The client can be placed in a variety of positions with the support of an upper frame. The client can gradually be raised to a standing position or can be placed in the prone position. Circular beds can be operated by one person, although it is strongly advised to use two people.

The recovery room bed is an adaptation of the basic hospital bed. This bed has the same features as the basic bed but is usually nonelectric. It is generally narrower and has side rails all the way around the bed instead of a head and footboard. It is easily movable and is occasionally used in intensive care units, labor rooms, and emergency rooms.

Two other special types of beds are air and artificial fluid beds. These beds are most commonly used for clients with poor wound healing or severe skin conditions, such as pressure ulcers or burns. These beds are frequently used in oncology and orthopedic units and in geriatric facilities. Instead of the standard mattress, a specially designed heavy plastic casing is filled with artificial fluid or air and serves as the mattress. They are used to create less pressure on weight-bearing areas of the body.

Bathing

Routine bathing is an essential component of daily care. It is essential to prevent body odor, because excessive perspiration interacts with bacteria to cause odor. Dead skin cells can lead to infection if impaired skin integrity occurs. Excessive bathing, on the other hand, can be dangerous to elderly patients. In the aged, the skin may become dry and cracked, which can also lead to infection.

Bathing promotes a feeling of self-worth by improving the person's appearance. Relaxation and improved circulation are benefits of bathing and play a therapeutic role in the care of clients on bedrest. The apocrine glands, found in the axillae and pubic areas, produce sweat, which leads to odor. Therefore, special bathing considerations should be given to these areas.

In addition to the therapeutic effects, the bath affords the nurse time to spend in communication and assessment. Assessment of skin conditions, mobility, and self-care deficits can be detected while bathing the client.

Bathing is accomplished in a variety of ways, according to the client's needs, condition, and personal habits. Bathing is necessary to cleanse the skin and to

TABLE 9–1. Potential Skin Problems

Skin Condition	Problem	Nursing Responsibility
Xeroderma, or dry skin	If skin is extremely dry, it could crack and become infected. May cause pruritus.	Maintain skin integrity. Bathe less frequently. Use superfatted soap. Use tepid, not hot, water and rinse well after bathing. Relieve discomfort. Use emollient or moisturizing lotion after bathing. Encourage nutritious diet. Increase fluid intake. Maintain cool, humid environment.
Skin rash or contact dermatitis. May be allergic or nonallergic reaction.	Erythema, flat or raised eruptions and inflammation. Could cause pruritis, discomfort, and infection if scratched.	Avoid soap and heat, and rubbing area. Bathe area: may use antiseptic soap with orders. Apply ordered lotion or spray (steroids) to prevent itching. Use cool, wet dressing.
Abrasions	Break in skin integrity could result in infection. Healing may be prolonged due to age (poor circulation, etc.)	Wash abrasions with soap and water. Apply lotion as ordered.

promote circulation. Baths may also be used as a treatment to promote healing for a client with burns. Various types of bathing include:

- Complete bed bath: The client, who is usually totally dependent, is bathed by the nurse due to physical or mental incapacity. The client is encouraged to complete as much of his or her bath as possible.
- Partial bath: Face, axilla, hands, back, and genital area are bathed. Partial bath may be completed by client or nurse.
- Therapeutic bath: This bath is used as part of a treatment regimen for specific conditions, such as skin disorders, burns, high body temperature, and muscular injuries. Medicinal substances, such as oatmeal, Aveeno, and cornstarch, may be included in the bath water.
- Shower: Preferred method of bathing if client is ambulatory or can be transported to use a shower chair.
- Tub bath: Used by ambulatory clients as well as those who must be assisted by a device such as the Hoyer lift.
- Cooling bath: the client is placed in a tub of tepid water to reduce body temperature.

Skin Problems

Skin types, colors, textures, and condition are as different and unique as each person. The condition of a client's skin is determined by his or her health status, age, activity level, and environmental exposure (Table 9–1). For example, the skin of an infant is often more sensitive and delicate than that of an adult because it has not been exposed to many of the elements of the environment. Most infants cannot tolerate strong soaps and lotions, and must be handled gently to avoid trauma. Adolescents are affected by acne and have areas of increased oil secretion. Adults may have drier skin, especially as they age. Older adults cannot always tolerate harsh soaps because their skin is more delicate. They require less frequent bathing and more lubrication with oil-rich creams and lotions.

Maintaining skin integrity is an integral part of providing nursing care; being aware of the client's skin condition and alterations in the integrity is a critical aspect of providing total client care.

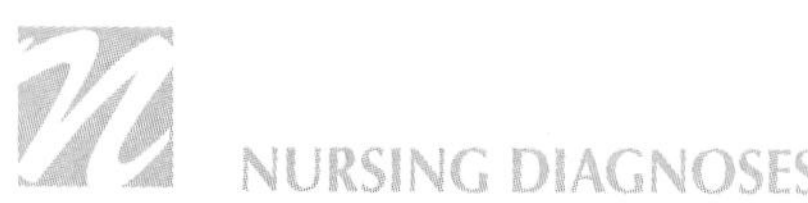

NURSING DIAGNOSES

The following nursing diagnoses are appropriate to include in a client care plan when the components are related to basic care of the client.

NURSING DIAGNOSIS	RELATED FACTORS
Activity Intolerance	Prolonged bed rest, surgery, pain, treatment schedule, weakness, fatigue
Altered Health Maintenance	Ineffective coping, lack of motivation, motor impairment, lack of financial resources
Bathing/Hygiene Self-Care Deficit	Lack of coordination, motor impairment, visual disorders, surgery, muscle weakness, pain
Impaired Skin Integrity	Surgery, immobility, prolonged bedrest, mechanical factors (shearing force, pressure)

unit 1

BEDMAKING

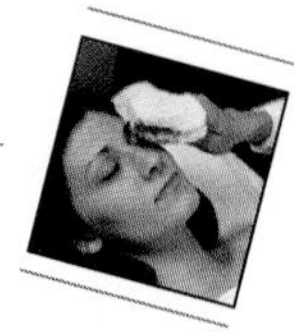

NURSING PROCESS DATA

ASSESSMENT Data Base

Assess the client's need to have linen changed.

Determine if the client's present condition permits a change of bed linen.

Determine how many and what type of linens are required.

Check client's unit for available linens.

Determine client's prescribed level of activity and any special precautions in movement.

Assess client's ability to get out of bed during linen change.

PLANNING Objectives

To provide a clean, comfortable sleeping and resting environment for the client

To eliminate irritants to skin by providing wrinkle-free sheets and blankets.

To avoid client exertion by making bed while occupied (Do not move client more than necessary)

To enhance client's self-image by providing a clean, neat, and comfortable bed

To properly dispose of soiled linens and prevent cross-contamination

To correctly align clients to assist in promoting a physically and emotionally safe and comfortable position

To prevent stress to the nurse's back or limbs during procedure

IMPLEMENTATION Procedures

Folding a Mitered Corner

Changing a Pillowcase

Making an Unoccupied Bed

Making a Surgical Bed

Changing an Occupied Bed

EVALUATION Expected Outcomes

Client is rested during and after bedmaking procedure.

Bed remains clean, dry, free of wrinkles or other skin irritants, and at a comfortable temperature.

Skin remains free of irritation caused by contact with linens.

The nurse feels no stress to back or limbs during the procedure.

FOLDING A MITERED CORNER

Equipment

Same as for an unoccupied bed

Procedure

1. Tuck sheet tightly and smoothly under mattress at top of the bed.
2. Grasp edge of sheet with hand and bring sheet onto mattress so that edge forms a right angle.

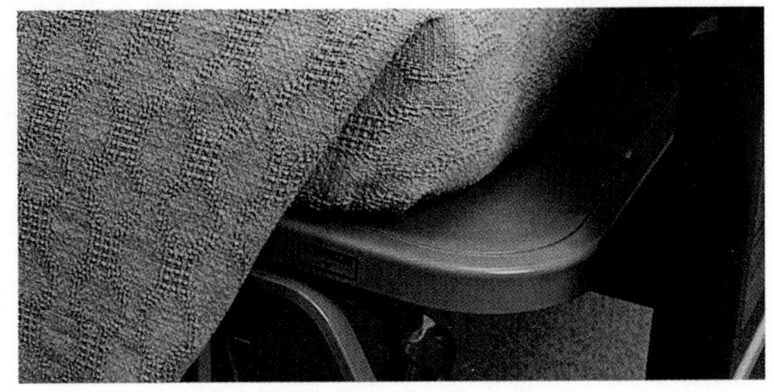

Mitered corners keep bed linens tight and wrinkle-free.

3. Tuck lower edge of sheet under mattress.
4. Place finger on sheet where it meets mattress and lower top of sheet over finger. **Rationale:** This action makes the mitered corner neat and tight.
5. Remove finger without disturbing folds.
6. Tuck sheet securely under mattress.

CHANGING A PILLOWCASE

Equipment

Clean pillowcase

Procedure

1. Pick up center of closed end of pillowcase.
2. Continue to firmly grip end of pillowcase; then with other hand gather pillowcase from open end and fold back (inside-out) over closed end.
3. Pick up center of one end of pillow with the hand holding the gathered pillowcase.
4. Pull pillowcase over pillow with other hand. Do not place pillow or case under arm, chin, or in teeth. **Rationale:** Contamination occurs from using these methods.
5. Adjust pillow corners in pillowcase by placing hand between case and pillow.

MAKING AN UNOCCUPIED BED

Equipment

Chair or table
Linen hamper
Linens (in order of use):
- Bath blanket
- Mattress pad
- Bottom sheet
- Drawsheet
- Incontinent pad, if needed
- Top sheet
- Blanket
- Bedspread
- Pillowcase

Preparation

1. Gather linen and hamper and bring to room.
2. Explain need for client to be out of bed during procedure.
3. Wash hands.
4. Assist client out of bed and into chair.
5. Arrange chair and hamper conveniently for use.
6. Wipe chair off before placing linen on chair.

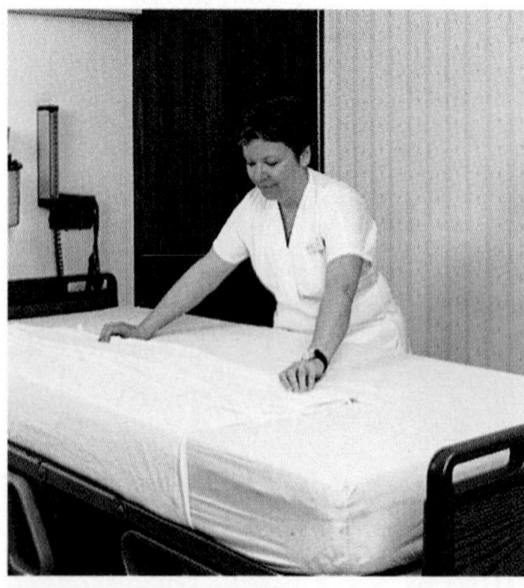
Tuck drawsheet in tightly.

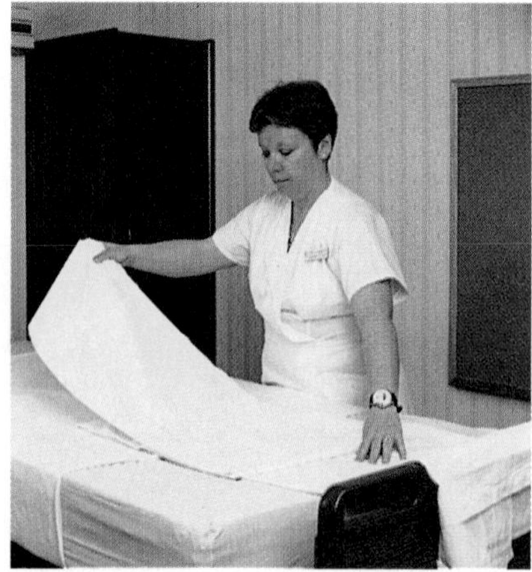
Unfold bottom sheet to cover mattress.

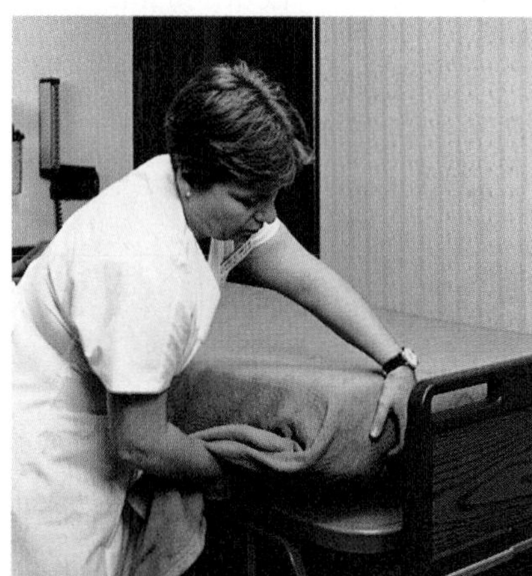
Smooth linen before mitering corners.

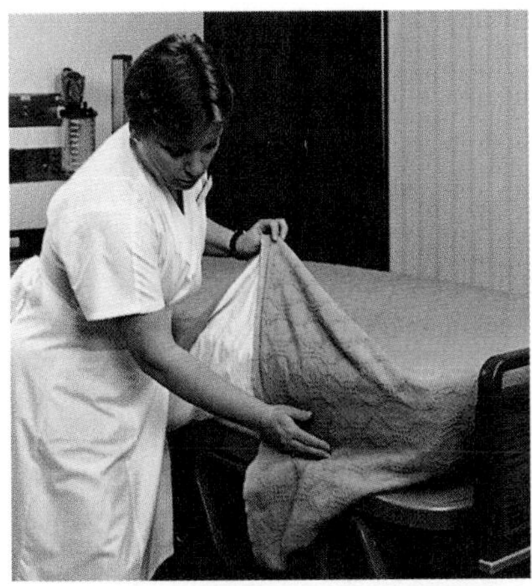
Form triangle and tuck in linen.

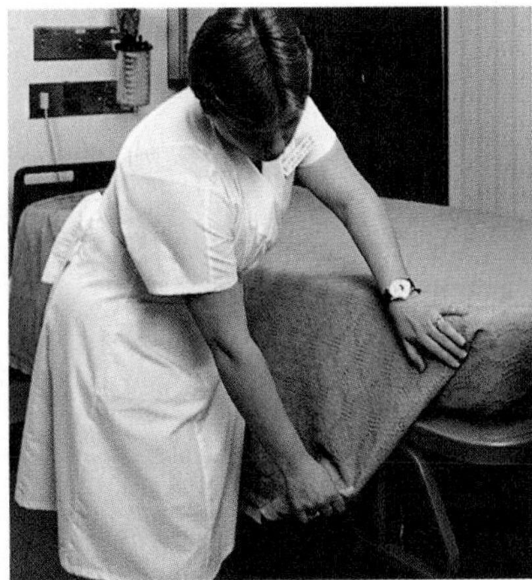
Pull down top linen while holding corner.

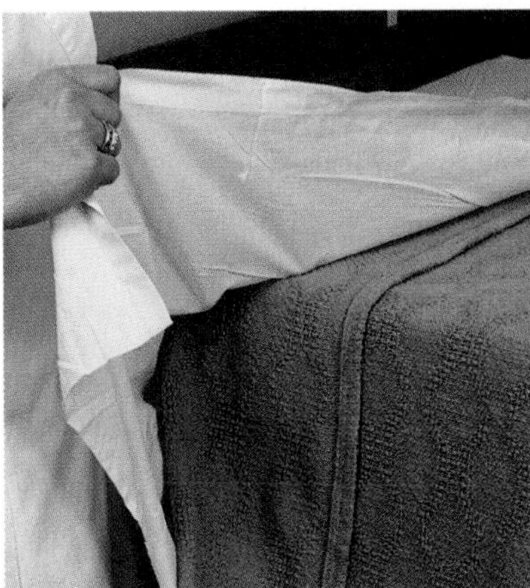
Fold cuff of sheet over spread.

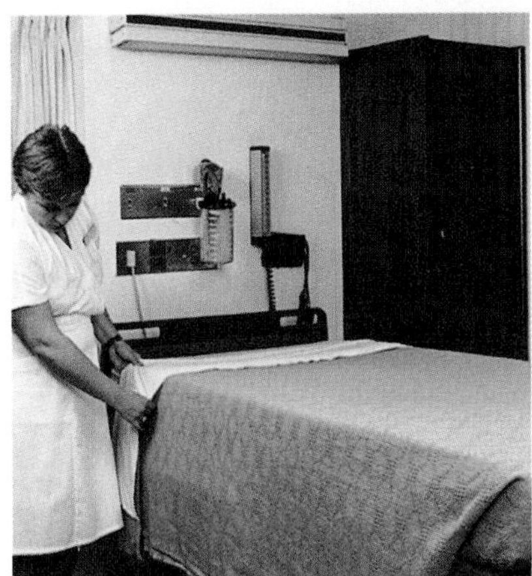
Fold sheet over spread and leave cuff.

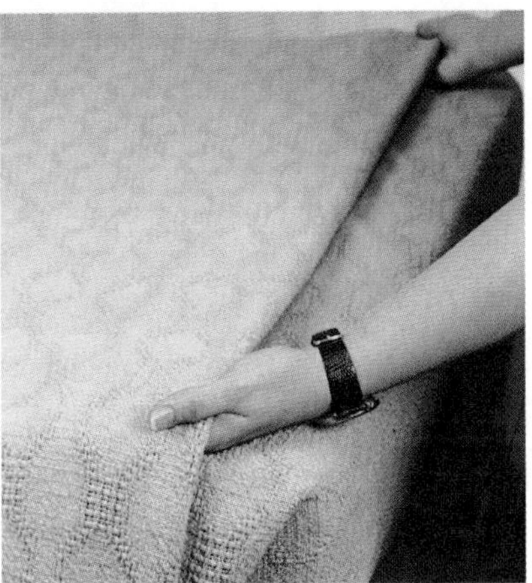
Pleat top linen to allow space for feet.

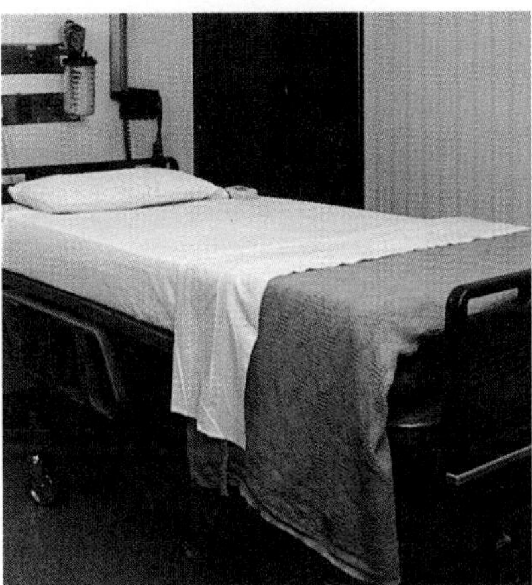
Fanfold linen to foot of bed.

Rationale: This action provides a clean surface and promotes infection control.

7. Place linen on chair.
8. Remove call signal from linen.
9. Adjust bed to a comfortable working height.

Procedure

1. Lower both side rails.
2. Loosen linen on all sides, including head and foot of the bed.
3. Remove spread and blanket. If they are to be reused, fold them and place on the chair.
4. Remove top, draw, and bottom sheet, and place in linen hamper. **Rationale:** Never place dirty linen on the floor as cross-contamination occurs from this action.
5. Push mattress to head of bed. Center the mattress if necessary.
6. If mattress pad is not changed, smooth out wrinkles and recenter pad on the bed surface.
7. Make up one side of the bed, then move to the other side of bed and make it. **Rationale:** This step saves time and energy.
8. Place contour bottom sheet on mattress, and continue making bed at Step 13. If using a flat bottom sheet, place the center fold of the sheet in the middle of the mattress with the end of the sheet even with the end of the mattress.
9. Unfold the bottom sheet, and cover the mattress.
10. Tuck the top of the sheet under the head of the bed.
11. Miter the corner of the bottom sheet at the head of the bed. (See procedure for mitered corner.) **Rationale:** A mitered corner is tighter and less likely to come apart.

12. Tuck the remaining side of the bottom sheet well under the mattress.
13. If the client needs a drawsheet, center the drawsheet on the bed and open drawsheet top to opposite side. Tuck the sheet under the mattress. Smooth out wrinkles.
    a. If a pull sheet is needed, fold drawsheet in half or quarters. Position sheet in middle of bed. **Rationale:** Pull sheets are used with heavy or difficult-to-move clients.
    b. If absorbent pad is needed, center it on bed over draw or pull sheet.
14. Move to the other side of the bed. Pull linen toward you and straighten out linen.
15. Tuck the top of the sheet under the head of the bed if using a flat sheet.
16. Miter the corner of the bottom sheet at the head of the bed if not using a contour sheet.
17. Tuck remaining bottom sheet well under the mattress. Gather sheet into your hand, lean away from the bed, and pull sheet downward. Tuck sheet under mattress.
18. If drawsheet is used, tighten and tuck the same as bottom sheet.
19. Straighten out absorbent pad and pull sheet if used.
20. Place top sheet, blanket, and spread full length on top of bed.
21. Leave a cuff of top sheet and spread at the head of the bed. **Rationale:** This prevents client's face from rubbing against blanket.
22. Tuck sheet, spread, and blanket well under foot of mattress, one side at a time.
23. Miter corners at the foot of the bed, one side at a time.
24. Make a small pleat to allow room for client's feet.

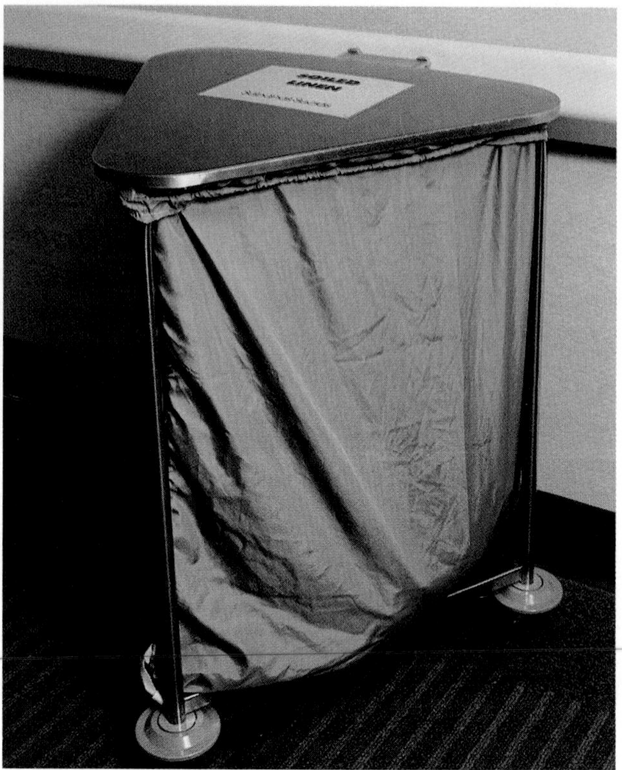

Keep linen hamper covered to prevent spread of microorganisms. Hamper can be taken into the client's room.

25. Fanfold linen to foot of bed.
26. Change pillowcase.
27. Return bed to lowest position. Reattach call signal to linens.
28. Pull side rail up on side furthest from client.
29. If the unit is unassigned, leave top linen pulled up, covering the bed.
30. Dispose of soiled laundry.
31. Wash your hands.

MAKING A SURGICAL BED

Equipment

Same as for an unoccupied bed

Procedure

1. Wash your hands.
2. Bring linens to the room.
3. Arrange chair and linen hamper conveniently for use.
4. Wipe off chair before placing linen on it.
5. Raise bed to highest position.
6. Place the bottom sheet on the bed, using the same method as for making an unoccupied bed.
7. Place a plastic or cloth drawsheet (or both) and absorbent pad on the bed.
8. Lay top sheet, blanket, and bedspread over top of bed.
9. Fold up linen from foot, head, and one side of the bed toward center of the bed.

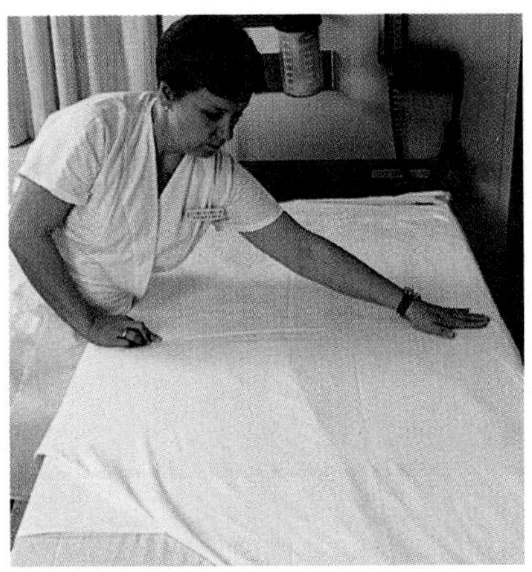

Place draw sheet and absorbent pad on bottom sheet.

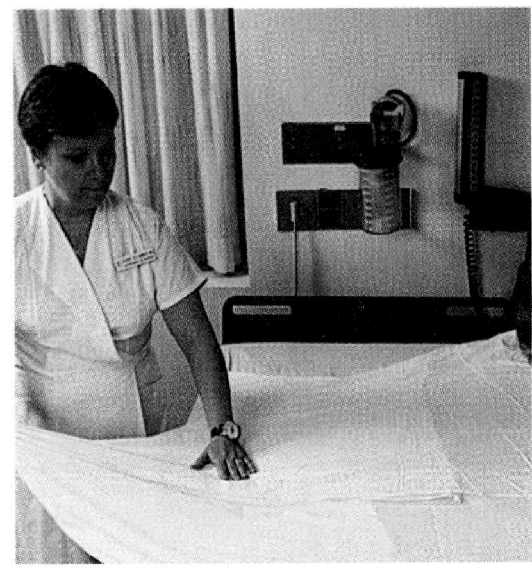

Fold bottom and top edges to opposite side forming a triangle.

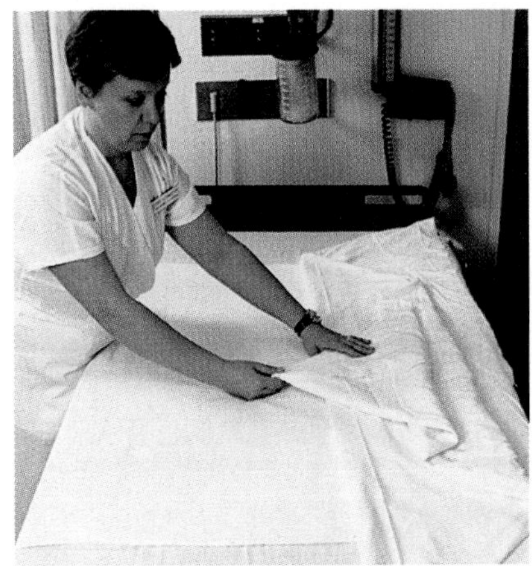

Fanfold linen to opposite side of bed for transferring client.

10. Fold bottom and top edges nearest you to the opposite side, forming a triangle. Pick up center point of triangle.
11. Fanfold linen to side of bed. **Rationale:** Folding linen at side of the bed facilitates moving surgical clients into the bed.
12. Leave bed in HIGH position to facilitate easy transfer of surgical client from gurney to bed.
13. Change pillowcase and leave on chair or at foot of bed.
14. Move all objects away from bedside area. **Rationale:** This allows surgical gurney to be placed close to bed for client transfer.

CHANGING AN OCCUPIED BED

Equipment

Chair or table
Linen hamper
Linens (in order of use):
- Bath blanket
- Mattress pad
- Bottom sheet
- Plastic drawsheet, if needed
- Cloth drawsheet
- Incontinent pad, if needed
- Top sheet
- Blanket
- Bedspread
- Pillowcase

Preparation

1. Talk with the client and explain how he or she can be involved in the procedure.
2. Explain the sequence for the procedure.
3. Arrange furniture and equipment (e.g., linen hamper and chair) for convenience of use.
4. Wipe chair or table before putting linen on it.
5. Wash your hands and collect the linen.
6. Place linen on chair or table after wiping it off.
7. Remove call signal from linens.
8. Pull curtain closed. **Rationale:** This provides privacy for the client.
9. Adjust the bed to a comfortable working height with side rails up. Help client into a supine position.
10. Don gloves if bed linen is soiled with body fluids.

Procedure

1. Lower side rail on your side of the bed, but make sure side rail on opposite side is in UP position. **Rationale:** This ensures client safety as client rolls to edge of bed.
2. Loosen top linens.
3. Remove spread, sheet, and blanket at the same time the bath blanket is pulled over client. **Rationale:** Blanket keeps client warm during bed

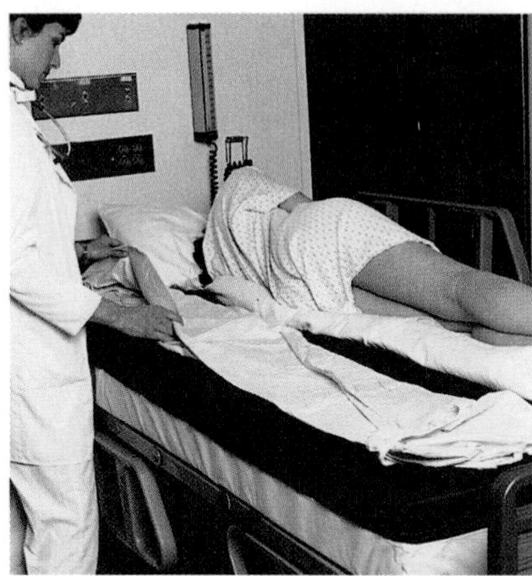
Place center of sheet in middle of bed.

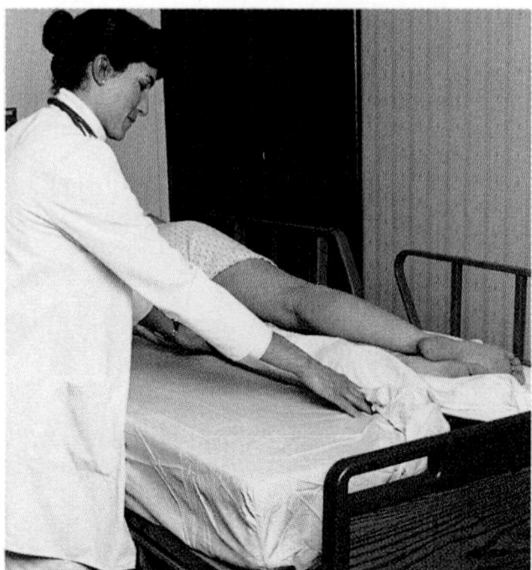
Tighten bottom sheet under mattress.

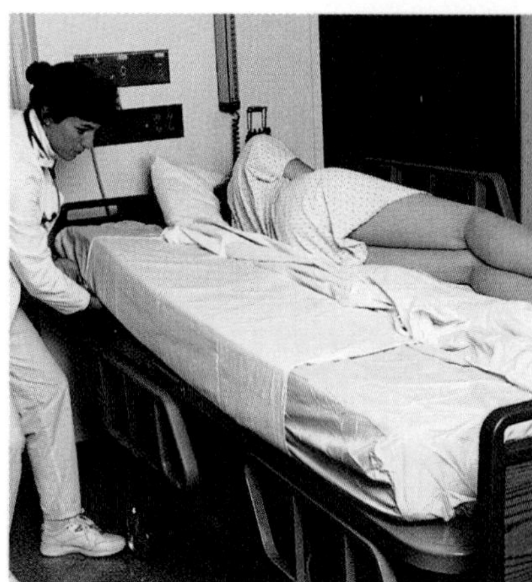
Place drawsheet in middle of bed.

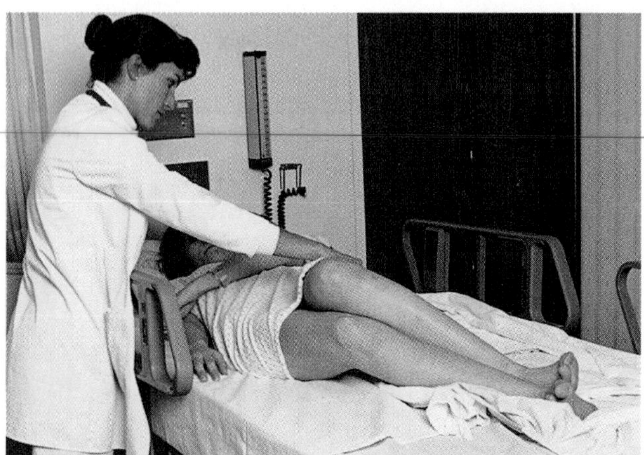
Assist client to roll over to other side of bed.

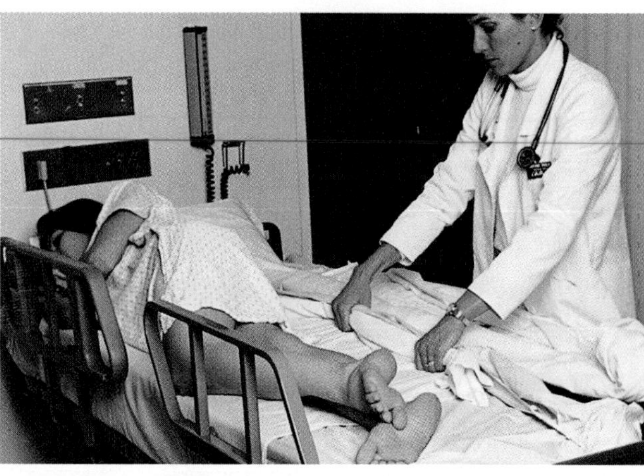
After raising side rail, pull linen toward you.

change. If they are to be reused, fold them and place on the chair.

4. Place top sheet in linen hamper.
5. Push mattress to head of bed. Center the mattress if necessary.
6. Assist client to the side of the bed, place in side-lying position facing away from you as near the far side rail as possible.
7. Loosen bottom linens on your side of the bed.
8. Push dirty linen under or as close as possible to client.
9. Smooth out wrinkles and recenter pad on the bed surface if mattress pad is not changed. **Rationale:** Wrinkles may cause skin irritation.
10. Place clean bottom sheet on mattress with client on the opposite side of the bed. Place the center fold of the sheet in the middle of the mattress with the end of the sheet even with the end of the mattress.
11. Unfold the bottom sheet and cover the mattress. Make sure the clean bottom sheet is underneath any used linen. **Rationale:** This keeps the clean linen uncontaminated.
12. Tuck the top of the sheet under the head of the bed, or position contour sheet around corner of mattress.
13. Miter the corner of the bottom sheet at the head of the bed.
14. Tuck the remaining bottom sheet well under the mattress from head to foot.
15. Center the plastic or cloth drawsheet on the bed, if the client requires a drawsheet, and fanfold half of the sheet under the client. Tuck side of the sheet under the mattress. Smooth out wrinkles.
    a. Fold cloth drawsheet in half or quarters if a pull sheet is needed. Position sheet in middle of bed. Fanfold half of the pull sheet under client.
    b. Fanfold absorbent pad and center it on bed

under client's buttocks. Place the pad close to the client for ease in pulling it through to the other side of the bed, absorbent side up and plastic side down.

16. Help the client roll over to the other side of the bed.
17. Tell the client why there is a hump of linen in the center of the bed. Make the client comfortable.
18. Raise the side rail. Move to other side of bed.
19. Move linens to the other side of the bed, by gently pulling linens toward you.
20. Lower side rail, and loosen bottom sheets.
21. Pull dirty linen to side of bed and roll into a bundle at the foot of the bed or place linen in linen hamper. **Rationale:** This reduces the spread of microorganisms.
22. Never place dirty linen on the floor. **Rationale:** Cross-contamination occurs from this action.
23. Pull clean linen across mattress and straighten under client.
24. Miter the top corner of the bottom sheet.
25. Gather bottom sheet into your hand, lean away from the bed, and pull linens downward at an angle. Tuck remaining bottom sheet well under the mattress. If drawsheet is used, tighten and tuck it in the same way.
26. Help the client into a supine position and adjust the pillow.
27. Place top sheet, blanket, and spread over the client. Leave at least a 6-inch cuff of top sheet at the head of the bed.
28. Remove bath blanket, and straighten top sheet and blanket.
29. Miter corners at foot of bed.
30. Pull up all layers of linen at client's toes. Make a small pleat. **Rationale:** This allows room for client's feet and prevents sheets from rubbing on client's toes.
31. Raise side rail.
32. Remove pillow from bed, and change pillowcase.
33. Return bed to lowest position. Reattach call signal to linens.
34. Position client for comfort.
35. Dispose of soiled laundry.
36. Wash your hands.

PRINCIPLES OF MEDICAL ASEPSIS

Place dirty linen in hamper.
Do not place dirty linen on floor.
Discard all unused linen from client area.
Do not transfer linen from one client area to another.
Do not allow dirty linen to touch uniform.

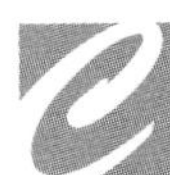

CHARTING for Bedmaking

- Specific linens or equipment that cause discomfort for the client
- Special requirements for linens (e.g., certain detergents or elimination of starch)
- Use of pull sheets, incontinent pads, or specified ways to keep bed dry

CRITICAL THINKING APPLICATION

CLINICAL PROBLEMS	CRITICAL THINKING OPTIONS
■ Client refuses to have bed made	• Assess reason for refusal. Client may be in pain or does not want to be disturbed. • Offer to make the bed at a later time. • Change only the pillowcase and drawsheet, if client allows. • Beds do not need to be changed unless soiled or damp so allow client's independence if possible.
■ Cross-contamination occurs from improper linen disposal.	• Provide adequate linen hampers for the nursing personnel. • Attend in-service education programs on infection control.
■ Client's skin becomes irritated from linen or begins to break down.	• Obtain hypoallergenic linen. • Place special mattress under client. • Use eggcrate mattress.
■ The nurse feels stress on back during bedmaking.	• Make sure bed is positioned for comfort of the nurse. • High position is generally used. • If client is heavy, ask for assistance with bedmaking, especially in moving side-to-side. • Attend in-service classes on "preventing back strain."

unit 2 BATH CARE

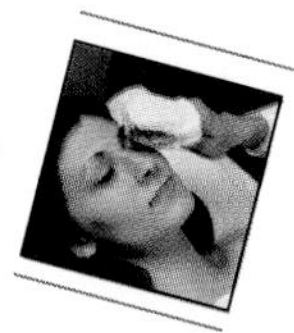

NURSING PROCESS DATA

ASSESSMENT Data Base

Assess client's need for bathing and other personal hygiene activities.

Check client's activity order. Note special precautions related to movement or exercise.

Assess client's ability to perform his or her own care and determine how much assistance he or she needs.

Discuss client's preferences for the bathing procedure, bath, and personal articles.

Check client's room for availability of bathing articles and linens.

Assess client's skin (see Unit 3 on skin integrity).

PLANNING Objectives

To decrease the possibility of infection by removing excessive debris, secretions, and perspiration from the skin

To promote circulation

To maintain muscle tone through active or passive movement during bathing

To alternate points of pressure on the body by changing client's position during the bath

To provide comfort for the client

To assess the client's overall status, skin condition, level of mobility, comfort

IMPLEMENTATION Procedures

Folding a Washcloth Mitt

Providing Morning Care

Bathing an Adult Client

Bathing an Infant

Bathing with a Hydraulic Bathtub Chair

Bathing the Critically Ill

EVALUATION Expected Outcomes

Client's skin is free of excessive perspiration, debris, secretions, and offensive odors.

Body positions have been changed and muscles and joints have been exercised actively or passively during the bath.

Client feels comfortable and does not complain of pain, fatigue, itching, irritated, or excessively dry skin.

Client participates in bath procedure to the best of his or her ability.

The nurse has assessed the integrity and condition of the client's skin and the level of mobility, comfort, or pain.

FOLDING A WASHCLOTH MITT

Procedure

1. Unfold the washcloth.
2. Place one corner of cloth in the palm of your hand, just above your fingers.
3. Wrap one edge of the cloth around the palm and fingers.
4. Anchor cloth with your thumb.
5. Bring far edge of cloth up and tuck under edge in palm of hand.

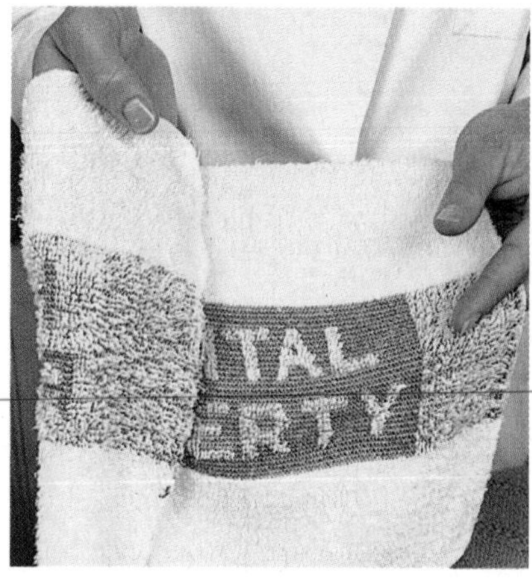

Wrap one edge of cloth around palm and fingers.

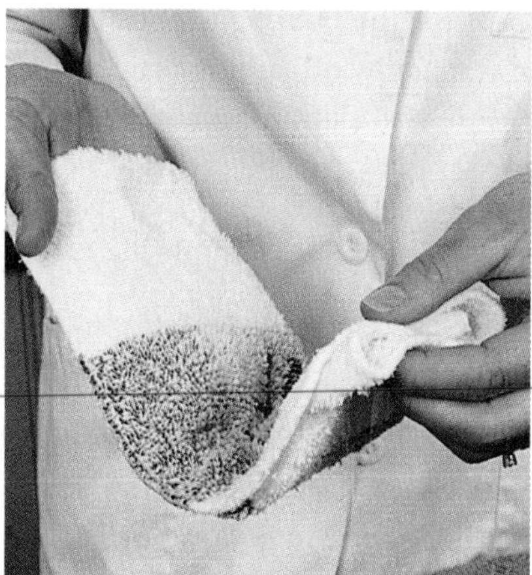

Wrap cloth around hand and anchor with thumb.

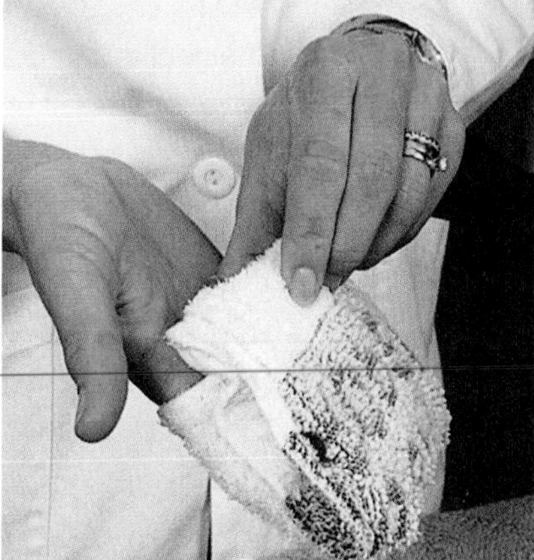

Tuck far edge of cloth under edge in palm of hand.

PROVIDING MORNING CARE

Equipment

Basin of warm water
Soap
Towel and washcloth
Emesis basin
Toothbrush and paste
Bedpan or urinal
Toilet tissue

Preparation

1. Determine if client wishes morning care. **Rationale:** Morning care is provided to "freshen" the client in preparation for breakfast, physicians' visits, and procedures occurring prior to bathing.
2. Wash your hands. **Rationale:** When providing morning care to several clients, it is important to wash your hands between clients so that microorganisms are not transmitted from one client to another.
3. Gather equipment and take it to client's room.
4. Explain that early morning care is available while client remains in bed. If client is able, assist him or her to the bathroom. Provide privacy.

Procedure

1. Offer bedpan or urinal and assist client as needed.
2. Wash your hands.
3. Move bed to comfortable working height, and lower side rail.
4. Put equipment on over-bed table within reach.
5. Wash client's face and hands or assist as needed. Dry face and hands.
6. Offer oral hygiene. Assist as needed.
7. Hold emesis basin so client can rinse after brushing teeth.
8. Assist client to comfortable position.
9. Reposition bed, and replace side rails.
10. Remove equipment and draw curtains.

BATHING AN ADULT CLIENT

Equipment

Basin or sink with warm water (110°–115°F)
Soap and soap dish
Personal articles (i.e., deodorant, powder, lotions)
Laundry hamper
Two to three towels
Washcloth
Bath blanket
Clean pajamas or hospital gown
Table for bathing equipment
Shaving equipment for male patients

Preparation

1. Provide a comfortable room environment (i.e., comfortable temperature, lighting).
2. Talk with client about plan for bathing to meet personal care needs.
3. Encourage client to bathe him or herself. **Rationale:**

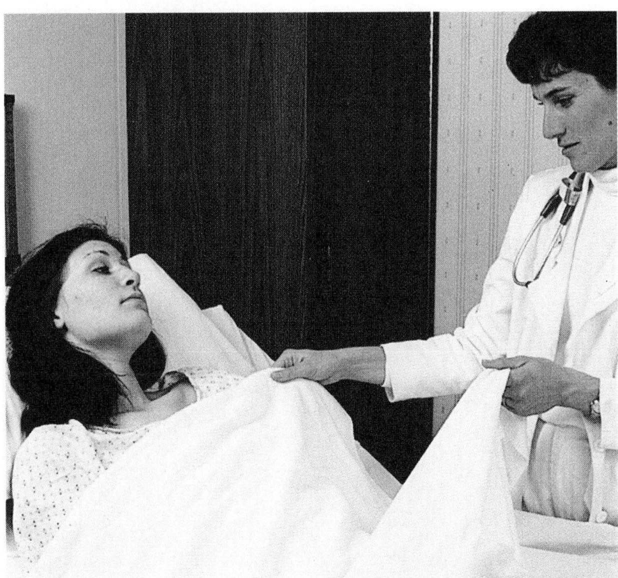

Remove top linen before bathing.

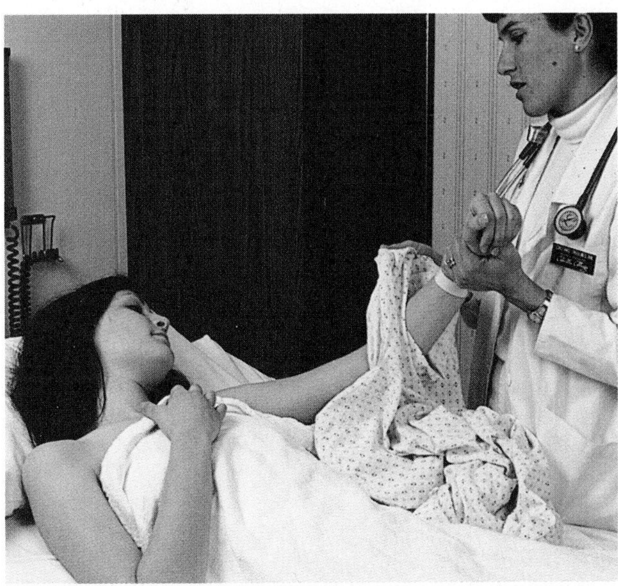

Remove gown maintaining client's modesty.

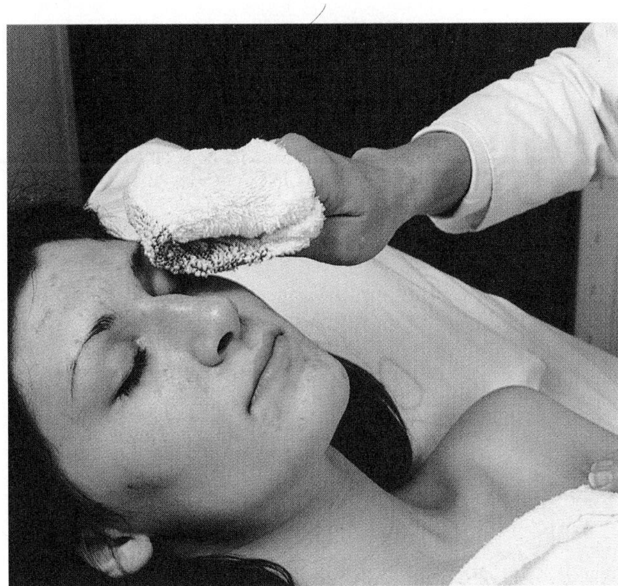

Wash eyes first, from inner to outer canthus.

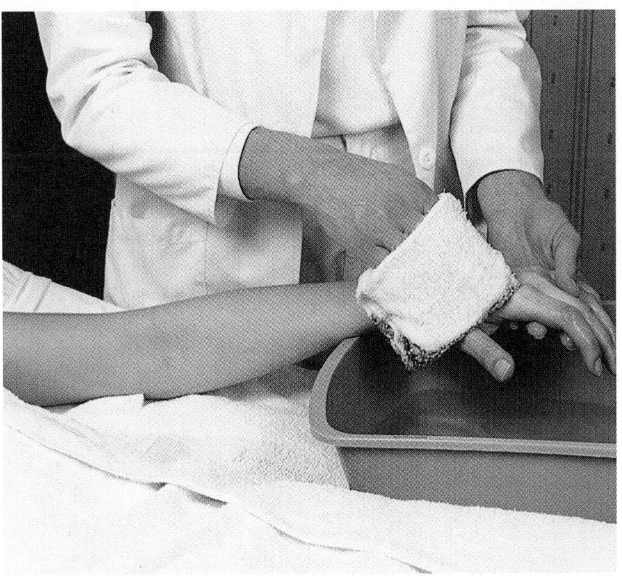

Wash hands by soaking them in a basin.

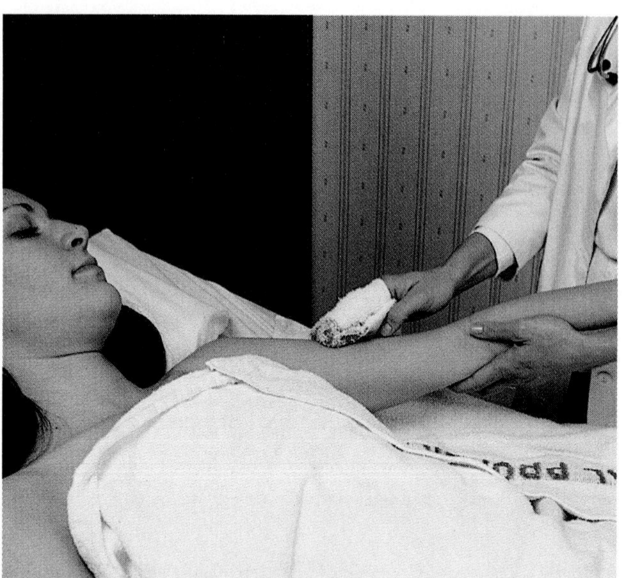

Support wrist when washing client's arm.

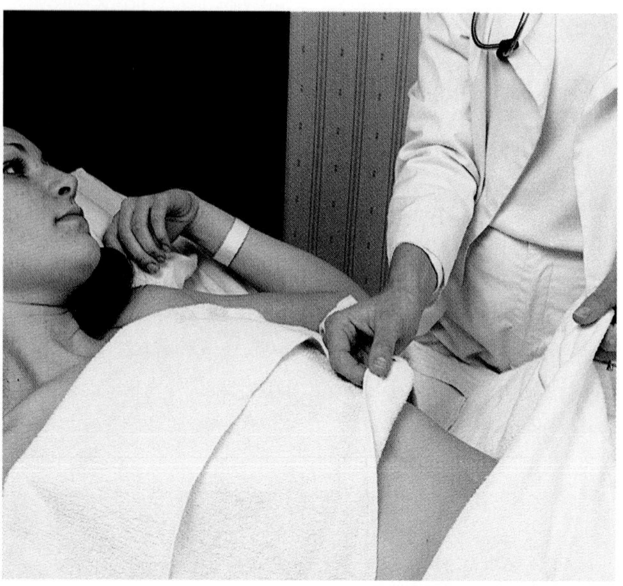

Keep client covered with towel or bath blanket during bath.

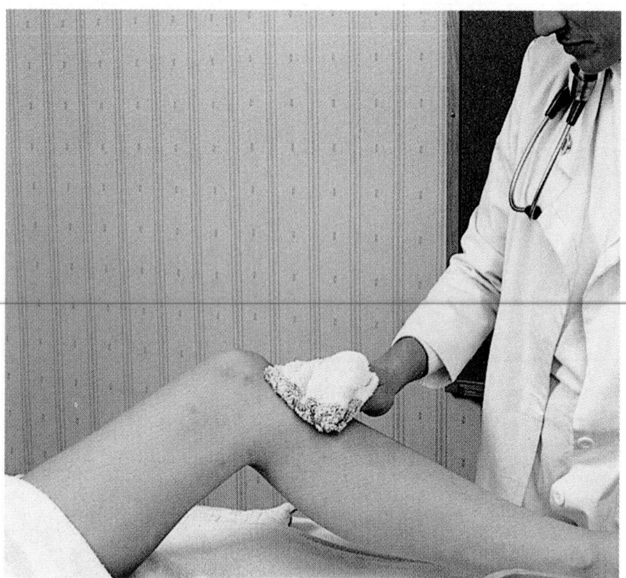

Wash client's legs and feet for a total bed bath.

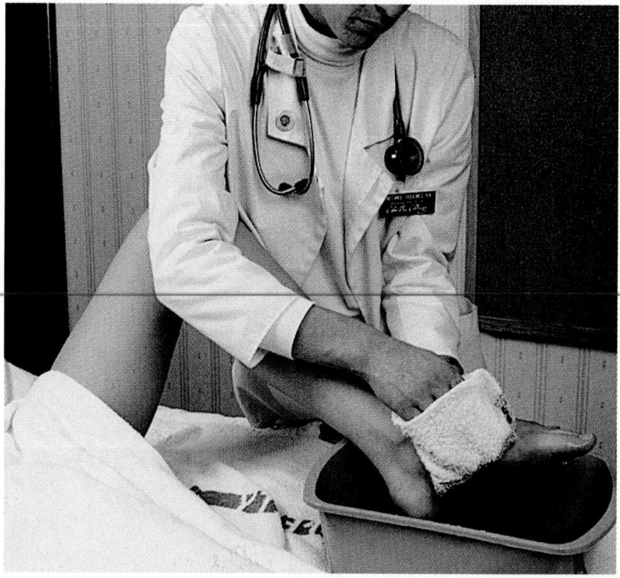

Place client's feet in basin while bathing to promote relaxation.

To increase independence, promote exercise and a sense of self-worth.

4. Explain any unfamiliar methods or procedures regarding bathing.
5. Wash your hands.
6. Collect necessary equipment, and place articles within reach on over-bed table.
7. Ask the client if he or she needs to void or defecate before starting the bath. **Rationale:** Warm water of the bath and movement can stimulate the client to void.
8. Position the bed at a comfortable working height.
9. Ensure privacy.

Procedure

1. Place bath blanket over client and over top linen. Loosen top linen at edges and foot of bed.

   a. Remove dirty top linen from under bath blanket, starting at client's shoulders and rolling linen down toward the client's feet.
   b. Ask client to grasp and hold top edge of bath blanket to keep it in place while you pull linen to foot of bed.
   c. Place dirty linen in laundry hamper.
2. Help client to the side of the bed closest to you. Keep the side rail on the far side of the bed in the UP position.
3. Remove client's hospital gown. Keep client covered with bath blanket. Place gown in laundry bag.
4. Remove pillow if client can tolerate.
5. Place towel under client's head.
6. Don clean gloves if risk of exposure to body fluids when bathing client. **Rationale:** To maintain universal precautions.
7. Make a mitt with a washcloth. Fold washcloth around your hand as illustrated previously. **Rationale:** This prevents wet ends of cloth from annoying client.
8. Bathe client's face. **Rationale:** Begin bath at cleanest area and work downward toward feet.
   a. Wash around client's eyes, using clear water. With one edge of facecloth, wipe from the inner canthus toward the outer canthus. **Rationale:** This prevents secretions from entering lacrimal duct. Using a different section of the washcloth, repeat procedure on other eye. Dry thoroughly.
   b. Wash, rinse, and dry client's forehead, cheeks, nose, and area around lips. Use soap with client's permission.
   c. Wash, rinse, and dry area behind and around the client's ears.
   d. Wash, rinse, and dry client's neck.
9. Remove towel from under client's head.
10. Bathe client's upper body and extremities. Place towel under area to be bathed.
    a. Wash both arms by elevating client's arm and holding client's wrist. Use gentle strokes from the wrist toward the shoulder, including the axillary area.
    b. Wash, rinse, and dry client's axillae. Apply deodorant and powder if desired.
    c. Wash client's hands by soaking them in the basin or with a washcloth. Nails can be cleaned now or after the bath.
    d. Keeping chest covered with the towel, wash, rinse, and thoroughly dry client's chest, (especially under breasts. Apply powder or cornstarch under breasts if desired).
11. Bathe client's abdomen. Using a towel over chest area and bath blanket, cover areas you are not bathing. Wash, rinse, and dry abdomen and umbilicus. Replace bath blanket over client's upper body and abdomen.
12. Bathe client's legs and feet. Place towel under leg to be bathed. Drape other leg, hip, and genital area with the bath blanket.
    a. Carefully place bath basin on the towel near the client's foot.
    b. With one arm under the client's leg, grasp the client's foot and bend knee. Place foot in basin of water.
    c. Bathe client's leg, moving toward hip. Rinse and dry client's leg.
    d. Wash client's foot with washcloth. Rinse and dry foot and area between toes thoroughly.
    e. Carefully move basin to other side of bed, and repeat procedure for client's other leg and foot.
13. Change bath water. Raise side rails when refilling basin. **Rationale:** This ensures client safety. Check the water temperature before continuing with the bath.
14. During the bath, continuously assess the client's skin and musculoskeletal system. Careful attention should be paid to the verbal statements and nonverbal expressions. **Rationale:** This data yields information about client's overall condition.
15. Help client turn to a side-lying or prone position. Place towel under area to be bathed. Cover client with a bath blanket.
16. Wash, rinse, and dry client's back, moving from the shoulders to the buttocks.
17. Provide back massage now or after completion of bath. (For procedure see Providing Back Care.)
18. Bathe client's genital area. Cover all body parts except area to be bathed. Place towel under client's hips.
    a. For a female client: Bathe from front to back. Use a different section of the washcloth for each stroke. Wash, rinse, and dry thoroughly between all skin folds.
    b. For a male client: Carefully retract the foreskin on the uncircumcised penis. Wash, rinse, and dry gently and replace foreskin to its original position. Continue to wash, rinse, and dry penis, scrotum, and remaining skin folds.

19. Remove gloves and place in receptacle.
20. Dress client in a clean hospital gown.
21. Clean and store bath equipment. Dispose of dirty linen.
22. Proceed with any other personal hygiene activities as needed.
23. Replace call light, lower bed, and place side rails in UP position before leaving client.
24. Wash your hands.

BATHING AN INFANT

Equipment

Tub or basin filled with warm water (100°F)
Two towels
Washcloth
Suction bulb
Mild soap
Cotton balls
Blanket
Clean clothing

Preparation

1. Provide a comfortable room environment (i.e., comfortable temperature, lighting.)
2. Wash your hands.
3. Collect necessary equipment, and place articles within reach.
4. Position the bed at a comfortable working height.
5. Place towel, laid out in diamond fashion, on bed next to basin.

Procedure

1. Test water temperature with your wrist or elbow.
2. Lift infant using football hold.
3. Remove all clothing except shirt and diaper.
4. Cover infant with towel or blanket. Never let go of the infant during the bath. **Rationale:** This is a safety intervention.
5. Clean infant's eyes, using a cotton ball moistened with water. Wipe from inner to outer canthus, using a new cotton ball for each eye. **Rationale:** This procedure prevents water and particles from entering the lacrimal duct.

■ CLINICAL ALERT

Discharge is present for 2 to 3 days due to prophylactic eye drops administered at birth.

6. Make a mitt with the washcloth.
7. Wash infant's face with water.
8. Suction nose, if necessary, by compressing suction bulb prior to placing it in nostril. **Rationale:** This prevents aspiration of moisture. Release bulb after it is placed in nostril.
9. Wash infant's ears and neck, paying attention to folds; dry all areas thoroughly.
10. Remove shirt or gown.

Most hospitals now use disposable rather than cloth diapers for the following reasons:

- Prevention of nosocomial infections
- Decreased skin irritation
- Safety of the infant (no pins for application)
- Simplified application and increased convenience

Environmental consideration in the mid-1990s, however, are influencing a trend away from disposable diapers and back to cloth diapers.

11. Remove and place closed safety pins in a safe area away from child if using cloth diaper. Remove diaper by picking up infant's ankles in your hand.
12. Pick up infant and place feet first into basin or tub. Immerse infant in tub of water only after umbilical cord has healed. Pick up infant by placing your hand and arm around infant, cradling the infant's head and neck in your elbow. Grasp the infant's thigh with your hand. **Rationale:** The umbilical cord is kept dry to prevent infection and encourage it to "fall off."
13. Wash and rinse the infant's body, especially the skin folds.
14. Wash infant's genitalia.
    a. For a female infant: Separate labia and with a cotton ball moistened with soap and water, cleanse downward once on each side. Use a new piece of cotton on each side.

b. For an uncircumcised male infant: Do not force foreskin back. Gently cleanse the exposed surface with a cotton ball moistened with soap and water.
c. For a circumcised male infant: Gently cleanse with plain water.

15. Wrap the infant in a towel and use a football hold when washing an infant's head. Soap your own hands and wash infant's hair and scalp, using a circular motion. Rinse hair and scalp thoroughly. **Rationale:** Football hold is the most secure for active infants.
16. Place infant on a clean, dry towel with head facing the top corner and wrap infant.
17. Use the corner of the towel to dry infant's head with gentle, yet firm, circular movements.
18. Replace infant's diaper and re-dress in a new gown or shirt.
19. Provide comfort by holding the infant for a time following the bath procedure.
20. Wash your hands.

BATHING WITH HYDRAULIC BATHTUB CHAIR

Equipment

Two towels and washcloth

Soap

Clean gown, robe, and slippers

Procedure

1. Bring client to tub room in wheelchair.
2. Fill tub with water and check temperature. **Rationale:** Temperature must not be over 105°F or client may burn skin.
3. Release chair to lowest point beside tub, and place towel on floor under chair.
4. Move client into bathtub chair, and attach seat belt.
5. Swing chair into position over tub.
6. Direct client to move legs down, then lower chair into low position in the tub filled with water.
7. When client is finished bathing, reverse chair out of tub.
8. Assist client to towel dry.
9. Put clean gown, robe, and slippers on client and transport to room.

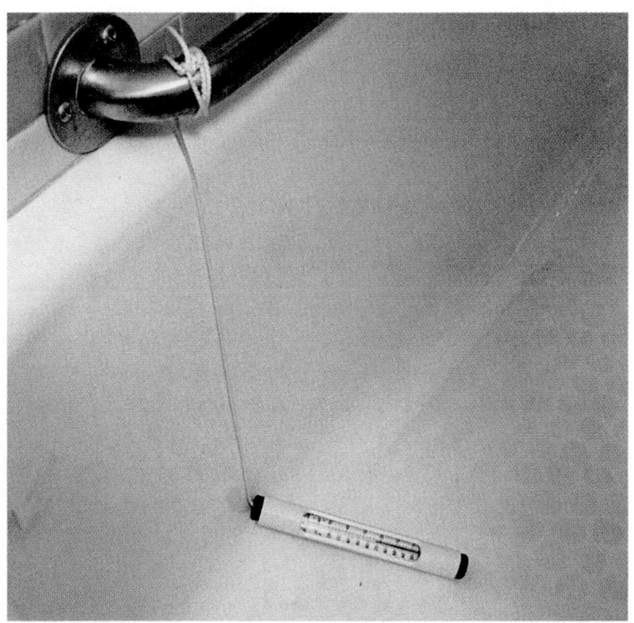

Check that water temperature is not above 105° for safety.

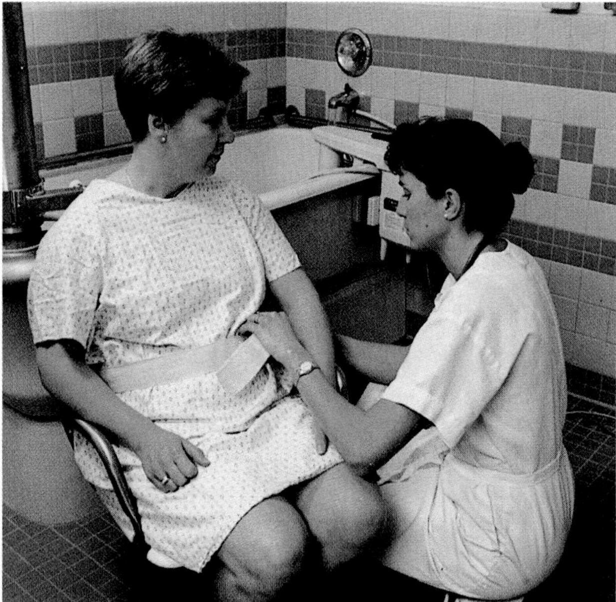

Attach seat belt before swinging chair over the tub.

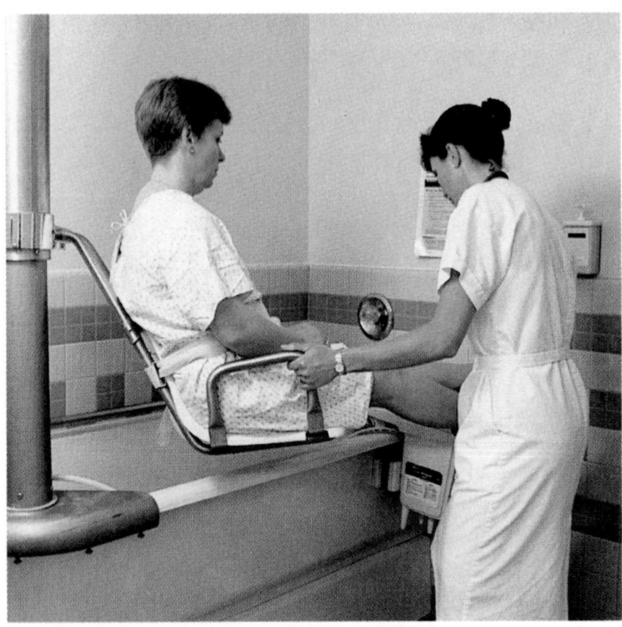
Support client in chair as chair is swung over tub.

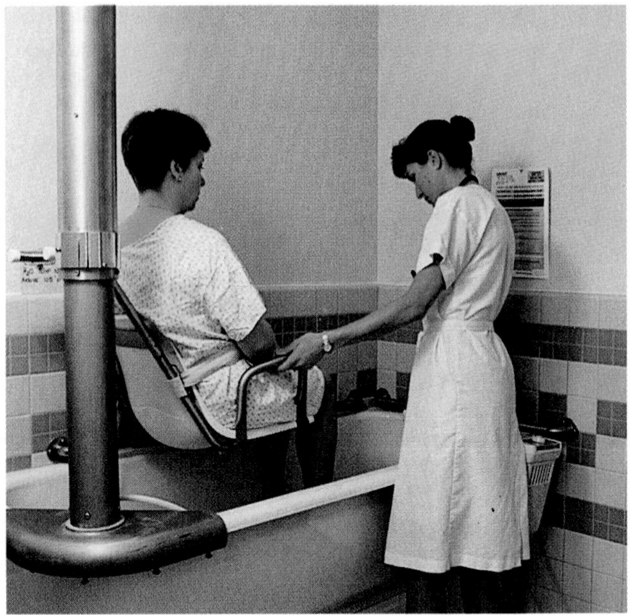
Lower chair into tub filled with water.

BATHING THE CRITICALLY ILL

Equipment

Two bath blankets
Septi-soft soap
Wash basin
Washcloth
Towel

Preparation

1. Provide a comfortable room environment (i.e., comfortable temperature, lighting).
2. Talk with client about plan for bathing to meet personal care needs if client is alert.
3. Encourage client to bathe hands and face if able. **Rationale:** This promotes exercise and sense of self-worth.
4. Explain any unfamiliar methods or procedures regarding bathing.
5. Wash your hands and collect necessary equipment; place articles on over-bed table within easy reach.
6. Position the bed at a comfortable working height, and lower side rail nearest you.

Procedure

1. Have client wash own face and hands if able; otherwise, wash them before starting Septi-soft bath.
2. Place bath blanket in basin and soak bath blanket with very warm water.
3. Pour Septi-soft soap into bath blanket and work soap into bath blanket.
4. Wring out bath blanket.
5. Remove top covers from client, and place wet bath blanket over client. Bath blanket extends from under client's chin down to feet.
6. Keep client covered with bath blanket while you rub anterior surfaces with your hands. Entire surfaces of legs and arms can be washed at this time. **Rationale:** This bath decreases the time it takes to bathe a client. Critically ill clients are not exposed to the long ordeal of a bath or to changes in temperature for long periods.
7. After all body surfaces are washed, place dry bath blanket under client's chin. As you pull dry bath blanket down over client, remove wet blanket.
8. Dry client thoroughly.
9. Turn client on side.

10. Wash and dry back and buttocks with towel.
11. Give back rub.
12. Change bed linen.
13. Position for comfort, and replace side rail to UP position.

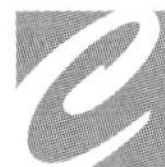

CHARTING for Bath Care

- Client's overall ability to participate in own care
- Type of bath given (i.e., complete or partial) and by whom (e.g., client, nurse, family member)
- Condition of client's skin and any interventions provided for the skin (e.g., lotion, massage)
- Client's educational needs regarding hygienic care
- Information shared with client or family

CRITICAL THINKING APPLICATION

CLINICAL PROBLEMS	CRITICAL THINKING OPTIONS
Client is unwilling to accept a complete bed bath.	• Respect client's wishes and take other opportunities for assessment. • Have client wash hands, face, and genitals. You should wash back and give back care. Reexplain the purpose of the bath to the client and request client participation.
Client is too shy to allow bath.	• Respect client's privacy and only wash areas client wishes you to do. • Give assistance so client can bathe him or herself. • Allow spouse or parent to give bath if this is more acceptable to client.
Client complains of dry, itching skin following the bath.	• Assess for cause of itching. • Ask physician for an order for special lotion. • Do not use soap for the bath.

unit 3

SKIN INTEGRITY

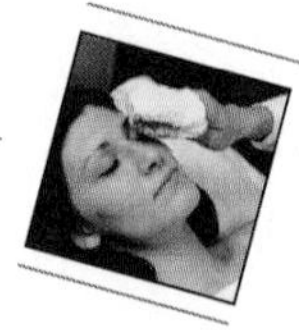

NURSING PROCESS DATA

ASSESSMENT Data Base

Assess for signs of skin breakdown or the eruption of lesions.

Assess color of skin.

Assess color of mucous membranes.

Check for alterations in skin turgor.

Evaluate for complaints of itching, tingling, or numbness.

Evaluate texture of skin.

Assess general hygienic state.

Observe skin for increased or decreased pigmentation and discoloration.

PLANNING Objectives

To maintain skin intact without signs of ischemia, hyperemia, or necrosis

To recognize a break in skin integrity

To avoid introduction of pathogens through break in skin

To prevent skin breakdown from pressure points or strain

To prevent excessive dryness, flaking, itching, or burning

IMPLEMENTATION Procedures

Monitoring Skin Condition

Preventing Skin Breakdown

EVALUATION Expected Outcomes

Client's skin remains intact without signs of ischemia, hyperemia, or necrosis.

Client is able to change position without evidence of pressure areas.

Client's skin does not show signs of dryness, flaking, itching, or burning.

MONITORING SKIN CONDITION

Equipment

Artificial light for observation if natural light is not available

Bath blanket

Gown

Lotion

Procedure

1. Explain monitoring process to client.
2. Provide privacy for client, and wash your hands.
3. Remove linens and gown if necessary. Cover client with bath blanket.
4. Compare color of client's skin with normal range of color within the individual's race. Observe for pallor (white color), flushing (red color), jaundice (yellow color), ashen (gray color), or cyanosis (blue color).
5. Place the back of your fingers or hand on client's skin to check temperature. *Consider the temperature of the room and of your hands.* **Rationale:** The back of the hand is more sensitive to changes in temperature than the palm.
6. Correlate abnormalities in skin color with changes in skin temperature. **Rationale:** Skin temperature reflects blood circulation in the dermis layer.
7. Observe for areas of excessive dryness, moisture, wrinkling, flaking, and general texture of skin.

8. Gently pick up a small section of the skin with your thumb and finger. Observe for ease of movement and speed of return to original position to check for skin turgor. **Rationale:** Hydration is reflected in the skin turgor.
9. Press your finger firmly against client's skin for several seconds (especially ankle area). After removing your finger, observe for lasting impression or indentation.
10. When checking skin temperature and texture of skin, note the client's response to heat, cold, gentle touch, and pressure.
11. Observe the amount of oil, moisture, and dirt on the skin surface.
12. Note presence of strong body odors or odors in the skin folds.
13. Use a disposable blunt-ended probe such as a comb to detect small moving white specks. Lice or white specks may be present on head as well as in pubic area when body lice are present.
14. Observe for areas of broken skin (lesions) or ulcers. Check if lesions are present over entire body or if they are localized to a specific area.
15. Check for skin discolorations (e.g., ecchymosis, petechiae, purpura, erythema, and altered pigmentation). **Rationale:** These signs are indications of generalized disease states, such as leukemia, vitamin deficiency, or hemophilia.

PREVENTING SKIN BREAKDOWN

■ CLINICAL ALERT

New guidelines from the U.S. Department of Health and Human Services advocate no skin massage on reddened skin or skin that has potential breakdown because massage causes friction and shearing.

Equipment

Skin lotion
Pressure-relieving mattress
Clean gloves if open lesions are present

Procedure

1. Observe the client's most vulnerable body surfaces for ischemia, hyperemia, or broken areas.
2. Change the client's body position at least once every 2 hours to rotate weight-bearing areas.

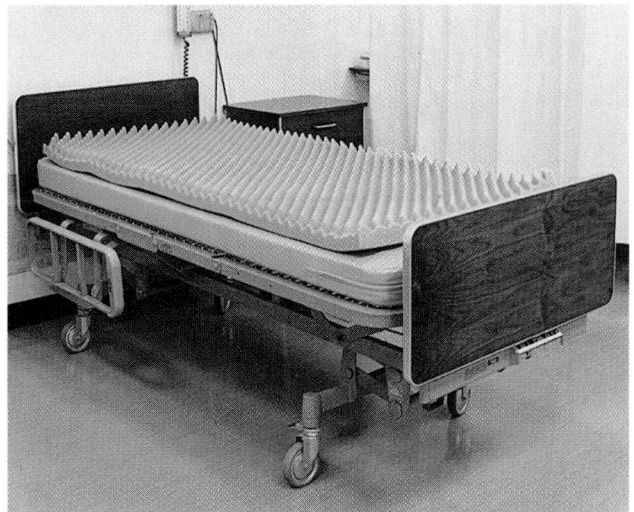

Eggcrate pressure mattress to prevent skin breakdown.

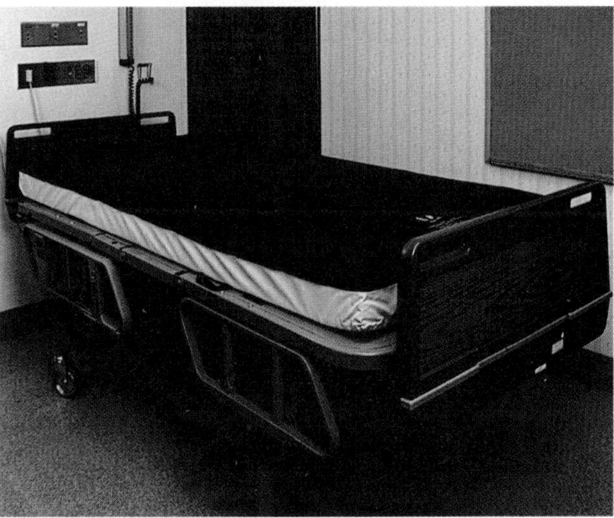

Special gel nonpressure mattress to preserve skin integrity.

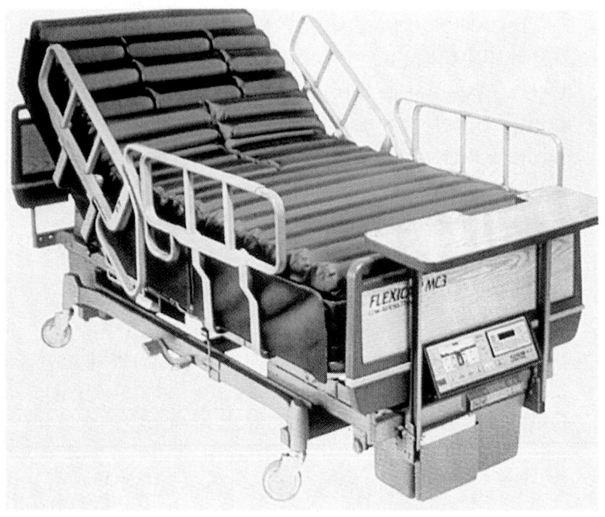

Low air loss therapy bed. Flexicair MC3. (Courtesy of Hill-Rom.)

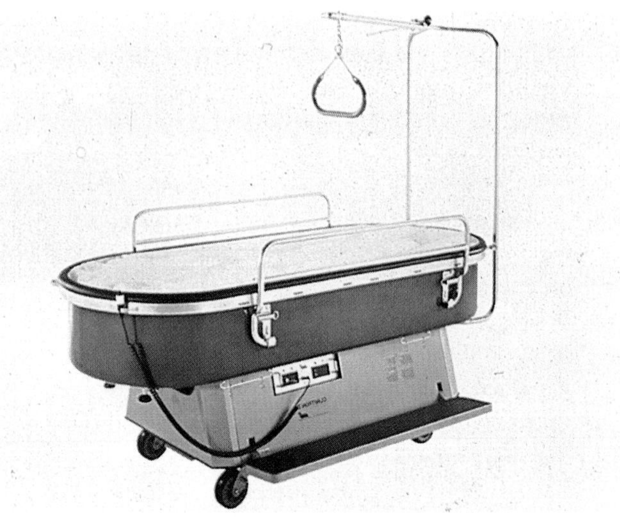
Air fluidized therapy bed-Clinitron. (Courtesy of Hill-Rom.)

TABLE 9–2. Therapeutic Beds

Type of Bed	Bed Features and Benefits	Client Recommendations
Static low air loss Flexicair (Mc3) illustrated KinAir Mediscus SMI 3000	Segmented cushions minimize shear and friction Automatic pressure adjustment Quick adjustment for CPR Built-in scale Bed-exit alarm Extended safetysides U-shaped cushions provide relief for head, sacral area, and heels	Clients at high risk for skin breakdown Clients with pulmonary problems—reduces risk of airbourn contamination Clients with external fixators, heavy casts, or who are obese
Air fluidized or static high-air-loss Clinitron illustrated Skytron Fluid Air SMI 5000	Fluid-like movement places minimum pressure on bony prominences Drying effect of beads prevents skin breakdown Offers softer surface than any other bed	Severe skin disorders Pressure ulcers Burns Generalized massive edema Poor wound healing Geriatric or orthopedic clients
Active low air loss Efica cc illustrated Biodyne Restcue Pulmonair 40	Built-in scale CPR deflation control Automatic pressure adjustment Gently pulsates or rotates side to side Protects skin integrity Promotes removal of pulmonary secretions Stimulates capillary blood flow	Massive edema Congestive heart failure Sepsis Critical care clients Pneumonia or other pulmonary problems with comprised skin integrity

Observe all vulnerable areas at this time. Include right and left lateral, prone, supine, and swimming-type positioning if possible.

3. Massage client's skin and pressure-prone areas, if skin is not reddened, when client changes position. **Rationale:** Massage increases risk of breakdown in clients with reddened areas over bony prominences.
4. Lubricate dry, unbroken skin to prevent breakdown.
5. Keep skin clean and dry. Prevent soap, urine, feces, and excessive moisture from irritating the skin.
6. Protect healthy skin from drainage secretions.

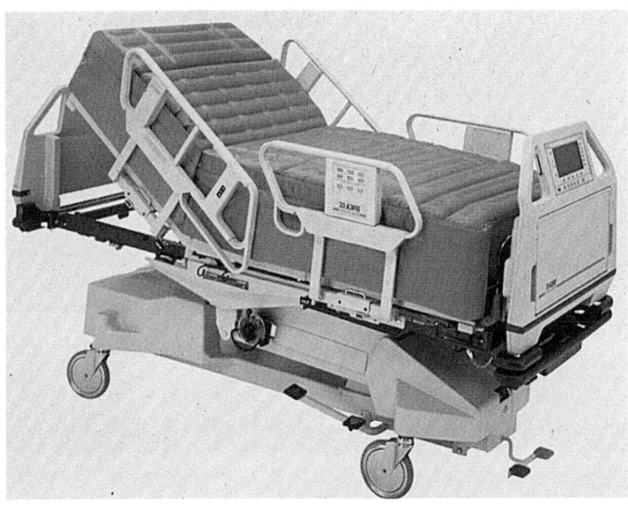

Air Fluidized–lowair loss combined–EFICA-CC. (Courtesy of Hill-Rom).

7. Apply lotion to bedridden client's sacrum, elbows, and heels several times during the day.
8. Keep linens clean, dry, and wrinkle-free.
9. Encourage active exercise or range-of-motion exercise.
10. Encourage client to eat a well-balanced diet with protein-rich foods and adequate fluids.
11. Teach client and family how to prevent pressure areas and pressure ulcer formation.

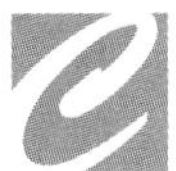

CHARTING for Skin Integrity

- Client's skin condition: odor, temperature, turgor, sensation, cleanliness, integrity
- Client's mobility
- Turning frequency and client positioning
- Type of care given (e.g., massage, bathing)
- Client's complaints about skin or pressure ulcer
- Time and method used to obtain wound specimen
- Type of lesion, location, size, shape, color
- Alterations in sensation in skin lesion area
- Skin or body odor

CRITICAL THINKING APPLICATION

CLINICAL PROBLEMS	CRITICAL THINKING OPTIONS
■ Skin is erythematous but remains intact.	• Monitor fluid balance and nutritional status. • Obtain eggcrate or pressure-relieving mattress. • Turn client every 2 hours.
■ Client cannot be positioned in a manner to avoid erythematous areas entirely.	• Turn at least every hour. • Do not turn on erythematous site. • Use protocol for stage 1 ulcer treatment on affected area.
■ Skin integrity is interrupted, even with skin care.	• Use aseptic technique in treating area to prevent spread of bacteria and promote wound healing. • Use appropriate skin care products. • If skin is sensitive and breakdown occurs over large area, the use of a CLINITRON unit or fluid bed might be indicated (Table 9–2). • Follow treatment for specific stages of decubitus ulcer.

unit 4

EVENING CARE

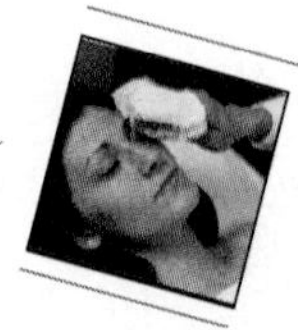

NURSING PROCESS DATA

ASSESSMENT Data Base

Review client's usual routines prior to sleep:

- Usual time of sleep and length of sleeping period
- Personal hygiene routines
- Temperature of room and number of blankets
- Anticipated elimination needs
- Religious or meditation needs

Evaluate client's understanding and acceptance of safety precautions, such as use of side rails.

Assess client's needs for comfort and security.

- Dressings
- Medication
- Linen change or adjustment
- Positioning
- Television, radio, light
- Communication needs

Assess physical and emotional status during evening care.

Assess condition of back, especially bony prominences.

PLANNING Objectives

To encourage a period of comfortable, uninterrupted rest

To evaluate the client's present health status

To make observations about the client's physical and emotional status

To provide time for the client and nurse to review the day's events

To provide time for the client to communicate needs and questions regarding health care

To provide the client with a clean, secure environment in which to sleep

IMPLEMENTATION Procedures

Providing Evening Care

Providing Back Care

EVALUATION Expected Outcomes

Client appears comfortable and ready for sleep in a safe, clean environment.

Client has the time to talk about concerns or ask questions.

The nurse is able to evaluate the client's health care status.

PROVIDING EVENING CARE

Equipment

Towels, washcloth

Clean linens if needed

Basin of warm water, soap

Dental items (i.e., toothbrush, dentifrice, denture cup)

Emesis basin, cup

Fresh pitcher of water if allowed

Skin care lotion and powder if desired

Personal care items (e.g., deodorant, skin moisturizers)

Bedpan, urinal, toilet paper

Miscellaneous supplies as needed (e.g., dressing, special equipment)

Preparation

1. Explain the needs and benefits of evening care; discuss how the client can be involved.
2. Collect and arrange equipment.
3. Adjust the bed to a comfortable working height, and assist the client into a comfortable position.
4. Ensure privacy.
5. Wash your hands.

Procedure

1. Offer bedpan or urinal if client is unable to use bathroom. Assist with handwashing.
2. If client needs or requests a bath, provide assistance as needed.
3. Assist with mouth and dental care as needed.
4. Remove equipment, extra linens, and pillows if possible. Remove stockings, ace wraps, and binders.
5. Change dressings. Perform any required procedural techniques.
6. Wash face, hands, and back. Provide back massage.
7. Assist with combing or brushing hair if desired.
8. Replace stockings and binders.
9. Replace soiled linen, or straighten and tuck remaining linen. Fluff pillow.
10. Straighten top linens. Provide additional blankets if desired.
11. Remove any additional equipment. Place call signal and water (if allowed) within client's reach.
12. Administer sleeping medication if ordered.
13. Assist client into a comfortable position.
14. Ensure that the client's environment is safe and comfortable.
15. Raise side rails, place bed in LOW position, and turn lighting to low.
16. Wash your hands.

PROVIDING BACK CARE

Equipment

Basin of warm water
Washcloth
Towel
Soap
Skin care lotion

Procedure

1. Check skin for reddened areas before beginning back rub.
2. Explain the purpose of a back rub, and ask client if he or she would like one.
3. Provide privacy.
4. Wash your hands with warm water.
5. Warm lotion by holding bottle under water.
6. Raise bed to comfortable height for you, and assist the client into a comfortable prone or semiprone position. Keep farthest side rail in UP position.
7. Drape bed clothes for warmth, and untie the client's gown. Wash back with warm water and soap if necessary.
8. Place lotion on your hands.
9. Once you place your hands on a client's back to begin a backrub, your hands should remain in

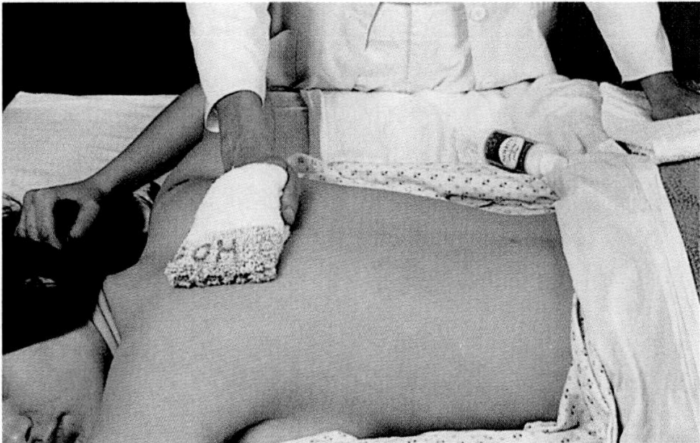

Wash back with soap and water, then dry thoroughly before beginning back rub.

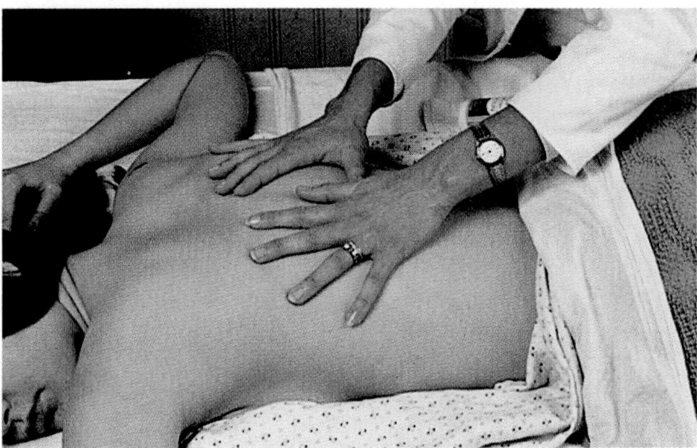

Without lifting hands from skin surface, massage in countinous motion.

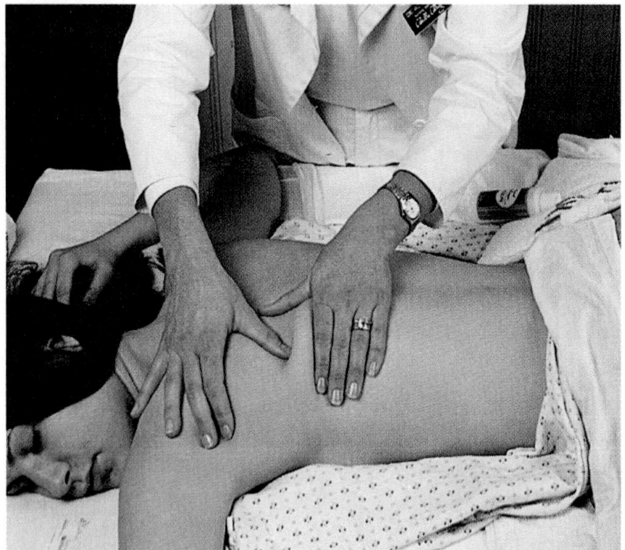

The petrissage, or kneading stroke, is used over the shoulders and along back.

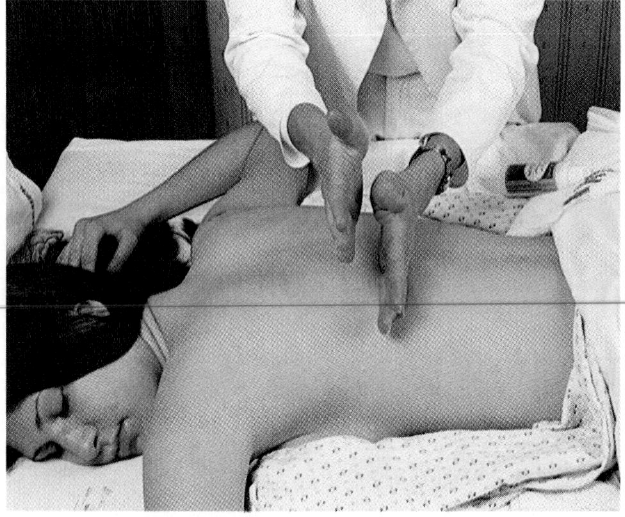

The tapotement stroke stimulates the skin as the hands move up and down the back.

constant skin contact with the client until backrub is complete. **Rationale:** To prevent "tickling" sensation.

10. Repeatedly move your hands up on either side of the client's spine, across shoulders, and down the lateral aspects of the back using the effleurage stroke, applying firm and steady pressure.
11. Then rub your hands over the scapular area, extending over the upper shoulders, using a circular motion.
12. Move your hands down the center of the client's back to sacral area.
13. Massage with a figure-eight motion from the sacrum out over each buttock.
14. Finally, rub lightly up and down the back a few strokes before lifting hands from client's back.
15. Assess skin for color, turgor, skin breakdown.
16. When stimulation is desired, the back and buttocks can be lightly struck with the fleshy sides of your hands, called tapotement. Using an alternating rhythm, move up and down the back several times. In addition, kneading can be accomplished by picking up the skin between the thumb and fingers as you move up the back. This movement is called petrissage.
17. Close client's gown, pull up bedcovers, and assist client to change position if desired. Place side rails in UP position. Place bed in LOW position.
18. Return lotion to the proper area.
19. Wash your hands.

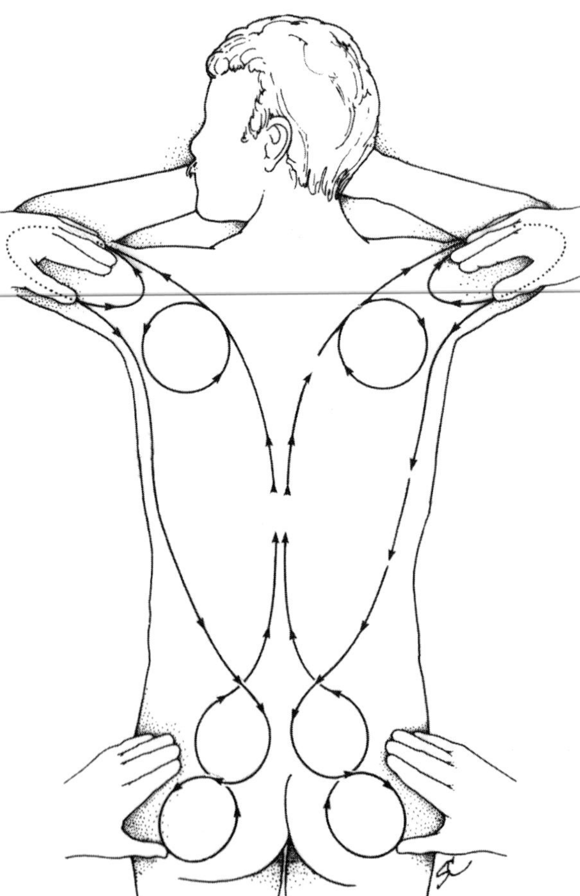

Maintain constant skin contact during back care by moving hands in figure-eight motion from shoulder to buttocks and back.

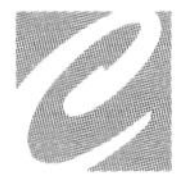

CHARTING for Evening Care

- Client's level of comfort or discomfort
- Type of care given (i.e., back care, evening care)
- Any significant complaints
- Nature of client teaching if done
- Medication required for discomfort or sleep
- Client's physical and emotional status after evening care completed

CRITICAL THINKING APPLICATION

CLINICAL PROBLEMS	CRITICAL THINKING OPTIONS
Client misinterprets back care from nurse and makes sexual advances.	• Set firm limits by explaining therapeutic purpose of back care. • Tell client that if he or she cannot accept back care as part of the therapeutic regimen, you will stop.
Client refuses back care because he or she thinks you are too busy or disinterested.	• Make sure you offer the back care in an unhurried and meaningful manner. Do not allow the client to misinterpret your offer for care. • Return to client and offer back care later in the evening.
Client is unable to sleep even after evening care is given.	• Encourage verbalization of fears. • Check to see if sleeping medication can be given. • Provide additional back care.

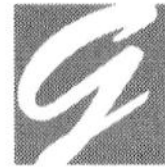

GERIATRIC CONSIDERATIONS

Skin changes with age.

- Skin is less effective as barrier and slow to heal.
- There is decreased protection from trauma.
- There is less ability to retain water.
- Geriatric skin is dry (osteotosis) due to decreased endocrine secretion and loss of elastin. This can cause pruritus, which could lead to skin ulceration.
- There is increased vascular fragility.

The skin of the elderly should be assessed

- Temperature, degree of moisture, dryness
- Intactness, open lesions, tears, pressure ulcers
- Turgor, dehydration
- Pigmentation alterations, potential cancer
- Pruritus—dry skin most common cause
- Bruises, scars

Bathing may minimize dryness

- Have client take complete bath only twice a week.
- Use superfatted or mild soap or lotions to aid in moisturizing.
- Use tepid, not hot, water.
- Apply emollient (lanolin) to skin after bathing.

10

Personal Hygiene

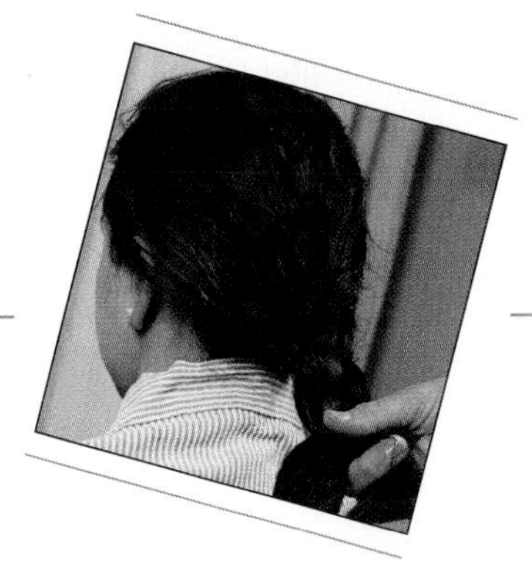

LEARNING OBJECTIVES

- Discuss oral hygiene needs of clients.
- Outline the procedure for flossing teeth.
- Compare and contrast oral hygiene for clients with natural teeth and dentures.
- Demonstrate safety awareness when providing oral care for unconscious clients.
- Identify the appropriate method of hair care according to client's condition.
- Outline the steps for shaving a male client.
- State the rationale for preventing prolonged scalp contact with solutions used to treat pediculosis.
- Discuss rationale for cutting nails straight across.
- Demonstrate proper draping technique for female clients.
- Demonstrate the skill of placing a bedpan for a bedridden client.
- Describe the steps in providing perineal care for male and female clients.
- List the steps in administering a vaginal irrigation.
- Describe nursing actions necessary to care for clients with a prosthetic eye or contact lenses.
- State two suggested solutions when hearing is not improved after cleaning a hearing aid.
- Demonstrate the procedure for replacing an artificial eye.
- State at least two nursing diagnoses pertinent to clients requiring assistance with personal hygiene.

TERMINOLOGY

Abrasion: the scraping away of a portion of skin or of a mucous membrane as a result of injury.

Adaptation: an alteration or adjustment by which an individual can improve his or her relationship to the environment.

Antibacterial: any substance that fights against or suppresses bacteria.

Anticoagulant: any substance that suppresses or counteracts coagulation of blood.

Aspiration: to draw in or out, as by suction.

b.i.d.: two times daily.

Canthus: the angle at either end of the slit between the eyelids.

Capillary: minute blood vessel carrying blood and forming the capillary system.

Cavitation: formation of a cavity.

Congenital: present at birth.

Cornea: the clear, transparent anterior portion of the fibrous coat of the eye.

Debilitated: to become feeble; tired; worn-out.

Decalcification: the act of removing calcium, the basic component of bones and teeth.

Decubitus: a bedsore.

Edema: a local or generalized condition in which there is excess fluid in the tissues.

Emesis: vomiting.

Epidermis: the outer layer of skin.

Eversion: a turning outwards.

Excoriation: the abrasion of the epidermis or of the coating of any organ of the body.

Expectoration: expulsion of mucus or phlegm from the throat or lungs.

Fissure: a groove, slit, or natural division; ulcer or crack-like sore.

Floss: a waxed or unwaxed tape or thread used to clean between teeth.

Fungus: a vegetable cellular organism that subsists on organic matter.

Genitals: organs of generation; reproductive organs.

Hemorrhage: abnormal internal or external discharge of blood.

Holistic: the philosophy that an individual must be looked at as a whole rather than a sum of the parts.

Hygiene: the study and observance of health rules.

Hypoallergenic: against allergy, as hypoallergenic tape.

Impetigo: inflammatory skin disease marked by isolated pustules that become crusted and rupture.

Incontinent: inability to retain urine or feces through loss of sphincter control.

Incurvate: curved, especially inward.

Intervention: the act of coming between, so as to hinder or modify.

Irritation: a source of annoyance; incipient inflammation, soreness or roughness, or irritability of a body part.

Labia: the lips of the vulva.

Lesion: an injury or wound; a single infected patch in a skin disease.

Metabolism: the sum of all physical and chemical changes that take place within an organism; all energy and material transformations that occur within living cells.

Microorganism: a minute living body such as a bacterium or protozoon not perceptible to the naked eye.

Mucosa: mucous membrane lining passages and cavities communicating with the air.

Nasolacrimal: pertinent to the nose and lacrimal apparatus.

Ophthalmic solution: solution designed especially for the eyes.

Oral: concerning the mouth.

Palate: the roof of the mouth.

Parotid gland: either of the largest of the paired salivary glands, located below and in front of each ear.

Pediculosis: infestation with lice.

Perineum: the external region between the vulva and anus in a female or between the scrotum and anus in a male.

Plaque: a patch on the skin or on a mucous surface; a blood platelet.

Pressure point: area for exerting pressure to control bleeding; an area of skin that can become irritated with pressure, especially over bony prominences.

Sclera: the tough, white, fibrous outer envelope of tissue covering all of the eyeball except the cornea.

Semi-Fowler's position: semisitting position.

Systemic: pertinent to the whole body rather than to one of its parts.

Thrush: fungus infection of mouth or throat, especially in infants and young children and in clients with AIDS.

Ulcer: an open sore or lesion of the skin or mucous membrane of the body.

Urethra: canal for the discharge of urine extending from the bladder to the outside.

Vascular: pertinent to or composed of blood vessels.

HYGIENIC CARE

Unfamiliar or life-threatening conditions affect the client's adaptation to the health care system. A holistic approach on the part of the nurse provides individualized care and assists the client to adapt. Basic hygiene care is an integral part of the total treatment program. Together with its role in enhancing the client's adaptation to the hospital environment and sense of self-worth, it provides an opportunity to do a total assessment and evaluation. This time also allows for establishing a working relationship with the client and offers an opportunity to reduce stress by discussing fears and concerns about being in the hospital or the care being received.

The manner in which hygienic care is provided by the nursing staff influences the client's perception of the staff. If the care is administered in a professional and efficient manner, the client's confidence in the health care system is increased. The need to provide personal hygiene depends on each client's physical state and ability to care effectively for him or herself. Your first responsibility is to assess the client's level of ability. After gathering this data, you should assist the client as necessary, providing any assistance or teaching he or she may require.

Oral Hygiene

The condition of the oral cavity has a direct influence on an individual's overall state of health. Dental diseases require a "host" (the tooth and gum), an "agent" (plaque), and an "environment" (e.g., the presence of saliva and food). When plaque comes in contact with bacterial enzymes, carbohydrates, and acids, cavitation begins as the enamel of the tooth is decalcified. As long as food and plaque remain in the oral cavity, the possibility of dental decay increases. In the hospital the incidence of caries (cavities) can be decreased by using a dentifrice containing fluoride, proper brushing and flossing, and adequate nutrition.

Hair Care

The appearance and condition of a client's hair can reflect his or her general physical and emotional status, individuality and feelings of worth, and the ability to care for him or herself. When complex medical care is required during illness or trauma, hair care is often neglected.

Hair care is an important aspect of regular hygiene. To prevent damage to the hair, scalp, and surrounding skin, and to promote the client's sense of well-being, you should assess the condition of a client's hair. Based on the assessment, provide hair and scalp care, shampooing, and shaving, and intervene to correct special problems.

Foot Care

The feet are especially susceptible to discomfort, trauma, and infection due to the amount of stress they must endure as well as to their distance from main blood supplies. Many conditions can be avoided if proper foot care is taken. The more common foot problems include

- Incurvated or ingrown toenails: The corners of the nail tend to press into skin, causing pain, ulceration, and infection.
- Cracks and fissures between toes: This problem often occurs as a result of excessively dry skin.
- Athlete's foot: Irritation characterized by itching, burning skin; caused by an easily transmitted fungus.
- Corns: High calluses caused by pressure on toes, joints, or bony prominences.
- Plantar warts: A virus manifested as a deep, often painful wart on the soles of the feet.
- Calluses: Thickened epidermis over areas of pressure.
- Decreased circulation to the feet: A problem that is often caused by diabetes, vascular diseases, or the constriction of major vessels to the lower extremities.

Perineal and Genital Care

The perineum consists of the area between the thighs and from the anterior pelvis to the anus. This area contains organs and structures related to sexual functioning, reproduction, and elimination.

Hygienic care involves cleaning the perineum and genitalia to prevent bacterial growth, which can rapidly increase in this warm, dark, moist environment. Perineal care is often provided as a routine part of bathing but may be required more frequently to prevent skin irritation, infection, discomfort, or odor.

All clients are susceptible to perineal irritation or infection. Clients who are especially vulnerable are those who are immobilized, incontinent, debilitated, postsurgical, or comatose; those who have indwelling catheters; those who have metabolic and fluid balance disorders; or those who require systemic medications.

Vaginal irrigations are not done as a routine hygiene measure, as odor from the perineal area is rarely due to a vaginal discharge. Perineal odor is usually a reflection of inadequate perineal care. Vaginal irrigations are used prior to radiation therapy, to apply antimicrobial solutions to the area, or to apply a heat or cold treatment to the vagina.

The normal vaginal pH and flora can be altered with vaginal irrigations; therefore, the irrigation should not be given 24 hours before a culture-and-sensitivity test of vaginal secretions or Pap smear is taken. White vinegar, salt, povidone-iodine, or tap water are solutions frequently used for vaginal irrigations.

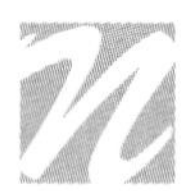

NURSING DIAGNOSES

The following nursing diagnoses are appropriate to include in a client care plan when a client is admitted and requires basic hygienic care.

NURSING DIAGNOSIS	RELATED FACTORS
Knowledge Deficit	Misinformation or lack of information, impaired cognitive function, lack of motivation
Altered Oral Mucous Membrane	Inadequate oral hygiene, chemotherapy, malnutrition, dehydration, infection, mechanical trauma
Noncompliance	Inability to perform tasks, disability, impaired memory
Bathing/Hygiene Self-care Deficit	Impaired motor or cognitive function, pain, disease condition, surgery
Self-esteem Disturbance	Impaired motor or cognitive function, chronic illness, chronic pain

unit 1

ORAL HYGIENE

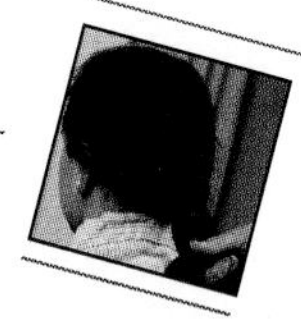

NURSING PROCESS DATA

ASSESSMENT Data Base

Assess whether client wears dentures.

Evaluate client's knowledge of oral hygiene techniques.

Assess condition of client's oral cavity, teeth, gums, and mouth.

Assess for color, lesions, tenderness, inflammation, intactness of teeth, and degree of moisture or dryness of the oral cavity.

Observe the external and internal lips.

Assess the palate (roof and floor of mouth), and inspect under the tongue.

Assess the entire oral mucosa, noting the inside of the cheek.

Observe the tongue. Note tip, sides, back position, and underside.

Evaluate the condition of gums and teeth.

Assess the condition of throat as client says "Ah."

If dentures or orthodontic appliances are used, observe the relationship of the appliances to the client's oral cavity (i.e., fit, irritation, condition of dentures).

PLANNING Objectives

To remove plaque and bacteria-producing agents from the oral cavity

To allow the nurse to assess the client's oral health status, knowledge, and routines of oral care

To decrease the possibility of irritation or infection of the oral cavity

To remove unpleasant tastes and odors from the oral cavity

To provide comfort for the client

To provide client teaching when appropriate

IMPLEMENTATION Procedures

Providing Oral Hygiene

Flossing Client's Teeth

Providing Denture Care

Providing Oral Care for Unconscious Clients

EVALUATION Expected Outcomes

The oral health status of the client has been assessed and documented by the nurse.

Oral hygiene care is provided without complications.

Plaque and bacteria-producing agents are removed.

PROVIDING ORAL HYGIENE

Equipment

Toothbrush: small enough to reach back teeth; soft and rounded with nonfrayed rows of nylon bristles

Dentifrice: client's choice, preferably one containing fluoride; special paste for dentures

Cup of water

Emesis basin or sink

Dental floss: regular or fine, waxed or unwaxed, depending on client's needs

Tissues or towel

Mouthwash if desired

Clean gloves

Preparation

1. Wash your hands.
2. Collect necessary equipment. Assist client with the arrangement of equipment if necessary.
3. Assist client to sink or provide privacy if care is to be given in bed.
4. Help client into a comfortable semi-Fowler's position or a sitting position.
5. If dentures are present, don clean gloves and help client remove them if necessary. Place dentures in denture cup.
6. Inspect surface of mouth for any abnormalities. Ask client about usual oral care routines.
7. Elicit any concerns, comments, or questions client may have about his or her oral health status.
8. Determine oral hygiene needs based on findings.
9. Assess client's need for teaching. Consider educational level, physical, emotional and mental state, previous experiences, cultural differences.
10. Assess client's physical condition. Consider diagnoses, treatments, fluid status, drugs, diet, level of comfort, or pain.
11. Assess client's ability to care for him or herself.

NURSE–CLIENT TEACHING

Begin teaching the client about oral care during your initial assessment. Focus the teaching on oral health needs and care. You may want to incorporate the following techniques:

- A demonstration and return demonstration to illustrate correct dental care techniques.
- Disclosure tablets or solution that temporarily stains dental plaque pink. This technique helps the client to see where plaque appears on the teeth. After applying tablets or solution, ask the client to brush and floss until plaque is removed.

Procedure

1. Wash your hands, and don clean gloves.
2. Request that client open mouth wide and hold emesis basin under chin.
3. Direct the bristles of the toothbrush toward the gum line for all areas to be brushed. **Rationale:** Action removes food particles from gum line and stimulates the gums.

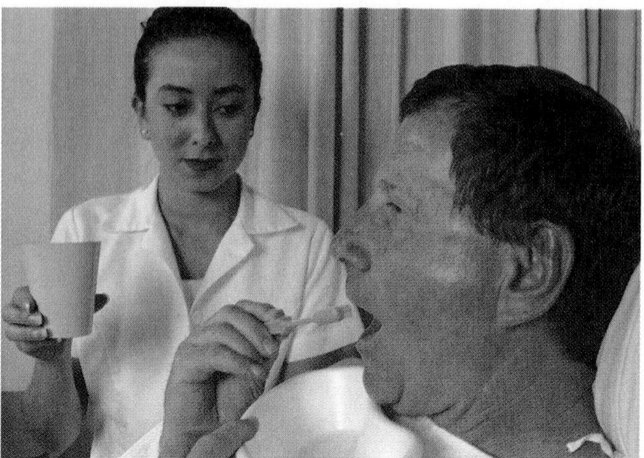

Providing oral hygiene is an essential component of client care, especially when client is on bed rest.

4. Keep the brush positioned over only two or three teeth at a time. Use small rotating movements to cover the outside surfaces of all teeth.
5. Using the brushing method described above, clean the inner surfaces of all back teeth.
6. To clean the flat chewing surfaces, use a firm back-and-forth motion.
7. To clean the inner surfaces of the front teeth, use the bristles on the end of the toothbrush and rotate the brush back and forth across the teeth.
8. Lightly brush all areas of the tongue—this improves the breath.
9. Rinse the client's mouth thoroughly with water.
10. Inspect oral cavity, and repeat brushing if necessary.
11. Floss thoroughly, using approximately 12–15 inches of floss loosely wrapped around one finger of each of your hands.
12. Floss between each tooth by looping floss around each edge of the tooth and sliding floss down to the gum line.
13. Rinse client's mouth thoroughly with water.
14. Wipe off client's mouth and chin.
15. Wash client's toothbrush, rinse and put it and paste away and return additional equipment.
16. Remove gloves and place in appropriate receptacle.
17. Wash your hands.
18. Check to see that client is comfortable.

FLOSSING CLIENT'S TEETH

Equipment

Dental floss 12–18 inches long–two pieces
Cup of water
Emesis basin
Towel
Clean gloves

Preparation

1. Discuss with client when he or she would prefer flossing teeth, after brushing or after morning care is completed.
2. Instruct client in procedure if he or she is able to floss; otherwise, you carry out procedure.
3. Gather necessary equipment.
4. Wash your hands, and don gloves. **Rationale:** This is an important step, as gloves prevent the transmission of microorganisms to the client's mouth and to the nurse.

Procedure

1. Place client in sitting position and move bed to HIGH position.
2. Place towel under client's chin and emesis basin within reach.
3. Cut dental floss into two 12- to 18-inch lengths.
4. Wrap one length around index fingers of both hands.
5. Hold floss taut between your two hands, and gently pull back and forth between each tooth.
6. Move floss up and down sides of teeth to clean plaque. Go as near gum line as possible without injury to gum. Pull floss back and forth gently, working back toward the biting surface of each tooth. Repeat other edge of each tooth, using a new section of floss. **Rationale:** Overly vigorous flossing can damage gums.
7. Floss each tooth several times until all particles of food are removed.
8. Assist client to rinse mouth and expectorate into emesis basin.
9. Remove basin and wipe client's mouth with towel.
10. Remove gloves and place in appropriate receptacle.
11. Lower bed and return client to comfortable position.

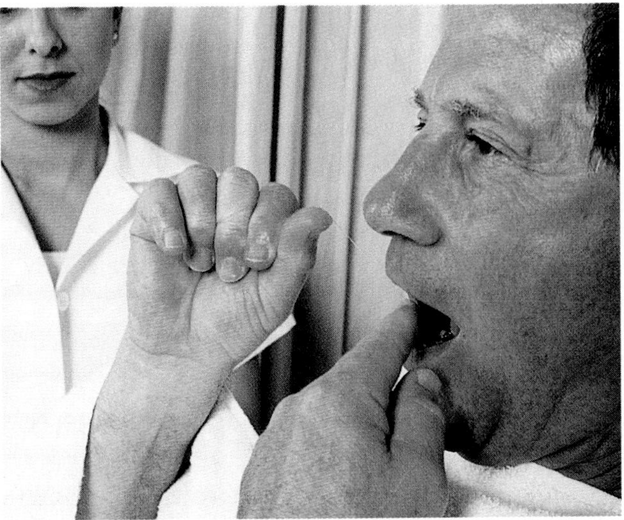

Instruct client to floss to prevent build-up of plaque and food particles between the teeth.

PROVIDING DENTURE CARE

Equipment

Denture toothbrush
Denture cup
Cleanser or effervescent tablets for dentures
Clean gloves

Procedure

1. Encourage client to use dentures. **Rationale:** Dentures improve speech, make eating easier, and improve the shape of the mouth, appearance, and self-image.
2. Wash your hands and don gloves.
3. Help client remove dentures. If client is unable to do this, carefully place your finger on the edge of the upper denture. **Rationale:** This action breaks the seal at the roof of the mouth and allows the denture to easily slide out. Lower denture generally lifts out easily.
4. If client is unable to clean own dentures, place them in an unbreakable container immediately and carry them to the sink. Place a paper towel or

washcloth on the bottom of the sink to cushion the surface in case you accidentally drop a denture.

5. Hold one denture in your hand. With your other hand, use a toothbrush or special denture brush and a cleaning agent, such as a commercially prepared paste or solution, to brush the denture. Use the same brushing motion as with natural teeth.
6. Rinse denture thoroughly in cold water.
7. If dentures are to remain out of the mouth for a period of time, as at night, store them in a clearly labeled, unbreakable container of cold water.
8. If dentures are to be worn immediately, help client to rinse oral cavity with warm water or mouthwash.
9. You may also gently brush client's gums and tongue.
10. Help client replace dentures.
11. Remove gloves, and place in appropriate receptacle.
12. Wash your hands.

PROVIDING ORAL CARE FOR UNCONSCIOUS CLIENTS

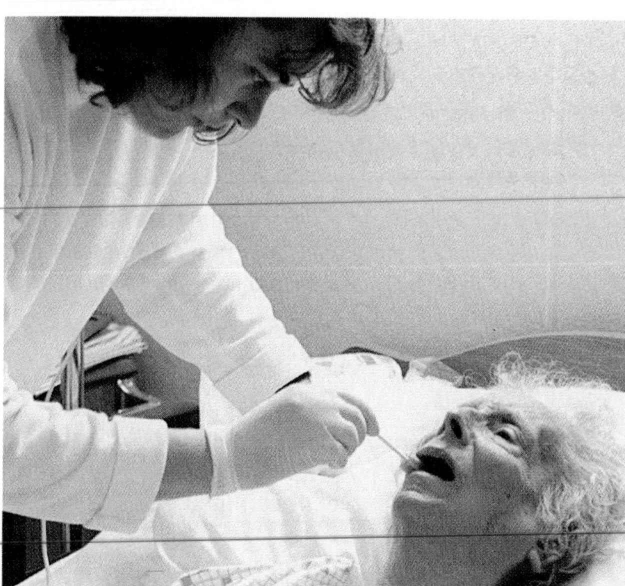

Provide frequent oral care with mouthswabs.

Equipment

Mouthswabs (lemon-glycerin type)
Lubricant for lips
Waterpik devices or brush
Bulb syringe
Tongue blades
Clean gloves

Procedure

1. Gather equipment.
2. Wash your hands and don gloves.
3. If possible, position client on side in a semi-Fowler's position. If this is not possible, turn client's head to the side. **Rationale:** Allows fluid to drain or be suctioned out of mouth and thus prevents aspiration.
4. Place a bulb syringe or suctioning equipment nearby to use for suctioning oral cavity as needed.
5. Brush the external surfaces of the teeth in the routine manner, using less water on the brush. You may use a tongue blade to move the cheeks and lips. Do not put your fingers in the client's mouth. **Rationale:** Accidental biting can cause serious injuries.
6. To clean the inner surfaces of the teeth, use a padded tongue blade to separate the upper and lower sets of teeth. Brush the teeth and tongue in the usual manner.
7. Rinse the client's mouth carefully, using very small amounts of water that can be suctioned.
8. Lubricate client's lips with petroleum jelly.
9. Provide oral care frequently—as often as every 2 hours if necessary. **Rationale:** Oral care maintains adequate oral health.
10. Remove gloves, and place in appropriate receptacle.
11. Wash your hands.

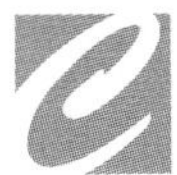

CHARTING for Oral Hygiene

- Findings of assessment of mouth, gums, mucous membranes, and teeth
- Assessment of client's oral hygiene needs
- Planning steps taken to meet client's oral hygiene needs
- Oral care given or observed
- Effectiveness of oral care on client's teeth, gums, mucosa
- Client's reaction and level of comfort
- Client's participation in nurse–client teaching

CRITICAL THINKING APPLICATION

CLINICAL PROBLEMS	CRITICAL THINKING OPTIONS
■ Even with increased oral hygiene, client still has odorous breath.	• Use antiseptic mouthwash between oral hygiene care. • Notify the physician, as this could be a symptom of systemic disease. • Obtain dental consultation to check for presence of dental caries or gum disease.
■ Client complains of extreme oral mucosal irritation or sensitivity.	• Request physician's order for one of the following solutions: Saline solutions: for soothing, cleansing rinses Anesthetic solutions: to dull extreme pain in the oral cavity Effervescent solutions (e.g., hydrogen peroxide or ginger ale) to loosen and remove debris from the mouth Coating solutions (e.g., Maalox) to protect irritated surfaces Antibacterial–antifungal rinses (e.g., nystatin [mycostatin]) to prevent the spread of organisms that cause thrush
■ Vigorous flossing results in bleeding and sore gums.	• Give client warm antiseptic mouthwash to relieve soreness. • Investigate gum condition and refer for consultation.
■ Client needs care after oral surgery or oral trauma.	• Oral care following surgery or trauma is always ordered by physician. No oral hygiene care should be attempted until physician has clearly defined the specific care. • Suctioning equipment should always be present. • Assessment of client's head, face, neck, and general status is critical at this time.

CLINICAL PROBLEMS	CRITICAL THINKING OPTIONS
Normal stimulation and cleaning is not sufficient to remove debris and plaque for the unconscious client.	• Use toothettes, lemon-glycerin swabs. • Provide mouth care with toothbrush and dentifrice at least b.i.d.
Parotid gland inflammation can occur with improper oral hygiene.	• Rinse mouth with mouthwash. • Use lemon-glycerin swab to reach back in oral cavity along mandible to temporomandibular area. • Floss teeth at least daily.

unit 2

HAIR CARE

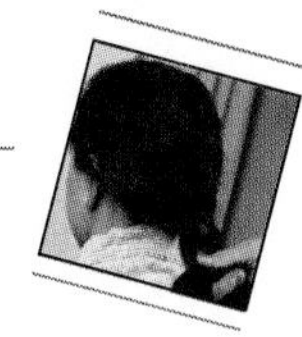

NURSING PROCESS DATA

ASSESSMENT Data Base

Review general physical assessment findings.

Elicit information regarding loss of hair, tenderness of scalp, or itching.

Determine client's ability to perform own hair care.

If unable to care for own hair find out who usually assists client.

Observe client's hair and scalp, noting the following:

- Texture
- Color
- Degree of thickness and hair distribution
- Degree of gloss or shine
- Dryness or oiliness
- Areas of irritation, rash, or scaliness on the scalp or surrounding skin
- Matting or snarls
- Pediculosis (lice)

Assess usual hair care routines, products, and appliances.

Assess method for providing hair care (e.g., in bed, on gurney, in wheelchair).

Determine client teaching needs regarding hair care.

PLANNING Objectives

To prevent irritation to the scalp and damage to the hair

To help maintain or improve client's existing condition of hair and scalp

To promote circulation to the hair follicle and growth of new hair

To distribute oils along the hair shaft

To promote self-esteem

IMPLEMENTATION Procedures

Providing Hair Care
- *for Routine Hair Care*
- *for Tangled Hair*
- *for Coarse or Curly Hair*

Shampooing Hair
- *for Client in a Chair*
- *for Client on a Gurney*
- *for Client on Bedrest*

Braiding Hair

Providing Hair Care for Beards and Mustaches

Shaving a Client

EVALUATION Expected Outcomes

Hair and scalp assessment are performed without complications.

Client's hair and scalp are clean, comfortable, and styled according to client's preference.

Client is comfortable and rested following shampooing.

Shaving is accomplished without discomfort.

PROVIDING HAIR CARE

Equipment

Blunt-ended comb or pick
Brush
Towel
Mirror
Hair care products and ornaments

Preparation

1. Determine client's hair care needs.
2. Wash your hands.
3. Help client into a comfortable position to perform hair care.
4. Collect and assemble equipment.

Procedure *for Routine Hair Care*

1. Place all hair care items within reach.
2. Place towel over client's shoulders.
3. Brush or comb client's hair from scalp to hair ends, using gentle, even strokes.
4. Style hair in a manner suitable to client.
5. Replace hair care items in appropriate place, and clean items as needed.
6. Wash your hands.

Procedure *for Tangled Hair*

1. Hold client's hair above the tangle to prevent discomfort.
2. Using a wide-toothed comb, gently comb tangle. Use short, gentle strokes. Work out the tangle from the end of hair shafts toward the scalp. Work on small amount of tangle at one time. **Rationale:** Working on large tangles results in broken ends and damaged hair shafts.
3. You may also apply small amounts of vinegar or alcohol to client's hair to make combing the tangle easier.
4. Style the client's hair in a manner that prevents further tangling (e.g., a loose braid placed in an area that does not put pressure on the head).

Procedure *for Coarse or Curly Hair*

1. Comb hair in small sections to remove tangles.
2. Use a comb or pick to comb hair in small sections.
3. Apply a small amount of oil to dry or flaking areas of the scalp.
4. Using a wide-toothed comb or pick, gently lift hair and smooth out evenly.
5. If corn-rowing is desired, make small rows of braids close to the scalp in the client's choice of design. (This type of braid is left in the hair for a longer time.)

SHAMPOOING HAIR

Equipment

Two bath towels
Washcloth
Shampoo
Conditioner, if desired
Hair dryer, if allowed in hospital
"Shampoo board" for clients confined to bed

Preparation

1. Determine client's hair care needs.
2. Wash your hands.
3. Collect and assemble equipment.
4. Help client into a comfortable position to perform hair care.
5. Shampooing the hair can be accomplished in a variety of ways depending on the client's usual routine and physical condition. In many institutions, a physician's order is necessary before shampooing a client's hair.
6. If possible, the easiest way to shampoo is to assist the client while he or she is in the shower. Caution should be taken to prevent the client from becoming overly tired or weak while in the shower.

Procedure *for Client in a Chair*

1. Have shampoo items readily available.
2. Drape one towel over client's shoulders and around neck. Place another towel within reach.
3. Face client away from sink. Lock wheels of wheelchair.

4. Pad the edge of the sink with a towel or bath blanket.
5. Ask client to lean head and neck against sink.
6. Using a washcloth to protect client's eyes, wet hair, and gently make a lather with shampoo.
7. Rinse thoroughly, and repeat if necessary.
8. Towel dry, add conditioner if desired, and rinse again.
9. Using a dry towel, pat hair dry, and wrap turban style to transport back to bed.
10. Use hair dryer if available.
11. Style as desired.
12. Replace equipment.

Procedure *for Client on a Gurney*

1. Have shampoo items readily available.
2. Position gurney with head end at sink.
3. Lock wheels on gurney. **Rationale:** This prevents the gurney from moving away from the sink.
4. Pad the edge of the sink with a towel or bath blanket.
5. Move the client's head just beyond the edge of the gurney to allow water to run off more easily.
6. Put a pillow or a rolled blanket under the client's shoulders to help elevate and extend the head.
7. Drape one towel over client's shoulders and around neck. Place another towel within reach.
8. Use a washcloth to protect client's eyes. Wet hair and gently make a lather with shampoo.
9. Rinse thoroughly and repeat if necessary.
10. Towel dry, add conditioner if desired, and rinse again.
11. Using a dry towel, pat hair dry, and wrap turban style to transport back to room.
12. Use hair dryer if available.
13. Style as desired.
14. Replace equipment.

Procedure *for Client on Bed Rest*

1. Place shampoo board, if available, under the client's head. This allows water and soap to run off into a basin at the side of the bed.
2. Drape one towel over client's shoulders and around neck. Place another towel within reach.
3. Place client's head on shampoo board.
4. Using a washcloth to protect client's eyes, wet hair, and gently make a lather with shampoo.
5. Rinse thoroughly, and repeat if necessary.
6. Towel dry, add conditioner if desired, and rinse again.
7. Using a dry towel, pat hair dry, and wrap turban style.
8. Remove equipment from bed.
9. Change gown and linen if wet.
10. Use hair dryer if available. Ensure that electrical equipment is checked by maintenance department before using. **Rationale:** This confirms that equipment is grounded and mechanically safe.
11. Style as desired.
12. Replace all equipment.
13. If a shampoo board is not available, follow these guidelines:
    a. Remove pillows so that client is flat on the bed.
    b. Place a plastic sheet or plastic bed protector under client.
    c. Roll a bath blanket or sheet, and form a trough under client's head. Be sure to have the trough directed over the edge of the bed.
    d. Cover entire trough with a plastic sheet.
    e. Adjust edge of trough to empty into a basin at the side of the bed.
    f. Using pitchers of water, proceed with the routine shampooing procedure.
    g. Change bed linens and clothes if they become wet.
    h. Replace all equipment.

BRAIDING HAIR

Equipment

Comb or brush
Barrette, ribbon, or covered elastic band

Procedure

1. Wash your hands.
2. Position client in a sitting position, if possible.
3. Comb or brush hair. Remove tangles, especially those close to scalp, before braiding.

4. Part hair into sections equal to the number of desired braids.
5. Divide each section into three equal strands.
6. Begin braid so that base is not in a pressure area of the head. **Rationale:** If braid is directly at base of scalp, it may be uncomfortable for client who is bedridden.
7. Weave each of the three strands, alternately placing right strand over the middle strand, then the left strand over the middle one. Move strands smoothly from one hand to the other and keep in hands at all times or the tension is released and hair unbraids.
8. Continue until ends of strands are reached.
9. Fasten ends with barrette or covered elastic. Put on a ribbon, if desired. **Rationale:** Avoid using rubber bands, as they damage the hair shaft.
10. Arrange braids as desired.
11. Reposition client for comfort.
12. Wash your hands.

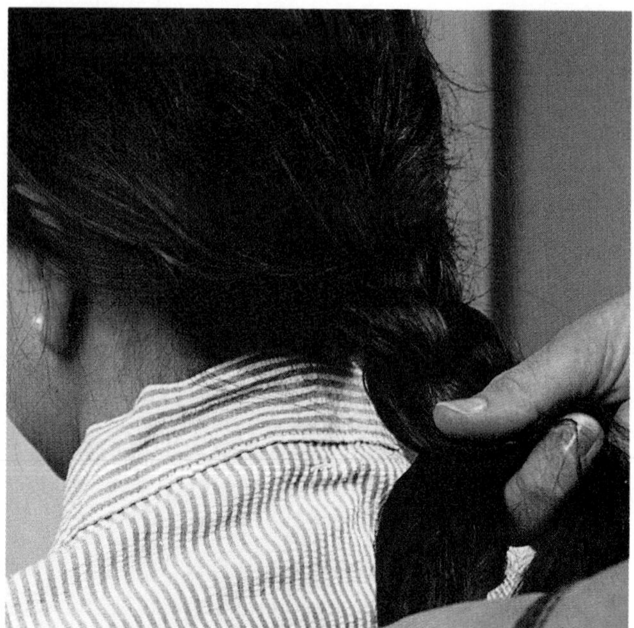

Braiding long hair will prevent tangles, especially for clients on bedrest.

PROVIDING HAIR CARE FOR BEARDS AND MUSTACHES

Equipment

Brush or comb
Towel
Mustache scissors

Preparation

1. Determine client's hair care needs and procedure for mustache or beard.
2. Wash your hands.
3. Help client to a comfortable position.
4. Collect and assemble equipment.

Procedure

1. Observe client's skin underneath beard or mustache.
2. If necessary, comb or brush the beard or mustache.
3. With client's or family's direction, periodically trim client's mustache or beard with sharp scissors.
4. Shampoo beard or mustache as needed.

SHAVING A CLIENT

Equipment

Safety or electric razor, specific to client's needs or wishes
Shaving cream
Aftershave lotion (optional)
Two towels
Basin of warm water

Preparation

1. Place client in sitting position.
2. Place towel over chest and under chin.
3. Provide mirror on overbed table.
4. Determine how the client usually shaves (i.e., use of safety edge or electric razor; use of special products).
5. Check to see if the client has excessive bleeding tendencies due to pathologic conditions (hemophil-

ia) or to the use of specific medications (anticoagulants or large doses of aspirin). **Rationale:** If client is accidentally cut, it could lead to serious loss of blood.

■ CLINICAL ALERT

According to the hospital policy, be sure to have the electric razor checked for safety aspects. Some hospitals do not allow clients to use their own electric razors.

Procedure

1. If using a safety edge razor, apply a warm, moist towel to client's skin to soften the hair.
2. Apply a thick layer of soap or shaving cream to the shaving area.
3. Holding skin taut, use firm but small strokes in the direction of hair growth.
4. Gently remove soap or lather with a warm, damp towel. Inspect for areas you may have missed.
5. Apply aftershave lotion or powder as desired.
6. Reposition client for comfort if needed.
7. Replace equipment.

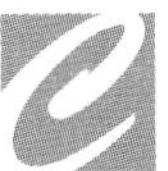

CHARTING for Hair Care

- Documentation of hair care assessment and needs
- Shampooing method, outcomes, problems encountered
- Client's tolerance to hair care
- Shaving done
- Unusual bleeding from shaving

CRITICAL THINKING APPLICATION

CLINICAL PROBLEMS	CRITICAL THINKING OPTIONS
■ Extreme matting, snarling, blood, or non-removable substances appear in client's hair.	• Never cut a client's hair unless it is absolutely necessary. Check hospital policy regarding hair cutting. • Secure permission of family or physician.
■ Client is cut during shaving procedure.	• Assess extent of cut, and place a clean towel on the area with pressure to stop bleeding. • If cut appears to be more than a nick, report to physician, and fill out unusual occurrence report.
■ Shaving is difficult and painful for the client.	• Place warm towels on area to be shaved for 15 minutes. • Apply more shaving cream. • Ensure that razor is sharp.

unit 3

PEDICULOSIS

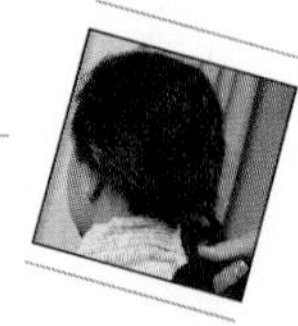

NURSING PROCESS DATA

ASSESSMENT Data Base

Observe head (scalp), body (beard, eyebrows, arms, legs), and pubic areas for the following signs:

Small, hemorrhagic areas on the skin

Scratches on the skin

Habitual itching and scratching

Insect-type bites or pustular eruptions behind the ears or hairline

Small, white dandruff-like particles

Assess client's personal hygiene, living conditions, contact or exposure to others with lice (e.g., school-aged children, sexual partners, siblings).

PLANNING Objectives

To remove lice from client's hair and prevent further skin problems such as impetigo or infection

To remove cause of itching and intense need to scratch scalp

To control spread to others

IMPLEMENTATION Procedure

Removing Lice

EVALUATION Expected Outcomes

Lice removed following treatment.

Client verbalizes cause of problem and preventive measures.

REMOVING LICE

Equipment

Isolation bags

Treatment solution as ordered (i.e., gamma benzene hexachloride (Kwell) or nonprescription drug)

Clean linen

Fine-tooth comb

Disinfectant for comb

Clean gloves

Procedure

1. Don clean gloves.
2. Remove and bag client's clothing and linens separately. Use isolation bags.
3. Notify physician and other health care providers.
4. Begin treatment as ordered by physician. Common treatment is gamma benzene hexachloride applied

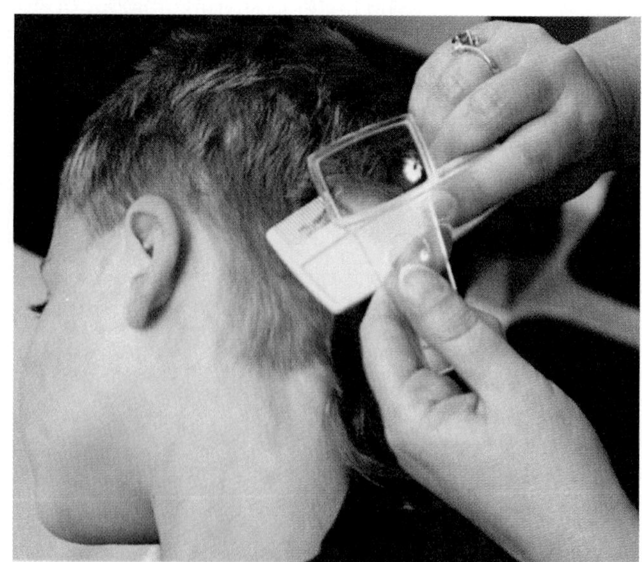

Use magnifying glass when inspecting for head lice.

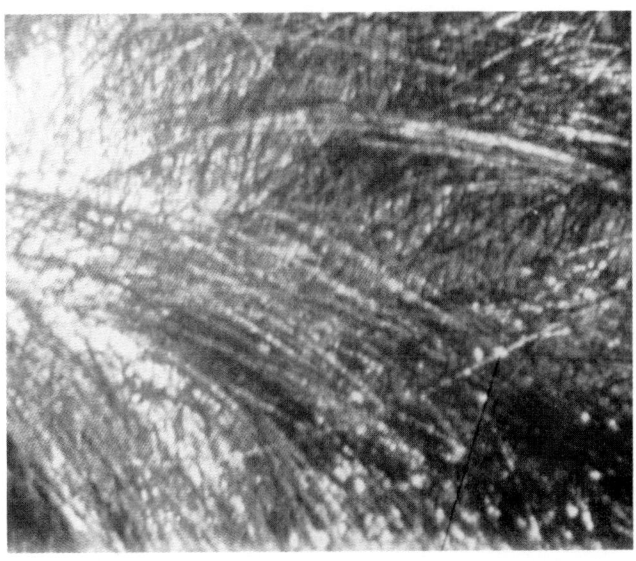

Examine hair closely for white nits on hair shaft.

as a cream, lotion, or shampoo. **Rationale:** Head lice requires shampoo. Body and pubic lice requires shower with soap followed by lotion application for 24 hours.

5. Apply solution, and leave in place several minutes. **Rationale:** Prolonged use of shampoo can burn scalp.
6. Rinse thoroughly.
7. Comb through hair with fine-tooth comb.
8. Disinfect comb and brushes with Kwell shampoo.
9. Remove gloves.
10. Wash hands.
11. Repeat in 24 hours if necessary.
12. Wash clothes and linens separately from other client's belongings.
13. Sterilize equipment as prescribed.
14. Discuss the cause, treatment, and preventive measures regarding lice infestation with client and family.

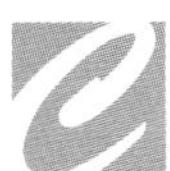

CHARTING for Removing Lice

- Location of lice infestation
- Notification of physician and health care providers
- Action taken and the results
- Client teaching activities

CRITICAL THINKING APPLICATION

CLINICAL PROBLEMS	CRITICAL THINKING OPTIONS
■ Kwell shampoo is left on too long.	• Observe for irritation or burning after rinsing out the shampoo. • If scalp is burned, notify physician for a medication order. • Do not repeat treatment until scalp is healed.
■ Other clients or staff become infested with lice.	• Isolate the client's linen and personal hair grooming equipment to prevent spread of lice. • Instruct client or staff on use of Kwell shampoo.
■ Lice are not eliminated with treatment.	• Obtain an order for shaving client's hair.

unit 4

FOOT CARE

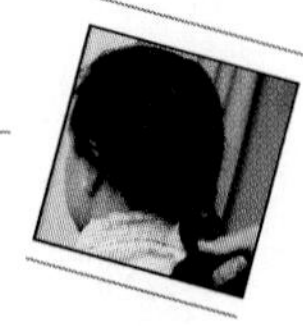

NURSING PROCESS DATA

ASSESSMENT Data Base

Review data from general physical assessment.

Observe the color of the client's feet and lower extremities.

Assess temperature of each foot.

Note color, shape, condition, contour, and length of toenails.

Assess speed of color return when nailbed is depressed (capillary refill).

Inspect skin of entire foot (including corner of toes, between toes, and heels) for irritation, cracking, lesions, corns, calluses, deformities, and edema.

Assess mobility of ankle and toes. Footdrop or plantar flexion and eversion of feet can occur during prolonged bed rest.

Assess cleanliness of feet.

Inspect client's shoes for excessive wear and proper fit.

During assessment, gather data from the client about level of comfort, pain, or tenderness.

PLANNING Objectives

To provide for specific foot care needs

To encourage self-care and prevention of future problems

To prevent infection, discomfort, deformities, circulatory problems, and odor

IMPLEMENTATION Procedures

Providing Foot Care

Providing Nail Care

EVALUATION Expected Outcomes

Foot care provided without complications.

Client's feet are clean and appear free of complicating conditions, such as excessive moisture, calluses, corns, blisters, abrasions, or infection.

Client and family understand the importance and techniques for proper foot care.

PROVIDING FOOT CARE

Equipment

Basin of warm water

Soap or emollient agent

Washcloth

Two towels

Toenail clippers

Nail file, emery board, pick, or orangewood stick

Skin care lotion or lanolin

Preparation

1. Determine foot care needs based on client's condition and assessment data.
2. Check physician's orders and client care plans.
3. Discuss procedure with client.
4. Wash your hands.
5. Collect necessary equipment.
6. Help client into a chair in a comfortable sitting position if possible.

Procedure

1. Place towel or bath mat on floor in front of client.
2. Place basin of warm water on towel.
3. Help client place feet in basin.
4. Add emollient agent to water, if desired.
5. Assist client with other personal hygiene activities while feet are soaking. Let feet soak for 10 minutes.
6. Using a washcloth, gently wash client's feet with soap and water.
7. Dry each foot thoroughly with a second towel. Dry between each toe.
8. Using nail clippers, cut straight across the nails. **Rationale:** Prevents trauma to surrounding tissue.
9. Clean underneath and on sides of nails using a file or orangewood stick.
10. If necessary, push back cuticles using an orangewood stick. Smooth rough edges with an emery board.
11. Apply lotion to entire foot focusing on callused or dry areas.
12. Assist client in putting on clean socks and shoes or slippers.
13. Replace equipment.
14. Assist client to bed or position for comfort in chair.
15. Wash your hands.

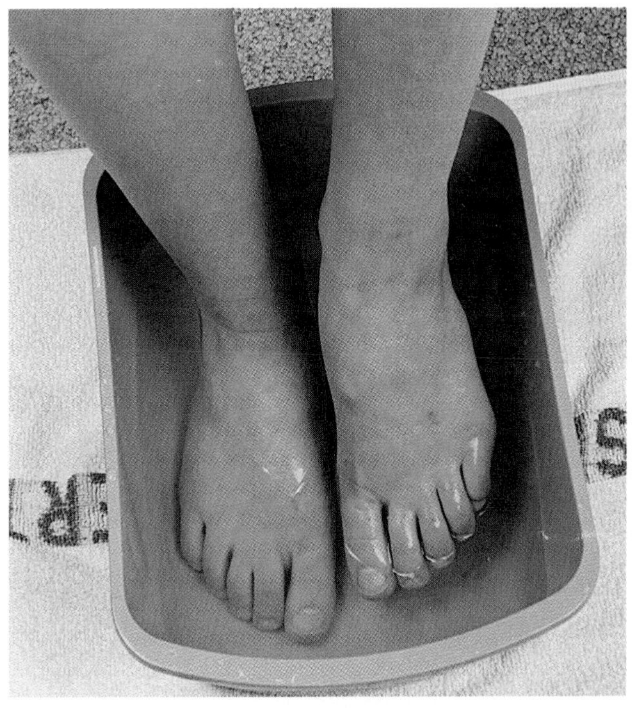

Place towel on floor in front of client and place feet in basin for soaking.

PROVIDING NAIL CARE

Equipment

Basin of warm water
Towel
Scissors or nail clippers
File or emery board
Orangewood stick

Procedure

1. Check hospital policy on nail cutting. Some institutions do not allow nurses to cut client's nails if the client has diabetes mellitus, peripheral vascular disease, or a localized condition such as a fungus infection. Thick, mycotic or ingrown toenails should not be cut by the nurse. Request that a podiatrist see the client.

> **CLINICAL ALERT**
>
> Check policy of hospital regarding cutting of nails. Some health care facilities require that only a podiatrist cut nails.

2. Wash your hands.
3. Position client for comfort.
4. Expose one extremity at a time.
5. Soak nails if softening is needed. Dry nails.
6. Cut toenails straight across with scissors or clippers. **Rationale:** Rounding off toenails may break the skin or cause ingrown toenails.

7. Smooth cut edges as necessary with file or emery board.
8. Clean under nail with orangewood stick to remove debris.
9. Reposition client.
10. Remove and clean equipment.
11. Wash your hands.

CHARTING for Foot and Nail Care

- Initial assessment findings and overall status of client's feet
- Foot and nail care needs and plans
- Care given and results of care
- Any abnormalities
- Involvement in client or family teaching

CRITICAL THINKING APPLICATION

CLINICAL PROBLEMS	CRITICAL THINKING OPTIONS
Client has excessively dry, scaly skin, even after routine foot care.	• Apply alkali solutions as ordered, such as Epsom salts or bicarbonate of soda, to soften skin and remaining scales. Repeated soakings are usually necessary. • Apply lanolin.
Client's feet are excessively moist.	• Give foot care twice a day. • Use moisture-absorbing powder.
Client has large calluses on feet	• After soaking, obtain an order to rub a pumice stone or an abrasive material on the callused area. Calluses are never cut from the skin due to possible scarring to the epidermis. • For diabetic clients, obtain services of a podiatrist.
Client has mycotic nails.	• Report to physician so podiatrist can be consulted.

unit 5 BEDPAN, URINAL, AND COMMODE

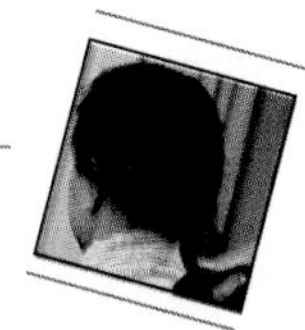

NURSING PROCESS DATA

ASSESSMENT Data Base

Determine client's usual voiding pattern.

Assess client's ability to assist with the procedure.

PLANNING Objectives

To assist the client to void when on bed rest or unable to urinate.

To help client void 200–500 mL of urine without discomfort or difficulty

IMPLEMENTATION Procedure

Using a Bedpan and Urinal

Assisting client to commode

EVALUATION Expected Outcomes

Client voids 200–500 mL of urine without discomfort or difficulty.

Bladder does not become distended.

Genitourinary system is free of infection.

USING A BEDPAN AND URINAL

Equipment

Bedpan or urinal
Toilet tissues
Absorbent pad, if needed
Clean gloves

Procedure

1. Wash your hands and don gloves.
2. Obtain bedpan or urinal and warm a metal bedpan or urinal by running warm water around the edges of the receptacle.
3. Provide privacy.
4. Elevate the head of the bed, or position client on the edge of the bed or in a chair.
5. Instruct the client to sit on the bedpan or urinal. If the client needs assistance, follow these steps:

   Using a bedpan

   a. Place absorbent pad under hips, if needed.
   b. Raise the client's hips and slip your arm under the client or turn the client on his or her side. Roll the client onto the pan.
   c. Place a rolled towel or blanket under the client's sacrum. **Rationale:** This provides comfort by padding the bony area.

   Using a urinal

   a. Place the base of the urinal flat on the bed between the client's thighs.
   b. Position the client's penis or vaginal opening over the urinal.

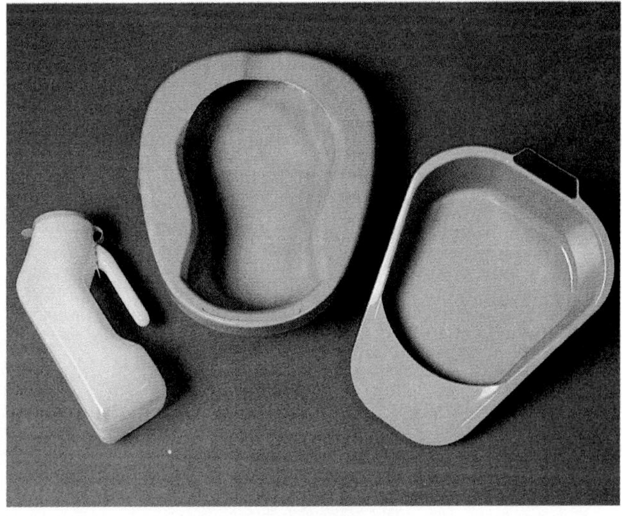

Urinal, bedpan and fracture pan used for clients on bedrest.

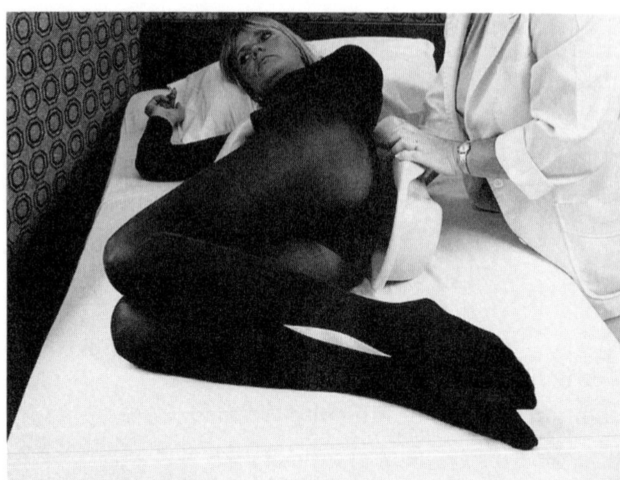
Turn client to side to place on bedpan.

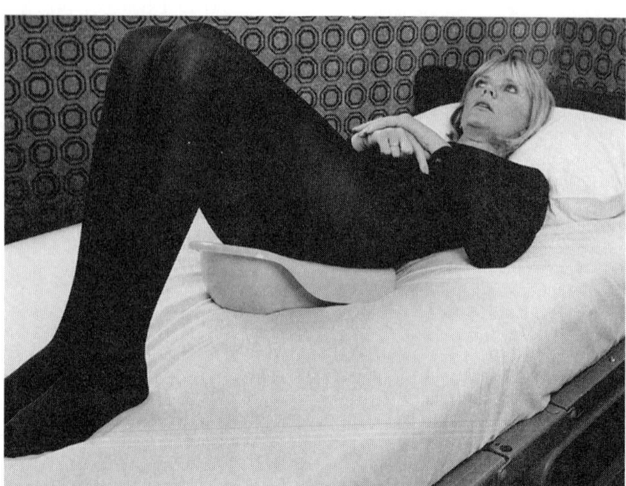
Roll client onto pan and make comfortable.

6. Place the signal light and toilet tissue within easy reach.
7. When the client has voided, remove the receptacle and assist with wiping as necessary.
8. Provide an opportunity for the client to wash his or her hands.
9. Reposition the client for comfort, pull back curtains.
10. Measure intake and output if required.
11. Empty bedpan or urinal, clean equipment, and return to proper area in client's room.
12. Remove gloves and wash your hands.

ASSISTING CLIENT TO COMMODE

Equipment

Commode with locking wheels or rubber tipped legs
Nurse's call bell
Slippers
Bath blanket

Procedure

1. Place commode at foot of bed. Be sure to lock wheels on commode if needed.
2. Place slippers on client.

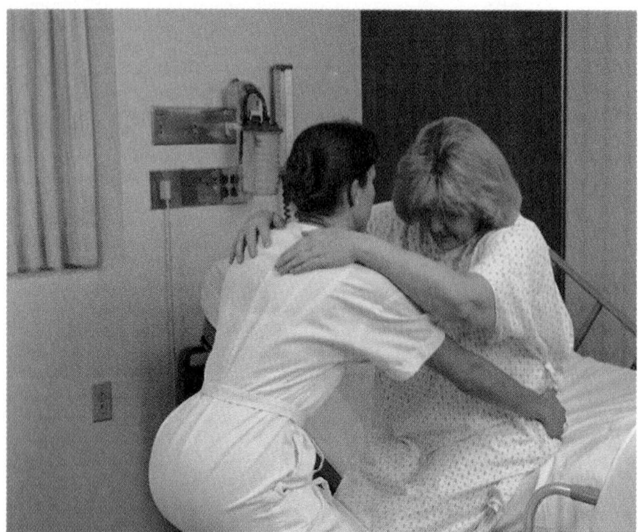
Use correct body mechanics when guiding client to commode.

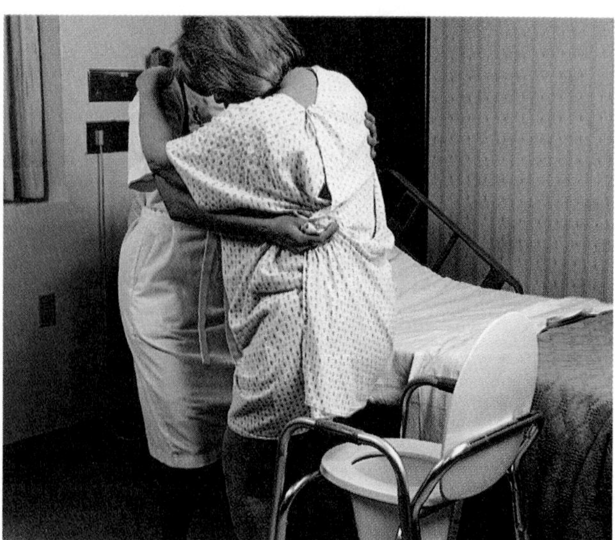
Pivot with client and bend knees when seating client.

3. Instruct client to grasp your shoulders.
4. Place your hands securely around client. **Rationale:** To stabilize client for transfer.
5. Pivot client in front of commode.
6. Lower client onto commode, using correct body mechanics; ensure client is securely positioned on commode.
7. Cover client with bath blanket for warmth and modesty.
8. Place call bell within easy access of client.
9. Provide privacy by closing curtains and shutting door.

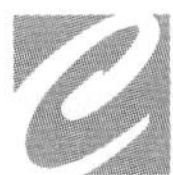

CHARTING for Bedpan, Urinal, and Commode

- Amount, color, appearance, and odor of urine.
- Techniques effective in stimulating voiding.
- Equipment used (e.g., commode, bedpan)

CRITICAL THINKING APPLICATION

CLINICAL PROBLEMS	CRITICAL THINKING OPTIONS
Client is unable to turn and has difficulty raising hips.	• Use a fracture pan rather than a bedpan. Powder the fracture pan. • Insert the fracture pan with the flat side toward the head, under the client's thighs.
Client is unable to void on bedpan.	• Run water in sink. • Massage the lower abdomen. • Place a hot washcloth on the abdomen. • Pour warm water over the perineum with client positioned on toilet or bedpan. • Give client a sitz bath after obtaining an order. • Put oil of wintergreen on a cotton ball in the bedpan or urinal.

unit 6

PERINEAL AND GENITAL CARE

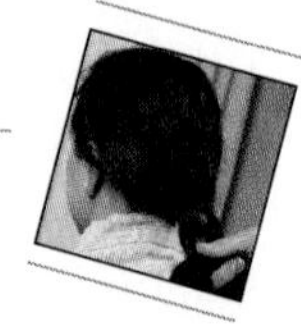

NURSING PROCESS DATA

ASSESSMENT Data Base

Review general assessment data about client.

Observe for signs of perineal itching, burning on urination, or skin irritation. Ask client if he or she experiences any of these problems.

Assess client's ability to bathe him or herself and to perform perineal care.

While providing privacy, assess the perineal–genital area for abnormal secretions, ulcerations, skin excoriations and sensitivity, drainage (amount, consistency, odor, color), swelling, enlarged lymph glands, catheter patency, and comfort.

Assess client's learning needs related to perineal and genital care.

PLANNING Objectives

To decrease the growth of bacteria

To remove excessive secretions

To promote healing after surgery and vaginal deliveries

To prevent the spread of microorganisms for clients with indwelling catheters

To increase client comfort

IMPLEMENTATION Procedures

Draping a Female Client

Providing Female Perineal Care

Administering a Vaginal Irrigation

Providing Male Perineal Care

EVALUATION Expected Outcomes

Perineal care has been comfortably and effectively provided.

Perineal area is clean, odor-free, and without irritation or discharge.

DRAPING A FEMALE CLIENT

Equipment

Bath blanket

Procedure

1. Bring bath blanket to bedside.
2. Identify client and explain procedure.
3. Provide privacy.
4. Wash your hands.
5. Place bed in HIGH position, and lower side rail nearest you.
6. Place bath blanket over client's top linen so that one corner of the blanket is pointed toward the

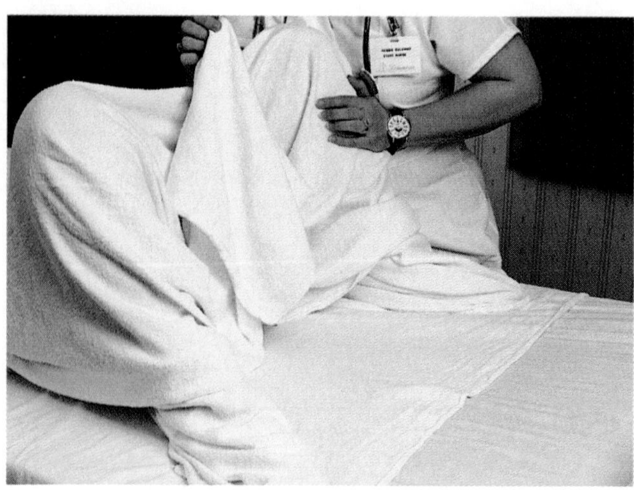

Drapery protects client's privacy when performing personal care.

client's head to form a diamond shape over the client.

7. Instruct client to hold onto bath blanket. Fanfold linen to foot of bed.
8. Request that client flex knees and keep them apart with feet firmly on bed.
9. Wrap lateral corners of bath blanket around feet in a spiral fashion until they are completely covered.
10. The corner of the blanket between knees and extending over perineum can later be folded back over the abdomen.

PROVIDING FEMALE PERINEAL CARE

Equipment

Bath blanket or sheet
Two bath towels
Protective pad
Washcloth
Three or more cotton balls (optional)
Clean surgical gloves
Bedpan (optional)
Pitcher of warm water (optional)
Antifungal–antibacterial solution as ordered

Preparation

1. Check to see if specific physician orders are to be followed.
2. Talk with client about how she can perform care or assist with procedure. **Rationale:** This gives client a sense of control.
3. Collect and arrange necessary equipment.
4. Provide privacy by closing door and pulling drapes.
5. Wash your hands.
6. Position client in a comfortable position. Perineal and genital care can be provided while client sits on a toilet or sitz bath, remains in bed in a supine position, or sits on a bedpan in a dorsal recumbent or semi-Fowler's position. **Rationale:** Adapting position to client's needs facilitates a positive outcome of procedure.
7. When care is given in bed, position patient comfortably. Drape according to procedure described above.
8. If possible, encourage the client to bend her knees and separate her legs. **Rationale:** The perineal area can be cleansed more efficiently in this position.

Procedure

1. Place a protective pad or towel and bedpan under the client's hips.

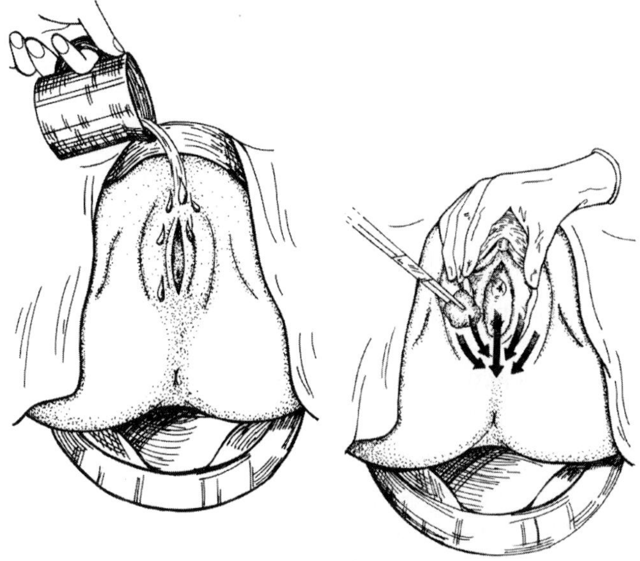

Cleansing the perineum with warm water and wiping front to back will provide effective perineal care and prevent contamination.

2. Pour warm water or a prescribed solution over the perineum while client is positioned on the bedpan. **Rationale:** The perineum is more comfortably and effectively cleansed by this method.
3. Tell the client what sensations she will feel as you perform the procedure.
4. Put on gloves. Separate the labia with one hand to expose the urethral and vaginal openings.
5. With your other hand, wipe from front to back in a downward motion, using warm water or soap and water and a washcloth or cotton balls. Be sure to use a different corner of the washcloth or a different cotton ball for each downward stroke. **Rationale:** This procedure prevents cross-contamination.
6. Wash the external labia and anus.
7. Thoroughly pat dry with second towel.
8. Remove equipment and cover client.
9. Remove gloves.
10. Position client for comfort.
11. Wash your hands.

ADMINISTERING A VAGINAL IRRIGATION

Equipment

Irrigation set
Douche tip
Solution
Bath blanket
Waterproof pad
Bedpan
Towel or toilet tissue
IV standard
"Clean" gloves

Preparation

1. Check physician's order and client care plan for type, amount, and temperature of irrigating solution (usually 1000–2000 mL of 105°F [40.5°C]).
2. Gather equipment and solution.
3. Identify client.
4. Explain procedure to client.
5. Provide privacy.
6. Have client void.
7. Wash hands.
8. Hang solution container on IV standard.
9. Raise bed to HIGH position, and lower head of bed.
10. Lower side rail nearest you.
11. Adjust IV standard so container base is 12–18 inches above vaginal orifice.

Procedure

1. With client in supine position, fanfold top bedding to foot of bed while replacing with bath blanket.
2. Don clean gloves.
3. Place waterproof pad under client.
4. Wash and dry perineum thoroughly if excess secretions or discharge present.
5. Position client with knees bent and feet flat on bed.
6. Drape client according to previously described Draping Procedure.
7. Place on bedpan.
8. Encourage client to relax and move knees apart. Cleanse external genitalia with soap and water.
9. Open clamp on tube from solution container and allow fluid to flow over perineum. **Rationale:** This procedure tests the water temperature and relaxes the client.
10. Spread labia with gloved hand and insert douche tip 3–4 inches.
11. Rotate douche tip while irrigating solution flows into vagina. **Rationale:** This promotes even flow of solution to all areas of the vagina.
12. Remove douche tip from vagina when solution flow ceases.
13. Assist client to sitting position. **Rationale:** A sitting position facilitates drainage from vagina.
14. Remove bedpan from client. Note amount of returned solution.
15. Dry perineum with toilet tissue or towel.
16. Remove waterproof pad from under client.
17. Remove gloves.
18. Replace top bedding, and remove drape.
19. Position client for comfort. Remove curtain.
20. Raise bed rails, and place bed in LOW position.
21. Remove and clean or discard irrigation equipment. Replace equipment to appropriate area. **Rationale:** Douche tips and bags are reusable for that client.
22. Wash your hands.

PROVIDING MALE PERINEAL CARE

Equipment

Bath blanket or sheet
Two bath towels
Protective pad or plastic sheet
Washcloth
Clean surgical gloves (optional)

Preparation

1. Collect and arrange necessary equipment.
2. Talk with client about how he can perform care or assist with procedure.
3. Ask client to attempt to empty bladder.
4. Provide privacy by closing door and pulling drapes.
5. Wash your hands and don gloves.

6. Cover client with bath blanket, exposing genital area as little as possible. **Rationale:** This contributes to client's comfort and privacy.

Procedure

1. If the client has not been circumcised, retract his foreskin carefully to expose the glans penis.
2. Gently but securely hold the shaft of the penis in one hand.
3. Using a circular motion, start at the tip of the penis and wash downwards toward the shaft with soap and water. Do not repeat washing over an area without using a clean area of the washcloth. **Rationale:** This procedure prevents cross-contamination.
4. Replace the foreskin over the glans penis.
5. Wash around the scrotum.
6. Wash the anus last.
7. Rinse and dry all areas thoroughly.
8. Remove articles and cover client.
9. Reposition client for comfort.
10. Remove gloves, and place in appropriate receptacle.
11. Wash your hands.

CHARTING for Perineal Care

- Assessment and care needs for perineal hygiene
- Client's level of understanding and teaching needs
- Perineal care provided and outcomes of care
- Time irrigation procedure performed
- Type, amount, and temperature of solution used for irrigation
- Description of returns from irrigation
- Response of client to procedure

CRITICAL THINKING APPLICATION

CLINICAL PROBLEMS	CRITICAL THINKING OPTIONS
Client has foul odor even after perineal care.	• Obtain order for sitz bath. • Request order for medicated solution. • Request culture of discharge so the appropriate treatment can be instituted.
Client develops urinary tract infection.	• Instruct client on proper technique for perineal care. • Instruct female clients to wash from anterior to posterior aspects of perineum, using different sections of cloth for each wipe. • Instruct male clients to wash from urethral opening down the shaft of the penis.

unit 7

EYE AND EAR CARE

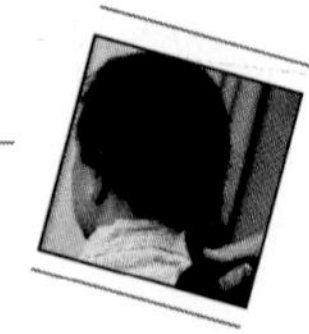

NURSING PROCESS DATA

ASSESSMENT Data Base

Assess if client is using eyeglasses or contact lenses, has an artificial eye, or is experiencing any eye problems.

Observe client's eyes for symmetry and clarity.

Assess the skin surrounding client's eyes for excessive dryness, scaling, and irritation.

Observe eyelids for irritation, edema, crustation, sties, and lesions.

Observe clent's tear ducts and sclera for inflammation and excessive tearing.

Assess client's pupils for response to light.

Observe client's eye movements or muscle action.

Evaluate ability to hear.

PLANNING Objectives

To ensure that the eyes and surrounding skin areas are clear, comfortable, and free of crustation

To improve or maintain the client's vision

To prevent irritation and infection

To maintain or improve the client's appearance and self-esteem

To increase ability to hear

IMPLEMENTATION Procedures

Providing Routine Eye Care

Providing Eye Care for Comatose Client

Providing Eye Care for Client with Glasses

Providing Eye Care for Client with Artificial Eye

Providing Eye Care for Client with Hard Contact Lenses

Providing Eye Care for Client with Soft Contact Lenses

Providing Ear Care for Client with Hearing Aid

EVALUATION Expected Outcomes

Eyes and surrounding area are clear and free of crustation.

Vision is maintained or improved.

Hearing is improved.

PROVIDING ROUTINE EYE CARE

Equipment

Small basin

Water or normal saline solution

Washcloth or cotton balls

Preparation

1. Determine client's eye care needs, and obtain physician's order if needed.
2. Explain the necessity for and method of eye care to the client. Discuss how client can assist you.
3. Collect necessary equipment.
4. Wash your hands.

Procedure

1. Use water or saline at room temperature.
2. Using the washcloth or cotton balls dampened in water or saline, gently wipe each eye from the inner to outer canthus. Use a separate cotton ball or corner of washcloth for each eye. **Rationale:** To prevent cross-contamination from one eye to the other.
3. If crusting is present, gently place a warm, wet compress over the eye(s) until crusting is loosened.

PROVIDING EYE CARE FOR COMATOSE CLIENT

Equipment

Water or normal saline solution

Washcloth, cotton balls, tissues

Sterile lubricant or eye preparations if ordered by the physician

Eye dropper or asepto bulb syringe

Eye pads or patches

Procedure

1. Cleanse the eyes using a dampened washcloth or cotton balls dampened in water or saline. Gently wipe each eye from the inner to outer canthus. Use separate cotton ball or corner of washcloth for each eye. **Rationale:** Wiping from the inner canthus to the outer prevents particles and fluid from entering the nasolacrimal duct.
2. Use a dropper to instill a sterile ophthalmic solution (liquid tears, saline, methylcellulose) every 3 to 4 hours as ordered by a physician. (See procedure for instilling eye drops.)
3. Keep client's eyes closed if blink reflex is absent. If eye pads or patches are used, explain their purpose to client's family. Do not tape eyes shut. **Rationale:** Corneal abrasions and drying occur when eyes lose blink reflex.

PROVIDING EYE CARE FOR CLIENT WITH GLASSES

Equipment

Towel

Water

Mild soap

Soft, dry cloth or lens paper

Procedure

1. Encourage client to wear eyeglasses as needed.
2. Clean glasses over a protected area (i.e., a towel). Holding glasses by the frame, gently wash the glass in tepid water. Use soap if necessary. Rinse thoroughly.
3. Dry and wipe lenses with a clean, soft cloth or lens paper.
4. Label eyeglasses with client's name.

PROVIDING EYE CARE FOR CLIENT WITH ARTIFICIAL EYE

Equipment

Rubber bulb or eyedropper

Water or normal saline solution

Mild soap

Washcloth

Towel

Preparation

1. If possible, encourage client or family member to care for client's artificial eye.
2. If assisting with artificial eye care, assess client's usual method for cleansing.
3. Gather equipment.

Procedure

1. Wash your hands.
2. Remove eye prosthesis by depressing lower lid and

sliding prosthesis out, or by using gentle suction with the rubber bulb of an eyedropper.

3. Flush empty socket with water or saline.
4. Clean the prosthesis with soap and water. Rinse thoroughly.
5. Lift upper eyelid and slide prosthesis into place.

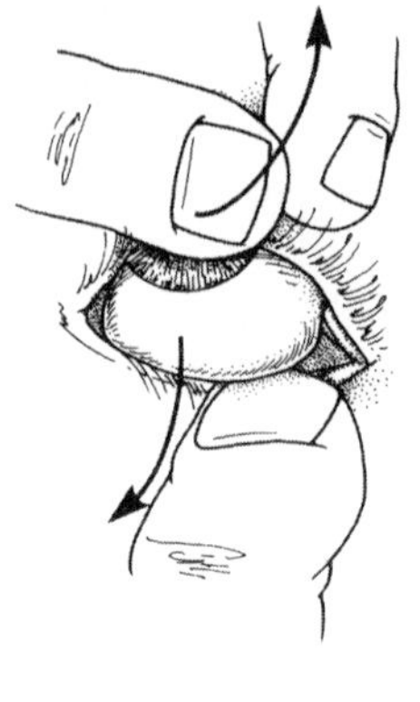
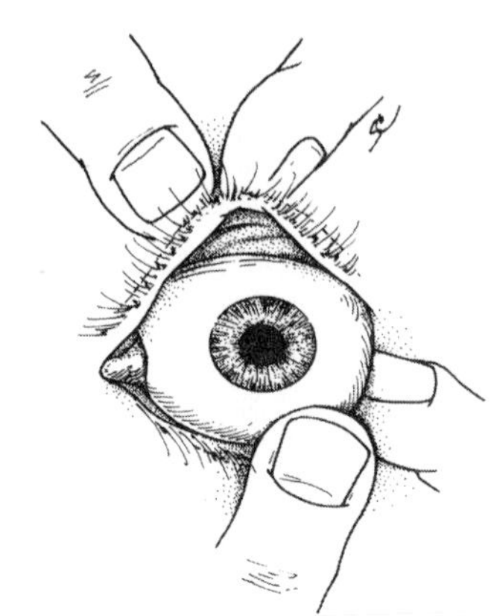

Removal of eye prosthesis.

PROVIDING EYE CARE FOR CLIENT WITH HARD CONTACT LENSES

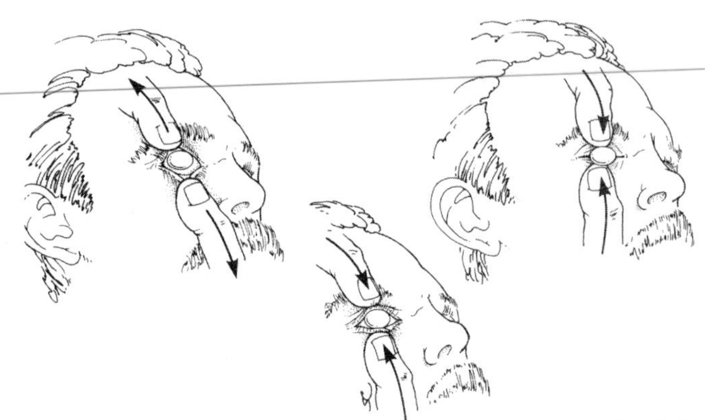

Removal of a hard contact lens.

Equipment

Towel
Commercial hard contact lens cleanser
Small container of water
Small empty basin

Preparation

1. If possible, encourage client or family member to care for client's lenses.
2. If assisting with contact lens care, assess client's usual method of cleansing.
3. Wash your hands.

Procedure

1. Place client in Fowler's position, and place a towel under the client's chin.
2. Place the tip of your forefinger across the lower lid below its margin.
3. Place the top of the forefinger of the other hand on the upper lid above its margin.
4. Assess for presence of lens.
5. Using a scissors motion, manipulate the two lids as the client closes, opens, and rolls eyes.
6. Observe carefully when lens pops out to ensure you don't lose it.
7. Drop a few drops of contact lens cleaner on lens while holding lens on tip of index finger.
8. Rub contact lens between fingertip and thumb for 1 minute or according to directions on lens cleaner container.
9. Hold lens gently between tips of index finger and thumb over empty basin, and rinse by pouring water from container over the lens.
10. Be sure lens is rinsed thoroughly before reinserting in eye.
11. If lens is not reinserted in eye, store in clean, dry contact lens storage case. Make careful note that each lens is placed in the properly marked side of container for that lens.

PROVIDING EYE CARE FOR CLIENT WITH SOFT CONTACT LENSES

Equipment

Towel
Contact lens container
Commercially prepared cleaning solution for soft lenses
Commercially prepared rinsing solution for soft lenses
Commercially prepared storing solution for soft lenses

Procedure

1. Place client in supine position, and place a towel under the client's chin.
2. Place the tip of your thumb across the lower lid below its margin.
3. Place the top of the forefinger of the same hand on the upper lid above its margin.
4. Spread eyelids apart as wide as possible.
5. Locate outer edges of soft lens which should appear as a rim around outer edge of iris.
6. Place thumb and forefinger directly on soft lens.
7. Gently remove soft lens from surface of eyeball by squeezing lens between thumbs and fingertip. (Lens bends like a piece of Saran wrap.)
8. Release eyelids.
9. Place lens in palm of hand.
10. Drop a few drops of special soft lens cleaner on lens.
11. Clean lens thoroughly by rubbing between fingertip and palm of hand for at least 2 minutes.
12. Clean other side of lens by repeating previous step.
13. Rinse lens thoroughly with special rinsing solution.
14. Place in lens container, and fill container with soft lens storage solution.
15. Repeat entire procedure for lens in client's other eye.

PROVIDING EAR CARE FOR CLIENT WITH HEARING AID

Equipment

Soap
Water
Petroleum jelly
Pipe cleaner
Cotton-tipped applicator
Hearing aid batteries

Procedure

1. Determine ability of client to perform all or part of cleaning procedure, and teach procedure when necessary.
2. Have client remove hearing aid if able to do so.
3. Remove ear mold from receiver before cleaning. Do not immerse receiver in water.
4. Wash ear mold, using soap and water. A pipe cleaner may be used to clean and dry the cannula. Reconnect receiver to dry ear mold.
5. Check batteries if hearing aid has not been functioning. Insert new batteries, matching positive (+) and negative (−) signs.
6. Examine cord for breaks; replace as necessary.
7. Before inserting ear mold, cleanse outer ear gently with cotton-tipped applicator.
8. Turn receiver switch to ON. Assist client to adjust volume control to desired level. If whistling or feedback noises occur, check for tightness of fit as ear mold probably has not been inserted properly.
9. Place hearing aid in container when not in use, and place in bedside stand.

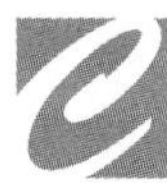

CHARTING for Eye and Ear Care

- Documentation of eye assessment and eye care needs
- Method and outcome of eye care provided
- Condition of eye and surrounding structure
- Condition of eye socket
- Response to using hearing aid
- Improved hearing after cleaning
- Client's ability to insert, remove, and clean hearing aid

CRITICAL THINKING APPLICATION

CLINICAL PROBLEMS	CRITICAL THINKING OPTIONS
Eyelids become crusted from exudate.	• Place warm, moist washcloth across eyes and leave in place for several minutes. • Moisten cotton applicator stick with sterile saline, and gently twist the applicator stick over crusted surface to assist in removing crust.
You are unable to replace the artificial eye or contact lens.	• If client is unable to assist, ask relatives for help. • Do not use force. Leave lens or eye out until someone who is able to replace it is available.
Wrong solution used on contact lens causes excessive tearing and burning sensation when lens is placed in eye.	• Immediately remove lens from eye, and place in proper storage container. • Immediately rinse client's eye with copious amounts of sterile water. • Have client checked immediately by ophthalmologist for emergency care of potentially burned cornea.
Hearing did not improve with cleaning of hearing aid.	• Check if receiver switch is ON. • Check if batteries are properly in place and that the poles match: positive (+) and negative (−).

GERIATRIC CONSIDERATIONS

Clients with dentures require special nursing care.

- Check for proper fit when replacing dentures. Ill-fitting dentures interfere with chewing and can lead to altered nutrition. Loss of teeth may limit meal planning and the nurse should assist the client to choose a balanced diet taking into account tooth loss.
- Monitor denture cleaning to ensure client has fresh-tasting mouth to encourage eating. Elderly client's have decreased sensitivity to sweet, sour, salty, and bitter tastes; thus, they may compensate by using extra salt. The nurse can counsel the client on alternative seasonings and request dietary consultation.

Nails and hair change with age.

- As client's age increases, nails become soft, fragile, and lusterless. Diabetic clients require a physician's order to cut nails.
- Nails should be kept trimmed (straight across with no jagged edges) so skin that is at risk is not scratched and opened.

A positive body image is enhanced with good personal hygiene. Nursing care should focus on assisting the client to maintain good personal hygiene.

11

Vital Signs

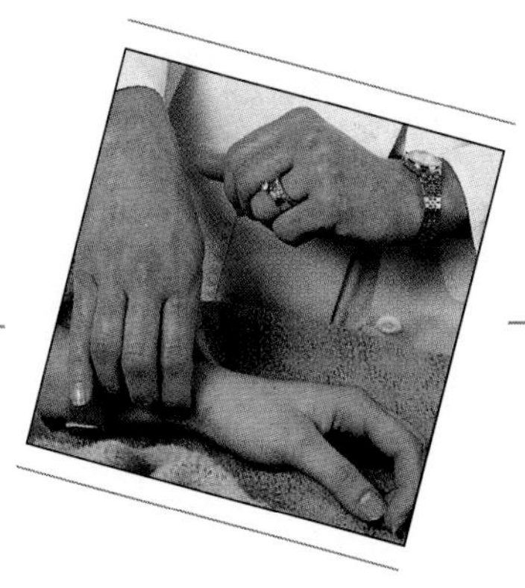

LEARNING OBJECTIVES

- State the defining characteristics and the related nursing diagnosis of hypovolemia.
- Identify the cardinal signs that reflect the body's physiologic status.
- List three mechanisms that increase heat production.
- Explain how disease alters the "set point" of the temperature-regulating center.
- Define hypothermia and list the symptoms of this condition.
- Differentiate between the oral, rectal, and axillary methods of taking temperature.
- Describe two nursing actions that can be performed when temperature is not within normal range.
- Describe at least three different types of pulses.
- Discuss the pulse, and indicate how it is an index of heart rate and rhythm.
- Compare normal heart rate for adults and children.
- Identify the characteristics of peripheral pulses.
- Define the term "respiration."
- List the normal respiratory rate for adults and children.
- Explain four types of abnormal respiratory patterns.
- Identify four factors that affect blood pressure.
- Demonstrate the method of palpating brachial systolic arterial blood pressure.

TERMINOLOGY

Pulse Terminology

Atrial fibrillation: a chaotically irregular pulse rhythm with a pulse deficit.

Bigeminal pulse: a regularly irregular pulse occurring with premature beats that is a disturbance in rhythm. The premature beat decreases the stroke volume for that beat and so is weaker than the normal beat.

Large, bounding pulse: pulse pressure in increased. It is felt as a slapping against the fingers because of the rapid upstroke and quick downstroke. It is seen in conditions of increased cardiac output, such as exercise, anxiety, alcoholic intake, and pregnancy. It is also noted in pathology with fever, anemia, hyperthyroidism, liver failure, complete heart block with bradycardia, and hypertension. When there is a rapid runoff of blood, such as with aortic insufficiency ("water-hammer" pulse) and patent ductus arteriosus, this type of pulse is characteristic. Increased rigidity in the aorta, which occurs with aging and arteriosclerosis, also causes this type of pulse.

Normal pulse: pulse pressure is about 30–40 mm Hg. It is smooth and rounded and is felt as a sharp upstroke and gradual downstroke.

Premature beats: a pacemaker outside the sinus node fires earlier than the sinus node, the normal pacemaker of the heart. Since the beat is early, the stroke volume is less because the ventricles do not have time to fill. This condition causes a pause in rhythm, which may result in a pulse deficit.

Pulse deficit: occurs when the heart rate counted at the apex by auscultation is greater than the heart rate counted by palpation of the radial pulse. The pulse wave is not transmitted to the periphery to produce a palpable radial pulse.

Pulsus alternans: rhythm is regular but the amplitude alternates from beat to beat.

Pulsus paradoxus: detected by blood pressure measurement. The disappearance of Korotkoff's sounds during inspiration phase of breathing with sounds appearing throughout the respiratory cycle (during inspiration and exhalation) at a pressure 10 mm Hg lower than heard during exhalation alone. This phenomenon occurs in COPD and with cardiac tamponade and should be further evaluated.

Sinus arrhythmia: common in children and young adults. The rate accelerates with inspiration and slows with expiration.

Small, weak pulse: pulse pressure is diminished. It is smooth and rounded but is felt as a gradual upstroke and prolonged downstroke. It is commonly seen in conditions resulting in decreased cardiac output, such as heart failure and shock, and with obstruction to left ventricular ejection, such as aortic stenosis.

Tachycardia: heart rate greater than 100 BPM.

Respiratory Terminology

Apnea: absence of breathing.

Biot's respirations: abrupt interruptions between a faster, deeper respiratory rate.

Bradypnea: slow, regular respirations. Rate is below 10 per minute.

Cheyne–Stokes: periods of apnea appear throughout cycle. Respirations become deeper and faster than normal followed by a slower rate and progressing to periods of apnea lasting up to 60 seconds.

Hyperpnea: abnormal increase in depth and rate.

Kussmaul's respirations: slow deep breathing. Attempt to blow off carbon dioxide as respiratory compensation for metabolic acidosis (e.g., diabetic ketoacidosis).

Sonorous: loud breathing.

Stertorous: loud, noisy breathing.

Tachypnea: respiratory rate increased above 24 breaths per minute. Rate remains regular but shallow in pattern.

General Terminology

Antipyretic: an agent that reduces febrile temperatures.

Apex: the pointed end of a cone-shaped part or organ (e.g., lower heart, upper lung).

Arteriosclerosis: an arterial disease characterized by inelasticity and thickening of the vessel walls with lessened blood flow.

Atherosclerosis: a form of arteriosclerosis in which there are localized accumulations of lipid-containing material within the internal surfaces of blood vessels.

Arthrosclerosis: stiffening or hardening of the joints.

Atrial: pertaining to the atrium, the upper cardiac chamber that receives blood from the lungs and systemic circulation.

Autoregulation: the intrinsic tendency of the heart to maintain constant blood flow despite changes in other factors.

Axilla: armpit.

Cardio: pertaining to the heart.

Cardiogenic: having origin in the heart itself.

Chemoreceptor: a sense organ or sensory nerve ending that is stimulated by and reacts to chemical stimuli.

Contractility: having the ability to contract or shorten muscle tissue or cells.

Diastole: the period in which the heart dilates and fills with blood; the period of relaxation.

Febrile: feverish, increased body temperature.

Fibrillation: quivering, involuntary contraction of individual muscle fibers.

Hyperpnea: increased respiratory rate with deeper breathing.

Hyperthermia: unusually high body temperature.

Hypervolemia: abnormal increase in the volume of circulating body fluid.

Hypothalamus: the part of the brain that lies below the thalamus; it maintains or regulates body temperature, certain metabolic processes, and other autonomic activities.

Hypothermia: a body temperature below the average normal range.

Hypovolemia: diminished blood volume.

Infarction: an area of tissue in an organ or part that undergoes necrosis following cessation of blood supply.

Ischemia: local and temporary hypoxia due to obstruction of the circulation to a part.

Myo: combining form pertinent to a muscle.

Myocardium: the middle muscle layer of the walls of the heart.

Palpate: to examine by touch; feel.

Peripheral: pertinent to the periphery, away from the central structure.

Peripheral vascular disease: indicates diseases of the arteries and veins of the extremities, especially those conditions that interfere with adequate flow of blood.

Pyrogen: any substance that produces fever.

Shock: state of inadequate tissue perfusion resulting from circulatory failure, precipitated by many factors and identified by various signs and symptoms.

Sphygmomanometer: instrument for indirectly determining arterial blood pressure.

Valsalva's maneuver: attempt to forcibly exhale with the glottis, nose, and mouth closed, producing an increased intrathoracic pressure.

Vaso: part meaning a vessel, such as blood vessel.

Vasoconstriction: constriction of the blood vessels.

VITAL SIGNS

Vital signs, also termed cardinal signs, reflect the body's physiologic status and provide information critical to evaluating homeostatic balance. Vital signs include four critical assessment areas: temperature, pulse, respiration, and blood pressure. The term "vital" is used because the information gathered is the clearest indicator of overall status. These four signs form baseline assessment data necessary for an ongoing evaluation of a client's condition. If the nurse has established the normal range for a client, deviations can be more easily recognized.

Routine vital signs are important to assess on every

TABLE 11–1. Vital Sign Chart for Children

Age	Normal Pulse Range	Normal Pulse Average	Blood Pressure Average	Respiration Average
Newborn	70–170	120	80/45	40–90
1 year	80–160	115	90/60	20–40
2 years	80–130	110	95/60	20–30
4 years	80–120	100	99/65	20–25
6 years	75–115	100	100/56	20–25
8 years	70–110	90	105/56	15–20
10 years	70–110	90	110/58	15–20

client. These parameters should be assessed by a staff member who is familiar with the client's health history so results can be evaluated against previous data. Vital signs should be taken at regular intervals. The more critical the client's condition, the more often these signs need to be taken and evaluated. They are not only indicators of a client's present condition but also cues to a positive or negative change in status.

Obtaining the total picture of a client's health status is a major objective of client care. Although vital signs yield important information in themselves, they gain even more relevance when compared with the client's diagnosis, laboratory tests, history, and records.

Temperature represents the balance between heat gain and heat loss and is regulated in the hypothalamus of the brain. Variations in temperature indicate the health status of the body; thermostatic function may be altered by pyrogens, nervous system disease, or injury.

The pulse is an index of the heart's action; by evaluating its rate, rhythm, and volume, one can gain an overall impression of the heart's action.

Respiration, the act of bringing oxygen into the body and removing carbon dioxide, yields data on the client's entire breathing process. When the pattern of respiration is altered, ongoing evaluation yields important cues to a client's changing condition.

Blood pressure readings provide information about the condition of the heart, the arteries and arterioles, vessel resistance, and the cardiac output. Serial readings provide the best indication of a client's cardiovascular status.

TEMPERATURE

Temperature control of the body is a homeostatic function, regulated by a complex mechanism involving the hypothalamus. The temperature of the body's interior (core temperature) is maintained within ±1°F except in the case of febrile illness. The surface temperature of the skin and tissues immediately underlying the skin rises and falls with a change in temperature of the surrounding environment. Core temperature is maintained when heat production equals heat loss. The temperature regulating center in the hypothalamus keeps the core temperature constant. Temperature receptors, which determine if the body is too hot or too cold, relay signals to the hypothalamus. When the body becomes overheated, heat-sensitive neurons stimulate sweat glands to secrete fluid. This enhances heat loss through evaporation. The vasoconstrictor mechanism of the skin vessels is reduced, thereby conducting heat from the core of the body to the body surface. Heat loss occurs through radiation, evaporation, and conduction.

Regulatory Mechanisms

When the body core is cooled below 98.6°F (37°C), heat conservation is affected. Intense vasoconstriction of the skin vessels results. There is also piloerection and a decrease in sweating to conserve heat. Heat production is stimulated by shivering and increased cellular metabolism.

The "set point" is the critical temperature level to which the regulatory mechanisms attempt to maintain the body's core temperature. Above the set point, heat-losing mechanisms are brought into play, and below that level heat-conserving and heat-producing mechanisms are set into action.

Disease can alter the set point of the temperature-regulating center to cause fever, a body temperature above normal. Inflammation, brain lesions, pyrogens from bacteria or viruses, or degenerating tissue (i.e., gangrenous areas or myocardial infarction) also increase the set point. Dehydration can cause fever due to lack of available fluid for perspiration and by increasing the set point, which brings more heat-conserving and heat-producing mechanisms into play. When the "thermostat" is suddenly set higher, the client complains of feeling cold, has cool extremities, shivers, and has piloerection. Hypoxia can occur due to increased oxygen use with the increased metabolism of heat production. When the "thermostat" returns to normal, heat-losing mechanisms again are activated. The client feels hot and starts perspiring. Other symptoms of fever the client may experience are perspiration over the body surface; body warm to touch; flushed face; feeling cold alternately with feeling hot; increased pulse and respirations; malaise and fatigue; parched lips and dry skin; and convulsions, especially with rapid temperature rise in children.

When the body temperature falls below the normal range, the client experiences hypothermia and complains of being cold, shivers, and has cool extremities. Hypothermia may be caused by accidental exposure, frostbite, or GI hemorrhage. Medically induced hypothermia is used for some surgical interventions. The ability of the hypothalamus to regulate body temperature is greatly impaired when the body temperature falls below 94°F (34.4°C) and is lost below 85°F (29.4°C). Cellular metabolism and heat production are also depressed by a low temperature.

Measuring Body Temperature

Oral or rectal temperatures reflect the body's core temperature. Ear canal and axillary temperatures are somewhat variable but are clinically acceptable for tracking important changes. The normal range of an oral temperature is 97°–99.5°F, or 36°–37.5°C. Rectal temperatures are approximately 1°F higher, ear canal 0.5° higher, and axillary temperatures are 1°F lower than oral readings. Body temperature may vary according to age (lower for the aged), time of day (lower in the morning and higher in the afternoon and evening), amount of exercise, or extremes in the environmental temperature.

The thermometer is the instrument used to measure body heat. Oral and rectal (also used for axillary temperature) thermometers are calibrated glass tubes with a bulb containing mercury. When exposed to heat, the mercury expands, moves up the glass, and records the body temperature. The thermometer is marked in degrees and tenths of degrees with either a Fahrenheit or Celsius (centigrade) scale and a range of 93°–108°F (34°–42.2°C).

Electronic thermometers, now widely used in hospitals, are more accurate than glass thermometers. In addition, they have disposable covers, which promote infection control, and therefore should be used when available. The electronic thermometer plugs into a receptacle and has a heat sensor that records the client's core temperature in seconds.

Heat-sensitive tapes are also used to record temperature. The tape is applied to the skin, and color changes indicate the temperature level. These tapes are both disposable and nonbreakable. They are most appropriate for use with normal newborns, small children, and in situations when proper cleaning of the thermometer is difficult. The ear canal provides another noninvasive site for temperature measurement using infrared thermometers.

PULSE

The pulse is an index of the heart's rate and rhythm. The apical pulse rate is the number of heart beats per minute. With each beat the heart's left ventricle contracts and forces blood into the aorta. Closure of the heart valves creates the sounds heard. The forceful ejection of blood by the left ventricle produces a wave that is transmitted through the arteries to the periphery of the body. The pulse is a transient expansion of peripheral arteries resulting from internal pressure changes. If cardiac output is reduced (such as with a premature or irregular heart beat) the peripheral pulse is weak, if felt, or skipped so that the radial pulse rate is less than the apical rate; the difference is called a "pulse deficit." The pulse wave is influenced by the elasticity of the larger vessels, blood volume, blood viscosity, and arteriolar and capillary resistance.

Circulatory System Control

The circulatory system is under the dual control of the autonomic nervous system and autoregulation (at the microcirculation level). This dual control allows the circulatory system to vary blood flow to meet the body's requirements. Local control of blood flow is called autoregulation. Blood flow is adjusted according to oxygen need based on changing metabolic activity of different tissues.

The autonomic nervous system regulates circulation through the vasomotor center in the medulla oblongata. Stimulation of the sympathetic nervous system causes vasoconstriction, increased heart rate and cardiac contractility, and a resulting increase in blood pressure. On the other hand, sympathetic inhibition causes vasodilation, reduced heart rate, and a reduction in blood pressure.

Pressure receptors, called baroreceptors, located in the walls of the carotid sinus and arch of the aorta also influence the vasomotor center. Decreased circulating volume (as in hemorrhage) stimulates these receptors, which then transmit signals to the vasomotor center to stimulate the sympathetic nervous system. Resulting cardiovascular responses divert blood flow to vital organs.

Heart Rate and Rhythm

A normal adult heart rate is from 60 to 100 beats per minute (BPM), the average rate is 72 BPM. Rates are slightly faster in women, and more rapid in children and infants (90–140 BPM: Table 11–1). The resting heart rate usually does not change with age. Tachycardia is a pulse rate over 100 BPM. Bradycardia is a pulse rate below 60 BPM.

When taking a client's pulse be aware that many pathologic conditions produce a bradycardia. Among the most common causes are decreased thyroid activity, hyperkalemia, Adams–Stokes disease, and increased intracranial pressure.

Tachycardia is associated with stressful conditions,

hypoxia, exercise, and fever. Client conditions, such as congestive heart failure, hemorrhage and shock, dehydration, and anemia produce a tachycardia as a compensatory response to poor tissue oxygenation.

Heart rhythm is the time interval between each heart beat. Normally, the heart rhythm is regular although slight irregularities do not necessarily indicate cardiac malfunction. An irregular cardiac rhythm, especially if sustained, requires cardiac evaluation because it may be indicative of cardiac disease.

Variance in heart rate, either increased or decreased, may be attributed to many factors, such as drug intake, lack of oxygen, loss of blood, exercise, and body temperature. When evaluating a pulse rate, it is important to ascertain the normal baseline for each client and then to determine variances from the normal for that particular client. The heart normally pumps about 5 L of blood through the body each minute. This cardiac output is calculated by multiplying the heart rate per minute by the stroke volume, the amount of blood ejected with one contraction. Increasing the heart rate is one of the first compensatory mechanisms the body employs to maintain cardiac output.

Evaluating Pulse Quality

The quality of the pulse is determined by the amount of blood pumped through the peripheral arteries. Normally, the amount of pumped blood remains fairly constant; when it varies, it is also indicative of cardiac malfunction. A so-called bounding pulse occurs when the nurse is able to feel the pulse by exerting only a slight pressure over the artery. If, by exerting firm pressure, the nurse cannot clearly determine the flow, the pulse is called weak or thready.

The arterial pulse can be felt over arteries that lie close to the body surface and over a bone or firm surface that can support the artery when pressure is applied. The radial artery is palpated most frequently since it is the most accessible. The femoral and carotid arteries are used in cases of cardiac arrest to determine the adequacy of perfusion. It is important to note characteristics of peripheral pulses: 0 = absent; 1+ = weak; 2+ = normal; and 3+ = full and bounding. (Use the system described in your hospital procedure manual.)

When peripheral pulses cannot be palpated, a Doppler ultrasound stethoscope is used by the nurse to confirm the presence or absence of the pulse. Remember, the pulse is not always an accurate indication of the force of cardiac contractions. If cardiac contractions are weak or ventricular filling is incomplete, the pulse is weak; however, in the case of aortic stenosis, the pulse may be weak in spite of forceful cardiac contraction.

The pulse should be taken frequently (every 5–15 minutes to 1–2 hours) on an acutely ill hospitalized client and less frequently (every 4–8 hours) on more stable hospitalized clients. Once a week or even once a month is adequate for clients in long-term care facilities. Do not wait until the next routine schedule if the client develops unexpected symptoms or has experienced a trauma.

RESPIRATION

Respiration is the process of bringing oxygen to body tissues and removing carbon dioxide. The lungs play a major role in this process. Another respiratory function is to maintain arterial blood homeostasis by maintaining the pH of the blood. The lungs accomplish this by the process of breathing.

Breathing consists of two phases, inspiration and expiration. Inspiration is an active process in which the diaphragm descends, the external intercostal muscles contract, and the chest expands to allow air to move into the tracheobronchial tree. Expiration is a passive process in which air flows out of the respiratory tree.

The respiratory center in the medulla of the brain and the level of carbon dioxide in the blood both control the rate and depth of breathing. Peripheral receptors in the carotid body and the aortic arch also respond to the level of oxygen in the blood. To some extent, respiration can be voluntarily controlled by holding the breath and hyperventilation. Talking, laughing, and crying also affect respiration.

The diaphragm and the intercostal muscles are the main muscles used for breathing. Other accessory muscles, such as the abdominal muscles, the sternocleidomastoid, the trapezius, and the scalene, can be used to assist with respiration if necessary.

Evaluating Respiratory Rate

The quality of breathing is important baseline information. Normal breathing is almost invisible, effortless, quiet, automatic, and regular. When the breathing pattern varies from normal, it needs to be evaluated thoroughly. For example, bronchial sounds heard over the large airways are fairly loud. There is normally a pause between inspiration and expiration. Softer sounds are heard over peripheral lung areas, and there are no pauses between inspiration, which is a long sound, and expiration, which is a short sound. If breathing is noisy, labored, or strained, an obstruction may be affecting the breathing pattern that could lead to major alterations in homeostasis.

In addition to evaluating the breathing pattern, it is also necessary to evaluate the rate and depth of breathing. The normal rate for a resting adult is 12–18 breaths per minute. A rate of 24 or above is considered tachypnea, and a rate of 10 or less is considered bradypnea. The rate for infants ranges from 24–30 breaths per minute and is often irregular. Older children average about 20–26. The ratio of pulse to breathing is usually 5:1 and remains fairly constant.

The depth of a person's breathing (tidal volume) is the amount of air that moves in and out with each breath. The tidal volume is 500 mL in the healthy adult. Alveolar air is only partially replenished by atmosphere air with each inspiratory phase. Approximately 350 mL (tidal volume minus dead space) of new air is exchanged with the functional residual capacity volume during each respiratory cycle. Accurate tidal volume can be measured by a spirometer, but a nurse can judge the approximate depth by placing the back of the hand next to the client's nose and mouth and feeling the expired air. Another method of estimating volume capacity is to observe chest expansion and to check both sides of the thorax for symmetrical movement.

After assessing the pattern, type, and depth of breathing, it is important to observe the physical characteristics of chest expansion. The chest normally expands symmetrically without rib flaring or retractions. In addition, observation of chest deformities should also be made, as all of these signs yield information about the respiratory process and overall health status of the client.

BLOOD PRESSURE

The heart generates pressure during the cardiac cycle to perfuse the organs of the body with blood. Blood flows from the heart to the arteries, into the capillaries and veins, and then flows back to the heart. Blood pressure in the arterial system varies with the cardiac cycle, reaching the highest level at the peak of systole and the lowest level at the end of diastole. The difference between the systolic and diastolic blood pressure is the pulse pressure, which is normally 30–50 mm Hg.

There are seven major factors that affect blood pressure.

Cardiac Output. The force of heart contractions, the amount of blood ejected by the heart, and the heart rate influence blood pressure, especially systolic pressure.

Peripheral Vascular Resistance. Resistance to the flow of blood is due to resistant vessels under the influence of the autonomic nervous system. Peripheral vascular resistance is the most important determinant of diastolic pressure.

Elasticity and Distensibility of Arteries. Elasticity refers to the action of the blood vessel walls to spring back after blood is ejected into them. When blood is ejected into the aorta and large arteries, the arterial vessel walls distend. Recoil during diastole propels blood through the arterial tree and maintains diastolic pressure. Both elasticity and distensibility decrease with age, resulting in increased systolic pressure and slightly increased diastolic pressure.

Blood Volume. Increased blood volume causes an increase in both systolic and diastolic blood pressure, whereas decreased blood volume causes the reverse effect. Hemorrhage decreases blood pressure whereas overhydration from excessive blood transfusions may cause an increase in blood pressure.

Blood Viscosity. Blood viscosity (thickness) influences blood flow velocity through the arterial tree. For example, increased viscosity, which occurs with polycythemia, increases resistance to blood flow, whereas decreased viscosity, resulting from anemia, decreases resistance.

Hormones and Enzymes. These substances have an important influence on blood pressure. For example, epinephrine and norepinephrine produce a profound vasoconstrictor effect on peripheral blood vessels (mediators of the sympathetic nervous system). Aldosterone (released by the adrenal cortex), renin (released by the juxtaglomerular apparatus of the kidney), and angiotensin (activated by the renin response) also produce effects that raise blood pressure. Histamine and acetylcholine (a parasympathetic mediator), causes vasodilation, therefore lowering blood pressure.

Chemoreceptors. Chemoreceptors in the aortic arch and carotid sinus also exert control over the blood pressure. They are sensitive to changes in $Pa{O_2}$, $Pa{CO_2}$, and pH. Decreased $Pa{O_2}$ stimulates the chemoreceptors, which stimulate the vasomotor center. Increased $Pa{CO_2}$ and decreased pH directly stimulate the vasomotor center, causing increased peripheral vascular resistance.

Measuring Blood Pressure

Measuring arterial blood pressure provides important information about the overall health status of the client. For example, the systolic pressure provides a data base about the condition of the heart and great arteries. The diastolic pressure indicates arteriolar or peripheral vascular resistance. The pulse pressure, or difference between the systolic and diastolic pressure, provides information about cardiac function and blood volume. A single blood pressure reading, however, does not provide adequate data from which conclusions can be drawn about all of these factors. Rather, a series of blood pressure readings should be taken to establish a baseline for further evaluation.

The *indirect method* of taking a blood pressure using a sphygmomanometer (mercury or anaeroid) and a stethoscope is accurate for most clients. New electronic blood pressure devices constantly monitor systolic, diastolic, and mean readings at preset time intervals and are helpful to measure blood pressure trends in clients who are at risk for hyper- or hypotension. These devices also provide a printout if needed for documentation. If a stethoscope is unavailable or the brachial artery amplitude is decreased, the brachial or radial artery can be palpated as the blood pressure cuff is inflated to determine the systolic blood pressure (palpated pulse disappears at this point). Alternatively, an inflated blood pressure cuff may be slowly deflated and the point at which distal pulsation is first palpated reflects systolic blood pressure. Those who are severely hypotensive or hypertensive (hemodynamically unstable), have low blood volume, or are on rapid-acting IV vasoconstricting or vasodilating drugs should have blood pressure measured by direct (intraarterial) method. The *direct method* is continuous and measures mean pressures. A needle or catheter is inserted into the brachial, radial, or femoral artery. An oscilloscope displays arterial pressure waveforms.

Normal blood pressure in an adult varies between 100 and 140 mm Hg systolic and 60–90 mm Hg diastolic. As blood moves toward smaller arteries and into arterioles, where it enters the capillaries, pressure falls to 35 mm Hg. It continues to fall as blood goes through the capillaries, where the flow is steady and not pulsatile. As blood moves into the venous system, pressure falls until it is the lowest in the venae cavae.

Blood pressures vary widely. A blood pressure of 100/60 mm Hg may be normal for one person but may be hypotensive for another. Hypotension (90–100 mm Hg systolic) in a healthy adult without other clinical symptoms is little reason for concern.

Blood pressure readings are recorded in association with Korotkoff's sounds. These sounds are described as "K" phases. The systolic, or first, pressure reading occurs with the advent of the first Korotkoff sound. The systolic reading represents the maximal pressure in the aorta following contraction of the left ventricle and is heard as a faint tapping sound.

According to American Heart Association standards, the diastolic, or second, reading should be taken at the time of the last Korotkoff sound (phase V) for adults. The diastolic reading represents the minimal pressure exerted against the arterial walls at all times. In children under age 13, pregnant women, and clients with high cardiac output or peripheral vasodilation, sounds are often heard to a level far below muffling and sometimes to levels near 0 mm Hg. In these individuals, muffling (phase IV) should be used to indicate diastolic pressure, but both muffling (phase IV) and disappearance (phase V) should be recorded (e.g., 110/80/20).

KOROTKOFF'S SOUND PHASES

Phase I: The pressure level at which the first faint, clear tapping sounds are heard. The sounds gradually increase in intensity as the cuff is deflated. This phase coincides with the reappearance of a palpable pulse.

Phase II: That time during cuff deflation when a murmur or swishing sounds are heard.

Phase III: The period during which sounds are crisper and increase in intensity.

Phase IV: That time when a distinct, abrupt, muffling of sound (usually of a soft, blowing quality) is heard.

Phase V: That pressure level when the last sound is heard and after which all sound disappears.

American Heart Association, 1993.

Frequency of blood pressure assessment should be individualized or as ordered. Blood pressure for an acutely ill client should be taken every 15 minutes to 1–2 hours and the blood pressure of more stabilized clients should be taken every 4–8 hours to once a day. Clients with severe hypotension or hypertension, with low blood volume, or those on vasoconstrictor or vasodilator drugs require checking every 5–15 minutes.

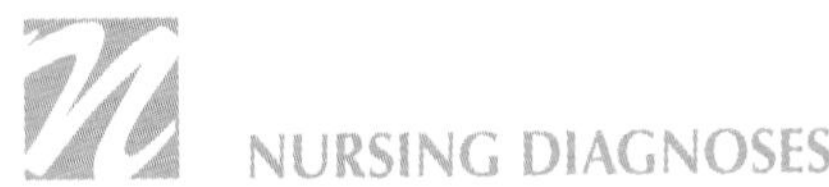

NURSING DIAGNOSES

The following nursing diagnoses are appropriate to use on client care plans when the components are related to vital signs.

NURSING DIAGNOSIS	RELATED FACTORS
Decreased Cardiac Output	Hypovolemia, rapid pulse, changes in breathing patterns, alteration in electric conduction or vascular tone
Fluid Volume Deficit	Excessive urinary output, abnormal fluid loss, infection, fever
Fluid Volume Excess	Decreased cardiac output, fluid retention, inflammatory process, low protein diet, increased fluid intake
Altered Tissue Perfusion	Vascular disorders, hypovolemia, medication

unit 1

TEMPERATURE

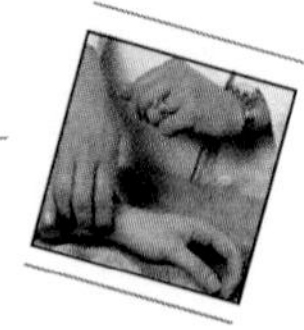

NURSING PROCESS DATA

ASSESSMENT Data Base

Determine the method most appropriate for obtaining temperature.

Oral Method

- Accurate method of determining body temperature
- Used only for alert and cooperative clients
- Not appropriate for use with tachypneic or mouth-breathing clients
- Not appropriate for clients with oral inflammatory processes
- Delivery of oxygen by nasal cannula does not affect oral temperature readings

Rectal Method

- Appropriate for tachypneic, uncooperative, confused, or comatose clients or for clients on seizure precautions.
- Used for clients with open mouth breathing, such as those with nasal or oral intubation.
- Appropriate for clients with wired jaws, facial fractures, or other abnormalities, or for clients with nasogastric tubes who cannot breathe easily with mouth closed.
- Contraindicated for infants or clients who have had abdominal perineal resection or hem orrhoidectomy.

Axillary Method

- Least accurate, but safe
- Preferred for infants and young children
- Used in recovery rooms to avoid turning clients.
- Time consuming

Electronic Thermometer

- Accurate for oral or rectal measurement, but inaccurate for axillary temperature measurement
- Prevents infection between clients
- Time efficient and easy to read

Infrared Ear Thermometer

- Measures body heat radiating from the tympanic membrane
- Noninvasive, safe, efficient
- Less sensitive in detecting fever in the very young child and infant

Determine number of times temperature needs to be taken daily.

Assess temperature in relationship to time of day and age of client.

Compare temperature with other vital signs to establish baseline data.

PLANNING Objectives

To determine if core temperature is within normal range

To provide baseline data for further evaluation

To determine alterations in disease conditions

IMPLEMENTATION Procedures

Taking an Oral Temperature

Taking a Rectal Temperature

Taking an Axillary Temperature

Using an Electronic Thermometer

Using an Infrared Thermometer for Ear Canal Temperature
Using a Chemical Strip Tape

EVALUATION Expected Outcomes

Temperature is within normal range.

Temperature readings are compared with age, time of day, and previous readings.

Alterations in temperature are detected early and treatment begun.

Appropriate method of temperature taking is determined for each client.

Correct length of time is used for thermometer insertion to obtain an accurate reading.

TAKING AN ORAL TEMPERATURE

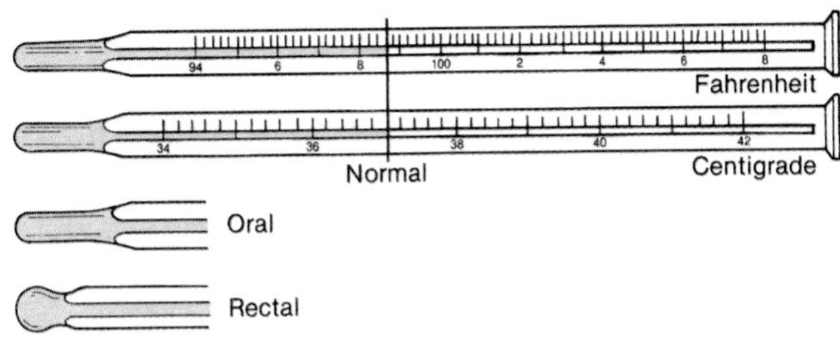

Comparison of thermometers calibrated to Fahrenheit and Centigrade.

■ CLINICAL ALERT

Temperature varies with time of day: it is highest between 5 and 7 PM and lowest between 2 and 6 AM. This variation is termed circadian thermal rhythm. A consistent method of body temperature measurement should be used so that readings are comparable.

Equipment

Oral glass mercury thermometer
Tissues

Procedure

1. Wash your hands. Wait 20–30 minutes to take an oral temperature if client has been eating, drinking, smoking, or exercising. **Rationale:** These activities may alter core temperature.
2. Rinse thermometer in cool water if kept in a chemical solution. **Rationale:** Chemical taste is bitter. Rinsing with cool water prevents expansion of the mercury.
3. Wipe thermometer dry with tissue from bulb end toward fingers. **Rationale:** Wipe from least to most contaminated area.
4. Grasp thermometer with thumb and forefinger and shake vigorously by flicking wrist in downward motion to lower mercury level to below 95–96°F.
5. Check temperature reading on thermometer.
6. Explain procedure to client.
7. Place thermometer in client's mouth under tongue and ask client to hold lips closed. **Rationale:** This location ensures contact with large vessels under tongue. Open-mouth breathing produces abnormally low readings.
8. Leave in place 3–5 minutes. **Rationale:** Optimum placement time varies in research studies. Use time recommended in agency procedure manual.
9. Remove thermometer, and wipe it with tissue from fingers down to bulb. Discard tissue. **Rationale:** Wipe from least contaminated to most contaminated area. Mucus on thermometer may interfere with the antiseptic solution's effectiveness.
10. Read temperature by rotating thermometer until the mercury level is clearly visible.
11. Shake thermometer down, rinse in cool water, and replace in bedside container.
12. Wash hands.
13. Record client's temperature according to hospital procedure.

TAKING A RECTAL TEMPERATURE

Equipment

Rectal (blunt bulb) glass mercury thermometer
Tissues
Lubricant on a paper wipe for rectal method
Clean gloves

Procedure

1. Wash your hands and don gloves.
2. Rinse thermometer in cool water if kept in a chemical solution. **Rationale:** Solution may be irritating to mucosa.
3. Wipe dry with tissue from bulb end toward fingers. **Rationale:** Wipe from least to most contaminated area.
4. Grasp thermometer with thumb and forefinger and shake vigorously, flicking wrist in downward motion. This method lowers mercury level.
5. Check temperature reading on thermometer—it should be below 95–96°F.
6. Explain procedure to client.
7. Provide privacy; instruct and assist client to turn on side facing away from you with knees slightly flexed.
8. Lubricate tip of thermometer with lubricant on a paper tissue.
9. Fold back bed linen to expose client's anal area.
10. Separate buttocks with one hand so anal sphincter opening is visible.
11. Insert thermometer into rectum approximately 1/2–1 1/2 inches depending on the age of the patient. **Rationale:** Inserting thermometer more than 1/2 inch in an infant may cause rectal perforation.
12. Hold in place 2–5 minutes. Use placement time recommended in agency procedure manual. **Rationale:** Holding thermometer prevents injury.
13. Remove thermometer, and wipe it with tissue from fingers down to bulb. Discard tissue in toilet.
14. Read temperature by rotating thermometer until the mercury level is clearly visible. Shake thermometer down.
15. Wipe anal area to remove lubricant or stool.
16. Assist client to a comfortable position.
17. Wash thermometer in warm, soapy water, rinse with cool water, and put away.
18. Dispose of gloves and wash your hands.
19. Record client's temperature according to hospital procedure.

TAKING AN AXILLARY TEMPERATURE

Equipment

Glass mercury thermometer (preferably blunt bulb)
Tissues

Procedure

1. Wash your hands.
2. Rinse thermometer in cool water if kept in a chemical solution, and wipe dry with tissue from bulb toward fingers. Wipe from least contaminated to most contaminated area. **Rationale:** Cool water prevents expansion of mercury.
3. Grasp thermometer with thumb and forefinger and shake vigorously, flicking wrist in downward motion, to lower mercury level.
4. Check temperature reading on thermometer—it should be below 95–96°F.
5. Explain procedure to client. Provide privacy.

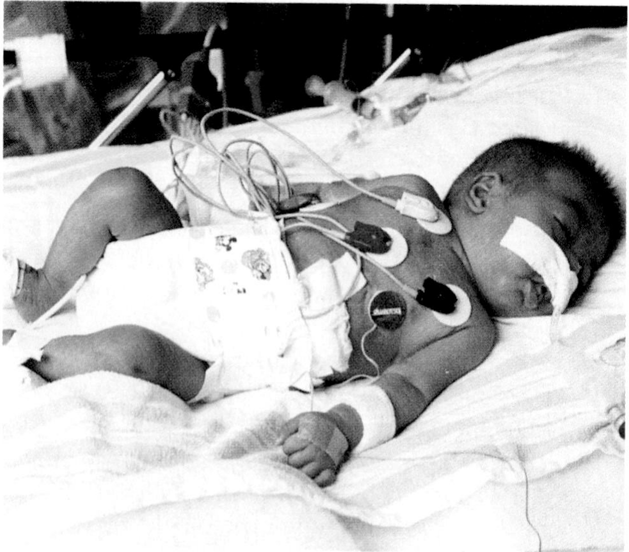

The axillary method is often used for children.

6. Assist client to a comfortable position, and expose axilla.
7. Dry axilla if necessary.
8. Place thermometer bulb in center of axilla. Lower client's arm down and across the chest. **Rationale:** This position ensures that thermometer remains in contact with large vessels of axilla.
9. Hold in place 6–8 minutes. (Optimum placement time varies among agencies.) **Rationale:** Axillary temperature recordings take a longer time to register accurately.
10. Remove thermometer, and wipe it with tissue from fingers down to bulb. Discard tissue. **Rationale:** Wipe from area of least to most contamination.
11. Read temperature by rotating thermometer until the mercury level is clearly visible, shake down, and replace in bedside container.
12. Assist client to a comfortable position.
13. Wash your hands.
14. Record client's temperature according to hospital procedure.

USING AN ELECTRONIC THERMOMETER

Equipment

Electronic thermometer unit with digital probe
Disposable cover for thermometer
Lubricant on tissue (for rectal temperature)

Procedure

1. Remove thermometer from charger unit.
2. Place carrying strap around your neck.
3. Grasp probe at top of stem using your thumb and forefinger. Do not put pressure on top because it is the ejection button.
4. Firmly insert probe in disposable probe cover.
5. Provide privacy if necessary.

for Oral Temperature

- Instruct client to open mouth and slide probe under front of client's tongue and along the gum line to the sublingual pocket at the base of the tongue. **Rationale:** The larger blood vessels in the pocket more accurately reflect the core temperature.
- Instruct client to close lips (not teeth). Lips should close at the ridge on the probe cover.

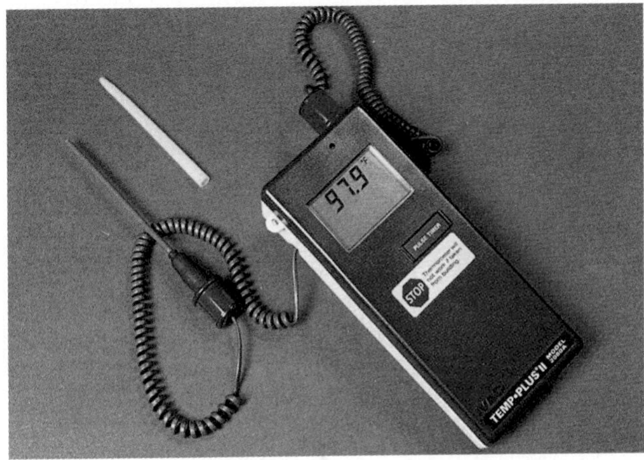

Electronic thermometer unit with digital probe.

for Rectal Temperature

- Position client on side facing away from you, separate buttocks, and insert covered and lubricated probe $1\frac{1}{2}$

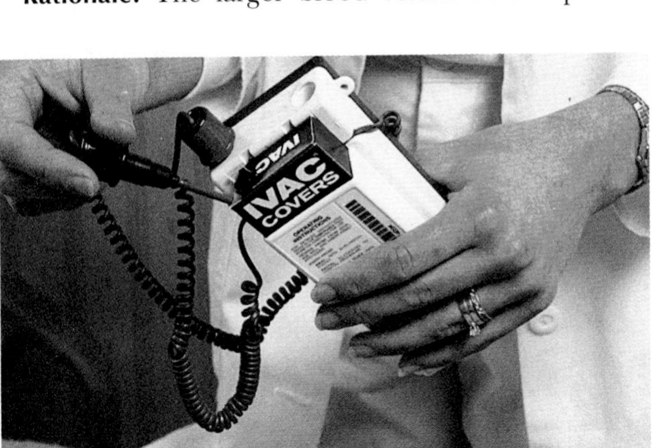

Cover probe of thermometer before taking temperature.

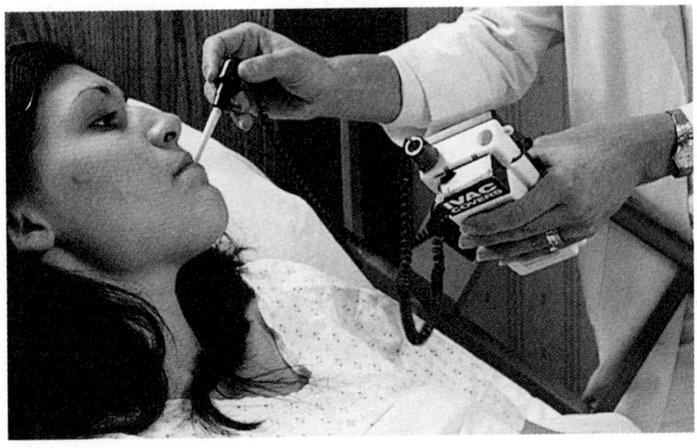

Slide probe under front of tongue to sublinqual pocket.

inches through anal sphincter. **Rationale:** Lubrication prevents tissue trauma.
- Position probe to side of rectum to ensure contact with tissue wall. **Rationale:** This ensures probe is in contact with large vessels of rectal wall.

6. Remove probe when audible signal occurs. Client's temperature is now registered on the dial.
7. Discard oral probe cover into trash by pushing ejection button. Discard rectal probe cover and tissue in bathroom. **Rationale:** Proper disposal prevents transmission of microorganisms.
8. Record temperature, and then return probe to storage well. **Rationale:** This ensures that system is ready for next use.
9. Return thermometer unit to charging base. Ensure charging base is plugged into electric outlet.

USING AN INFRARED THERMOMETER FOR EAR CANAL TEMPERATURE

Equipment

Infrared thermometer unit
Disposable probe cover

> **CLINICAL ALERT**
>
> Do not use ear thermometer in infected or draining ear, or if adjacent lesion or incision exists.

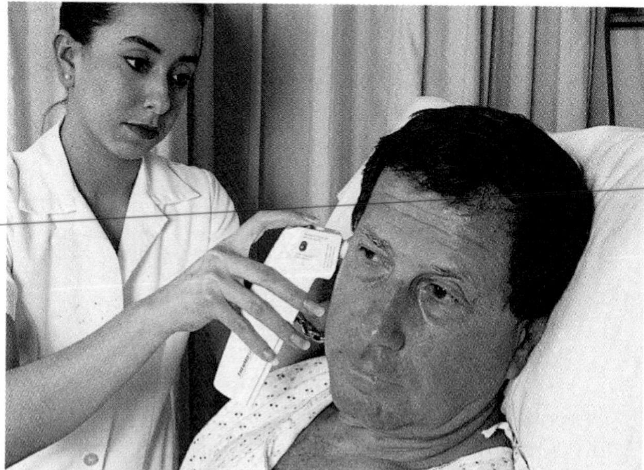

The tympanic route for taking a temperature is advised for clients over 3 months old.

Procedure

1. Wash hands.
2. Attach disposable cover centering probe on film and press firmly until backing frame of probe cover engages base of probe. **Rationale:** Cover protects client from transmission of microorganisms.
3. Stabilize the client's head.
4. Center probe and advance into ear canal to make a firm seal, directing probe toward tympanic membrane. **Rationale:** Pressure close to the tympanic membrane seals ear canal and allows for accurate reading.
5. Press and hold temperature switch until green light flashes and temperature reading displays (approximately 3 seconds). **Rationale:** Method records core body temperature.
6. Remove thermometer. Discard probe cover.
7. Return thermometer to home base or storage unit for recharge.
8. Keep lens clean using lint-free wipe or alcohol swab, then wipe dry. Do not use povidone-iodine (Betadine).
9. Wash hands.

USING A CHEMICAL STRIP TAPE

Equipment

Temperature tape
Soft cloth

Preparation

1. Obtain temperature tape from central supply.
2. Use tape indoors at room temperature and out of direct sunlight.
3. Do not use temperature tape if the client has been eating, drinking, or exercising within the last 30 minutes.
4. Check orders or client care plan that this method is appropriate for client.
5. Explain procedure to client.

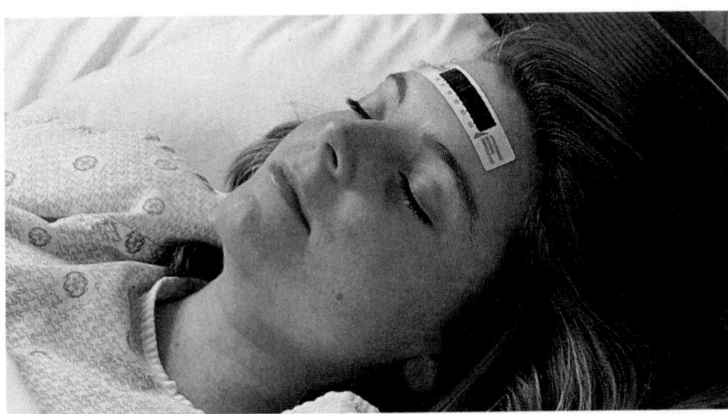

Place liquid crystal thermometer against lower forehead for 15 seconds for temperature reading.

Procedure

1. Position client comfortably with head slightly reclined. **Rationale:** This position facilitates getting an accurate temperature reading.
2. Grasp temperature tape firmly at both ends and press flush against a dry forehead.
3. Leave in place at least 15 seconds.
4. Read temperature while it is still on client's forehead.
5. Read temperatures as follows:
   a. The black demarcations that are numbered change color according to the client's temperature.
   b. Green appears over the correct temperature.
   c. If the center portion (between the black stripes) turns blue and tan, the temperature is half-way between the two numbered stripes.
6. Remove strip from client's forehead, and clean with a soft cloth.
7. Store at client's bedside in its protective case.
8. Reposition client for comfort.
9. Document temperature reading in appropriate record.

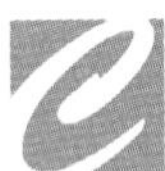

CHARTING for Temperature

- Site designated: "O" (oral), "R" (rectal), or "A" (axillary)
- Temperature recorded on temp sheet and graph
- Nursing interventions used for alterations in temperature
- Condition of skin related to alterations from normothermia (e.g., diaphoresis)
- Signs and symptoms associated with alterations in temperature (e.g., shivering, dehydration)

CRITICAL THINKING APPLICATION

CLINICAL PROBLEMS	CRITICAL THINKING OPTIONS
Fever develops.	• Check possible sources of infection, and take preventative measures. • Employ cooling methods if temperature is dangerously high, such as tepid sponge bath, cool oral fluids, ice packs, alcohol sponge bath, or antipyretic drugs.
Despite initial cooling measure, temperature remains elevated due to hypothalamus damage from brain disease or injury.	• Notify physician, and request cooling blanket. • Monitor temperature every 15–30 minutes. • Continue to administer antipyretic drugs as ordered.
Temperature remains elevated because of bacterial produced pyrogens.	• Check for order to obtain culture of possible sources of infection. • Give antipyretic drugs as ordered. • Decrease room temperature and remove excess covers. • Give tepid sponge bath.

unit 2 PULSE RATE

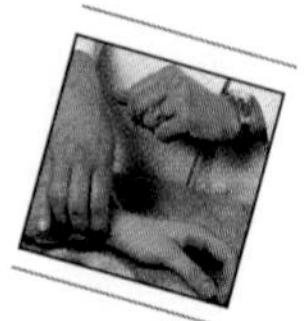

NURSING PROCESS DATA

ASSESSMENT Data Base

Assess appropriate site to obtain pulse.

Check pulse with health status changes.

Assess for rate, rhythm, pattern, and volume.

Take an apical pulse on clients with irregular rhythms or those on heart medications.

Obtain baseline peripheral pulses in any client going for cardiac or vascular surgery or medical clients with diabetes, arterial occlusive diseases, such as Raynaud's or Buerger's disease, atherosclerosis, or aneurysm.

Take an apical–radial pulse when deficits occur between apical and radial measurements.

Assess the need to monitor pulses with an ultrasound or electronic device.

PLANNING Objectives

To determine if the pulse rate is within normal range and if the rhythm is regular

To evaluate the equality of corresponding arterial pulses

To determine presence of peripheral pulses with ultrasound device when palpation is ineffective

To monitor and evaluate changes in the patient's health status

To determine apical pulse rate before heart medications are administered

IMPLEMENTATION Procedures

Taking a Radial Pulse

Taking an Apical Pulse

Taking an Apical–Radial Pulse

Taking a Peripheral Pulse

Monitoring Peripheral Pulses with Doppler Ultrasound Stethoscope

EVALUATION Expected Outcomes

Pulse is palpated without difficulty.

Pulse rate is within normal range and rhythm is regular.

All peripheral pulses are equal in amplitude when compared to the corresponding pulse on the other side and when compared to the next proximal site.

Apical pulse is easily detected and counted.

TAKING A RADIAL PULSE

Equipment

Watch with sweep second hand

Procedure

1. Wash your hands.
2. Place client in comfortable position.
3. Ask about activity level within last 15 minutes. **Rationale:** Pulse rate increases with activity, then returns to preactivity rate.
4. Palpate arteries by using pads of the middle three fingers of your hand. **Rationale:** The nurse may feel own pulse if palpating with the thumb.
   a. Radial artery is usually used because it lies close to the skin surface and is easily accessible at the wrist.
   b. Press the artery against the bone or underlying firm surface to occlude vessel, and then gradually release pressure. **Rationale:** Too much pressure obliterates the pulse.

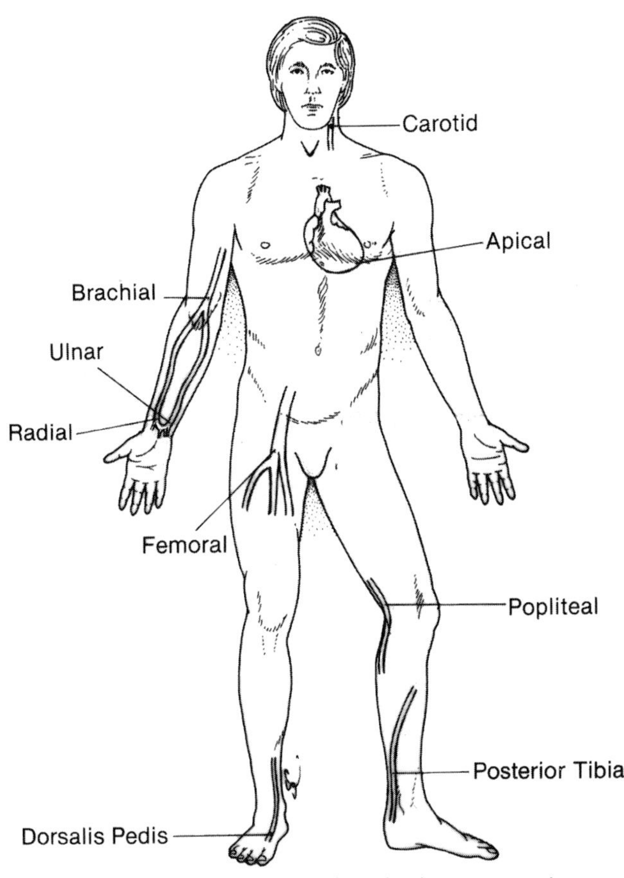

Radial artery is most commonly used site for determining pulse rate.

c. Note quality (strength) of pulse. **Rationale:** Strength of the pulse is an indication of stroke volume.

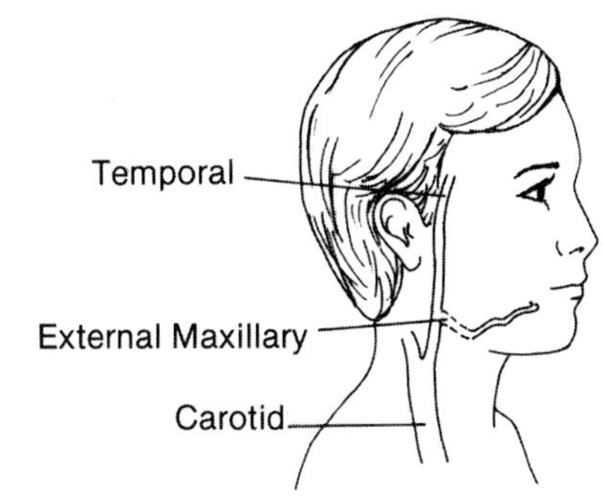

Carotid artery is used when other sites are inaccessible.

d. If pulse is difficult to palpate, try exerting more pressure on the most distal palpating finger. **Rationale:** This amplifies the pulse wave against the two more proximal palpating fingers.

5. Count pulse for 15 seconds, and multiply by four to obtain pulse rate. **Rationale:** This is sufficient time for rate determination if pulse rhythm is regular.
6. Count an apical pulse for at least 1 minute if rhythm is irregular or difficult to count. An apical–radial pulse measurement provides additional information regarding cardiac function if pulse is irregular. **Rationale:** It may take a minute or so to detect the irregularity. This method assists you to count the pulse more accurately.
7. Check to see that client is comfortable.
8. Wash your hands.
9. Record pulse rate, rhythm, and strength (volume).

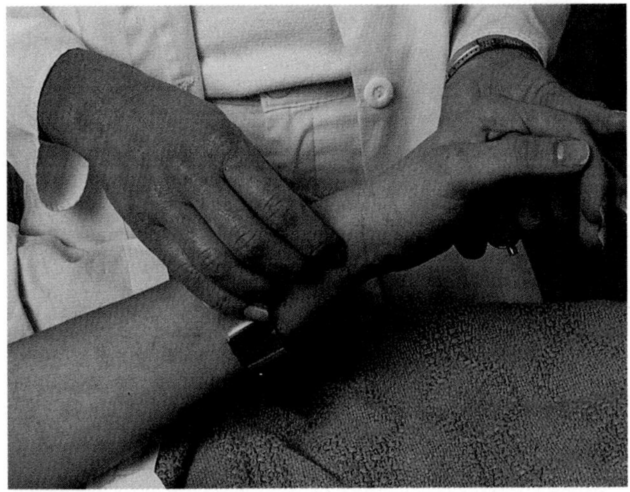

Palpate radial pulse by using tips of fingers, not thumb for accurate results.

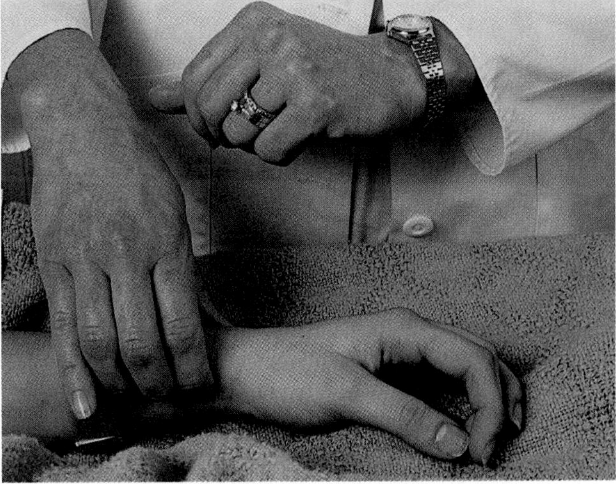

Count pulse beats for at least 30 seconds and multiply by two for rate.

TAKING AN APICAL PULSE

Equipment

Watch with sweep second hand
Stethoscope

Procedure

1. Gather equipment.
2. Wash your hands.
3. Check client's identaband. Provide privacy.
4. Explain procedure to client.
5. Place client in a supine position and expose chest area. If possible, stand at client's right side. **Rationale:** Ausculation of heart sounds is often enhanced when examiner is at client's right side.
6. Count client's apical pulse.
   a. Place diaphragm of stethoscope firmly over apex of the heart. The apex is normally located in the fifth intercostal space left of the sternum in the midclavicular line. **Rationale:** Heart sounds are high pitched and most clearly heard with diaphragm of stethoscope.
   b. Count the rate for 1 minute when taking an apical pulse. **Rationale:** More accurate readings are obtained over 1 minute, especially if pulse is irregular.
   c. Determine if there is a regular pattern to any irregularity or if it is chaotically irregular. **Rationale:** This finding helps describe the rhythm disturbance.
   d. Auscultate the apical pulse and palpate the radial pulse simultaneously (preferably using two nurses, one at each site) to note a pulse deficit when rhythm is irregular. **Rationale:** Atrial dysrhythmias and premature ventricular beats generally produce pulse deficits (apical greater than radial rate).
   e. Assess pulse volume by feeling the pressure of the beat.
7. Check to see that client is comfortable.
8. Wash your hands.
9. Record apical pulse rate, rhythm, and strength (volume).

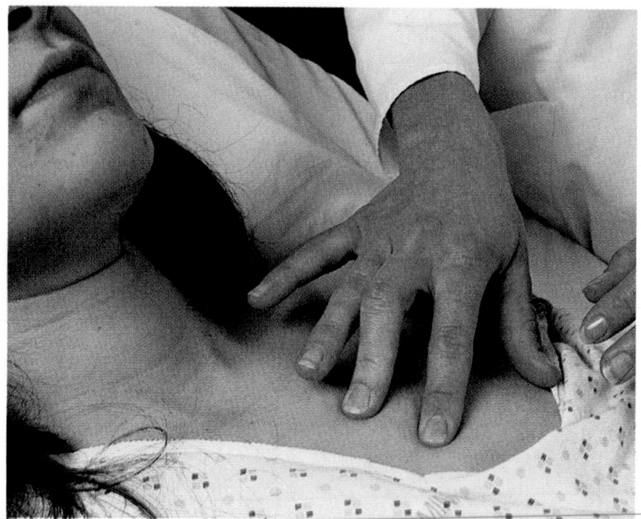

Determine fifth intercostal space by accurate palpation before taking apical pulse.

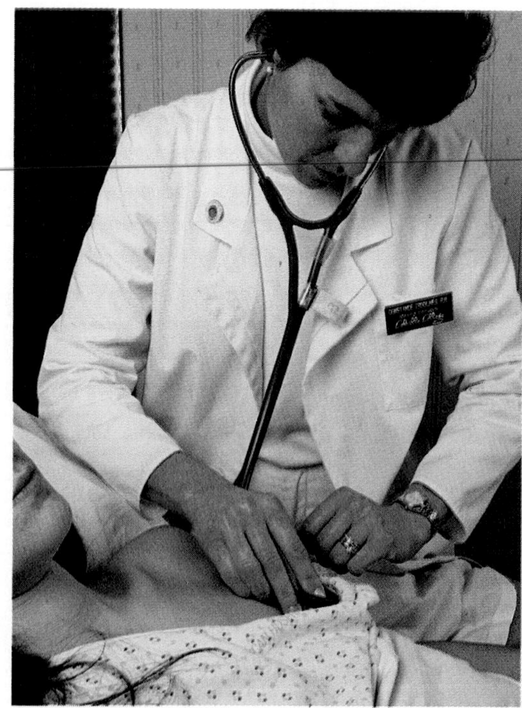

Ausculate tricuspid area, or Erb's point, to take accurate apical pulse.

TAKING AN APICAL–RADIAL PULSE

Equipment

Watch with sweep second hand

Stethoscope

Another nurse to assist with procedure

Note: An experienced nurse may be able to assess apical and radial rates simultaneously without an assistant.

Procedure

1. Gather equipment.
2. Wash your hands.
3. Check client's identaband.
4. Provide privacy.
5. Explain procedure to client especially if two nurses are taking the pulse. **Rationale:** Clients may be apprehensive when two nurses are at the bedside, so a full explanation helps allay fears.
6. Assist client to a supine position and expose chest area.
7. Place watch where clearly visible to both nurses. **Rationale:** Both nurses count pulse rates within the same time span, preferably using one watch.
8. Locate radial pulse. The second nurse locates apical pulse at the fifth intercostal space and midclavicular line, and firmly places diaphragm of stethoscope on the site. **Rationale:** Firm application helps transmit high-pitched heart sounds.

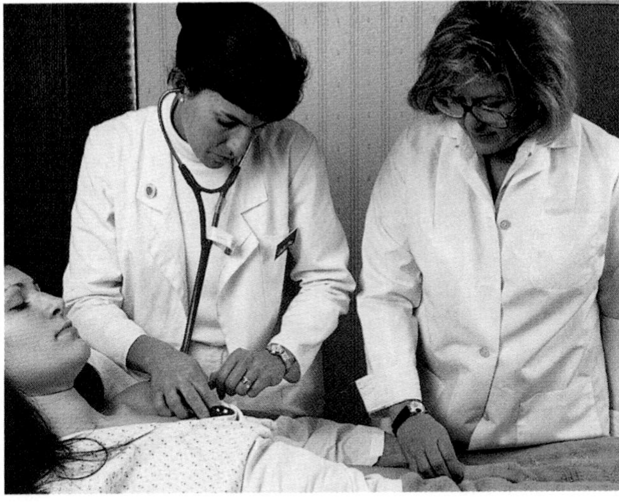

Use two nurses to take apical-radial pulse for accurate reading.

9. With assistant, select number on watch to start counting pulse (e.g., 12:00).
10. Signal to the other nurse with your hand when to start taking the pulse and when to stop. Both nurses simultaneously count pulse for 1 full minute.
11. Position client for comfort.
12. Wash your hands.
13. Subtract radial rate from apical rate to obtain pulse deficit. **Rationale:** The pulse deficit represents the number of ineffective or nonperfused heartbeats.
14. Chart apical and radial rate and pulse deficit.

TAKING A PERIPHERAL PULSE

Equipment

Felt-tipped pen

Watch with second hand

> ■ **CLINICAL ALERT**
>
> If palpating the carotid pulse, avoid pressing on the carotid sinus in the upper neck area near the jaw. *Do not* palpate both carotids simultaneously because this decreases blood flow to the brain.

Procedure

1. Gather equipment.
2. Wash your hands.
3. Check client's identaband.
4. Provide privacy. Explain procedure.
5. Place client in a reclining position with the trunk of the body at a 30° angle.
6. Palpate peripheral pulses: radial, brachial, femoral, popliteal, dorsalis pedis, posterior tibial. (For special cases, after carotid surgery, palpate temporal pulse also.)
7. Compare pulse sites bilaterally by palpating with pads of the middle three fingers of your hand.
8. Press artery against the bone or underlying firm

surface to occlude vessel and then gradually release pressure.

9. Palpate weak pulses gently. **Rationale:** Too much pressure obliterates a weak pulse.
10. Assess if bilateral pulses are equal in amplitude (strength).
    a. If pulse is not immediately palpable, examine adjacent area. **Rationale:** This action identifies where interruption or alteration in circulation occurs in an extremity.
    b. Since pulse locations differ, mark pulse locations with felt-tipped pen, especially when they are difficult to palpate. **Rationale:** Marking site allows the next nurse to find location without spending extra time.
    c. Compare presence and characteristic of peripheral pulses with previous findings. **Rationale:** This action allows early identification of alterations in peripheral circulation.
11. Check to see that client is comfortable.
12. Wash your hands.
13. Record pulse rate, rhythm, pattern, and volume.

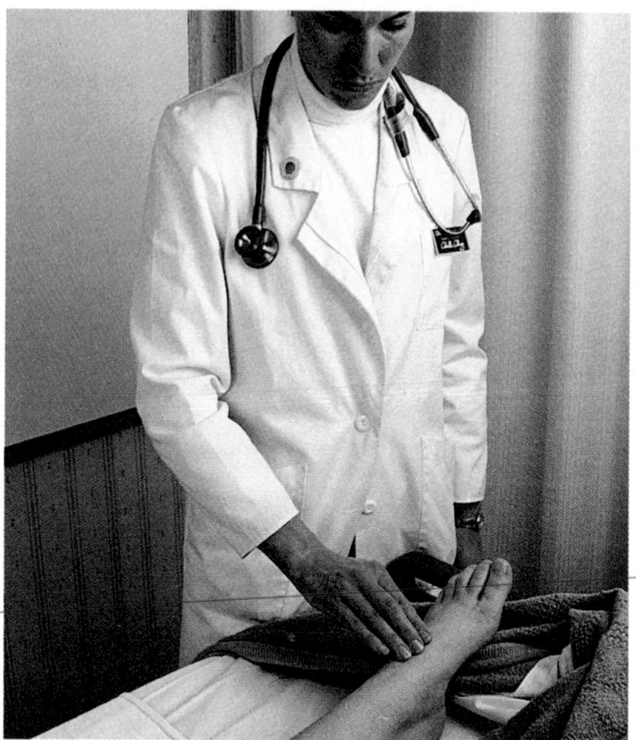

Press artery against bone to find peripheral pulse.

MONITORING PERIPHERAL PULSES WITH DOPPLER ULTRASOUND STETHOSCOPE

Equipment

Doppler ultrasound stethoscope
Conductive jelly (not K-Y)

Procedure

1. Gather equipment.
2. Wash your hands.
3. Explain procedure to client.
4. Provide privacy.
5. Uncover extremity to be assessed.
6. Place extremity in a comfortable position.
7. Plug headset (stethoscope) into one of the two outlet jacks located next to the volume control.
8. Apply conductive gel to client's skin. **Rationale:** The ultrasound beam travels best through gel and requires an airtight seal between the probe and the skin.
9. Hold probe (at tapered end of plastic core) against

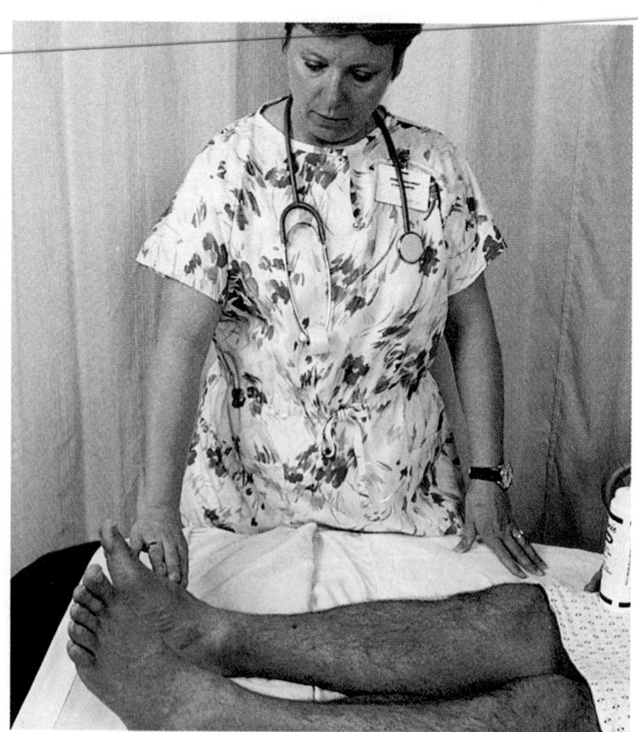

Find peripheral pulse with fingers before applying gel.

skin at a 90° angle to the blood vessel being examined.

10. Turn on Doppler stethoscope by pressing down the "ON."
11. Move probe over site if pulse is not detected. Keep it in direct contact with skin, and adjust volume to detect blood flow. **Rationale:** This action should facilitate detection of swooshing pulse sounds.
12. Reapply new gel if pulse is still not detected and, with light pressure, place probe over site and turn switch ON. Increase volume control, or check if batteries are weak.
13. Mark site where pulsations were heard. **Rationale:** This facilitates future assessments.
14. Clean gel from skin and probe. Replace cover over extremity.
15. Position client for comfort.
16. Replace Doppler stethoscope to appropriate location.
17. Wash your hands.
18. Document pulse findings.

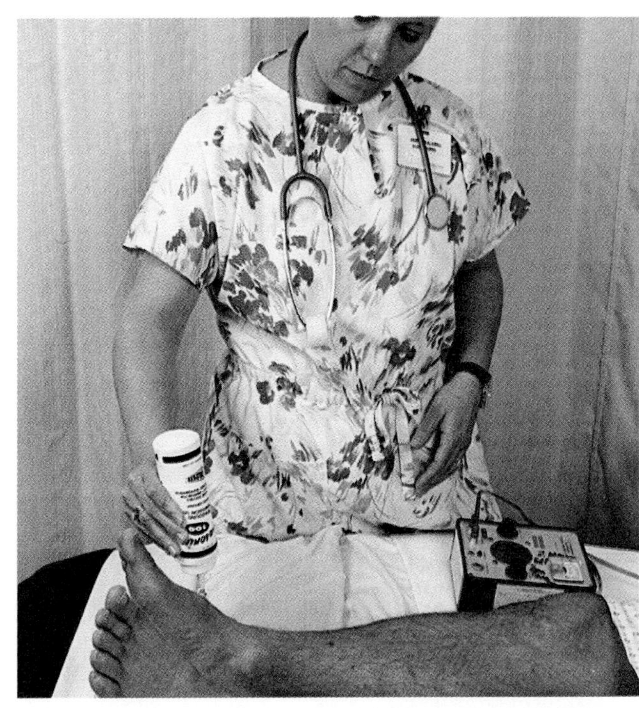

Apply gel to skin to facilitate beam transmission.

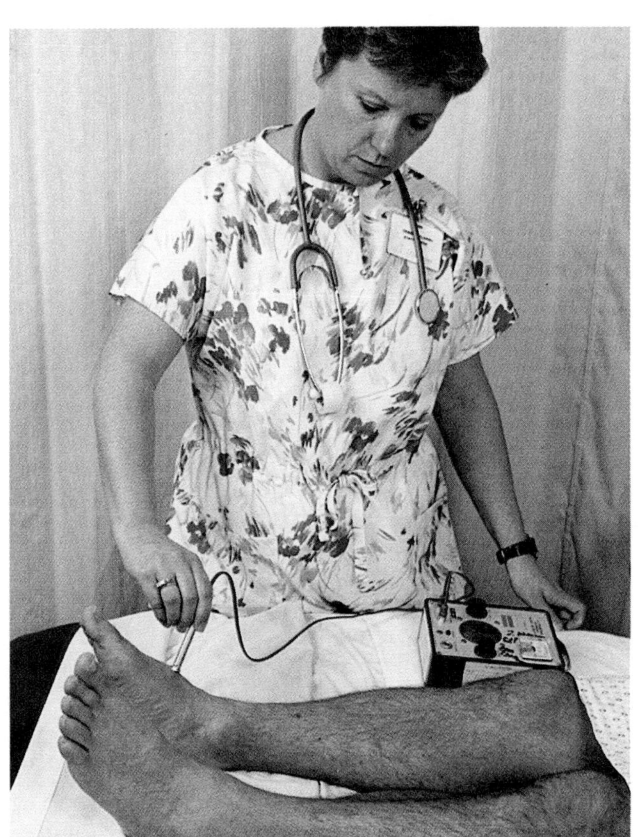

Hold probe against skin at 90° angle.

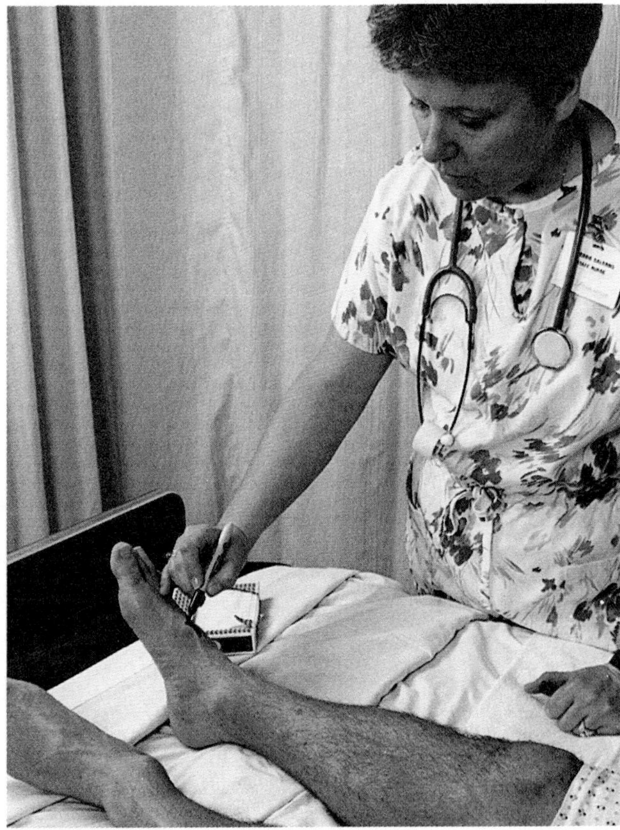

Mark site where pulsations were heard.

CHARTING for Taking a Pulse

- Type of pulse taken
- Rate and rhythm of pulse
- Pulse volume
- Pulse deficit if any present
- Characteristics of all peripheral pulses—use rating scale
- Use of Doppler stethoscope if needed
- Effects of nursing or medical treatments on abnormal pulse rates or rhythms

CRITICAL THINKING APPLICATION

CLINICAL PROBLEMS	CRITICAL THINKING OPTIONS
■ Apical, femoral, and carotid pulse is absent.	• Immediately repeat procedure to validate findings and call a Code. • Initiate CPR immediately, and continue to assess the femoral or carotid pulse during resuscitation. • For absent femoral pulse, assess for systemic circulation and presence of disorders affecting circulation to extremities. • Use Doppler stethoscope to assess for presence of pulse.
■ Irregular heart beats are present. ***Tachycardia*** (pulse rate over 100 BPM in adults or 140 in children):	• Relieve anxiety, fear, or stress through communication and pertinent information. • If client has pain, relieve with change of position, back rub, and analgesic. • Decrease heart rate by reducing an elevated temperature to normal. • Take vital signs every 15 minutes to 2 hours until condition stabilizes and pulse rate is within normal limits. • Determine significance of pulse rate as it affects blood pressure, sensorium, and client comfort.
■ ***Bradycardia*** (pulse rate less than 60 in adults or less than 70 in children):	• Notify physician for electrocardiogram request to determine if heart block is present. • If client is on digitalis, hold the drug and notify the physician. • Have atropine and temporary pacemaker available for physician if pulse is consistently slow (less than 50). • Continue monitoring pulse rate every 15 minutes to 2 hours until pulse is within normal limits.
■ ***Ectopic Beats*** (premature or atrial fibrillation):	• Relieve pain if irregularity is due to premature beats associated with pain. • Administer oxygen if client has an order to do so.

CLINICAL PROBLEMS	CRITICAL THINKING OPTIONS
	• If associated with stimuli from noise, visitors, caffeinated beverages, or smoking, eliminate the cause of the stimulation. • Notify physician to request a medical order for an electrocardiogram since premature beats in a client with myocardial infarction may be potentially harmful. • Obtain order from physician to draw serum electrolytes, especially potassium. Low potassium levels can cause premature ventricular contractions. • Continue monitoring pulse rate every 15 minutes to 2 hours until irregularity is controlled.
■ Doppler stethoscope unable to detect sounds.	• Check that K-Y jelly is not used because salt in it can damage the probe. • Check that batteries are less than 6 months old. The date should be indicated on all batteries. • Use alkaline batteries; they last longer.
■ Client is in isolation and requires vascular assessment.	• Clean with gas sterilization after discontinuing use of Doppler stethoscope. • Do not clean with alcohol or autoclave.

unit 3

RESPIRATIONS

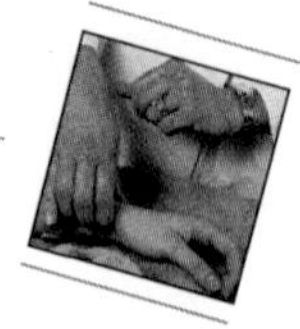

NURSING PROCESS DATA

ASSESSMENT Data Base

Assess client's respiratory rate, depth, and position.

Evaluate any abnormalities noted during inspection and palpation or by percussion and auscultation.

Assess presence of dyspnea or cyanosis.

Assess for presence of abnormal sounds, such as stertorous or sonorous breathing.

Assess if accessory muscles are used for breathing.

PLANNING Objectives

To note respiratory rate, rhythm, and depth

To establish baseline information on admission to the unit

To note labored, difficult, or noisy respirations or cyanosis

To identify alterations in respiratory pattern resulting from disease condition

To compare if respiratory rate is within normal range with pulse and blood pressure readings

IMPLEMENTATION Procedure

Obtaining the Respiratory Rate

EVALUATION Expected Outcomes

Regular rate of breathing and symmetrical respiratory excursion is established.

Client exhibits quiet, effortless breathing.

OBTAINING THE RESPIRATORY RATE

Equipment

Watch with a second hand

Procedure

1. Wash your hands.
2. Explain procedure to client.
3. Check lighting to ensure it is adequate for procedure.
4. Maintain client's privacy.
5. Place hand on chest or observe chest rise and fall and count respirations.
6. Note relationship of inspiration to expiration. Note also depth and effort of breathing.
7. Count respirations for 30 seconds and multiply by 2. **Rationale:** This is adequate for normal breath-

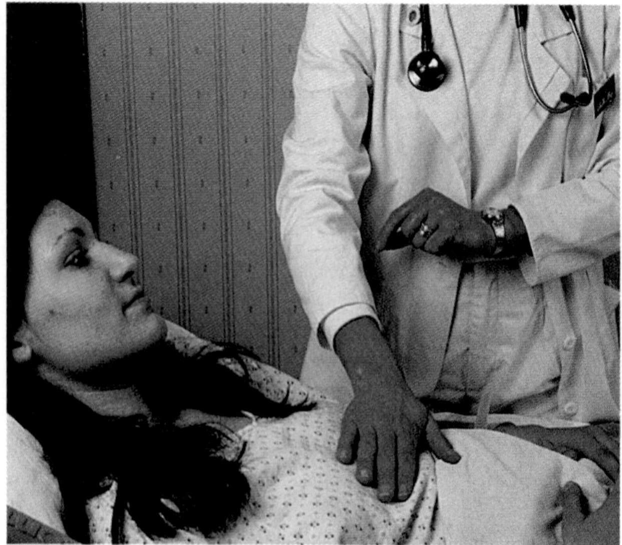

Place hand on chest when respirations are difficult to count.

ing. One full minute is more accurate for abnormal breathing patterns.

8. Wash your hands.
9. Compare respiratory rate with previous recordings.
10. Record respiratory rate. Record if rhythm or depth altered from normal.

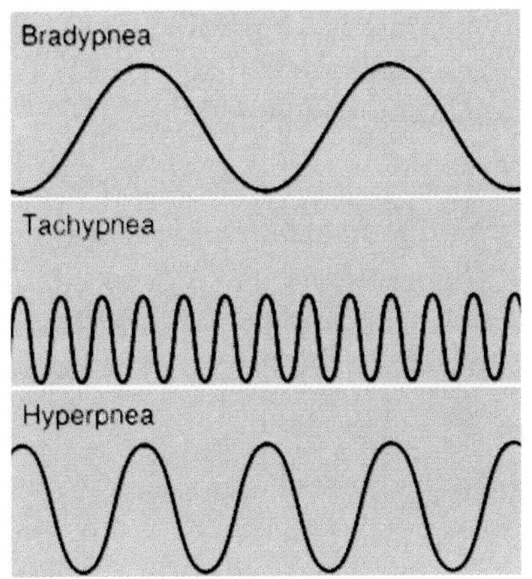

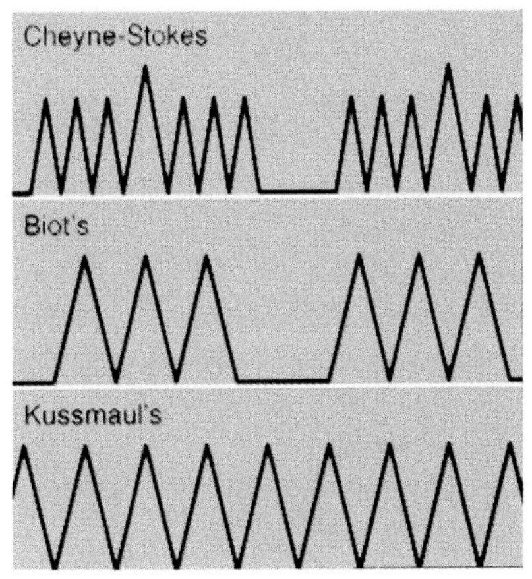

Apnea

Examples of abnormal respiratory wave patterns.

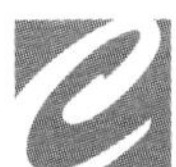

CHARTING for Respirations

- Rate and rhythm of respirations
- Abnormal sounds associated with breathing
- Effectiveness of therapy if needed to correct respiratory problems
- Alterations from baseline respiratory patterns

CRITICAL THINKING APPLICATION

CLINICAL PROBLEMS	CRITICAL THINKING OPTIONS
■ Apnea (absence of breathing) occurs, may be intermittent	• Begin artificial ventilation by mouth-to-mouth, mouth-to-nose, or other airway adjunct method at the rate of 12 per minute for an adult or 20 per minute for a child. • Summon help immediately.
■ Tachypnea (rate faster than normal and more shallow >24) occurs.	• Relieve anxiety, fear, and stress through communication and pertinent information. • Relieve fever if that is the cause. • Correct respiratory insufficiency with low-flow oxygen administration, good pulmonary toilet, and deep breathing and coughing exercises.
■ Bradypnea (rate slower than normal <10) occurs.	• If due to respiratory depressant drugs, such as opiates, barbiturates, and tranquilizers, be prepared to assist respirations or administer mouth-to-mouth resuscitation. • Administer oxygen at 6 L/min via nasal cannulae as ordered. If client has COPD use 2 L/min. • Stimulate client to take breaths at least 10 times per minute.
■ Hyperpnea (increased depth of respiration) occurs.	• Rest after period of exertion. • Relieve fear, anxiety, or stress. • May be indicative of respiratory compensation for metabolic acidotic state (Kussmaul pattern).
■ Cheyne–Stokes respirations (respiratory cycle in which respirations increase in rate and depth, then decrease, followed by a period of apnea) occur.	• Follow physician's orders to treat underlying disease state (e.g., heart failure, increased intracranial pressure). • Monitor respirations every 15 minutes to hourly, depending on client's status. • Be prepared to administer CPR if apnea occurs. • One of the indicators that death is approaching.
■ Biot's (irregular pattern—slow and deep or rapid and shallow, followed by apnea respirations) occur.	• Assess for central nervous system (CNS) abnormalities (increased intracranial pressure, meningitis).
■ Kussmaul's (slow, deep, and regular—more than 20 breaths/minute) respirations occur.	• Follow orders to treat for renal failure, septic shock, or diabetic ketoacidosis.

unit 4

BLOOD PRESSURE

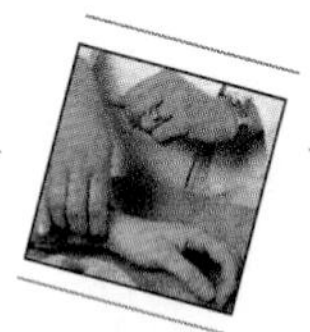

NURSING PROCESS DATA

ASSESSMENT Data Base

Assess blood pressure initially and whenever client's status changes.

Assess size of cuff needed for accurate reading.

Assess the beginning, and disappearance of Korotkoff's sounds during a blood pressure reading.

Assess presence of factors that can alter blood pressure readings.

Note any changes from prior assessments.

PLANNING Objectives

To determine if arterial blood pressure reading is within normal range for the individual client

To assess condition of heart, arteries, blood vessel resistance, and stroke volume

To establish a baseline for further evaluation

To identify alterations in blood pressure resulting from a change in disease condition

To correlate blood pressure readings with pulse and respirations

IMPLEMENTATION Procedures

Taking a Blood Pressure

Palpating Systolic Arterial Blood Pressure

Measuring Leg Blood Pressure

Measuring Blood Pressure by Flush Method in Small Infant

Using a Continuous Noninvasive Monitoring Device

EVALUATION Expected Outcomes

Blood pressure is within normal range (100/60–140/90 mm Hg).

Alterations in blood pressure are identified early and appropriate treatment initiated.

Severely altered blood pressure readings are rechecked with different equipment or validated by another nurse.

Unstable blood pressure readings are monitored frequently for trend recognition.

TAKING A BLOOD PRESSURE

Equipment

Sphygmomanometer with proper sized cuff

Stethoscope

Procedure

1. Gather equipment. Be sure the cuff is an appropriate size for the client. **Rationale:** A cuff that is too narrow results in erroneously high readings.
2. Provide quiet environment.
3. Wash your hands.
4. Check client's identaband.
5. Explain procedure to client.
6. Place client in relaxed reclining or sitting position.

CLINICAL ALERT

When a client moves from recumbent to standing position, systolic pressure can fall 10–15 mm Hg and diastolic may rise by 5 mm Hg.

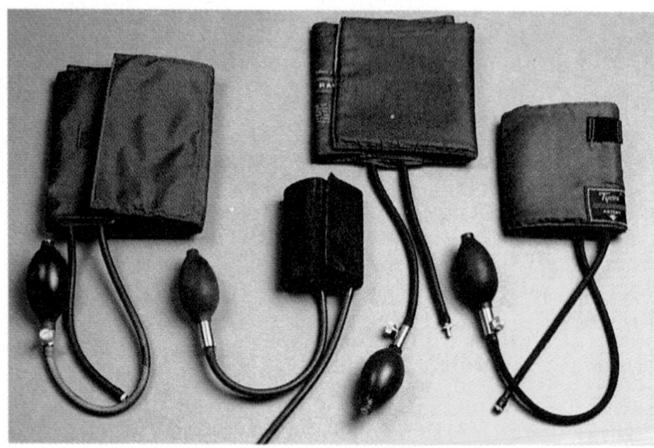

Blood pressure cuffs are available in various sizes.

BLOOD PRESSURE CUFF SIZES

- Standard (12–14 cm wide) for the average adult arm.
- Narrower cuff for infant, child, or adult with thin arms.
- For children (younger than 13 years) the bladder should be large enough to encircle the arm completely (100%).
- Wider cuff (18–22 cm) for client with obese arms or thigh pressure readings.

The cuff's inflatable bladder width should be 40% of the circumference of the limb on which it is used. The length of the bladder should be twice its width.

7. Allow client to rest several minutes before beginning a reading. Client should be instructed not to cross legs or talk during the procedure. **Rationale:** Client activities and a slouched position yield false high readings.
8. Expose upper part of client's arm and position it with palm upward, arm slightly flexed with the whole arm supported at heart level. **Rationale:** If arm is below level of heart, the blood pressure reading is higher than normal.
9. Wrap totally deflated cuff snugly and smoothly around upper part of arm (lower border of cuff 1 inch above antecubital space) with center of cuff bladder over brachial artery (pressure dial or mercury meniscus at zero).
10. Locate brachial artery with fingertips (medial aspect of antecubital fossa).
11. Position stethoscope ear pieces in ears.
12. Close valve on sphygmomanometer pump.
13. Palpate radial artery pulsations on arm that is cuffed.
14. Inflate cuff rapidly (while palpating radial artery) to a level 30 mm Hg above level at which radial pulsations are no longer felt. **Rationale:** This level ensures that cuff is inflated to a pressure exceeding the client's systolic pressure. Slow inflation can yield gaps in pressure readings.
15. Place bell (or diaphragm) of stethoscope lightly on the medial antecubital fossa where brachial artery pulsations are located. **Rationale:** Korotkoff sounds are low frequency and can be heard more clearly with bell of stethoscope, but diaphragm is commonly used.

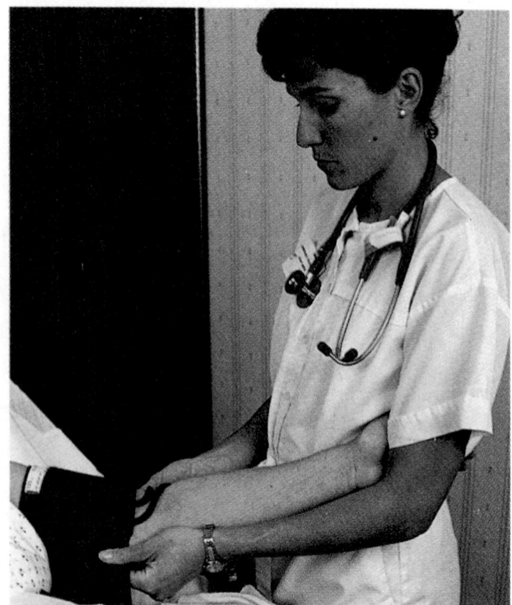

Wrap blood pressure cuff snugly around upper arm.

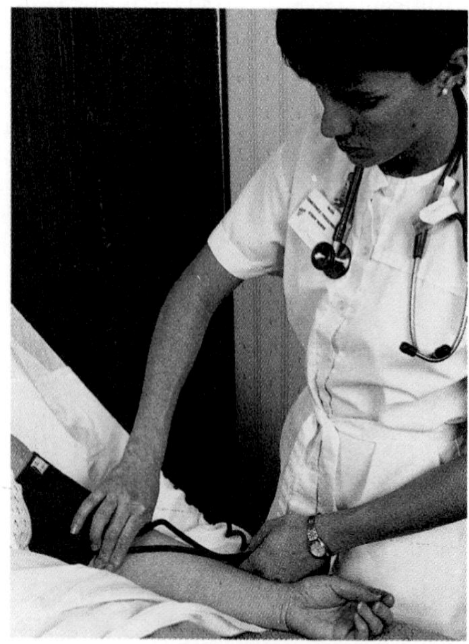

Palpate brachial artery on medial antecubital fossa.

16. Deflate cuff gradually at a constant rate by opening valve on pump (2 mm Hg/second) until the first Korotkoff sound is heard. This is the systolic pressure, or phase I, of Korotkoff's sounds. **Rationale:** Slower or faster deflation yields false readings.
17. Read pressure with mercury at eye level when using manometer filled with mercury. **Rationale:** If the mercury meniscus is below eye level, the reading is a false low.
18. Continue to deflate cuff at a rate of 2 mm Hg/second, do not reinflate without letting cuff totally deflate. **Rationale:** Reinflating cuff results in erroneously high readings.
19. Note point at which Korotkoff's sounds begin (phase I), and when they disappear completely (phase V). Disappearance of sounds (phase V) is regarded by the American Heart Association as the best index of diastolic blood pressure in individuals over age 13. The best indication of diastolic pressure in children is the distinct muffling of sounds at phase IV.
20. Do not leave cuff inflated for a prolonged period. **Rationale:** Leaving cuff inflated produces patient discomfort.
21. Deflate cuff completely and wait at least 30 seconds before rechecking the blood pressure. **Rationale:** This allows time for blood vessels to return to normal.
22. Remove cuff from client's arm.
23. Check that client is comfortable.
24. Compare blood pressure reading with previous recordings.

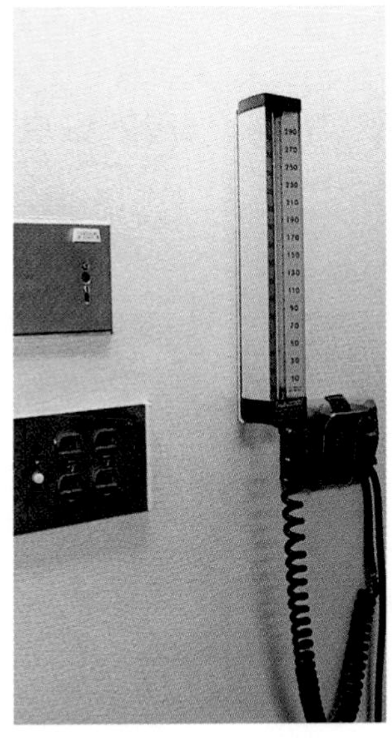

Example of wall-mounted mercury manometer.

25. Wash your hands.
26. Record blood pressure readings using two or three phases (120/80, 110/80/20). If appropriate, record blood pressure site, client position, and cuff size used (if other than standard).

■ CLINICAL ALERT

The American Heart Association recommends routine use of the *bell* of the stethoscope for blood pressure (Korotkoff's sounds) auscultation.

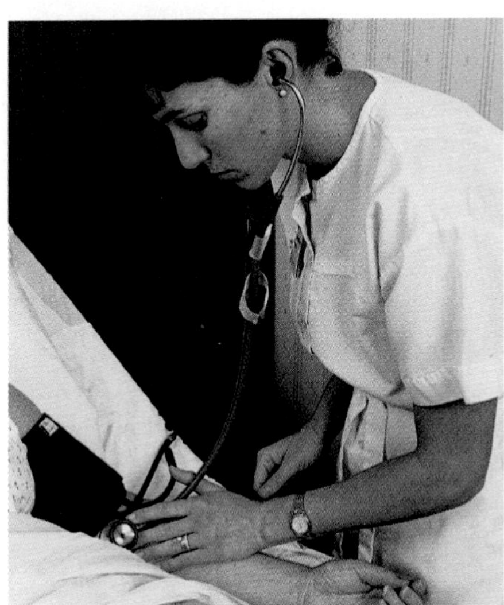

Place bell of stethoscope on medial antecubital fossa.

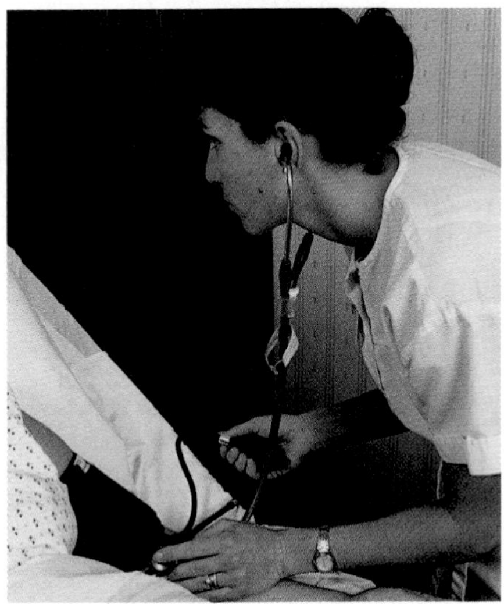

Read manometer at eye level.

PALPATING SYSTOLIC ARTERIAL BLOOD PRESSURE

Equipment

Sphygmomanometer with proper size cuff

Procedure

1. Gather equipment. Check that cuff is appropriate size for patient. **Rationale:** A cuff that is too narrow results in erroneously high readings.
2. Wash your hands.
3. Check client's identaband.
4. Explain procedure to client.
5. Place client in relaxed position, and support arm at heart level.
6. Wrap cuff snugly and smoothly around the upper part of the arm (1 inch above antecubital space) with center of bladder over brachial artery.

> **CLINICAL ALERT**
>
> - Avoid measuring blood pressure in an arm with extensive axillary node dissection (e.g., radical mastectomy) or an arteriovenous fistula (e.g., for dialysis).
> - Ultrasound techniques such as that using a Doppler stethoscope can be used to measure systolic blood pressure when auscultatory sounds are too faint to be heard.

7. Keep pressure level in cuff at zero.
8. Locate radial artery pulsations on cuffed arm.

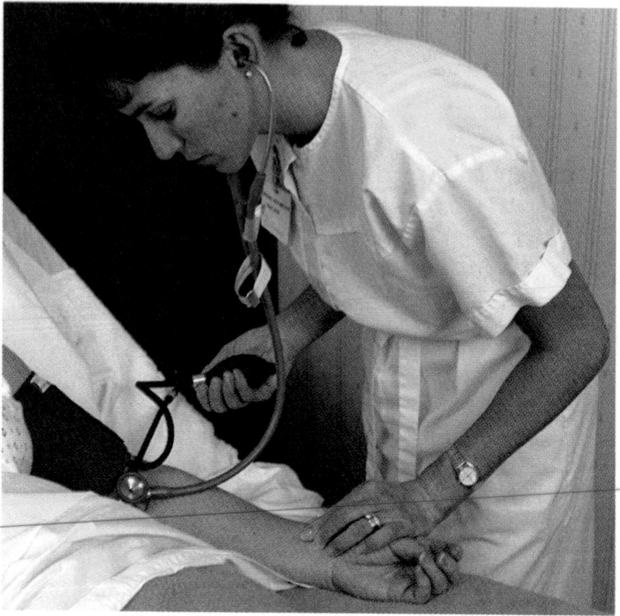

Palpate radial artery while inflating cuff and releasing pressure from cuff.

9. Inflate cuff rapidly (while palpating radial artery), to a level 30 mm Hg above level at which radial artery pulsations are no longer felt. **Rationale:** This level ensures that cuff is inflated to a pressure exceeding client's systolic pressure.
10. Continue to palpate artery and release pressure from cuff slowly (2 mm Hg/second). The first palpated beat is the systolic pressure. This should be the same point at which the last pulsation was felt during inflation of cuff.
11. Remove cuff and return equipment.
12. Wash your hands.
13. Record systolic blood pressure reading as "palpated systolic pressure."

MEASURING LEG BLOOD PRESSURE

Equipment

Stethoscope
Sphygmomanometer with standard size cuff

Procedure

1. Gather equipment.
2. Wash your hands.
3. Check client's identaband.
4. Explain procedure to client.
5. Wrap cuff snugly and smoothly around lower leg with cuff's distal edge at the malleolus.
6. Locate either the dorsalis pedis or posterior tibial artery pulsations.
7. Inflate cuff rapidly while palpating foot artery, to a level 30 mm Hg above level at which artery pulsations are no longer felt.

8. Place bell (or diaphragm) of stethoscope quickly on pulse site.
9. Deflate cuff slowly (2 mm Hg/second) while auscultating sounds over the selected artery.
10. Remove cuff and return equipment.
11. Check to see that client is comfortable.
12. Record readings for first (systolic) and last (diastolic) sounds, noting site and client position.

Alternative Methods

13. Measure blood pressure in thigh by using a large cuff with bladder placed over posterior mid-thigh. Listen with bell of stethoscope at popliteal fossa with client in prone position, or supine with knee flexed enough for stethoscope placement.
14. Measure blood pressure in forearm by placing appropriate size cuff around forearm 13 cm from elbow; listen for Korotkoff's sounds over radial artery at wrist.
15. Compare blood pressures measured indirectly in the arm, leg, and thigh to reveal similar values. Measurements may be difficult to obtain in clients with peripheral vascular disease.

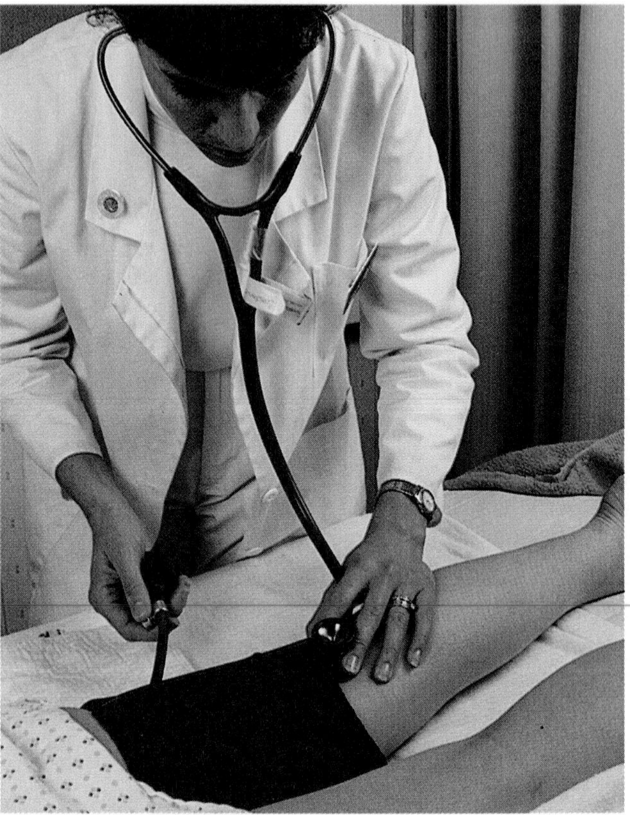

Use a large size cuff to measure blood pressure in clients thigh.

MEASURING BLOOD PRESSURE BY FLUSH METHOD IN SMALL INFANT

Equipment

Sphygmomanometer with appropriate cuff
Elastic bandage
Assistant for observing flush
Well-lighted room

> **■ CLINICAL ALERT**
>
> Flush pressures are taken on small infants or on adults when unable to auscultate or palpate blood pressure readings.

Procedure

1. Gather equipment.
2. Wash your hands.
3. Check client's identaband.
4. Wrap cuff snuggly and smoothly just above wrist or ankle.
5. Elevate extremity above heart level.
6. Wrap elastic bandage firmly around exposed hand or foot. **Rationale:** Bandage compression empties the veins.
7. Lower extremity to heart level when compression is complete.
8. Inflate cuff rapidly to 200 mm Hg.
9. Remove elastic bandage.
10. Deflate cuff slowly (not exceeding 5 mm Hg/second).
11. Instruct assistant to watch for appearance of flush in the extremity distal to cuff. **Rationale:** An assistant is necessary so that pressure at which flush appears can be precisely noted. This reading more clearly reflects the *mean* blood pressure than the systolic pressure.
12. Document that blood pressure was taken by flush method.

USING A CONTINUOUS NONINVASIVE MONITORING DEVICE

Equipment

Blood pressure cuff
Display monitor
Readout paper for monitor

Procedure

1. Wash hands.
2. Gather equipment. Select proper size blood pressure cuff. Attach the cuff to the air hose by firmly pushing the valve from the cuff into the air hose and twisting to secure fit.
3. Squeeze the air from the cuff.
4. Wrap the cuff securely around the extremity (usually the arm).
5. Turn power switch ON.
6. Position the extremity at the level of the heart.
7. Set arterial pressure alarm limits by pushing *Alarm* to ON and set both HIGH and LOW parameters by depressing the *Alarm* button until the parameters read out on the digital display. **Rationale:** The alarm parameters provide a safety factor by alerting the nurse when the readings exceed the parameters.
8. Test time cycles by turning wheel (found above alarm button) to 1 minute and check for cycling effects. Then, to set automatic cycle time, move the wheel to desired time increments.
9. Press *Start* button for approximately 4 seconds to activate printer for readout of blood pressure. Systolic, diastolic, mean arterial pressures, and heart rates can be monitored with this system.
10. Press *Start* button to begin timed blood pressure reading.
11. Alternate extremities if device is used for a polonged period of time.

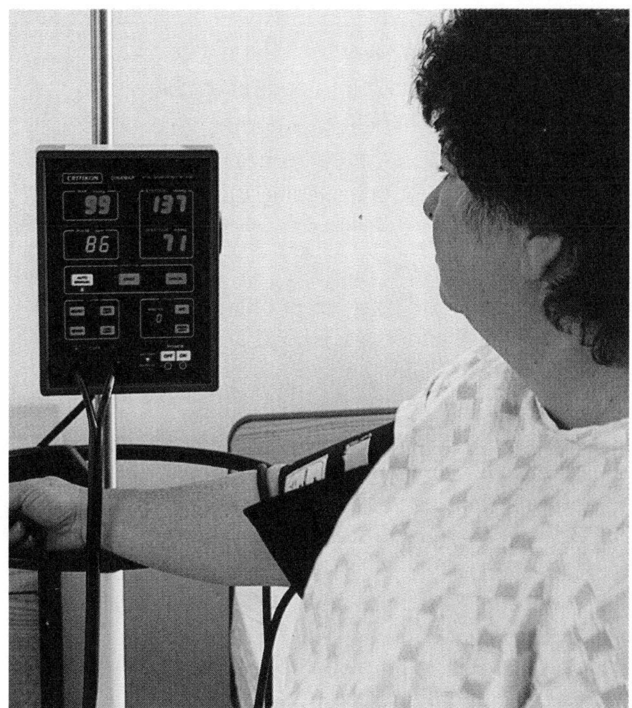

Continuous monitoring of blood pressure is done by attaching cuff to display monitor.

CHARTING for Blood Pressure

- Two phases of Korotkoff's sounds (e.g., 120/80) and site
- Response to alternative nursing actions
- Response to position changes

CRITICAL THINKING APPLICATION

CLINICAL PROBLEMS	CRITICAL THINKING OPTIONS
■ Blood pressure reading is abnormally high without apparent physiologic cause.	• Check if cuff was too narrow. • Check if cuff was not snug. • Check if cuff was deflated too slowly or reinflated during deflation causing venous engorgement and abnormally high diastolic readings. • Observe if mercury column, if used, was above eye level. • Ask if client was anxious or had just exercised or eaten. • Check blood pressure on both arms. The normal difference from arm to arm is usually no more than 5 mm Hg.
■ Blood pressure reading is very low in absence of significant clinical findings.	• Assess if cuff is too wide. • Check if mercury column was below eye level. • Check if client's arm was above heart level. • Check if inflation was too slow. This reduces intensity of Korotkoff's sounds. • Assess if Korotkoff's sounds were barely audible. Raise client's arm, and then recheck. Sounds should be louder. • Identify if stethoscope was misplaced and was not on brachial artery. • Take blood pressure 3 minutes after client rises from supine to standing if postural hypotension is suspected.
■ Hypotension (systolic pressure is less than 90 mm Hg) develops.	• Take vital signs more frequently (every 15 minutes to 2 hours) until condition has stabilized. • Place client in supine position with lower extremities elevated 45° and head on pillow. • Assess cause of hypotension, and notify physician. • Increase or administer fluids as ordered by physician. • Observe postoperative clients for signs of bleeding. • Administer oxygen.
■ Blood pressure cannot be measured on upper extremity due to casts, or other causes of inaccessibility.	• Use lower extremity to obtain blood pressures. Systolic pressure in thigh is usually 10–40 mm Hg higher than in arms, but diastolic pressure is equivalent to arm readings.
■ Korotkoff's sounds cannot be heard due to hypotension.	• Use the palpation method or ultrasound technique. Client may be candidate for intraarterial (direct method) pressure monitoring.
■ Hypertension (blood pressure consistently over 140/90 mm Hg) develops.	• For clients with severe, acute hypertension, take vital signs more frequently (every 15 minutes to 2 hours) until condition has stabilized.

CLINICAL PROBLEMS	CRITICAL THINKING OPTIONS
	• If client is anxious or excited, institute relaxation techniques to lower blood pressure. • Allow client to rest after strenuous exercise. • Relieve pain with reassurance, change of position, and analgesia as ordered by physician. • For clients with essential hypertension, administer antihypertensive and diuretic drugs as ordered by the physician. Evaluate response by checking blood pressure in reclining, sitting, and standing position. Instruct client in diet therapy, such as low salt, low fat, and inclusion of vitamins and garlic. • For client with hypoxia, relieve with oxygen administration by most effective mode.
■ Continuous BP monitoring system displays 00 instead of blood pressure reading. (00 indicates the unit is unable to determine parameters.)	• Check cuff placement and size to determine if appropriately placed.

GERIATRIC CONSIDERATIONS

Cardiac status—changes

- Changes in cardiovascular status with aging are often insidious and may become apparent when system is stressed and there is increased demand for cardiac output (which may occur with illness and hospitalization). Nursing care assessment should focus on client's cardiovascular status, even when diagnosis does not include a cardiac condition.
- Blood pressure measurement should take age into account. If client has severe arthrosclerosis, pseudohypertension may be present. If this is suspected, raise the cuff pressure above the systolic blood pressure and, if the radial pulse remains palpable, the reading may show 10 to 15 mm Hg in error.
- Postural hypotension is common in the elderly; nurses should take note when helping a client out of bed. Hypertension is also common in this age group.

Respiratory status—changes

- Changes in the respiratory system may be subtle and gradual with the elderly: oxygen saturation is decreased to 93–94%; there is often poor cough response and incomplete lung expansion—all of which leads to increased risk of pulmonary infection when the elderly client is hospitalized.

Temperature—changes

- With the elderly, temperature may be as low as 95°F. Because they may be easily dehydrated with increased temperature, nursing assessment should include baseline temperature at admission and continued monitoring during hospitalization.

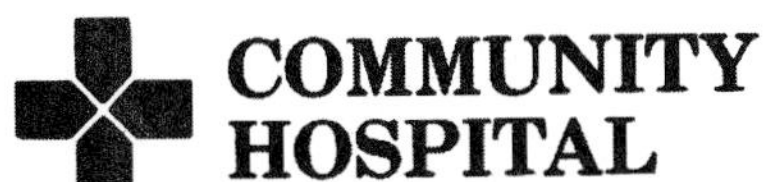

CLINICAL RECORD

KEY	PULSE	TEMP C	TEMP F																		
DATE																					
HOSP DAY/POSTOP DAY																					
TIME				0200	0600	1000	1400	1800	2200	0200	0600	1000	1400	1800	2200	0200	0600	1000	1400	1800	2200
BLACK – PULSE & RESPIRATIONS RED – TEMPERATURE	140	40.6	105																		
	130	40.0	104																		
	120	39.4	103																		
	110	38.8	102																		
	100	38.3	101																		
	80	37.7	100																		
	80	37.2	99																		
	70	36.6	98																		
	60	36.1	97																		
	50	35.5	96																		
	RESPIRATIONS																				
	BLOOD PRESSURE																				

HEIGHT	WEIGHT			WEIGHT			WEIGHT		
	BREAKFAST	LUNCH	DINNER	BREAKFAST	LUNCH	DINNER	BREAKFAST	LUNCH	DINNER
DIET – TYPE									
% CONSUMED									
INTAKE & OUTPUT INTAKE HOURS	0600-1400	1400-2200	2200-0600	0600-1400	1400-2200	2200-0600	0600-1400	1400-2200	2200-0600
Oral									
IV									
Blood - Plasma									
Other									
8 Hr. Total									
Output									
Urine									
Emesis									
Stools									
GI Suction									
8 Hr. Total									
24 Hr. Intake									
24 Hr. Output									
SIGNATURE									

DATE:

CLINICAL RECORD

12

Body Mechanics and Positioning

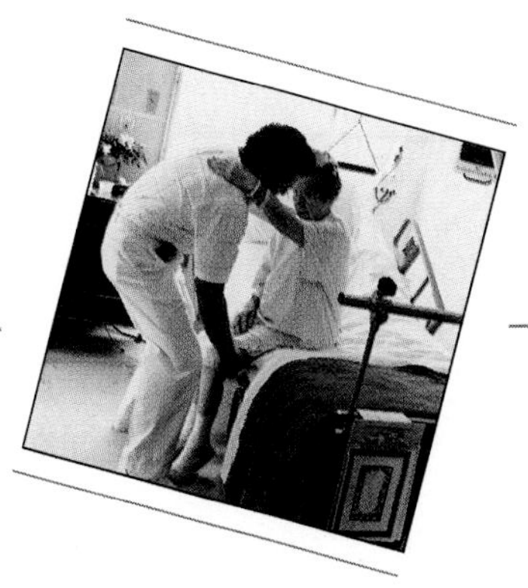

LEARNING OBJECTIVES

- Discuss the primary function of the skeletal muscles, joints, and bones.
- Describe nursing measures that assist in preserving joints, bones, and skeletal muscles.
- Describe a minimum of two principles of correct body mechanics.
- State two expected outcomes of using proper body mechanics.
- Discuss the objectives for moving and turning clients.
- Compare and contrast the methods used in moving clients up in bed for a single nurse and when assistants are available.
- Demonstrate passive range-of-motion exercises using all muscle groups.
- Explain the rationale of assisted ambulation for clients.
- Demonstrate the procedures for moving a client to the side of the bed and dangling a client.
- Outline the steps in logrolling a client.
- Demonstrate a three-man lift.
- List the pertinent data that should be charted when moving a client from the bed.
- Write a client care plan using at least three nursing diagnoses for a client requiring moving and turning interventions.

TERMINOLOGY

Alignment: referring to posture, the relationship of body parts to one another.

Ambulate: walking; able to walk.

Amphiarthrotic joint: a joint that has limited movement.

Appendicular skeleton: composed of 126 bones, which include the shoulder, girdle, arm bones, pelvic girdle, and leg bones.

Axial skeleton: includes the head and trunk, which form the central axis to which the appendicular skeleton is attached.

Base of support: surface area on which an object rests (e.g., for a client lying in prone position, the base of support is the entire undersurface of the body).

Body mechanics: movement of the body in a coordinated and efficient way so that proper balance, alignment, and conservation of energy is maintained.

Brachial plexus: network of spinal nerves supplying arm, forearm, and hand.

Cartilage: bone-like tissue of the very young that is replaced by bone tissue through the process of ossification. In adults cartilage is found in such areas as the nose, ears, and knees.

Center of gravity: midpoint or center of the body weight. In an adult it is the midpelvic cavity between the symphysis pubis and umbilicus.

Compact bone layer: dense, hard layer of bone tissue.

Dangle: to have a client sit on the edge of the bed with feet in a dependent position.

Diarthrotic joint: type of joint that allows for free movement; a cavity enclosed by a capsule lined with synovial membrane that secretes a lubricant.

Dorsiflexion: flexion of the foot at the ankle joint; the act of turning the foot and toes upward, as in standing on the heel.

Flexion: the act or condition of being bent.

Footdrop: a falling or dragging of the foot from paralysis of the flexors of the ankle.

Fowler's position: head of bed is at a 45° angle; client's knees may or may not be flexed.

Gravity: the force that pulls objects toward the earth's surface.

High-Fowler's position: head of bed is at a 90° angle; often used to achieve maximum chest expansion.

Hoyer lift: a mechanical device that enables one person to safety transfer a client from bed to chair.

Joint: the portion of the body where two or more bones join together.

Leverage: the use of a lever to apply force.

Ligament: a band or sheet of strong fibrous connective tissue connecting the articular ends of bones serving to bind them together and to facilitate or limit motion.

Line of gravity: an imaginary line that goes from the center of gravity to the base of support.

Marrow: soft tissue that is contained in the compact bone hollow.

Mobility: state or quality of being mobile; facility of movement.

Musculo: pertaining to muscles.

Musculoskeletal: pertaining to the muscles and bones.

Paralysis: temporary or permanent loss of function, especially loss of sensation or voluntary motion.

Periosteum: the thin, tough membrane of fibrous tissue that forms the outer or exterior layer of bone.

Posture: attitude or position of body.

Prone: lying horizontal with face downward.

Reverse Trendelenburg's position: mattress remains unbent, but head of bed is raised and foot is lowered.

Semi-Fowler's position: head of bed is at a 30° angle; often used for clients with cardiac and respiratory problems.

Skeletal system: system of separate bones (206) bound together by ligaments and responsible for supporting, moving, and giving shape to the body.

Sprain: injury caused by wrenching or twisting of a joint that results in tearing or stretching of the associated ligaments.

Stable: when the center of gravity is close to the base of support.

Strain: injury caused by excessive force or stretching of muscles or tendons around the joint.

Synarthrotic joint: type of joint that is immovable (e.g., suture lines of the skull).

Trendelenburg's position: mattress remains unbent but the head of the bed is lowered and the foot is raised. "Shock blocks" may be used under the legs of the bed to achieve this position.

Trochanter: either of the two bony prominences below the neck of the femur.

MUSCULOSKELETAL SYSTEM

The musculoskeletal system protects the body, provides a structural framework, and allows the body to move. The primary structures in this system are muscles, bones, and joints.

Skeletal Muscles

Skeletal muscles move the bones around the joints by contracting and relaxing so that movement can take place. Each muscle consists of a body, or belly, and tendons, which connect the muscle to another muscle or to bone.

When skeletal muscles contract, they cause two bones to move around the joint between them. One of these bones tends to remain stationary while the other bone moves. The end of the muscle that attaches to the stationary bone is called the origin. The end of the muscle that attaches to the movable bone is called the insertion.

Muscles are designated flexors or extensors according to whether they flex the joint (decrease the angle between the bones) or extend the joint (increase the angle between the bones). For example, when the deltoid muscle contracts, it abducts the arm and raises it laterally to the horizontal position. The anterior fibers aid in flexion of the arm, and the posterior fibers aid in extension of the arm.

Joints

Joints are the places where bones meet. Their primary function is to provide motion and flexibility. Although the internal structure of joints varies, most joints are composed of ligaments, which bind the bones together, and cartilage, or tissue, which covers and cushions the ends of the bones.

Bones

Bones provide the major support for all the body organs. Bone is composed of an organic matrix, deposits of calcium salts, and bone cells. The organic matrix provides the framework and tensile strength for the bone. The calcium salts, which are about 75% of the bone, provide compressional strength by filling in the matrix. As a result, it is very difficult to damage a bone by twisting it or by applying direct pressure.

Bone cells include osteoblasts, osteocytes, and osteoclasts. Osteoblasts deposit the organic matrix; osteocytes and osteoclasts reabsorb this matrix. Because this process is usually in equilibrium, bone is deposited where it is needed in the skeletal system. If increased stress is placed on a bone, such as the stress of continued athletic activity, more bone is deposited. If there is no stress on a bone, as is often the case with clients on prolonged bed rest, part of the bone mass is reabsorbed, or lost.

SYSTEM ALTERATIONS

Alterations in mobility can result from problems in the musculoskeletal system, the nervous system, and the skin. A primary cause for alterations in muscles is inactivity. With forceful activity muscles increase in size. With inactivity muscles decrease in size and strength. When clients are in casts or in traction, on prolonged bed rest, or unable to exercise, their muscles become weak and atrophied.

Alterations in joints result when mobility is limited by changes in the adjacent tissues. When muscle movement decreases, the connective tissue in the joints, tendons, and ligaments becomes thickened and fibrotic.

Chronic flexion and hyperextension can also cause alterations in the joints. Chronic flexion can cause joints to become contracted in one position so that they are unmovable. Hyperextension occurs when joints are extended beyond their normal limits, which is usually 180°. The results of hyperextension are pain and discomfort to the client and abnormal stress on the ligaments and tendons of the joints.

Alterations in bone are caused by disease processes, decalcification and breaks caused by trauma, or twisting. Encouraging clients to stand and to walk is important because the body functions best when it is in a vertical position. When a person is horizontal, the abdominal organs press on the diaphragm and inhibit its movement, thus decreasing respiratory efficiency. Physical activity forces muscles to move and increases blood flow, which improves metabolism and facilitates such body functions as gastrointestinal peristalsis.

Nursing Measures

Nursing care measures to preserve the joints, bones, and skeletal muscles should be carried out for all clients who require bed rest. Positions in which clients are placed, methods of moving, and turning should all be based on the principles of maintaining the musculoskeletal system in proper alignment. The nurse must also use good body mechanics when moving and turning clients to preserve her or his own musculoskeletal system from injury.

BODY MECHANICS

Knowledge of a client's body and how it moves is important. Knowledge of your own body and what happens to it when you care for clients with altered mobility is also important. Before you lift or move a client, determine the causes and consequences of the client's illness. This knowledge enables you to move the client without causing additional discomfort. Before you begin, thoroughly explain the procedures you will be completing so that you obtain the client's cooperation.

Trying to lift or move too much weight forces you to use your body incorrectly and frequently causes injuries. Incorrect lifting puts most of the pressure on the muscles of your lower back. Because these muscles are not strong enough to handle the stress, you can sustain severe injuries. If you do not follow guidelines for promoting proper body mechanics, you are putting yourself in jeopardy.

Proper use of body mechanics prevents injuries to clients and all members of the health team. Guidelines that underly the implementation of body mechanics appear below.

- Assume a proper stance before moving or turning clients.
- Distribute workload evenly before moving or turning clients.
- Establish a comfortable height when working with clients.
- Push and pull objects when moving them to conserve energy.
- Use large muscles for lifting and moving, not the back muscles.
- Avoid leaning and stretching.
- Request assistance from others when working with heavy clients to avoid strain.
- Avoid twisting your body.

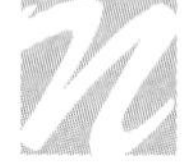

NURSING DIAGNOSES

The following nursing diagnoses are appropriate to use on client care plans when the components are related to body mechanics.

NURSING DIAGNOSIS	RELATED FACTORS/RISK FACTORS
Activity Intolerance	Impaired motor function, pain
Risk for Disuse Syndrome	Debilitated state, immobility, muscle weakness, decreased motor agility
Risk for Injury	Altered mobility, impaired sensory function, prolonged bed rest
Impaired Physical Mobility	Trauma or musculoskeletal impairment, surgical procedure, muscle weakness, pain, decreased strength

unit 1

PROPER BODY MECHANICS

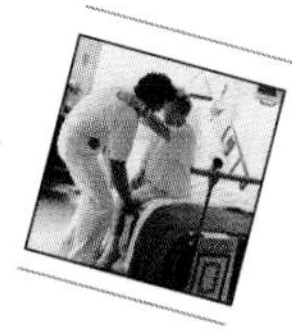

NURSING PROCESS DATA

ASSESSMENT Data Base

Evaluate personnel's knowledge of the principles of body mechanics.

Evaluate personnel's knowledge of how to use correct muscle groups for specific activities.

Assess knowledge and correct any misinformation about body alignment and how to maintain it with each position.

Assess knowledge of physical science and application to balance and body alignment.

Assess the competency of spinal cord and associated musculature.

Assess the muscle mass of the long, thick, and strong muscles of the shoulders and thighs.

PLANNING Objectives

To promote proper body mechanics while caring for clients

To maintain good posture, thereby promoting optimum musculoskeletal balance

To provide knowledge of the musculoskeletal system, body alignment, and balance in order to assist the nurse in caring for clients

To correct body mechanics, promote health, enhance appearance, and assist body function.

IMPLEMENTATION Procedures

Establishing Body Alignment

Maintaining Proper Body Alignment

Using Coordinated Movements

Using Basic Principles

EVALUATION Expected Outcomes

Correct body mechanics are used in caring for clients.

Injuries are prevented to both the nurse and the client.

Proper body mechanics facilitate client care.

Coordinated movements prevent client discomfort.

Center of gravity is maintained when lifting objects.

ESTABLISHING BODY ALIGNMENT

Procedure

1. Establish a firm base of support by placing both feet flat on the floor, with one foot slightly in front of the other.
2. Distribute weight evenly on both feet.
3. Slightly bend both knees.
4. Hold abdomen firm and tuck buttocks in so that spine is in alignment.
5. Hold head erect, and secure firm stance.

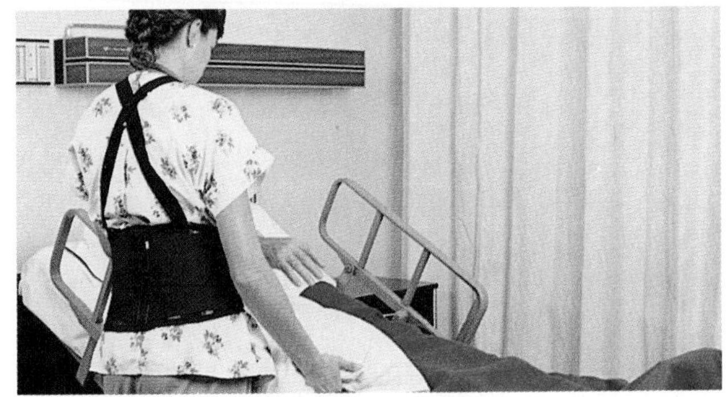

Wear a back brace to support back and keep body in alignment.

6. Use this stance as the basis for all actions in moving, turning, and lifting clients.
7. Wear a back brace to protect and support back and keep body in alignment.

MAINTAINING PROPER BODY ALIGNMENT

Procedure

1. Begin with the proper stance established in the previous intervention.
2. Evaluate working height necessary to achieve objective.
   a. Test parameters of possible heights (i.e., bed moves within an approximate range of 18 inches from floor).
   b. Establish a comfortable height in which to work; usual height is between waist and lower level of hip joint.
3. Test that this level minimizes muscle strain by extending your arms and checking that your body maintains proper alignment.
4. If you need to work at a lower level, flex your knees. **Rationale:** Bending over at the waist results in back strain.
5. Make accommodations for working at high surface levels. **Rationale:** Reaching up may result in injury to the back through hyperextension of muscles.
6. Work close to your body so that your center of gravity is not misaligned and your muscles are not hyperextended.
7. Use your longest and strongest muscles (biceps, quadriceps, and gluteal) when moving and turning clients.
8. Whenever possible, roll, push, and pull objects instead of lifting.

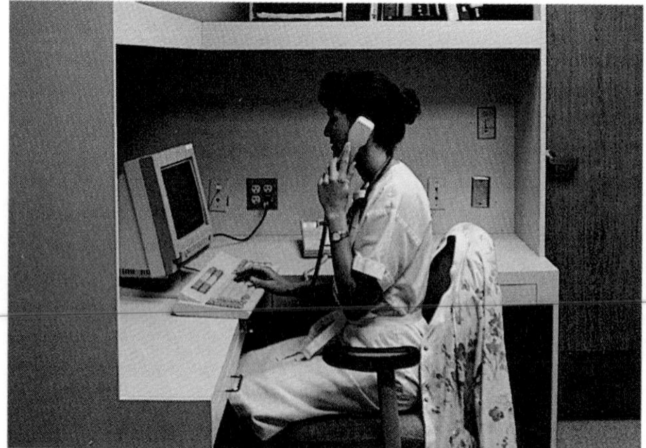

Correct: Work close to the body so that center of gravity is not misaligned.

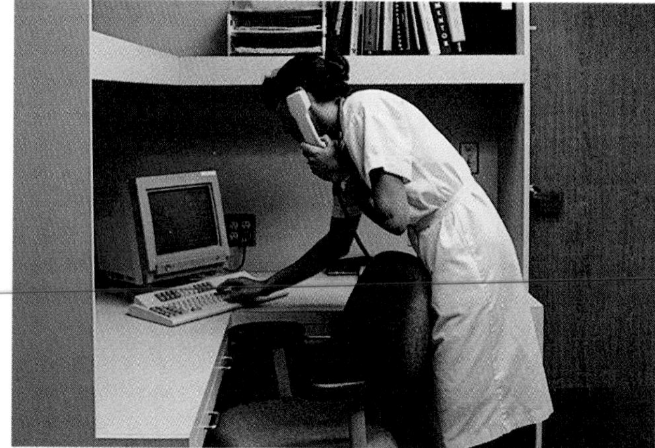

Incorrect: Bending over incorrectly could injure back muscles and cause undue strain.

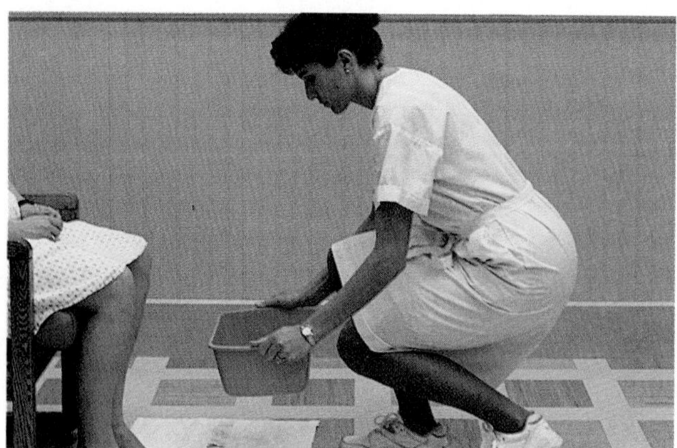

Correct: Keep body in proper alignment by bending knees and keeping back straight when lifting objects.

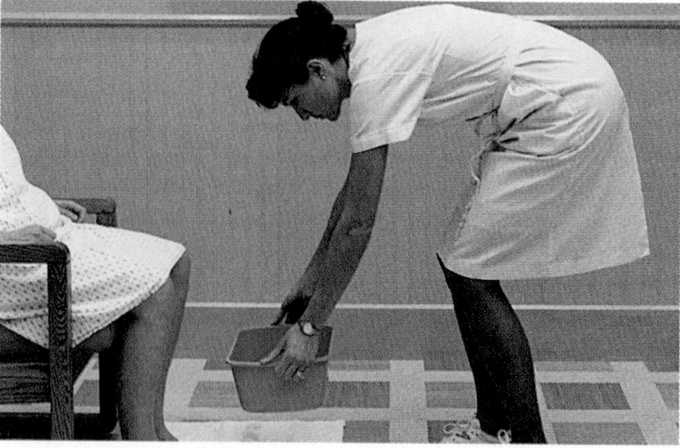

Incorrect: Prevent injury to back muscles; for proper alignment, bend at knees and use leg muscles.

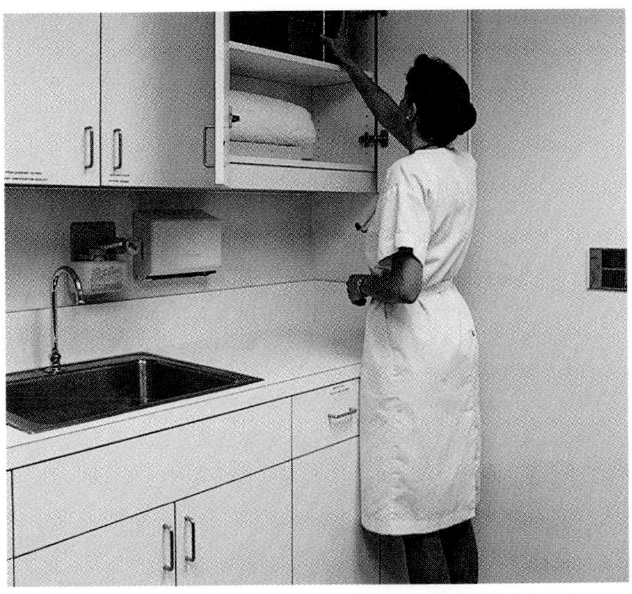
Correct: Keep body in correct alignment when turning and reaching for objects to prevent muscle strain or back injury.

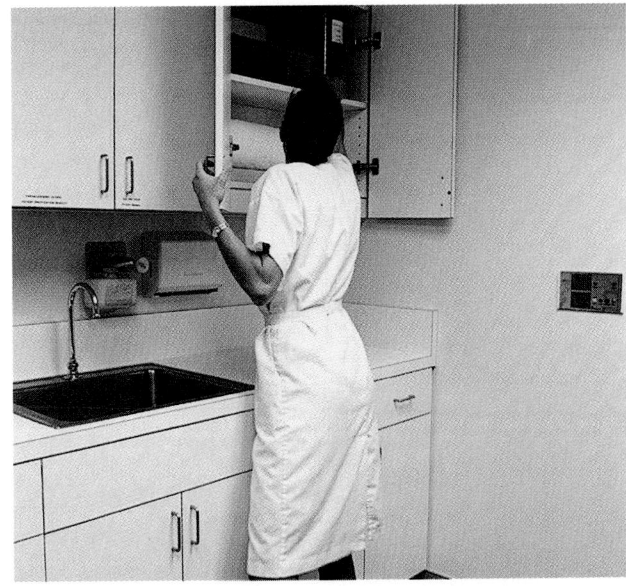
Incorrect: Do not use stretching or twisting movements when you reach for objects out of close proximity to your body.

USING COORDINATED MOVEMENTS

Procedure

1. Plan muscle movements to distribute workload before you actually begin turning, moving, or lifting clients.
   a. Establish a clear plan of action before you begin to move.
   b. Take a deep breath so oxygen is available for energy expenditure.
   c. Tense antagonistic muscles (abdomen) to those you will be using (diaphragm) in preparation for the movement.
   d. Release breath and mobilize major muscle groups (abdominal and gluteal) to do the work.
2. Move muscles in a smooth, coordinated manner.
   Rationale: This avoids putting strain on one muscle and is more efficient.
3. Do not make jerky, uncoordinated movements.
   Rationale: This may cause injury or frighten the client.
4. When you are working with another staff member, coordinate plans and movements before implementing them.

USING BASIC PRINCIPLES

Procedure

1. Move an object by pushing and pulling to expend minimal energy.
   a. Stand close to the object.
   b. Place yourself in proper body alignment stance.
   c. Tense muscles, and prepare for movement.
   d. Pull toward you by leaning away from the object and letting arms, hips, and thighs (*not back*) do the work.
   e. Push away from you by leaning toward object, using body weight to add force.
2. When changing direction, use pivotal movement-moving muscles as a unit and in alignment, rather than rotating or twisting upper part of body.
3. When working at lower surface levels, do not stoop by bending over. Flex body at knees and, keeping back straight, use thigh and gluteal muscles to accomplish task.
4. Use the muscles of arms and upper torso in an extended, coordinated movement parallel to body

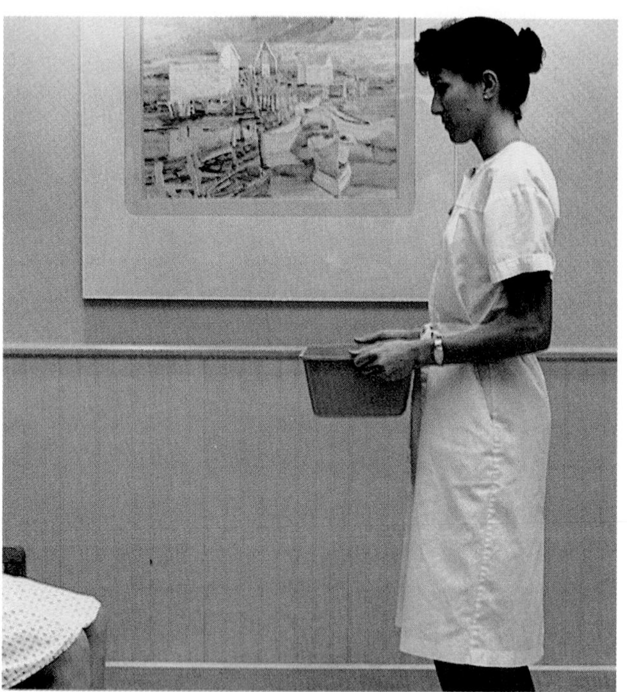

Correct: Hold objects close to the body to prevent muscle strain and possible back injury.

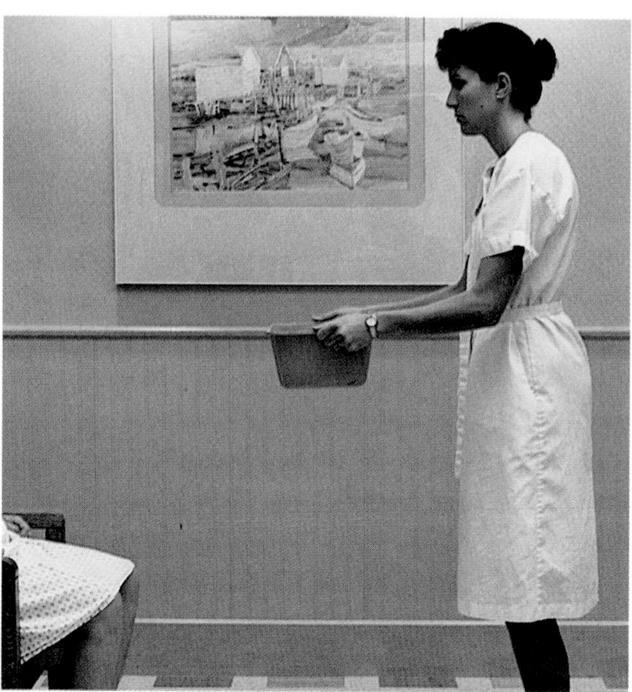

Incorrect: Holding objects away from the body may cause back strain or injury.

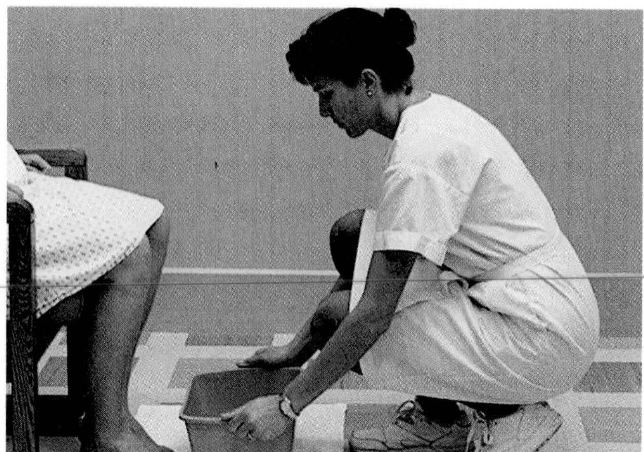

Correct: Move muscles as a unit and in alignment rather than twisting.

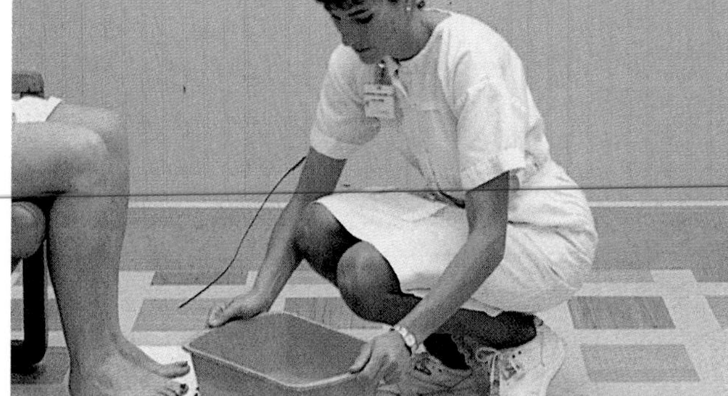

Incorrect: Do not twist or rotate upper body when working at lower surface levels.

stance when reaching to prevent twisting or hyperextension of muscles.

5. Lift or carry clients or objects with the maximum use of these body alignment principles:
   a. Determine that the movement is within your capability to perform without injury.
   b. Place yourself in proper body alignment stance.
   c. Stand close to and grasp the object or person near the center of gravity.
   d. Prepare muscles by taking a deep breath, and set muscles.
   e. Lift object with arms or by stooping and using leg and thigh muscles.
   f. Carry the object or person close to your body to prevent strain on your back.
   g. Take frequent rest periods to prevent additional strain.

CHARTING for Body Mechanics

- Injury to client resulting from poor body mechanics
- Devices needed for turning and moving
- Number of personnel required for turning and moving
- Ways in which client assists in moving
- Special requirements of client for proper body alignment
- Special turning and moving requirements

CRITICAL THINKING APPLICATION

CLINICAL PROBLEMS	CRITICAL THINKING OPTIONS
■ Incorrect body mechanics are used while giving client care.	• Identify areas of your body where you feel stress and strain. • Evaluate the way you use body mechanics. • Attend an in-service program on using body mechanics appropriately. • Concentrate on how you are using your body when moving and turning clients. • Position bed and equipment at a comfortable height and proximity to working area. • Use your longest and strongest muscles to prevent injury.
■ Nurse injures self while giving client care.	• Report any back strain immediately to supervisor. • Complete incident report. • Go to health service or emergency room for evaluation and immediate care. • Evaluate any activities that led to injury to determine incorrect use of body mechanics. • Prevent additional injury by obtaining assistance when needed. • Use devices such as turning sheets to assist in turning difficult clients.
■ Nurse uses poor body mechanics and injures client.	• Assess the extent of client's injury. • Notify client's physician. • Complete incident report. • Carry out physician's orders for follow-up treatment.
■ Due to staffing shortage, nurse is unable to obtain sufficient assistance with turning and moving clients.	• Place turning sheets on all clients who are difficult to move. • Use principles of leverage in moving clients. • Until adequate staff is available, turn and position client from side to side at least every 2 hours. • Use Hoyer lift.

unit 2

MOVING AND TURNING CLIENTS

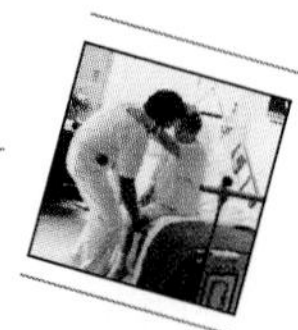

NURSING PROCESS DATA

ASSESSMENT Data Base

Observe the client and identify ways to improve the client's position and alignment.
Determine the client's physical ability to assist you with positioning.
Note the presence of tubes and incisions that alter the positioning and alignment procedures.

PLANNING Objectives

To provide increased comfort
To provide optimal lung excursion and ventilation
To prevent contractures due to constant joint flexion
To promote optimal joint movement
To help maintain intact skin
To prevent injury due to improper movement

IMPLEMENTATION Procedures

Turning to Side-Lying Position
Turning to a Prone Position
Moving the Client Up in Bed
Moving the Client with Assistance
Preparing to Move Client from Bed
Dangling at the Bedside
Moving from Bed to Chair
Using a Hoyer Lift
Logrolling the Client
Using a Footboard
Placing a Trochanter Roll

EVALUATION Expected Outcomes

Client's comfort is increased.
Skin remains intact without evidence of breaking down.
Breathing is adequate and unlabored.
Joint movement is maintained.
Foot drop is prevented.
Alignment is maintained.

TABLE 12–1. Bed Positions for Client Care

Positions	Placement	Use
High-Fowler's	Head of bed 60° angle	Thoracic surgery, severe respiratory conditions
Fowler's	Head of bed 45° angle; hips may or may not be flexed	Postoperative, gastrointestinal conditions, promotes lung expansion
Semi-Fowler's	Head of bed 30° angle	Cardiac, respiratory, neurosurgical conditions
Low-Fowler's	Head of bed 15° angle	Necessary degree elevation for ease of breathing, promotes skin integrity, client comfort
Knee-Gatch	Lower section of bed (under knees) slightly bent	For client comfort; contraindicated for vascular disorders
Trendelenburg's	Head of bed lowered and foot raised	Percussion, vibration, and drainage (PVD) procedure; promotes venous return
Reverse Trendelenburg's	Bed frame is tilted up with foot of bed down	Gastric conditions, prevents esophageal reflux

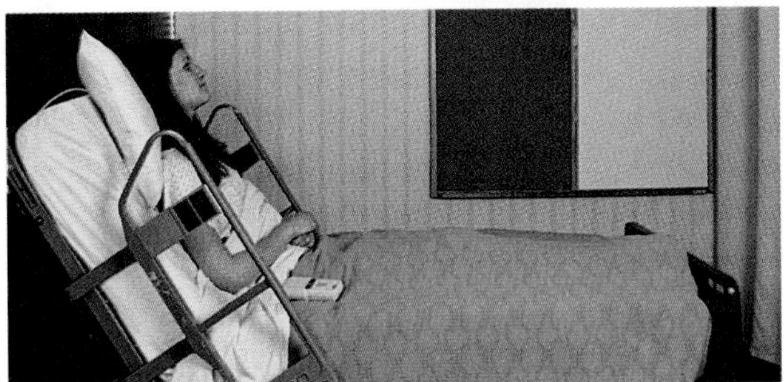

High-Fowler's position −60°.

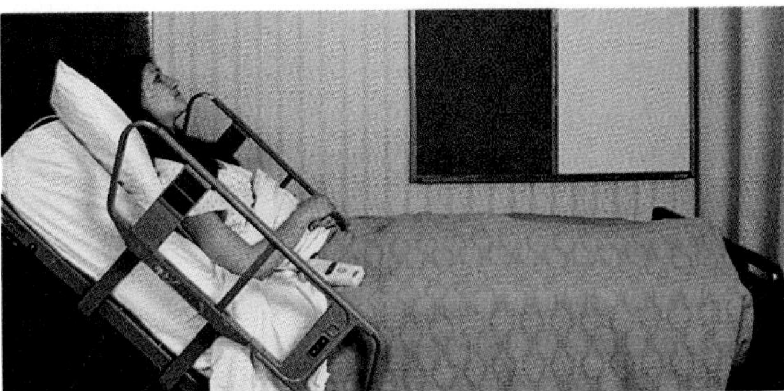

Fowler's position −45°.

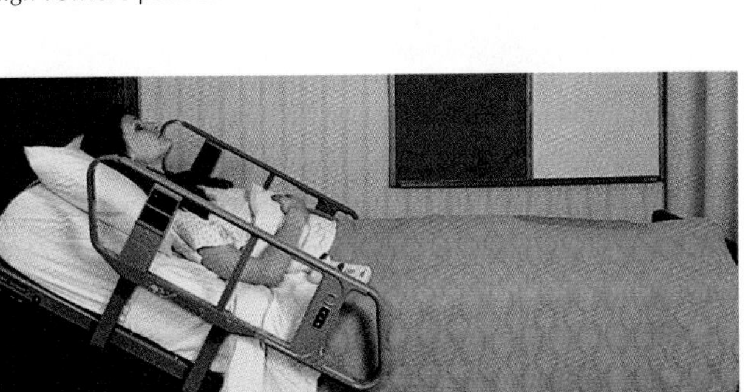

Semi-Fowler's position −30°.

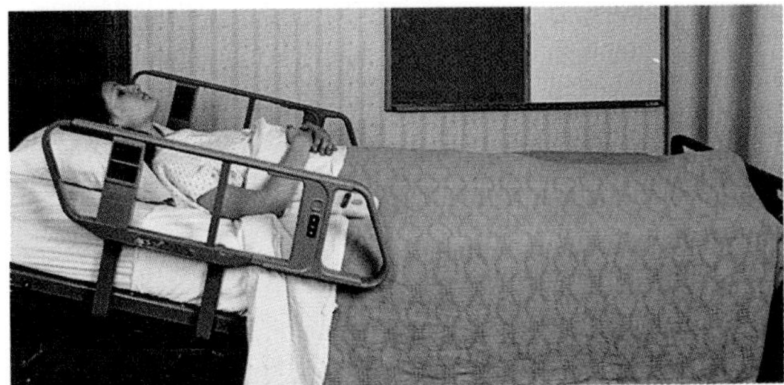

Low-Fowler's position −15°.

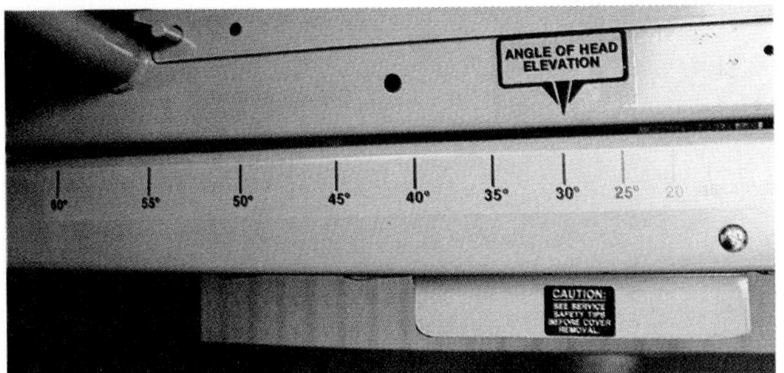

Angle gauge on bed.

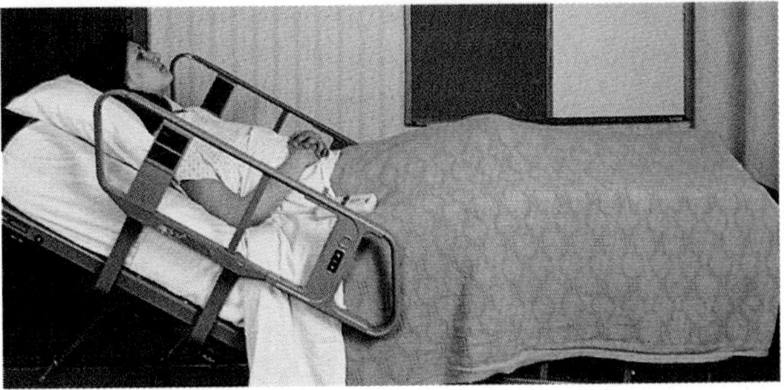

Elevated knee gatch.

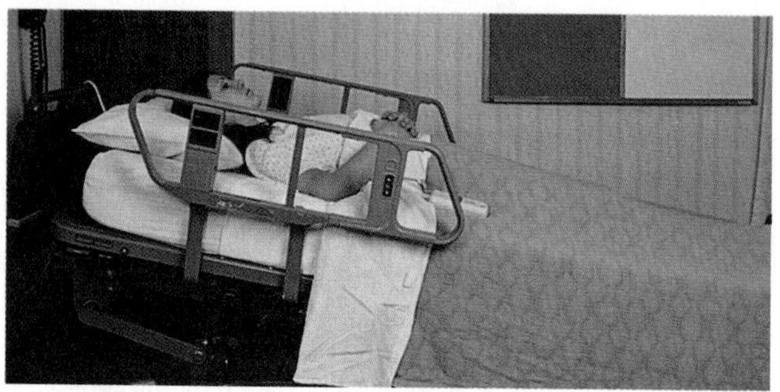
Reverse Trendelenburgs' position.

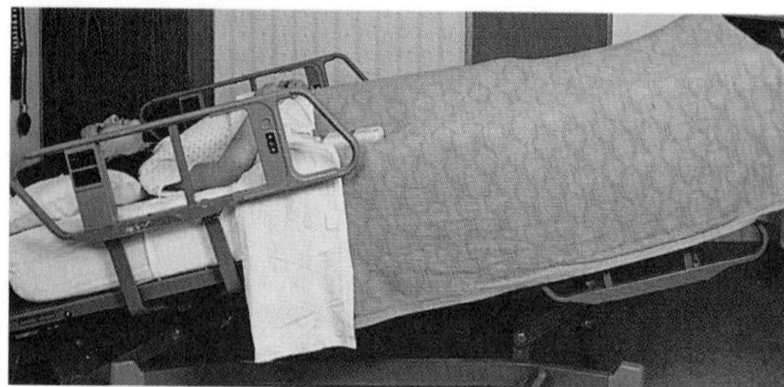
Trendelenburg's position.

TURNING TO SIDE-LYING POSITION

Equipment

Pillows for positioning
Turning sheet
Drawsheet for trochanter roll

Procedure

1. Identify the client.
2. Explain the rationale for the procedure to the client.
3. Lower the head of the bed completely or to a position that is as low as the client can tolerate.
4. Elevate the bed to a comfortable working height.
5. Move the client to your side of the bed. Put siderails up, and move to other side of bed.
6. Flex the client's knees.
7. Place one hand on client's hip and one hand on the client's shoulder; roll onto side.
8. Position pillow to maintain proper alignment.
9. Be sure to position the client's arms so that they are not under the body.

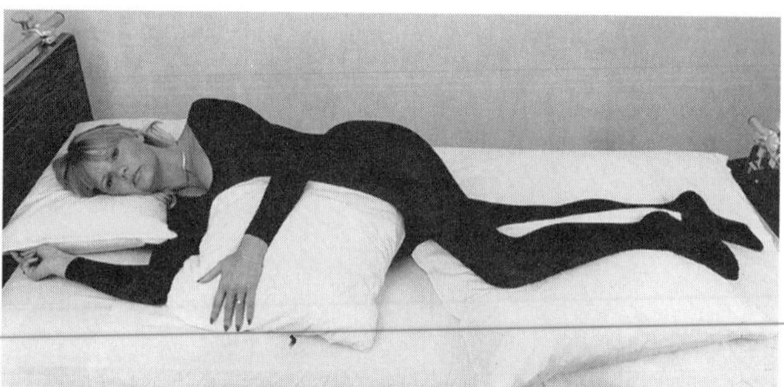
Lateral (side-lying) position.

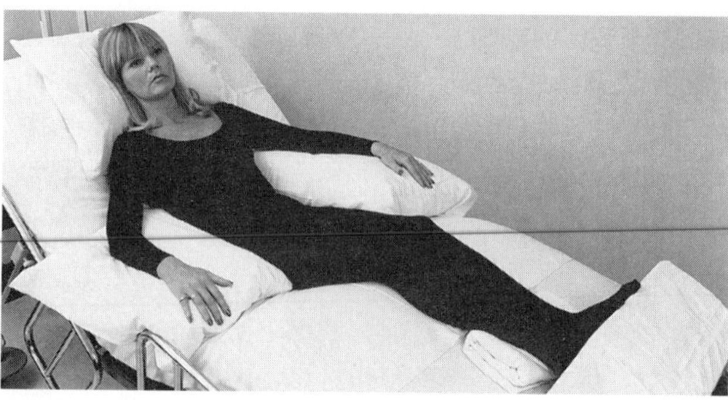
Semi-Fowler's position.

TURNING TO A PRONE POSITION

Equipment

Pillows for positioning
Turning sheet

Procedure

1. Identify the client.
2. Explain the rationale for the procedure to the client.
3. Lower the head of the bed completely or to a position that is as low as the client can tolerate.
4. Elevate the bed to a comfortable working height.
5. Move the client to the side of the bed away from the side where he or she will finally be positioned.
6. Position pillows on the side of the bed for the client's head, thorax, and feet.
7. Roll the client onto the pillows, making sure that the client's arms are not under his or her body.
8. Reposition pillows as necessary for client's comfort.

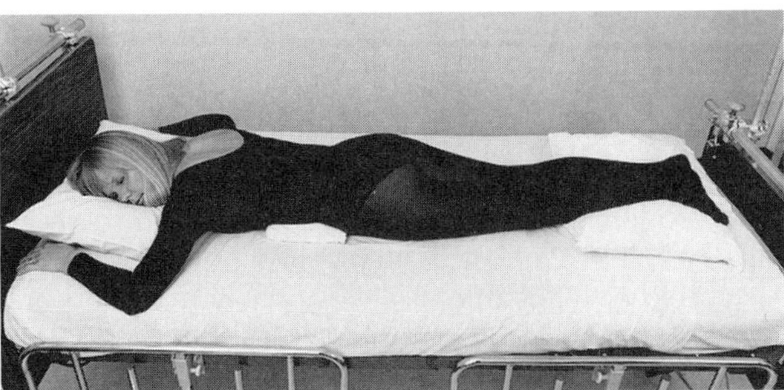

Prone position.

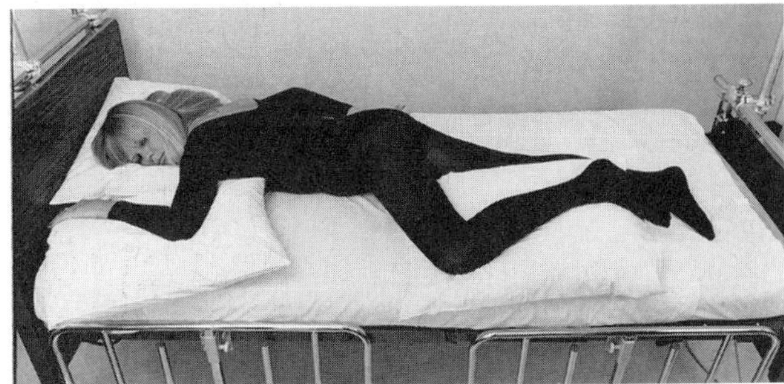

Semi-prone position.

MOVING THE CLIENT UP IN BED

Procedure

1. Identify the client.
2. Explain the rationale for the procedure to the client.
3. Lower the head of the bed so that it is flat or as low as the client can tolerate.
4. Raise the bed to a comfortable working height.
5. Remove the pillow and place it at the head of the bed to prevent striking the client's head against the bed.
6. Place one arm under the client's shoulders and the other arm under the client's thighs.
7. Instruct the client to put arms across chest.
8. Instruct the client to bend legs and to put feet flat on the bed.
9. Lift and pull the client as client pushes with feet. There are several other methods of moving a client up in bed—including using client's elbows, lifting under the back, and having client use the trapeze.
10. Position the client comfortably, replacing the pillow and arranging bedding as necessary.

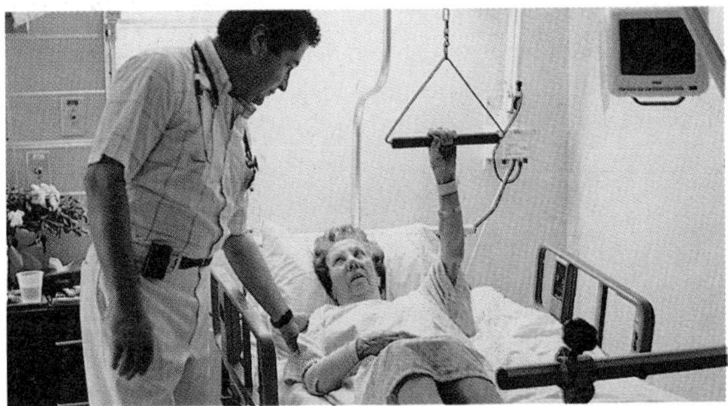

Encourage client to help when moving up in bed.

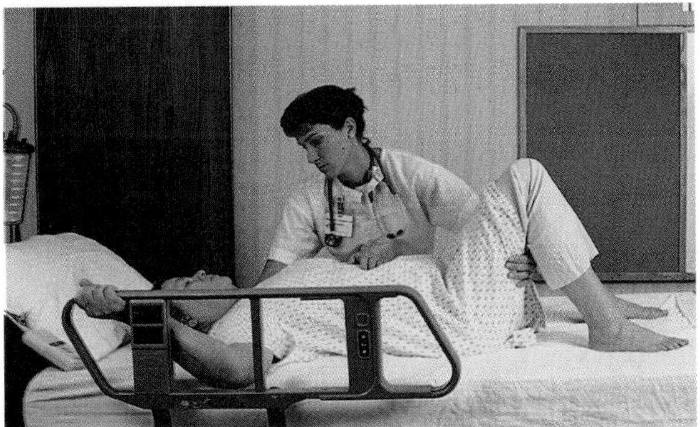

Assume proper body alignment when moving client up in bed.

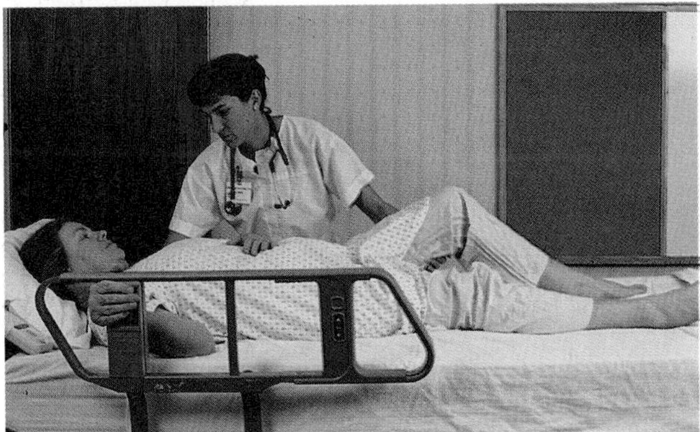

Use large leg muscles for leverage when moving client.

MOVING THE CLIENT WITH ASSISTANCE

Equipment

Drawsheet folded to use as lift sheet

Procedure

1. Identify the client.
2. Explain the rationale for the procedure to the client.
3. Lower the head of the bed so that it is flat or as low as the client can tolerate.
4. Raise the bed to a comfortable working height.
5. Remove the pillow, and place it at the head of the bed.
6. Positioning with two nurses or staff members.
   a. First position: Position one nurse on each side of the client. Each nurse should have one arm under the client's shoulders and one arm under the client's thighs.
   b. Alternate position: Position one nurse at the client's upper body. The nurse's arm nearest the head of the bed should be under the client's head and opposite shoulder. The other arm should be under the client's closest arm and shoulder. Position the other nurse at the client's lower torso. The nurse's arms should be under the client's lower back and thighs.
   c. Alternative position: Place folded drawsheet under client's body extending from shoulder line to just below buttocks. Position one nurse on each side of bed. Roll up sides of lift sheet as close as possible to sides of client. Assist client to flex knees, if possible. Each nurse firmly grasps sheet at level of client's upper back with one hand and at level of buttocks with other hand. Then with one firm, coordinated, rocking movement, lift client toward head of bed.
7. Positioning with three staff members.
   a. Position two nurses so that each one is supporting the client's shoulders as described above. Position the third nurse at the client's lower torso.
   b. Position three staff at the same side of the bed for a three-man lift.
8. Positioning with four staff members.
   a. Position two nurses, one on each side of the client, so that each one is supporting the client's shoulders.
   b. Position the other two nurses, one on each side of the client's hips or legs.
9. Coordinate the movements of all nurses. **Rationale:** One nurse is responsible for stating when to move client.
10. Place client in a comfortable position.

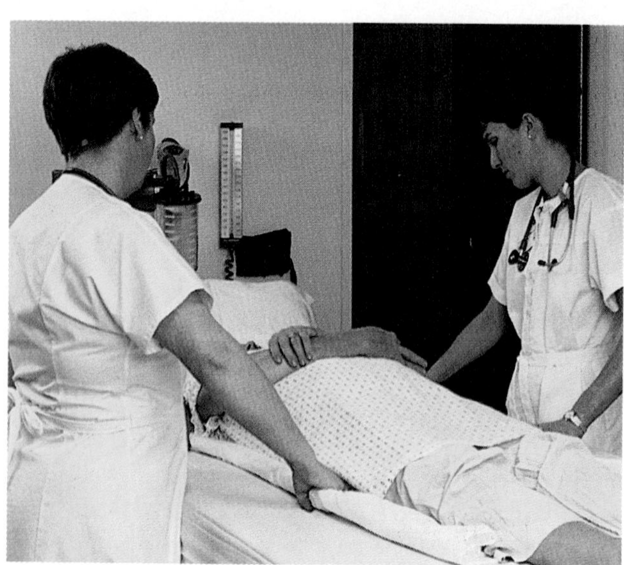

Hold drawsheet firmly and close to client for proper support.

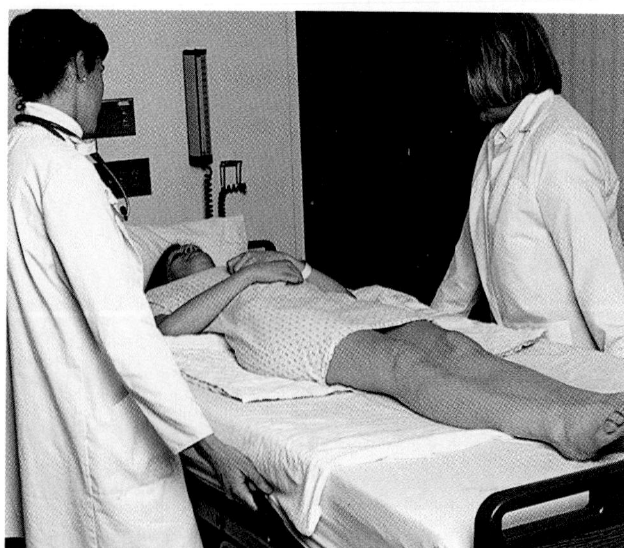

Shift weight from back to front leg when moving client up.

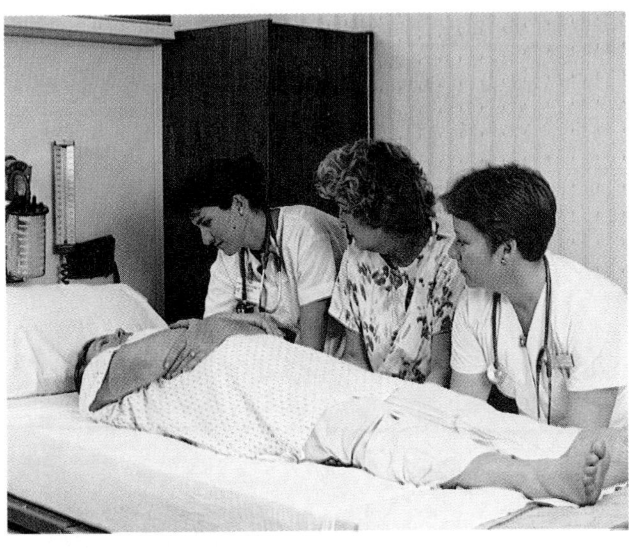
Position staff on same side of bed with three-man lift.

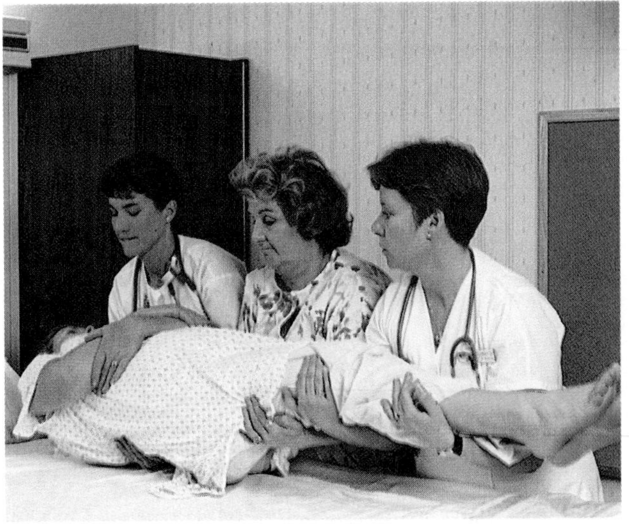
Move client to the side of the bed before lifting to a transfer.

PREPARING TO MOVE CLIENT FROM BED

Procedure

1. Elevate the bed to a comfortable working height.
2. Place the bed in a flat position. Lower the side rail on the side nearest you.
3. Position yourself at the head of the client's bed on the side toward which the client will move.
4. Place the client's arms across the chest.
5. Place one foot in front of the other. **Rationale:** This stance gives you a broad base of support.
6. Flex your knees.
7. Place your arm closest to the head of the bed under the client's head and shoulder farthest from you.
8. Place your other arm under the small of the client's back.
9. Rocking backward and shifting your weight from the front foot to the back foot, pull the upper part of the body toward you.
10. Move your arms to the client's middle section. Place one arm under the client's waist and the other arm under the thighs.
11. Repeat step 9.
12. Move to the foot of the client, and place one arm under the thighs and the other arm under the calves.
13. Repeat step 9.
14. Proceed as ordered: transfer client to gurney by using three-nurse lift, or assist client to dangle at bedside.

DANGLING AT THE BEDSIDE

Procedure

1. Identify the client.
2. Lower the bed to the lowest position.
3. Raise the head of the bed until the client is sitting upright.
4. Stand at the client's waist with one of your arms under the client's arm and around upper back. Put your other arm over the client's legs.
5. Bend the client's legs and grasp them at the knees.
6. In one motion, swing the legs over the side of the bed and pull the client's torso upright. Use thigh muscles for leverage when pulling.
7. Stabilize the client by pushing your knees against

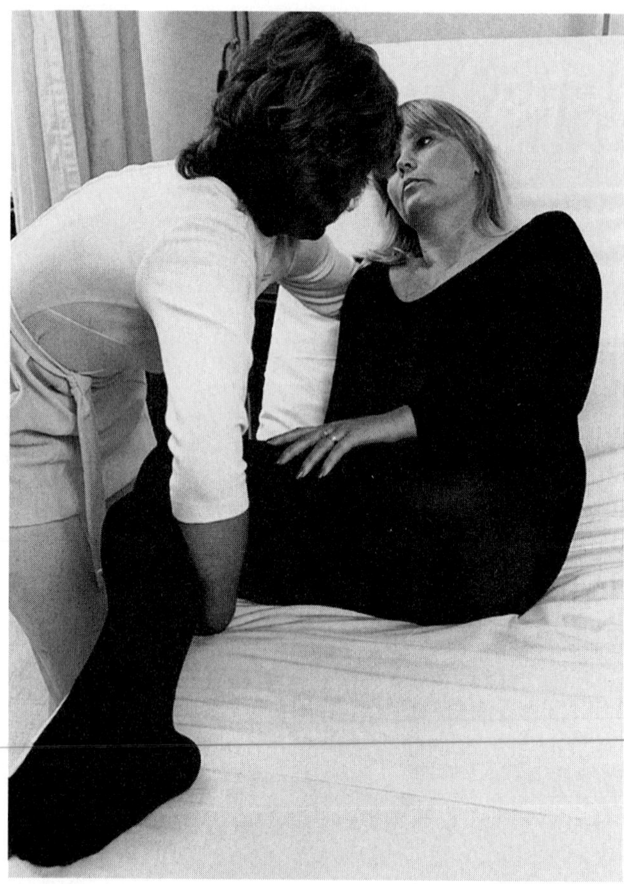

Place arm around shoulders and grasp knees with other arm.

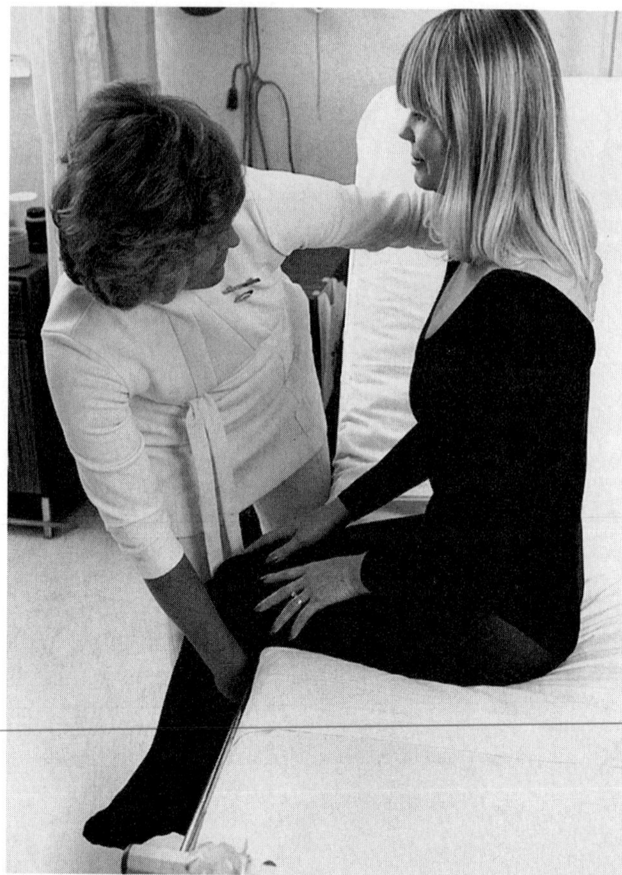

Swing client's legs over bedside to sitting position.

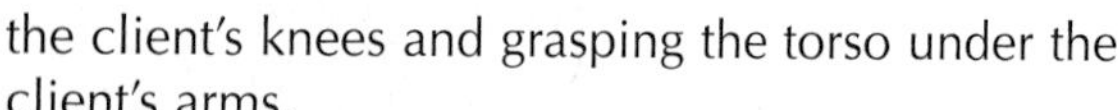

the client's knees and grasping the torso under the client's arms.

8. Assess the client for dizziness or lightheadedness.
9. Dangle client for a few minutes before transferring to a chair or ambulating.

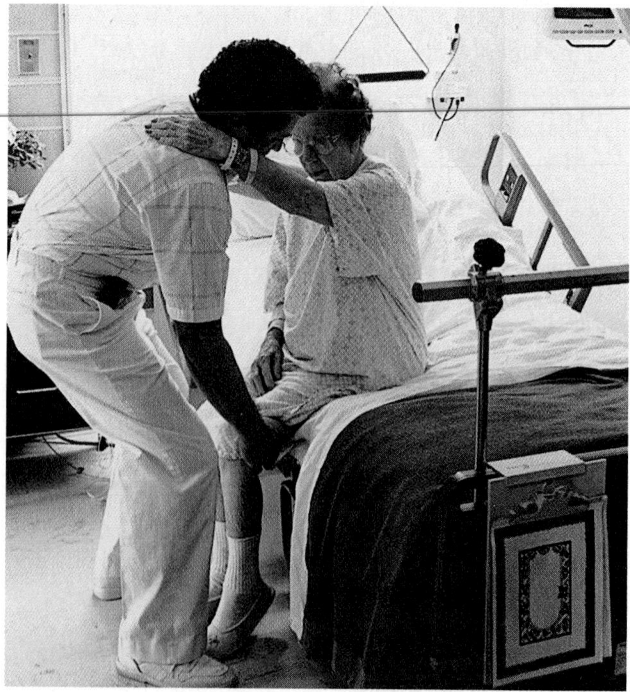

Stabilize clients by having them hold onto nurse.

MOVING FROM BED TO CHAIR

Equipment

Chair
Bath blanket

Procedure

1. Identify the client.
2. Lock the bed in place.
3. Place the chair at the head of the bed. Be sure to lock chair wheels or have someone hold the chair as you move the client.
4. Dangle the client until he or she is stable.
5. Give the client nonslip shoes or slippers.
6. Have the client reach across the chair and grasp the chair arm, if possible.
7. Place your hands under the client's axilla or around client's back.

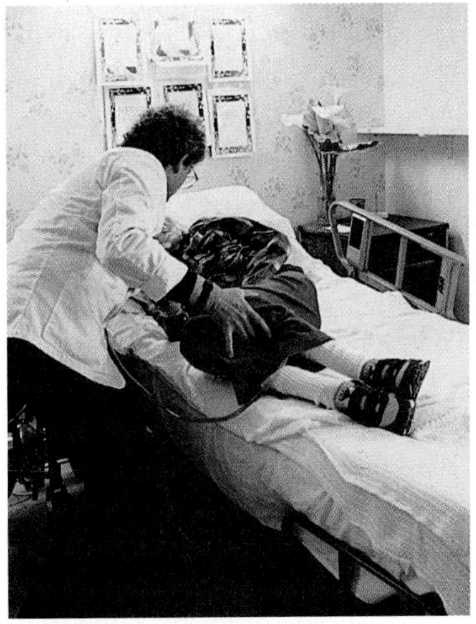

Move client to the side of bed before positioning.

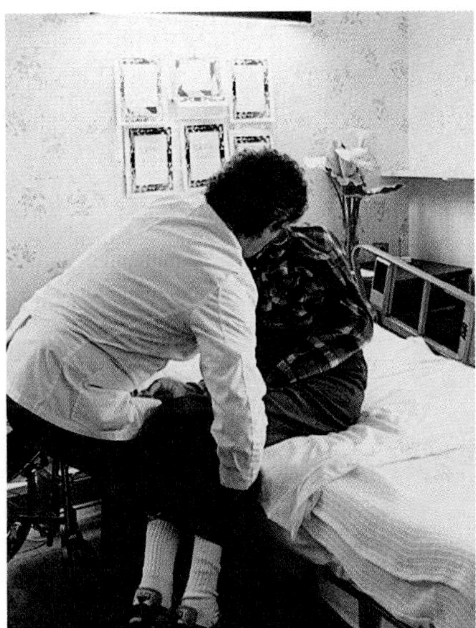

Pivot client and dangle feet before placing feet flat on floor.

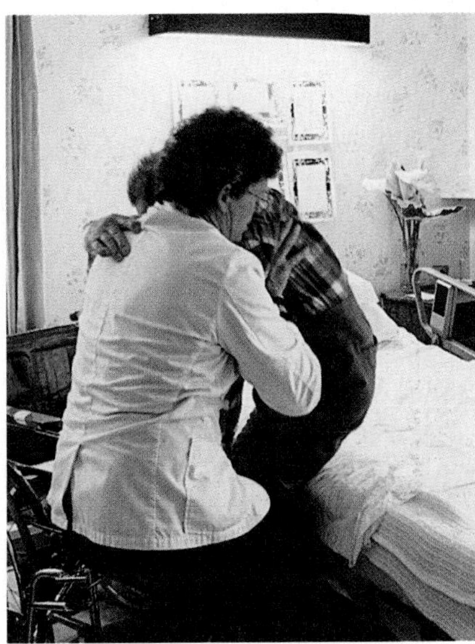

Have client reach arm across shoulder for balance.

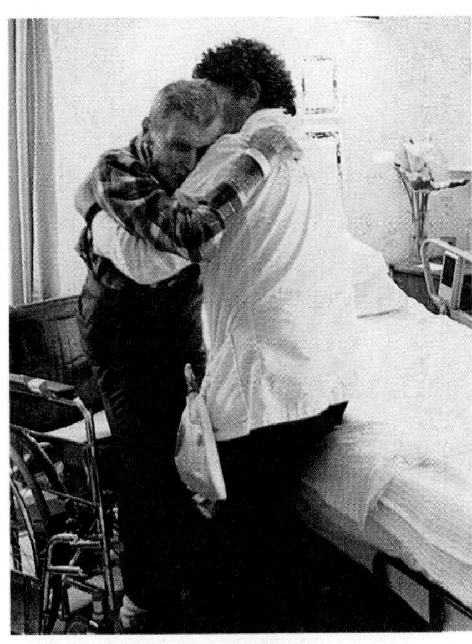

Stabilize client by positioning nurse's foot at the outside edge of client's foot.

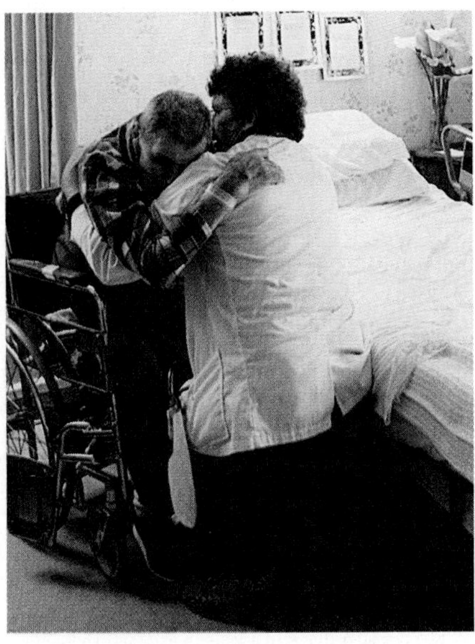

Pivot client into chair using leg muscles instead of back muscles.

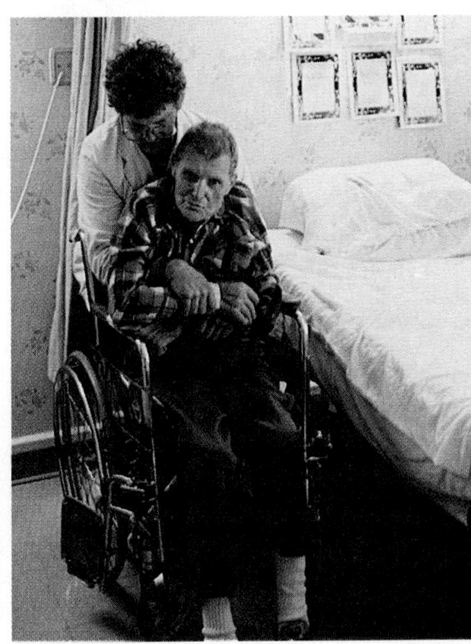

Pull client back and up in wheelchair for better posture.

8. Place your feet slightly to the side and in front of the client.
9. Rock the client and, on the count of three, pivot the client into the chair.
10. Position the client in the chair to prevent pressure areas. If the client has circulatory impairment, elevate legs while out of bed. **Rationale:** This promotes venous return.

USING A HOYER LIFT

Equipment

Hoyer lift base
2 canvas pieces: 1 large, 1 small
2 sets of canvas straps

Procedure

1. Check orders and client care plan. Determine that lift can safely move the weight of the client.
2. Explain the procedure to the client. **Rationale:** Clients may be frightened by the use of a mechanical device.
3. Wash your hands.
4. Bring Hoyer frame to bedside.
5. Provide privacy for client.
6. Lock wheels of bed.
7. Place client's chair by the bed. Allow adequate space to maneuver the lift.
8. Raise the bed to HIGH position and adjust head and knee gatch so that mattress is flat.
9. Keep side rail on opposite side in UP position.
10. Roll client away from you.
11. Place the lower edge of the wide canvas piece under the client's thighs.
12. Place the upper edge of the narrow canvas piece under the client's shoulders.
13. Raise side rail on your side of bed.
14. Move to opposite side of bed, and lower side rail.
15. Roll client away from you to opposite side, and straighten out canvas pieces. Turn client to supine position.
16. Place U base of the frame under the bed on side where chair is positioned.
17. Lock wheels of frame. Lower side rail.
18. Attach canvas straps from swivel bar to each canvas piece using the hooks.
19. Be sure straps are evenly placed on canvas pieces.
20. Elevate head of bed.

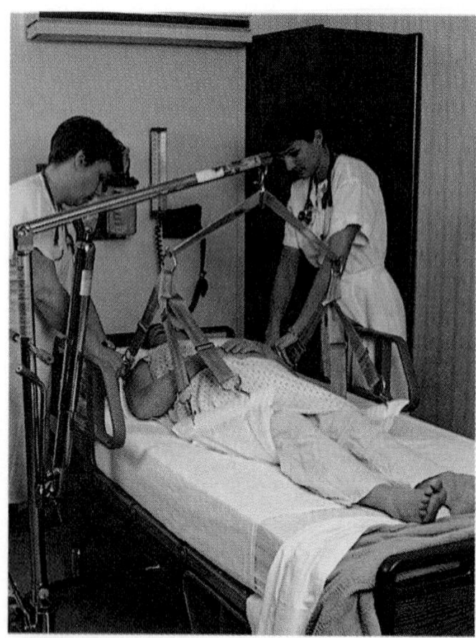
The Hoyer lift is a device used to move immobilized clients.

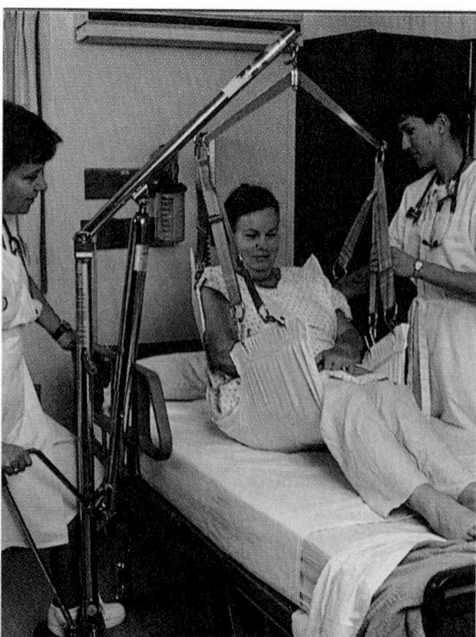
Place canvas pieces under client's thighs and shoulders.

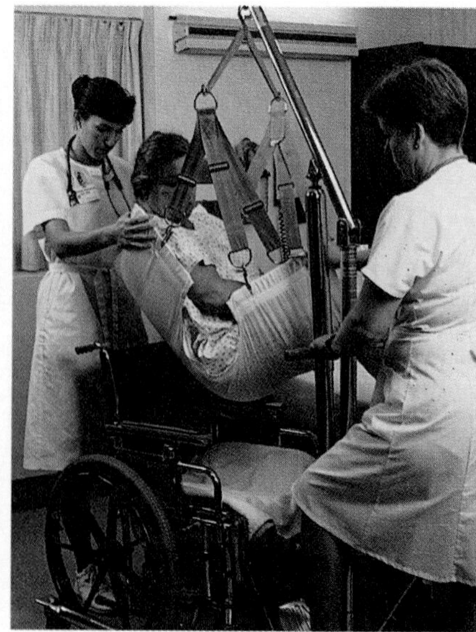
Use one nurse to stabilize client as second nurse guides client into chair.

21. Raise client by turning release knob clockwise to close pressure valve.
22. Pump the lift handle until client is lifted clear of the bed.
23. Maneuver the client over the chair.
24. Lower the client by turning release knob *slowly* counterclockwise.
25. Guide client into the chair.
26. Align client into chair.
27. Remove the straps from the bar, and move the lift out of the way.
28. Check for client's comfort in chair; place call bell close at hand.
29. Wash your hands.
30. Return client to bed using the same method.

LOGROLLING THE CLIENT

Equipment

Pillows, towels, blankets for positioning
Turning sheet

Procedure

1. Check order for logrolling client.
2. Check Kardex and client care plan as to exactly why the client needs to be logrolled.
3. Obtain sufficient assistance to complete the procedure with ease. Three nurses are preferable.
4. Before moving the client, place a pillow between the client's knees.
5. Position two nurses on side of the bed to which the client will be turned. Position third nurse on the other side of the bed.
6. Designate the person at the head of the bed to be in charge of coordinating move.
7. Assume the correct position for client move:
   a. Nurse at head: one arm supports client's head, second arm supports shoulders and neck.
   b. Second nurse: one hand grasps client's other shoulder, the other hand and arm around knee.
   c. Third nurse: on the opposite side of the bed, nurse holds drawsheet firmly to support torso in alignment.
8. Move the client in one coordinated movement when the nurse at the head of bed signals. **Rationale:** To maintain proper alignment, all of the body parts must be moved at the same time. If not, injury to the client's neck and spinal column may occur.

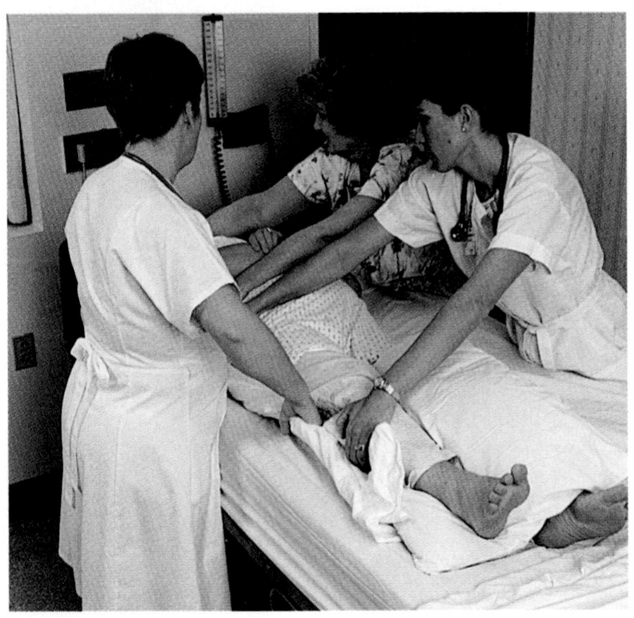

Position nurses on each side of client.

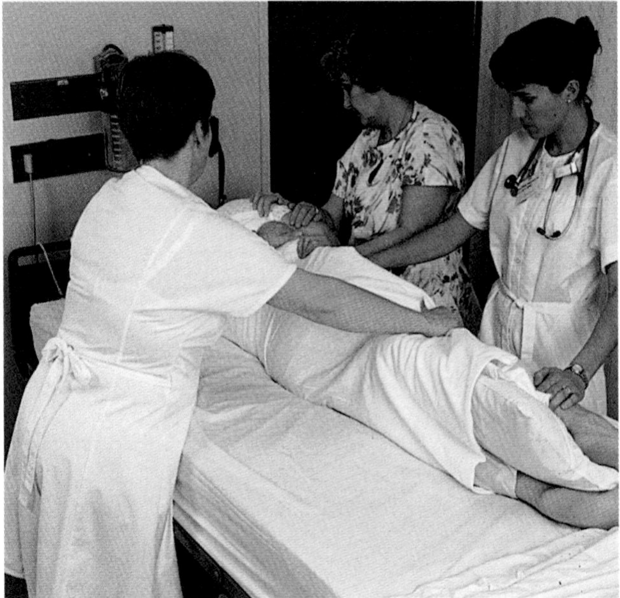

Maintain proper alignment while turning client.

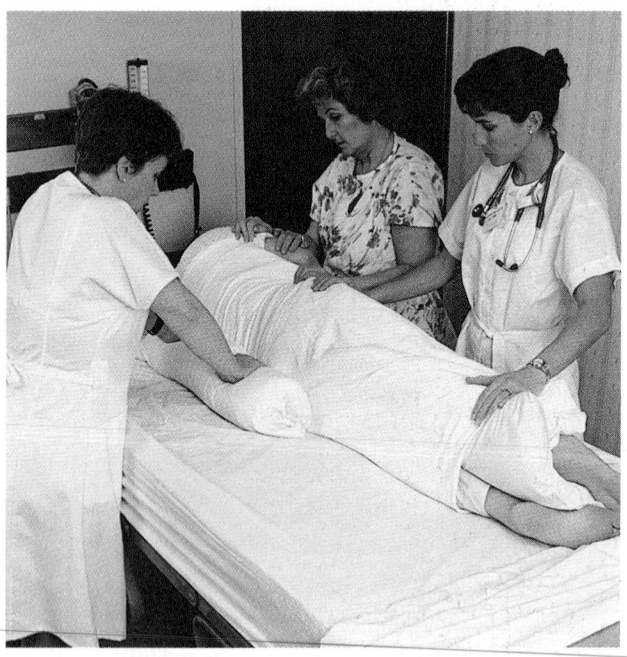

Maintain client's position with pillow support under client's back.

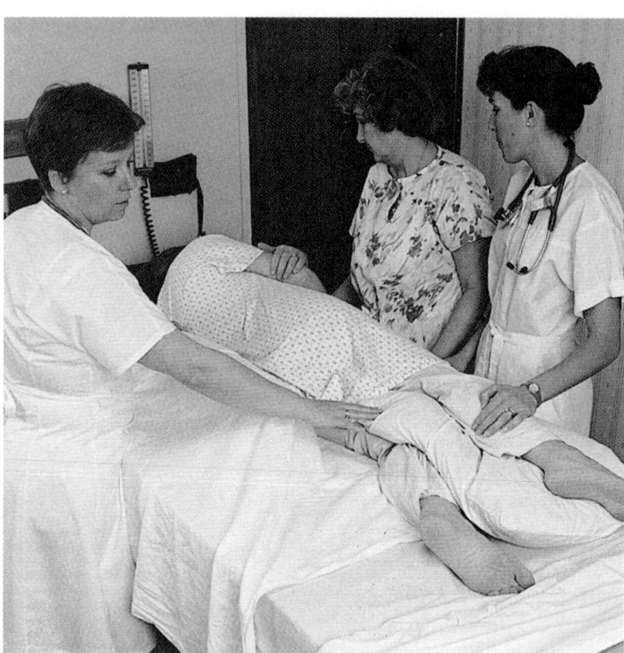

After positioning pillow, allow client to lean back for support.

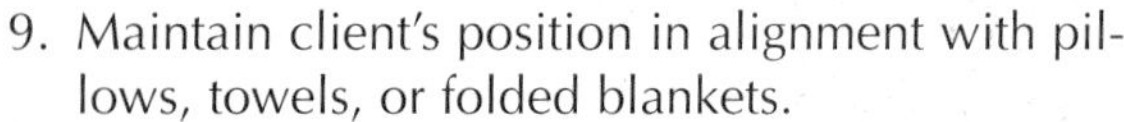

9. Maintain client's position in alignment with pillows, towels, or folded blankets.
10. Change client's position frequently (minimum 2 hours) according to physician's orders.

USING A FOOTBOARD

Equipment

Footboard

Procedure

1. Assess client's ability to place feet in dorsal flexion. If unable to do so, or plantar flexion is continuous, provide a footboard.
2. Cover footboard with a bath blanket to protect feet from rough surfaces.
3. Place footboard on the bed in a place where client's feet can firmly rest on it without sliding down in bed.
4. Observe legs to ensure that they are not in a flexed position when feet are against the board.
5. Tuck top linen under mattress at foot of bed, and bring linen up over the footboard to the top of the bed. Do not drape top linen over footboard as it can easily be pulled off the bed.
6. Put feet and ankles through range-of-motion exercises every 4 hours for clients on prolonged bed rest.
7. Observe heels and ankles frequently for signs of breakdown.

■ CLINICAL ALERT

Footboards are used to prevent plantar flexion. Ensure proper positioning to prevent footdrop.

PLACING A TROCHANTER ROLL

Equipment

Bath blanket

Procedure

1. Place client in supine or prone position.
2. Place folded bath blanket on bed next to client.
3. Extend blanket from client's waist to knee.
4. Place blanket edge under leg and buttocks to anchor.
5. Roll bath blanket toward client by rolling it under.
6. Rotate affected leg to slight internal hip rotation. **Rationale:** The purpose is to prevent external rotation of the head of the femur in the acetabulum.
7. Tighten the roll by tucking the roll under the hip joint.
8. Allow affected leg to rest against trochanter roll. Hip should be in normal alignment, not internally or externally rotated. **Rationale:** This is used most commonly for clients who have a muscle weakness or paralysis of that side of the body.

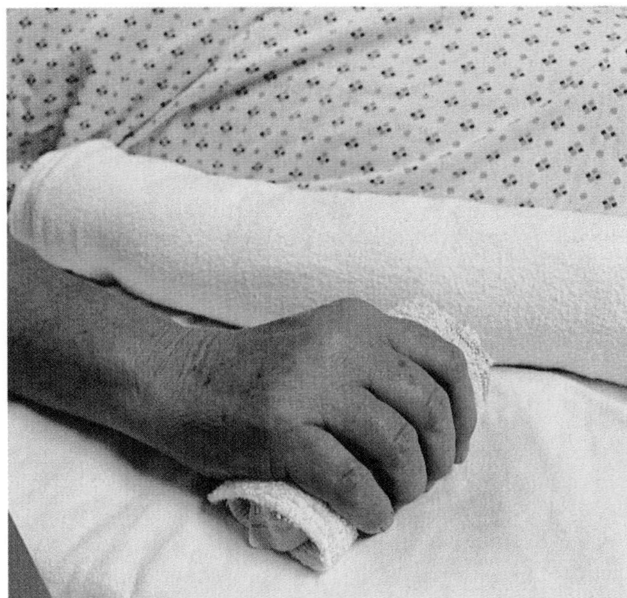

Use trochanter rolls made from bath blankets to align client's hips and handrolls to position hand and wrist.

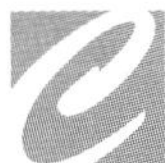

CHARTING for Moving and Turning Clients

- How often client turned or moved
- Condition of skin and joint movement
- Unexpected problems with moving or positioning client and solutions to problems
- Client's acceptance of and feelings about the procedure
- Number of staff needed to complete the procedure
- Transferred by Hoyer lift from bed to chair, if appropriate
- Time client was in chair or dangling at bedside
- Use of a footboard or trochanter roll

CRITICAL THINKING APPLICATION

CLINICAL PROBLEMS	CRITICAL THINKING OPTIONS
Client unwilling to move due to fear of pain or discomfort.	• Explain rationale and need for the procedure more thoroughly. • If possible, check if client can be medicated before the procedure. • Obtain additional assistance to decrease client's apprehension.
Client unable to assist with movement.	• Use a draw sheet to provide more support for client. • Obtain additional assistance to help with moving "dead" weight.
Client unable to maintain any type of position without assistance.	• Use trochanter roll to prevent external rotation of client's hip. • Use foam bolsters to maintain side-lying positions. • Using folded towels, blankets, or small pillows, position client's hands and arms to prevent dependent edema.
Skin begins to break down.	• Change client position every 2 hours. • Check with physician for therapeutic mattress or medications for decubitus care.

GERIATRIC CONSIDERATIONS

Physiologic age changes in the musculoskeletal system that affect nursing care of the elderly

- Contractures—muscles atrophy, regenerate slowly; tendons shrink and sclerose.
- Range of motion of joints decreases—lack of adequate joint motion, ankylosis.
- Mobility level is limited—muscle strength lessens and gait may be unsteady.
- Kyphosis occurs—cervical vertebrae may be flexed; intervertebral discs narrow.
- Bone changes—loss of trabecular bones and bones become brittle.

Nursing care for positioning elderly clients

- Ambulate within limitations of age.
- Alter position every 2 hours; align correctly.
- Prevent osteoporosis of long bones by providing exercises against resistance as ordered.
- Provide active and passive exercises—rest periods necessary and exercise paced throughout the day for the elderly.
- Provide range-of-motion exercises to all joints three times a day.
- Educate family that allowing the client to be sedentary is not helpful.
- Encourage walking, which is best single exercise for the elderly.

13

Exercise and Ambulation

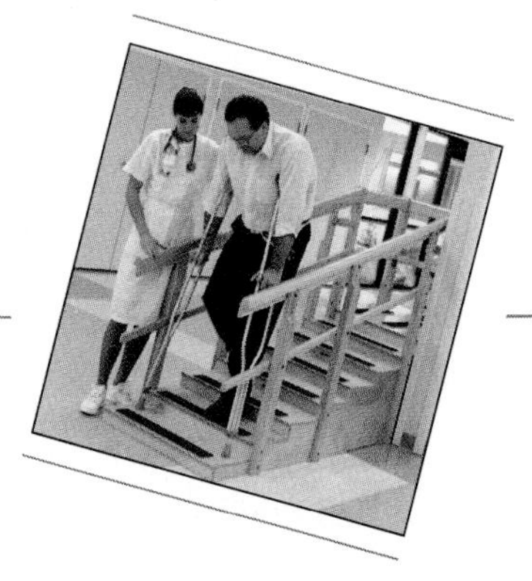

LEARNING OBJECTIVES

- Define rehabilitative nursing.
- Compare and contrast preservative and restorative methods of care.
- Identify the joints and the type of movement they allow.
- Compare and contrast passive and active range of motion.
- Demonstrate passive range-of-motion exercises using all muscle groups.
- Explain the rationale of assisted ambulation for clients.
- Complete a client-teaching guide for clients requiring muscle-strengthening exercises.
- Demonstrate the proper method for measuring crutches.
- Name and discuss four crutch-walking gaits.
- Demonstrate four crutch-walking gaits.
- List the components of crutch walking that require documentation.
- Write three nursing diagnoses that are appropriate for clients requiring exercise and ambulation activities.

TERMINOLOGY

Abduction: movement of a bone away from the midline of the body or body part, as in raising the arm or spreading the fingers.

Adduction: movement of a bone toward the midline of the body or part.

Alignment: arranged in a straight line.

Ambulate: walking; able to walk.

Antagonists: muscles that exert an action opposing that of prime mover.

Atrophy: a wasting of any organ or body part due to lack of nutrients or oxygen.

Cardiovascular: pertaining to heart and blood vessels.

Circumduction: movement of a bone in a circular direction so that the distal end scribes a circle while the proximal end remains stationary, as in "winding up" to throw a ball.

Contractility: ability of muscle to shorten, tighten, and contract.

Dorsiflexion: flexion of the foot at the ankle joint; the act of turning the foot and toes upward, as in standing on the heel.

Elasticity: ability of strained muscle to regain original size and shape when applied force is removed.

Eversion: turning outward; movement of the foot at the ankle joint so that the sole faces outward.

Excitability: capacity of muscle to respond to stimulus without intervention of motor nerves.

Extensibility: ability of muscle to stretch in response to applied force.

Extension: a movement that increases the angle between two bones, straightening a joint.

Fibrotic: pertinent to fibrosis, the formation of fibrous material.

Flexion: a movement that decreases the angle between two bones; the act of bending a joint.

Fracture: any break or crack in a bone.

Hyperextension: continuation of extension beyond the anatomic position, as in bending the head backward.

Inversion: turning inward; movement of the foot at the ankle joint so that the sole faces inward.

Ligament: a band or sheet of strong fibrous connective tissue connecting the articular ends of bones serving to bind them together and to facilitate or limit motion.

Mobility: state or quality of being mobile; facility of movement.

Musculoskeletal: pertaining to the muscles and bones.

Paralysis: temporary or permanent loss of function, especially loss of sensation or voluntary motion.

Plantar flexion: extension of the foot at the ankle joint; the foot and toes are turned downward toward the sole of the foot, as in standing on tiptoe.

Posture: attitude or position of body.

Prime movers: muscles responsible for the primary movement of contraction.

Pronation: rotation of the forearm so that the palm faces backward or downward; movement of the whole body so that the face and abdomen are downward.

Prone: lying horizontal with face downward.

Protraction: movement of the clavicle (collar bone) or mandible (lower jaw) forward on a plane parallel to the ground.

Proximal: nearest the point of attachment or reference point.

Retraction: movement of the clavicle or mandible backward on a plane parallel to the ground.

Rotation: movement of a bone around its own axis, as in moving the head to indicate "no" or turning the palm of the hand up and then down.

Sprain: injury caused by wrenching or twisting of a joint that results in tearing or stretching of the associated ligaments.

Strain: injury caused by excessive force or stretching of muscles or tendons around the joint.

Supination: rotation of forearm so that the palm faces forward or upward; movement of the whole body so that the face and abdomen are upward.

Synergists: muscles that enhance action of prime mover.

Tendons: fibrous connective tissue serving for the attachment of muscles to bones and other parts.

Tonicity: ability of muscle to maintain steady contraction, which determines its firmness.

Ulcer: an open sore of the skin or mucous membrane.

REHABILITATION CONCEPTS

Rehabilitative nursing involves the prevention and correction of alterations in the musculoskeletal system. In fact, the definition of rehabilitative nursing is the process of restoring a person's ability to live and work in as normal a manner as possible. To assist clients to achieve and maintain optimal mobility, both preservative and restorative methods are used.

Preservative methods, such as exercises and assisted ambulation, include those interventions that are needed to help clients maintain their normal mobility. Because the changes that occur in the human body when a person is hospitalized are varied and subtle, preservative methods are used with every client. Restorative methods, such as crutch walking and splinting, are used with clients who have decreased mobility caused by such factors as debilitating illness or major surgery. The purpose for applying restorative methods is to assist the client in achieving the level of mobility he or she enjoyed before becoming ill.

The general goals for using these methods are to assist the client to strive for optimal function, to prevent further injury, and to restore normal function. To achieve these goals of care, it is important for the nurse to accept the philosophy underlying rehabilitative nursing: that every illness is accompanied by the intrinsic threat of disability and that this part of total client care must begin with the initial client contact. Finally, it is important to accept that the principles of rehabilitation are basic to the care of all clients and that rehabilitation must be begun early in the client's hospitalization.

Being hospitalized and immobile seriously affects a person's body image, behavior, and overall adaptation and adjustment. The greater the disability, the more these aspects of a person's life are affected. The nurse's responsibility in providing total client care is to be aware of these responses and to take them into account when developing a client care plan.

MUSCULOSKELETAL SYSTEM

The muscular system is a system of more than six hundred fibers that are attached to bones. The system allows for body movement under the control of the voluntary nervous system. Muscles provide for body movement or locomotion, support the body, and perform several body functions, such as the partial production of heat. The fibers of the voluntary muscles are grouped together in a sheath of connective tissue. Each bundled group of muscle fibers is surrounded by a connective tissue sheath. The sheath tissue may be continuous with fibrous tissue that extends from the muscle as a tendon.

There are several properties of muscle fibers. The first is excitability, or the capacity of a muscle to respond to stimulus without intervention of the motor nerves. Another property is contractility, the ability of a muscle to shorten, tighten, or contract. Muscles are also able to maintain steady contraction (tonicity), stretch in response to applied force (extensibility), and regain their original size and shape when applied force is removed(elasticity).

Muscle Function

Skeletal muscles produce body movements by pulling on the bones. Bones serve as levers, and joints serve as fulcrums of these levers. Each muscle has a point of origin and a point of insertion that are usually attached to the bone. Muscles that move a body part usually do not extend over that part. These muscles usually perform with group action; some contract, and others relax. Prime movers are muscles responsible for the primary movement of contraction. Antagonists are muscles that exert an action opposing that of the prime movers.

Synergists are muscles that enhance action of the prime mover. The accessory parts to muscles are the ligaments and the tendons.

JOINT MOVEMENTS

Abduction: Movement of a bone away from the midline of the body or body part, as in raising the arm or spreading the fingers.

Eversion: Turning outward; movement of the foot at the ankle joint so that the sole faces outward.

Flexion: A movement that decreases the angle between two bones; the act of bending a joint.

Protraction: Movement of the clavicle (collar bone) or mandible (lower jaw) forward on a plane parallel to the ground.

Pronation: Rotation of the forearm so that the palm faces backward or downward; movement of the whole body so that the face and abdomen are downward.

Circumduction: Movement of a bone in a circular direction so that the distal end scribes a circle while the proximal end remains stationary, as in "winding up" to throw a ball.

Adduction: Movement of a bone toward the midline of the body or part.

Inversion: Turning inward; movement of the foot at the ankle joint so that the sole faces inward.

Extension: A movement that increases the angle between two bones, straightening a joint.

Hyperextension: Continuation of extension beyond the anatomic position, as in bending the head backward.

Retraction: Movement of the clavicle or mandible backward on a plane parallel to the ground.

Supination: Rotation of forearm so that the palm faces forward or upward; movement of the whole body so that the face and abdomen are upward.

Rotation: Movement of a bone around its own axis, as in moving the head to indicate "no" or turning the palm of the hand up and then down.

Joints

A joint of the body is the point at which two or more bones join together. The function of a joint is skeletal flexibility and motion. Joints are classified according to structural variations that allow for different kinds of movements. There are three main types of classification: synarthrotic, amphiarthrotic, and diarthrotic joints.

Synarthrotic joints are immovable and include those areas where tissue grows between articulating surfaces, such as the suture lines of the skull. Amphiarthrotic joints have limited movement.

Diarthrotic joints are freely movable. This type of joint is a cavity enclosed by a capsule lined with synovial membrane, which secretes a lubricant. The following types of joint movement allow for structural variations.

- Hinge type allows single directional movement (elbow).
- Ball-and-socket type allows bending (hip).
- Saddle type allows multidirectional shifting (thumb).
- Pivot type allows rotary movement.
- Gliding type allows limited sliding of bones against each other (wrist, ankle, invertebral joints).

Each of these types of joints have specific kinds of movements they can perform. These movements can be described in relationship to the three body planes: sagittal, transverse, and coronal. The sagittal plane divides the body into two portions with a straight vertical line between the two parts. The transverse plane divides the body into upper–lower portions with a horizontal line. The coronal plane divides the body into anterior–posterior portions at right angles to the sagittal plane. The synovial joints accomplish a variety of movements that range from flexion–extension to rotation and circumduction. For definitions of joint movements through the planes of the body refer to the following chart.

EXERCISE

Muscles that are not used become weak and shortened. During prolonged bed rest, strength and endurance decrease rapidly. Clients can regain muscle strength and mobility by practicing specific groups of exercises daily. Promoting exercise, both passive and active, is one of the most important nursing functions. The purpose of exercises is to promote good alignment, prevent contractures, stimulate circulation, and prevent thrombophlebitis and decubiti. Exercise also prevents edema of the extremities and promotes lung expansion.

The nurse both performs and teaches several types of exercises as a component of providing total client care. Passive exercises are carried out by the therapist or nurse without assistance from the client. These exercises enable the client to retain as much joint range of motion as possible as well as stimulating circulation.

Active exercises, although supervised by the nurse, are performed by the client. These exercises increase muscle strength when the client is partially immobile.

Resistive exercises, another rehabilitative measure, provide resistance in order to increase muscle power. These active exercises are performed by the individual working against resistance. Isometric or muscle-setting activities are similar to resistive exercises. These exercises maintain strength in a muscle when the joint is immobilized. They are performed by the individual without assistance.

Range-of-motion (ROM) exercises are the most common form of exercises for maintaining joint mobility and increasing maximal motion of a joint when the client is totally or partially immobilized. These exercises are completed by the nurse or physical therapist. The therapist puts an extremity through its full range so that the joint is moved through all the appropriate planes. Before beginning these exercises, it is important that the nurse assess the client's condition, the baseline ROM capabilities, establish the extent of ROM to be carried out, and ensure that the client is comfortable. Be aware that clients might be fearful of this type of exercise and that a full explanation of what you are going to do is helpful to allay fears. Enlist the cooperation of the client for maximum benefit. Discontinue all range-of-motion exercises if the client complains of pain, for it is at this point that the exercises become counterproductive.

AMBULATION

Ambulation, or walking, is an important function that most of us accomplish automatically, that is, without thinking or conscious effort. When a person has been immobilized, confined to bed following surgery or an injury, or unable to ambulate, this seemingly simple activity can become a major hurdle to overcome. The longer a person is immobilized, the more difficult it is to regain ambulatory ability; likewise, the sooner a person begins to ambulate after being bedridden, the more easily he or she will regain preimmobilization status. Early ambulation decreases hospitalization time and prevents complications, such as paralytic ileus or thrombophlebitis.

The human body functions best when it is placed frequently in a vertical position. Ambulation improves physical and mental well-being. Ambulation increases muscle strength and joint mobility. It also increases respiratory exchange, gastrointestinal muscle tone, and circulation. Without stress on bones, calcium deposits occur and renal problems increase from calcium-based calculi.

Balance, coordination, and good body alignment are aspects important to walking. One must be able to move forward and maintain an upright balance; use muscles, bones, and joints correctly for coordination; and keep the head erect and vertebral column fairly straight with feet and knee caps pointed forward in order to maintain good body alignment.

The major muscle groups used for walking are the thigh and leg muscles. If these muscles have not been used or exercised because the client has been in bed for a long time, ambulation must be accomplished step by step. Weak muscles cannot support a human frame for the mechanics of walking. It is important, then, to begin the process of ambulation by administering muscle-strengthening exercises. Several different types of exercises were described previously; however, the most important preambulatory preparation is a quadriceps-setting and gluteal-setting exercises. Carried out several times a day, these exercises restore muscle strength and prepare the legs for weight bearing.

Before actually assisting the client to walk, explain exactly what you are going to do, and prepare the client by doing the ambulatory procedure in stages. For example, begin with the muscle-strengthening exercises. Then assist the client to sit up in bed to determine if he or she is experiencing vertigo. Have the client move to the side of the bed with legs down, and only when he or she is ready and feels comfortable in doing so, assist the client to stand beside the bed. Allow the client to remain there with the bed as support until he or she feels totally secure. Finally, and with the assistance of one or two nurses (depending on the assessment of the client's ability and readiness to ambulate), have the client walk by taking short steps and walking only as long as he or she can tolerate. Do this several times a day, and it will not be long before the client's legs are strengthened, and he or she can graduate to one assistant, a walker, or cane. Throughout this procedure, do not allow the client to lose confidence in the ability to walk or your ability to support and assist while regaining his or her independence of action.

A variety of assistive devices are available to give the client support when ambulating. Such devices may give the client confidence (especially important with the elderly), stability, support for a weak limb, or reduce the pressure on a limb. These devices may include canes (standard cane, T-handled cane, tripod cane, and quad cane) and walkers (standard, with wheels, or a hemiwalker). Other assistive devices include crutches, used to lesson or remove weight from one or both legs.

CRUTCHES

Crutches are an aid to walking by providing support during ambulating when the lower extremities are unable to support the body weight. It is hoped that this situation is temporary, but even if it is permanent, crutches do allow independence of movement that otherwise could not occur.

There are three main types of crutches: the axillary (most common for short-term use), the Lofstrand, or Canadian (a forearm crutch with a metal band and handle), and the platform, for clients who are unable to use their wrists to bear weight.

Several safety factors should be taken into account before assisting the client to use crutches. The measurement from the axillary fold to the crutch bar should be $1\frac{1}{2}$ to 2 inches (4 inches in front and 6 inches to the side of the toes). The handpiece should be adjusted to allow 30° elbow flexion, and rubber suction tips should be placed on the bottom of the crutches. Finally, the client should be informed that he needs well-fitting shoes with nonslip soles.

The type of crutch used by the client depends on the ability to ambulate, the muscle strength needed for support, and the individual needs of the client.

NURSING DIAGNOSES

The following nursing diagnoses are appropriate to use on client care plans when the components are related to exercise and ambulation needs of clients.

NURSING DIAGNOSIS	RELATED FACTORS
Activity Intolerance	Nutritional disorders, surgery, disease states, impaired motor function, pain
Impaired Home Maintenance Management	Chronic debilitating disease, injury, surgery, lack of knowledge, insufficient funds, lack of support or community resources
Pain	Altered body function (muscle spasms or rigidity), musculoskeletal disorders, inflammation, immobility
Impaired Physical Mobility	Neuromuscular impairment, musculoskeletal impairment, surgical procedure, trauma
Self-Care Deficit (specify)	Neuromuscular impairment, surgery, musculoskeletal impairment, visual disorders, external devices

unit 1

RANGE OF MOTION

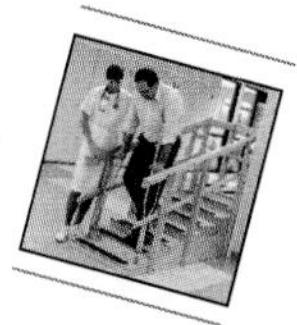

NURSING PROCESS DATA

ASSESSMENT Data Base

Determine client's physical ability to perform exercises (i.e., level of consciousness, presence of casts, traction).

Ascertain client's baseline level of joint movement and muscle strength.

Note amount of spontaneous movement shown by the client.

Assess client's understanding of ROM exercises.

PLANNING Objectives

To improve or maintain joint function

To improve or maintain muscle tone and strength

To counteract effects of prolonged bed rest or immobilization

To prevent contractures

To increase client comfort

To prepare the client for ambulation

IMPLEMENTATION Procedures

Performing Passive Range of Motion

Using Continuous Passive Motion Machine

Teaching Active Range of Motion

EVALUATION Expected Outcomes

Client experiences improved range of motion and muscle tone.

Client is comfortable following range-of-motion exercises.

Client is able to ambulate without difficulty following a period of bed rest.

PERFORMING PASSIVE RANGE OF MOTION

Equipment

Hospital bed

Procedure

1. Wash hands.
2. Explain the rationale for the procedure to the client.
3. Position the client on his or her back with the bed as flat as possible.
4. Expose limb to be exercised.
5. Put all joints through range of motion slowly and gently (Tables 13–1 and 13–2).
6. Protect against gravity and detrimental movement when performing range-of-motion exercises.
7. Provide support above and below the joint using a cradling or cupping support while performing the exercises.
8. Follow sequence of exercises for upper and lower body according to chart.
9. All joints should be put through exercises at least twice daily and five full-range motions to each joint.
10. Encourage client to do active exercises as soon as possible. **Rationale:** Passive exercises only help prevent contractures. They do not maintain the muscle.
11. Discontinue exercises if client complains of pain or discomfort.
12. Reassess client's ability to perform ROM exercises and adjust schedule accordingly.

TABLE 13–1 Range of Motion: Upper Body

	Neck	Shoulder	Elbow	Forearm	Wrist	Finger and Thumb
Flexion	Move head forward 90° with chin on chest	Raise arm 180° from side to above head	Bend elbow so arm moves up toward shoulder		Bend hand 90°toward inner arm	Make a fist so fingers are all bent inward
Extension	Move head up from chest 90°—resting position	Move arm to side of body	Straighten elbow and return to position		Move hand straight pointed out	Move fingers 90° to straight position
Hyperextension	Move head backwards 90°	Move arm to back of body 50° angle			Bend hand up and back 90° toward arm	Move fingers up toward back of hand
Abduction		Hold arm away from side 180° to above head			Bend wrist out away from arm	Spread fingers as much as possible
Adduction		Move arm from side across chest			Bend wrist inward toward radius	Move fingers and thumb together
External Rotation		Hold arm out to side with elbow bent 45°; move forward so palm faces forward				
Internal Rotation		Move arm to side at shoulder level with elbow bent 45°. Lower arm so palm faces back				
Rotation	Move head in circular motion—90° left, then 90° right					
Circumduction		Move arm in full circle				
Supination				Rotate forearm 90° so palm is up		
Pronation				Rotate forearm 90° so palm is down		

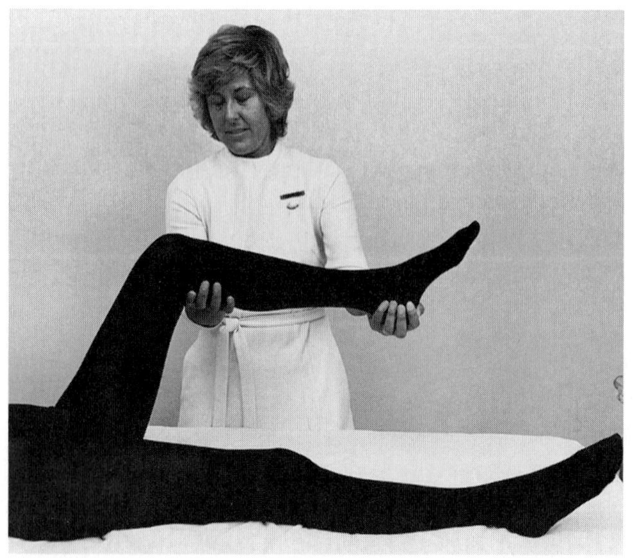
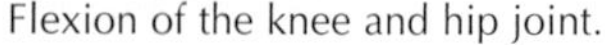
Flexion of the knee and hip joint.

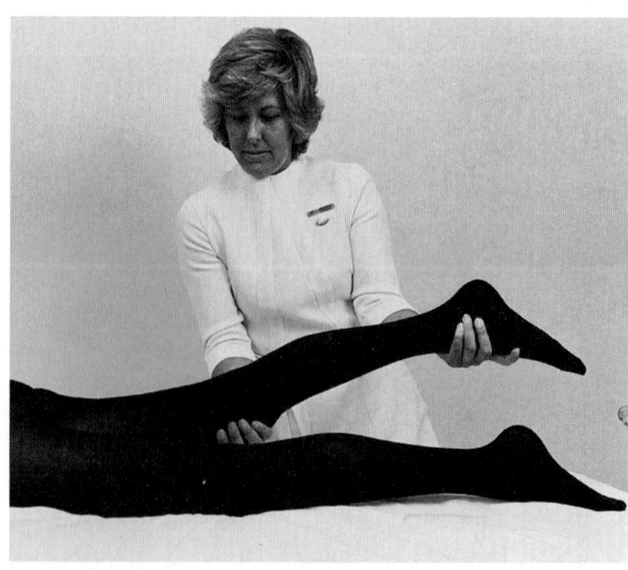
Range of motion from prone position.

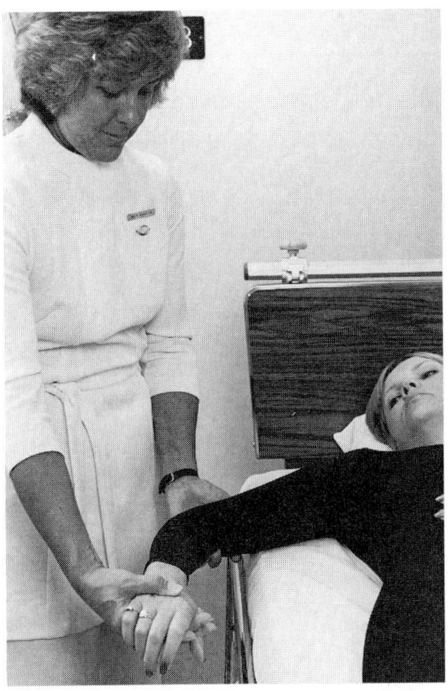
Internal rotation of shoulder.

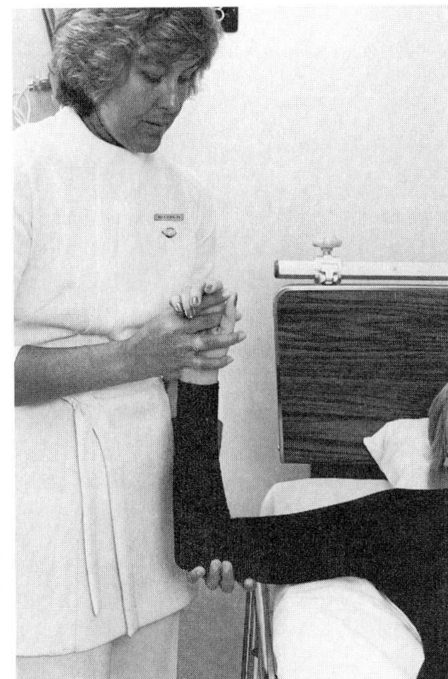
Rotation midpoint.

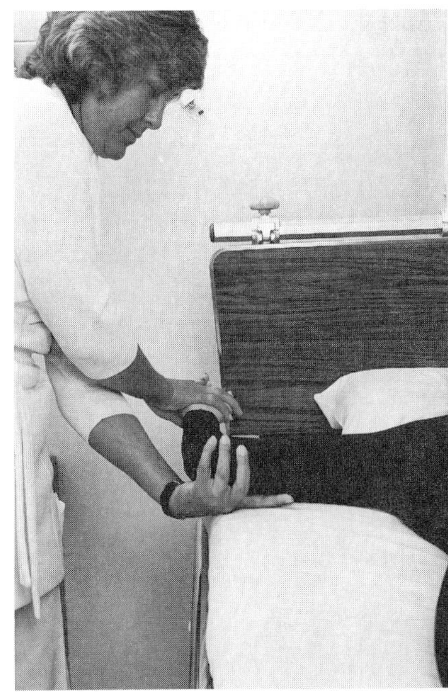
External rotation of shoulder.

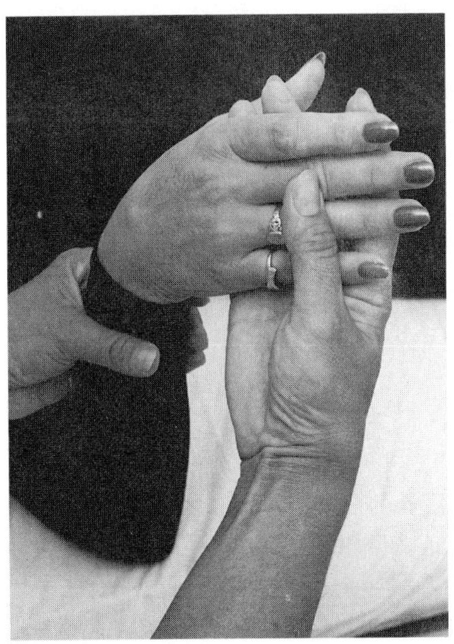
Rotation of the wrist.

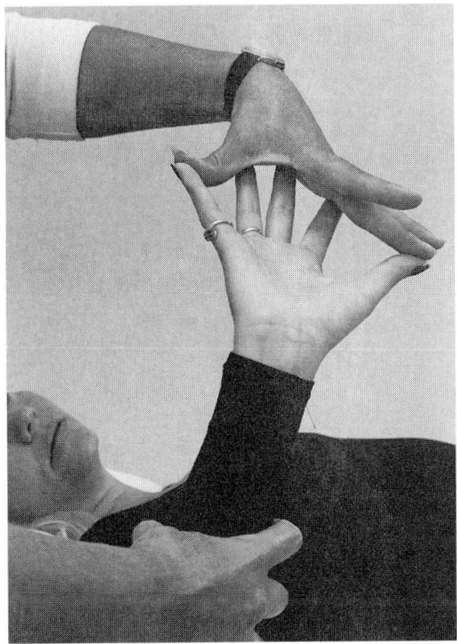
Extension of finger joints.

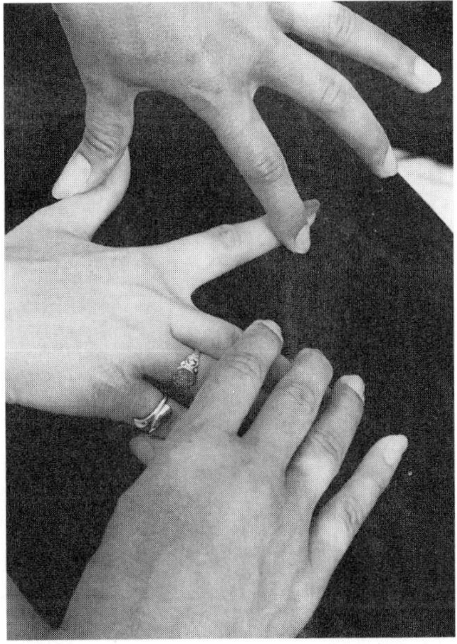
Adduction—abduction finger exercise.

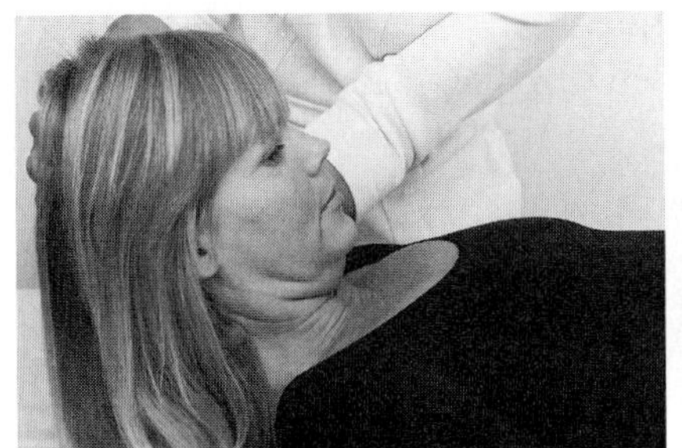
Flexion of the neck.

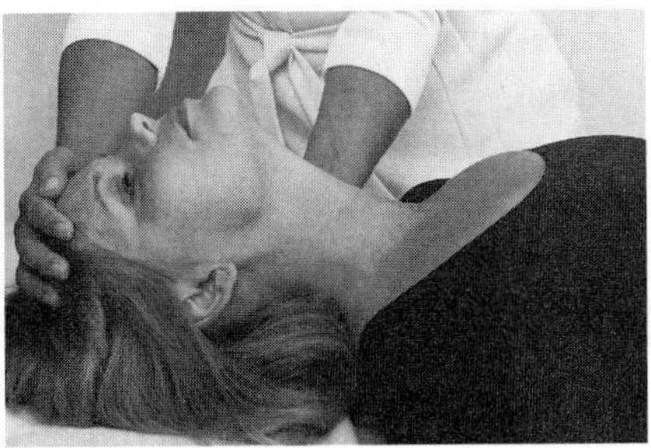
Extension of the neck.

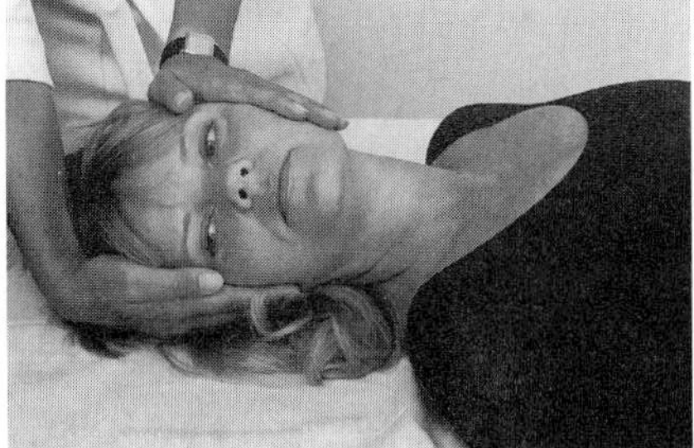
Rotation of the neck.

TABLE 13–2 Range of Motion: Lower Body

	Trunk	Hip	Knee	Ankle	Toes
Flexion	Bend forward 90°	Move leg forward and up 90°	Bend knee 90°; foot moves back and up		Point down 90°
Extension	Stand in straight position	Move leg in straight alignment with trunk	Move foot 90° with knee straight and leg in line with body		Straight out from foot
Hyperextension	Bend backward 30°	Move leg backward 50°			Point up 45°
Lateral Flexion	Bend to both sides 45°				
Plantar Flexion				Move foot down 45°	
Internal Rotation		Turn leg and foot inward 90°			
External Rotation		Turn leg and foot outward 90°			
Circumduction		Move leg in circle 360°			
Abduction		Move leg away from body 45°			Spread apart 15°
Adduction		Move leg toward body 45°			Bring together in normal position
Rotation	Move in circle 360° from waist				
Dorsiflexion				Raise foot up 45°	
Eversion				Move sole of foot lateral to outside	
Inversion				Move sole of foot medial to inside	

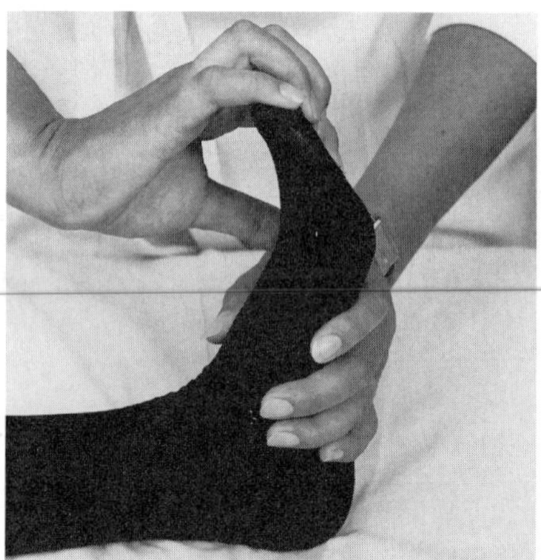

Dorsiflexion.

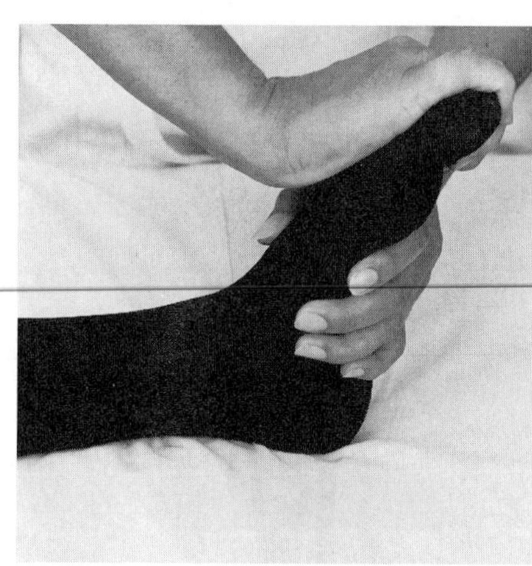

Plantar flexion.

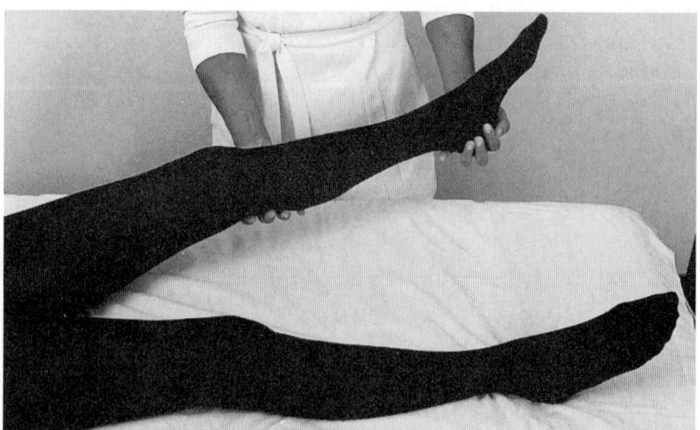

Abduction (moving away from body).

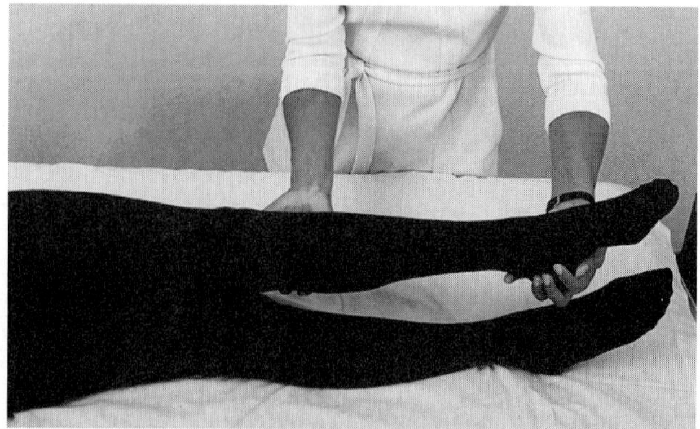

Adduction (moving toward the body).

USING CONTINUOUS PASSIVE MOTION MACHINE

Equipment

Continuous passive motion (CPM) machine specific for joint involved
Balkan frame or traction equipment
Sheepskin mattress

Procedure

1. Read physician's orders for flexion and extension limits and limb involved.
2. Select appropriate device for involved joint.
3. Read manufacturer's instruction manual.
4. Check date machine was tested for electrical safety.
5. Remove egg crate mattress, if used, from the bed. **Rationale:** This provides a stable surface.
6. Place machine on bed.
7. Attach machine to bed using traction equipment like the Balkan frame.
8. Turn off electric bed controls. **Rationale:** This prevents client from using bed controls that could change client's alignment.
9. Connect control box to CPM machine.
10. Set limits of flexion and extension. Usually physician orders 10°–45° of flexion and 0°–10° of extension.
11. Set speed control to slow or moderate range.
12. Put machine through one full cycle. **Rationale:** This ensures CPM is working properly.
13. Stop machine when in extension. Place sheepskin on CPM.
14. Place client's extremity in CPM.
15. Adjust machine to client's extremity. Lengthen and shorten appropriate sections of frame.
16. Center client's extremity on frame. **Rationale:** This avoids pressure areas on extremity.
17. Align client's joints with machine joints.
18. Secure extremity on CPM with straps attached to machine.
19. Start machine. When it reaches fully flexed position, stop machine and check degree of flexion. **Rationale:** This prevents possible complications.

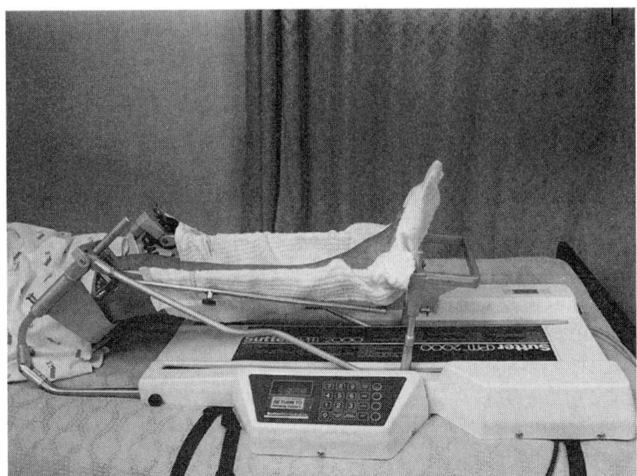

Place leg in CPM cradle and set machine for degree of flexion according to physician's orders.

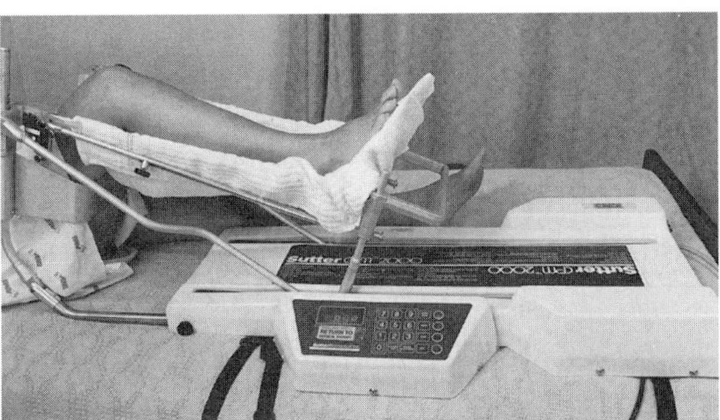

Set cycle rate, usually 2-10 cycles per minute, for 12-14 hours per day or as ordered.

20. Start machine and observe at least two full cycles.
21. Set cycle rate as ordered, usually 2–10 cycles/minute.
22. Raise side rails to keep machine in place.
23. Keep bed flat. (Raise head of bed only 20° if necessary.)
24. Assess client's comfort level. **Rationale:** Discomfort leads to resistance to increases of speed and flexion.
25. Keep machine on for 12–14 hours each day or as ordered.
26. Increase flexion 5°–10° per shift or not more than 20° in 24 hours. Follow physician's orders.
27. Assess operative site every 2–4 hours for bleeding.
28. Evaluate alignment of extremity, placement of straps and CMS checks every 2–4 hours.

Rationale: This prevents complications and promotes client's compliance to therapy.

29. Evaluate skin condition over bony prominences and provide skin care every 2 hours. **Rationale:** This assists in preventing pressure ulcers from developing.
30. Administer analgesics as ordered for discomfort.
31. Remove extremity from machine when machine is in full extension six times each day and provide quadriceps-setting exercises.

TEACHING ACTIVE RANGE OF MOTION

Equipment

Hospital bed
Sturdy nonslip shoes or slippers

Procedure

1. Explain the rationale for the procedure to the client.
2. Demonstrate the exercises that the client should perform.
3. Watch as the client does the exercises.
4. Assist with the exercises as needed.
5. Correct any problems you notice in the client's performance.
6. Encourage client to perform as much of the exercises as possible.
7. Instruct client to do range-of-motion exercises every 4 hours, exercising all joints.

CHARTING for CPM

- Client's tolerance for CPM
- Rate cycles per minute of CPM
- Degree of flexion and extension used
- Condition of extremity
- Condition of skin and nursing actions provided
- Condition of operative site
- Time extremity in CPM

CHARTING for ROM Exercises

- Amount of time needed to complete exercises
- Any changes in condition of joint or joint mobility
- Movements that caused unusual pain or discomfort
- Amount of client participation
- Specific joints put through range of motion
- Alterations in usual procedure

CRITICAL THINKING APPLICATION

CLINICAL PROBLEMS	CRITICAL THINKING OPTIONS
Client continues to lose mobility and strength despite nursing intervention.	• Discuss the need for additional measures to improve joint range with the health team. • Assess the client for the need to use splints and braces to maintain the best physiologic position between exercise periods, and discuss your findings with the physician.
Client experiences pain and discomfort during range-of-motion exercises.	• Assess amount and type of pain and report findings to physician. • Reevaluate your technique to ensure you are performing the exercises correctly. • Check with physician about premedicating the client before exercises are initiated.

unit 2 AMBULATION

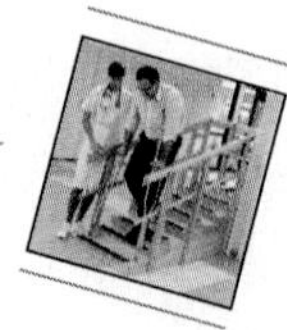

NURSING PROCESS DATA

ASSESSMENT Data Base

Assess client's previous activity level.

Check physician's orders for activity.

Assess vital signs and physical ability to ambulate.

Assess need for safety belt.

Assess client for dizziness when moved into an upright sitting position.

Determine if client feels pain from operative site.

Observe client's balance.

Assess any sensory deficits (visual, perceptual)

PLANNING Objectives

To promote increased feelings of physical and mental well-being

To develop increased tolerance for exercise

To decrease hospitalization time

To regain independence of action by regaining ability to walk

To prevent paralytic ileus by increasing abdominal wall and gastrointestinal tract muscle tone

To prevent thrombophlebitis by increasing circulation in the legs

To promote healing by increasing circulation and muscle contraction

IMPLEMENTATION Procedures

Ambulating with Two Assistants

Ambulating with One Assistant

Ambulating with a Walker

Ambulating with a Cane

EVALUATION Expected Outcomes

Feelings of physical and mental well-being increased.

Balance and muscle tone improve.

Client progresses from needing assistance with ambulation to becoming independent in ambulation.

Complications of immobility are prevented with ambulation.

AMBULATING WITH TWO ASSISTANTS

Equipment

Robe or second hospital gown (put on backwards so that client is not exposed)

Shoes or slippers that fit well and have nonslip soles

Procedure

1. Explain the rationale for the procedure to the client.
2. Help the client sit on the side of the bed after placing bed in LOW position.
3. Assess the client for dizziness or faintness. Keep the client in this position until he or she is able to stand without becoming dizzy. **Rationale:** Orthostatic

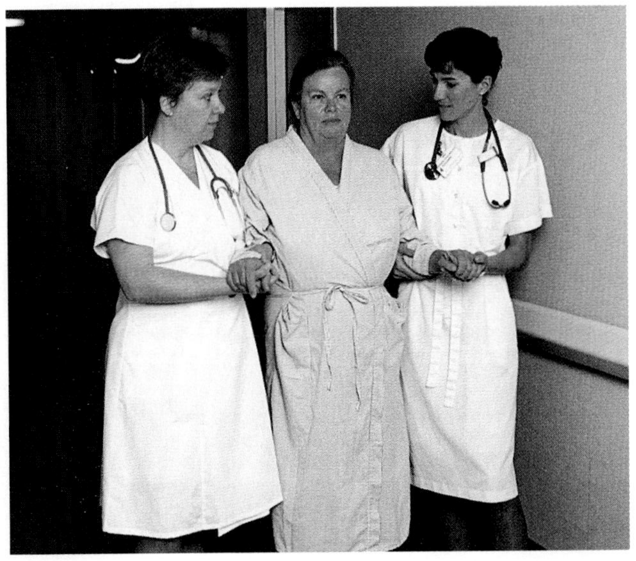

Support is provided by two nurses when client's condition requires.

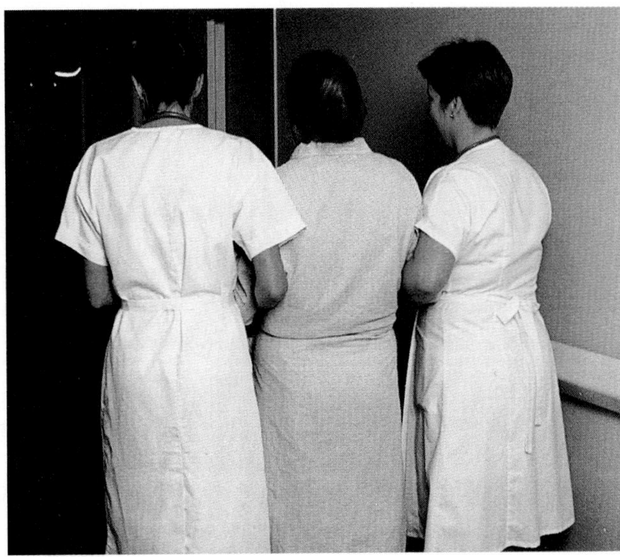

Grasp client's arms firmly on both sides to provide support.

hypotension can occur with prolonged bed rest.

4. Position one nurse on each side of the client.
5. Have each nurse grasp the client's upper arm with the hand that is closest to the client.
6. Have each nurse grasp the client's hand with the other hand.
7. Encourage the client to maintain good posture and look straight ahead, not down.
8. Ask the client to lift each foot to take a step. The client should not shuffle. Walk the client only as far as he or she is capable of walking and returning without exhaustion.

AMBULATING WITH ONE ASSISTANT

Equipment

Robe or second hospital gown (put on backward so that client is not exposed)

Shoes or slippers that fit well and have nonslip soles

Safety belt if indicated

Procedure

1. Explain the rationale for the procedure to the client.
2. Help the client sit on the side of the bed after placing bed in LOW position.
3. Assess the client for dizziness or faintness. Keep the client in this position until he or she is able to stand without becoming dizzy.
4. Apply safety belt if client is unsteady. **Rationale:** Provides support if client is weak and prevents injury.
5. Help the client to stand and observe balance.
6. Grasp client around waist to stabilize, and grasp arm with other hand to guide client.

■ CLINICAL ALERT

If the client is collapsing, try to break the fall with your body and guide client to the floor.
If the client is unsteady or appears to be falling, support his or her body, especially the head and trunk, maintaining your body in good alignment with line of gravity within your base of support. This alignment prevents injury to yourself, while giving the client adequate support. If necessary, guide the client all the way to the floor.

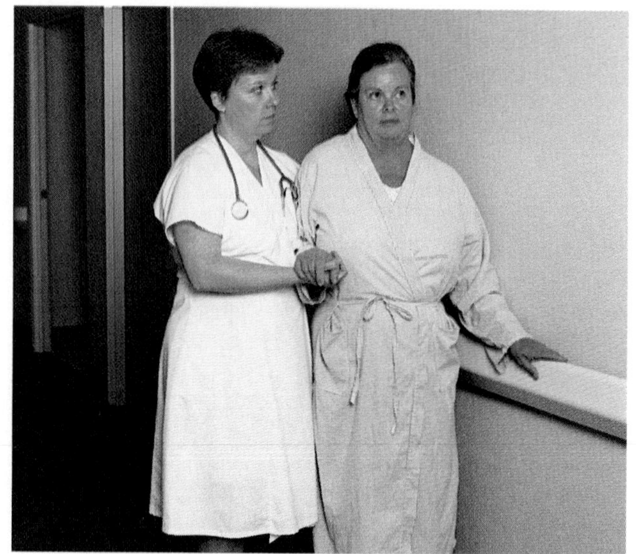
Grasp client around waist and stabilize, holding other arm.

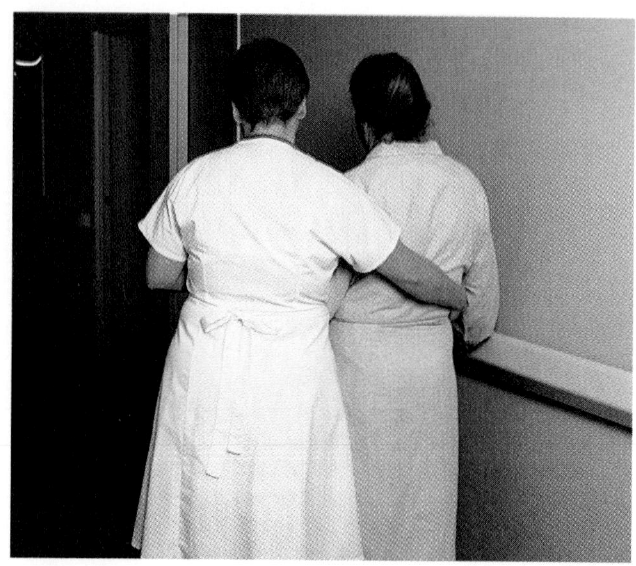
Use wall rail if available to support client.

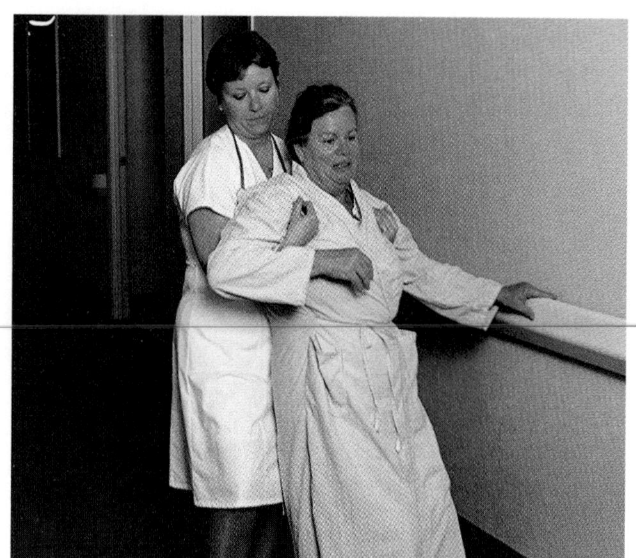
Grasp client under both arms when she begins to fall.

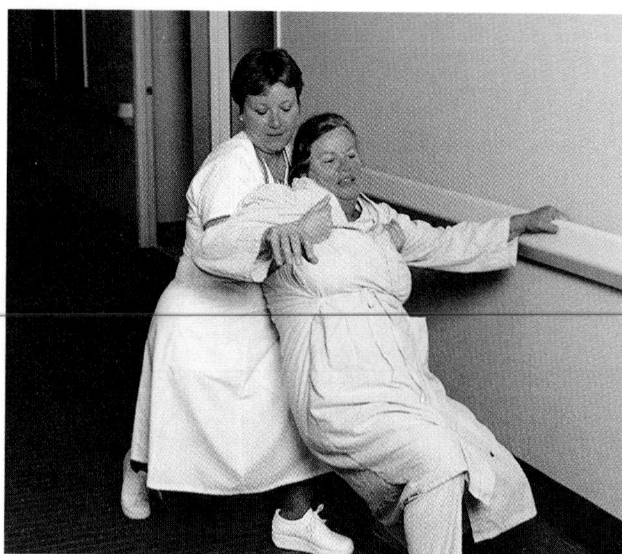
Break client's fall using your body to prevent injury.

7. Stand on weaker side, except for cerebrovascular accident (CVA) client—then stand on unaffected side. **Rationale:** Flaccid muscles on affected side do not provide sufficient muscle strength for you to grasp and support client.
8. Encourage client to maintain good posture and to look straight ahead. **Rationale:** Tendency is for client to look down, which may increase vertigo.
9. Instruct client to lift each foot to take a step, not to shuffle.
10. Walk client as far as he or she is capable of walking without becoming exhausted.

AMBULATING WITH A WALKER

Equipment

Robe or second hospital gown (put on backward so that client is not exposed)
Shoes or slippers that fit well and have nonslip soles
Walker

Procedure

1. Explain the rationale for the procedure to the client.
2. Help the client stand.
3. Tell client to grasp the upper handles of the walker.
4. Have the client move the walker forward, keeping all four feet of the walker on the floor.
5. When the walker is stable, tell the client to walk into it.
6. Make sure the client lifts his or her feet to walk.

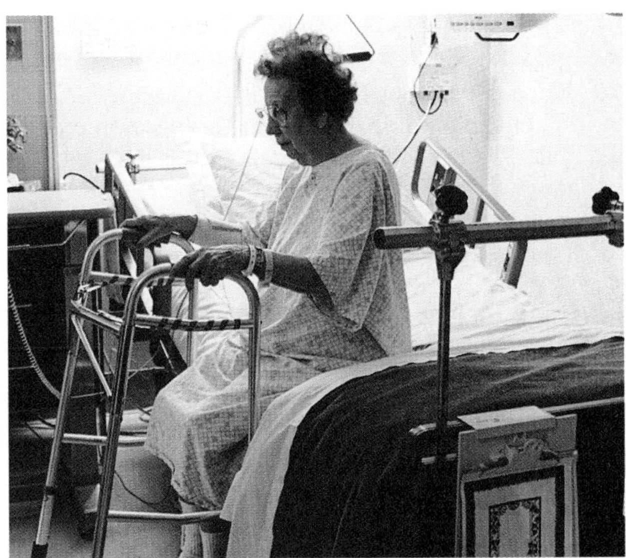

Instruct client how to use walker before ambulation.

AMBULATING WITH A CANE

Equipment

Appropriate type of cane
- Straight-legged or standard cane
- Tripod or three-pronged cane
- Quad cane

Sturdy shoes with nonskid soles

Procedure

1. Check physician's orders and client care plan to ensure client is ready to use a cane for ambulation.
2. Ascertain that cane provides sufficient support for the client.
3. Explain the purpose of using a cane for ambulation, and answer client questions.
4. Check that cane extends from greater trochanter to floor with 20°–30° for elbow flexion. **Rationale:** If cane is too short, client cannot support weight and may injure back.
5. Demonstrate use of cane if client is unfamiliar with its use.
6. Assist client to put on appropriate shoes and socks for walking.
7. Assist client to standing position with feet firmly on the floor.

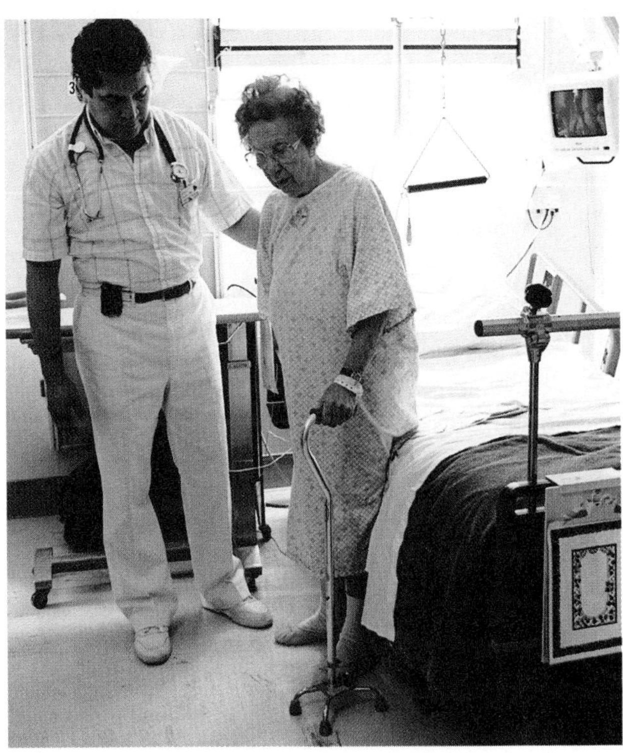

Direct client to hold cane on stronger side of body.

8. Instruct client to hold cane on the stronger side of the body. **Rationale:** This offers the most support.
9. Place cane about 12 inches in front of the foot and slightly to the side. **Rationale:** This position provides the best balance, because the client's center of gravity is within the base of support.
10. Determine that client can maintain balance and does not feel dizzy before taking the first step.
11. Assist client to move unaffected (or stronger) leg forward to the cane. **Rationale:** This procedure allows the weight to be distributed first to the unaffected leg and cane, then to the affected leg and cane.
12. Accompany client by walking beside him or her on the affected side. **Rationale:** If the client loses his or her balance, supporting client on affected side is most effective. Simply insert your hand and arm underneath the client's axilla and support his or her arm with your other hand.
13. Evaluate client's ability to use the cane, and instruct about its use as needed.
14. Reinforce the client's achievement to assist him or her to gain confidence in ambulating.
15. Continue to accompany client until the time for walking is completed.
16. Assist client to return to the room and to bed if indicated.
17. Position client for comfort.

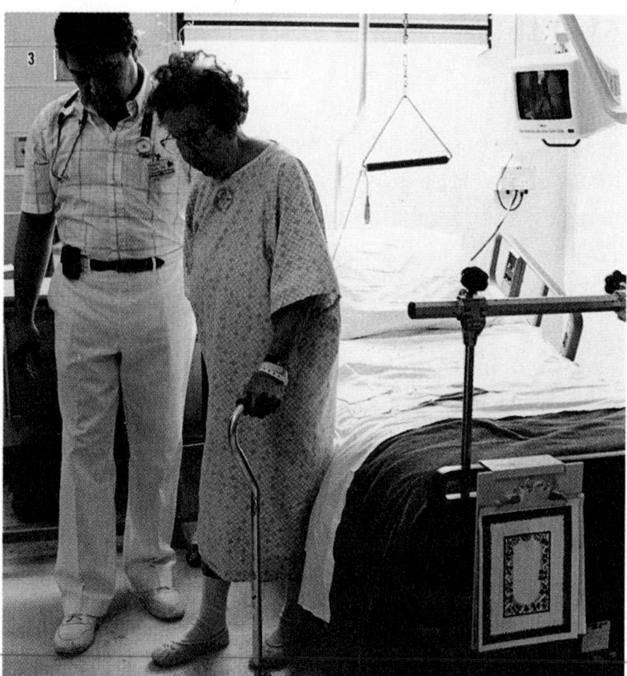

Instruct client to move unaffected leg forward first.

18. Assess client's response to ambulation.
19. Wash hands.
20. Chart client's progress, and evaluate plan for increased periods of ambulation in terms of client's capability.

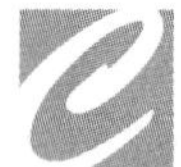

CHARTING for Ambulation

- Client's ability to balance
- Time and distance of ambulation
- Use of correct procedure for walker or cane
- Client's perceptions of ambulation

CRITICAL THINKING APPLICATION

CLINICAL PROBLEMS	CRITICAL THINKING OPTIONS
■ Client becomes dizzy or feels faint.	• If in the client's room, help the client return to the chair or bed. • If in the hall, ease the client down the wall to the floor. Do not attempt to hold the client. • Summon help if possible.
■ Client is too weak to ambulate.	• Provide action and passive ROM. • Begin ambulation protocol as soon as possible.
■ Client is heavy or has poor balance.	• Ask other nurses or staff to help you ambulate the client until able to walk on his or her own. • If necessary, enlist the aid of a stronger assistant whose presence may give the client additional psychologic as well as physical support. • Gradually increase ambulation as muscle tone improves and balance improves.
■ Client feels unable to ambulate.	• Ambulate more frequently for shorter periods and with more assistance to increase confidence. • Medicate at least 1 hour before ambulation to decrease pain. • With abdominal surgery, check with physician for an order for a binder to decrease fear of dehiscence and pain. • Establish rapport with the client so you can discuss fears about ambulation.

unit 3

CRUTCH WALKING

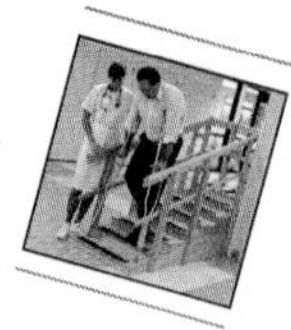

NURSING PROCESS DATA

ASSESSMENT Data Base

Assess physical ability to use crutches and strength of the client's arm back, and leg muscles.
Observe client's ability to balance self.
Note any unilateral or unusual weakness or dizziness.
Assess which gait is appropriate for client.
Assess client's understanding of crutch-walking technique.

PLANNING Objectives

To improve client's ability to ambulate when he or she has lower extremity injury
To increase muscle strength, especially in the arms and legs
To increase feeling of well-being when client can ambulate
To promote joint mobility

IMPLEMENTATION Procedures

Teaching Muscle-Strengthening Exercises
Measuring Client for Crutches
Teaching Crutch Walking: Four-Point Gait
Teaching Crutch Walking: Three-Point Gait
Teaching Crutch Walking: Two-Point Gait
Teaching Swing-To Gait and Swing-Through Gait
Teaching Upstairs and Downstairs Ambulation with Crutches

EVALUATION Expected Outcomes

Client's ability to ambulate is improved.
Muscle strength of client's arms and legs is improved.
Client experiences a feeling of well-being.

TEACHING MUSCLE-STRENGTHENING EXERCISES

Equipment

Books, boards, or other firm surface for each hand

Procedure

1. Explain the rationale for the exercises to the client.
2. Check the client care plan for orders.
3. Demonstrate the exercises that client will practice.

Quadriceps-setting exercises:

a. Try to hyperextend the client's leg by pushing the popliteal area (the area behind knee) into the bed and lifting heel off the bed.
b. Instruct client to contract muscle for a count of 5, then relax for a count of 5.
c. Have client repeat exercise two to three times, gradually working up to 10–15 times an hour.

Gluteal-setting exercises:

a. Tell client to pinch his or her buttocks together for a count of 5 and then to relax for a count of 5.
b. Have client repeat exercise 10–15 times an hour.

Pushups in sitting position:

a. Tell client to sit up in bed with arms at sides.
b. Put books, boards, or something firm under the client's hands and have the client push down, raising hips off the bed. (This exercise may also be practiced while sitting in a chair.)

c. Have client repeat exercise until he or she can do 10–15 pushups an hour.

Pushups in prone position:

a. Tell client to lie prone in bed.
b. Ask client to place hands on the bed, close to the shoulders.
c. Tell client to extend arms and to push the upper part of the body into an upright position.
d. Have client repeat exercise until he or she can do 10–15 pushups an hour.

4. Monitor as the client performs the exercises, and correct any problems that may occur.
5. Assess the client for increasing strength as he or she continues to practice the exercises.

MEASURING CLIENT FOR CRUTCHES

Equipment

Measuring tape
Hardsoled street shoes

Procedure

1. Explain the rationale for the procedure to the client.
2. Tell client to put on the shoes she or he will be wearing when using the crutches.
3. Ask client to lie flat in bed with arms at sides.
4. Measure the distance from the client's axilla (armpit) to a point 6–8 inches out from heel.
5. Adjust hand bars on the crutches so that the client's elbows are always slightly flexed.
6. Tell the client to stand with the crutches under the arms.
7. Measure the distance between the client's axilla and the arm pieces on the crutches. You should be able to put two of your fingers in the space between the axilla and the crutch bar. **Rationale:** Crutches that do not fit the client correctly or crutches that are used incorrectly can damage the brachial plexus and cause paralysis of the arms.

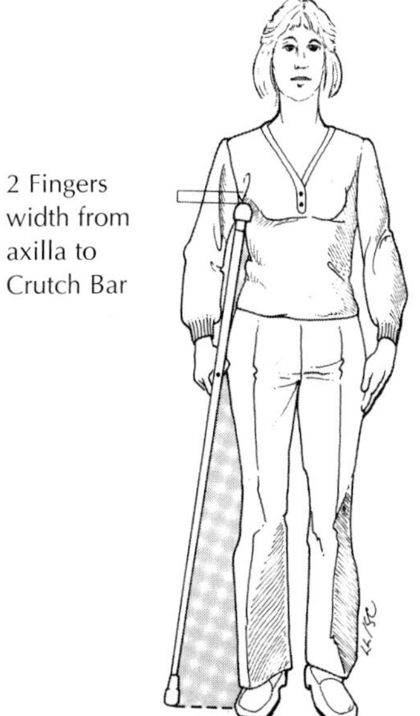

Measure from axilla to heel for crutch height.

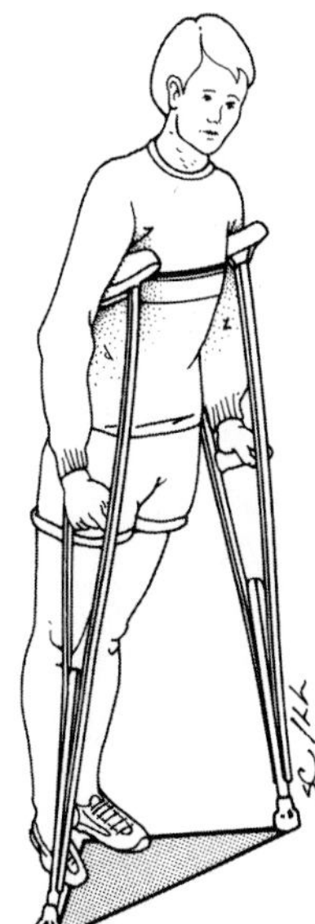

Tripod crutch stance for balance in crutch walking.

TEACHING CRUTCH WALKING: FOUR-POINT GAIT

Equipment

Properly fitted crutches
Regular, hardsoled street shoes
Safety belt, if needed

Procedure

1. Explain the rationale for the procedure to the client.
   a. The gait is rather slow but very stable.
   b. The gait can be performed when the client can move and bear weight on each leg.
2. Demonstrate the crutch-foot sequence to the client.
   a. Move the right crutch.
   b. Move the left foot.
   c. Move the left crutch.
   d. Move the right foot.
3. Help the client practice the gait. Be ready to help with balance if necessary.
4. Assess client's progress, and correct mistakes as they occur.

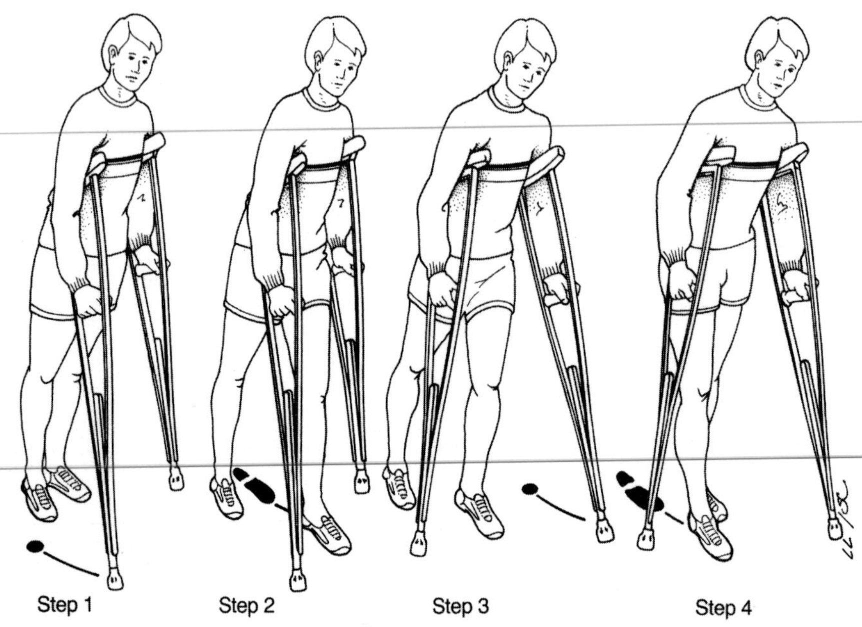

Four-point gait.

TEACHING CRUTCH WALKING: THREE-POINT GAIT

Equipment

Properly fitted crutches
Regular, hardsoled street shoes
Safety belt, if needed.

Procedure

1. Explain the rationale for the procedure to the client.
   a. The gait can be performed when the client can bear little or no weight on one leg or when the client has only one leg.
   b. This gait is fairly rapid and requires strong upper extremities and good balance.
2. Demonstrate the crutch-foot sequence to the client.
   a. Two crutches support the weaker extremity.
   b. Balance weight on the crutches.
   c. Move both crutches and affected leg forward.
   d. Move unaffected leg forward.
3. Assess the client's progress, and correct any mistakes as they occur.
4. Remain with client until crutch safety is ensured.

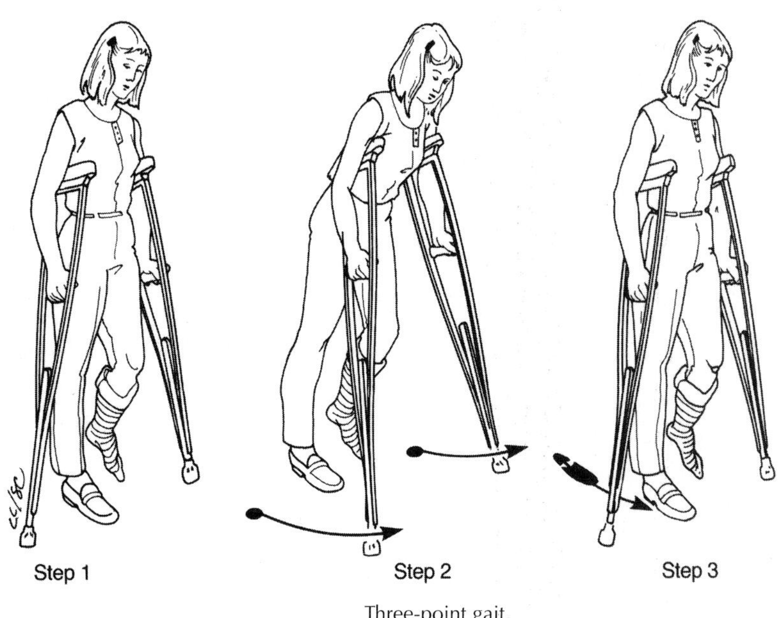

Three-point gait.

TEACHING CRUTCH WALKING: TWO-POINT GAIT

Equipment

Properly fitted crutches
Regular, hardsoled street shoes
Safety belt, if needed

Procedure

1. Explain the rationale for the procedure to the client.
   a. This procedure is a rapid version of the four-point gait.
   b. This gait requires more balance than the four-point gait.
2. Demonstrate the crutch-foot sequence to the client.
   a. Advance the right foot and the left crutch simultaneously.
   b. Advance the left foot and the right crutch simultaneously.
3. Help the client practice the gait.
4. Assess the client's progress, and correct any mistakes as they occur.

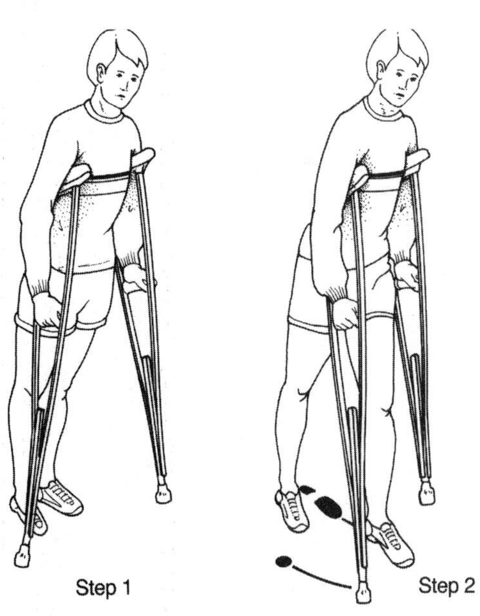

Two-point gait.

TEACHING SWING-TO GAIT AND SWING-THROUGH GAIT

Equipment

Properly fitted crutches
Regular, hardsoled street shoes

Procedure

1. Explain the rationale for the procedure to the client.
   a. These gaits are usually performed when the client's lower extremities are paralyzed.
   b. The client may use braces.
2. Demonstrate the crutch-foot sequence to the client.
   a. Move both crutches forward.
   b. Swing-to gait: Lift and swing the body to the crutches.
   c. Swing-through gait: Lift and swing the body past the crutches.
   d. Bring crutches in front of the body and repeat.
3. Help the client practice the gaits.
4. Assess the client's progress, and correct any mistakes as they occur.

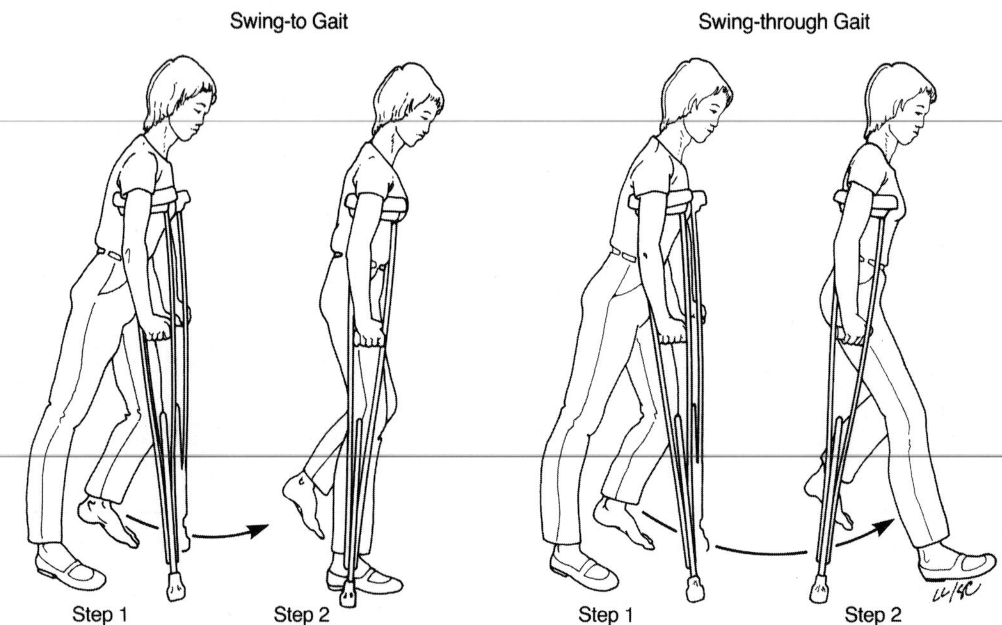

TEACHING UPSTAIRS AND DOWNSTAIRS AMBULATION WITH CRUTCHES

Equipment

Properly fitted crutches
Regular, hardsoled street shoes
Safety belt, if needed

Procedure

1. Explain the rationale for the procedure to the client.
2. Apply safety belt if client is unsteady or requires support.
3. Demonstrate the procedure using a three-point gait.

Going downstairs:

   a. Start with weight on the uninjured leg and crutches on the same level.
   b. Put crutches on the first step.
   c. Put weight on the crutch handles and transfer unaffected extremity to the step where crutches are placed.
   d. Repeat until client understands the procedure.

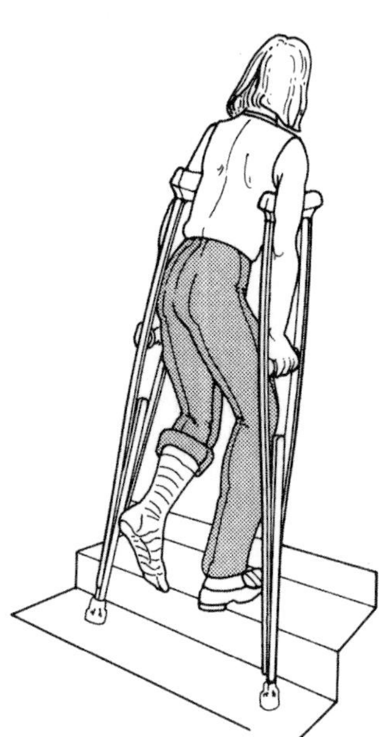

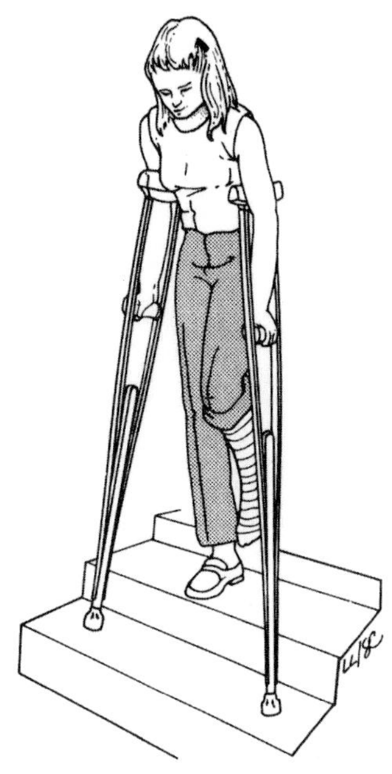

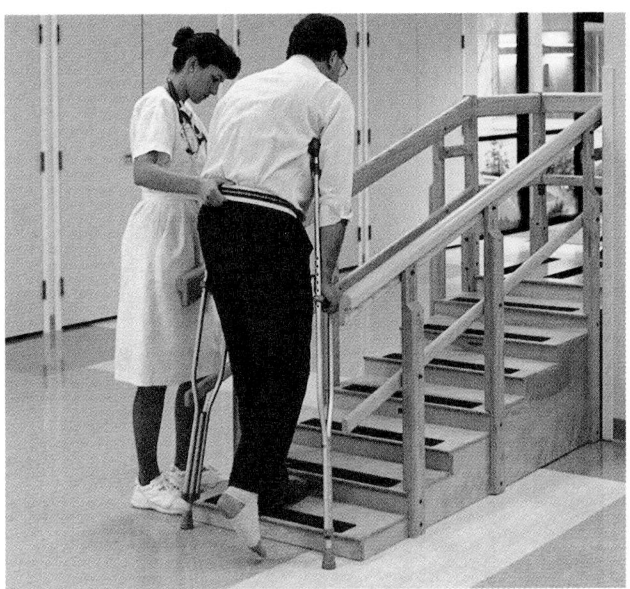

Use safety belt when client is first learning to manipulate stairs.

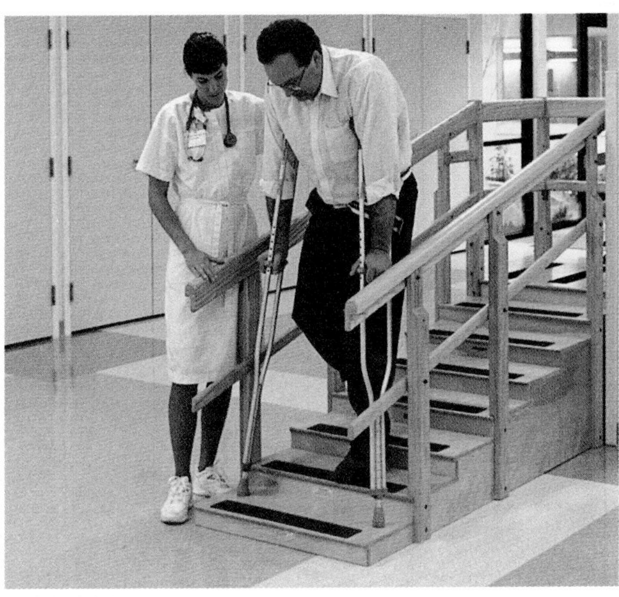

Demonstrate going up or down stairs using a three-point gait.

Going upstairs:

a. Start with the crutches and unaffected extremity on the same level.
b. Put weight on the crutch handles and lift the unaffected extremity onto the first step of the stairs.
c. Put weight on the unaffected extremity and lift other extremity and the crutches to the step.
d. Repeat until client understands the procedure.

4. Help the client practice.
5. Make sure that the client has adequate balance. Be ready to assist if necessary.
6. Assess the client's progress, and correct any mistakes as they occur.

CHARTING for Crutch Walking

- Time and distance of ambulation on crutches
- Balance
- Problems noted with technique
- Remedial teaching
- Client's perceptions of ambulation with crutches

CRITICAL THINKING APPLICATION

CLINICAL PROBLEMS	CRITICAL THINKING OPTIONS
Client states he or she is frightened of the crutches.	• Observe as the client practices the procedures to make sure that he or she is completing the steps correctly for each gait. • Explain that it takes time to become proficient. • Reassure the client that he or she will improve with continued practice. • Assess the client's ability to use the crutches and evaluate level of confidence. • Check with physician about obtaining an order for a walker until the client feels more confident.
Client fears falling while dependent on crutches.	• Slow down crutch protocol until client gains confidence at every level of mastery (e.g., four-point gait to two-point gait). • Remain with client and give verbal reassurance and feedback for improvement.
Shoulder girdle is too weak to bear client's weight for crutch support.	• Increase exercise of shoulder (biceps and triceps setting) to gain strength. • Request that physician write order for overhead frame with trapeze for shoulder exercise sets.
Slipping occurs with crutch walking.	• Check crutch tips to ensure they cover all metal or wood. • Observe the client's stance or gait to determine if it is too broad. • Be sure that floor surface is dry and free of scatter rugs.
Client complains of numbness and tingling in fingers when crutch walking.	• Remeasure distance between axilla and crutch bars to determine if two finger breadths can be inserted. • Observe client's gait to determine if he or she is leaning on crutch inappropriately.

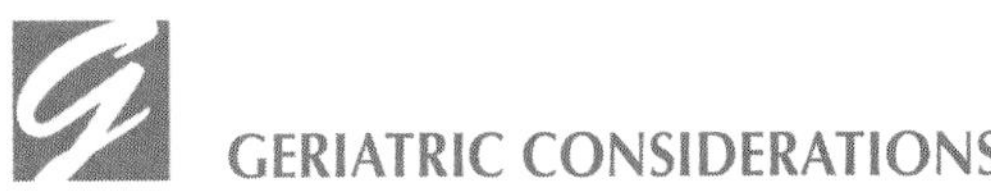

GERIATRIC CONSIDERATIONS

The elderly can suffer impaired mobility and disability due to decreased physical function or accidents.

- Nearly 23% of older people living in the community have some degree of disability.
- Persons 85 and older constitute 27% of those who have impaired mobility.
- Impaired mobility can lead to many subsequent problems, including depression, negative self-image, dependent behavior, and loss of independence.
- Effects of disability can influence the individual's body image, physical appearance, and bodily sensations.

Special assessment parameters are important for the elderly.

- Specific source of disability or impaired mobility.
- Presence of accompanying disease state: arthritis, stroke, dementia, diabetes, CHF, COPD
- Strength and function of limbs and joints; stability of gait; history of falls
- Presence of pain
- Condition of skin
- Drug effects: sedation, incontinence, orthostatic hypotension
- Motivation for rehabilitation
- Nutritional status
- Best assistive aid for client

Develop nursing care plan to meet elderly client's needs.

- Focus on disability or impaired mobility.
- Establish supportive relationship.
- Teach activities of daily living. Determine activities that must be accomplished each day for individual to care for own needs and be as independent as possible.
- Increase activities as individual progresses and is able to assume activity.
- Give positive reinforcement for all effort expended.

14

Basic Physical Assessment

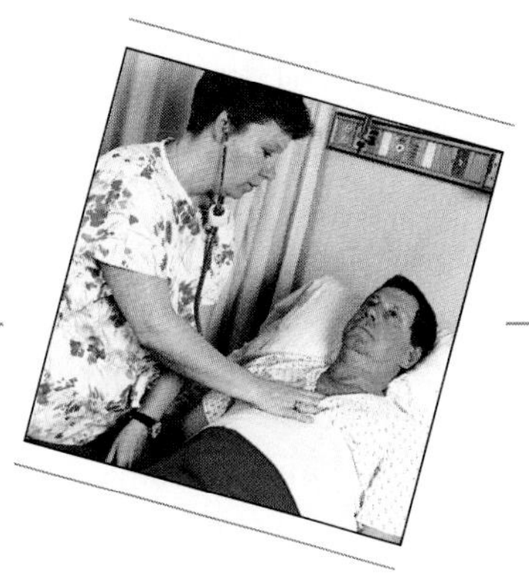

LEARNING OBJECTIVES

- Outline the essential elements obtained from a health history.
- List the four techniques of physical assessment.
- Describe the abnormal manifestations associated with each specific body system for one patient with whom you are familiar.
- List four normal responses that determine the patient's level of consciousness.
- Describe four abnormal responses in pupil assessment.
- State three assessment components of the skin.
- Describe normal and abnormal lung sounds.
- Outline the steps of breast assessment.
- Identify the four areas for heart sound auscultation.
- List at least five essential elements included in a mental status assessment.

ASSESSMENT TECHNIQUES

Basic assessment discussed in this chapter can be performed in less than 10 minutes using a stethoscope, penlight, reflex hammer, your hands, and observational skills. Although you may not be able to perform assessment rapidly at first, you will have many opportunities to practice your skills, because every client should be assessed at least once a shift.

While interviewing the client, note such characteristics as hair, skin, posture, facial expression, and body language—in other words, the general appearance of the client. Then proceed with a head-to-toe systems assessment using the four techniques of assessment: inspection, palpation, percussion, and auscultation. This IPPA sequence is used for all systems except for the abdominal assessment, which requires auscultation *before* palpation and percussion. Palpation and percussion are performed using fingers and hands to assess abnormalities of sound, such as vocal fremitus, enlarged organs, organ displacement, and chest expansion. Auscultation is accomplished by using a stethoscope to listen to breath, heart, and bowel sounds. Observe the client's response as each system is assessed.

Equipment

The stethoscope is the primary instrument used for assessment. Remember that any movement of the tubing or chest piece by clothing or hands can cause extraneous noise that obliterates the sounds you want to hear. The diaphragm piece should be applied firmly to the skin. It enhances high-pitched sounds (breath sounds, normal heart sounds, bowel sounds). The bell piece should be placed very lightly to pick up low-pitched sounds, such as vascular sounds and abnormal heart sounds. If the bell is pressed firmly, it stretches the skin and acts as a diaphragm. Other instruments used include the penlight, reflex hammer, ophthalmoscope, otoscope, and tuning fork.

HEALTH HISTORY

A total client assessment begins with a nursing health history. Using open-ended questions such as "tell me about. . . ," collect data about past health conditions, current problems, and present needs. The information is obtained through objective (observed) and subjective (stated by client) data collection.

Information obtained from the interview and the physical assessment constitutes the basis for identifying nursing diagnoses and establishing the individualized client care plan. A complete health history includes the following elements:

- *Biographic information*: age, sex, educational level, marital status, living arrangements
- *Chief complaint*: condition that brought client to health care facility
- *Present health status or illness*: onset of the problem; clinical manifestations, including severity of symptoms; pain characteristics if present
- *Health history*: general state of health, past illnesses, surgeries, hospitalizations, allergies, current medications, and general habits such as smoking
- *Family history*: age and health status of parents, siblings, and children; cause of death for immediate family members
- *Psychosocial factors, lifestyles*: cultural beliefs that influence health management; religious or spiritual beliefs
- *Nutrition*: dietary habits, preferences, or restrictions

NEUROLOGIC ASSESSMENT

The neurologic examination begins with the initial contact with the client. Evaluation of verbal responses, movement, and sensation is carried out throughout the examination. In addition, functions of the cerebrum, cerebellum, cranial nerves, spinal cord, and peripheral nerves are assessed. The level of consciousness is the most sensitive and reliable index of cerebral function.

LEVEL OF CONSCIOUSNESS

ASSESSMENT	NORMAL	ABNORMAL
Evaluate **verbal responses** If client seems awake and alert but does not respond properly, check to see if client is blind, deaf, or speaks another language	Alert Mood appropriate to situation Responds to verbal command Answers questions appropriately Speaks clearly Oriented to time, person, place and purpose Recent and remote memory intact	Drowsy Difficult to awaken Unable to give date, month, place Irritable Memory defect Difficulty finding words Does not recognize family Does not respond to own name
Observe and test **motor responses** on both sides of body	Eyes open Follows command to stick out tongue, squeeze fingers, move extremities	Eyes closed Does not follow directions to stick out tongue, squeeze fingers, or move extremities
Exert pressure on nailbed with pen Apply pressure to supraorbital ridge Pinch Achilles tendon	Responds to painful stimuli by reaching out or trying to stop pressure	Does not localize or withdraw from painful stimulus Assumes *decorticate posturing* (legs extended; feet extended with plantar flexion; arms internally rotated and flexed on chest): due to lesion of corticospinal tract near cerebral hemisphere Assumes *decerebrate posturing* (arms stiffly extended and hands turned outward and flexed; legs extended with plantar flexion): may be due to lesion in diencephalon, pons, or midbrain Assumes *flaccid posturing* (no motor response): may be due to extreme brain injury to motor area of brain *Involuntary movements* Choreiform (jerky and quick): present in Sydenham's chorea Athetoid (twisting and slow): present in cerebral palsy Tremors: hyperthyroidism, cerebellar ataxia, parkinsonism Spasms: cord-injured patients Seizures: brain injury, heat stroke, electrolyte imbalance

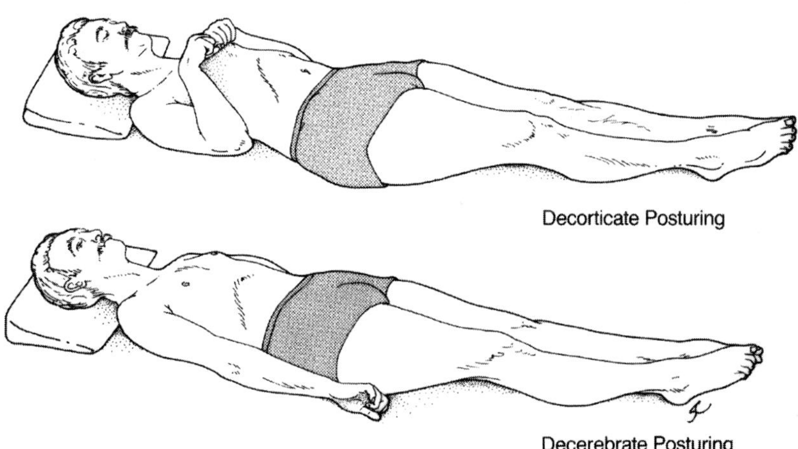

Decorticate and decerebrate posturing.

ASSESSMENT	NORMAL	ABNORMAL
		Asterixis: metabolic encephalopathy due to liver or kidney failure
PUPIL ASSESSMENT Observe **appearance of pupils** by holding eyelids open and checking for:		
Size of pupils	Diameter: 1.5–6 mm	Unilateral dilation: sign of third cranial nerve involvement Bilateral dilation: sign of upper brainstem damage Unilateral dilation and nonreactive: sign of increased intracranial pressure or ipsilateral oculomotor nerve (III) compression from tumor or injury
Shape of pupils	Round and midposition	Midposition and fixed: sign of midbrain involvement Pinpoint and fixed: sign of pontine involvement or opiate effect
Equality of pupils	Equal	Unequal: sign that parasympathetic and sympathetic nervous systems are not in synchronization
Observe **reaction to light** by using pen light in darkened room Open eyelid being tested; cover opposite eye Move light toward client's eye from side position 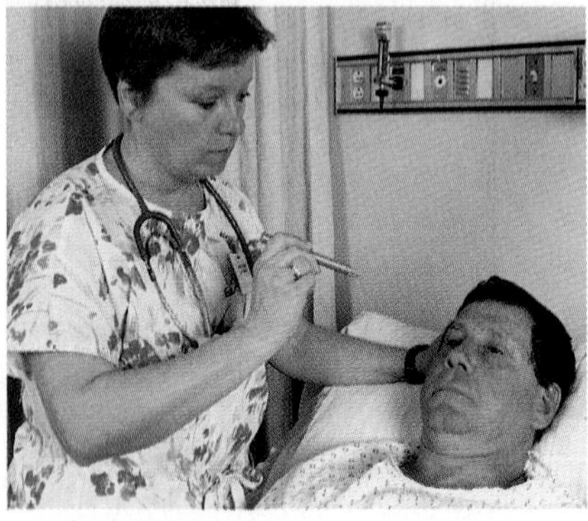	Pupil constricts promptly	Sluggish reaction: early warning of deteriorating condition Light reflex is the most important sign differentiating structural (cranial involvement) from metabolic coma due to extracranial cause (e.g., diabetic coma), which does not alter light reflex
Observe consensual **light reflex** Hold both eyelids open Shine light into one eye only Observe opposite eye	Pupil constricts	Pupil does not constrict: sign that connection between brainstem and pupils is not intact

MOTOR FUNCTION ASSESSMENT

ASSESSMENT	NORMAL	ABNORMAL
Assess bilateral **muscle strength** Test hand grip by asking client to squeeze your fingers (muscle strength is equal bilaterally)		Absent or weak muscle function on one side may be sign of hemiplegia (paralysis of one side of the body); or hemiparesis (weakness on one side); paraplegia (paralysis of the legs or lower part of the body); quadriplegia (paralysis of arms and legs)
Test arm strength by asking client to close eyes and hold arms out in front with palms up	Maintain position for 20–30 seconds	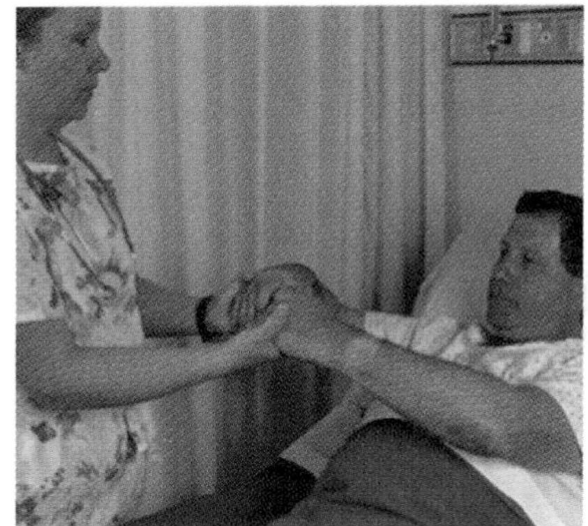
Assess **flexion** and **extension** strength in extremities Stand in front of client, place your hand in front of client, and ask client to push your hand away Place your hand on client's forearm and ask client to pull arm upward	Equal response in both arms	
Position client's leg with knee flexed and foot resting on bed; as you try to extend leg, ask client to keep foot down Place one hand on client's knee and one hand on client's ankle; ask client to straighten leg as you apply resistant force to knee and ankle	Equal response in both legs	
Assess **muscle tone** Flex and extend client's upper extremities to assess how well client resists your movements Flex and extend client's lower extremities to assess resistance	Client resistance is apparent	Increased resistance: sign of increased muscle tone from muscle rigidity or spasticity in upper motor neuron (UMN) lesions, such as with CVA and parkinsonism Decreased resistance to leg extension and arm flexion in UMN lesion (CVA) Weakness in lower motor neuron (LMN) and cerebellar lesion

ASSESSMENT	NORMAL	ABNORMAL
Assess **coordinat on** *Hand coordination* Ask client to pat both thighs as rapidly as possible Ask client to turn hands over and back in quick succession	Client able to perform coordinated movements on request	Uncoordinated movements: may be due to cerebellum or basal ganglia involvement
Ask client to touch thumb with each finger in rapid succession—repeat with other hand		Clumsy movement with cerebellar involvement
Foot coordination Place your hands close to client's feet Ask client to tap your hands alternately with the balls of feet		
Hand positioning coordination With client's eyes open, extend your hand in front of client's face Ask client to touch nose with index finger several times in rapid succession		Tremor as nose approached indicates cerebellar involvement
Repeat test with client's eyes closed		Inability to perform task with eyes closed: may be due to loss of positioning sense
Leg positioning coordination Ask client to put heel on opposite knee and to slide heel down leg to foot		
Assess **reflexes** *Blink reflex* Hold client's eyelid open Approach client's eye unexpectedly from side of head, or brush client's cornea with cotton wisp	Eyes close immediately	Absence of blink response; eyelid continuously in open position: due to fifth or seventh cranial nerve (pons) involvement
Gag and swallow reflex Open client's mouth and hold tongue down with tongue blade Touch back of pharynx on each side with applicator stick		Absence of gag and swallow reflex; inability to swallow food or liquid: due to nineth or tenth cranial nerve (medulla) involvement

ASSESSMENT	NORMAL	ABNORMAL
Plantar response Run top of pen along outer lateral aspect from heel to little toe of client's foot Continue tracing a line across ball of foot toward great toe	Toes are pointed down	Babinski response: great toe dorsiflexes; other toes fan on foot of paralyzed side in CVA, and bilaterally in spinal cord injury (SCI)
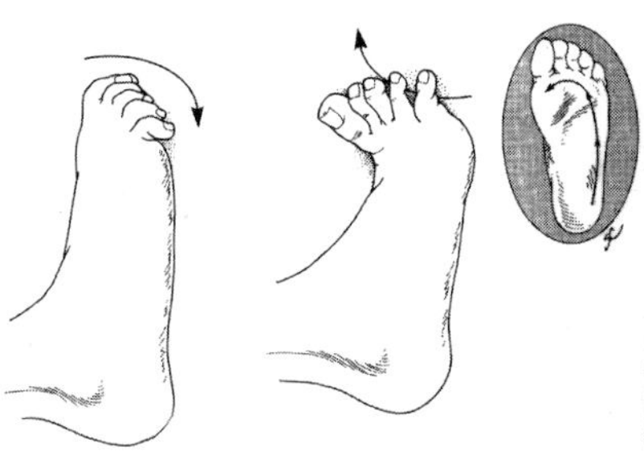	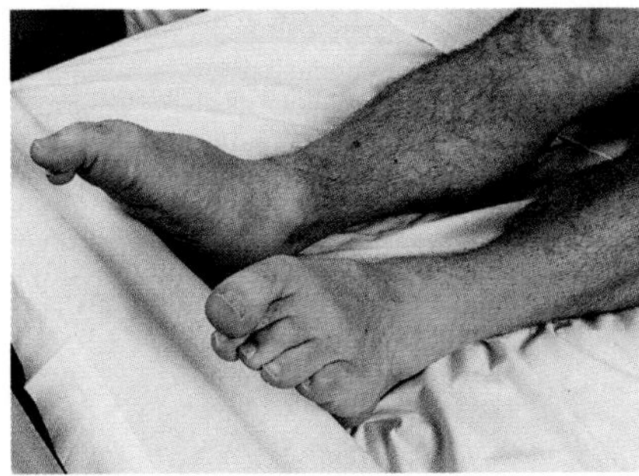	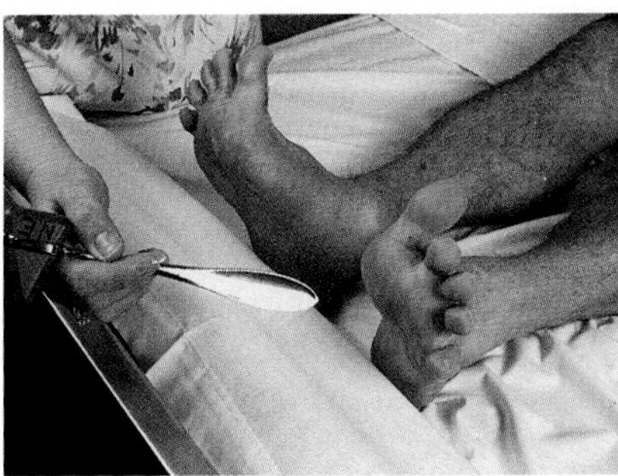
Deep tendon reflex Ask client to relax Position limb to be assessed so that muscle is somewhat stretched Using reflex hammer, strike tendon quickly	Biceps reflex: flexion at elbow and contracting of biceps muscle Triceps reflex: extension at elbow and contraction of triceps muscle	Absent or diminished: sign of cervical cord (C-5 or C-6) involvement Absent or diminished: C-7 or C-8 involvement
Assess according to scale	Knee reflex: extension of knee and contraction of quadriceps	Absent or diminished: L2-3, or L3-4 cord involvement
Grading Scale 4+ Hyperactive or exaggerated 3+ More brisk than usual but not indicative of disease state 2+ Average or normal 1+ Slightly diminished, low normal 0 No response		Indicates UMN lesion or SCI Seen with LMN lesion
SENSORY FUNCTION Assess **superficial sensations** *Pain* Ask client to close eyes Stroke or touch skin with safety pin, alternating blunt end and sharp end of pin Ask client to distinguish sharp and dull pain	Ability to distinguish between sharp and dull sensations	Alterations in pain or temperature sensations: indicate lesion in posterior horn of spinal cord or spinothalamic tract of cord
Temperature Fill two test tubes with water, one hot, one cold Ask client to close eyes and touch client's skin with test tubes	Ability to distinguish between hot and cold	

ASSESSMENT	NORMAL	ABNORMAL
Touch Ask client to close eyes Stroke cotton wisp over client's skin	Ability to identify light touch—equal bilaterally	Anesthesia = loss of light touch Hypaesthesia = decreased light touch Analgesia = loss of pain Hypalgesia = decreased pain sensation Hyperalgesia = exaggerated response to pin prick Hyperaesthesia = exaggerated response to light touch
Positioning Ask client to close eyes Grasp client's finger with your thumb and index finger Move client's finger up and down Ask client to identify direction finger is moving	Ability to identify position or mimic position with other hand	Inability to determine direction of movement: may be due to posterior column or peripheral nerve disease
VITAL SIGNS Assess Respiration Assess rate and pattern of breathing	Regular rate: 12–20 breaths per minute	Cheyne–Stokes (rhythmic increase in depth of breathing followed by period of apnea) may be due to deep cerebral or cerebellar lesion or condition altering cerebral perfusion Central neurogenic (sustained) hyperventilation due to upper brainstem involvement Ataxic (Biot's) breathing unpredictably irregular, due to lower brainstem involvement
Monitor **arterial blood gases** if signs of respiratory imbalances occur	pH: 7.35–7.45 P_{CO_2}: 35–45 mm Hg HCO_3: 22–26 mEq/L	Alterations in pH and P_{CO_2} values indicate respiratory imbalances: pH below 7.35 and P_{CO_2} above 45: sign of respiratory acidosis (hypoventilation) pH above 7.45 and P_{CO_2} below 35: sign of respiratory alkalosis (hyperventilation) HCO_3 above 26 indicates metabolic compensation for chronic respiratory acidosis (hypoventilation)
Assess temperature If client is semiresponsive or nonresponsive, take rectal or tympanic temperature.	Ability to maintain normal body temperature (approximately 98.6°F, or 37°C)	Inability to maintain normal temperature: may be due to damage to hypothalamus No sweating below level of injury: due to spinal cord injury Hypothermia

ASSESSMENT	NORMAL	ABNORMAL
Assess apical and radial pulses. Note character of pulses Count heart rate Count radial pulse rate	Regular rhythm Rate 60–100 BPM Apical and radial rates are equal	Fast heart rate due to decreased blood volume, arrhythmia, heart failure Irregular rhythm with premature beats due to hypoxia, cardiac irritability, or electrolyte imbalance
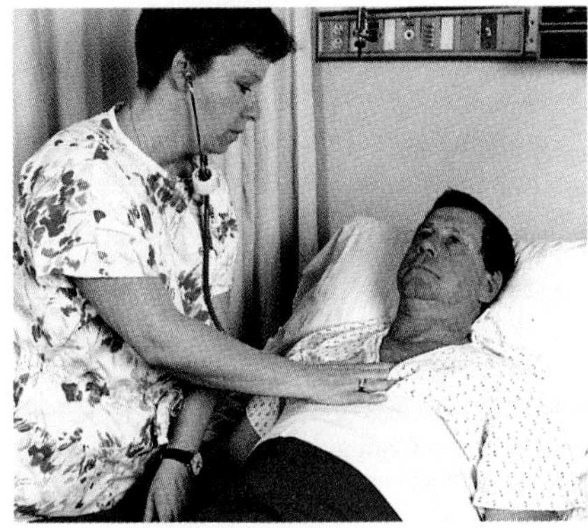		
Assess **blood pressure** Position neurologic clients in low to semi-Fowler's position	Normal pressure (range 120/80–140/90)	Systolic blood pressure rises with diastolic pressure remaining same (widening pulse pressure): sign of increased intracranial pressure Blood pressure over 140/90 mm Hg: sign of hypertension Blood pressure below 95/60 mm Hg: sign of hypotension

ASSESSMENT OF THE HEAD AND NECK

The names of the regions of the head are derived from the bones that form the skull. Knowing the names of the bones and regions of the skull can assist in describing the location of the physical findings.

An understanding of the function of each lobe of the brain allows the nurse to be able to identify potential client problems when an injury occurs to that portion of the brain.

The brain comprises three segments: the brainstem, cerebrum, and the cerebellum. There are 12 cranial nerves, which are discussed later in this chapter, and 31 spinal nerves with the respective dorsal and ventral roots.

The brainstem is divided into four sections: The *diencephalon* comprises the thalamus, which screens and relays sensory impulses to the cortex, and the hypothalamus, which regulates the autonomic nervous system, stress response, sleep, appetite, body temperature, water balance, and emotions. The *midbrain* is responsible for motor coordination and conjugate eye movements. The *pons* controls involuntary respiratory reflexes and contains projection tracts between the spinal cord, medulla, and brain. The *medulla* contains cardiac, respiratory, vomiting, and vasomotor centers. In addition, all afferent and efferent nerve tracts must pass between the spinal cord and brain through the medulla.

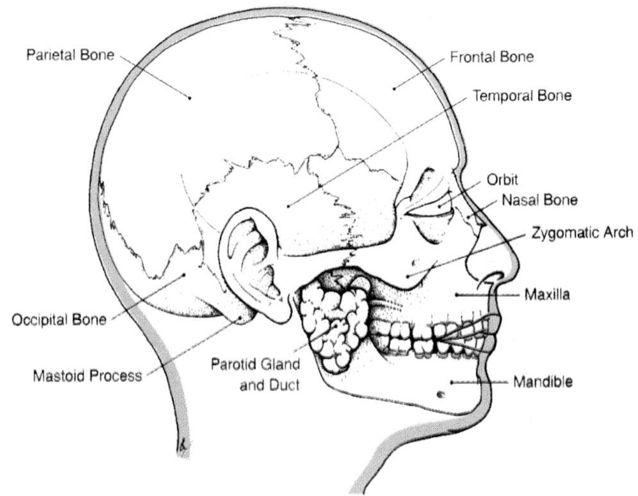

The cerebral hemispheres have an outer layer formed by cellular gray matter, called the cerebral cortex. The two cerebral hemispheres are divided into four

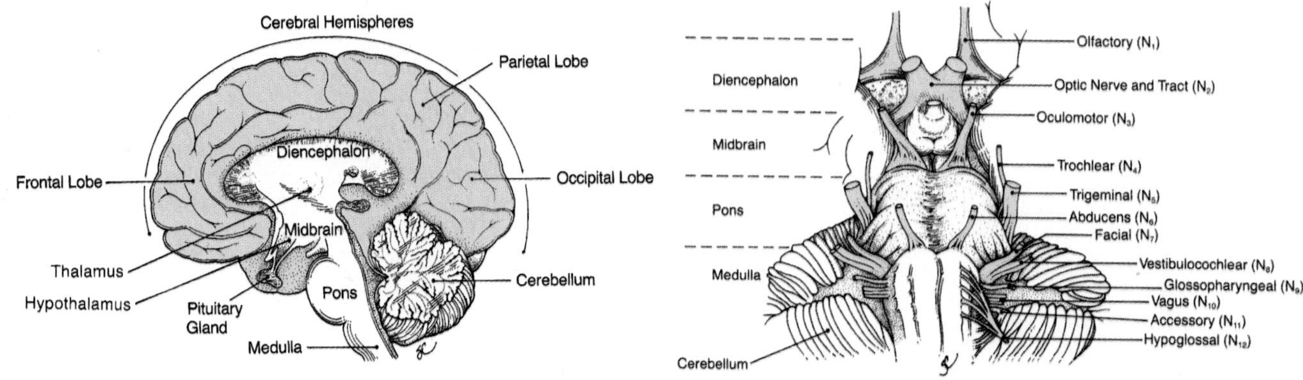

TABLE 14–1. Cranial Nerves and Their Function

	Cranial Nerve	Function	Testing Cranial Nerves
I	Olfactory	Sensory nerve	Recognizes odor in each nostril separately (e.g., coffee)
II	Optic	Sensory nerve: conducts sensory information from the retina	Demonstrates visual acuity: can read newsprint
III	Oculomotor	Motor nerve: controls four of the six extraocular muscles; raises eyelid and controls the constrictor pupillae and ciliary muscles of the eyeball	Responds to light: pupils constrict
IV	Trochlear	Motor nerve: controls the superior oblique eye muscle	Follows moving object horizontally and vertically
V	Trigeminal	Mixed nerve with three sensory branches and one motor branch: the ophthalmic branch supplies the corneal reflex	Demonstrates normal facial sensation; clenches teeth with no lateral jaw deviation; blinks as wisp touched to cornea
VI	Abducens	Motor nerve: controls the lateral rectus muscle of the eye	Moves eyes laterally
VII	Facial	Mixed nerve: anterior tongue receives sensory supply, motor supply to glands of nose, palate lacrimal submaxillary, and sublingual; motor branch supplies hyoid elevators and muscles of expression and closes eyelid	Elevates eyebrows; puffs cheeks; recognizes tastes (sugar, salt)
VIII	Acoustic	Sensory nerve with two divisions: hearing and semicircular canals	Hears whisper with each ear separately
IX	Glossopharyngeal	Mixed nerve: motor innervates parotid gland; sensory innervates auditory tube and posterior portion of taste buds	Demonstrates gag reflex to tongue blade when touched to back of tongue
X	Vagus	Mixed nerve: motor branches to the pharyngeal and laryngeal muscles and to the viscera of the thorax and abdomen; sensory portion supplies the pinna of the ear, thoracic, and abdominal viscera	Same as IX
XI	Accessory	Motor nerve: innervates the sternocleidomastoid and trapezius muscles	Shrugs shoulders
XII	Hypoglossal	Motor nerve: controls tongue muscles	Sticks tongue out in midline without deviation

major lobes. The frontal lobe controls emotions, judgments, motor function, and the motor speech area. The parietal lobe integrates general sensations; interprets pain, touch, and temperature; and governs discrimination. The temporal lobe contains the auditory center and sensory speech center. The occipital lobe controls the visual area. The cerebellum coordinates muscle movement, posture, equilibrium, and muscle tone.

The 12 cranial nerves are summarized in Table 14–1. The 2nd through 12th nerves arise from the brainstem.

The cranial nerves are 12 pairs of parasympathetic nerves with their nuclei along the brainstem.

ASSESSMENT	NORMAL	ABNORMAL
EYE ASSESSMENT		
Note **visual acuity** by observing client performance of activities of daily living	Adequate performance of activities of daily living	Hyperopia (farsightedness) Myopia (nearsightedness)
Factors influencing visual acuity include client's previous status and age	Appropriate responses to environment	Cataract (opacification of the lens) Enucleation (loss of an eye): may have prothesis in place
Note exact location, size, and color of any **external lesions** Palpate for mobility and firmness	No external lesions	Circumocular ecchymosis: may be sign of basal skull fracture Xanthalasma (small, yellowish, well-circumscribed plaques): may appear on eyelids of clients with lipid disorders *Example*: atherosclerosis

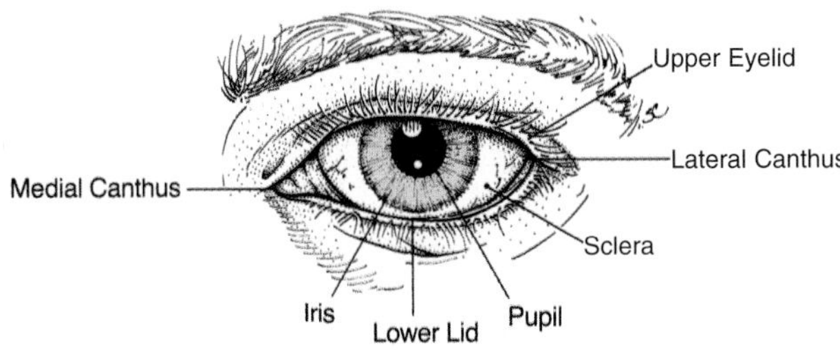

ASSESSMENT	NORMAL	ABNORMAL
Note **equality of eyelid movement**	Eyelids are equal in movement	Ptosis (paralytic drooping of the upper eyelid)
Note color, consistency, amount, and origin of **discharge** from eyes	No discharge	Sty, or hordeolum Thick white discharge: may be due to conjunctivitis
Note **internal lesions**	No internal lesions	Conjunctival or ciliary injection (dilatation of the blood vessels)
Assess differences between **pupil size and reaction** Note presence of hemorrhage	Both pupils are the same size	Anisocoria (indicates unequal pupil size): may be indicative of neurologic trauma or deficit Corneal edema (very soft, movable mass that looks like raw egg white): frequently occurs in clients who have increased intracranial pressure Arcus senilis (partial or complete whitish circle near the outer edge of the cornea): usually due to aging

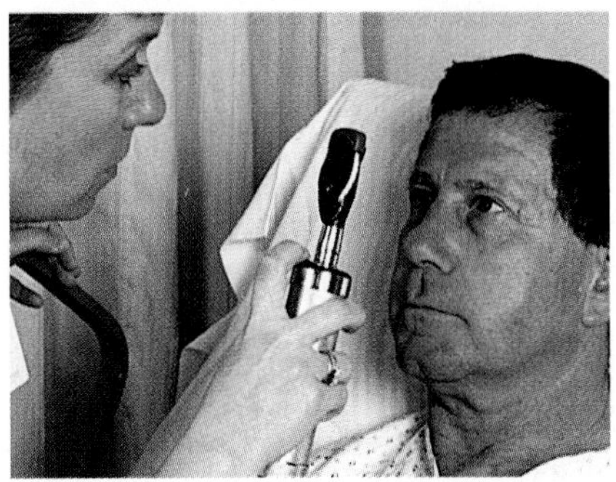

ASSESSMENT	NORMAL	ABNORMAL
EAR ASSESSMENT		
Note **auditory acuity** by asking client to indicate if he or she hears normal sounds as you make them	Adequate responses to normal sounds Auditory changes due to aging	Deafness or impaired hearing: excess cerumen in auditory canal Abnormal sounds in the ears (ringing or buzzing) may be caused by ototoxic drugs
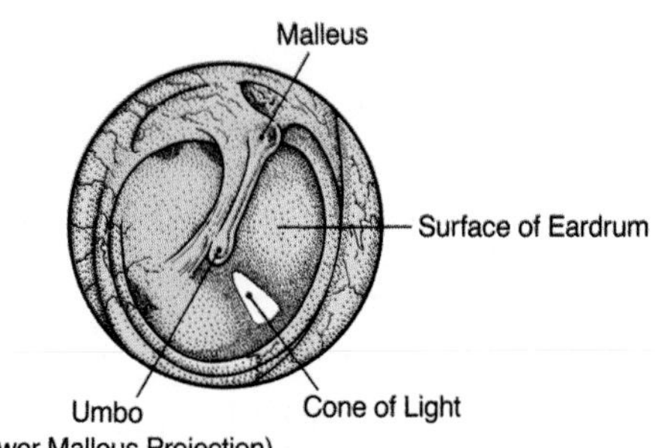		
Note exact size, color, and location of any **external** lesions Palpate lesions for mobility and firmness	No external lesions	Battle's sign (ecchymosis behind the ear): may be sign of basilar skull fracture
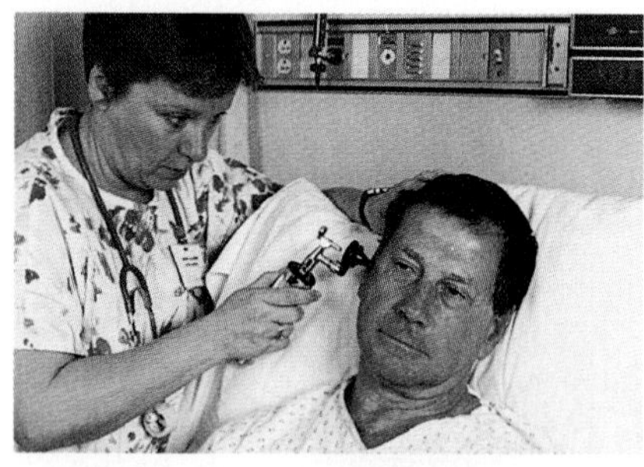		
Note color, quantity, and consistency of any **discharge** from the ears Test clear fluid for glucose using a Labstix	No discharge Glucose test negative	Cerebrospinal fluid leak: may be due to head injury. If drainage is blood and CSF, it will develop a "halo" with a reddish area in the center surrounded by a whitish circle if placed on white material Perforation of tympanic membrane: serosanguineous or purulent drainage Glucose test of clear drainage is positive if CSF
NOSE ASSESSMENT		
Note any **structural changes** in the nose by observing client breathe Gently occlude one nostril at a time; ask client to breathe through the nonoccluded nostril	Regular breathing with mouth closed Breathing through nonoccluded nostril	Breathing through the mouth only: furuncles may occlude breathing Obstruction in the nose due to deviated nasal septum or excessive mucus secretions
Note color, quantity, and consistency of any **discharge** from the nose	Minimal discharge	Cerebrospinal fluid leak (fluid tests positive for glucose with Labstix) Copious, watery-to-thick, mucopurulent discharge: may be due to acute rhinitis

ASSESSMENT	NORMAL	ABNORMAL
MOUTH AND LIP ASSESSMENT Note size, color, and location of any **external lesions** Palpate for mobility and firmness	No external lesions	Excessive build-up of mucous secretions Dehydrated mouth or lips Fissures Pressure sores Necrosis
Note size, color, and location of any **internal lesions** Palpate for mobility and firmness	No internal lesions	Candidiasis (a fungal infection indicated by adherent, white patches)
NECK ASSESSMENT Note any **lesion or swelling** in the neck Ask client to relax and flex neck slightly Palpate the neck, using the pads of your fingers to move the skin and underlying tissues	Occasional small, mobile discrete, nontender lymph nodes	Enlarged, tender immobile nodes

ASSESSMENT OF THE SKIN

The skin is the body's first line of defense against disease and injury. It is made up of three layers: the epidermis, the dermis, and the subcutaneous tissues.

The epidermis is divided into two avascular, or bloodless, layers: an outer layer that consists of dead keratinized cells and an inner layer that consists of live cells where keratin and melanin are formed. The dermis contains blood vessels, connective tissue, sebaceous glands, and some of the hair follicles. The subcutaneous tissues contain the remainder of the hair follicles, fat, and the sweat glands.

Hair, nails, sweat glands, and sebaceous glands are appendages of the skin. There are two types of sweat glands: eccrine and apocrine. Eccrine glands are distributed over most of the body except for the palms and soles. These glands help control body temperature through their sweat production. The apocrine glands are found mainly in the axillary and genital areas and are stimulated by emotional stress. Bacterial decomposition of aprocrine sweat glands causes adult body odor.

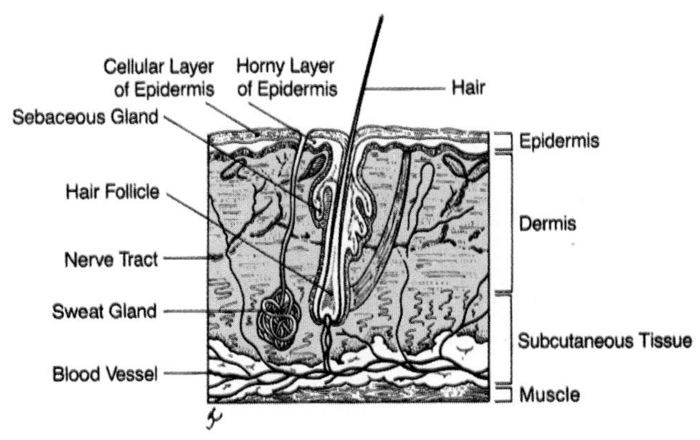

ASSESSMENT	NORMAL	ABNORMAL
Note **color** of the skin by assessing the oral mucous membranes, the conjunctiva, and the nail beds	Pink, tan, or brown, depending on the client's basic skin color	Pallor (decrease in color) *Example*: anemia from acute blood loss (hemorrhage), renal failure, dietary deficiencies, or arterial insufficiency

ASSESSMENT	NORMAL	ABNORMAL
		Jaundice (icterus): due to the presence of conjugated or unconjugated bilirubin in the blood and tissues; appears most frequently in the face and sclerae; seen best under natural light *Example*: liver disease Cyanosis (blue, bluegray, or purple discoloration of the skin and mucous membranes): caused by hypoxia, a result of an increased amount of reduced hemoglobin Peripheral: seen in nail beds and earlobes *Example*: vasoconstriction, venous insufficiency Central: seen in nail beds, lips (circumoral), and oral mucosa Erythema (redness of the skin): caused by capillary congestion; occurs with inflammation or infection; usually a local finding
Note **pigmentation** 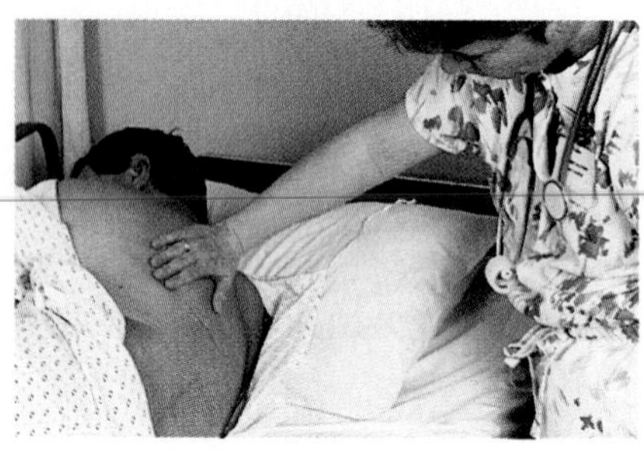		Hyperpigmentation (especially in skin creases) *Example*: use of oral contraceptives, pregnancy, Addison's disease, and hyperthyroidism
Note **turgor** and **mobility**	Smooth and elastic	Tight or stretched and difficult to move: due to local or generalized edema
Pinch skin over the sternum If the fold persists, skin turgor is poor	Resilient and supple	Wrinkled: due to dehydration caused by rapid weight loss; appears as folds of skin on upper arms or abdomen Thin and translucent (parchment) *Example*: chronic steroid use Thin, shiny, and smooth with alopecia on lower extremities

ASSESSMENT	NORMAL	ABNORMAL
		Example: chronic arterial insufficiency
Press finger firmly for 5 seconds into skin on top of foot or inner ankle bone 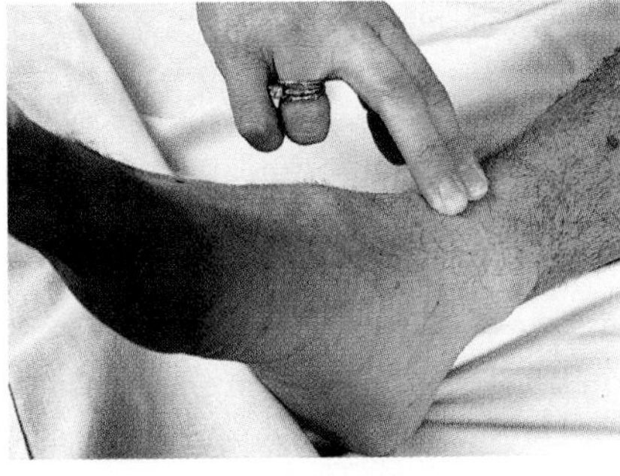	Resilient and no depression remains after pressure released	Pitting edema: excess interstitial fluid *Example:* congestive heart failure, renal failure, cirrhosis of the liver, venous stasis
Note **moistness** and **temperature** of the skin	Warm and dry	Warm (hot) and moist due to temperature elevation Cool and moist (cold and clammy): may be due to shock states Abnormally dry: may be due to dehydration, decreased sebaceous gland secretions, or the excessive use of soap
Assess for **sensation**—response to external stimuli	Feels touch, sensitive to heat and cold and pressure	Absence of touch or pain sensation *Example:* spinal cord injury or nerve damage Diminished heat and cold sensation *Example:* peripheral vascular disease Itching and tingling *Example:* peripheral vascular disease, peripheral neuropathy, allergy
Note **lesions** on the skin Physical characteristics include color, elevation, shape, mobility, and contents	No lesions present	Macules (flat localized changes in color) *Example:* petechiae, first-degree burns, purpura Papules, plaques, nodules (solid, elevated, varying in size) *Example:* psoriasis, xanthomas Wheals (elevated, circumscribed, transient) *Example:* urticaria, insect bites Vesicles and bullae (clear, fluid-filled pockets between skin layers) *Example:* second-degree burns Pustules (vesicles or bullae filled with exudate) *Example:* furuncles, acne

ASSESSMENT OF THE CHEST: LUNGS, BREASTS, AND HEART

The chest, or thorax area, extends from the base of the neck to the diaphragm. The overall shape of the thorax should be elliptical, although deformities such as barrel chest, pigeon chest, or funnel chest do occur. Total assessment includes the external aspect: the nurse should observe for movement, posture, shape, and symmetry, especially of the breast and axilla area, and the internal components of the lungs and the heart.

The lungs anteriorly extend from 2 to 4 cm above the inner third of the clavicle to the eighth rib at the midaxillary line and the sixth rib at the midclavicular line.

Posteriorly the lungs extend from the third thoracic spinous process and descend to the tenth process or, on deep inspiration, to the twelfth process.

Chest assessment begins with inspection, proceeds to palpation, and then to auscultation. Breath sounds of clients differ due to the depth of breathing, underlying disease, or obesity. Because of these differences, it is difficult to compare the breath sounds of one client with another. The basic principle to remember when auscultating the lungs is to do a comparison between the right and left lung. To make these comparisons, begin auscultating at the apices of one lung, alternating sides as you work down through both lungs. By comparing similar areas in both lungs, you can note changes and determine causes for these changes more easily.

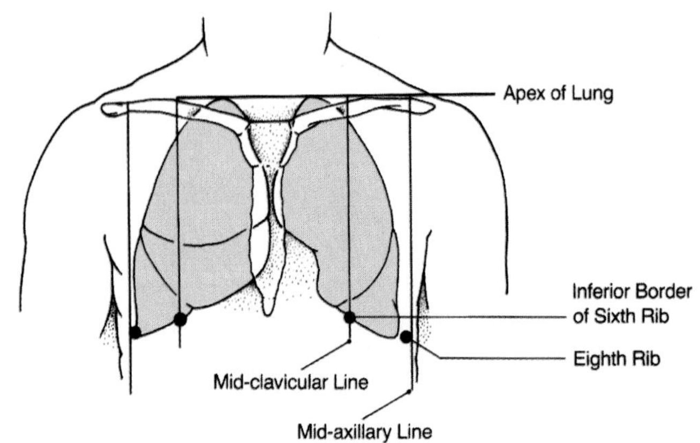

Anterior anatomical relationship of lungs to skeletal structure.

Examination of the chest usually proceeds from posterior to anterior. For posterior assessment of the lungs, place the client in an upright sitting position with shoulders pulled forward. For anterior assessment, the client can be sitting or supine (especially if female). If the client is lying on his or her side, the lung closest to the bed is mechanically compressed, and true lung sounds cannot be heard.

Ask the client to breathe a little deeper than usual through the mouth. Breathing through the nose produces extra sounds that mask true lung sounds.

The heart is located directly behind the sternum, with the left ventricle projecting into the left chest. The heart is usually thought to be in the left chest for two reasons: the left ventricle produces the most movement

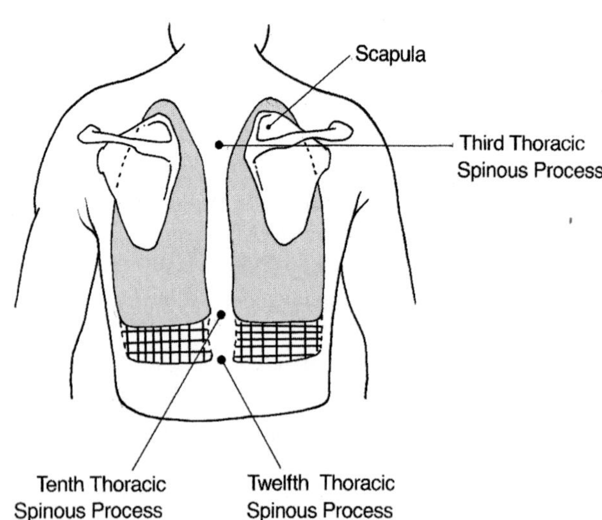

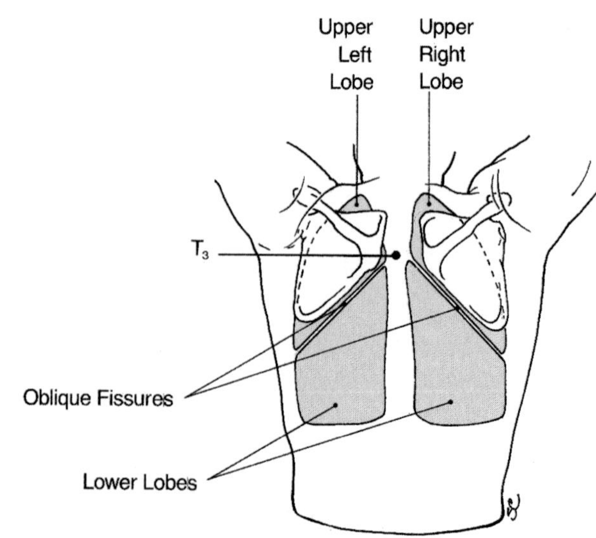

Posterior relationship of lung lobes to skeletal structures.

(ventricular contraction), and three of the valve sound areas are located to the left of the sternum.

The action of the heart should be assessed both proximally and distally. Proximal assessment involves evaluating heart sounds, heart rate, and rhythm to obtain information about the mechanical activity of the heart. Distal assessment involves evaluating the peripheral pulses to obtain information about the effectiveness of the heart's pumping action.

One method for assessing heart sounds is to start at the aortic area, moving slowly across to the pulmonic area, down to the tricuspid area, and over to the mitral area. This same general progression can also be used in reverse, starting at the mitral area and progressing up to the aortic area. Most clinicians begin the assessment at the mitral area, which is the point of maximum impulse and where the apical pulse is the loudest.

The most important point to remember in heart assessment is to use the same method every time, repeating the same steps in the same sequence. By using one systematic approach, you learn how to compare the different sounds more easily and not neglect to listen to all areas on the chest.

ASSESSMENT	NORMAL	ABNORMAL
CHEST INSPECTION		
Increased respiratory rate may be due to fever, pain	A normal or increased rate does not assume a normal tidal volume	Clients may have an increased rate to compensate for decreased tidal volume, but the resultant minute volume is still not sufficient. (Normal minute volume is 6–8 L/minute.) Increased depth: due to neurologic disease, intracranial pressure (ICP) from trauma, drug overdose, exertion, fear, or anxiety Decreased depth: due to neurologic disease, ICP from trauma, drug overdose, respiratory disease, or pneumothorax
Note the **general appearance** of the chest and movement when client breathes	Straight spine, level shoulders	Breathes sitting forward with arms on pillows or overbed table (present with emphysema)
	Relaxed breathing; rib cage moves symmetrically with respirations	Uses accessory muscles (i.e., scalene, trapezius, sternocleidomastoid, or pectoralis)
Estimate the anterior–posterior diameter		Intercostal or sternal retractions (present with obstruction and increased effort with atelectasis)
Note **shape of chest**	Anterior–posterior dimension is half of lateral dimension	Anterior–posterior dimension increased in emphysema (barrel chest) Deformities such as scoliosis (lateral curvature), kyphosis (forward curvature), or kyphoscoliosis

ASSESSMENT	NORMAL	ABNORMAL
Note **position of ribs**	Slant downward	Horizontal is common in COPD Bulging of interspaces during exhalation with retraction on inhalation (present with asthma and emphysema) Chest tilted to one side when client sits or stands: may be due to pain in ribs or chest wall or trauma (i.e., fractured ribs or surgery such as a thoracotomy) Flail chest: occurs when four or more ribs are broken; area collapses inward during inhalations and outward on exhalation

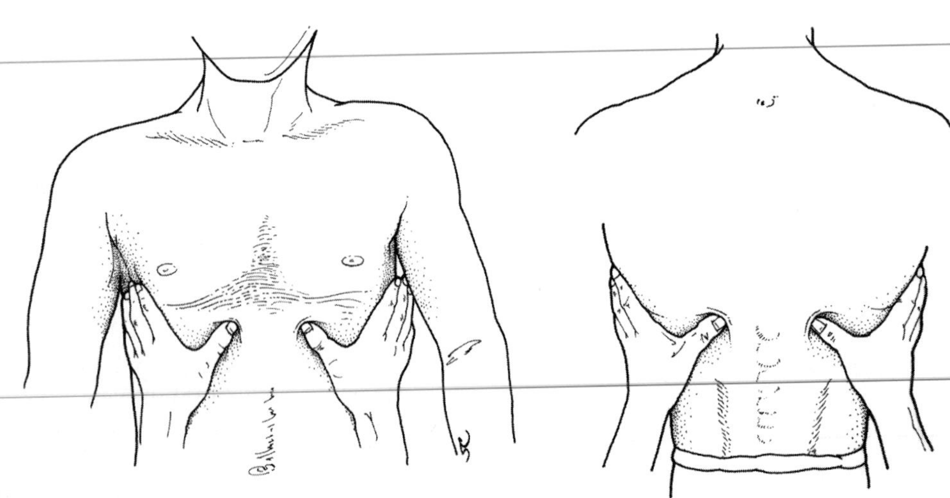

Measure chest excursion while client takes deep breath

ASSESSMENT	NORMAL	ABNORMAL
CHEST PALPATION Measure chest excursion: place hands parallel to 10th rib (under scapulae) with thumbs beside spine. Bunch up fold of skin pushing thumbs medially. Ask client to inhale. For anterior assessment, place hands over lower thorax, push medially, then have client inhale. Note equidistant lateral movement of hands	On inhalation, the thumbs move equidistant away from midline indicating equal expansion	Asymmetrical (unequal) chest expansion occurs with pneumothorax, fractured ribs, atelectasis, or when client's chest splints due to pain

ASSESSMENT	**NORMAL**	**ABNORMAL**
BREAST ASSESSMENT Inspect **size, symmetry** and **contour** of breasts, comparing one side with the other Place client in sitting position Have client remove clothing from waist up Have client raise arms over her head	Size varies with each client Breasts should be fairly equal in size and contour and symmetric in position	Masses, skin thickening, dimpling, or flattened areas: indicate possible cancer
Color, edema, and **venous pattern of skin**	Normal skin color with darker area surrounding nipples No edema or prominent vessels	Erythema: indicates infection or inflammatory carcinoma Edema or increased venous prominence: indicates carcinoma
Inspect **size and shape of nipples** Note direction in which they point, and any **rashes** or **discharge** To palpate breasts, position client supine or on side	Simple inversion of nipples is common	Flattening, nipple retraction, or axis deviation of nipple points: may be due to fibrosis associated with cancer Ulcerations of nipples and areola: may be due to Paget's disease Discharge: may not be malignant but should be observed closely
Place a pillow under the shoulder of the side being examined Using three fingers in a circular motion, compress breast tissue gently against chest wall Systematically examine entire breast, top to bottom, moving medially to laterally into the axilla	Soft, elastic tissue with mobile nodules: indicates cystic disease 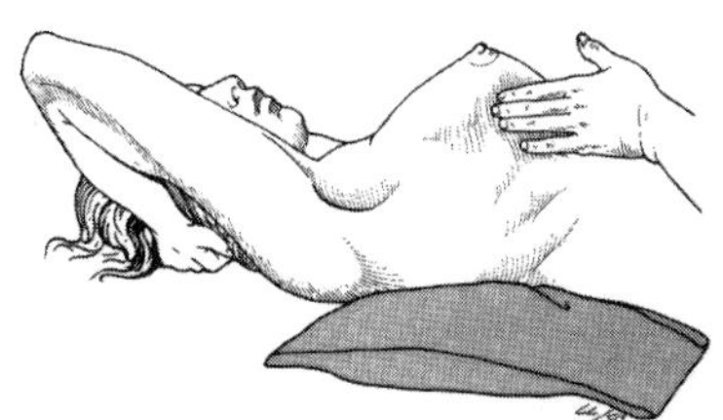	Hard nodules fixed to skin or underlying tissue may indicate cancer When nodules are present Describe location and quadrant of breast where found Note size in centimeters Describe consistency and shape Note tenderness and mobility of nodule in relationship to underlying tissue
Palpate nipples Compress nipple and areola between thumb and index finger to inspect for discharge	No discharge or small amount of milky discharge in previously nursing mother	Bloody discharge: may indicate papilloma
Note **elasticity** Observe for erection of nipple with palpation	Elastic, no retraction of nipple	Loss of elasticity: indicates possible cancer Inversion, flattening, or retraction: may indicate cancer
LUNG ASSESSMENT Complete a **general assessment** of the lungs *Respiratory rate* *Respiratory depth or volume*	12–20 respirations/minute Normal depth is equal to about 500 mL	Increased respiratory rate: may be due to increased metabolic needs (fever), mechanical injury, surgery, or trauma to chest wall

ASSESSMENT	NORMAL	ABNORMAL
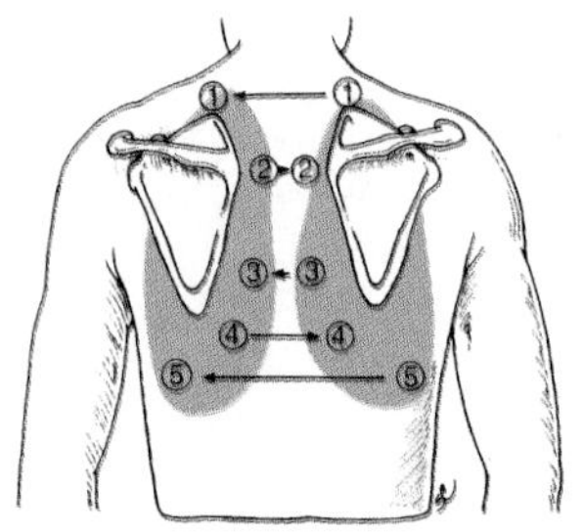	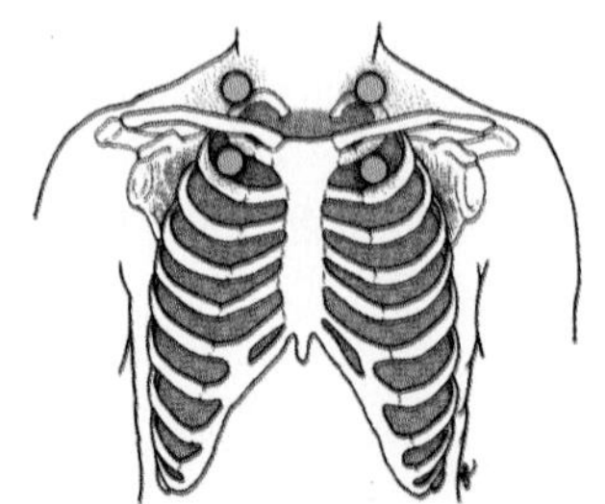 Stethoscope placement sites for posterior (left) and anterior (right) auscultation of breath	
CHEST AUSCULTATION Note location and quality of **lung sounds**		
Bronchial sounds Heard over the trachea above the sternal notch Note presence of adventitious (extra) sounds, such as crackles, wheezes, and rhonchi, or friction rub 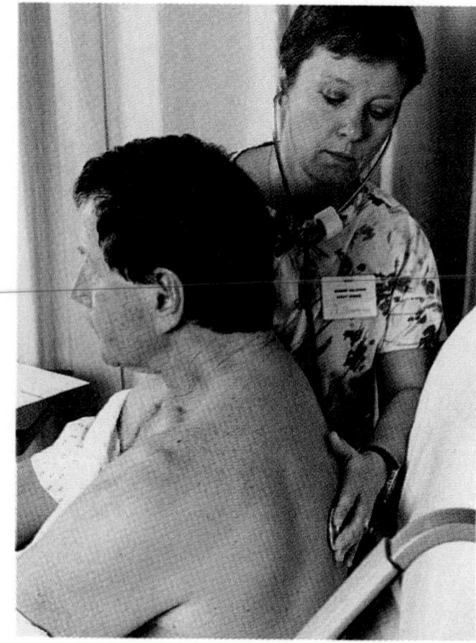	High pitch and amplitude Harsh, loud, tubular quality Expiration longer than inspiration No extra sounds heard	*Discontinuous Sounds:* *Crackles* are due to sudden opening of closed airways, indicating hypoventilation; usually heard at end of inspiration in dependent areas of bedridden clients or in early CHF. Simulate by rubbing hair together in front of your ear. *Continuous Sounds:* *Wheezes* are produced by air passing through airways narrowed by edema, spasm or mucus; may be heard in inspiration but more often heard on expiration in the chest and at the mouth; are high-pitched and musical; may clear on coughing. *Rhonchi* are similar to wheezes but louder and coarser, usually heard on expiration *Pleural friction rub* produced when inflamed pleurae rub together in the absence of normal pleural fluid; localized, high-pitched, jerky, and scratchy; frequently transient; may be heard on inspiration and expiration *Stridor* is an inspiratory wheeze heard in the neck due to partial obstruction at the tracheal or laryngeal level
Bronchovesicular breath sounds Heard over the mainstem bronchi below the clavicles and adjacent to the sternum, between scapulae	Moderate to high pitch, with moderate amplitude Hollow, muffled quality Inspiration and expiration equal in duration	Bronchial or bronchovesicular sounds heard in the perimeter where vesicular sounds are expected indicate consolidation such as pneumonia. The client's

ASSESSMENT	NORMAL	ABNORMAL
		spoken and whispered words are also clearly heard by the examiner over consolidated lung areas.
Normal (Vesicular) breath sounds Heard over lung parenchyma (Heart will mask breath sounds on the left side.) Lungs extend anteriorly to the sixth intercostal space Lungs extend posteriorly to T-10 on expiration, to T-12 on deep inspiration	Low to medium pitch, with low amplitude Soft, whooshing quality Inspiration two to three times longer than expiration	Breath sounds may be absent over areas of atelectasis, pneumothorax, or pleural effusion Breath sounds are decreased (faint) with hypoventilation, early atelectasis, and COPD
HEART ASSESSMENT Evaluate **atrioventricular heart sounds** (S_1 heart sound). Use diaphragm of stethoscope *Mitral valve sounds* Heard best at left, fifth intercostal space at, or medial to, the midclavicular line	S_1 (the first heart sound, a combination of the mitral and tricuspid closure) heard best over the mitral and tricuspid areas. S_1 louder than S_2 in this area	Heart sounds not heard in the area prescribed (e.g., with left ventricular hypertrophy, mitral sound moves laterally)
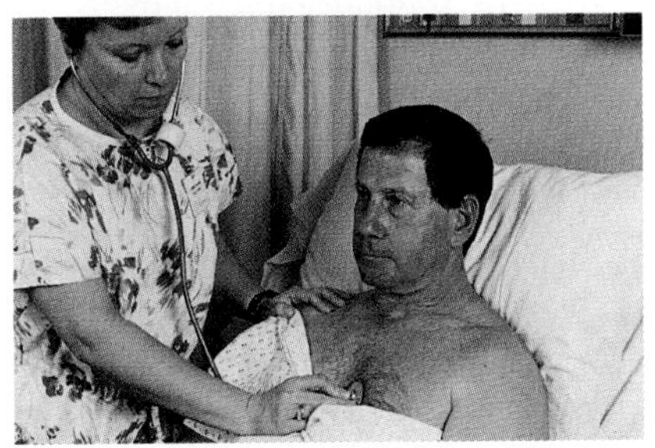		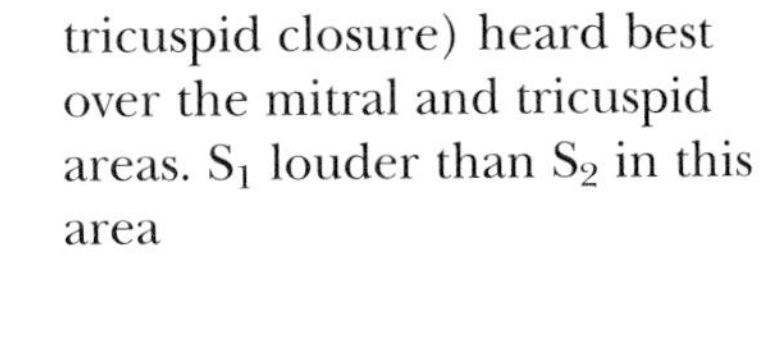
Tricuspid valve sounds Heard best at fifth intercostal space, left sternal border	S_1 also heard at this area and is louder than S_2	
Evaluate **semilunar heart sounds** (S_2 heart sounds) *Aortic valve sounds* Heard best at second intercostal space, right sternal border	S_2 (the second heart sound, a combination of the aortic and pulmonic closure): heard best over the aortic and pulmonic areas	Sounds altered with aortic stenosis and hypertension (accentuated sound)
Pulmonic valve sounds Heard best at second intercostal space, left sternal border	Part of S_2. Is louder than S_1 in this area. May be heard separately from aortic closure if client inhales deeply	Accentuated with pulmonary hypertension
Evaluate presence of **diastolic heart sounds** Use bell of stethoscope—place lightly on chest with client in left side lying position	Quiet and low-pitched	
S_3 (ventricular gallop) Heard just after S_2, at the apex or at lower, left sternal border	May be a physiologic finding in children and young adults Abnormal finding in older clients	Almost always signifies heart failure

ASSESSMENT	NORMAL	ABNORMAL
S_4 (atrial gallop) Heard just before S_1, at the apex or at lower, left sternal border; occurs when blood flow from atrial contraction meets increased resistance in ventricle	Normal finding in elderly	Heard in older individual with hypertension
Assess for **heart murmurs**, heard between heart sounds Produced by atypical flow of blood through the heart (e.g., irregularity or partial obstruction, increased flow in normal area, flow into dilated chamber, flow through abnormal passage); regurgitant flow Occurs during systole (between S_1 and S_2) or during diastole (between S_2 and S_1)	Faint sound More common during systole Often found in children and young adults	Faint or loud enough to be heard without a stethoscope Occurs during systole or diastole (diastolic murmurs are almost always pathologic)—found in older clients with heart disease or infants and children with congenital heart defects
Evaluate the **apical pulse** when assessing for general heart rate and rhythm of contractions Palpate and view pulse on chest wall if client's chest wall is thin enough Auscultate at the apex of the heart (left, fifth intercostal space at the midclavicular line)	Regular rhythm Heart rate: 60–100 beats/minute Moderate bradycardia common in well-trained athletes Mild tachycardia possible with stress, infection, or fever	Irregular rhythm (dysrhythmia) may be regularly irregular or irregularly irregular (i.e., atrial fibrillation) Bradycardia (less than 60 beats/minute) Tachycardia (more than 100 beats/minute)
Assess for **irregular apical pulse** With another nurse, take apical and radial pulses *simultaneously* Compare beats per minute for both pulses	Equal apical and radial pulses	Fewer beats at the radial area may indicate an irregular apical pulse, producing ineffective pumping
Palpate **peripheral pulses**: radial, brachial, femoral, popliteal, dorsalis pedis, posterior tibial (For special cases, after carotid surgery, palpate temporal pulse also.) Follow these guidelines for palpating peripheral pulses: If pulse is not immediately palpable, examine adjacent area Pulse locations differ with clients	Easily palpated Equally strong on both sides Posterior tibial pulse usually weaker than femoral 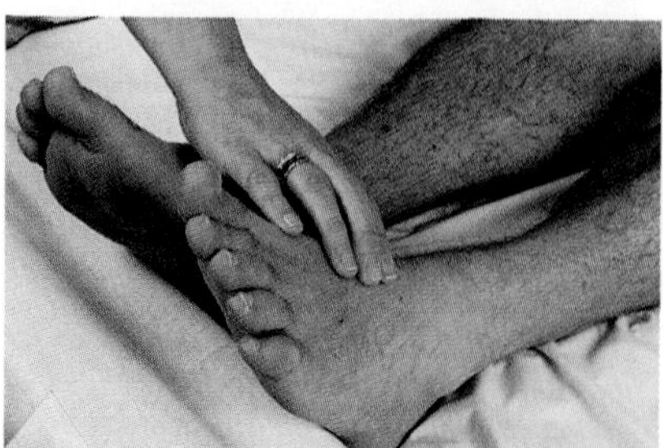	Difficult to palpate Unequal pulses Weak pulses Absent pulses

ASSESSMENT	NORMAL	ABNORMAL
Palpate weak pulses gently so that you do not obliterate pulse with too much pressure If you cannot differentiate your pulse from client's pulse, check your radial pulse, or observe monitor pattern Weak pulses may be difficult to feel		

ASSESSMENT OF THE ABDOMEN AND GENITOURINARY TRACT

The abdomen extends from the diaphragm to the pelvis. Generally speaking, there are two body systems present in this area: the gastrointestinal system and the genitourinary system.

The gastrointestinal system begins at the mouth and consists of the stomach, the small and large intestines, and associated organs that include the liver, pancreas, and spleen.

The urinary tract consists of the kidneys, ureters, bladder, and the urethra. The urinary tract should be assessed frequently and accurately because changes in urine production reflect changes in other body systems.

The most common way to assess the urinary tract is to note the quantity and quality of the urinary output. Some medications or foods produce unusual odors and colors in urine (e.g., sulfasalazine (Azulfidine) turns urine a yellow-orange color; asparagus gives urine a musty odor.

External male genitalia include the penis, the scrotum, and the testicles. External female genitalia include the vulva, the urethral orifice, and the vagina.

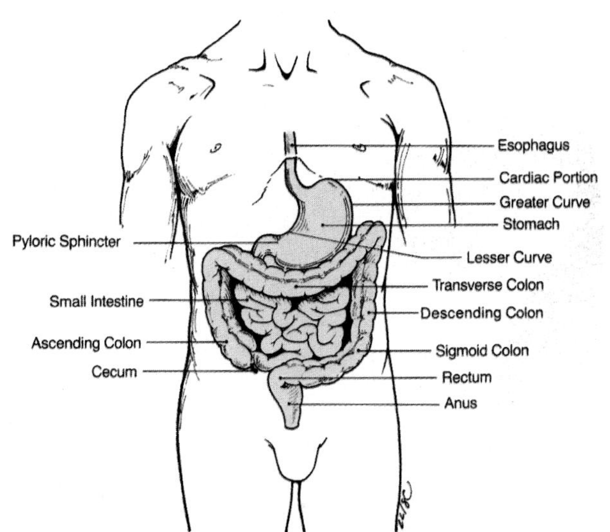

Assessment requires knowledge of abdominal organ anatomy.

ASSESSMENT	NORMAL	ABNORMAL
ABDOMEN Have client lay flat in bed. At the client's abdominal level, inspect the **general contour** of the abdomen	Abdomen flat from chest to pubis with concave indentation at umbilicus	Scaphoid (concave) abdominal contour: due to inadequate nutritional intake to meet caloric need or inadequate food absorption. Distended abdomen: caused by gas and fluid accumulation due to lack of peristalsis, hemorrhage, or intestinal leakage after trauma (e.g., auto accident or surgery), or ascitic fluid (e.g., liver or cardiac failure)

ASSESSMENT	NORMAL	ABNORMAL
Observe for scars, stretch marks, dilated veins, presence of hernia	Correlate with health history	Dilated veins caused by liver disease Bulge seen with defect in abdominal wall
Assess **circumference** for intraabdominal hemorrhage by placing a tape measure around the largest circumference of the abdomen and drawing two lines around client's entire abdomen, one line at the top of the tape measure, one line at the bottom of the tape measure; perform measurement when client exhales	No increase in abdominal circumference	Abdominal circumference increases steadily within 1–2 hours
Auscultate abdomen to assess presence and quality of **bowel sounds**		
Place diaphragm of stethoscope firmly on right lower quadrant and count sounds for 1 minute	Bowel sounds gurgle, about 5 to 30 per minute	Increased bowel sounds: due to blood in GI tract, diarrhea, or to partial bowel obstruction (sounds become high-pitched and tinkling or come in "rushes," followed by silence as obstruction progresses)
Listen at all quadrants for several minutes if sounds not heard initially	Varying frequency of sounds with clients and time of day (i.e., more sounds right before and after eating)	
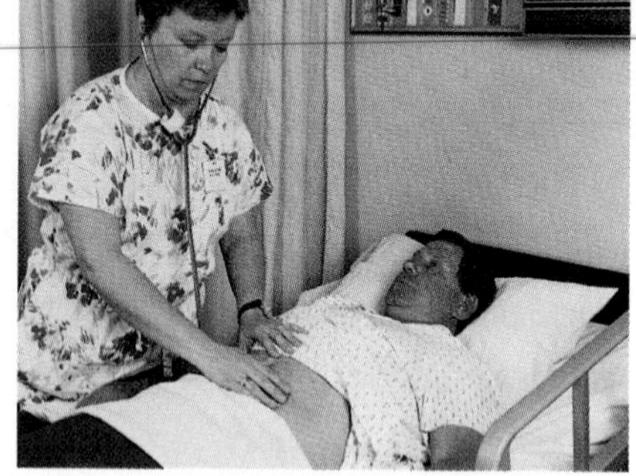	Decreased or absent bowel sounds after surgery After general anesthesia, normal sounds in 1–2 days After abdominal surgery, normal sounds in 3–5 days	Bowel sounds hypoactive, quiet, and infrequent: may be due to peritonitis, paralytic ileus, or no obvious cause Absent bowel sounds: may be due to complete bowel obstruction or systemic illness
Palpate abdomen to determine condition of **abdominal muscles** and organs beneath muscles		
Assist client to relax, lie flat in bed, and flex knees. Have client mouth-breathe		
Place your hand flat on client's abdomen, holding your four fingers together and depressing $\frac{1}{2}$ inch	Soft, pliant musculature when relaxed	Rigid, tender muscles/pain produced with cough, may be due to presence of muscle spasm, inflammation or infection (peritonitis)

ASSESSMENT	NORMAL	ABNORMAL
Have client cough to determine any areas of abdominal tenderness	Cough does not produce pain in abdomen	
Begin palpation at the pubis, moving upward. Palpate any problem areas last to minimize effects of discomfort	No bulges felt	Pain with quick release of pressure indicates rebound tenderness suggesting peritoneal inflammation
Palpate all quadrants of abdomen to assess organs contained in each quadrant	No masses felt	If hernia is suspected, have client raise head and shoulders and observe for abdominal bulge
Superficial palpation: use slight pressure only		
Deep palpation: indent the abdominal wall 4–5 cm—may use one hand over the other to apply pressure	No masses felt	Masses felt with colon disease, vascular aneurysm, dilated bowel, distended bladder, or cancer
URINARY TRACT ASSESSMENT		
Assess the **external urethra**	Orifice is pink and moist; clear, minimal discharge	Burning or pain at urethral orifice: may indicate urinary infection
Assess the quantity, color, odor, specific gravity, and pH of **urine output**	Output: 1200–1500 mL/24 hours, or 30–50 mL/hour—should equal oral and IV intake	Increased output: may indicate increased intake, diuresis, potential diabetes mellitus, or inappropriate antidiuretic hormone (ADH) response (e.g., head injury) Frequent small amounts of urine output indicate urinary retention. Decreased output: may indicate dehydration, acute nephritis, cardiac disease, or renal failure
	Clear, yellow-amber color (Vegetarians may have slightly cloudy urine)	Cloudy (turbid): may indicate possible urinary tract infection Dark amber: may indicate very concentrated urine due to dehydration Dark amber to green: may indicate hepatitis or obstructive jaundice
	Slight odor (ammonia-like odor indicates that specimen has been sitting for some time)	Foul-smelling: may indicate urinary tract infection, drug or specific food ingestion (e.g., asparagus) Sweet odor: may indicate acetone from ketoacidosis (i.e., diabetes mellitus)
	Specific gravity: 1.003–1.030	Specific gravity of more than 1.030: indicates dehydration Constant specific gravity of 1.010, regardless of fluid intake: indicates renal failure

ASSESSMENT	NORMAL	ABNORMAL
	pH range from 4.5–7.5; average is 6–7	Acidic pH is common Alkaline pH greater than 7.0: indicates metabolic alkalosis or alkaline ash diet (e.g., vegetarian)
Assess for **blood** in urine using Hemastix or Labstix	No blood present	Smokey to mildly pink-tinged to grossly red-colored urine: indicates blood in urine
Palpate for **bladder distension**	Not normally palpated	Distended bladder (firm, round mass) accompanied by discomfort and urge to void: indicates distention (common following surgery, where catheter is not used)
Assess for **pain**	No pain	Severe pain in the flank region (below ribcage posteriorly and lateral to spine): indicates kidney infection or stones
GENITAL ASSESSMENT		
Visually examine the **male genitalia** Retract the foreskin of the uncircumcised penis to note cleanliness, any **lesions**, and **discharge**	Clean No odor No lesions	Unclean Odor Lesions and discharge: may indicate venereal disease
Lift scrotum to inspect for rash	No discharge Size of penis and scrotum vary	Oval and round, dark erosion: may indicate syphilitic chancre
Noting groin area, ask client to strain down	Urethra opens midline of the tip of the glans No bulges in groin area	Hypospadias: due to congenital displacement of the urethral meatus Bulge or straining seen with hernias Indurated nodule or ulcer: may indicate carcinoma
Using thumb and first two fingers, gently palpate each testicle for size, shape, and consistency	Two testicles in the scrotum No nodules felt, no swelling or tenderness	Mass in scrotum: indicates possible hernia, hydrocele, testicular tumor, or cyst Pain indicates inflammatory disease
Visually examine **female genitalia**	Clean No odor	Unclean Odor (musty with bacterial infection)
Assess for **lesions** or **discharge** or complaints of itching	Minimal, clear discharge Menstrual flow Lochia (normal discharge after delivery) No lesions No pruritus	Thick; thin, white, yellowish, or green discharge: may indicate trichomoniasis Thick, white, and curdy discharge with pruritus may indicate candidiasis Lesions: could indicate syphilitic chancre, herpes infection, venereal wart, or carcinoma of vulva

MENTAL–SPIRITUAL ASSESSMENT

The mental assessment is completed throughout the physical assessment during the history taking. It is not generally considered a separate entity. Mood, memory, orientation, and thought processes can be evaluated while obtaining the health history. A spiritual assessment can be obtained as a part of the health history, although specific sociocultural beliefs may need to be ascertained separately. Nutritional preferences and restrictions can be determined as a part of a client care plan and may or may not be included in the general client assessment.

The purpose of a spiritual assessment is to facilitate the client adapting to the hospital environment and to help the staff understand stressors the client may be experiencing as a result of belief systems.

The purpose of a mental status assessment is to evaluate the present state of psychologic functioning. It is not designed to make a diagnosis; rather it should yield data that contribute to the total picture of the client as he or she is functioning at the time the assessment is made.

The specific rationale for completing a mental status assessment is:

- To collect baseline data to aid in establishing the cause, diagnosis, and prognosis
- To evaluate the present state of psychologic functioning
- To evaluate changes in the individual's emotional, intellectual, motor, and perceptual responses
- To determine the client's ability to cope with the present situation
- To assess the need and availability of support systems
- To ascertain if some seemingly psychopathologic response is, in fact, a disorder of a sensory organ (i.e., a deaf person appearing hostile, depressed, or suspicious)
- To determine the guidelines of the treatment plan
- To document altered mental status for legal records

The initial factors that the nurse must consider in completing a mental status assessment are to correctly identify the client, the reason for admission, record of previous mental illness, present complaint, any personal history that is relevant (living arrangements, role in family, interactional experience), family history if appropriate, significant others and available support systems, assets, and interests.

The actual assessment process begins with an initial evaluation of the appropriateness of the client's behavior and orientation to reality. The assessment continues by noting any abnormal behavior and ascertaining the client's chief verbalized complaint. Finally, the evaluation determines if the client is in contact with reality enough to answer particular questions that further assess the client's condition.

MENTAL STATUS ASSESSMENT

ASSESSMENT	NORMAL	ABNORMAL
GENERAL APPEARANCE, MANNER, AND ATTITUDE		
Assess **physical appearance**	General body characteristics, energy level	Inappropriate physical appearance, high or low extremes of energy
Note **grooming**, mode of dress, and **personal hygiene**	Grooming and dress appropriate to situation, client's age, and social circumstance Clean	Poor grooming Inappropriate or bizarre dress or combination of clothes Unclean
Note **posture**	Upright, straight, and appropriate	Slumped, tipped, or stooped Tremors
Note speed, pressure, pace, quantity, volume, and diction of **speech**	Moderated speed, volume, and quantity Appropriate diction	Accelerated or retarded speech and high quantity Poor or inappropriate diction

ASSESSMENT	NORMAL	ABNORMAL
Note relevance, content, and organization of **responses**	Questions answered directly, accurately, and with relevance	Inappropriate responses, unorganized pattern of speech Tangential, circumstantial, or out-of-context replies
EXPRESSIVE ASPECTS OF BEHAVIOR		
Note **general motor activity**	Calm, ordered movement appropriate to situation	Overactive (e.g., restless, agitated, impulsive) Underactive (e.g., slow to initiate or execute actions)
Assess **purposeful movements and gestures**	Reasonably responsive with purposeful movements, appropriate gestures	Repetitious activities (e.g., rituals or compulsions) Command automation Parkinsonian movements
Assess style of **gait**		Ataxic, shuffling, off-balance gait
CONSCIOUSNESS		
Assess **level of consciousness**	Alert, attentive, and responsive Knowledgeable about time, place, and person	Disordered attention; distracted, cloudy consciousness Delirious Stuporous Disoriented in time, place, and person
THOUGHT PROCESSES AND PERCEPTION		
Assess **coherency, logic**, and **relevance** of thought processes by asking questions about personal history (e.g., "Where were you born?" "What kind of work do you do?")	Clear, understandable responses to questions Attentiveness	Disordered thought forms Autistic or dereistic (absorbed with self and withdrawn); abstract (absent-mindedness); concrete thinking (dogmatic, preaching)
Assess **reality orientation**: time, place, and person awareness	Orderly progression of thoughts based in reality Awareness of time, place, and person	Disorders of progression of thought: looseness, circumstantial, incoherent, irrelevant conversation, blocking Delusions of grandeur or persecution: neologisms, use of words whose meaning is known only to the client Echolalia (automatic repeating of questions) No awareness of day, time, place, or person
Assess **perceptions** and reactions to personal experiences by asking questions, such as "How do you see yourself now that you are in the hospital?" "What do you think about when you're in a situation like this?"	Thoughtful, clear responses expressed with understanding of self	Altered, narrowed, or expanded perception illusions Depersonalization

ASSESSMENT	NORMAL	ABNORMAL
THOUGHT CONTENT AND MENTAL TREND		
Assess degree of anxiety Ask questions to determine general themes that identify **degree of anxiety** (e.g., "How are you feeling right now?" "What kinds of things make you afraid?")	Mild or 1+ level of anxiety in which individual is alert, motivated, and attentive	Moderate to severe (2+ to 4+) levels of anxiety
Assess **ideation** and **concentration**	Ideas based in reality Able to concentrate	Ideas of reference Hypochondria (abnormal concerns about health) Obsessional Phobias (irrational fears) Poor or shortened concentration
MOOD OR AFFECT		
Assess prevailing or **variability in mood** by observing behavior and asking questions, such as "How are you feeling right now?" Check for presence of abnormal **euphoria**	Appropriate, even mood without wide variations high to low	Cyclothymic mood swings; euphoria, elation, ecstasy, depressed, withdrawn
If you suspect **depression**, continue questioning to determine depth and significance of mood (e.g., "How badly do you feel?" "Have you ever thought of suicide?")	May be sad or grieving but mood does not persist indefinitely	Flat or dampened responses Inappropriate responses Ambivalence
MEMORY		
Assess **past and present memory** and **retention** (ability to listen and respond with understanding or knowledge); ask client to repeat a phrase (e.g., an address)	Alert, accurate responses Able to complete digit span Past and present memory appropriate	Hyperamnesia (excessive loss of memory); amnesia; paramnesia (belief in events that never occurred) Preoccupied Unable to follow directions
Assess **recall** (recent and remote) by asking questions, such as "When is your birthday?" "What year were you born?" "How old are you?"	Good recall of immediate and past events	Poor recall of immediate or past events
JUDGMENT		
Assess **judgment, decision-making ability**, and interpretations by asking questions, such as "What should you do if you hear a siren while you're driving?" "If you lost a library book, what would you do?"	Ability to make accurate decisions Realistic interpretation of events	Poor judgment, poor decision-making ability, poor choice Inappropriate interpretation of events or situations

ASSESSMENT	NORMAL	ABNORMAL
AWARENESS		
Assess **insight**, the ability to understand the inner nature of events or problems, by asking questions, such as "If you saw someone dressed in a fur coat on a hot day, what would you think?"	Thoughtful responses indicating an understanding of the inner nature of an event or problem	Lack of insight or understanding of problems or situations Distorted view of situation
INTELLIGENCE		
Assess **intelligence** by asking client to define or use words in sentences (e.g., recede, join, plural)	Correct responses to majority of questions	Incorrect responses to majority of questions indicate possible severe psychiatric disorders
Assess **fund of information** by asking questions, such as "Who is president of the United States?" "Who was the president before him?" "When is Memorial Day?" "What is a thermometer?" (Consider client's cultural and educational background and his or her grasp of English)	Correct responses to majority of questions	Deteriorated or impaired cognitive processes
SENSORY ABILITY		
Assess the **five senses** (e.g., vision, hearing, taste, feeling, and smell)	Able to perceive, hear, feel, touch appropriate to stimulus	Lack of response Suspicious, hostile, depressed Kinesthetic imbalance
DEVELOPMENTAL LEVEL		
Assess **developmental level** compared with normal	Behavior and thought processes appropriate to age level	Wide span between chronologic and developmental age Mentally retarded
LIFESTYLE PATTERNS		
Identify **addictive patterns** and effect on individual's overall health	Normal amount of alcohol ingested Smoking habits Prescriptive medications Adequate food intake for physical characteristics	High quantity of alcohol taken frequently Heavy smoker Addicted to illegal drugs Habituative medication; user of over-the-counter or legal medications Anorexic eating patterns Obese or overindulgence of food

ASSESSMENT	NORMAL	ABNORMAL
COPING DEVICES		
Identify **defense-coping mechanisms** and their effect on individual	Conscious coping mechanisms used appropriately, such as compensation, fantasy, rationalization, suppression, sublimation, or displacement	Unconscious mechanisms used frequently, such as repression, regression, projection, reaction formation, insulation, or denial
	Mechanisms effective, appropriate, and useful	Mechanisms inappropriate, ineffective, and not useful

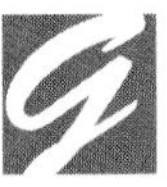

GERIATRIC CONSIDERATIONS

HEAD AND NECK AND NEUROLOGIC ASSESSMENT

Physiologic Changes with Age

- Decreased speed of nerve conduction and delay in response and reaction time, especially with stress.
- Diminution of sensory faculties: decreased vision, loss of hearing, diminished sense of smell and taste, greater sensitivity to temperature changes with low tolerance to cold.
- Tooth loss.
- Poor dentition, inadequate chewing, poor swallowing reflex.
- Condition of teeth, gums, buccal cavity.
- Peridontal disease.

Taste sensation decreases.

- Chronic irritation of mucous membranes.
- Atrophy of up to 80% of taste buds.
- Lose sensitivity of those on tip of tongue first: sweet and salt.
- Lose sensitivity of those on sides later: salt, sour, bitter.

Assessment

- Facial symmetry.
- Poor reflex reactions.
- Level of alertness—presence of organic brain changes: memory impairment.
- Motor function—strength.

SKIN

Physiologic Changes with Age

Skin less effective as barrier.

- Decreased protection from trauma.
- Less ability to retain water.
- Decreased temperature regulation.

Skin composition changes.

- Dryness (osteotosis) due to decreased endocrine secretion.
- Loss of elastin.
- Increased vascular fragility.
- Thicker and more wrinkled on sun-exposed areas.
- Melanocyte cluster pigmentation.

Sweat glands

- Decreased number and size.
- Decreased function of sebaceous glands.

Hair

- General hair loss.
- Decreased melanin production.
- Facial hair increases in women.

Nails more brittle and thick.

Assessment

Skin

- Temperature, degree of moisture, dryness.
- Intactness, open lesions, tears, decubiti.
- Turgor, dehydration.
- Pigmentation alterations, potential cancer.
- Pruritus—dry skin most common cause.

Bruises, scars.

Condition of nails (hard and brittle).

- Presence of fungus.
- Overgrown or horny toenails, ingrown.

Condition of hair.

Infestations (scabies, lice)

CHEST ASSESSMENT

Physiologic Changes with Age

Respiratory muscles lose strength and become rigid.

Ciliary activity decreases.

Lungs lose elasticity.

- Residual capacity increases.
- Larger on inspiration.
- Maximum breathing capacity decreases; depth of respirations decreases.

Alveoli increase in size, reduce in number.

- Fewer capillaries at alveoli.
- Dilated and less elastic alveoli.

Gas exchange is reduced.

- Arterial blood oxygen PaO_2 decreases to 75 mm Hg at age 70.
- Arterial blood carbon dioxide $PaCO_2$ unchanged.

Coughing ability is reduced—less sensitive mechanism.

More dependent on the diaphragm for breathing.

System less responsive to hypoxia and hypercardia.

Assessment

- Shape of chest excursion.
- Lung and breath sounds.
- Quality of cough, if present; sputum.

Rib cage deformity.

Dyspnea, hypoxia, and hypercarbia

Breast—size, symmetry, contour.

- Presence of lumps.
- Size and shape of nipples.

HEART ASSESSMENT

Physiologic Changes with Age

Mitral and aortic valves thicken and become rigid.

Cardiac output decreases 1% per year after age 20 due to decreased heart rate and stroke volume.

Vessels lose elasticity.

- Less effective peripheral oxygenation.
- Position change from lying-to-sitting or sitting-to-standing can cause blood pressure to drop as much as 65 mm Hg.

Increased peripheral vessel resistance

- Blood pressure increases: systolic may normally be 170 mm Hg, diastolic may normally be 95 mm Hg.
- Smooth muscle in arteries is less responsive.

Blood clotting increases.

Assessment

Heart sounds—murmurs.

Peripheral circulation, color, warmth.

- Apical pulse.
- Jugular vein distention.

Orthostatic hypotension.

- Dizziness.
- Fainting.

Edema.

Activity intolerance.

Dyspnea.

Transient ischemic attacks (TIAs).

ABDOMEN

Physiologic Changes with Age

Esophagus dilates, decreased motility.

Stomach.

- Hunger sensations decrease.
- Secretion of hydrochloric acid decreases.
- Emptying time decreases.

Peristalsis decreases and constipation is common.

Absorption function is impaired.

- Body absorbs less nutrients due to reduced intestinal blood flow and atrophy of cells on absorbing surfaces.

- Decrease in gastric enzymes affects absorption.

Hiatal hernia common (40–60% of elderly).

Diverticulitis common (40% over age 70).

Liver.

- Fewer cells, with decreased storage capacity.
- Decreased blood flow.
- Enzymes decrease.

Impaired pancreatic reserve.

Decreased glucose tolerance.

Assessment

- Indications of possible hiatal hernia.
- Bowel distention.
- Bowel sounds.

URINARY TRACT—GENITAL ASSESSMENT

Physiologic Changes with Age

Kidneys.

- Smaller due to nephron atrophy.
- Renal blood flow decreases 50%.
- Glomerular filtration rate decreases 50%.
- Tubular function diminishes: less able to concentrate urine; lower specific gravity; proteinuria 1+ is common; blood urea nitrogen (BUN) increases 21 mg%.

Renal threshold for glucose increases.

Bladder.

- Muscle weakens.
- Capacity decreases to 200 mL or less, causing frequency.
- Emptying is more difficult, causing increased retention.

Prostate enlarges to some degree in 75% of men over age 65; hypertrophy.

Menopause occurs by mean age of 50.

Perineal muscle weakens.

Vulva atrophies.

Vagina.

- Mucous membrane becomes dryer.
- Elasticity of tissue decreases, so surface is smooth.
- Secretions become reduced, more alkaline.
- Flora changes.

Sexuality.

- Older people continue to be sexual beings with sexual needs.
- No particular age at which a person's sexual functioning ceases.
- Frequency of genital sexual behavior (intercourse) may tend to decline gradually in later years, but capacity for expression and enjoyment continue far into old age.

Assessment

- Condition of skin—dehydration.
- Urinary output; blood in urine; color; specific gravity; prothrombin time (PT).
- Incontinence.
- Bladder distention.
- Genital assessment.

MUSCULOSKELETAL SYSTEM

Physiologic Changes with Age

Contractures.

- Muscles atrophy, regenerate slowly, strength lessens.
- Tendons shrink and sclerose.

Range of motion of joints decreases.

- Lack of adequate joint motion, ankylosis.
- Slight flexion of joints.

Assessment

Mobility level.

- Ambulate with more difficulty.
- Limitation to movement.
- Muscle strength cramps.
- Gait becomes unsteady.

Presence of kyphosis.

Pain in joints.

15

Infection Control

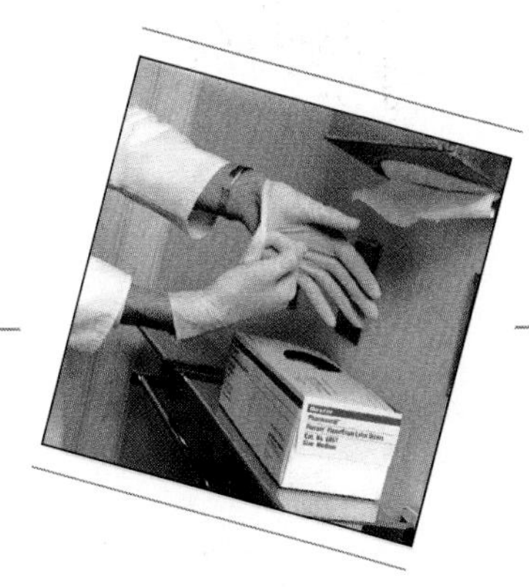

LEARNING OBJECTIVES

- Describe three methods the body uses to resist infection.
- Explain what is meant by the body's natural defenses.
- List and describe eight conditions that predispose clients to infection.
- State the main purpose of handwashing.
- Compare and contrast category-specific and disease-specific isolation.
- Demonstrate putting on and removing a gown.
- Define the terms "infection control" and "medical asepsis."
- Outline the steps in putting on isolation clothing before entering the room.
- Outline the steps in taking off isolation clothing before leaving the room.
- State the isolation procedure for removing specimens and equipment from an isolation room.
- Define HIV infection according to the CDC criteria.
- Describe the modes of transmission of HIV.
- List at least four infection control guidelines for the hospital setting.
- List blood and body fluid protection protocol.
- Describe the preventive measures for caring for the maternity patient with AIDS.
- Describe appropriate techniques for caring for the newborn.

TERMINOLOGY

AIDS: acquired immunodeficiency syndrome—a serious condition characterized by a defect in natural immunity against disease. When the immune system is suppressed, the individual is vulnerable to a host of opportunistic infections.

Antibody: protein substance developed by the body to fight disease organisms. Not effective against a virus that is inside the cells.

Antimicrobial: an agent that prevents the development or pathogenic action of microbes.

Antiseptics: agents that are applied to body tissues, such as skin or mucous membrane, to destroy or retard the growth of microorganism.

ARC: AIDS related complex—characterized by a prolonged history of fever, unexplained weight loss, swollen lymph nodes, or fungus infection of the mouth and throat. A certain but unknown percentage of persons with ARC will develop AIDS.

Asepsis: the absence of disease-producing microorganisms.

Aseptic technique: a method to eliminate contamination, germs, or infection.

Autoinfections: infections that arise from an individual's own body flora.

AZT: also called compound S, an antiviral drug in the experimental stages currently being used and evaluated for potential effectiveness against HIV.

Bacteriostatic: a substance that prevents the growth or multiplication of bacteria.

Barrier nursing: any technique that reduces the risk of cross-contamination.

Carrier: a person or animal without signs of illness but who carries pathogens on or within his or her body that can be transferred to others.

Cell-mediated immunity: reactions to antigens by cells rather than antibody molecules present in body fluids.

Chemotaxis: attraction and repulsion of living protoplasm to a chemical stimulus.

Cofactors: existing characteristics in the individual which may make them more susceptible to the AIDS virus.

Colonization: organisms present in body tissue but not multiplying or invading the tissue.

Contagious disease: a disease conveyed easily to others.

Contamination: introduction of disease, germs, or infectious materials into or on normally sterile objects.

Depilatory: agent that removes hair from skin surfaces.

Disinfectants: chemical agents that are used to destroy or reduce microorganisms on inanimate surfaces and objects.

Disinfection: a process that employs physical and chemical means to remove, control, or destroy most of the organisms that may be present on equipment or materials.

Duration of the infectious challenge: sustained exposure to even a relatively small number of organisms that poses a significant risk to the client (e.g., intravenous catheters become colonized with microorganisms).

Endogenous: organisms natural to an individual's own body.

Enteric precautions: isolation practices designed to prevent transmission of pathogens through contact with fecal matter and vomitus.

Exogenous: organisms external to an individual's own body.

False negative: a negative test in someone who in fact has been infected by a microorganism but for some reason has not developed antibodies.

False positive: a positive test for an antibody. Usually the result of an artifact of the laboratory test; the person has not in fact been exposed to the microorganism. All persons who test positive should have the test repeated.

Granulation: formation of granules (roughened prominences). Each granulation represents an outgrowth of new capillaries and enriched blood supply.

Host: an animal or person on which or within which microorganisms live.

HTLV-III: human T-lymphotrophic virus type. One label of the virus that causes AIDS.

Humoral immunity: acquired immunity in which the circulating antibody is predominant.

Hygiene: study of health and observance of rules pertinent to health.

Incubation period: the time between infection from a microorganism and the onset of symptoms. Seems to range from 6 months to 7 years for AIDS. Not everyone who is exposed to the virus develops the disease.

Infection: establishment of a disease process that involves invasion of the body tissue by microorganisms and the reaction of the tissues to their presence and to the toxins generated by them.

Involved cells: the HIV virus changes the protein layer on the surface of the T4 lymphocytes (helper cells) in such a way as to prevent them from activating B cells (antibody-producing cells) and killer T cells.

Isolation technique: practices designed to prevent the transmission of communicable diseases.

Kaposi's sarcoma: a type of cancer usually occurring on the surface of the skin or in the mouth. Kaposi's sarcoma may also spread to internal organs of the body and may be responsible for death.

LAS: lymphadenopathy syndrome is a disease of the lymph nodes and evidenced as a part of the ARC syndrome.

LAV: lymphodenopathy associated virus: This is the same as the HTLV-III virus, also called the HIV virus.

Microorganism: minute living body, such as a bacterium, protozoan, or virus, not perceptible to the naked eye.

Nosocomial infection: an infection acquired while in the hospital that was not present or incubating at the time of admission.

Opportunistic infections: illness or diseases that would not be a threat to anyone whose immune system is functioning normally, but in a person with AIDS may be responsible for death.

Opsonin: a substance in blood serum that acts on microorganisms and other cells and facilitates phagocytosis.

Outbreak: a critical incident in which infections occur above an established level and are caused by the same infective agent.

Pneumocystis carinii pneumonia: PCP is a parasitic infection of the lungs. This is one of the two rare diseases that affect 85% of AIDS clients. PCP has symptoms similar to other severe forms of pneumonia.

Populations at risk for HIV infection: in descending order of risk they are: sexually active homosexual men with multiple partners; sexually active bisexual men with multiple partners; present or past abusers of IV drugs; prostitutes; female partners of bisexual men; and heterosexual men and women with multiple partners.

Primary immune response: response that occurs when the B cell recognizes an antigen, becomes activated, and divides into more memory cells.

Protective isolation: practices designed to protect a highly susceptible person from contagious diseases, reverse isolation.

Protocol: description of steps taken in exact order.

Resident (normal) flora: organisms natural to an individual's own body. Organisms multiply in the environment, not merely survive there.

Retrovirus: a virus with a life cycle in which the genetic information is in reverse of that in an ordinary virus: the RNA code is transcribed backward into DNA.

Safe sex: practices that need to be taught to the population at large to prevent transmission of sexually transmitted diseases such as AIDS. These practices refer to the use of a condom and spermicidal foam for all sexual activity so that there is no exchange of blood or body fluids.

Sepsis: condition resulting from the presence of pathogenic bacteria and their products.

Sterile: free from any living microorganisms.

Subungual: an area beneath a fingernail or toenail.

Surgical asepsis: practice to keep area free from microorganisms, as by a surgical scrub.

Susceptible sites: an area that is sensitive to or can be invaded by a bacterium or other infectious agent.

Virulence: recognized pathogenic organisms designated because of their ability to invade and propagate in normal, intact, uncompromised individuals. Some organisms that are avirulent for normal individuals become pathogenic when defense mechanisms are impaired.

Virus: minute, parasitic organism that depends on nutrients inside cells for its metabolic and reproductive needs. These organisms cause a variety of infectious diseases and stimulate host antibodies. Unlike a bacteria, viruses are unable to survive long on their own and are not affected by antibodies.

INFECTION CONTROL

Clients may enter the health care facility with an infection or develop an infection while in the facility. Clients in health care settings are at risk for acquiring what is termed nosocomial infections. These infections occur because hospitals harbor many different types of microorganisms, some of which are resistent to antibiotics. Clients come into contact with many different health care workers over the course of a day. They are subjected to invasive procedures, and the longer their hospital stay, the more at risk they are for developing an infection. Infection control principles prevent the spread of infection or disease by maintaining medical asepsis and Standard Precautions in the delivery of client care. Infection control involves monitoring the client, the environment, and health care workers to prevent the spread of infection. Immediate procedures are instituted when infection is present. These procedures involve the handling of linen, food trays, equipment, and supplies used in client care.

Chain of Infection

For an infection to occur a chain of events must take place. If the chain is broken through the implementation of infection control measures, the infection is less likely to occur. The chain of infection involves six steps.

Infectious Agent (Microorganism). The first step in the chain involves the presence of an infectious agent, or microorganism. Whether the microorganism is capable of producing an infection depends on a number of circumstances. The virulence and number of organisms present, the susceptibility of the host, the existence of a portal of entry, and the affinity of the host to harbor the microorganism.

Reservoir. A reservoir must provide a favorable environment for growth and multiplication of the microorganism. These reservoirs include the respiratory, gastrointestinal, reproductive and urinary tract, and blood.

Portal of Exit. The third link in the chain must be a portal of exit, which allows the microorganism to move from the reservoir to the host. Without a portal of exit an infection cannot occur. The portal of exit is directly associated with the reservoir. For example, if the reservoir is the respiratory tract, the portal of exit is through sneezing, coughing, breathing, or talking. If the reservoir is blood, the portal of exit is through an open wound, needle puncture site, or intact skin surface.

Mode of Transmission. The fourth step involves either direct, indirect, or airborne method of transmission of the microorganism to the susceptible host. Direct transmission involves the transfer of a microorganism from one source to another. For example, through sexual intercourse, kissing, or in some cases touching. Spread of microorganisms through droplet sources is a means of direct transmission through coughing or sneezing. Indirect transmission can be vehicle-borne, such as from eating utensils, soiled clothing, used needles, soiled dressings, or via surgical instruments. Contaminated water, food, milk, and blood are also examples of vehicle-borne transmission. Indirect

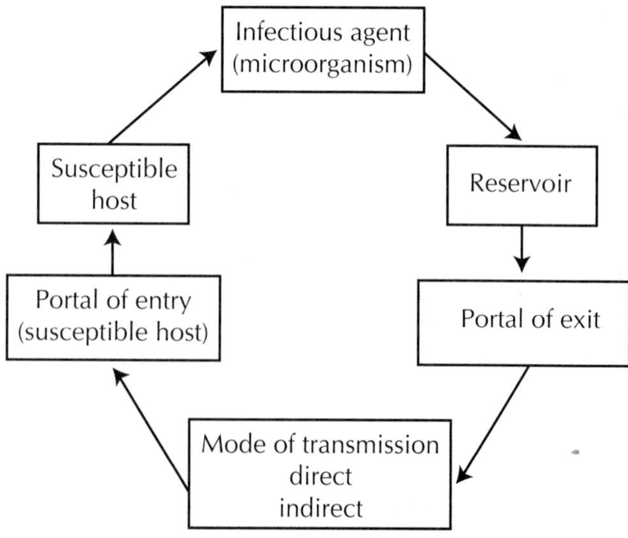

transmission can be vector-borne; vectors include insects or animals. Airborne transmission occurs when the droplet nuclei enters the susceptible host via the respiratory tract. Tuberculosis and one type of clostridium infection are spread through this mechanism.

Portal of Entry. The most effective barrier to transmission of microorganism is an intact skin. For an infection to occur it must have a means of entering the body. A disruption in the integrity of the skin provides such a portal of entry for microorganisms. Microorganisms also enter the body the same way they leave the body. The respiratory system provides a viable portal of both exit and entry.

Susceptible Host. For an infection to occur a susceptible host is needed—someone who is "at risk." This includes clients who are immunosuppressed, fatigued, stressed, anemic, not immunized, poorly nourished, or those who have underlying diseases. Hospitalized clients with wounds, catheters, and IVs are at high risk for developing infections. Clients who require invasive procedures, blood specimen collections, and surgery are also in the high risk category.

BARRIERS TO INFECTION

An individual's ability to resist infection is determined by the status of the body's defense mechanisms and by the person's general health. Factors that contribute to susceptibility to infection include altered nutritional status, stress, fatigue, disease, drugs, metabolic functions, and age. Clients with severe underlying diseases are most likely to develop nosocomial infections. The body is protected against infection by immunities, by the inflammatory process, and by anatomic barriers that include the skin and mucous membranes.

When the integrity of the skin or mucous membrane is broken, both resident and transient flora or bacteria have a direct route to the internal tissues of the body. To prevent the spread of infection, the body's internal defense mechanisms mobilize and begin clearing and repairing the damaged site. How quickly a wound heals depends on the degree of vascularization in the injured area, the location and cleanliness of the wound, and the degree of tissue damage.

The second way the body resists infections is through immunity, antitoxins, and vaccines. Natural immunity is inherited. Acquired immunity occurs after an individual has been exposed to a disease or infection or has been vaccinated.

The third way the body resists infection is through the inflammatory process. Inflammation involves use of metabolic energy, increased blood flow to the inflamed area, and, in many cases, drainage of inflammatory debris to the external environment.

When an area becomes inflamed, cells at the site activate the plasmin system, the clotting system, and the kinin system. The result of the activation of these systems is the release of histamine, which creates increased vascular permeability around the injured site, and the release of chemotaxic agents, which summon phagocytes into the vascular and tissue spaces. Phagocytes are white blood cells that combat and prevent infection by ingesting harmful microorganisms.

The Body's Natural Defenses

Any alteration in the body's natural defenses increases the probability that an infection will occur. Given the proper circumstances, almost any organism can be the cause of a significant nosocomial infection. Some of the variables that help determine which organism emerges as the pathogen are the virulence and number of organisms, the exposure and attachment of the organism to a susceptible site, and the duration of the client's exposure to the infectious challenge. The following formula illustrates these variables.

$$\frac{\text{Dose} \times \text{Virulence}}{\text{Host Resistance}} = \text{Infection}$$

Using this formula, the client's risk factors can be evaluated. The inherent health and immunologic status of the client are also major factors in determining whether an infection occurs.

Alterations in the skin barrier include any physiologic break in the integrity of the skin. Intentional breaks are caused by the use of percutaneous catheters and needles and by surgical procedures. Unintentional causes of skin breakdown include the development of decubitus ulcers and traumatic wounds.

CONDITIONS PREDISPOSING TO INFECTION

Certain conditions and invasive techniques predispose clients to infection because the integrity of the skin is broken or the illness itself establishes a climate favorable for the infectious process to occur. Among the most common are surgical wounds, changes in the antibacterial immune system, or alterations to the body.

Surgical Wounds

It has been documented that the longer a person is hospitalized prior to the surgical procedure the greater the risk of postsurgical infection. Other factors that influence infection rates are duration of time in the operating room, time surgery is done (between midnight and 8:00 AM is period of greatest risk), whether the client has postsurgical drains in place, and if the surgery enters a colonized or infected part of the body.

It is useful for the nurse to be aware of conditions that increase the risk of postoperative infection. Risk reduction measures include preoperative showering with an antiseptic solution; the use of depilatory creams or the clipping of hair in lieu of shaving the surgical site, and keeping the incision site covered with a dry sterile dressing. A wet dressing, through osmosis and diffusion, pulls organisms down into the wound from the surface. This is particularly important during the first 45 hours before the wound becomes "watertight." Research shows that preoperative shaving results in disruption of normal flora on the surface of the skin.

Antibacterial Immune Mechanisms

There are three categories of abnormalities in antibacterial immune mechanisms: those affecting inflammatory responses, those affecting phagocytic functions, and those affecting opsonins (humoral immunity).

Anything that interferes with the migration of phagocytic cells to the area of contamination or with the physical contact of phagocytes and bacteria enhances the development of an infection. Examples of such interferences include deficient blood supplies, the presence of ischemic or dead tissue, sutured material, foreign bodies, and hematomas. Vasopressor agents, radiation injury, uremia, severe nutritional deficiencies, and steroid therapy inhibit the synthesis of antibodies and other essential proteins.

Clients with severe thermal injuries and severe nutritional deficiencies have abnormalities involving the number of neutrophils collected at the site of an inflammatory response and defects of bactericidal chemotaxic capacity. Clients with Hodgkin's disease have a specific defect in cell-mediated immunity.

Genetic inabilities to synthesize complement components or specific antibodies can cause abnormalities in opsonins. Burn clients may have complement inactivated by a circulating substance released by the damaged tissue. Without complement, lysis of cells and destruction of bacteria cannot take place.

Respiratory Tract

Common alterations in the respiratory tract that facilitate the development of an infection include endotracheal intubation, tracheostomy, bronchotracheal suctioning, and stasis due to poor respiratory excursion for clients on bed rest.

The bronchi and trachea are so sensitive to foreign matter that they initiate the cough reflex whenever irritation occurs. Ciliated, mucus-coated epithelium lining the trachea and lungs aids in clearing the respiratory tract of bacteria and mucus by the beating motion of the cilia. Intubation bypasses the cough reflex and compromises the effectiveness of this action. Although the trachea is usually considered sterile, it does not remain sterile after 48–72 hours of intubation. Infections associated with endotracheal intubation include pneumonia, tracheitis, and purulent bronchitis.

Catheters placed directly in the trachea can force pathogenic microorganisms into the respiratory system. In addition, catheters can damage the mucous lining of the respiratory tract, further compromising the effectiveness of its clearing mechanisms.

Genitourinary Tract

Instrumentation, including catheterization of the bladder, and complicated obstetric delivery after prolonged confinement in bed are two procedures that introduce potentially pathogenic bacteria into the genitourinary tract. Acute urinary tract infection and pyelonephritis often occur after the use of a catheter or cystoscope.

The most common alteration is the placement of an indwelling urinary catheter. Research has demonstrated that significant bacteriuria develop in only 2% of the clients who have a single "straight" catheterization (in and out) to empty a distended bladder. Although bacteriuria may be considered benign and usually resolve after removal of the catheter, bacteriuria following catheterization may result in symptomatic cystitis and, occasionally, in acute pyelonephritis, chronic pyelonephritis, and persistent asymptomatic bacteriuria. Lack of adequate fluid intake, improper positioning of the catheter and bag, use of an open versus a closed drainage system, and inadequate emptying of the bladder all serve to increase the risk of infection in the catheterized client.

Invasive Devices

Most nosocomial septicemias occur as a result of significant alterations in normal host defenses. These infections may be primary (caused by direct introduction of microorganisms into the bloodstream) or secondary (arising from an infection at another site such as the urinary tract).

The use of IV therapy greatly increases the risk of introducing harmful microorganisms. The incidence of septicemia in clients receiving IV therapy varies from 0 to 8%.

Septicemia may also be caused by the introduction of microorganisms from contaminated fluids, infected venipuncture sites, or foci of septic thrombophlebitis as a complication of using an indwelling IV catheter.

Infusion-related sepsis is associated with contaminated infusion fluid, which may be contaminated either during manufacturing (intrinsic contamination) or during hospital use (extrinsic contamination).

Venipuncture Sites

The wounds made by a percutaneous stick at the venipuncture site may become colonized or infected. This opening provides a reservoir for bacteria that could move along the catheter into the bloodstream.

Organisms that travel down the catheter ultimately reside in the thrombus, which is usually present on the catheter tip. Around the thrombus, bacteria are shielded from the immune response and antibiotics. When these microorganisms attain a critical level, they seed the bloodstream and cause bacteremia. Site infections can be reduced by several methods: selecting a catheter appropriate to the size of the vein; avoiding sites near joints; the performance of proper site preparation; maintaining a regimen for site care; and changing the site every 48–72 hours as well as maintaining a closed system of therapy. Discontinuing IVs started in emergency situations like codes or "field starts" in which proper site hygiene wasn't carried out also reduces IV-related infections.

Total Parenteral Nutrition Therapy

Total parenteral nutrition therapy (TPN) is a means of achieving an anabolic state in clients who would otherwise be unable to maintain normal nitrogen balance. Problems with IV-related sepsis in TPN are the same as those seen in conventional IV therapy, only greatly magnified. The hypertonic solution used with these clients supports the growth of a wide variety of organisms, especially fungus, to a greater extent than conventional IV solutions. Clients on TPN are critically ill and malnourished. Peripheral inserted central catheter (PICC) lines are usually inserted for TPN infusions. These lines are not changed for months. Meticulous site care must be done at least every 3 days to preserve the site.

Implanted Prosthetic Devices

Commonly used implanted devices include artificial cardiac valves, synthetic vascular grafts, orthopedic prosthetic joints, neurosurgical shunts, and cerebrospinal fluid pressure monitoring devices. Most infections associated with prosthetic devices require long-term IV antibiotic therapy. If the infection is not controlled removal and replacement of the prosthesis is indicated.

ISOLATION PROCEDURES

In 1983, the Centers for Disease Control and Prevention (CDC) revised the infection control guidelines that had been in use since 1975. At that time hospitals were experiencing new endemic nosocomial infections, some caused by multidrug-resistent microorganisms and others by newly recognized pathogens, which required different isolation precautions from those currently in practice. As a result, two separate systems for isolation were established: category-specific and disease-specific. The disease-specific category was instituted so as not to overisolate clients. Prior to 1983, there were seven categories of isolation precautions, including contact isolation, respiratory, enteric precautions, drainage and secretion precautions, blood and body fluid precautions, strict isolation, and tuberculosis isolation. In the new category, the epidemiology of the infectious disease was considered individually and only those precautions that were needed to interrupt transmission of the infection was initiated. The precautions

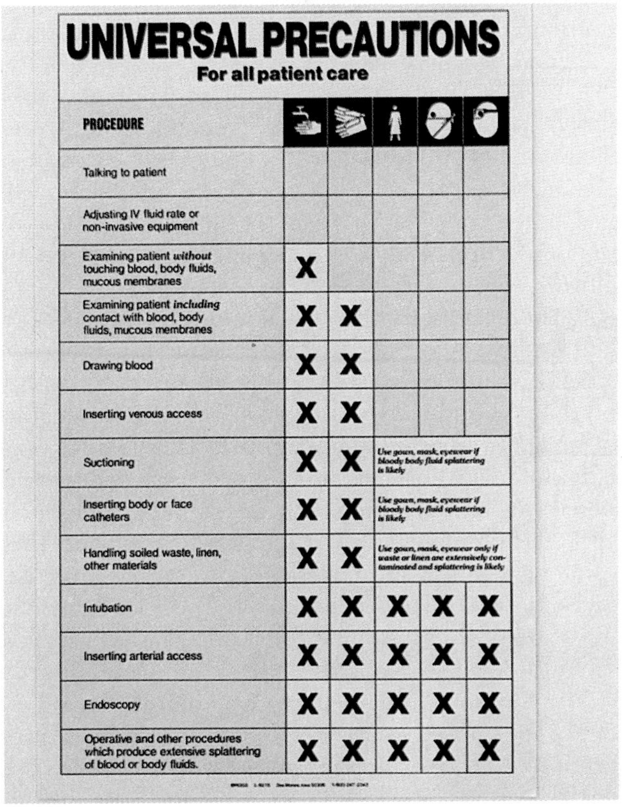

UNIVERSAL PRECAUTIONS

For all patient care

PROCEDURE					
Talking to patient					
Adjusting IV fluid rate or non-invasive equipment					
Examining patient *without* touching blood, body fluids, mucous membranes	X				
Examining patient *including* contact with blood, body fluids, mucous membranes	X	X			
Drawing blood	X	X			
Inserting venous access	X	X			
Suctioning	X	X	*Use gown, mask, eyewear if bloody body fluid splattering is likely*		
Inserting body or face catheters	X	X	*Use gown, mask, eyewear if bloody body fluid splattering is likely*		
Handling soiled waste, linen, other materials	X	X	*Use gown, mask, eyewear only if waste or linen are extensively contaminated and splattering is likely*		
Intubation	X	X	X	X	X
Inserting arterial access	X	X	X	X	X
Endoscopy	X	X	X	X	X
Operative and other procedures which produce extensive splattering of blood or body fluids.	X	X	X	X	X

TABLE 15–1. Category-Specific Isolation Precautions

Disease	Infective Category	Material	Apply Precautions: Time Period	Comments
Gastroenteritis				
Dientamoeba fragilis	Enteric precautions	Feces	Duration of illness	
Escherichia coli (enteropathogenic, enterotoxic, or enteroinvasive)	Enteric precautions	Feces	Duration of illness	
Giardia lamblia	Enteric precautions	Feces	Duration of illness	
Rotavirus	Enteric precautions	Feces	Duration of illness or 7 days after onset, whichever is less	
Salmonella species	Enteric precautions	Feces	Duration of illness	
Shigella species	Enteric precautions	Feces	Until three consecutive cultures of feces taken after ending antimicrobial therapy are negative for infecting strain	
Unknown cause	Enteric precautions	Feces	Duration of illness	

included the use of gowns, gloves, mask, and a private room.

In 1985, universal precautions were instituted as a result of the human immunodeficiency virus (HIV) epidemic in the United States. Blood and body fluid precautions were practiced on all clients regardless of their potential infectious state.

In 1987, body substance isolation (BSI) was proposed. The intent of this isolation system was to isolate all moist and potentially infectious body substances (blood, feces, urine, sputum, saliva, wound drainage, and other body fluids) from all clients, regardless of their infectious status, primarily through the use of gloves.

There has been a great deal of confusion in the use and interpretation of universal precautions, category-specific, and body substance isolation. This was probably due to hospitals adopting one or the other category of isolation. Interpretation and use of the systems varied, with many hospitals adopting parts of each system. Based on the difficulties with the various systems the CDC has developed new guidelines for isolation precautions in hospitals. Tables 15–1, 15–2, and 15–3 depict the category-specific, disease-specific, and BSI information that has been common isolation practice since 1987.

In the late fall of 1994, the CDC drafted new guidelines. The revised guidelines contain two tiers of precautions. The first tier, **standard precautions**, blends the major features of universal precautions, (blood and body fluids precautions) and body substance isolation into a single set of precautions to be used for the care of all clients in hospitals. The new standard precautions apply to blood, all body fluids, secretions, and excretions, whether or not they contain visible blood; nonintact skin; and mucous membranes. These precautions are designed to reduce the risk of transmission of both recognized and unrecognized sources of infection in hospitals. As a result of the new category of standard precautions, clients with diseases or conditions that previously required category-specific or disease-specific precautions are now covered under this category and do not require additional precautions.

The second tier, **transmission-based precautions**, reduces the disease-specific precautions into three sets of precautions based on routes of transmission. These categories are designed for clients documented or suspected to be infected or colonized with highly transmissible or epidemiologically important pathogens for which additional precaution must be used to interrupt transmission to others in the hospital. The three types of transmission-based precautions include airborne precautions, droplet precautions, and contact precautions. Airborne precautions reduce the risk of airborne transmission of infectious agents, such as measles, varicella, and tuberculosis. Droplet precautions are used to prevent the transmission of diseases, such as meningitis, pneumonia, scarlet fever, diphtheria, rubella, and pertussis. Contact precautions are used for clients known or suspected to have serious illnesses easily transmitted

TABLE 15–2. Disease-Specific Isolation Precautions

Disease	Private Room?	Mask?	Gowns?	Gloves?	Infective Material	Apply Precautions: Time Period	Comments
Gastroenteritis							
Salmonella species	Yes, if client hygiene is poor	No	Yes, if soiling is likely	Yes, for touching infective material	Feces	Duration of illness	
Shigella species	Yes, if client hygiene is poor	No	Yes, if soiling is likely	Yes, for touching infective material	Feces	Unit Three consecutive cultures of feces taken after ending antimicrobial therapy are negative for infecting strain	
Unknown cause	Yes, if client hygiene is poor	No	Yes, if soiling is likely	Yes, for touching infective material	Feces	Duration of illness	
Vibrio parahaemolyticus	Yes, if client hygiene is poor	No	Yes, if soiling, is likely	Yes, for touching infective material	Feces	Duration of illness	
Viral	Yes, if client hygiene is poor	No	Yes, if soiling is likely	Yes, for touching infective material	Feces	Duration of illness	
Yersinia enterocolitica	Yes, if client hygiene is poor	No	Yes, if soiling is likely	Yes, for touching infective material	Feces	Duration of illness	

TABLE 15–3. Body Substance Isolation Precautions

1. Body substance isolation (BSI) is an alternative to category-specific and disease-specific isolation protocols. BSI consists of six components:
   - Gloves are worn for all anticipated contact with blood, secretions, mucous membranes, nonintact skin, and moist body substances; must be changed between clients.
   - Handwashing is indicated for other types of client contact or if gloves are torn and hands become soiled.
   - Gowns, plastic aprons, masks, or goggles are worn to prevent soiling of skin or clothing or contamination of mucous membranes.
   - Soiled reusable articles, linen, and trash should be contained securely to prevent leaking.
   - Needles and sharp instruments should be placed in puncture-resistant, rigid containers; needles should be recapped.
   - Private rooms are indicated for those clients with diseases transmitted by the airborne route.
2. BSI uses a single, universal reminder sign for each client's room and at the bedside of clients in intensive care units.
3. "Stop Sign Alert" is added to the doors of clients with airborne diseases. The sign instructs persons to check with the floor nurse prior to entering the client's room.

TABLE 15–4. HICPAC* Recommendations for Transmission-Based Precautions

	Contact	Droplet	Airborne
Purpose	Prevent transmission of known or suspected infected or colonized microorganisms by direct hand or skin-to-skin contact that occurs when providing direct client care. Conditions in which contact precautions are required: diphtheria, herpes simplex, scabies, staphyloccus infection, hepatitis A, and respiratory syncytial virus wound or skin infection	Prevent transmission of large-particle droplets, larger than 5 microns (μm) (i.e., diphtheria, pertussis, streptococcal pharyngitis, pneumonia, scarlet fever, meningitis, rubella)	Prevent transmission of small-particle residue of 5 microns (μm) or smaller droplets (i.e., measles, varicella, tuberculosis)
Client Placement	• Private room • Can be placed in room of client with same microorganism	• Private room • Can be placed in room of client with same diagnosis	• Private room • Can be placed in room of client with same diagnosis • Monitor negative air pressure • Keep door closed • Keep client in room
Respiratory Protection	• Mask not necessary	• Use mask when working within 3 feet of client	• Respiratory protective equipment • Do not enter room of clients with rubeola or varicella if susceptible to these infections
Gloves and Gown	• Wear gloves when entering room • Change gloves after contact with infective material, such as wound drainage or fecal material • Wash hands immediately after removing gloves • Wear gown when working with clients with diarrhea, ostomies, or wound drainage not contained in dressing • Wear gown if contact with client or environment will occur	• Follow standard precautions	• Follow standard precautions
Client Transport	• Transport only if essential • Ensure precautions are maintained to minimize risk of transmission	• Transport only if essential • Place mask on client when outside room	• Transport only if essential • Place mask on client when outside room
Client Care Items	• Client care items and environmental surfaces are cleaned daily • Dedicate equipment to single client use (i.e., stethoscope, thermometer)		

* Hospital Infection Control Practices Advisory Committee
Adapted from Department of Health and Human Services: CDC, *Federal Register* "Draft Guidelines for Isolation Precautions in Hospitals," November 7, 1994.

by direct contact, such as herpes simplex, staphylococcal infections, hepatitis A, respiratory syncytial virus, and wound or skin infections.

All three types of precautions may be used at one time when multiple routes of transmission are suspected in a client. These precautions are always used in conjunction with standard precautions. Table 15–4 outlines recommendations for transmission-based precautions.

Isolation Fundamentals

Some fundamental isolation precautions should be used with all clients. The first is handwashing. Handwashing is the single most important means of preventing the spread of infection. A second fundamental precaution involves the use of gloves. Gloves are worn to provide a protective barrier, prevent gross contamination of the hands when touching body substances or blood, and reduce the risk of exposure to blood pathogens. Gloves also prevent the spread of microorganisms to other clients and to health care personnel.

The proper placement of clients in the hospital prevents the spread of microorganisms to others or to the client. Clients may not always be placed in private rooms when they are infected. They can be placed in a room where the second client has the same infectious process.

The fourth fundamental principle of isolation precautions is the appropriate use of isolation paraphernalia to prevent the spread of microorganisms to health care workers and other clients. The equipment required is based on the specific transmission route of the microorganism. Specific handling of client care items needs to be considered in preventing the spread of infection.

Standard Precautions

Standard precautions are used in the care of all clients.

Handwashing. Wash hands with nonantimicrobial soap after touching blood, body fluids, secretions, excretions, and contaminated items. This is done whether or not gloves are worn. Wash hands immediately after gloves are removed and between client contact.

Gloves. Clean, nonsterile gloves are worn when touching blood, body fluids, secretions, excretions, and contaminated items. Put gloves on just before touching mucous membranes and nonintact skin. Remove gloves immediately after use, and wash hands before touching noncontaminated items and environmental surfaces or giving care to another client. Gloves should be discarded immediately and not reused.

Mask, Eye Protection, Face Shield. Wear mask and eye protection during procedures in which splashes or sprays could come in contact with eyes and mucous membranes. Face shields protect the mucous membranes of the eyes, nose, and mouth from splashes of blood, body fluids, secretions, and excretions. Suctioning clients and assisting physicians in insertion of hemodynamic monitoring lines are examples of situations in which this type of protection is required.

Gown. Nonsterile disposable gowns are used to protect the skin and clothing from contamination while providing client care. Gowns should be worn whenever there is a risk of contamination from blood, body fluids, secretions, or excretions. Soiled gowns should be removed immediately and hands washed to prevent the spread of microorganisms.

Linen. Transport soiled linens in a manner that prevents skin and mucous membrane exposures or contamination of clothing and avoids transfer of microorganisms to other clients and environments. This is usually accomplished through double-bagging linen before taking it to the laundry facility.

Occupational Health and Bloodborne Pathogens. Take precautions to prevent injuries caused by needles, scalpels, or other sharp instruments or devices. Never recap used needles, purposely bend or break needle by hand, remove needles from disposable syringes, or otherwise handle needles directly. All such instruments should be placed in puncture-resistant containers for disposal. The use of needleless systems for IV management has decreased needle sticks dramatically.

Mouth pieces, resuscitation bags, or other ventilation devices should be used as an alternative to mouth-to-mouth resuscitation.

Client Placement. Clients who are at risk for contaminating the environment or who are unable to maintain appropriate hygiene or environmental control should be placed in a private room. If this is not possible, other arrangements need to be made in consultation with the hospital's infection control department.

In addition to health care workers following standard precautions the following guidelines should be considered when providing client care:

- Health care workers who have open lesions, upper respiratory infections, or weeping dermatitis should refrain from all direct client contact and from handling client care equipment.
- Because of the risk of transmission of HIV and hepatitis B virus (HBV) from mother to fetus, pregnant health workers should be especially familiar with, and strictly adhere to, precautions to minimize risk of these viruses. Currently, pregnant health care workers are not known to be at greater risk of contracting HIV or HBV than other workers.

ACQUIRED IMMUNODEFICIENCY SYNDROME

Epidemiology and Modes of Transmission

The incidence of acquired immunodeficiency syndrome (AIDS) has grown exponentially since it was first recorded in 1981. The statistics are chilling: by June 1994, the number of U.S. victims of AIDS was 401,749. AIDS has become the second leading killer of young men 24–44 years old and the fifth leading killer of U.S. women. The World Health Organization estimates that 8–10 million adults and 1 million children are infected with HIV and by the year 2000, 40 million persons will be infected with HIV. AIDS will be the third most common cause of death in the United States. Cases have been reported from all 50 states and three U.S. territories. AIDS is perhaps the most serious epidemic facing the modern world, making knowledge about it and techniques for caring for the AIDS client mandatory learning for all nurses. No one is immune to AIDS. The two major risk groups continue to be homosexual or bisexual men and IV drug abusers, which make up 85% of all AIDS cases. All other groups, hemophiliacs (1%), blood transfusion recipients (2%), heterosexuals (7%), and those for whom the cause is undetermined (4%), make up the remainder. Young adults and women are the fastest growing population of HIV-positive individuals. Although the number of youths diagnosed with HIV is still relatively low, the numbers are likely to increase dramatically in the next decade because of the virus' long latency period.

Definitions

Acquired Immunodeficiency Syndrome. AIDS is the most severe form of a continuum of illnesses associated with HIV infection. AIDS is defined by the CDC as an HIV infection in a person with a CD4+ T-lymphocyte count of less than 200 cells/microliter (μL) of blood or a CD4+ percentage of less than 14. Twenty-six clinical conditions are listed in the CDC AIDS surveillance case definition in category C. Once clients have a condition listed in category C they remain in that surveillance category. Among those 26 conditions listed in the category are cytomegalovirus (CMV) retinitis; Kaposi's sarcoma; **Mycobacterium avium** complex (MAC) (which includes the m. avium and m. intracellulare organisms) or *M. kansasii; Mycobacterium tuberculosis*, any site; *Pneumocystis carinii*; and recurrent pneumonia.

Human Immunodeficiency Virus. HIV is a bloodborne infective retrovirus that invades the CD4+ T-lymphocyte (immunity) cell, renders it useless, and then duplicates itself by means of that cell. With loss of the client's immune function, the disease becomes clinically manifested. Infection with HIV progresses to AIDS in at least 35% of those infected. Once a client has been diagnosed with HIV, the usual approach to care includes evaluation of the immune system and classification by CDC grouping, (A) asymptomatic, acute (B) symptomatic, and (C) AIDS-indicator conditions. Identification and treatment of infectious and neoplastic complications, initiation of approved antiretroviral therapy, and consideration of experimental measures are also included in the evaluation.

HIV is transmitted through high-risk behaviors or other contact with the virus, including

- Sexual contact with HIV-infected individuals
- Sharing needles with HIV-infected individuals
- Transfusions of blood or blood products from infected individuals (not common today, but new cases are still reported)
- Babies who become infected from the mother before or during birth, or through breast feeding
- Contact with contaminated needles, blood, secretions, or excretions from an HIV-infected client

OTHER INFECTIOUS DISEASES

Tuberculosis

Tuberculosis is an infectious disease caused by the tubercle bacillus *Mycobacterium tuberculosis.* The main reservoir for the organism is the human respiratory tract, and transmission occurs between individuals through respiratory contact. The tubercle bacillus enters the respiratory tract on droplets transmitted through productive coughing from the infected individual. Symptoms may occur in 4–12 weeks after exposure or may go unnoticed for many years. Active pulmonary tuberculosis has a slow, insidious onset. Without treatment tuberculosis progresses to other body sites. Disseminated tuberculosis occurs in many of the body areas, not just the lungs. The incidence of tuberculosis cases in this country has increased greatly, due in large part to the AIDS epidemic. Immunosupressed hosts are very vulnerable to the bacillus. In addition to immunosuppressed individuals others considered at high risk for infection include alcoholics; IV drug abusers; individuals who share a closed environment with the infected individual; residents of institutions such as long-term care and correctional facilities; foreign-born individuals from countries with a high prevalence of tuberculosis, such as Asia, Latin America, and Africa; and low-income populations who are medically underserved. Health care workers who come in contact with any of the high-risk populations are at risk for infection.

Early recognition and treatment of tuberculosis must be initiated promptly and isolation measures instituted to prevent the spread of the disease. The CDC describes effective tuberculosis control requirements as early identification, isolation, and treatment of persons with active tuberculosis. The PPD skin test is the only method available to quickly identify the infection in the absence of clinical symptoms. A client who is known to be HIV-positive with a 5 mm or larger induration at the site of the PPD injection should be considered positive for tuberculosis.

The CDC recommendation for tuberculosis isolation includes a directional air-flow, negative-pressure ventilation system in the room of tuberculosis clients. Negative-pressure ventilation pulls air away from hallways and exhausts it out of the room to areas away from air intake vents. Six air changes each hour is required to provide microbial dilution within the room. Ultraviolet irradiation lamps can be used to supplement ventilation systems when the risk of tuberculosis transmission is high.

Anyone entering the client's room should wear a mask that forms a tight-fitting seal against particulates 1–5 microns (μm). Two examples of tuberculosis masks are the high-efficiency particulate air (HEPA) mask used for suspected or confirmed multidrug-resistant (MDR) tuberculosis and the disposable submicron mask used for confirmed tuberculosis. Disposable particulate respirators are suggested by the CDC when adequate ventilation is not available in the room. All treatments and procedures should be performed in the client's room if at all possible. If the client must leave the room, a valveless particulate respirator must be used.

Hepatitis B

Hepatitis B is caused by a highly infectious virus that involves the liver. Approximately 5% of the U.S. population contracts HBV (about 240,000 individuals) each year, including adults and children. Hepatitis B virus (HBV) causes severe illness, liver damage, and can lead to death in some clients.

Transmission of HBV is through contact with body fluids, serum, semen, vaginal secretions, and saliva of infected individuals. It is not transmitted through sweat, tears, urine, or respiratory secretions. HBV is spread through unprotected sex, from mother to child during pregnancy, by contact with blood or body fluids, by sharing personal items with infected individuals, and through unclean needles. Isolation guidelines for hepatitis B include the use of standard precautions.

STANDARD PRECAUTIONS

The following standard precautions are recommended for use with clients to prevent transmission of infectious agents. Please follow these guidelines when caring for clients.

- Wear gloves when there is direct contact with blood, body fluids, secretions, excretions, and contaminated items. This includes a neonate before first bath. Wash as soon as possible if unanticipated contact with these body substances occurs.
- Protect clothing with gowns or plastic aprons if there is a possibility of being splashed or direct contact with contaminated material.
- Wear masks, goggles, or face shield to avoid being splashed; includes during suctioning, irrigations, and deliveries.
- Wash hands thoroughly after removing gloves and before and after all client contact.
- Do not break or recap needles, discard them intact into containers.
- Place all contaminated articles and trash in leakproof bags. Check hospital policy regarding double-bagging.
- Clean spills quickly with a 1:1000 solution of bleach if spill occurs in an HIV/AIDS client's room.
- Place clients at risk for contaminating the environment in a private room or with another client with same infectious organism.

NURSING DIAGNOSES

The following nursing diagnoses may be appropriate in a client care plan when the components are related to clients requiring isolation protocol or sterile procedures.

NURSING DIAGNOSIS	RELATED FACTORS
Altered Health Maintenance	Participation in high-risk activities, substance abuse, infectious states, religious or cultural beliefs
Knowledge Deficit	Lack of access to health care facilities, lack of education, cognitive limitation
Noncompliance	Lack of motivation, education or readiness, information misinterpretation, cultural or religious beliefs
Social Isolation	Medical condition (communicable disease, HIV-positive), hospitalization, terminal illness
Risk for Infection	Immunosuppressed hospitalized clients, HIV/AIDS clients, invasive procedures

unit 1

BASIC MEDICAL ASEPSIS

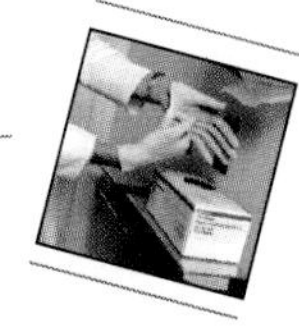

NURSING PROCESS DATA

ASSESSMENT Data Base

Assess need for handwashing.

Identify clients at risk for infection.

Assess availability of equipment for frequent handwashing.

Evaluate health status of the nurse.

Check agency policy for handwashing protocol.

Assess need for use of unsterile gloves.

PLANNING Objectives

To deliver client care with pathogen-free hands

To prevent pathogenic microorganisms from spreading from client to client

To protect clients from cross-contamination

To protect the nurse

IMPLEMENTATION Procedures

Handwashing (Medical Asepsis)

Cleaning Washable Articles

Donning and Removing Clean Gloves

EVALUATION Expected Outcomes

Infection is prevented from spreading.

Cross-contamination is prevented.

Nurse is protected from infection.

HANDWASHING (MEDICAL ASEPSIS)

Equipment

Soap containing a germicide

Orangestick for cleaning nails

Running warm water

Paper towels

Trash basket

> ■ **CLINICAL ALERT**
>
> Nurses must wash hands for 30 seconds before and after each direct contact with a client or each use of client care items.

Procedure

1. Stand in front of but away from sink. **Rationale:** Uniform should not touch sink to avoid contamination.
2. Crank towel out of holder before washing. **Rationale:** Crank is considered contaminated.
3. Turn on water faucet so that flow is adequate, but not splashing.
4. Adjust temperature to warm. **Rationale:** Cold does not facilitate sudsing and cleaning; hot is damaging to skin.
5. Wet hands under running water.
6. Place a small amount, one to two teaspoons, of liquid soap on hands. Soap should come from a dispenser, not bar soap. **Rationale:** This prevents spread of microorganisms.

7. Rub vigorously, using a firm, circular motion, while keeping your fingers pointed down, lower than wrists. Start with each finger, then between fingers, then palm and back of hand.
8. Wash your hands for at least 30 seconds.
9. Clean under your fingernails with an orangewood stick. (This should be done at least at start of day and if hands are heavily contaminated.)
10. Rinse your hands under running water, keeping fingers pointed downward.

■ CLINICAL ALERT

Aseptic technique, especially handwashing, prevents the spread of infection in hospitalized clients.

11. Resoap your hands, rewash, and rerinse if heavily contaminated.
12. Dry hands thoroughly with a paper towel or crank towel, while keeping hands positioned with fingers pointing up. **Rationale:** Moist hands tend to gather more microorganisms from the environment.
13. Turn off water faucet with dry paper towel.
14. Restart procedure at step 5 if your hands touch the sink any time between steps 5 and 13.

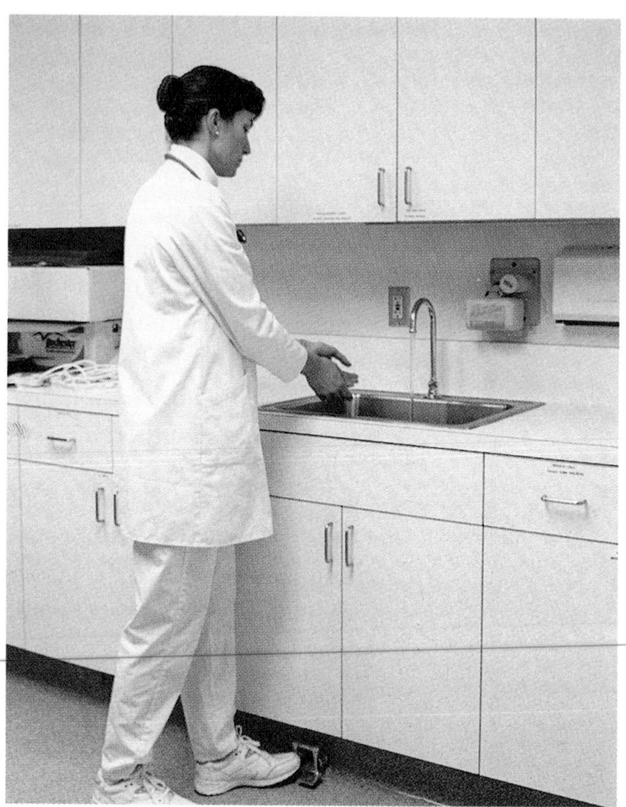

Use foot pedals when available to prevent contamination of hands.

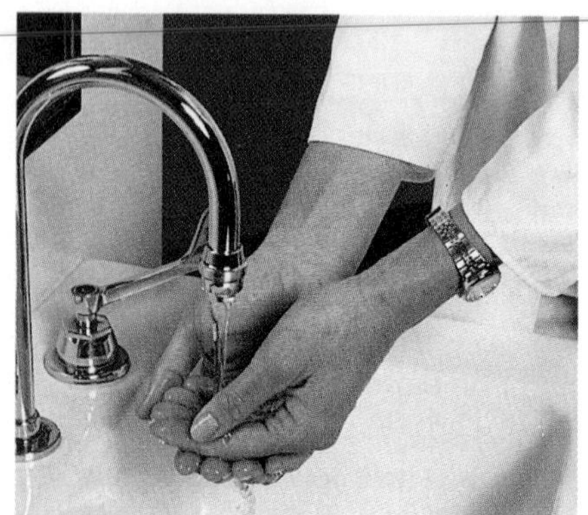

Wet hands thoroughly before applying soap to facilitate removal of pathogens.

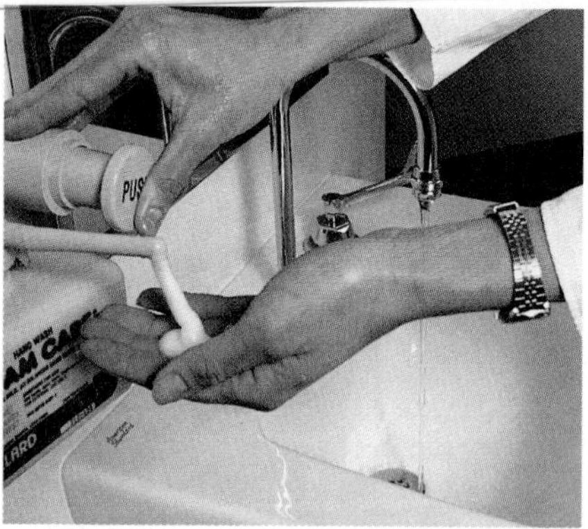

Use a generous amount of soap and friction during hand washing procedure.

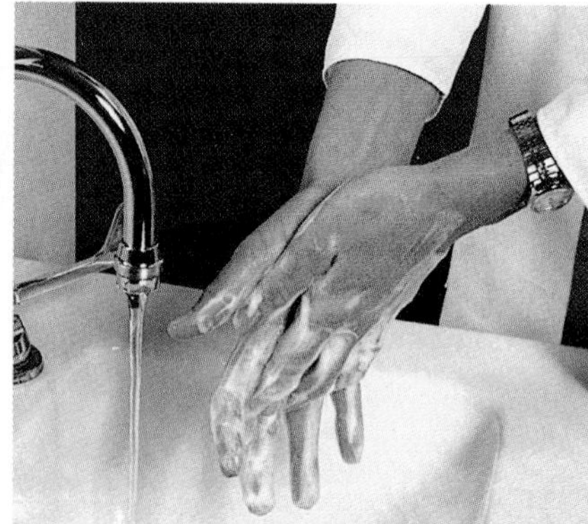

Keep fingers pointed down during hand washing to prevent contamination of arms.

CLEANING WASHABLE ARTICLES

Equipment

Article to be washed
Soap
Running warm water
Paper towels
Trash basket
Clean gloves

Procedure

1. Wash your hands and don clean gloves.
2. Rinse under cold running water.
3. Wash with warm, soapy water using friction or follow hospital protocol for cleaning equipment.
4. Rinse well with clear water.
5. Dry thoroughly.
6. Return to proper place or prepare for sterilization or disinfection if indicated.
7. Remove gloves and wash your hands.

DONNING AND REMOVING CLEAN GLOVES

Equipment

Clean gloves
Trash receptacle

Procedure

1. Wash your hands.
2. Pick up first glove at wrist edge and slip fingers into openings. Pull glove up to wrist.
3. Repeat step 2 for second glove.
4. Remove glove by pulling off, touching only outside of glove at cuff, so that glove turns inside out.

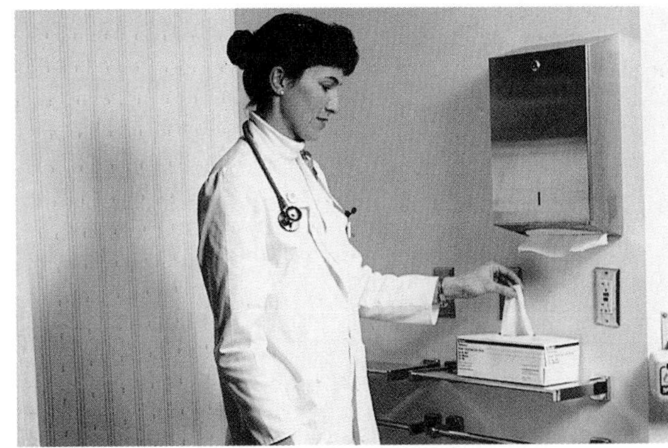

Clean gloves need to be easily accessible for health care wokers.

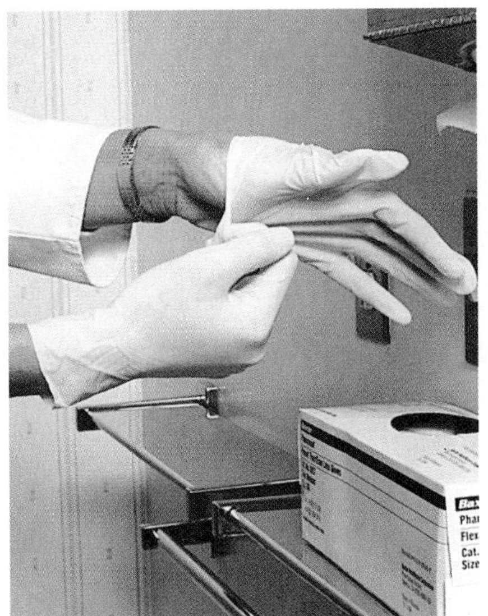

Pick up glove at wrist edge and slip fingers into openings.

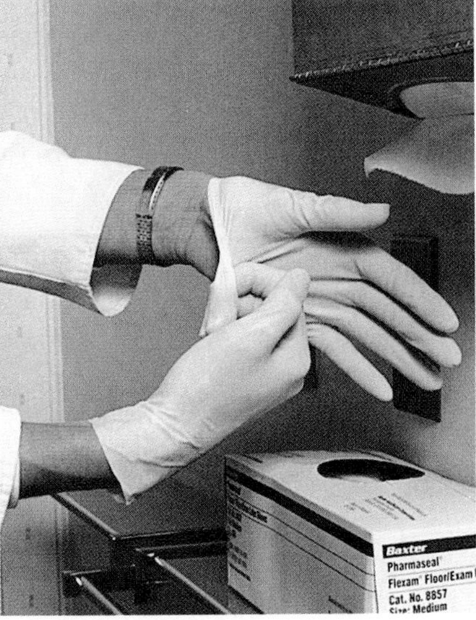

Remove glove by pulling off without touching hand with soiled glove.

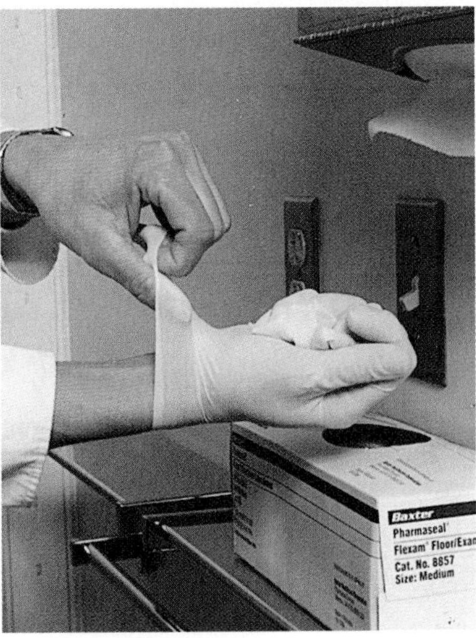

Place rolled up glove in palm of second hand and then remove glove.

GLOVE SELECTION

- Use sterile gloves for procedures involving contact with normally sterile areas of the body.
- Use examination gloves for procedures involving contact with mucous membranes, unless otherwise indicated, and for client care or procedures that do not require use of sterile gloves.
- Change gloves between clients.
- Do not wash, disinfect, or reuse surgical or examination gloves.
- Use general purpose utility gloves (rubber household gloves) for housekeeping tasks that involve potential blood contact and for instrument cleaning and decontamination procedures.

5. Place rolled-up glove in palm of second hand.
6. Remove second glove by slipping one finger under glove edge and pulling down and off so that glove turns inside out. Both gloves are removed as a unit.
7. Dispose of gloves in proper container, not at bedside.
8. Wash your hands.

CHARTING for Basic Asepsis

- Infection control measures used
- Clean gloves used for procedure

CRITICAL THINKING APPLICATION

CLINICAL PROBLEMS	CRITICAL THINKING OPTIONS
Infection occurs in client.	• Administer antibiotics specific to microorganism as ordered. • Review handwashing technique. • Attend in-service program on infection control procedures.

unit 2 ISOLATION

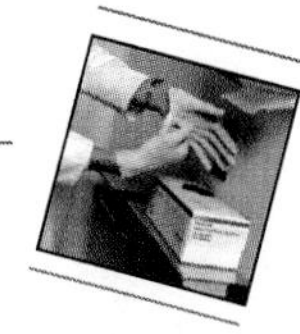

NURSING PROCESS DATA

ASSESSMENT Data Base

Identify appropriate times for handwashing.

Identify type of protective clothing required for barrier nursing.

Identify epidemiology of the disease to determine how to prevent infection from spreading.

Identify equipment needed to prevent spread of organisms.

Assess method of terminal cleaning and disposing of equipment.

PLANNING Objectives

To prevent the spread of endogenous and exogenous flora to other clients

To reduce potential for transferring organisms from the hospital environment to the client

To protect hospital personnel from becoming infected

IMPLEMENTATION Procedures

Preparing for Isolation

Putting on and Removing a Gown

Using a Mask

Assessing Vital Signs

Removing Items from Isolation Room

Removing a Specimen from Isolation Room

Transporting Isolation Client Outside the Room

Removing Soiled Large Equipment from Isolation Room

EVALUATION Expected Outcomes

Isolation environment is maintained to prevent contamination of surrounding area.

Personnel working with isolation clients remain free of infection.

PREPARING FOR ISOLATION

Equipment

Specific equipment depends on isolation precaution system used

Soap and running water

Isolation cart containing masks, gowns, gloves, plastic bags, isolation tape

Linen hamper and trash can, when needed

Paper towels

Door card indicating precautions

Procedure

1. Check physician's order for isolation.
2. Obtain isolation cart from central supply, if needed.
3. Check that all necessary equipment to carry out the isolation order is available.
4. Place isolation card on the client's door.
5. Ensure that linen hamper and trash cans are available, if needed.
6. Explain purpose of isolation to client and family.
7. Instruct family in procedures required.

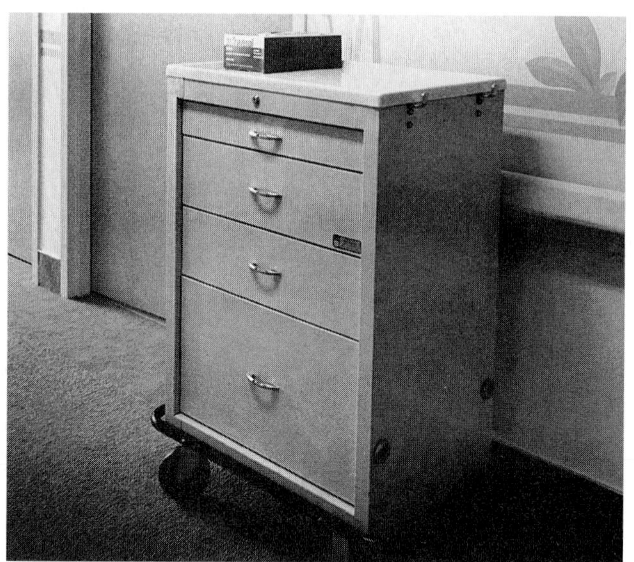

Place isolation cart outside client's door when cart is required.

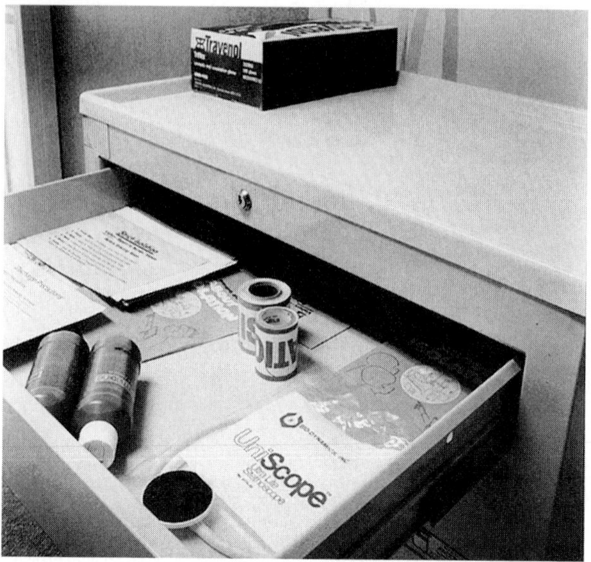

Check that all supplies are restocked at the end of each shift.

PUTTING ON AND REMOVING A GOWN

Procedure

1. Take gown from isolation cart. Put on a new gown each time you enter an isolation room.
2. Hold gown so that opening is in back when you are wearing the gown.
3. Put gown on by placing one arm at a time through sleeves. Pull gown up and over your shoulders.
4. Wrap gown around your back, tying strings at your neck.
5. Wrap gown around your waist, making sure your back is completely covered. Tie strings around your waist. Don gloves.
6. To remove soiled gown, take gloves off, then untie waist strings.
7. Next, untie neck strings, bringing them around your shoulders so that gown is partially off your shoulders.
8. Using your dominant hand and grasping clean part of wristlet, pull sleeve wristlet over your nondominant hand. Use your nondominant hand to pull sleeve wristlet over your dominant hand.
9. Grasp outside of gown through the sleeves at shoulders. Pull gown down over your arms.
10. Hold both gown shoulders in one hand. Carefully draw your other hand out of gown, turning arm of gown inside out. Repeat this procedure with your other arm.
11. Hold gown away from your body. Fold gown up inside out.

> **CLINICAL ALERT**
>
> Some isolation gowns do not tie at the neck, they slip over the head. When removing these gowns, pull shoulders forward to tear the neck area. Remove gown in same manner as those which tie at the neck.

12. Discard gown in appropriate place.
13. Wash your hands. **Rationale:** This prevents cross-infection to other clients.

Hospitals in the United States may use plastic aprons instead of long-sleeved gowns. This alternative is acceptable for infection control as long as gloves are worn, skin on arms is intact, and rigorous handwashing includes the arms.

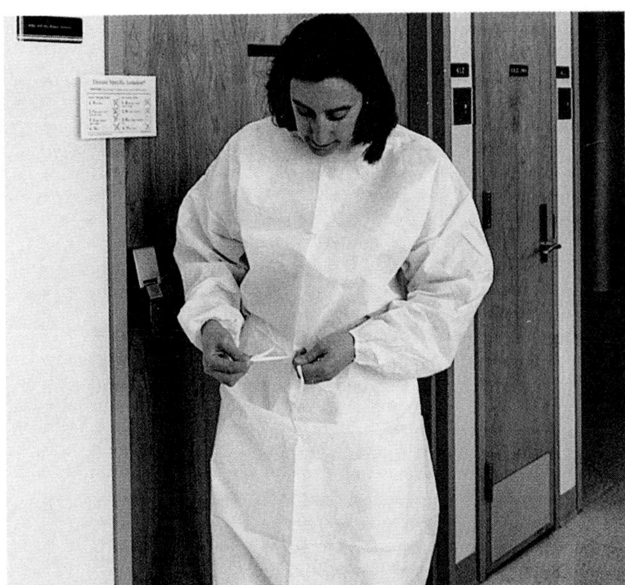

Isolation gown is put on before mask or gloves.

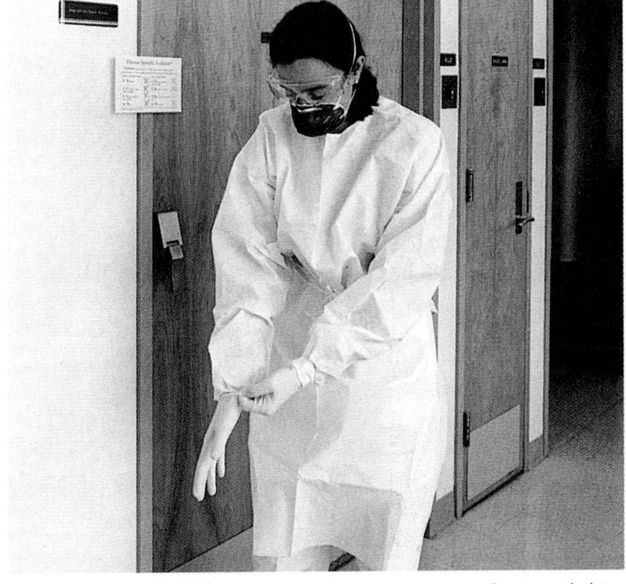

Cover wristlets completely to prevent contamination of exposed skin.

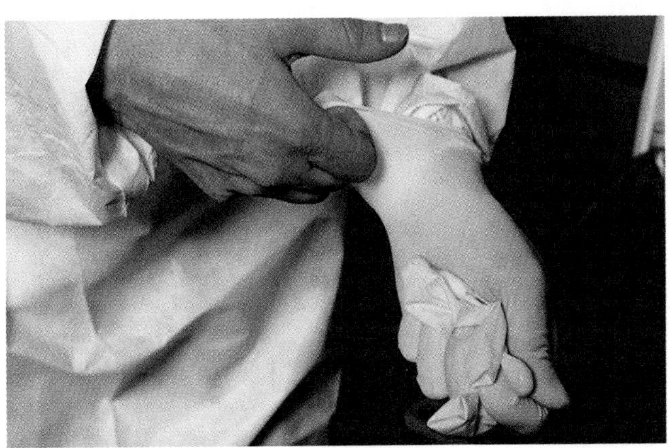

Remove gloves before gown or mask are taken off.

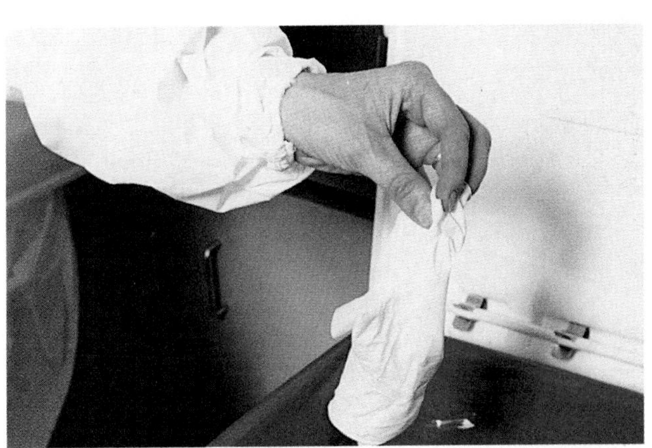

Dispose of gloves in appropriate receptacle.

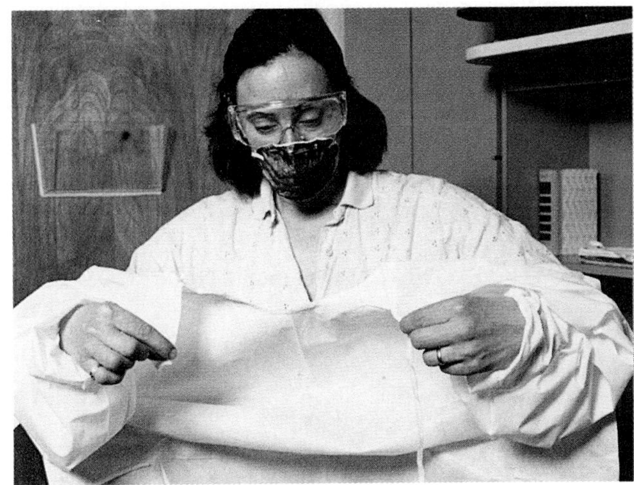

Pull gown down shoulders first and then arms.

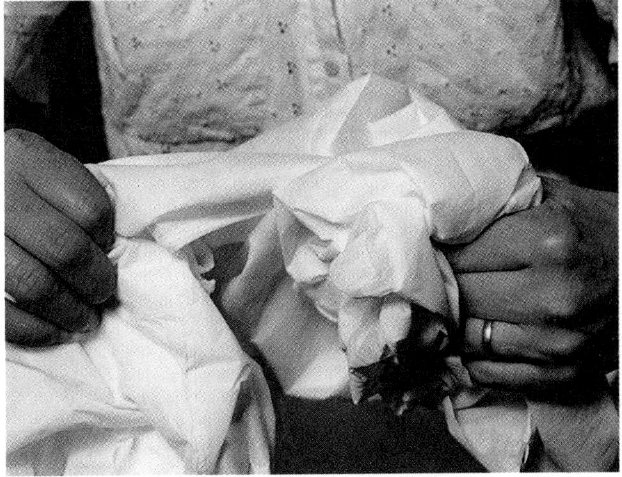

Hold gown away from body when rolling inside out.

USING A MASK

Equipment

Clean mask

> **■ CLINICAL ALERT**
>
> HEPA (High-efficiency particulate air) masks are recommended for suspected or confirmed multidrug-resistant tuberculosis.
> - Masks are fitted to worker.
> - Wear mask until it becomes difficult to breathe. This indicates mask is clogged.
> - When not in use, store mask in zip-lock bag in safe area.
> - Masks are expensive and can be used repeatedly.

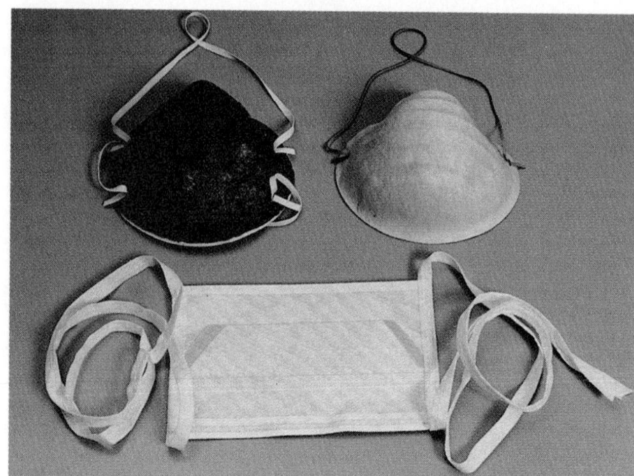

Sample masks used for isolation protocol.

Procedure

1. Obtain mask from box.
2. Position mask to cover your nose and mouth.
3. Bend nose bar so that it conforms over bridge of your nose.
4. If you are using a mask with string ties, tie top strings on top of your head to prevent slipping. If you are using a cone-shaped mask, tie top strings over your ears.
5. Tie bottom strings around your neck to secure mask over your mouth. There should be no gaps between the mask and your face.
6. Wash your hands before removing mask.
7. To remove mask, untie strings without touching mask. **Rationale:** Only strings are considered clean.
8. Discard mask in a trash container.
9. Wash your hands.

Protective eye wear such as goggles and face shield are worn when there is a risk of splashes or sprays from blood, secretions, excretions, or body fluids.

ASSESSING VITAL SIGNS

Equipment

Thermometer
Stethoscope
Blood pressure cuff and sphygmomanometer
Thermometer stand
Watch with sweep second hand

Procedure

1. Wash your hands.
2. Don isolation clothing as required by type of isolation.
3. Proceed to take vital signs as you would for any client.
4. Place equipment in appropriate area if it is to be left in room.
5. Remove isolation clothing according to protocol.
6. Wash hands.
7. Wipe watch if accidentally contaminated. Use appropriate solution.

> **PROTOCOL FOR LEAVING ISOLATION ROOM**
>
> Take off gloves.
> Untie gown at waist.
> Untie gown at neck.
> Pull gown off and place in laundry hamper.
> Take off goggles or face shield.
> Take off mask.
> Wash hands.

REMOVING ITEMS FROM ISOLATION ROOM

Procedure

1. Close isolation bag when it is one-half to three-fourths full. Close bag inside the isolation room.
2. Set up a new bag for continued use inside room. Bag is usually red with the word "Biohazard" written on outside of bag.
3. Before removing from room, enclose top of bag and tie off the top of bag. If outside of bag is contaminated, if the bag could be easily penetrated, or if contaminated material in the bag is heavy and could break, the bag should be double-bagged for safety.
4. Place bag from inside room into a bag held open by a second health care worker outside room if double-bagging is required. Second health care worker makes a cuff with the top of the bag and places hands under cuff. **Rationale:** This prevents hands from becoming contaminated.
5. Place bag into second bag without contaminating outside of the bag. Secure top of bag by tying a knot in top of bag.
6. Take bag to designated area where biohazard material is collected, usually "dirty" utility room.

■ CLINICAL ALERT

Linen and burnable trash are disposed of in same manner. Ensure that when placing bags in containers in "dirty" utility room you place in correct container according to bag contents.

THREE REQUIREMENTS FOR DOUBLE-BAGGING

Outside of bag is contaminated.
Bag could easily be penetrated.
Contaminated material is too heavy and could break bag.

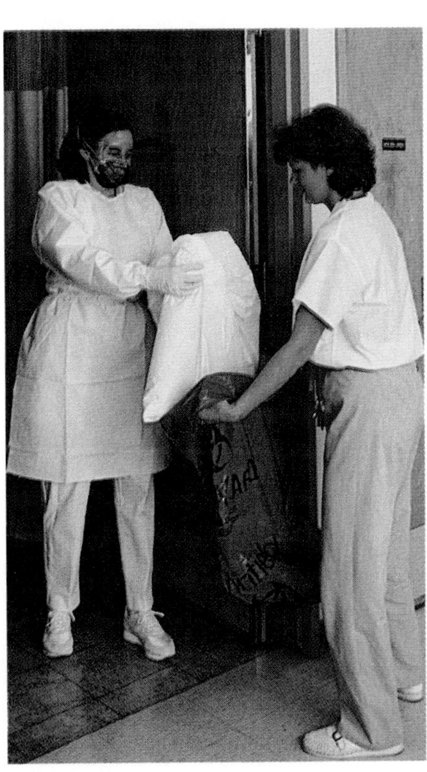
Place bag into second bag without contaminating outside of bag.

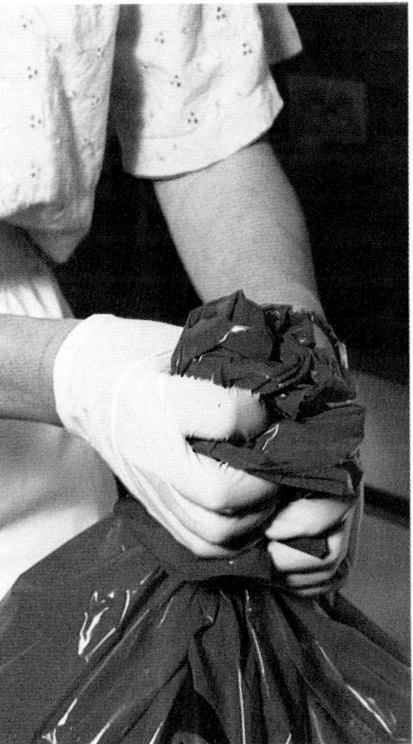
Close bag securely and label contents, if necessary.

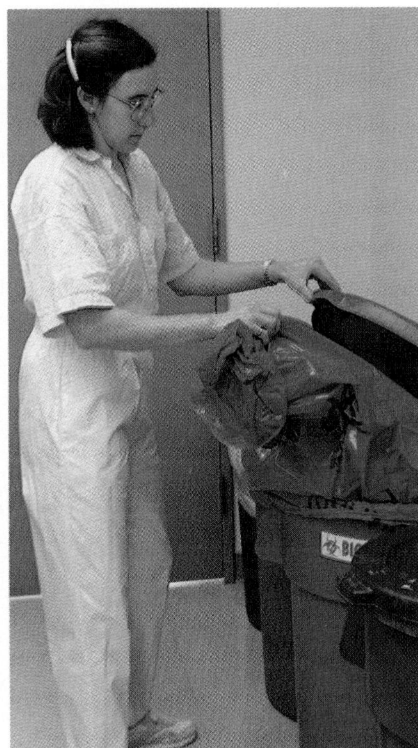
Place isolation bag in appropriate collection area.

REMOVING A SPECIMEN FROM ISOLATION ROOM

Procedure

1. Mark a specimen container with the client's name, type of specimen, and the word "isolation" before entering an isolation room.
2. Collect specimen, and place container in a clean plastic biohazard bag outside the room. Use clear bags so that laboratory personnel can see the specimen easily.
3. Wash your hands.
4. Send specimen to laboratory with appropriate laboratory request form.

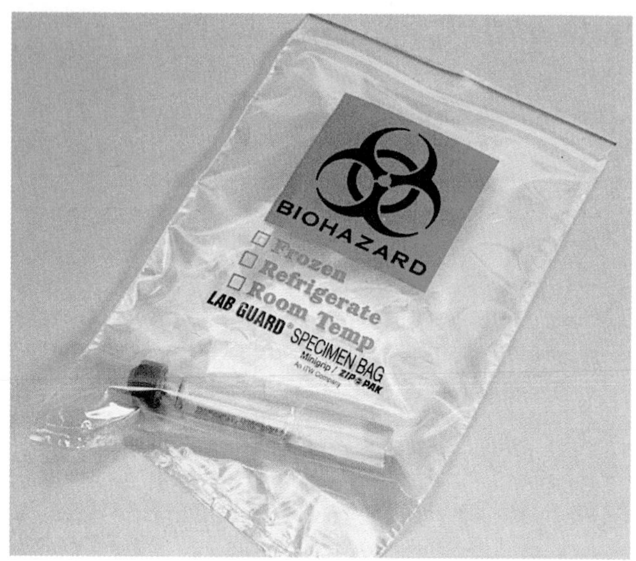

Biohazard bag for transportation of specimens from isolation room.

TRANSPORTING ISOLATION CLIENT OUTSIDE THE ROOM

Procedure

1. Explain procedure to client.
2. If client is being transported from a respiratory isolation room, instruct him or her to wear a mask for the entire time out of isolation. **Rationale:** This prevents the spread of airborne microbes.
3. Cover the transport vehicle with a bath blanket if there is a chance of soiling when transporting a client with a draining wound or diarrhea.
4. Help client into transport vehicle. Cover client with a bath blanket.
5. Tell receiving department what type of isolation client needs and what precautions hospital personnel should follow.
6. Remove bath blanket, and handle as contaminated linen when client returns to room.
7. Instruct all hospital personnel to wash their hands before they leave the area.
8. Wipe down transportation vehicle with a germicidal-virucidal solution if soiled.

REMOVING SOILED LARGE EQUIPMENT FROM ISOLATION ROOM

GUIDELINES FOR DISPOSING OF CONTAMINATED EQUIPMENT

Disposable glass: Place in isolation bag separate from burnable trash and direct to appropriate hospital area for disposal.

Glass equipment: Bag separately from metal equipment and return to CSR.

Metal equipment: Bag all equipment together, label, and return to CSR.

Rubber and plastic items: Bag items separately and return to CSR for gas sterilization.

Dishes: Require no special precautions unless contaminated with infected material; then bag, label, and return to kitchen.

Plastic or paper dishes: Dispose of these items in burnable trash.

Soiled linens: Place in laundry bag, and send to separate area of laundry room for special care. If possible, place linens in hot-water–soluble bag. This method is safer for handling, as bag may be placed directly into washing machine. (Double-bagging is usually required because these bags are easily punctured or torn. They also dissolve when wet.)

Food and liquids: Dispose of these items by putting them in the toilet—flush thoroughly.

Needles and syringes: Do not recap needles; place in puncture-resistant container.

Sphygmomanometer and stethoscope: Require no special precautions unless they are contaminated. If contaminated, disinfect using the appropriate cleaning protocol based on the infective agent.

Thermometers: Dispose of electronic probe cover with burnable trash. If probe or machine is contaminated, clean with appropriate disinfectant for infective agent. If reusable glass thermometers are used, disinfect with appropriate solution.

Procedure

1. Don isolation garb as recommended.
2. Wash equipment with an antimicrobial agent.
   Rationale: Washing is preferred to spraying to ensure all surfaces are cleaned.
3. Cover equipment with a plastic bag.
4. Remove garb, and wash your hands outside the room. Take equipment to the decontamination area of CSR.

CHARTING for Isolation

- Type of isolation protocol being practiced
- Client's reactions to sensory deprivation
- Specimens sent to laboratory

CRITICAL THINKING APPLICATION

CLINICAL PROBLEMS	CRITICAL THINKING OPTIONS
Outbreak of disease occurs in isolation environment.	• Identify cause of outbreak, and contact the infection control practitioner for consultation. • Examine handwashing and infection control practices among staff. • Attend in-service education program on isolation techniques to increase your awareness of appropriate procedures.

unit 3

STANDARD PRECAUTIONS

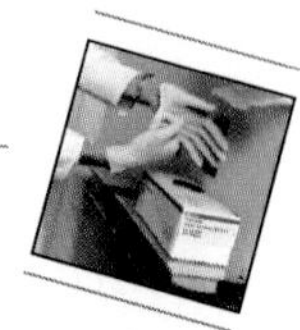

NURSING PROCESS DATA

ASSESSMENT Data Base

Assess for skin integrity.

Assess for presence of drainage from lesions or body cavity.

Assess for ability to deal with oral secretions.

Assess for compliance to hygiene measures (i.e., covering mouth when coughing, ability to control body fluids).

Assess ability to carry out activities of daily living (ADLs).

Assess extent of barrier techniques needed (i.e., gloves, gown, mask, protective eyewear).

Assess need for special equipment (i.e., hazardous waste bags, plastic bags for specimens).

PLANNING Objectives

To prevent the spread of the microorganism to health professionals

To reduce potential for the transmission of microorganisms

To protect hospital personnel and others from contamination

To provide appropriate equipment and techniques for preventive measures

IMPLEMENTATION Procedures

Caring for Isolation Clients

EVALUATION Expected Outcomes

The microorganism is not transmitted to other individuals.

The health care worker is protected from the microorganism.

Appropriate nursing interventions are carried out for the client.

CARING FOR ISOLATION CLIENTS

Equipment

Disposable gloves

Gown

Mask

Protective eyewear

Specimen container, plastic bag, biohazard label if needed

Red plastic container for sharp articles

Laundry bag, large plastic bag

Heavy gloves if bagging trash, plastic bag

Cleaning articles

UNIVERSAL PRECAUTIONS

For all patient care

PROCEDURE					
Talking to patient					
Adjusting IV fluid rate or non-invasive equipment					
Examining patient *without* touching blood, body fluids, mucous membranes	X				
Examining patient *including* contact with blood, body fluids, mucous membranes	X	X			
Drawing blood	X	X			
Inserting venous access	X	X			
Suctioning	X	X	*Use gown, mask, eyewear if bloody body fluid splattering is likely*		
Inserting body or face catheters	X	X	*Use gown, mask, eyewear if bloody body fluid splattering is likely*		
Handling soiled waste, linen, other materials	X	X	*Use gown, mask, eyewear only if waste or linen are extensively contaminated and splattering is likely*		
Intubation	X	X	X	X	X
Inserting arterial access	X	X	X	X	X
Endoscopy	X	X	X	X	X
Operative and other procedures which produce extensive splattering of blood or body fluids.	X	X	X	X	X

CLIENT CARE PROTECTION PROTOCOL

Entering Room of Client

Put on protective garments before entering client's room
Put on gown, tie at neck and back
Put on mask
Put on protective eyewear
Don disposable latex gloves

Leaving Room of Client Following Care

Remove protective garments before leaving client's room
Take off gloves, turning them inside out when removing
Take off protective eyewear
Take off gown, turning back into front so that inside of gown is on outside
Take off mask

Procedure

1. Wear gloves. **Rationale:** Worn for any anticipated contact with client's blood, body fluid, secretion, or excretion. Not worn for contact with unsoiled articles or intact skin.
2. Don gown. **Rationale:** Worn when it is likely that personal clothing will be soiled with blood, body fluids, secretions, and excretions.
3. Wear mask. **Rationale:** Worn for anticipated contact with respiratory droplet secretions (e.g., client with suspected or known tuberculosis) coughing client who does not cover mouth or nose, suctioning client; any potential splatter into mouth or nose while performing procedures.
4. Wear protective eyewear. **Rationale:** Worn in situations where blood or other body substances such as blood or sputum may splatter into the eyes.
5. Handle laboratory specimens with care. **Rationale:**

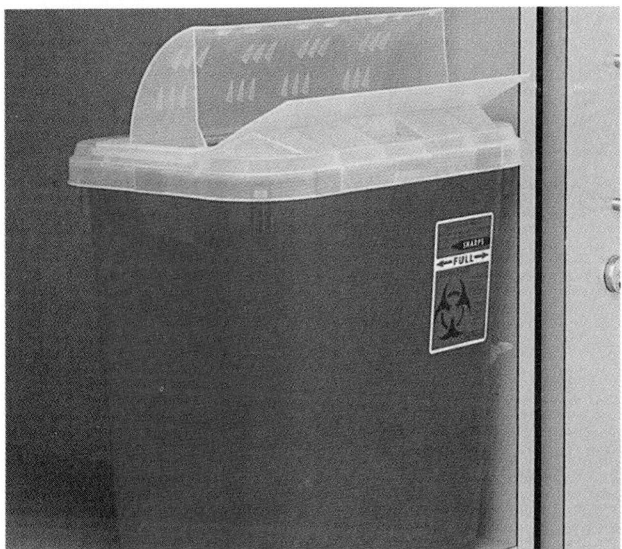

Larger sharps containers are available for areas where usage is greater.

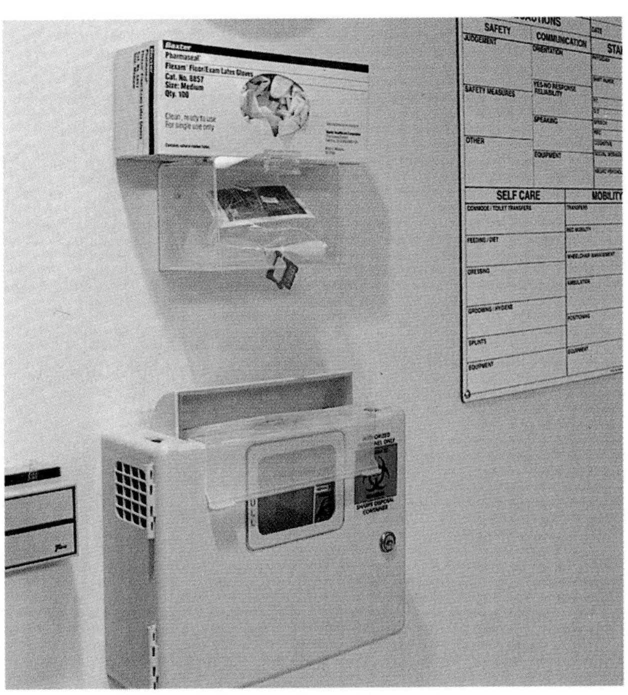

Sharps container needs to be placed in area for easy access.

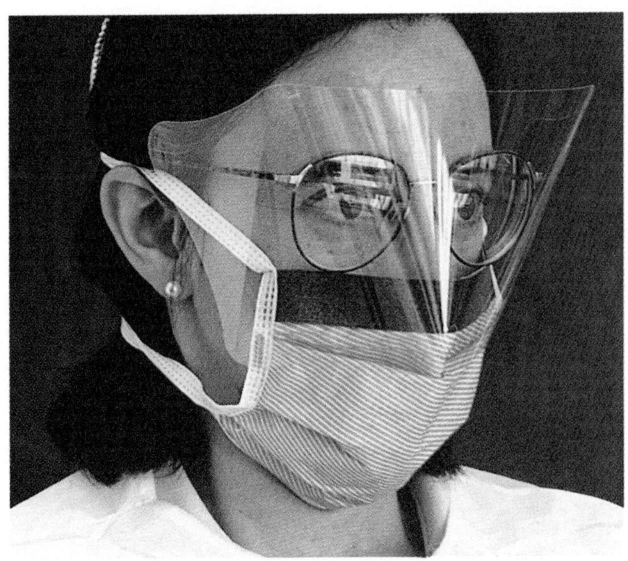

Face shield should be used when there is a risk of splashing from body fluids or blood.

All specimens are potentially infected. Place specimen in biohazard bag outside room. Be careful to not contaminate outside of plastic bag.

6. Take specimens to laboratory.
7. Bag reusable soiled articles. **Rationale:** This prevents leakage and identifies the contents as soiled so that central supply personnel will glove to handle them.
8. Place soiled instruments in marked containers located in "dirty" utility rooms.
9. Place all used syringes, needles, and disposable sharps in the red heavy plastic needle container. Do not recap or break off used needles under any circumstances. There is considerable danger of injury when recapping used needles.

■ CLINICAL ALERT

Disposal Precautions

Secretion: Client should be instructed to expectorate into tissue held close to mouth. Suction catheters and gloves should be disposed of in impervious, sealed bags.

Excretion: Excrement should be disposed of by flushing into sewage system. Strict attention should be paid to careful handwashing; disease can be spread by oral–fecal route.

Blood: Needles and syringe should be disposable. Used needles should *not* be recapped. They should be placed in a puncture-resistant container that is prominently labeled "isolation." Specimens should be labeled "blood precaution."

10. Place soiled linen in a laundry bag in room and then in the biohazard container in "dirty" utility room. **Rationale:** This prevents leakage.
11. Bag trash and disposable articles soiled with body substances. Check hospital policy for double-bagging protocol.
12. Perform cleaning of client's room consistently and thoroughly. Promptly clean up body substances using gloves, gown, and approved germicide.

■ HIV–HBV CLINICAL ALERT

Sample protocol for accidental contact with blood or body fluids.

1. Any percutaneous or mucocutaneous exposure should receive immediate first aid.
   a. Percutaneous exposure—a break in the skin caused by contaminated needle or sharp instrument, broken glass container holding blood or body fluids, or human bite.
   b. Mucocutaneous exposure—body fluid contact to open wounds, nonintact skin (eczema), or body fluid splash to mucous membranes (mouth, eyes).
2. Apply immediate first aid to site.
   a. Needlestick or puncture wound: Express blood from wound; scrub area vigorously with soap and water for 5 minutes.
   b. Oral mucous membrane exposure: Rinse area several times with oxygenating agent such as half-strength hydrogen peroxide. Do not swallow agent.
   c. Ocular exposure: Irrigate immediately with water or normal saline solution.
   d. Human bite: Cleanse wound with povidone-iodine (Betadine) and sterile water.
3. Report unusual occurrence to the charge nurse or supervisor.
4. Complete an unusual occurrence form and, if appropriate, a worker's compensation form.
5. Follow facility protocol for emergency care including HIV antibody testing; if HIV risk is a consideration, case will be evaluated for prophylactic AZT. (Usually this protocol involves massive or serious exposure.)

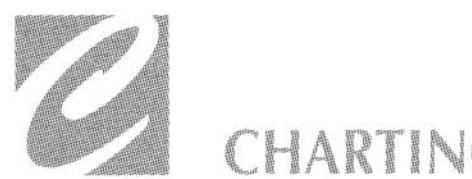

CHARTING for Standard Precautions

- Isolation protocol maintained
- Type of isolation procedures implemented
- Client's response to care

CRITICAL THINKING APPLICATION

CLINICAL PROBLEMS	CRITICAL THINKING OPTIONS
Contaminated blood or body fluid comes in contact with your skin or mucous membranes.	• Wash area that is spattered immediately with germicidal soap. • Report incident, and complete unusual occurrence report. (Very important for follow-up legal and medical implications.) • HIV exposure should be immediately reported, as most hospitals offer AZT preventive therapy. This therapy should be administered within 1 hour, not more than 24 hours after exposure. • Obtain AIDS antibody test in ensuing months. • Continue to monitor own health status and carry out specific activities to build immune system. Do not smoke or drink excessively. Eat well-balanced meals with reduced fat intake. Take vitamin supplements designed to boost immune system (vitamin C, beta-carotene, vitamin A, Coenzyme Q 10, zinc). Check with nutritionist or holistic physician for complete protocol. Exercise frequently. Obtain adequate sleep and rest. Learn and practice stress reduction activities (stress is known to lessen effectiveness of immune system).
Working with AIDS patients becomes extremely stressful, and you experience burn-out.	• Request consultation therapy to handle feelings and learn new methods of coping with stress. • Leave this type of work temporarily. • Change other aspects of your life to reduce stress. • Follow above-mentioned regimen to enhance immune system.
Clients you are caring for frequently die and you have difficulty handling grieving process.	• Request assistance from skilled professional to work through own feelings about death. • Request that a support group be formed for health care workers of AIDS clients.

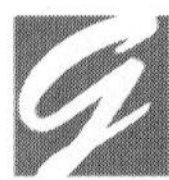

GERIATRIC CONSIDERATIONS

- Social isolation resulting from infection control requirements is more intense with the elderly. They need frequent contact with health care workers. Sometimes being ill is the only attention they receive.
- Elderly clients can become confused in the hospital and when placed in isolation, there is an even greater risk. Frequent monitoring for safety issues is necessary.
- Frequent explanations of why isolation is necessary is important for the elderly. They may have a lapse of memory and forget earlier discussion about isolation.
- Ensure that call lights are easily accessible and the client understands how to call for assistance. They may have impaired hearing and sight, which can interfere with communications.

16

Medication Administration

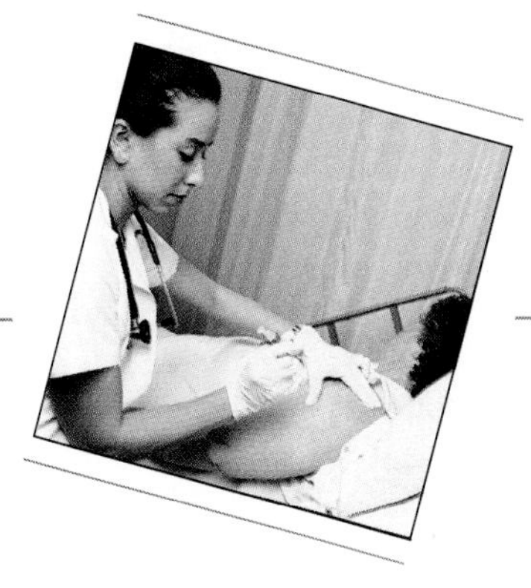

LEARNING OBJECTIVES

- Explain the concepts of absorption, transportation, biotransformation, and excretion.
- State the "five rights" for administering medications.
- List the seven parts of a drug order.
- Differentiate between unit dose and the more traditional method of medication administration.
- Describe the medication cart and its purpose.
- Identify three nursing actions that prevent drug injuries.
- Outline the method of calculating oral dosages of drugs.
- List at least four assessment factors important for administering parenteral medications.
- Outline the steps in preparing for injecting parenteral medications.
- State the rationale for using the Z-track method of injection.
- Compare insulin types, their action, onset, peak, and duration.
- Describe the assessment factors used before applying medications to the skin and mucous membranes.
- Outline the steps in applying a transdermal medication.
- State four techniques for alleviating client pain during injections.
- Describe the information that should be included in charting injections.
- Outline the steps for instilling eye drops.
- Differentiate between the positions for instilling ear medications in adults and children.
- List the steps for inserting a rectal suppository.
- Demonstrate the ability to mix two medications.

TERMINOLOGY

Absorption: the passage of a substance through some surface of the body into body fluids and tissues.

Addictive: alcohol or drug that causes enslavement to some habit.

Allergy: an antigen–antibody reaction or sensitivity to a substance.

Anaphylaxis: a hypersensitive shock state due to a foreign substance, protein, or drug.

Anesthesia: partial or complete loss of sensation with or without loss of consciousness as a result of injury, disease, or administration of a drug.

Aseptic: sterile; condition free from germs and infection.

Aspirate: to remove by suction.

Biotransformation: the biologic process of changing a substance so that it may be metabolized or excreted.

Bronchodilatation: dilatation of a bronchus.

Cardiotonic: increasing tonicity of the heart.

Cathartic: an active purgative for the bowels.

Circulation: having to do with the movement of blood in a circular course, exiting from the aorta and coming back into the heart via the vena cava.

Compatible: able to mix with another substance without destructive changes.

Congestion: the presence of an excessive amount of blood or tissue fluid in an organ or in tissue.

Contaminate: to soil, stain, or pollute; to render impure.

Contraindication: any symptom or circumstance indicating the inappropriateness of a form of treatment otherwise advisable.

Dosage: the amount of medicine to be administered to a client at one time.

Drug: any substance that when taken into the living organism may modify one or more of its functions.

Dyspnea: labored or difficult breathing.

Ecchymosis: a form of macula appearing in large, irregularly formed hemorrhagic areas of the skin.

Emetic: medicine that produces vomiting.

Generic: general; pertinent to a genus; distinctive.

Hydration: the chemical combination of a substance with water.

Hypnotic: an agent that induces sleep or which dulls the senses.

Infection: condition in which the body or body part is invaded by a pathogenic agent (microorganism or virus) that may multiply and produce effects that are injurious.

Instillation: slowly pouring or dropping a liquid into a cavity or onto a surface.

Intradermal: within the dermal layer of the skin.

Intravenous: within or into a vein.

Medicine: a drug or remedy.

Metabolism: all energy and material transformations which occur within living cells.

Narcotic: a drug that, in moderate doses, depresses the central nervous system, thus relieving pain and producing sleep; most narcotics are addictive and in excess may produce coma or death.

Ointment: a medicated, fatty, soft substance having antiseptic, cosmetic, or healing properties.

Parenteral: injection of substances into the body through any route other than alimentary; outside the intestines.

Peristalsis: a progressive, wavelike movement that occurs involuntarily in the intestines of the body.

Salve: an ointment applied to a wound; any ointment made with a base of fat, oil, petrolatum, or resin.

Subcutaneous: third tissue layer; introduced beneath the skin.

Sublingual: beneath the tongue.

Synthetic: artificially prepared.

Systemic: pertinent to a whole body rather than one specific area.

Therapeutic: having medicinal or healing properties.

Tonicity: state of normal tension, especially muscular, as with muscular tone.

Vasodilator: an agent that causes blood vessels to dilate.

THERAPEUTIC AGENTS

Therapeutic agents are drugs or medications that, when introduced into a living organism, modify the physiologic functions of that organism. The term "therapeutic agent" usually refers to a chemical compound. If this substance has an effect on body functions, it can also be a vitamin, mineral, herb, or even a natural food. In this chapter, however, the term "therapeutic agent" refers to drugs and their actions.

DRUG METABOLISM

Drug metabolism in the human body is accomplished in four basic stages: absorption, transportation, biotransformation, and excretion. For a drug to be completely metabolized, it must first be given in sufficient concentration to produce the desired effect on body tissues. When this "critical drug concentration" level is achieved, body tissues change.

Routes for Absorption

The first stage of metabolism refers to the route a drug takes from the time it enters the body until it is dissolved and absorbed in the circulating fluids. Drugs are absorbed by the mucous membranes, the gastrointestinal tract, the respiratory tract, and the skin. The mucous membranes are one of the most rapid and effective routes of absorption because they are highly vascular.

Oral drugs (drugs that are given by mouth) are absorbed in the gastrointestinal tract. Portions of these drugs dissolve and are absorbed in the stomach. The rate of absorption depends on the pH of the stomach's contents, the food content in the stomach at the time of ingestion, and the presence of disease conditions. Most of the drug concentrate dissolves in the small intestine where the large vascular surface and moderate pH level enhance the process of breaking down the drug.

Parenteral methods are the most direct, reliable, and rapid route of absorption. This method of administration includes intradermal, subcutaneous (Sub Q), intramuscular (IM), and intravenous (IV). The actual administration site depends on the type of drug, its action, and the client. For example, a client with a severe allergic reaction receives epinephrine IV, since this is the fastest route for drug absorption in an emergency situation.

Another route of medication administration that is faster than the gastrointestinal tract but not as rapid as parenteral injections is inhalation through the respiratory system. Drugs are administered by a pressure device such as a nebulizer and are reduced to small particles that can reach the lower respiratory tract where they have a local therapeutic effect. Little systemic absorption occurs.

The mucous membranes provide a variety of routes for medication administration and absorption. Sites include sublingual and buccal areas, the eye, nose, vagina, and rectum. Local or systemic effects can be achieved by these routes.

Medications can be applied topically to the eye (ophthalmic), ear (otic), or skin (dermal) for a local effect. The skin is also used for transdermal administration of drugs via patches, which release a medication continuously for a systemic effect.

Transportation

The second stage of metabolism refers to the way in which a drug is transported from the site of introduction to the site of action. When a drug enters or is absorbed by the body, a portion of the drug binds to plasma protein and may compete with other drugs for this storage site. Another portion is transported in "free" form through the circulation to all parts of the body. It is the "free" drug that is pharmacologically active. As the free drug moves from the circulatory system, it crosses cell membranes to reach its site of action. As the drug is metabolized and excreted, protein-bound drug is freed for action. Lipid-soluble drugs are distributed to and stored in fat and then released slowly into the bloodstream when drug administration is discontinued. The amount of the drug that is distributed to body tissues depends on the permeability of the membranes and the blood supply to the absorption area.

Biotransformation

The third stage of metabolism takes place as the drug, which is a foreign substance in the body, is converted by enzymes into a less active and harmless agent that can be easily excreted. Most of this conversion occurs in the liver, although some conversion does take place in the lungs, kidney, plasma, and intestinal mucosa.

Excretion

The final stage in metabolism takes place when the drug is changed into an inactive form or excreted from the body. The kidneys are the most important route of excretion because they eliminate both the pure drug and the metabolites of the parent drug. During excretion, these two substances are filtered through the glomeruli, secreted by the tubules, and either reabsorbed through the tubules or directly excreted. Other routes of excretion include the lungs (which exhale gaseous drugs), feces, saliva, tears, and mother's milk.

Factors That Affect Drug Metabolism

Many factors affect drug metabolism, including personal attributes, such as body weight, age, and sex; physiologic factors, such as state of health or disease processes; acid–base and fluid and electrolyte balance; permeability; diurnal rhythm; and circulatory capability. Genetic and immunologic factors play a role in drug metabolism, as do psychologic, emotional, and environmental influences; drug tolerance; and cumulation of drugs. Responses to drugs vary, depending on the speed with which the drug is absorbed into the blood or tissues and the effectiveness of the body's circulatory system.

DRUG ADMINISTRATION

The route of drug administration influences the action of that drug on the body. To obtain a systemic effect, a drug must be absorbed and transported to the cells or tissues that respond to them. How a drug is administered depends on the chemical nature and quantity of the drug, as well as on the desired speed of effect and the overall condition of the client.

Individual drugs are designed to be administered by specific routes—be sure to check drug labels for the appropriate route of administration. Common routes of administration to obtain systemic effects include the following: oral, sublingual, rectal, transdermal, and parenteral. Parenteral injections are commonly administered in these sites: intradermal, subcutaneous, IM, and IV.

Source and Naming of Drugs

The primary natural sources from which drugs are compounded are roots, bark, sap, leaves, flowers, and seeds of plants. Other natural sources include animal organs or organ cells, secretions, and mineral sources. Synthetic drugs, such as sulfonamides, are made in a laboratory from chemical substances.

Most drugs are given chemical, generic, and trademark names. The chemical name, for example, 1-methyl-4-phenyl-4-piperidinecarboxylic acid ethyl ester hydrochloride, refers to the chemical derivation of the drug. The generic name, meperidine hydrochloride, is shorter and simpler and reflects the chemical family to which the drug belongs. Demerol is one of the trademark names for this compound; and this is the most common way in which this drug is known. Once a drug is registered with a brand name (Demerol), that drug can be manufactured only by its legal owners.

Safety Procedures

When you administer drugs, you must follow certain safety rules, which are also known as "The Five Rights." These rules should be carried out each time you give a drug to a client.

The Five Rights

- Right medication. Compare drug card, medication sheet, or drug Kardex (client's medication record) three times, with label on drug container. Know action, dosage, and method of administration. Know side effects of the drug.
- Right client. Check the client's identaband and door number.

- Right time
- Right method of administration
- Right amount. Check all calculations of divided doses with another nurse. Check heparin, insulin, and IV digitalis doses with another nurse.

Documenting the Medication

A medication must have a physician's order or prescription before it can be legally administered to a client. The physician's order is a verbal or written order, which is recorded in a book or file or in the client's chart. If an order is given verbally over the telephone, you must write a verbal order in the client's chart for the physician to sign within 24 hours. Written orders are safer because they leave less room for potential misunderstanding or error.

A drug order should consist of seven parts:

1. The name of the client
2. The date the drug was ordered
3. The name of the drug
4. The dosage
5. The route of administration and any special rules of administration
6. The time and frequency the drug should be given
7. The signature of the individual who ordered the drug

There are two basic types of drug orders: routine and one-time only drug orders. A routine medication is administered according to instructions until it is canceled by another order. Routine medication orders can also be used for p.r.n. drugs. These drugs are administered when the client needs the medication, not necessarily on a routine time schedule. Medication for bowel elimination is a type of p.r.n. drug that is not necessarily administered every day. When you administer medications, you should assess the continued validity of any routine order. Physicians occasionally forget to cancel an order when it is no longer appropriate for a client's condition. One-time only orders are administered as stated, only one time. These orders may be given at a specified time or "stat," which means immediately.

If you prepare a medication, you must also give it to the client and chart it after the client has taken the required dosage. If a client refuses a medication, you should chart that the medication was refused and report this information to the physician. When you chart medications, be sure to use the correct abbreviations and symbols.

If you find an error in a drug order, such as an inaccurate dose or method of administration, it is your responsibility to question the order. If you cannot understand or read the order, verify it with the physician. Do not guess or have someone other than the originator of the order interpret it—this constitutes gross negligence. In many hospitals it is the pharmacist's responsibility to contact physicians when medication orders are unclear.

Always report medication errors to the physician immediately so that potential danger to the client is minimized. Although no nurse or doctor would intentionally commit an error, errors do occur. When they do, it is important that measures be taken immediately to assess and evaluate the client's status and to institute a plan of action to reverse the effects of the medication.

Errors in medication should also be documented in a medication incident report and on the client's record. This documentation is necessary for both legal reasons and nursing audits. Nursing audits are conducted to determine if an error in medication indicates one primary problem, a particular source of problems, or a range of problems that seem to have no connection.

Each hospital has its own policies and protocols for administered medications. Before administering any drugs, you must find out what these policies are and perform them accordingly.

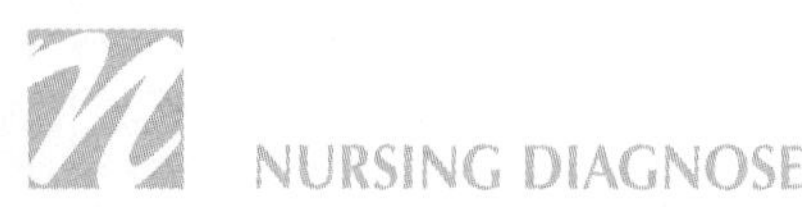

NURSING DIAGNOSES

The following nursing diagnoses may be appropriate to include in a client care plan when the components relate to a client who requires treatment with medications.

NURSING DIAGNOSIS	RELATED FACTORS
Altered Health Maintenance	Lack of education or readiness to learn, cognitive impairment, lack of equipment, inadequate support systems, inadequate financial resources, religious beliefs, cultural beliefs
Knowledge Deficit	Inadequate understanding of condition, misinformation, cognitive impairment
Noncompliance	Impaired ability to perform tasks, side effects of therapy, nontherapeutic environment, denial of condition, lack of information, poor self-esteem, nonsupportive family

unit 1

DRUG ADMINISTRATION

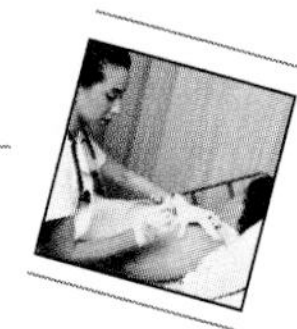

NURSING PROCESS DATA

ASSESSMENT Data Base

Assess route for drug administration.

Assess specific drug action for client.

Observe for signs and symptoms of side effects or adverse reactions.

Assess need for and accuracy of drug calculations.

PLANNING Objectives

To administer medications using correct route

To determine appropriate drug actions

To identify when side effects or adverse reactions occur

To accurately calculate drug dosages

IMPLEMENTATION Procedures

Preparing for Drug Administration

Converting Medications

Calculating Dosages

Using the Unit Dose System

Using the Narcotic Control System

EVALUATION Expected Outcomes

Medications are administered by correct route.

Medication actions and side effects are identified.

Drug dosages are calculated accurately.

PREPARING FOR DRUG ADMINISTRATION

Equipment

Reference resource (e.g., a pharmacology textbook)

Physician's Desk Reference

The hospital formulary

Medication administration record (MAR)

Client's drug Kardex

Procedure

Preclinical Preparation

1. Check all medications your client is receiving.
2. Determine which drugs are unfamiliar to you.
3. Research unfamiliar drugs using appropriate reference.
4. Bring drug handbook, or write out drug information on an index card if required. Include the following information.
   a. Generic and trade name
   b. Drug classification
   c. Pharmacologic actions
   d. Usual dosage, route of administration
   e. Major uses
   f. Side effects
   g. Nursing implications
5. Review procedure for medication administration (e.g., IM, Sub Q, oral).

CONFIDENTIAL INFORMATION

FROM TO

UNIVERSITY MEDICAL CENTER

MEDICATION ADMINISTRATION RECORD

INTRAMUSCULAR/SUBCUTANEOUS SITE CODES		PAIN SCALE	SEDATION SCALE
		0-No Pain	1-Wide Awake
		1-Mild Pain	2-Drowsy
A-Right Arm	F-Right Thigh	2-Discomforting	3-Dozing Intermittently
B-Left Arm	F-Left Thigh	3-Distressing	4-Mostly Sleeping
C-Right Hip	G-Right Abdomen	4-Horrible	5-Awakens Only When Aroused
D-Left Hip	H-Left Abdomen	5-Excruciating	

MEDICATIONS AND DIRECTIONS	RT	2301-0700	0701-1500	1501-2300

MESSAGE MAR CHECKED

Time																						
Pain Rating																						
Sedation Level																						
Respiration Rate																						

NURSE INITIALS AND SIGNATURE	NURSE INITIALS AND SIGNATURE	NURSE INITIALS AND SIGNATURE

CONFIDENTIAL INFORMATION

Rm & Bed # Name **CHART COPY** Med Rec # Page____ of____

Example of a medication administration record (MAR).

> ■ **CLINICAL ALERT**
>
> Individual drugs are designed to be administered by specific route—be sure to check drug labels for appropriate route of administration.

6. Calculate dosages if necessary.
7. Review safety procedures of "The Five Rights."

During Clinical Practice

1. Check client's MAR or Kardex and drawer in medication cart for drugs to be given during your clinical practice.
2. Check MAR for drug dose, route, and time before beginning client care.
3. Start with medication listed first on the MAR. Find the appropriate medication card.
4. Check if the client has allergies to drugs or food by reading the history and physical findings, client care plan, and MAR. Check the client's ID band for allergies.
5. Develop a drug time flowsheet. **Rationale:** This ensures that a client's medications are given on time.
6. Take medication cart and prepare to administer medications. Only set up the drugs to be administered for the specific time period. Do not set up drugs for the entire day.

CONVERTING MEDICATIONS

Procedure

1. To make conversions from the metric to apothecaries' or household systems, it is necessary to memorize or refer to equivalency tables.
2. To convert milligrams to grains, use the following formula:

$$\frac{1\text{ gr}}{\text{milligrams per grain}} = \frac{\text{Dose desired}}{\text{Dose on hand}}$$

$$\frac{1}{60} = \frac{x}{180}$$

$$60x = 180$$
$$x = 3\text{ gr}$$

3. You may also make this conversion as a ratio:

$$1\text{ gr}:60\text{ mg}: :x\text{ gr}:180\text{ mg}$$
$$60x = 180$$
$$x = 3\text{ gr}$$

4. Check equivalency tables in the drug supplement.
5. To convert milligrams to milliliters, you can set up a direct proportion and, following the algebraic principle, crossmultiply.
6. Check equivalency tables in the drug supplement.

CALCULATING DOSAGES

Equipment

Orders for dosage of medication needed

Dosage of medication on hand

Procedure

1. To calculate oral dosages, use the following formula. (D and H must be in same unit of measure.)

$$\frac{D}{H} = X$$

where D = dose desired; H = dose on hand; and X = dose to be administered.

Example: Give 500 mg of ampicillin sodium when the dose on hand is in capsules containing 250 mg.

$$\frac{500\text{ mg}}{250\text{ mg}} = 2\text{ capsules}$$

2. To calculate dose when in liquid form, use the following formula:

$$\frac{D}{H} \times Q = X$$

where D = dose desired; H = dose on hand; Q = quantity; and X = amount to be administered

Example: Give 375 mg of ampicillin when it is supplied as 250 mg/5 mL.

$$\frac{375\text{ mg}}{250\text{ mg}} \times 5$$

$$1.5 \times 5 = 7.5\text{ mL}$$

3. To calculate parenteral dosages, use the following formula:

$$\frac{D}{H} \times Q = X$$

Example: Give client 40 mg gentamicin C complex sulfate. On hand is a multidose vial with a strength of 80 mg/2 mL.

$$\frac{40}{80} \times 2 = 1\text{ mL}$$

4. Check your calculations before drawing up the medications.
5. See Calculations of Solutions in the Drug Supplement at the end of the chapter.

USING THE UNIT DOSE SYSTEM

Equipment

Medication administration record or drug Kardex

Medication cart

Medication keys

Preparation

for Oral Medications

1. Validate client's orders for consistency regarding drug, dose, time intervals, route of administration.
2. Check physician's orders for any discrepancy on medication record.

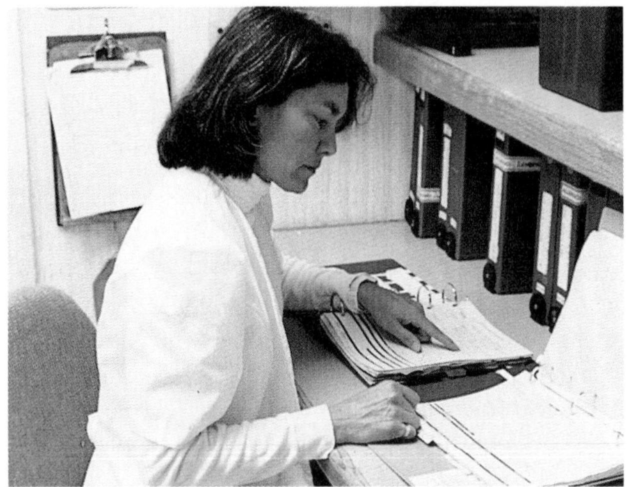

Check physicians order against MAR.

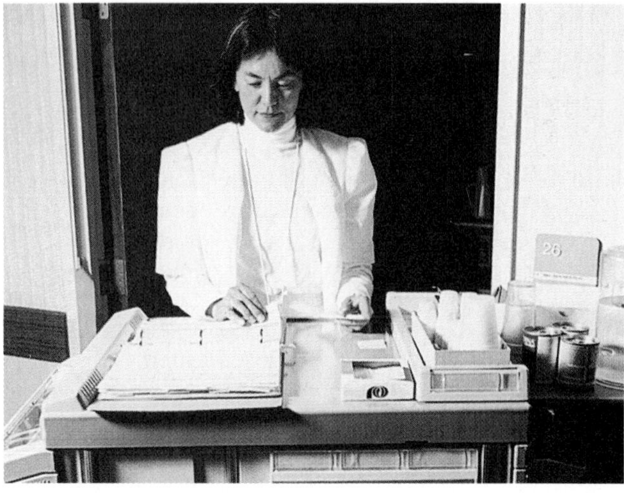

Take medication cart to client's room.

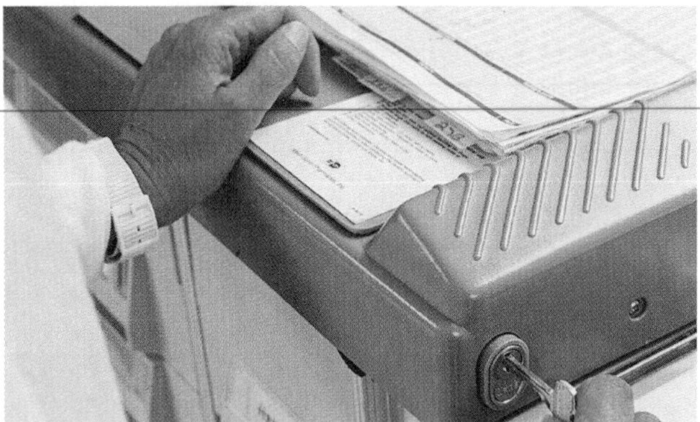

Unlock medication cart to access drugs.

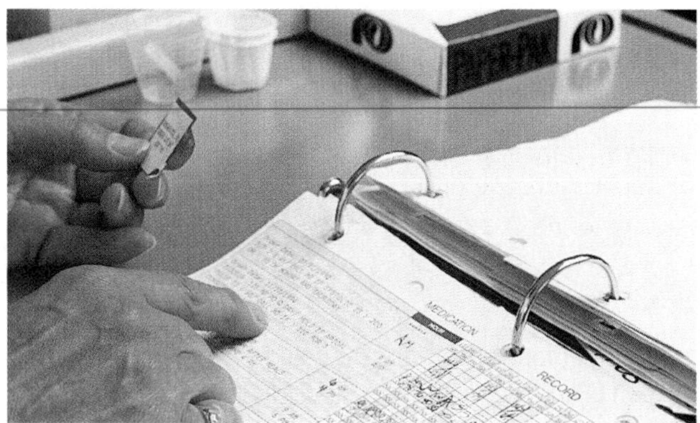

Find each medication to be given at one time.

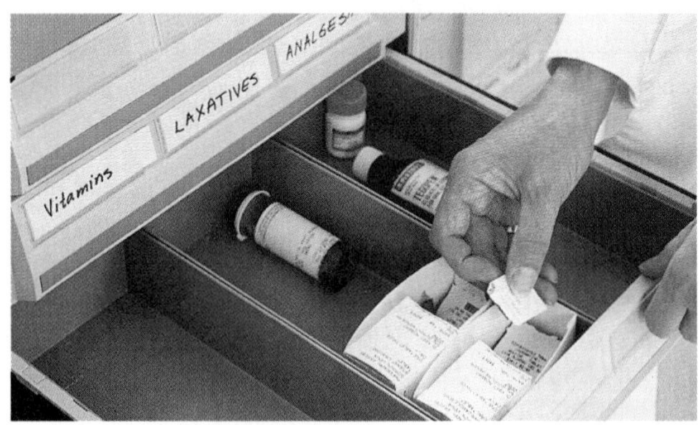

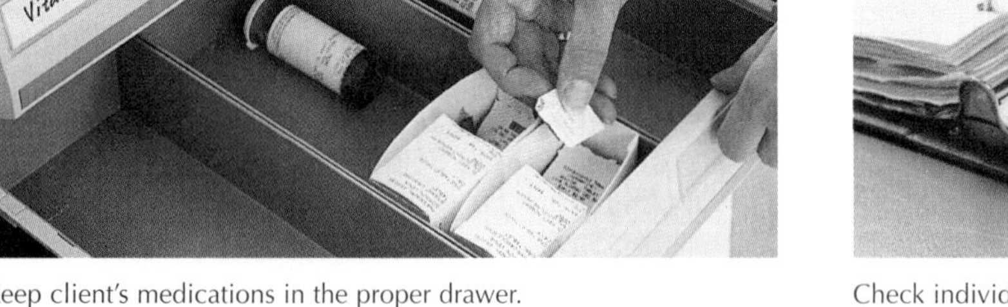

Keep client's medications in the proper drawer.

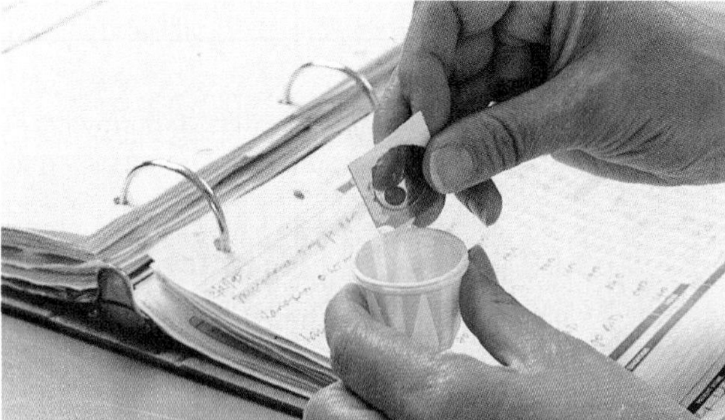

Check individually wrapped medication with record.

3. Wash your hands.
4. Take medication cart to the client's room.
5. Open medication cart; take out client's medication drawer.
6. Starting at the top of the medication record, check each medication in order against the medication packages in the drawer. Ensure that all doses for your shift are there. Pharmacy restocks cart every 24 hours. **Rationale:** If a dose is missing, or too many doses remain, check medication record for possible error in administration.
7. Check each drug with medication record for dose, time, and route of administration.
8. Start at top of medication record, and find each

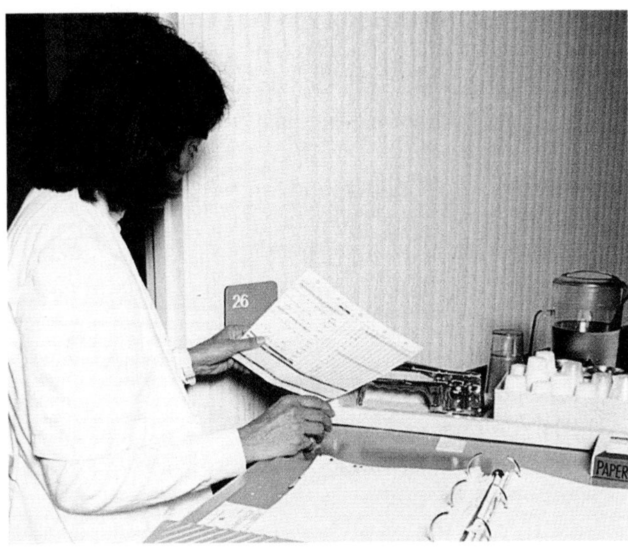

Check room number against medication.

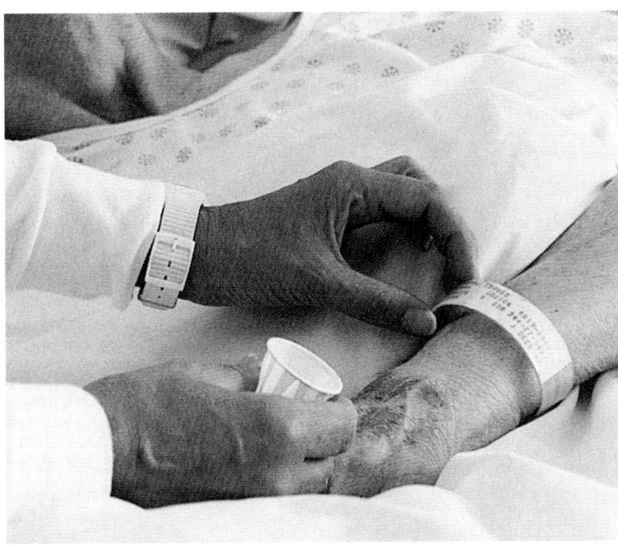

Check client's identaband and ask client to state name.

drug to be given at that time. Compare drug label with medication record. **Rationale:** This is a safety check to ensure the right medication is given.

9. Place the individually wrapped drugs in a medication cup or open package, and place drug in cup according to hospital policy. Compare the drug label with the medication record. **Rationale:** This is a second safety check.
10. Check the room number against the medication record, and lock the medication cart before entering the room. **Rationale:** Locking the cart is a safety measure because cart is frequently left unattended in hallway.
11. Check client's identaband, and ask client to state name.

> **■ CLINICAL ALERT**
>
> Assess vital signs, lab data, and so forth as indicated according to drug's action to ensure safe parameters for drug administration.

12. Assist client to sitting position. Hand medication cup and glass of water to client. Name drug, describe its use, and answer any questions.
13. Ensure that client swallows medications.
14. Position client for comfort.
15. Dispose of medication wrappers and cup.
16. Wash your hands.
17. Chart medications in medication record and any unusual findings in nurse's notes.
18. Take medication cart to next client room or medication room.

MEDICATION SAFETY MEASURES

- Keep all medicines in locked carts or cupboards.
- Remove drugs from bedside unless there is a physician's orders.
- Keep narcotics in double-locked cabinets. Count all narcotics at the end of each shift.
- Keep all poisonous solutions and materials in a secure area away from medicines.
- Clearly label and separate topical medicines from parenteral or oral medicines.
- Provide complete instructions to clients regarding medicines to be used at home. Make sure every physician involved with a client is aware of the medications the client is taking home.
- Have another nurse check mathematical calculations for dosages of drugs such as insulin before administering to clients.
- Report any errors in the administration of medicines to the charge nurse immediately. Document drug given, and complete a written unusual incident report.

for Parenteral Medications

1. Open medication cart, take out client's medication drawer, and open binder to client's medication record (MAR).

2. Starting at the top of the medication record, check each medication in order against the medication packages in the drawer. Ensure that all doses for your shift are there.
3. Check each drug and medication record for dose, time, and route of administration.
4. Check physician's orders for any discrepancy between medication record and drug package.
5. Take medication cart to the client's room.
6. Wash your hands.
7. Start at top of medication record, and find each drug to be given at that time. Compare the drug label with the medication record. **Rationale:** This is the first safety check to ensure the right medication is being given.
8. Prepare parenteral medications according to procedure.
9. Place syringe and alcohol swab on tray (if hospital policy) or carry in your hand to room.
10. Check the drug name and dosage again. Compare the drug label with the medication record. **Rationale:** This is the second safety check.
11. Check the room number against the medication record, and lock the medication cart before entering the room.
12. Check client's identaband, and ask client to state his or her name.
13. Provide privacy, and place client in appropriate position for type of parenteral medication to be administered.
14. Follow procedure for administering parenteral medications.
15. Position client for comfort.
16. Discard syringe in puncture-proof container. (Do not recap needle).
17. Wash your hands.
18. Chart medications in medication record.
19. Take medication cart to next client's room or to medication room.

USING THE NARCOTIC CONTROL SYSTEM

Equipment

Narcotic sign-out sheet
Medication record (MAR) or Kardex
Medication

Procedure

for Unit Stock

1. Check MAR or sheet for narcotic orders.
2. Check time last narcotic was administered.
3. Open narcotic box or cupboard, and find appropriate narcotic container.
4. Count the number of pills, ampules, or injectable cartridges in container.
5. Check the narcotic sign-out sheet, and check that the number of narcotics matches the number on sign-out sheets. **Rationale:** Laws on controlled substances require careful monitoring of narcotics.
6. Correct the situation before proceeding with nar-

Lock narcotic drawer after removing medication.

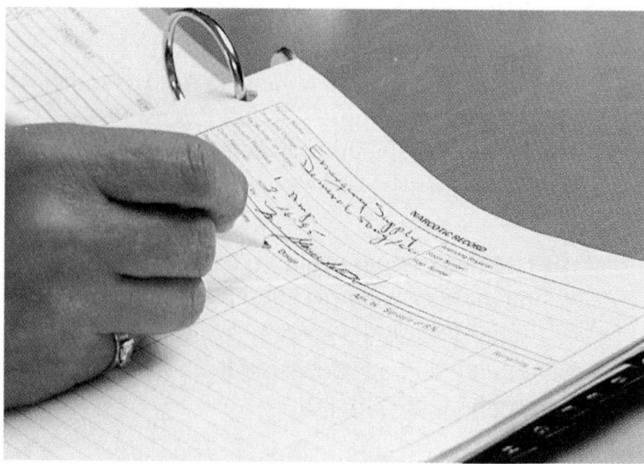

Chart medication in record immediately after administration.

cotic administration if narcotics and sign-out sheets do not agree.

7. Sign out for the narcotic on the narcotic sheet after taking narcotic out of drawer or cupboard.

■ **CLINICAL ALERT**

A licensed person must sign for each narcotic dispensed from the medication drawer.

8. Lock drawer or cupboard after taking out medication.
9. Administer medications according to specific procedure.
10. Sign out narcotics on client's medication record according to usual procedure.
11. Check narcotics every 8 hours. One off-going and one on-coming nurse check the narcotics. The number on sign-out sheets must match the remaining number of narcotics. Each narcotic sheet is checked for accuracy.
12. Return the empty counter (if used) to the pharmacy with the completed narcotic sign-out sheet when the sheet is filled. A new narcotic supply and narcotic check sheet are signed out in the pharmacy.
13. Sign the narcotic record receipt if you are the nurse receiving the narcotics.

COMPUTERIZED ACCESS SYSTEMS

Computerized access systems are now available for dispensing and recording drugs, an example of which is the PYXIS system. The purpose of these systems is to

- Control access to drugs and narcotics

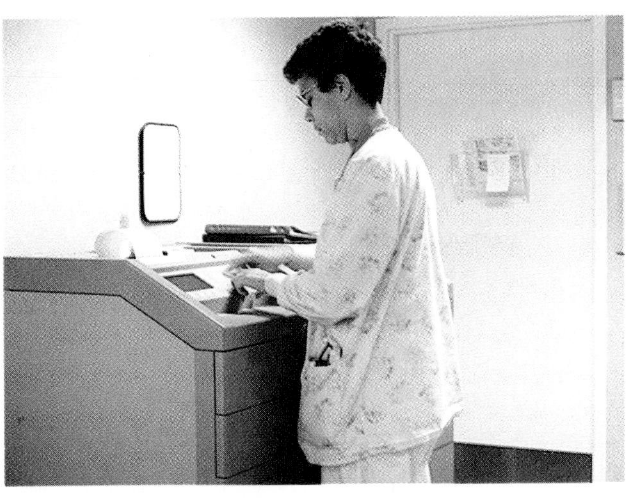

Obtain code number (user ID) from the pharmacy.

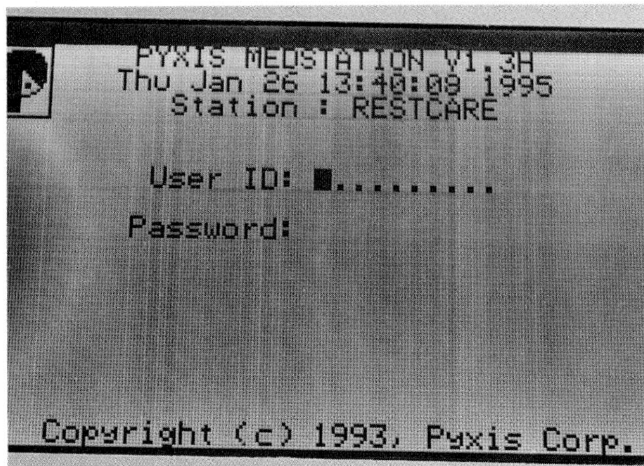

Check client's ID number on screen.

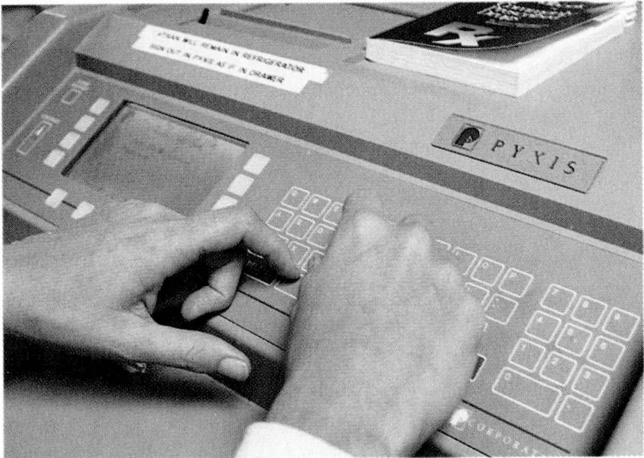

Enter code to open specific drawer for client's drug.

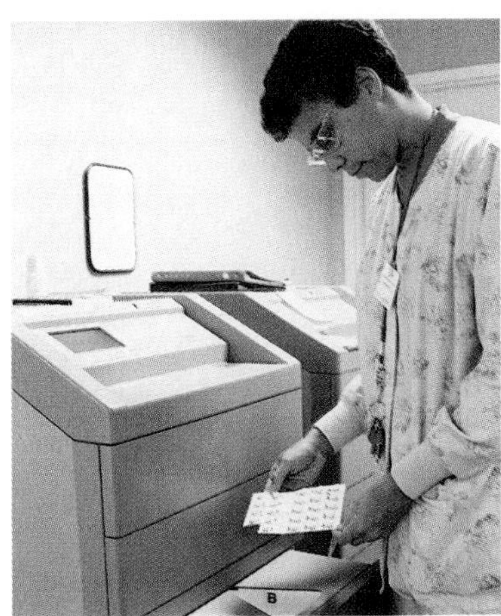

Check number of drugs remaining.

- Record drugs from the source
- Directly bill the appropriate client

Accessing the system is simple and straightforward:

- Obtain code number (user ID or password) from the pharmacy.
- Enter code, and drawer that contains the specific drug ordered opens.
- Check number of drugs remaining.
- Sign out drug, and proceed to administer to client.

CRITICAL THINKING APPLICATION

CLINICAL PROBLEMS	CRITICAL THINKING OPTIONS
Nurse is unsure of correct answer when calculating or converting drug dose.	• Request that another nurse check calculation or conversion.
Computer access system does not open.	• Recheck client ID number or password, or check with pharmacy.
Narcotic and sign-out sheets do not agree.	• Check Kardex and MAR for narcotics signed out to specific clients. • Check with other nurses who may have administered drug. • Submit report if sign-out sheets cannot be verified.

unit 2

ORAL MEDICATIONS

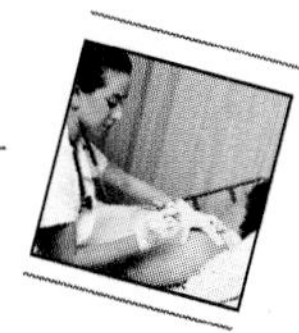

NURSING PROCESS DATA

ASSESSMENT Data Base

Assess that oral route is the most efficient means of medication administration.

Check medication orders for completeness and accuracy.

Assess that five rights for medication administration are followed.

Determine client's physical ability to take medication as ordered.

- Swallow reflex present.
- State of consciousness.
- Signs of nausea and vomiting.
- Uncooperative behavior.

Check to make sure you have the correct medication for the client.

Evaluate correct dosage when calculation is needed.

Observe that client swallows medications when administered.

PLANNING Objectives

To ensure that client metabolizes medication without feelings of nausea or vomiting

To offer the most common, easiest, and least expensive route of administering medications

To provide a sustained drug action and increased absorption time

IMPLEMENTATION Procedures

Preparing Oral Medications

Administering Oral Medications to Adults

Administering Oral Medications to Children

EVALUATION Expected Outcomes

Client is able to ingest and metabolize medication without feeling nauseated or vomiting.

Client emotionally accepts medication.

Client experiences a sustained action of drug and a positive effect on the body.

PREPARING ORAL MEDICATIONS

Equipment

Medication: tablet, capsule, or liquid

Water, juice, or milk (if not contraindicated by drug absorption) to prevent gastric irritation

Mortar and pestle for crushing pills (if needed)

Medication record (MAR) or Kardex

Medication cart, if unit dose system is used

Procedure

1. Obtain client's medication record.
2. Compare the medication record with the most *recent* physician's order.
3. Wash your hands.
4. Gather necessary equipment.
5. Remove medication from the drug drawer on medication cart.
6. Compare label on bottle or drug package to the medication record.
7. Correctly calculate dosage if necessary, and check dosage to be administered.
8. Take drug package from medication drawer when using unit dosage, and place in medication cup. Do not remove drug from drug package. Compare

■ **CLINICAL ALERT**

Medications that cannot be altered

- Check with pharmacy for liquid medication or call the physician if crushing medication is contraindicated.
- Do not crush *sustained-release tablets* or open *sustained-release capsules.* **Rationale:** The client may receive too much drug too soon.
- Do not crush *enteric-coated tablets,* which are not meant to be absorbed by the stomach
- Do not alter *carcinogenic* or *teratogenic tablets or capsules.* This could expose the nurse to harmful substances that might be inhaled or absorbed through the skin.

drug label or drug package with medication record. **Rationale:** This is a safety check.

9. Place medication in separate cup for drugs that require assessment before administration (i.e., digoxin). **Rationale:** This is a safety precaution for drugs that may be held following assessment.
10. Place lid upside down to avoid contamination and pour with label facing up to avoid obliterating label.
11. Pour liquid by setting medicine cup on a firm surface. At eye level read fluid level at the lowest point of the meniscus. **Rationale:** This reading ensures accurate dose of drug.
12. Wipe bottle off before replacing. Check medication label again. **Rationale:** This safety check ensures correct drug and dosages.
13. Return a multidose bottle to the storage area. If medication to be given is a narcotic, sign out the narcotic sheet with your name.
14. Remember, check label three times:
    a. When taking medication from drawer
    b. Before placing medicine into medicine cup
    c. Before returning to storage place

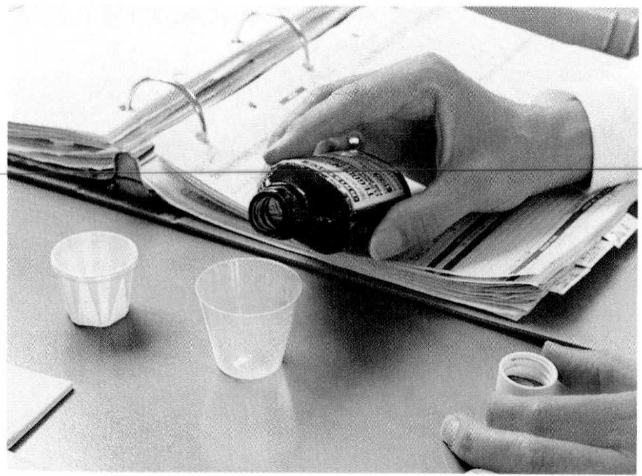

Pour liquid with label up, using firm surface.

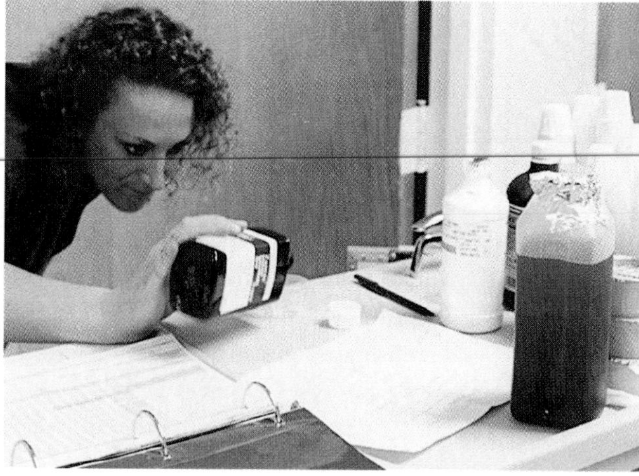

Pour liquid at eye level to read dose correctly.

ADMINISTERING ORAL MEDICATIONS TO ADULTS

Equipment

Medication: tablet, capsule, or liquid

Liquid (e.g., water, juice, or milk [if not contraindicated by drug absorption]) for washing down medication

Medication record (MAR)

Preparation

See *Preparing Oral Medications.*

Procedure

1. Take medication tray or cart to client's room; check room and bed number against medication record.

2. Place client in sitting position, if not contraindicated by his condition.
3. Check the client's identaband, and ask client to state name so that you are sure you have correct client.
4. Explain to client what type of medication you are going to give, and explain the actions this medication will produce.
5. If prepackaged medication is used, read label, take medication out of package, and put into medication cup. Determine if assessment parameters are indicated before administering (e.g., blood pressure and pulse).
6. Give the medication cup to the client.
7. Offer a fresh glass of water or other liquid. **Rationale:** Aids swallowing and camouflages taste of bitter medications.
   - Tablets and capsules are given with water to prevent antagonism of chemical properties of the drug.
   - Cough syrups that are demulcents and antacids are not followed by water because it would dilute the topical effect.
   - Crushed pills or liquids may be mixed with a small quantity of food, if not contraindicated by the client's diet.
8. Make sure the client swallows the medication.
9. Discard used medicine cup.
10. Position client for comfort.
11. Record the medication on the appropriate forms.
12. Assess client for drug action and side effects.

ADMINISTERING ORAL MEDICATIONS TO CHILDREN

Equipment

Medication: tablet, capsule, or liquid

Water, juice, or milk (if not contraindicated by drug absorption) to prevent gastric irritation

Medication record (MAR) or drug Kardex

Drug cart

Preparation

See *Preparing Oral Medications.*

Procedure

1. Follow the procedure for Preparing and Administering Oral Medications. Keep the following guidelines in mind:
   a. Play techniques may help to elicit a young child's cooperation.
   b. Remember: the smaller the quantity of diluent (food or liquid), the greater the ease in eliciting the child's cooperation.
   c. Never use a child's favorite food or drink as an enticement when administering medication because the result may be the child's refusal to eat or drink anything.

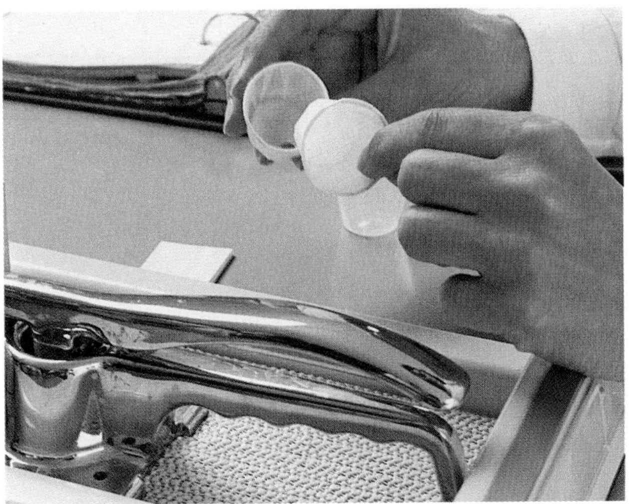

Place tablet in cup and put second cup on top.

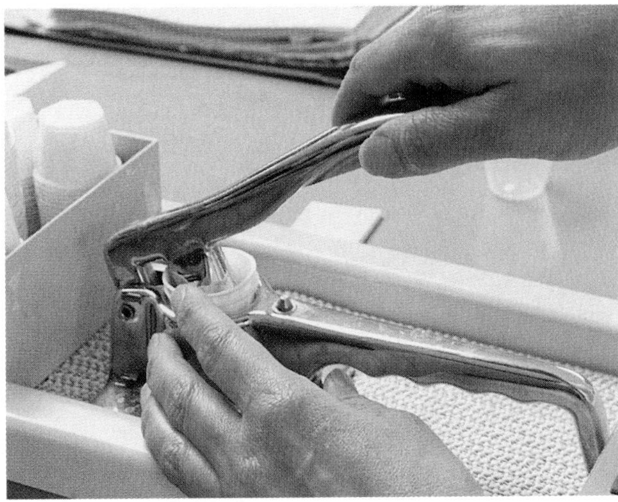

Place in pill crusher to crush tablet for a child.

d. Be honest and tell the child that you have medicine, not candy.
e. When crushing a medication, place tablet in cup, put second cup on top, and place in pill crusher.

2. Assess child for drug action and possible side effects.
3. Explain medication action and side effects to parents.

CHARTING for Oral Medications

Client's Medication Record

- Name of medication
- Dosage
- Route
- Site
- Time administered
- Initials of nurse administering medication
- Signature of nurse identifying initials

Nurses' Notes

- Client's assessment parameters
- Record p.r.n., stat, and experimental medications
- Name of medication, dosage, route, site, time administered
- Client's response
- Signature of nurse

CRITICAL THINKING APPLICATION

CLINICAL PROBLEMS	CRITICAL THINKING OPTIONS
■ Client has an allergic or anaphylactic response to the medication.	• Immediately stop or hold medication. • Notify physician at once; prepare to administer antihistamine. • If reaction is severe, Keep client flat in bed with head elevated. Take vital signs every 10–15 minutes. Assess for hypotension or respiratory distress—if latter is present, administer oxygen via nasal prongs at 6 L/minute (unless contraindicated). Have emergency equipment available. Provide psychologic support to client to alleviate fears. Record type and progression of allergic reactions.
■ Client has difficulty swallowing tablets or capsules.	• Use mortar and pestle to crush medications and administer to client mixed with juice or a food, such as applesauce or jelly. • If totally unable to swallow medications, do not attempt administering by mouth. Ask physician to order same or comparable medication by a more appropriate route (e.g., parenteral, rectal).

unit 3

SUBLINGUAL MEDICATIONS

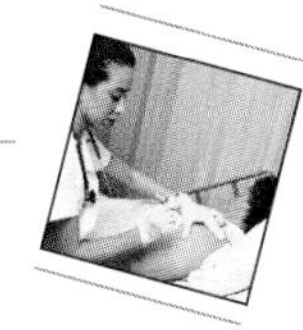

NURSING PROCESS DATA

ASSESSMENT Data Base

Assess that the drug can be administered sublingually.

Assess client's ability to understand and follow verbal directions.

Check to see if the area underneath client's tongue is excoriated or painful. If so, do not give medication.

PLANNING Objectives

To provide a fast route of absorption for drugs such as nitroglycerin and glucose

To provide the most efficient method of absorption

IMPLEMENTATION Procedure

Administering Sublingual Medications

EVALUATION Expected Outcomes

Therapeutic effect is achieved as chest pain is relieved following administration of nitroglycerin given sublingually.

Therapeutic effect is experienced within minutes of administration of quick-acting glucose.

ADMINISTERING SUBLINGUAL MEDICATIONS

Equipment

Medication is kept in dark bottle (nitroglycerin loses potency when exposed to light)

Medication record (MAR) or appropriate method for correctly identifying client and medication

Procedure

1. Follow the procedures for preparing and administering oral medications, with these exceptions:
   a. Explain that client must not swallow drug or eat, smoke, or drink until the drug is completely absorbed.
   b. Ask client to place drug under the tongue or to hold tongue up so that you can place medication under the tongue. **Rationale:** Absorption is enhanced by the thin layer of epithelium underneath the tongue, as well as by the vast network of capillaries in that area.
2. Evaluate client for drug action and possible side effects.
3. Document actions of drug or client's response in nurses' notes to monitor effects closely.

■ CLINICAL ALERT

Sublingual medications such as nitroglycerin can be administered to non-responsive clients. These medications dissolve rapidly and quickly with minimal chance of aspiration.

CHARTING for Sublingual Medications

Client's Medication Record

- Name of medication
- Dosage
- Route
- Site
- Time administered
- Initials of nurse administering medication
- Signature of nurse identifying initials

Nurses' Notes

- Client' assessment parameters
- Record p.r.n., or stat
- Name of medication, dosage, route, site, time administered
- Client's response
- Signature of nurse

CRITICAL THINKING APPLICATION

CLINICAL PROBLEMS	CRITICAL THINKING OPTIONS
■ Client's condition is unchanged with administration of nitroglycerin.	• Check bottle for expiration date—potency decreases 3 months after opening bottle. • Administer second tablet in 5 minutes. (You may give client three tablets in a 15-minute period unless client is hypotensive.) If three tablets do not relieve discomfort, client may be having a myocardial infarction and should seek emergency assistance.
■ Comatose condition is unaltered with administration of fast-acting glucose sublingually.	• Give rapid-acting glucose sublingually or glucagon intravenously if ordered to determine if glucose dose increases blood glucose level and reverses insulin reaction. • Assess for conditions other than hypoglycemia or insulin reaction that may have brought on coma.

unit 4

PARENTERAL MEDICATIONS

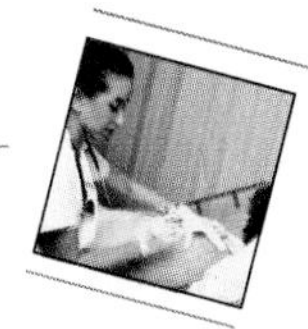

NURSING PROCESS DATA

ASSESSMENT Data Base

Check that appropriate method for administration of drug was ordered.

Assess condition of administration site for presence of lesions, rash, inflammation, lipid dystrophy, ecchymosis.

Assess for tissue reaction from previous injections.

Assess client's level of awareness.

Check client's written history and ask for verbal history for past allergic reactions. Do *not* rely solely on client's chart.

Review client's chart noting previous injection sites, especially insulin and heparin administration sites.

PLANNING Objectives

To perform the injection as painlessly as possible

To ensure proper drug administration

To observe and report side effects of the drugs administered

To alternate injection sites according to protocol

IMPLEMENTATION Procedures

Preparing Injections

Administering Intradermal Injections

Administering Subcutaneous (Sub Q) Injections

Preparing Insulin Injections

for One Insulin Solution

for Two Insulin Solutions

Teaching Use of Insulin Pump

Administering Sub Q Heparin

Administering Intramuscular (IM) Injections

Using Z-Track Method

EVALUATION Expected Outcomes

Injection is completed without technical complications.

Injection is as painless as possible.

Injection sites are rotated.

Types of Injections

Intradermal or Intracutaneous Injections

- Injection sites: inner aspect of forearm or scapular area of back; upper chest, medial thigh.
- Purpose: for antigens for skin or for tuberculin tests
- Amount injected: ranges from 0.01 to 0.1 mL
- Absorption rate: slow

Subcutaneous Injections

- Injection sites: abdomen, lateral and posterior aspects of upper arm or thigh, scapular area of back, upper ventrodorsal gluteal areas
- Purpose: for medications that are absorbed slowly, to produce a sustained effect
- Amount injected: variable—small amount of fluid, no

more than 1 mL. If repeated doses are necessary, alter site accordingly.

Intramuscular Injections

- Injection sites: anterolateral aspect of thigh (vastus lateralis), dorsogluteal (gluteus maximus), ventrogluteal (gluteus medius), upper arm (deltoid)
- Purpose: to promote rapid absorption of the drug; to provide an alternate route when drug is irritating to subcutaneous tissues
- Amount injected: variable—may be large amount of fluid. If more than 5 mL for adult or 3 mL for child, use two syringes
- Absorption rate: depends on circulatory state of client

PREPARING INJECTIONS

Equipment

Medication tray
Alcohol wipes
Vials or ampules of medications
Vial of diluent (when necessary)
Syringe with appropriate needles
Sterile 2×2 gauze pads
Band-Aid (optional)

Procedure

1. Obtain client's medication record.
2. Compare the medication record with the most recent physician's order. **Rationale:** This is a safety check against medication errors.
3. Calculate correct volume to be given.
4. Wash your hands. **Rationale:** This prevents transmission of microorganisms.
5. Obtain equipment for injections. Compare medication record with label on drug container. **Rationale:** This is the first safety check.
6. Assemble the syringe and needle, maintaining sterility. Select the appropriate size needle by considering the client's muscle mass and the viscosity of the medication. **Rationale:** The larger the gauge number, the smaller the diameter of the cannula. Smaller gauges produce less tissue trauma but larger gauges are required for viscous solutions such as paraldehyde.

Selecting the Appropriate Needle

- *Intradermal injections:* 1 mL tuberculin syringe with short bevel, 25–27 gauge, $\frac{3}{8}$–$\frac{1}{2}$ inch needle.
- *Subcutaneous injections:* .05–3 mL syringe with 25–29 gauge, $\frac{3}{8}$–$\frac{5}{8}$ inch needle.
- *Intramuscular injections:* 1–5 mL syringe with needle gauge and length appropriate for muscle site; deltoid muscle requires 23–25 gauge, $\frac{5}{8}$–1 inch needle; needle sizes for the vastus lateralis and gluteus muscles vary from 18 to 23 gauge, needle lengths, 1–1$\frac{1}{2}$ inch.

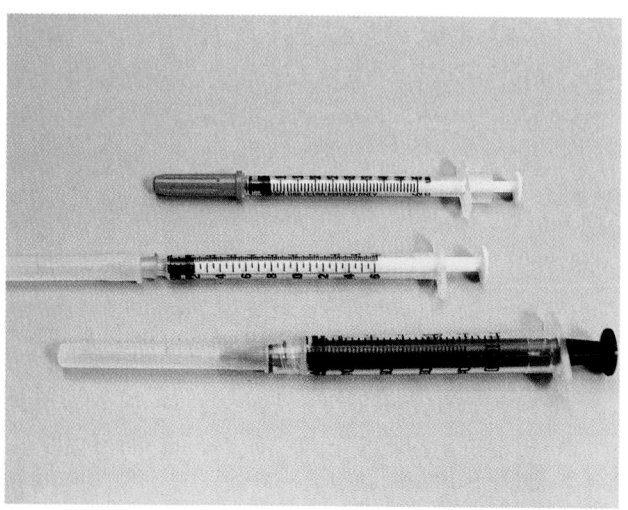

Three types of syringes: Tuberculin, Insulin, and 3-mL.

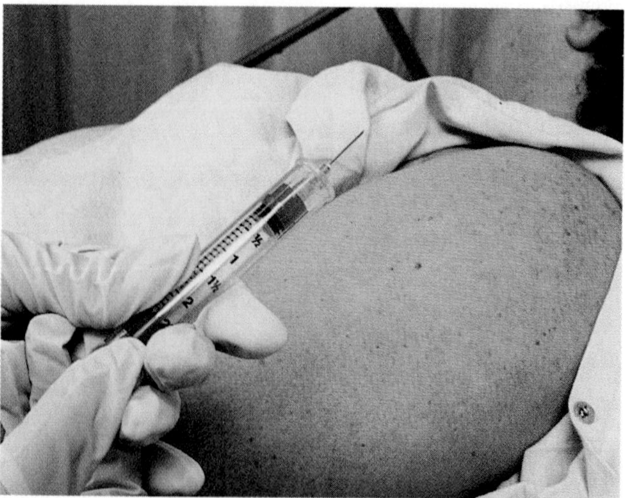

Safety syringe with retractable sheath.

7. Break the seal on the syringe by pulling down on the plunger.
8. Fill syringe with medication as follows:

for Withdrawing Medication from a Vial

1. Remove the vial cap.
2. Open the alcohol wipe, and cleanse the rubber top of the vial. **Rationale:** Manufacturer does not guarantee sterility of rubber top.
3. Tighten needle on syringe. Remove needle guard and place on alcohol wipe, medication tray, or inside of syringe wrapper.
4. Pull back on plunger to fill syringe with an amount of air equal to amount of solution to be withdrawn. **Rationale:** The displacement of solution with air is necessary to prevent the formation of a vacuum in the sealed vial.
5. Insert needle into upright vial. Inject air into vial keeping bevel above surface of medication. **Rationale:** Air creates positive pressure within vial allowing accurate withdrawal of medication.
6. Invert vial, and extract the desired amount of medication. Touch only syringe barrel and plunger tip. **Rationale:** This prevents contamination of the plunger, inside of barrel, and medication.
7. Expel any air bubbles from syringe at this time by tapping the side of syringe sharply with your finger or pen. **Rationale:** Air bubbles always form in syringe due to dead air space in needle hub. Removing air bubbles while needle remains within the inverted vial avoids accidental contamination of needle and facilitates easy removal of air and accurate withdrawal of solution.
8. Recheck amount of medication in syringe.
9. Turn vial to upright position and remove needle. **Rationale:** Removing needle from inverted vial may cause leaking of medication from needle insertion site.
10. Cover needle with guard.
11. Compare medication label and dosage against medication record and calculation. **Rationale:** Safety check two.

Reconstituting Powdered Medication

- Insert needle into upright powdered medication vial.
- Remove the amount of air equal to desired quantity of diluent; this provides for adequate displacement of air.
- Insert diluent into upright powdered medication vial.
- Remove needle and cover with guard.
- Rotate powdered medication vial with diluent between palms of your hands. Do not shake vial because shaking creates excess air bubbles. This may cause inaccurate measurement of medication.
- Withdraw medication from vial.

Note: Most drugs that previously required reconstituting from powder form now come from the pharmacy.

for Withdrawing Medication from an Ampule

1. Move solution from neck to body of ampule by tapping stem sharply or holding neck of ampule between thumb and forefinger and flicking wrist.

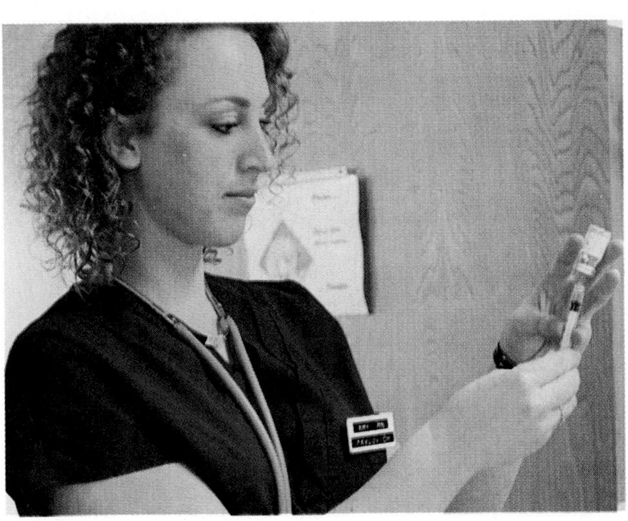

Insert needle into upright vial, inject air, then invert vial.

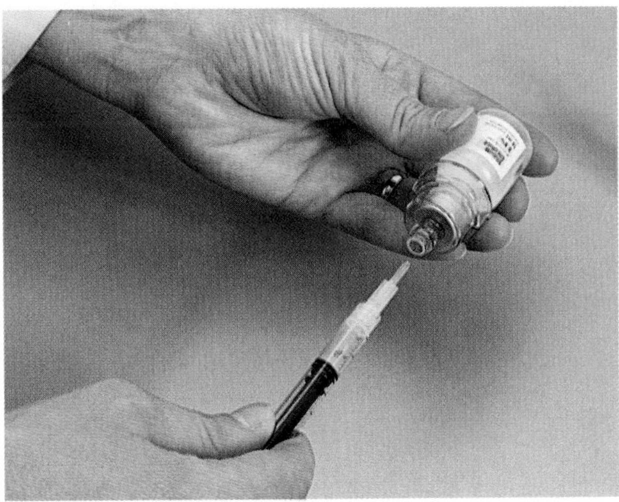

Extract ordered amount of drug by pulling on plunger tip.

2. Grasp top of ampule between thumb and forefinger of one hand and grasp body of ampule with other hand. Using a pad, break ampule away from you. (If ampule is not scored, partially file neck of ampule). **Rationale:** Gauze pad protects hands and breaking away from you prevents injury from glass fragments.
3. Set the ampule upright. It is not necessary to add air prior to withdrawing the medication.
4. Use a special filter needle to withdraw solution. **Rationale:** filter needle prevents aspiration of glass when withdrawing solution from ampule.
5. Remove needle guard and set aside. Insert needle into ampule without touching sides of neck. If needle is sufficiently long, medication may be withdrawn with ampule in upright position. When a short needle is used, invert ampule and withdraw appropriate amount of medication. **Rationale:** Surface tension prevents solution from leaking out of inverted ampule. Also, the calibration on syringe can be more easily read in this position. (A break in surface tension and contamination of the medication may occur if hub of needle is inserted into ampule opening.)
6. Return ampule to an upright position and withdraw syringe.
7. Tap barrel to dislodge air bubbles to hub of syringe.
8. Eject air with syringe in an upright position. If amount of solution is overdrawn, invert syringe and remove excess solution into a nearby receptacle.
9. Cover needle with guard.

for Combining Medications in One Syringe Using Two Vials

1. Prepare both vials by removing cap and cleansing tops with separate alcohol wipes.
2. Draw into syringe the amount of air equal to amount of solution to be removed from *second* vial. Inject air into *second* vial. Do not withdraw medication at this time. **Rationale:** Air creates positive pressure within the vial allowing withdrawal of solution.
3. Draw into syringe amount of air equal to amount of solution to be removed from *first* vial and inject it into *first vial.*

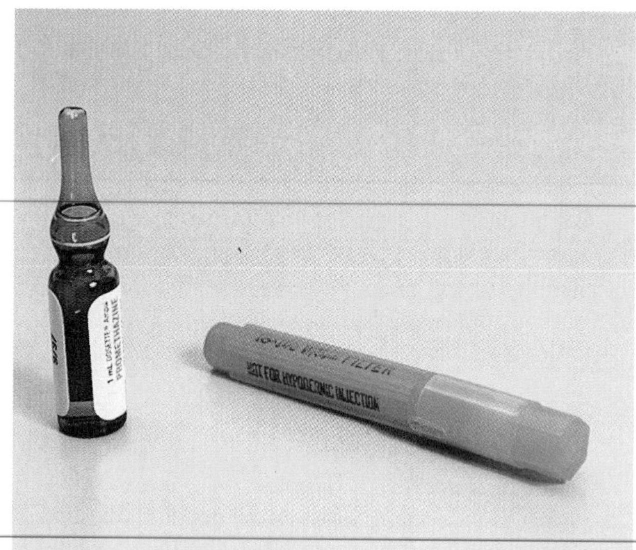

Ampule with medication and filter needle.

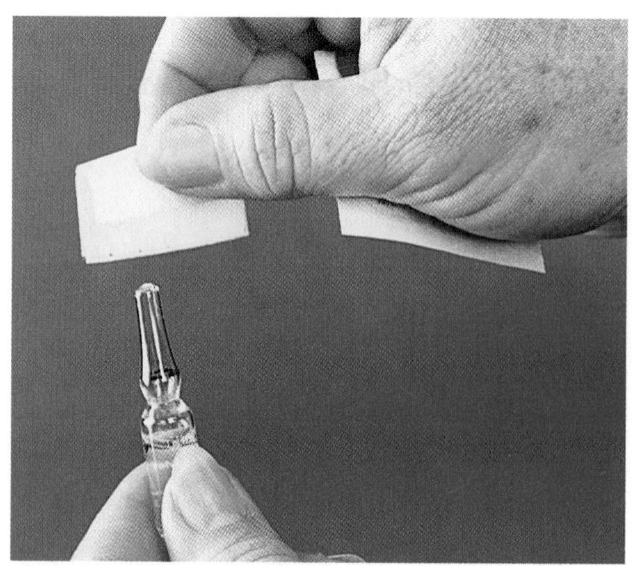
Use pad to protect hand when breaking ampule.

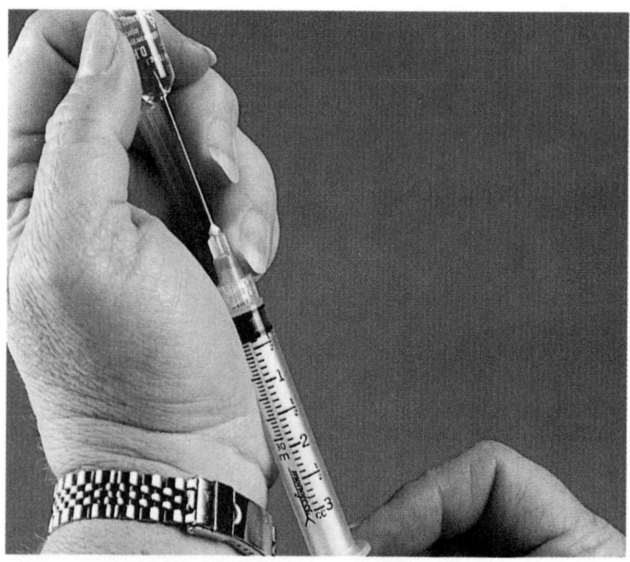
Filter needle prevents aspiration of glass when using ampule.

4. Invert vial and withdraw ordered amount of medication without removing syringe.
5. Expel all air bubbles from syringe.
6. Recheck amount of solution and remove syringe from vial.
7. Insert needle into *second* vial, invert, and withdraw exact amount of solution ordered. **Rationale:** Withdrawing excess solution from second vial results in an inaccurate dosage of medication. If this occurs, syringe must be discarded and procedure begun again.

Alternative Method for Combining Medications

- Draw up ordered dose from each vial into two separate syringes.
- Pull back plunger of first syringe, removing air equal to volume of second medication to be added.
- Remove needle from first syringe.
- Insert needle of second syringe into barrel of first syringe.
- Inject solution from second syringe slowly into first syringe.
- Withdraw needle from first syringe.
- Attach new sterile needle to first syringe.
- Discard needles and second syringe.

for Preparing Prefilled Medication Cartridges

1. Hold barrel of tubex in one hand and pull back on plunger with the other hand.
2. Insert prefilled medication cartridge, needle first, into barrel.
3. Twist cartridge until it is secure.
4. Bring plunger back into place and twist plunger until it fits firmly and tightly into rubber stopper.
5. Check amount of solution in tubex.

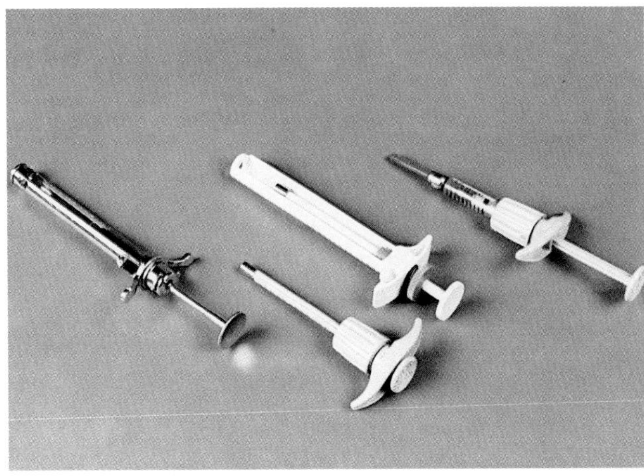

Examples of prefilled cartridges.

6. Determine if dosage in cartridge is greater than required amount; if so, remove needle guard and any air bubbles, invert tubex, and gently expel the excess medication. Be especially alert to maintain the sterility of needle. **Rationale:** If permanent needle is contaminated, the cartridge becomes contaminated and must be discarded.
7. Replace needle guard.
8. Compare medication label and dosage against medication record. **Rationale:** Safety check for correct drug and dosage.
9. Place the syringe, alcohol wipes, 2×2 gauze pad and Band-Aid (optional) on the medication tray.

If prefilled cartridge has separate cylinder vial and needle, the needle can be broken away from the cylinder. The cylinder has a rubber stopper from which the medication can be withdrawn into a second syringe or prefilled cartridge.

ADMINISTERING INTRADERMAL INJECTIONS

Equipment

Medication record
Medication tray
Syringe with medication
Alcohol wipes
2×2 gauze pads; Band-Aid (optional)
Clean gloves

Procedure

1. Take equipment to client's room. Check room and bed number against the client's medication record. Provide privacy.
2. Wash your hands and don gloves. **Rationale:** There is a possibility of encountering blood.
3. Check client's identaband and ask client to state name.
4. Explain the medication action and the procedure for administration to the client. **Rationale:** This

action encourages client's cooperation during procedure and decreases anxiety.

5. Select the site of injection using appropriate anatomic landmarks where skin is not damaged or discolored. Remember to alternate sites when multiple injections are given. **Rationale:** Alternating sites is less traumatizing to the body.
6. Cleanse area with an alcohol wipe. Using a circular motion, cleanse from inside to outside. **Rationale:** Cleanse from most clean to least clean area.
7. Take off the needle guard and place on tray while waiting for alcohol to dry.
8. Grasp the client's dorsal forearm and gently pull the skin taut on ventral forearm.
9. Insert needle at a 10–15° angle with the bevel of the needle facing up. Needle point should be visable under skin. Do not aspirate. **Rationale:** Bevel up enables medication to enter intradermal tissue layer rather than subcutaneous tissues.
10. Inject medication slowly. Observe for signs of wheal formation and blanching at the site. **Rationale:** This indicates that the medication was injected within the dermis.
11. Withdraw needle. Pat area gently with a dry 2 × 2 gauze pad. Do *not* massage area. **Rationale:** Massaging could disperse medication.
12. Return client to a comfortable position.
13. Discard needle–syringe unit in puncture-proof container. Do *not* recap needle.
14. Chart medication and site used.

TUBERCULIN TESTING

- Inject 0.1-mL solution.
- Observe for wheal.
- Instruct client to have site checked in 48–72 hours.

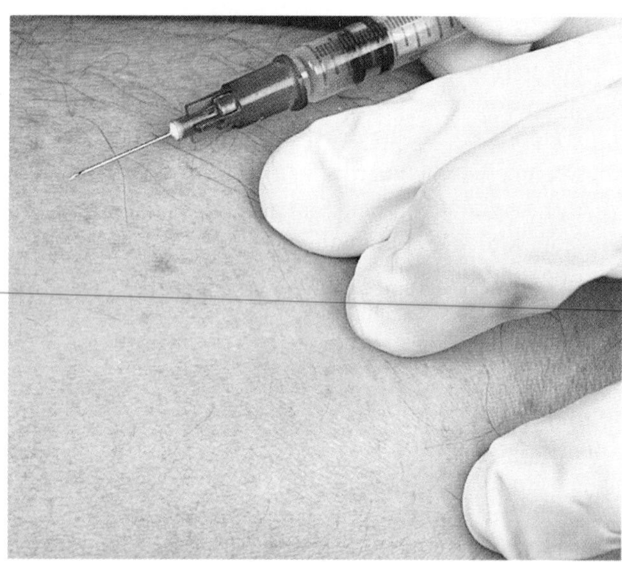

Insert needle with bevel up for intradermal injection.

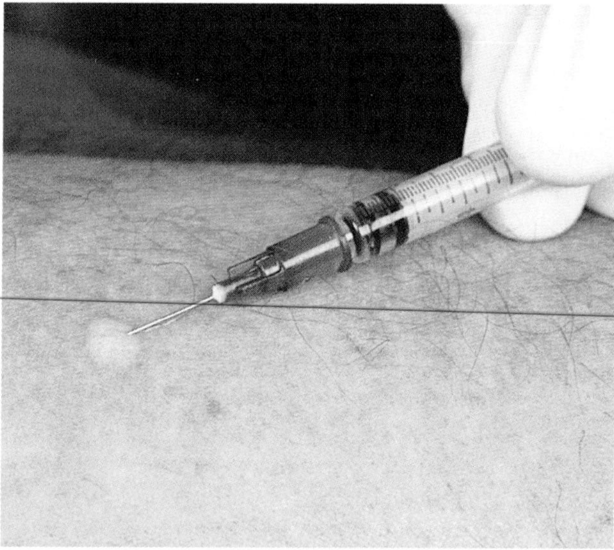

Inject solution to form wheal on skin.

ADMINISTERING SUBCUTANEOUS (SUB Q) INJECTIONS

Equipment

3-mL syringe with $\frac{5}{8}$-inch needle
Medication vial or ampule
2 alcohol swabs
Clean gloves

Preparation

See *Preparing Injections.*

Procedure

1. Take medication to client's room.
2. Set tray on a clean surface, not the bed.
3. Check client's identaband, and ask client to state name.

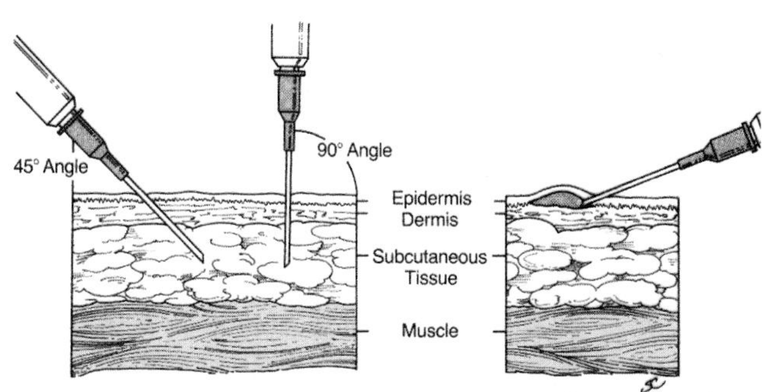

Insert needle at 45° or 90° angle into tissue for subcutaneous injection.

Insert needle at 15° angle just under the epidermis for intradermal injection.

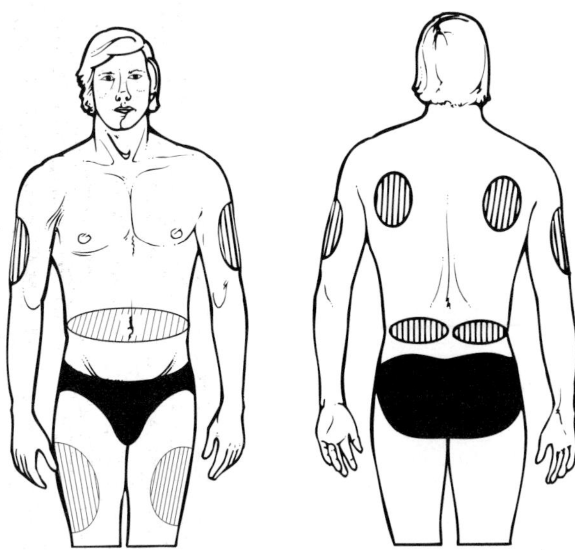

Sites for subcutaneous injections given routinely. Avoid umbilicus area.

4. Explain action of medication and procedure of administration.
5. Provide privacy.
6. Wash your hands and don gloves.
7. Select site for injection by identifying anatomic landmarks. Remember to alternate sites each time injections are given. **Rationale:** This allows time for area to heal between injections.
8. Cleanse area with alcohol wipe. Using a circular motion, cleanse from inside outward. **Rationale:** This action supports the principle of moving from clean to dirty area.
9. Take off needle guard.
10. Express any air bubbles from syringe.
11. Grasp subcutaneous tissue between the thumb and forefinger, lateral aspect, middle third of arm. **Rationale:** This position ensures insertion of medication within subcutaneous tissue, *not muscle*. (*Note*: Spreading the skin is acceptable when there is substantial subcutaneous tissue.)
12. Hold syringe like a dart or between the thumb and forefinger.
13. Insert the needle at a 45° or 90° angle. A 90° angle is used more commonly due to short needles on prepackaged syringes. **Rationale:** Angle varies with the amount of subcutaneous tissue and selected site.

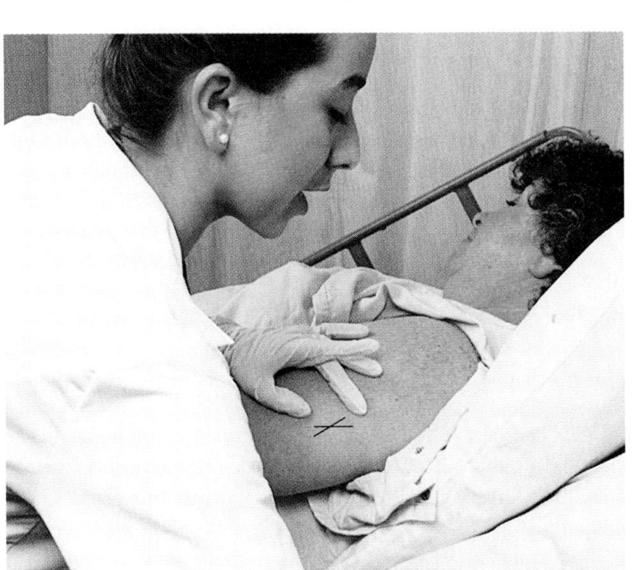

Select site on lateral aspect of upper arm.

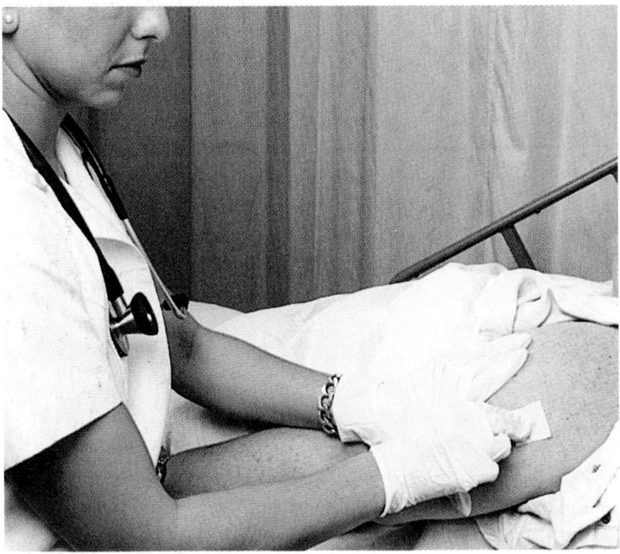

Cleanse area with alcohol wipe before injecting.

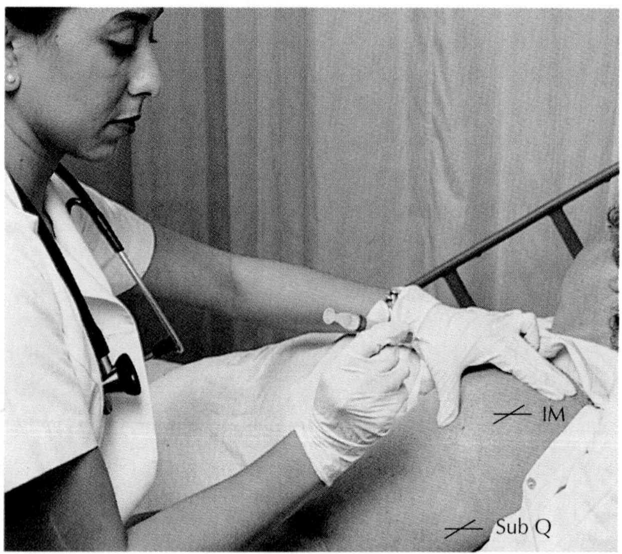

The upper arm can be used for both IM and Sub Q injections.

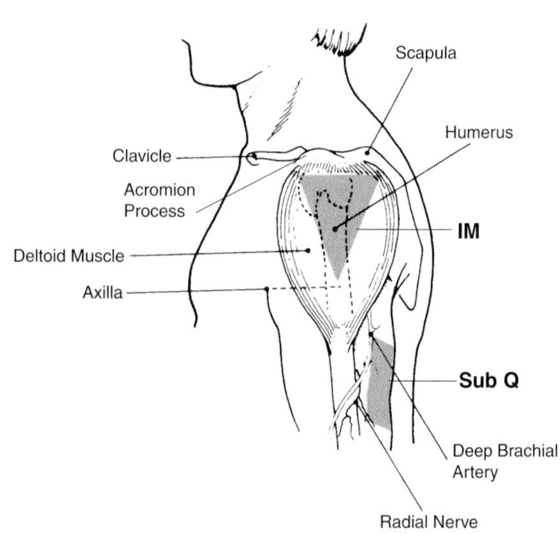

Administer IM injection in upper arm. Lower area is used for Sub Q injection.

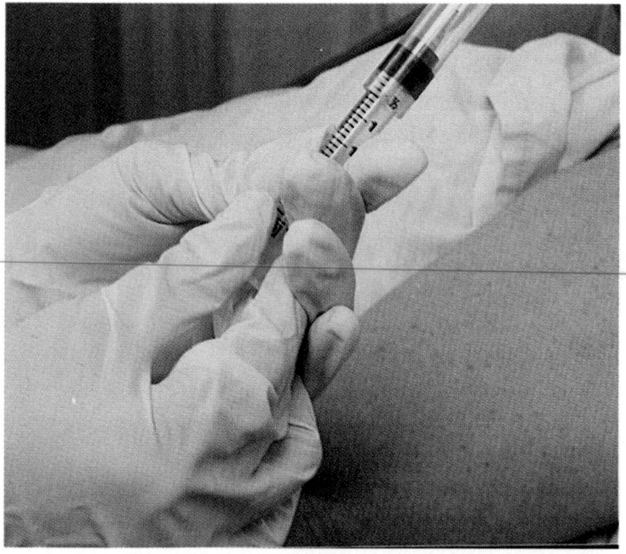

Push cap to cover needle when using safety syringe.

14. Release subcutaneous tissue.
15. Hold syringe barrel with one hand and aspirate by pulling back on the plunger according to agency policy. If blood does not appear, continue the injection. If blood appears, withdraw the syringe, discard, and prepare a new injection. **Rationale:** Blood indicates needle has entered a blood vessel. Injecting the drug IV increases the absorption rate of the medication and may be dangerous.
16. Inject medication slowly. Limit medication volume to 1.5 mL.
17. Withdraw needle quickly and massage area with the alcohol swab. **Rationale:** Massaging area aids absorption.
18. Return client to position of comfort.
19. Discard needle–syringe unit in puncture-proof container. Do *not* recap needle. When using safety syringe push cap to cover needle.
20. Chart medication and site used.

PREPARING INSULIN INJECTIONS

Equipment

Insulin(s)
100-unit or 50 unit insulin syringe with needle
Medication sheet or card
2 alcohol wipes

Procedure

for One Insulin Solution

1. Check medication orders, injection site, and rotation chart. Insulin does not need to be refrigerated.
2. Gather equipment.
3. Wash your hands.
4. Rotate intermediate or long-acting insulin bottle

between hands. **Rationale:** This brings cloudy insulin solution into suspension Regular (rapid-acting) insulin is clear and requires no rotation.

5. Wipe top of insulin bottle with alcohol swab.
6. Take off needle guard, and place on tray.
7. Pull plunger of syringe down to desired amount of medication (e.g., 30 units). Inject amount of air into air space, not solution. **Rationale:** Injecting air directly into insulin solution causes bubbles. Bubbles can confuse drug amount withdrawn.
8. Draw up ordered amount of insulin into syringe.
9. Validate medication record, insulin bottle, and syringe with an RN for accuracy. **Rationale:** Checking insulin by two nurses promotes accurate dosage.
10. Remove needle from vial, and expel air from syringe.
11. Replace needle guard.
12. Take medication to client's room.
13. Follow protocol for administration of medications by subcutaneous injections, noting Special Considerations for Insulin Administration.

TABLE 16. Insulin Types and Action (in hours)*

Types	Onset	Peak	Duration
Rapid Acting	$\frac{1}{2}$–1 hr.	2–4 hrs.	6–8 hrs.
Regular Iletin			
Semilente			
Humulin R			
Intermediate Acting	1–4	6–12	12–18
NPH			
Lente			
Humulin N			
Long Acting	8	(18) many small peaks	24–36
Ultralente Humulin			
Mixture of NPH/Regular 70/30 Humulin (H) 50/50 Humulin (H)	combination short and intermediate action	combination short and intermediate action	combination short and intermediate action

Abbreviations: NPH = neutral protamine Hagedorn.
*Insulin is produced by two companies—Lilly and Novo Nordisk. The types listed above are Lilly. Onset and duration differ according to different brands and different individuals.

Special Considerations for Insulin Administration

- Rotating injection areas is not recommended due to variation in insulin absorption and action. A body area should be used consistently. The injection site should be 1 inch from the previous injection site (see chart).
- Absorption is most predictable in the abdomen.
- Avoid injection into area to be actively used because absorption is enhanced.
- Wait 30 seconds after slowly injecting insulin before withdrawing needle to prevent insulin leakage.
- Aspirating before and massaging after injecting the insulin are not recommended due to the potential for tissue damage.

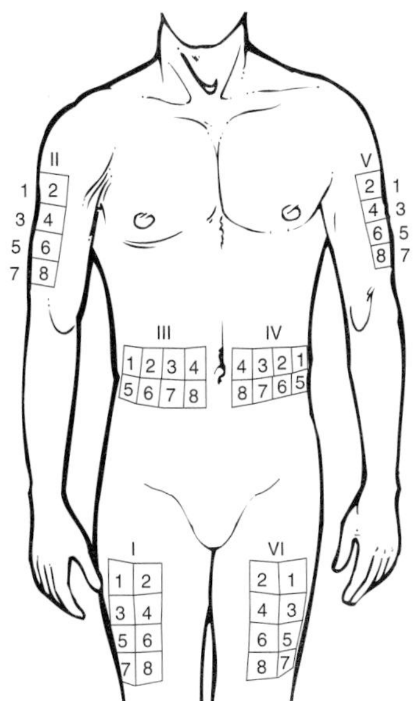

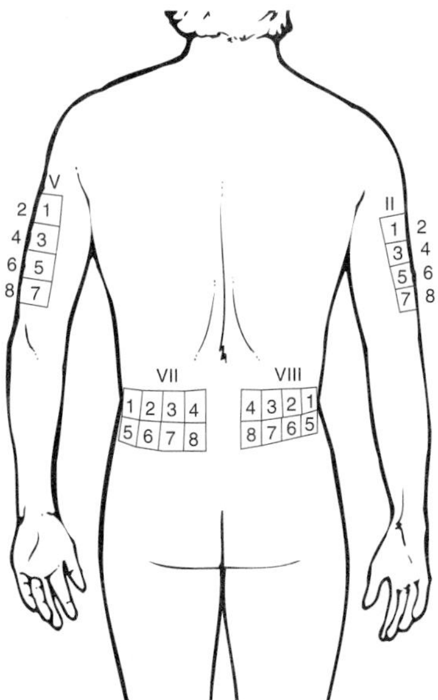

Insulin injection sites. To avoid overuse of injection sites and dramatic changes in daily insulin absorption, use an approved method of site rotation. One method is to begin with site I (right thigh), give injections consecutively at points 1 to 8, then move to site II (right arm) (e.g., a client on one injection daily would inject insulin into the right thigh for 8 days, then into the right arm for 8 days).

for Two Insulin Solutions

1. Check medication orders, injection site, and rotation chart. Insulin does not need to be refrigerated.
2. Wash your hands.
3. Gather equipment.
4. Rotate intermediate or long-acting insulin bottle between hands. **Rationale:** This brings cloudy solution into suspension for insulins other than regular.
5. Wipe top of insulin bottles with alcohol.
6. Take needle guard off and place on tray.
7. Pull plunger of syringe down to desired units of intermediate or long-acting insulin.
8. Bottle A: Insert needle and inject prescribed amount of air into intermediate-acting (NPH, lente) or long-acting (PZI, ultralente) bottle. Do not touch insulin with the needle. **Rationale:** This method prevents contamination of the second bottle (B).
9. Bottle B (regular insulin): Inject air into insulin, invert bottle, and withdraw medication. **Rationale:** Withdrawing regular insulin first prevents inadvertent injection of intermediate-acting insulin into the regular insulin bottle, which would inactivate its rapid action.
10. Check dose with another nurse. **Rationale:** This

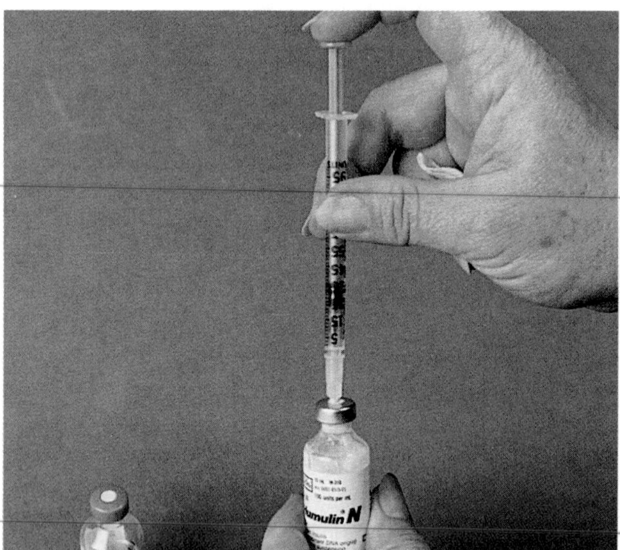

Step 1: Inject prescribed amount of air into long-acting (cloudy) vial without needle touching solution.

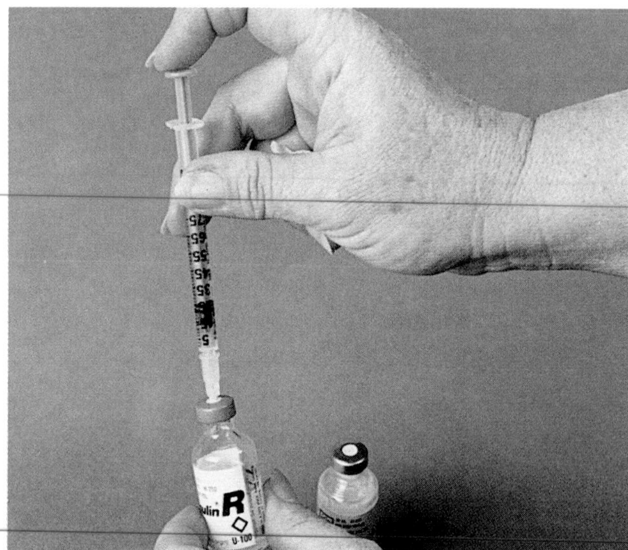

Step2: Inject prescribed amount of air into Regular (clear) insulin. Do not withdraw needle.

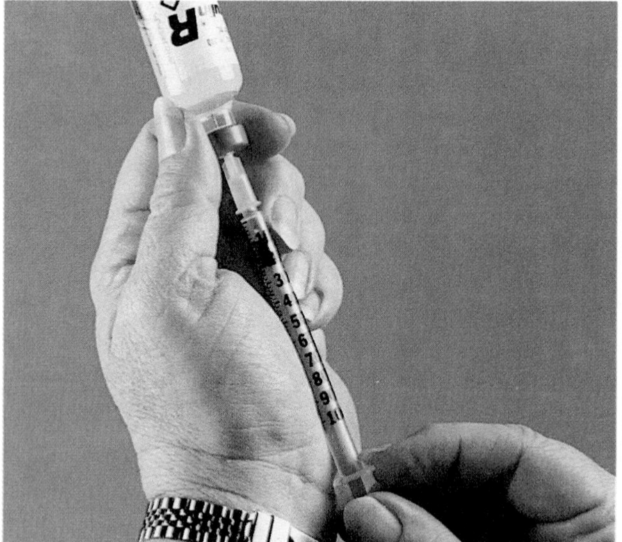

Step 3: Invert vial of Regular insulin and withdraw prescribed amount of medication.

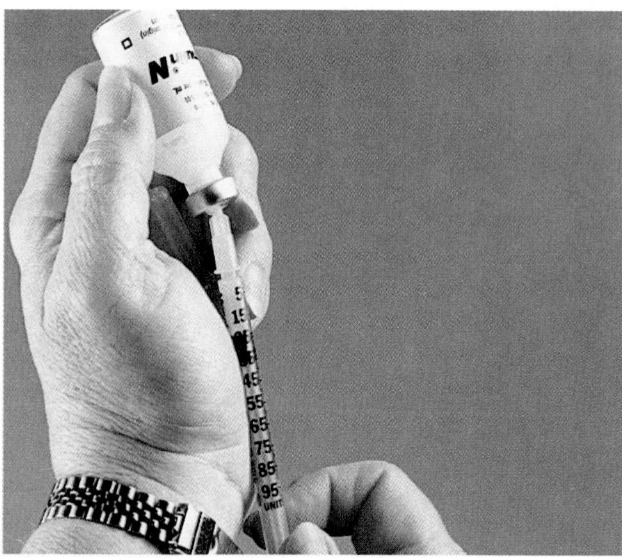

Step 4: Invert NPH bottle and withdraw exact amount without injecting Regular insulin into bottle.

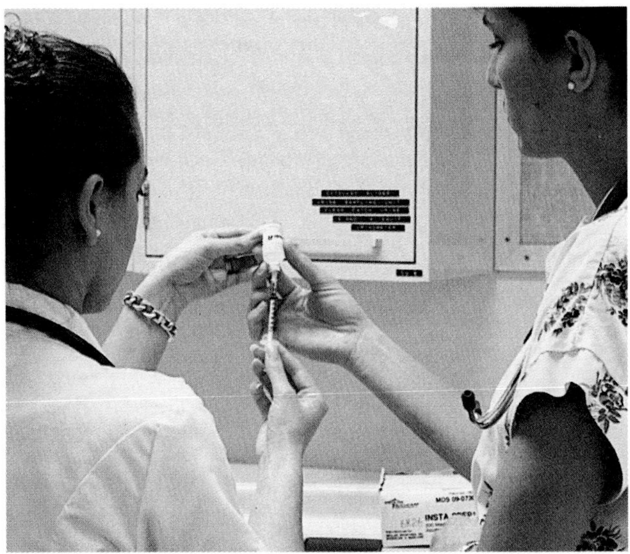

Double check insulin dose with a second nurse to ensure accurate dosage.

checking procedure by two nurses ensures accurate dosage.

11. Withdraw needle from bottle and expel all air bubbles.
12. Invert Bottle A and insert needle. Take care not to push any regular insulin into bottle. This can be avoided by holding steady pressure on plunger with your small finger when inserting needle into bottle.
13. Pull back on plunger to obtain exact prescribed amount of intermediate or long-acting insulin. The total insulin dose now includes both the regular insulin, previously drawn up into syringe, and the intermediate or long-acting insulin you have just drawn up. (Do not rotate syringe to mix insulins.)
14. Expel air from syringe.
15. Replace needle guard.
16. Follow protocol for administration of medications by subcutaneous injections, noting special Considerations for Insulin Administration.

CLINICAL ALERT

Do not massage site following insulin injection. Hold alcohol wipe over injection site for several seconds. This hastens absorption and drug action.

TEACHING USE OF INSULIN PUMP

Equipment

Insulin pump
Regular insulin and diluting fluid
26- to 27-gauge needle or 24-gauge over-needle catheter
Insulin syringe
Tubing
Batteries
Alcohol wipe
Povidone-iodine (Betadine) or bacitracin
Tape

Procedure

1. Inform client of advantages of using insulin pump. **Rationale:** In teaching a new method, this enhances acceptance.
   a. Mimics release of insulin by pancreas.
   b. Continuous delivery of fixed small amounts of regular insulin.
   c. Larger doses delivered before meals.
   d. Lifestyle advantages: fast-acting, provides tighter control of blood sugar, client does not have to adjust life and eating habits to coincide with peak action time of intermediate-acting insulin, since only regular (rapid-acting) insulin used.
   e. Clients report feeling physically better.
2. Client disadvantages.
   a. Requires conscientious client commitment to learn blood sugar monitoring and pump use.
   b. Requires extensive client teaching for self-monitoring.
3. Remind client that amount of insulin is based on results of blood glucose monitoring.
   a. Client does finger sticks for blood glucose monitoring.
   b. Insulin requirements are monitored and adjusted according to blood glucose levels.
4. Teach client how to determine basal rate of insulin. **Rationale:** This indicates to client how much insulin should be delivered over a 24-hour period.
   a. Use as a guideline for basal rate, 50% of usual daily dose.

   b. Take remaining 50% and divide into three premeal bolus doses (example: 15% before breakfast, 15% before both lunch and dinner, and 5% before snacks).
5. Instruct client how to care for insulin pump. (Once a client begins using this external delivery system, self-management procedures are necessary.)
   a. Mechanics of pumps, battery changes, and alarm system. (See manufacturer's guide.)
   b. How to load syringe and strap on chest or belt.
6. Cleanse abdominal site with alcohol prior to needle insertion. **Rationale:** Abdomen is usually chosen as a site because the fat tissue minimizes variations in absorption and it is a convenient needle site to attach the insulin pump to waist.
7. Place small amount of povidone-iodine (Betadine) or bacitracin on site.
8. Insert 26- or 27-gauge needle or 24 gauge catheter into subcutaneous tissue.
9. Tape needle into place using technique similar to taping IV needle.
10. Check that tubing is attached to needle and insulin pump.
11. Teach client how to dilute insulin.
    a. Usual diluting fluid is normal saline or insulin-diluting fluid.
    b. Regular insulin is diluted to proper unit per milliliter ratio as ordered.
12. Teach client to change needle catheter site and tubing every 48–72 hours. **Rationale:** To prevent infection at the site and tissue trauma.
13. Teach client to change syringe and insulin every 24 hours at same time each day. **Rationale:** Even though most pumps hold a 36-hour supply, changing at the same time every day establishes a routine.

■ CLINICAL ALERT

Insulin type and brand should remain consistent for an individual client.

14. Teach client how to administer premeal bolus.

Nasal Spray Insulin

- Intranasal insulin may soon replace regular insulin boluses for mealtimes. A single puff of 30 units replaces 8 units sub Q.
- *Advantages*: It has rapid physiologic action and can be used either before or after meals.
- *Disadvantages*: It requires higher doses and thus be more expensive. A potential side effect might be nasal irritation.

ADMINISTERING SUB Q HEPARIN

Equipment

See *Subcutaneous Injection.*
Medication vial
1-mL tuberculin syringe
2 needles: $\frac{5}{8}$-inch 25 gauge
Alcohol swab
Clean gloves

Preparation

See *Preparing Injections.*

Procedure

1. Follow steps 1 through 6 for Administering Subcutaneous Injections. Validate dose with another nurse.
2. Change needles after drawing up prescribed amount of medication. **Rationale:** This prevents tracking of heparin and bruising of tissue.
3. Don gloves. **Rationale:** Follow universal precautions for all injections to prevent potential contact with blood.
4. Select site on client's lower abdominal fat pad at least two fingerbreadths from umbilicus and above

■ CLINICAL ALERT

Assess for preexisting conditions that contraindicate heparin injections (e.g., kidney or liver disease, blood dyscrasias, chronic ulcerative colitis). Minor bleeding can lead to serious consequences.

Check partial thromboplastin (PTT) time. If PTT time is double the control time, check with physician before implementing heparin injection orders.

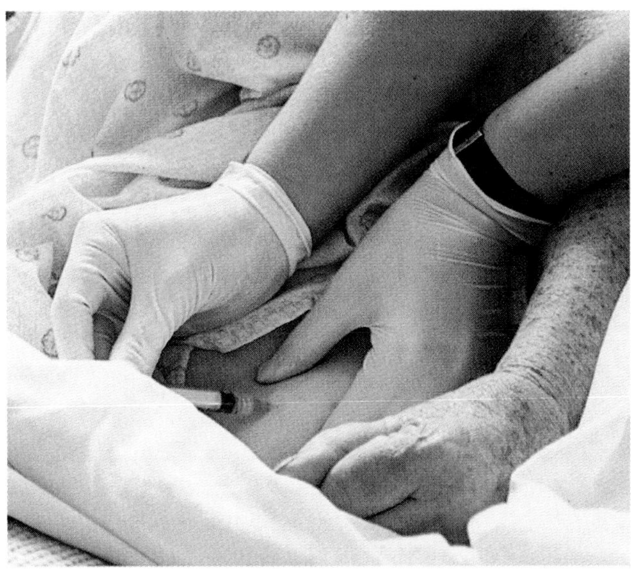

Do not aspirate or massage area when administering heparin.

iliac crest. **Rationale:** This location avoids umbilical veins.

5. Avoid ecchymotic areas, scars, or lesions. Do not use extremities. **Rationale:** Heparin injections can traumatize tissue and cause bleeding.
6. Cleanse site gently with antiseptic swab, using circular motion from inside outward. Dry thoroughly before injecting drug. **Rationale:** If skin is wet, you may inject antiseptic under skin.
7. Gently pinch an inch of subcutaneous tissue (fat roll) between thumb and forefinger of one hand.
8. Hold syringe between thumb and forefinger of other hand, and insert needle into skinfold at a 90° angle.
9. Inject medication slowly without aspirating first.
10. Wait 10 seconds before gently withdrawing needle at same angle in which it entered skin. **Rationale:** This allows heparin to absorb into tissue and minimizes bruising.
11. Press and hold alcohol swab over injection site. **Rationale:** This prevents oozing of medication.
12. Do not massage area. **Rationale:** Bleeding and bruising may result from massage following a heparin injection.

■ CLINICAL ALERT

Do not aspirate or massage heparin injections, as these actions may cause tissue damage and bruising.

13. Return client to position of comfort.
14. Do not recap needle. Discard needle–syringe unit in puncture-proof container at bedside.
15. Document injection and site. **Rationale:** Rotating sites is important to prevent hematomas.

ADMINISTERING INTRAMUSCULAR (IM) INJECTIONS

Equipment

Medication vial or ampule
3-mL syringe with 1–1½-inch needle
2 alcohol swabs
Clean gloves

■ CLINICAL ALERT

If client is obese, use a 2–3-inch needle so that medication is absorbed into muscle (not fat) tissue and blood level of drug is achieved.

Preparation

See *Preparing Injections.*

Procedure

1. Take medication to client's room. Check room number against medication card or sheet.
2. Set tray on a clean surface, not the bed.
3. Check client's identaband, and have client state name.
4. Explain the procedure to client.
5. Provide privacy for client.
6. Wash your hands, and don gloves.
7. Select the site of injection by identifying anatomic landmarks. Consider amount and viscosity of solution being injected when choosing site. Remember to alternate sites each time injections are given.
8. Cleanse the area with alcohol wipe. Using a circular motion cleanse from inside outward.
9. Hold the syringe; take off needle cover.

IM ABSORPTION VARIES

- Absorption rates in muscle tissue vary site to site. Studies show blood flow in deltoid is 7% greater than vastus lateralis and 17% greater than gluteal muscles.
- Technique affects absorption
  A study showed $1\frac{1}{2}$-inch needle absorbed $2\frac{1}{2}$ times faster than $1\frac{1}{4}$ inch—which probably hit the subcutaneous tissue rather than the muscle.

10. Express air bubbles from syringe. Some clinicians suggest leaving a small air bubble at the top so that all medicine is expelled.
11. Spread skin taut between thumb and forefinger. (Grasping muscle is acceptable in pediatric and geriatric clients to increase muscle mass and to ensure needle placement in muscle belly rather than striking bone.)
12. Insert needle at a 90° angle using a quick, darting motion. **Rationale:** This angle facilitates medication reaching muscle.

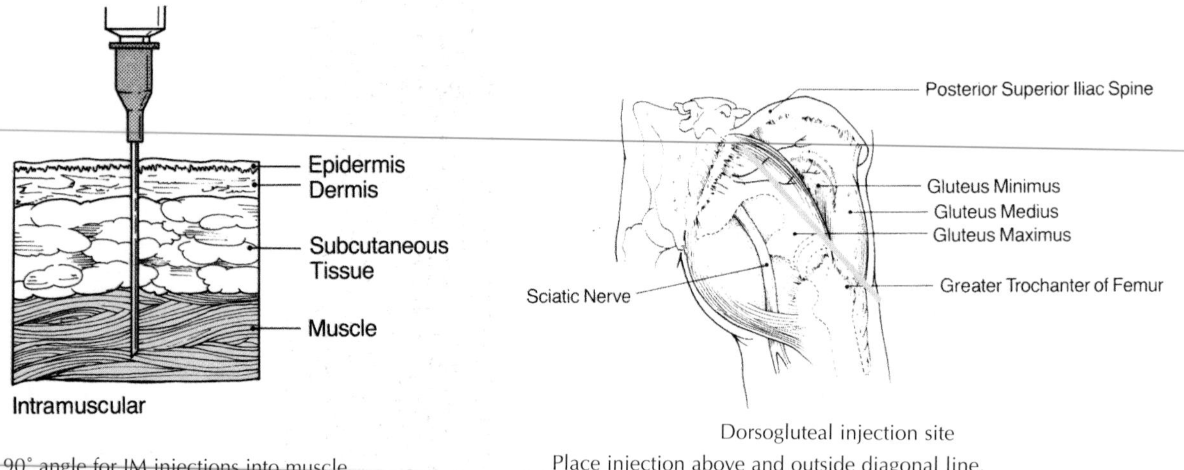

Insert needle 90° angle for IM injections into muscle.

Dorsogluteal injection site
Place injection above and outside diagonal line.

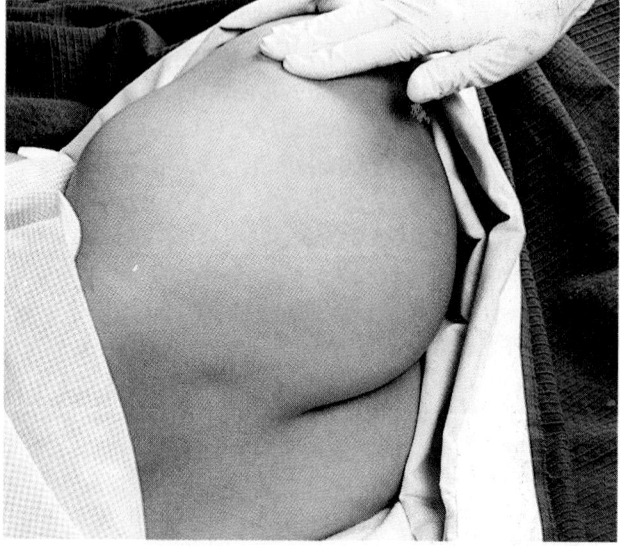

Place hand on greater trochanter to identify dorsogluteal site.

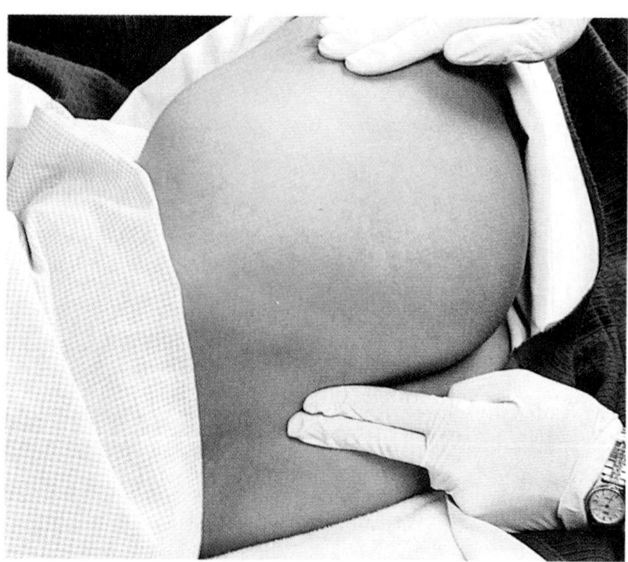

Place hand on iliac crest and locate posterosuperior iliac spine.

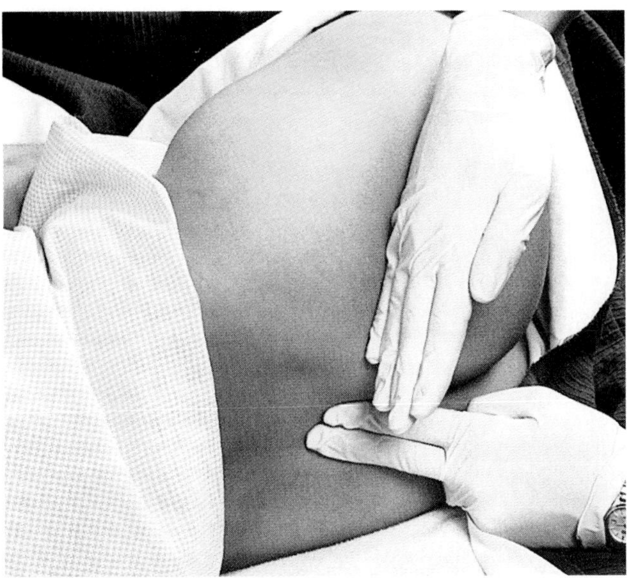
Draw imaginary line between trochanter and iliac spine.

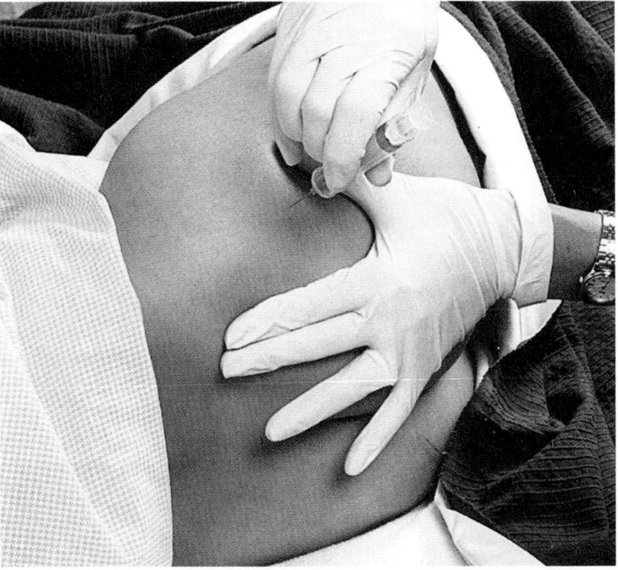
Inject medication directly into dorsogluteal site at 90° angle.

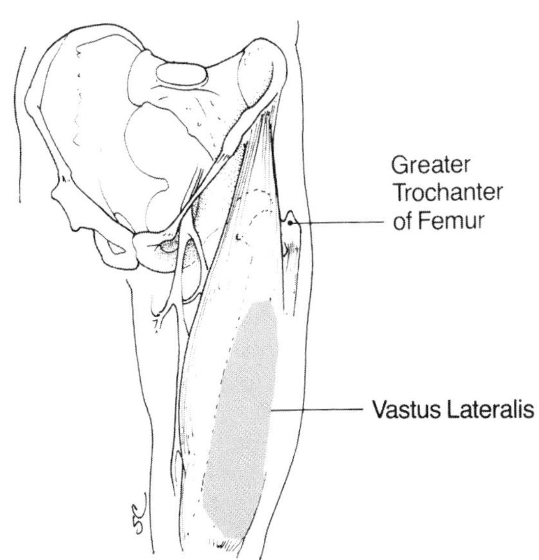

Shaded area indicates site location for vastus lateralis injection.

13. Pull back on plunger. If blood returns, you know that you have entered a blood vessel and need to discard and prepare a new injection. **Rationale:** The appearance of blood indicates needle has entered a blood vessel, and medication injected directly into bloodstream may be dangerous.
14. Inject medication slowly. **Rationale:** This allows medication time to disperse through tissue.
15. Withdraw needle quickly, and massage area with an alcohol wipe.
16. Put on Band-Aid, if needed.
17. Return client to comfortable position.
18. Discard supplies in appropriate area.
19. Chart medication and site used.

Techniques for Minimizing Pain During Injections

- Encourage client to relax.
- If you must draw needle through rubber stopper or if medication is irritating, use a new needle for injection.
- Place client on side with upper knee flexed for ventrogluteal, or flat on abdomen with toes turned inward for dorsogluteal injection.
- Avoid injecting into sensitive or hardened tissue.
- Stretch skin between landmark areas.
- Prevent antiseptic from clinging to needle during insertion by waiting until skin antiseptic is dry.
- Reduce puncture pain by "darting" needle.
- Inject medication slowly.
- Maintain grasp on syringe; do not move needle once inserted.
- Withdraw needle quickly after injection.

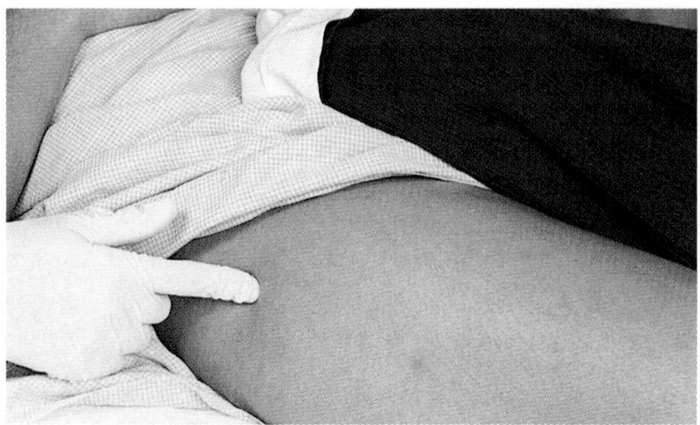

Vastus lateralis site: identify greater trochanter.

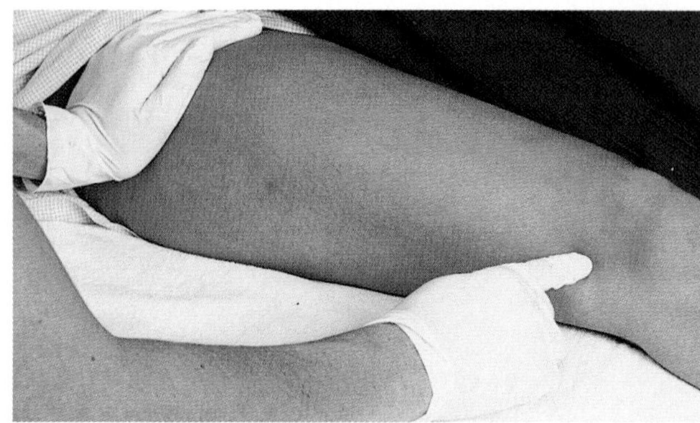

Place hand at lateral femoral condyle.

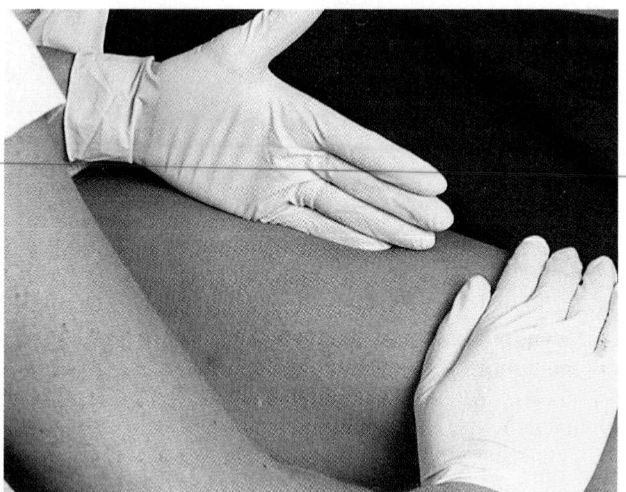

Select site using middle third and anterior lateral aspect.

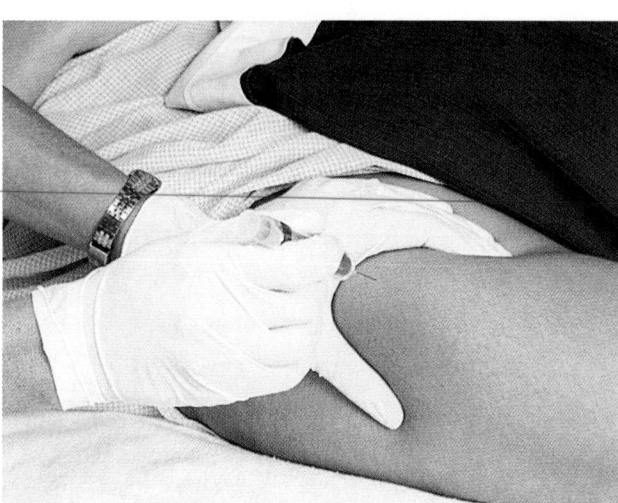

Inject medication at 90º angle directly into muscle.

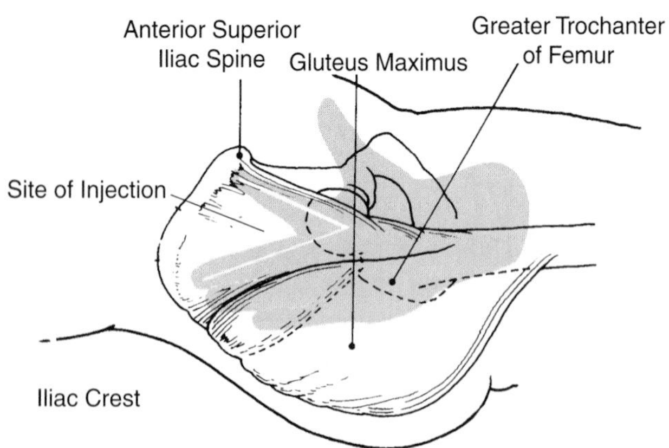

Overlay of hand shows area of injection into ventrogluteal site.

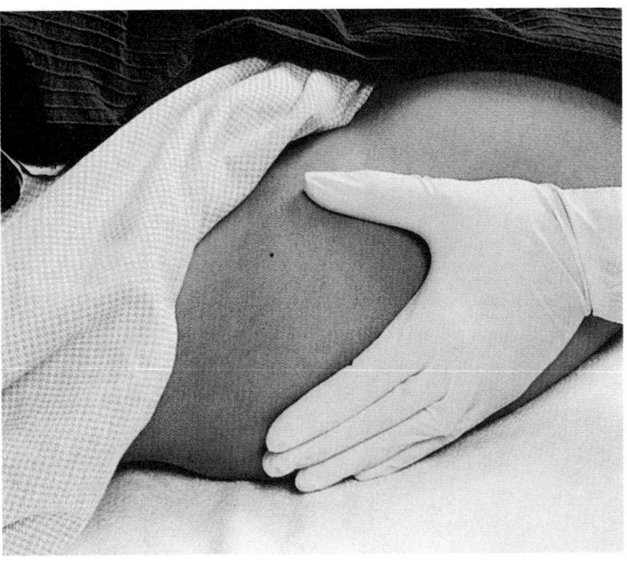

Place heel of hand over greater trochanter to locate injection area.

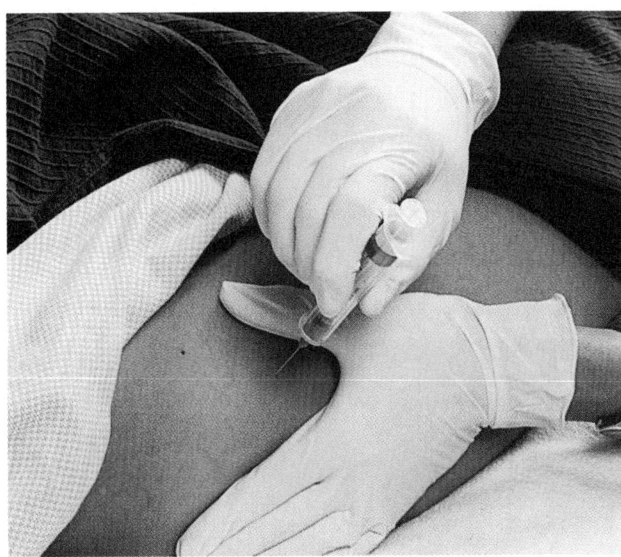

Inject medication at 90° angle into ventrogluteal muscle.

USING Z-TRACK METHOD

Equipment

Syringe
2 needles (one 2–3-inch needle)
Alcohol swabs
Medication
Clean gloves

Preparation

See *Preparing Injections.*

Procedure

1. Check the medication record with physician's order.
2. Gather equipment.
3. Wash your hands.
4. Draw up prescribed medication into syringe.
5. Add 0.3–0.5 mL of air to syringe. **Rationale:** Air clears needle and prevents medication from leaking back into the subcutaneous tissue after medication has been injected.
6. Attach a new $1\frac{1}{2}$–2-inch sterile needle to syringe. **Rationale:** A new needle prevents introducing medication that could be irritating to tissue.
7. Take medication to client's room; check room number against MAR.
8. Check identaband, and ask client to state his or her name.
9. Explain reason for injection.
10. Provide privacy.
11. Don clean gloves.
12. Place client in prone position, if possible. **Rationale:** This position provides the best perspective for identifying landmarks: posterosuperior iliac crest and greater trochanter (upper outer quadrant of buttock).
13. Cleanse site with alcohol.

■ CLINICAL ALERT

The Z-track is used for administering medications that are especially irritating to subcutaneous and nerve tissue (e.g., imferon).

■ CLINICAL ALERT

Ventrogluteal site is preferred over dorsogluteal whenever possible, because dorsogluteal area is especially vulnerable to nerve and vascular injury.

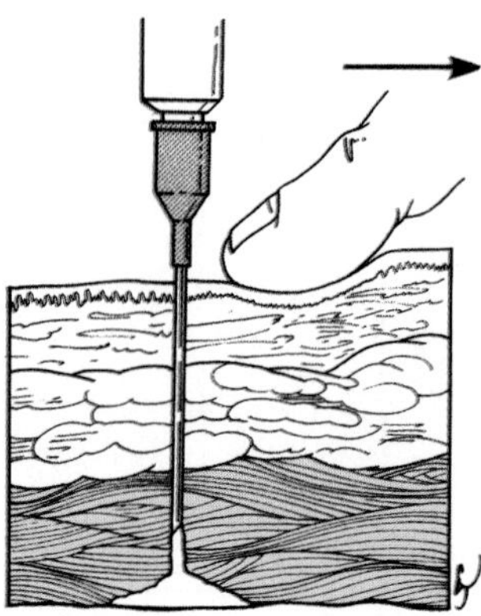

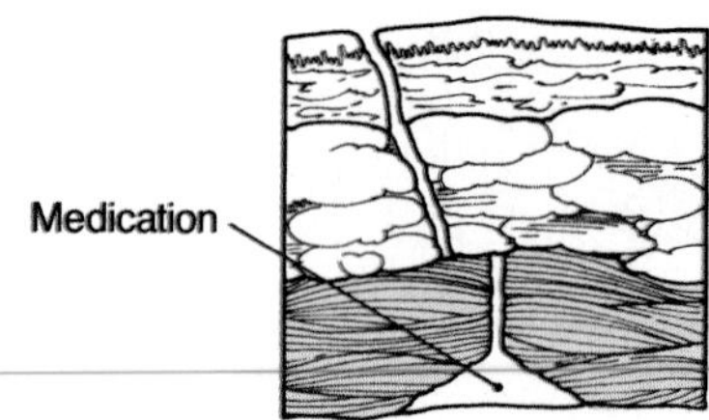

Z-track is used to prevent tracking of medications into subcutaneous tissue.

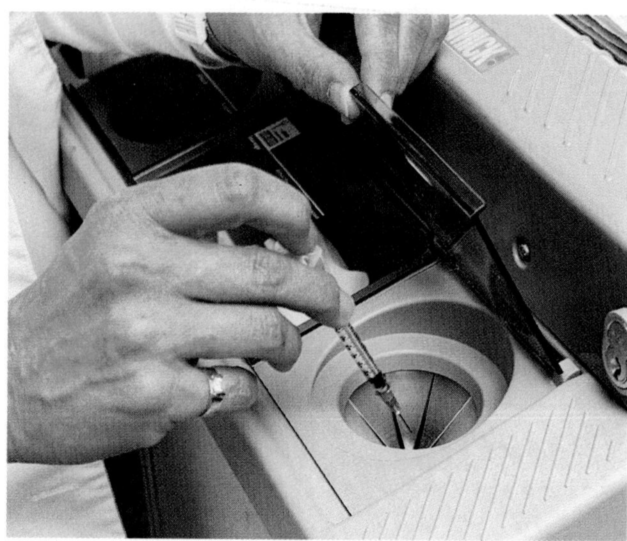

Dispose of syringe without recapping needle.

14. Pull skin 1–1½ inch laterally away from injection site. **Rationale:** This tissue displacement creates a track that keeps medication from seeping into subcutaneous tissue.
15. Insert needle at a 90° angle. Aspirate by pulling back on plunger and checking to see if needle is in blood vessel. If so, discard and prepare new injection.
16. Inject medication slowly and wait 10 seconds keeping skin taut. **Rationale:** Permits muscle relaxation and absorption of medication.
17. Withdraw needle and release retracted skin. **Rationale:** Lateral tissue displacement interrupts needle track and seals medication in the muscle when the tissue is released.
18. Apply light pressure with 2×2 gauze pad. Do not massage. **Rationale:** Massage may disperse medication into subcutaneous tissue and cause tissue irritation.
19. Return client to a position of comfort and safety.
20. Discard equipment in appropriate area.
21. Document administration of medications in the medication record.

CHARTING for Parenteral Medications

Client's Medication Record

- Name of medication
- Dosage
- Route
- Site
- Time administered
- Initials of nurse administering medication
- Signature by nurse (to identify initials)

Nurses' Notes

- Record p.r.n., stat, intradermal, and experimental medications
- Name of medication, dosage, route, site, time administered
- Client's response, pain relief, side effects
- Signature of nurse

CRITICAL THINKING APPLICATION

CLINICAL PROBLEMS	CRITICAL THINKING OPTIONS
■ Sciatic nerve is injured by needle or medication when administering IM injection.	• Notify physician. • Fill out incident report. • Take greater care to identify anatomic landmarks. Use dorsogluteal site only when necessary. • Locate a line from posterosuperior iliac spine to the greater trochanter of the femur; injection lateral and slightly superior to midpoint of line. Use Z-track technique. Inject muscle at a 90° angle. • Obtain order for warm, moist packs. • Assess need for pain medication.
■ Medication is administered using wrong parenteral route.	• Notify physician, and initiate incident report. • Medications may need to be administered to reverse the action of the medication. • Insulin or heparin administered IM rather than sub Q leads to faster absorption rates; therefore an assessment needs to be done to determine action of medication (blood glucose to determine effectiveness of insulin and PTT level for heparin injection)
■ Ecchymosis occurs following heparin injection.	• Rotate injection site. Do not inject medication into ecchymotic area. • Do not aspirate before injection or massage site following needle withdrawal. • When forming fat pad in preparation for injection site, do not pinch tightly. • Administer medication at room temperature to prevent tissue trauma with injections.
■ Client has an anaphylactic allergic response.	• Maintain patent airway. • Position client for optimal cerebral perfusion—flat or 30° elevation if dyspneic. • Notify physician immediately. • Be prepared to carry out the following actions following physician's orders. Administer oxygen 6 L/minute via nasal prongs as ordered after epinephrine for bronchodilation. Insert IV line for fluid resuscitation. Monitor client for alterations in signs and symptoms to determine client status. Monitor vital signs frequently until the client's status is stabilized.

unit 5

TOPICAL MEDICATIONS

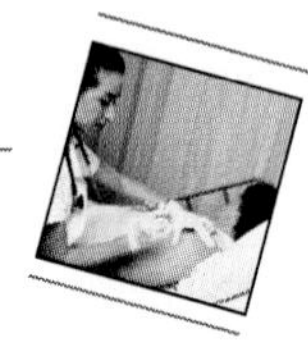

NURSING PROCESS DATA

ASSESSMENT **Data Base**

Observe for open lesions, rashes, or areas of erythema and skin breakdown.
Assess for known allergies as related by the client or as noted in the chart.
Observe local changes in the skin occurring from the use of the drug.
Assess for proper medication administration.

PLANNING **Objectives**

To provide continuous absorption of medication
To protect the skin
To stop, slow, or prevent the growth of microorganisms
To provide a local anesthetic to specified parts of the body

IMPLEMENTATION **Procedures**

Applying Dermal Ointments and Salves
Applying Ointment to Burns
Applying Transdermal Medications

EVALUATION **Expected Outcomes**

Skin returned to normal state.
Alleviation of symptoms for which medication was administered.
Decreased pain.
Control of microorganisms.

APPLYING DERMAL OINTMENTS AND SALVES

Equipment

Medication container
Application tube (if needed)
2×2 gauze pads for cleansing
Sterile tongue blade
Gloves
Sterile gauze

Preparation

1. Obtain client's medication record.
2. Compare the medication record with the most *recent* physician's order.
3. Wash your hands.
4. Gather necessary equipment, including gloves or tongue blade as needed.
5. Remove the medication from the drug box or tray on medication cart.
6. Compare the label on the medication tube or jar to the medication record. **Rationale:** First safety check.
7. Place medication tube or jar (include a tongue blade with jar) on a tray if not using medication cart. Compare label on medication tube or jar with medication record. **Rationale:** Second safety check.

Procedure

1. Take medication to client's room; check room and bed number against medication record.
2. Check client's identaband and ask client to state name.

3. Provide privacy.
4. Wash your hands. Don gloves if indicated.
5. Cleanse skin surface with soap and water unless contraindicated by client's condition. Dry thoroughly.
6. Compare label on medication jar or tube with medication record. **Rationale:** Third safety check.
7. Squeeze medication from a tube, or using a tongue blade, take ointment out of jar.
8. Spread a small, smooth, thin quantity of medication evenly over client's skin surface following direction of hair follicles. Use a tongue blade or your fingers to facilitate smooth application of ointment. **Rationale:** Softened medication applied with fingers ensures even distribution of medication.
9. Protect skin surface with a dressing, unless contraindicated. **Rationale:** Dressing ensures that medication cannot rub off.
10. Check to see that client is comfortable before leaving room.
11. Return medication to appropriate storage area.
12. Wash your hands.

APPLYING OINTMENT TO BURNS

Equipment

Medication container
Application tube (if needed)
Sterile 2×2 gauze pads for cleansing
Sterile tongue blade
Sterile gloves
Sterile gauze (for burn dressing)
Commercially prepared burn dressings
Stretch body net

Preparation

See *Applying Dermal Ointments and Salves.*

Procedure

1. Take medication to client's room; check room and bed number against medication record.
2. Check client's identaband, and ask client to state name.
3. Provide privacy.
4. Wash your hands.
5. Squeeze medication from a tube, or using a tongue blade, take ointment out of jar.
6. If *no dressing is ordered,* apply medication directly to burn area; using sterile gloves and tongue blade, cover entire burn area with medication. **Rationale:** To provide an occlusive effect.
7. If *dressing is ordered,* use sterile gloves or sterile tongue blade to rub drug directly into sterile gauze. Then apply medicated gauze to burn area. (Commercially prepared premedicated gauze dressings can be applied directly to burn area, using sterile technique.) Cover medicated dressings with sterile Kerlix.
8. Apply body net if large area is involved.
9. Check to see that client is comfortable before leaving room.
10. Remove gloves and wash your hands.
11. Return drug and equipment to appropriate storage area.

APPLYING TRANSDERMAL MEDICATIONS

Equipment

Medication container patch
Gloves
Premeasured paper

Preparation

See *Applying Dermal Ointments and Salves.*

Procedure

1. Take medication to client's room, check room and bed number against medication record.

2. Check identaband, and ask client to state name.
3. Provide privacy.
4. Wash your hands.
5. Put on gloves. **Rationale:** Gloves prevent absorbing medication through fingertips.

> **■ CLINICAL ALERT**
>
> Considerations for Applying Vasodilator Patches
> - Check client's blood pressure before applying vasodilator.
> - Wear gloves to prevent medication being absorbed.

6. Obtain transdermal patch or premeasured paper that accompanies medication tube.
7. Place prescribed medication directly on paper (usually $\frac{1}{2}$–1-inch strip) or remove protective covering from patch.
8. Apply medicated paper or patch to anterior surface of chest. You may apply medicated paper or patch to any area of body. **Rationale:** Most clients feel medication works better if applied to chest surface; therefore it is most frequently used area.
9. Alternate areas with each dose of medication. Be sure to remove previous medicated paper and cleanse skin prior to applying new dose. Secure paper, if necessary, with adhesive tape.
10. Remove gloves.
11. Label patch with date, time, and your initials.
12. Return medication to appropriate storage area.
13. Wash your hands.

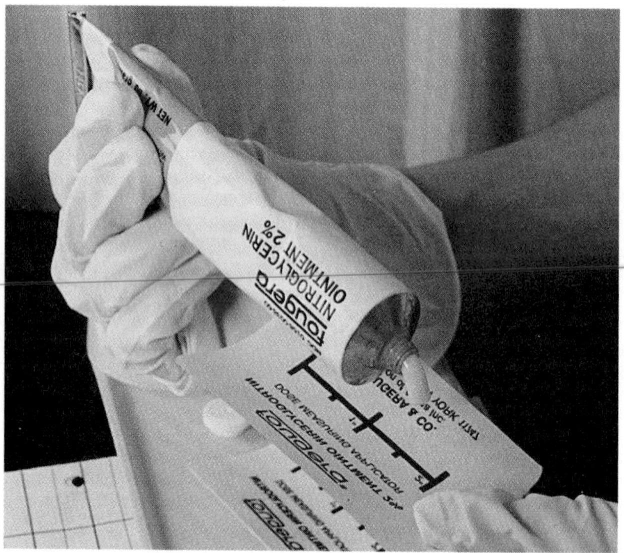

Use premeasured paper to measure medication.

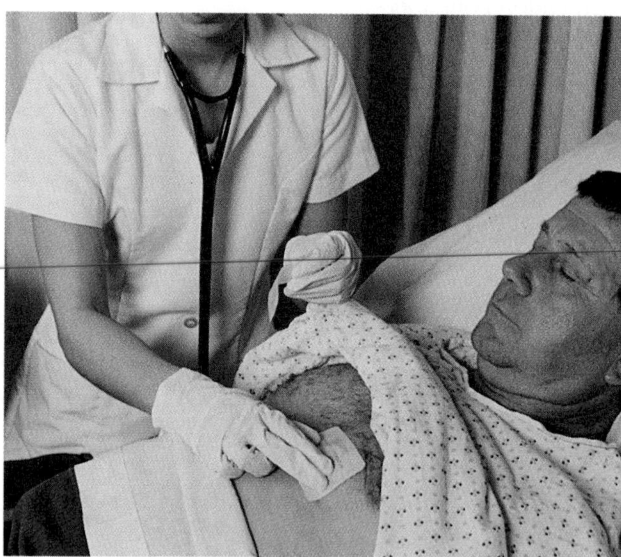
Use gloves to prevent drug absorption through fingertips.

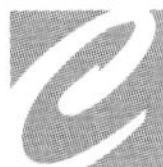

CHARTING for Dermal or Transdermal Medications

Client's Medication Record

- Name of medication
- Dosage
- Route
- Site
- Time administered
- Initials of nurse administering medication
- Signature by nurse which identifies initials

Nurses' Notes

- Record p.r.n., stat, and experimental medications
- Name of medication, dosage, route, site, time administered
- Client's response, skin condition, any areas of irritation, erythema
- Signature of nurse

CRITICAL THINKING APPLICATION

CLINICAL PROBLEMS	CRITICAL THINKING OPTIONS
Skin irritation due to medication.	• Notify the physician so that medication may be discontinued.
Client has allergic response (hives, rash, or itching).	• Hold medication; notify physician. • Obtain order for antihistamine if necessary.
Headache occurs after nitroglycerine ointment applied to skin.	• Notify physician. Dosage may be lowered. • Administer analgesic if ordered.
Patch does not stay on skin.	• Cover with plastic wrap and/or tape in place.

unit 6

EYE MEDICATIONS

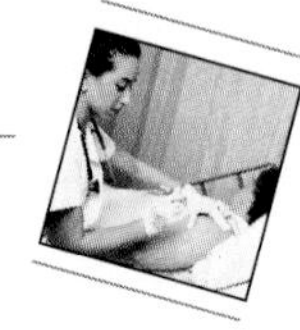

NURSING PROCESS DATA

ASSESSMENT Data Base

Assess client's ability to cooperate during administration, since medications are instilled into the lower conjunctival sac.

Check medication expiration date.

Assess condition of eye and surrounding areas.

PLANNING Objectives

To provide direct route for local effect

To decrease intraocular pressure

To provide pupillary dilation to facilitate eye examination

IMPLEMENTATION Procedures

Instilling Eye Drops

Administering Eye Ointment

EVALUATION Expected Outcomes

Client cooperates with instillation of eye medication.

Desired therapeutic effect is obtained.

Eye surgery or evaluation is accomplished.

Intraocular pressure is reduced.

INSTILLING EYE DROPS

Equipment

Eye medication in ocumeter container
Cotton ball or tissue

Preparation

1. Obtain client's medication record. Medication record may be a drug card, medication sheet, or drug Kardex, depending on the method of dispensing medications in your facility.
2. Compare the medication record with the most *recent* physician's order.
3. Wash your hands.
4. Gather necessary equipment.
5. Remove the medication from the drug box or tray on medication cart.
6. Compare the label on the medication bottle to the medication record. **Rationale:** Safety check.
7. Place medication on a tray if not using medication

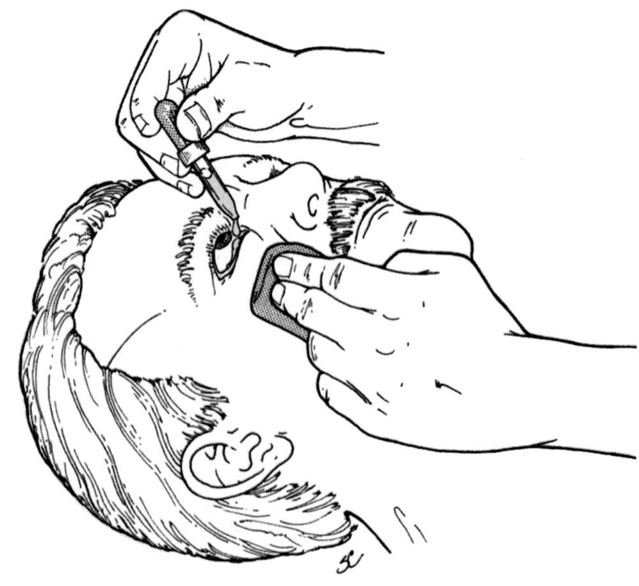

Drop eye medication in the center of lower conjunctival sac.

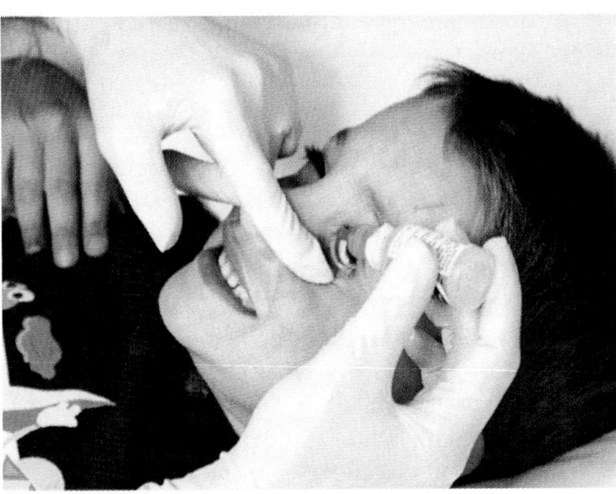
Use nondominant hand to pull child's lower lid down.

cart. Compare label on medication bottle with medication record. **Rationale:** Safety check.

Procedure

1. Take medication to client's room, and check room and bed number against medication record.
2. Check identaband, and ask client to state name.
3. Wash your hands.
4. Explain procedure to client.
5. Tilt head slightly backward and ask client to look up. **Rationale:** The cornea is protected as client looks up.
6. Uncap ocumeter, placing cap on its side or squeeze the prescribed amount of medication into eye dropper. Hold dropper with bulb in uppermost position.
7. Give tissue to client for wiping off excess medication.
8. Place eye dropper $\frac{1}{2}$–$\frac{3}{4}$-inch above eyeball with dominant hand. **Rationale:** This position reduces risk of dropper touching eyeball and thereby causing injury.
9. Stabilize hand holding dropper as necessary. Place nondominant hand on cheekbone and hand holding dropper on top.
10. Expose lower conjunctival sac by pulling down on cheek.
11. Drop prescribed number of drops into center of conjunctival sac. **Rationale:** Placing medication directly on cornea could cause injury to cornea.

> **■ CLINICAL ALERT**
>
> Apply pressure to inner canthus to prevent rapid absorption if eye drops have potential systemic effects (e.g., bradycardia due to timolol maleate [Timoptic] drops for glaucoma).

12. Ask client to gently close eyelids and move eyes. **Rationale:** This distributes solution over conjunctival surface and anterior eyeball.
13. Remove excess medication with tissue.
14. Wash your hands.
15. Replace medication in appropriate place.

ADMINISTERING EYE OINTMENT

Equipment

Ointment
Cotton ball or tissue
Cotton-tipped applicator

Preparation

1. Obtain client's medication record.
2. Compare the medication record with the most *recent* physician's order.
3. Wash your hands.
4. Gather necessary equipment.
5. Remove the medication from the drug box or tray on medication cart.
6. Compare the label on the medication tube to the medication record. **Rationale:** Safety check.

O.S. = Left eye
O.D. = Right eye
O.U. = Both eyes

Procedure

1. Place medication on a tray if not using medication cart. Compare label with medication record. **Rationale:** Safety check.

2. Take medication to client's room, and check room and bed number against medication record.
3. Check identaband, and ask client to state name.
4. Wash your hands.
5. Explain procedure to client.
6. Take protective guard off medication tip, and lay on its side.
7. *For lower lid*:
   a. Gently separate client's eyelids with your thumb or two fingers, and grasp lower lid near the margin of the lower lid immediately below the lashes. Exert pressure downward over the bony prominence of the cheek.
   b. Instruct the client to look upward. **Rationale:** To keep cornea out of way of medication.
   c. Apply eye medication along the inside edge of the entire lower eyelid, from inner to outer canthus.
8. *For upper lid*:
   a. Instruct client to look down.
   b. Grasp client's lashes near center of upper lid with your thumb and index finger. Draw lid up and away from eyeball.
   c. Squeeze ointment along upper lid starting at inner canthus.
9. Ask client to close eyelids and move eyes to assist in spreading ointment under the lids and over the surface of the eyeball.
10. With a cotton ball or soft tissue, remove the excess medication from client's eye and cheek.
11. Recover and replace medication.
12. Wash your hands.

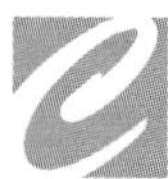

CHARTING for Eye Medications

Client's Medication Record

- Name of medication
- Dosage
- Route
- Site
- Time administered
- Initials of nurse administering medication
- Signature by nurse which identifies initials

Nurses' Notes

- Condition of eye and surrounding tissue
- Signature of nurse

CRITICAL THINKING APPLICATION

CLINICAL PROBLEMS	CRITICAL THINKING OPTIONS
■ Infection is introduced because of break in aseptic technique.	• Medication dropper is contaminated. Discard dropper and obtain new one. • Review the recommended procedures for administering the medication, and have another nurse observe until you perfect the skill of administering eye medications.
■ Irritation of eye occurs.	• Notify physician for new orders. • Obtain orders for sterile soaks to ease pain and discomfort.

unit 7

EAR MEDICATIONS

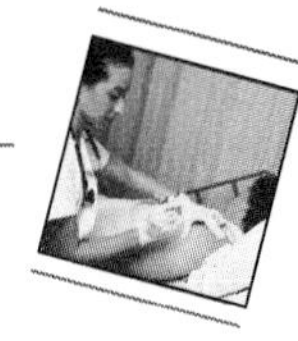

NURSING PROCESS DATA

ASSESSMENT Data Base

Assess client's ability to cooperate with instillation.

Assess client's ability to be positioned on side.

PLANNING Objectives

To soften ear wax

To relieve pain and obtain desired therapeutic effect

To apply anesthetic agent

To provide route for antibacterial medications

IMPLEMENTATION Procedure

Administering Ear Medications

EVALUATION Expected Outcomes

Client cooperates with instillation.

Desired therapeutic effect is obtained.

ADMINISTERING EAR MEDICATIONS

Equipment

Medication

Dropper for instilling medication

Cotton wick

Preparation

1. Obtain client's medication record.
2. Compare the medication record with the most *recent* physician's order.
3. Wash your hands.
4. Gather necessary equipment.
5. Remove the medication from the drug box or tray on medication cart.
6. Compare the label on the medication bottle to the medication record. **Rationale:** Safety check.
7. Before preparing medication for administration, warm medication bottle to body temperature.

Procedure

1. Place medication on a tray if not using medication cart.

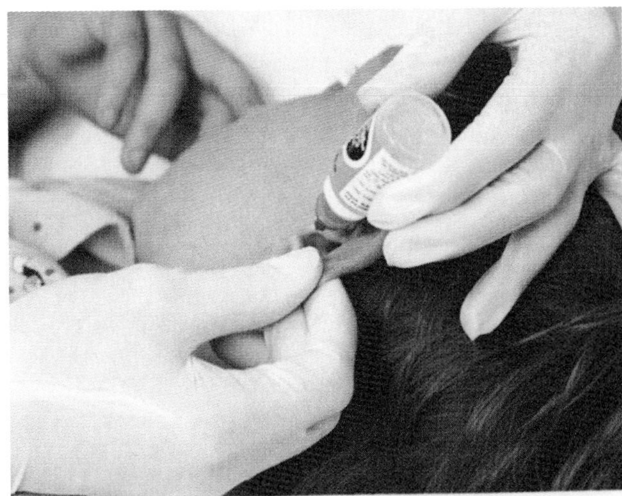

Gently pull pinna back and upward to instill medication in an older child.

2. Take medication to client's room, and check room number against medication card or sheet.
3. Check identaband, and ask client to state name.
4. Explain procedure to client.
5. Wash your hands.

6. Position client on side, with ear to be treated in the uppermost position. **Rationale:** This position allows medication to enter external ear canal.
7. Compare label on medication bottle with record. **Rationale:** Safety check.
8. Fill medication dropper with prescribed amount of medication.
9. Prepare client for instillation of ear medication as follows:
   a. *Infant.* Draw the auricle gently downward and backward. **Rationale:** This separates the drum membrane from the floor of the cartilaginous canal.
   b. *Adult.* Lift pinna upward and backward. **Rationale:** This position straightens out the ear canal.
10. Instill medication drops, holding dropper slightly above ear. **Rationale:** This position does not contaminate dropper.
11. Insert a loose cotton wick into outer canal if ordered. **Rationale:** Prevents medication from draining out.
12. Instruct client to remain on side for 5–10 minutes following instillation. **Rationale:** Prevents medication from escaping and facilitates distribution.
13. Place client in comfortable position.
14. Dispose of used supplies and wash hands.

CHARTING for Ear Medications

Client's Medication Record

- Name of medication
- Dosage
- Route
- Site
- Time administered
- Initials of nurse administering medication
- Signature by nurse which identifies initials

Nurses' Notes

- Color, consistency of drainage
- Comfort level of client
- Signature of nurse

CRITICAL THINKING APPLICATION

CLINICAL PROBLEMS	CRITICAL THINKING OPTIONS
Client moves unexpectedly, causing medication to run down client's neck.	• Repeat explanation of procedure to client. • Readminister medication while holding client in the correct position. Keep client positioned on side for 15 minutes after instillation.
Client complains medication is too warm.	• Check to ensure medication is heated only to 98.6°F. • Observe client for any untoward effects.
Client complains of nausea or vertigo following ear medication instillation	• Warm medication to body temperature. Cold medication may cause these effects.

unit 8

RESPIRATORY MEDICATIONS

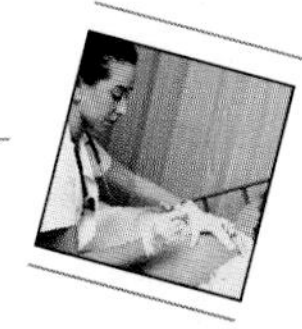

NURSING PROCESS DATA

ASSESSMENT Data Base

Assess for dyspnea, labored breathing, and breath sounds.

Assess vital signs for alterations.

Assess for known allergies as related by the client or as noted in the chart.

Observe local changes in the mucous membranes.

Assess for proper medication administration.

Assess for side effects of aerosol therapy (tremors, nausea, tachycardia, dysrhythmias).

PLANNING Objectives

To improve breath sounds

To apply an agent that stops, slows, or prevents infection or inflammation

To provide local anesthesia to specified parts of the body to relieve pain or discomfort

To provide relief of nasal congestion

To provide appropriate surface for effective absorption

To provide relief for bronchospasms, asthma, or allergic reactions

To confine drug actions to the airway when using aerosol therapy

To facilitate ease and consistency of self-administration

IMPLEMENTATION Procedures

Administering Respiratory Medications

Instilling Nose Drops

Administering Metered-Dose Inhaled Drugs

Using Spacer for Aerosol Therapy

EVALUATION Expected Outcomes

Alleviation of symptoms for which medication was administered.

Increased comfort and relief.

Infection or inflammation controlled.

Breath sounds improved.

ADMINISTERING RESPIRATORY MEDICATIONS

Equipment

Medication container

Medication dropper for nasal drops

Appropriate medication device for administration

Tissues

Gloves

Preparation

1. Obtain client's medication record. Medication record may be a medication sheet or drug Kardex, depending on the method of dispensing medications in your facility.
2. Compare the medication record with the most recent physician's order.
3. Wash your hands.
4. Gather necessary equipment.
5. Remove the medication from the drug box or tray on medication cart.

6. Compare the label on the medication container to the medication record.
7. Place medication container on a tray if not using medication cart.

Procedure

1. Take medication to client's room; check room number against medication card or sheet.
2. Identify client by name; check identaband.
3. Wash your hands.
4. Provide client privacy.
5. Complete application according to specific directions.

INSTILLING NOSE DROPS

Equipment

Medication

Dropper

Preparation

See *Administering Respiratory Medications.*

Procedure

1. Take medication to client's room; check room number against medication card or sheet.
2. Wash your hands.
3. Place client in sitting position with head tilted back or in supine position with head tilted back over pillow.
4. Fill dropper with prescribed amount of medication.
5. Place dropper just inside the nares and instill correct number of drops. Repeat procedure in other nares.
6. Instruct client not to sneeze and to keep head tilted back for 5 minutes to prevent medication from escaping.
7. Check to see that client is comfortable before leaving room.
8. Return medication to appropriate storage area.

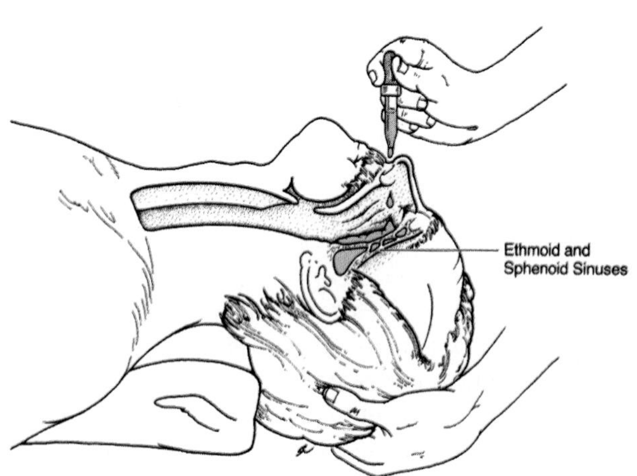

Instruct client to tilt head backwards and place dropper inside nares when instilling nose drops.

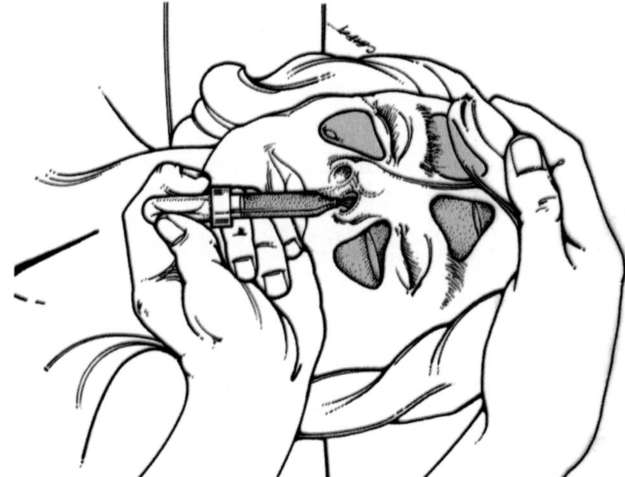

Tilt client's head back for nose drops to reach maxillary and frontal sinuses.

ADMINISTERING METERED-DOSE INHALED DRUGS

Equipment

Metered-dose inhaler device
Medication canister
Spacer if indicated

Preparation

1. Obtain client's medication record.
2. Compare the medication record with the most recent physician's order.
3. Wash your hands.
4. Gather necessary equipment.
5. Compare label of drug canister to the medication record.

ASSESSING LEVEL OF MEDICATION CANISTER

- To determine the amount left in the inhaler, fill a container with cold water and observe the position canister takes in the water.

Canister level	Position in water
Full	Sinks flat to bottom
Empty	Floats flat on top
Three-quarters full	Sinks to bottom; stands upright
Half full	Floats upright on top
One-quarter full	Floats on top at an angle

Procedure

1. Take medication canister and inhaler to room.
2. Check room number against medication card or sheet.
3. Identify client by name; check identaband.
4. Explain procedure to client.
5. Provide privacy.
6. Wash your hands.
7. Assist client to comfortable sitting position.
8. Insert canister (stem down) into longer part of dispenser.
9. Remove mouthpiece (short end) cap.
10. Shake canister to mix medication and propellant.
11. Instruct client to hold inhaler 2 inches away from mouth (following manufacturer's instructions). **Rationale:** When inhaler is held in mouth large droplets go to back of throat and are swallowed. Goal is to have mist inhaled so that it goes directly to the airway.
12. Instruct client to exhale deeply through nose.
13. Instruct client to depress inhalation device releasing a puff of medication and inhale slowly and deeply through mouth. **Rationale:** With inhalation, medication goes to lower respiratory tract.
14. Tell client to hold breath for 10 seconds and slowly exhale through pursed lips. **Rationale:** Holding the breath allows time for the medication to be absorbed.

CLINICAL ALERT

If several types of medications are used, follow this sequence: Quick-acting bronchodilator (e.g., albuterol sulfate); slower acting bronchodilator (e.g., ipratropium bromide [Atrovent]); antimediators (e.g., steroids).

15. Assess client's breathing and reaction to medication. **Rationale:** With certain drugs, pulse may increase indicating cardiac dysrhythmias.
16. Instruct client to use inhaler only as directed and according to prescribed dose. **Rationale:** A specific amount of medication is delivered with each depression of the canister.
17. Instruct client to wait 2 minutes between puffs if more than one puff is ordered.
18. Caution client not to increase dose without physician's order. **Rationale:** Potential side effects of an increased dose could be severe.
19. Teach client how to clean device according to manufacturer's instructions. **Rationale:** These devices are sites for bacterial growth.
20. Review possible side effects with client. **Rationale:** Client usually uses this device at home and must be able to evaluate side effects of medication.

Inhaled Medications

- Inhaled medications are rapidly absorbed in bronchioles and provide relief for bronchospasms, wheezing, asthma, or allergic reactions.

- Medications used in inhalers may be bronchodilators, antibiotics, steroids, or mucolytic agents. When using steroids, instruct client to rinse with water and expectorate following inhalation.
- Most common side effects are tremors, nausea, tachycardia, palpitations, nervousness, and dysrhythmias.

USING SPACER FOR AEROSOL THERAPY

Procedure

1. Insert metered dose inhaler (MDI) mouthpiece into spacer. **Rationale:** Latest research indicates a spacer fitted on an inhaler is a safer method of delivering medication because large drops do not fall into the mouth.
2. Remove mouthpiece cover from spacer.
3. Shake MDI with spacer.
4. Hold MDI with spacer with drug canister upright.
5. Instruct client to exhale slowly through pursed lips.
6. Instruct client to close lips around spacer mouthpiece. **Rationale:** Spacer eliminates need for simultaneous hand-to-eye inspiration coordination.
7. Activate MDI canister with thumbs, pushing it further into plastic adapter.
8. After activation, instruct client to then inhale slowly and deeply through mouth.
9. Hold breath 10 seconds.
10. Exhale and relax.
11. Wipe mouthpiece after use.
12. Remove rubber end of spacer, rinse with warm water, and dry thoroughly.

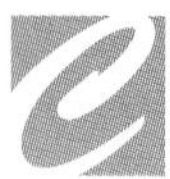

CHARTING for Respiratory Medication Administration

Client's Medication Record

- Appropriate medication form for facility used
- Name of drug
- Dosage
- Side effects noted
- Method of administration
- Times ordered
- Time administered
- Initials of nurse administering drug

Nurses' Notes

- Changes in breath sounds
- Client tolerance of medication
- Observed effects of medication
- Results of teaching client use of device

CRITICAL THINKING APPLICATION

CLINICAL PROBLEMS	CRITICAL THINKING OPTIONS
■ Client complains that breathing has not improved.	• Validate that mist is inhaled and medication is not swallowed. • Validate that device is functioning correctly.

7. Place client in the Sims' (left lateral) position.
8. Remove the foil wrapper from the suppository.
9. Moisten suppository tip with warm water or use lubricant on tip of suppository to facilitate its insertion.
10. Using a clean glove, insert the suppository into the rectal canal beyond the anal sphincter. **Rationale:** Prevents suppository from slipping out.
11. Instruct the client to lie quietly for 15 minutes while the medicine is absorbed.
12. Dispose of equipment and wash your hands.
13. Return after 15 minutes to ensure client is comfortable.
14. Chart medication and results obtained.

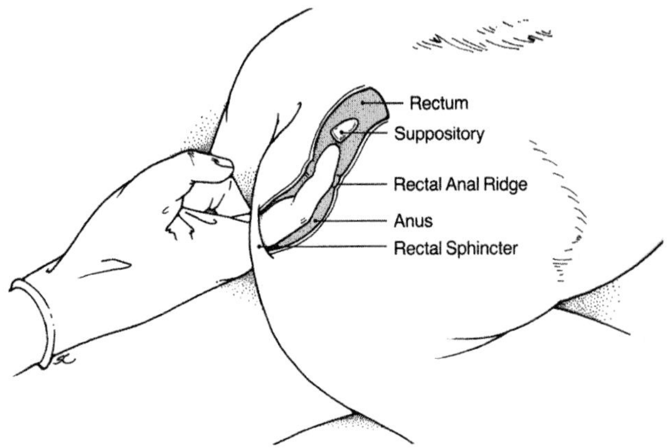

After donning a clean glove, insert rectal suppository beyond the anal-rectal ridge to ensure it is retained.

INSERTING VAGINAL SUPPOSITORIES

Equipment

Suppository
Applicator (should be kept in client's room)
Disposable glove

Preparation

1. Obtain client's medication record. Medication record may be a drug card, medication sheet, or drug Kardex, depending on the method of dispensing medications in your facility.
2. Compare the medication record with the most recent physician's order.
3. Wash your hands.
4. Gather necessary equipment.
5. Remove the medication from the drug box or tray on medication cart.
6. Compare the label on the medication to the medication record.
7. Place medication jar on a tray if not using medication cart. Include applicator to be left in client's room.
8. Check drug information to determine if appropriate for application to mucous membranes.

Procedure

1. Take medication to client's room, and check room number against medication card or sheet.
2. Check client's identaband and ask client to state name.
3. Check medication route and dosage.
4. Provide privacy.
5. Wash your hands.
6. Place client in the dorsal recumbent or Sims' position.
7. Remove the foil wrapper from the suppository. Insert into applicator.
8. Using a disposable glove, insert the suppository into the vaginal canal at least 2 inches. **Rationale:** Prevents suppository from slipping out.

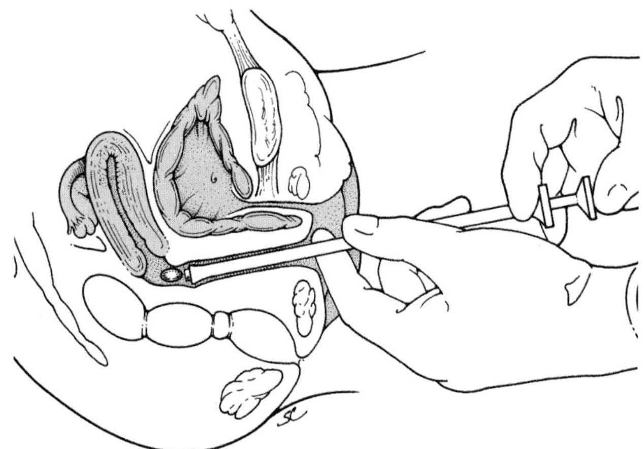

Insert vaginal suppositories at least two inches using glove or applicator as shown.

unit 9 SUPPOSITORY MEDICATIONS

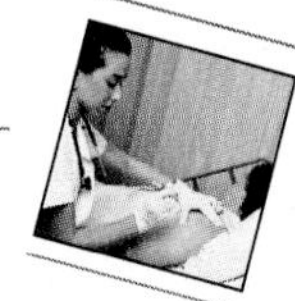

NURSING PROCESS DATA

ASSESSMENT Data Base

Observe for signs of rectal irritation or bleeding.

Observe for hemorrhoids.

Check sphincter control.

Observe for presence of vaginal irritation or secretions.

PLANNING Objectives

To provide alternative route when upper GI tract is malfunctioning (i.e., vomiting)

To offer alternative route when drug has offensive taste or odor

To maintain chemical integrity of drug when digestive enzymes change the chemical properties of the drug

To obtain high blood concentration of the drug

To assist in bowel elimination

IMPLEMENTATION Procedures

Inserting Rectal Suppositories

Inserting Vaginal Suppositories

EVALUATION Expected Outcomes

Medication is inserted without technical complications.

Medication enters the bloodstream and is effective.

Medications are retained without expulsion.

Bowel elimination is achieved.

INSERTING RECTAL SUPPOSITORIES

Equipment

Suppository as ordered

Disposable glove

Vaginal–rectal lubricant (K-Y jelly)

Preparation

1. Obtain client's medication record. Medication record may be a drug card, medication sheet, or drug Kardex, depending on the method of dispensing medications in your facility.
2. Compare the medication record with the most recent physician's order.
3. Wash your hands.
4. Gather necessary equipment.
5. Remove the medication from the drug box or tray on medication cart.
6. Compare the label on the medication bottle.
7. Place medication and lubricant on a tray if not using medication cart.
8. Check drug information to determine if appropriate for application to mucous membranes.

Procedure

1. Take medication to room.
2. Check room number against medication card or sheet.
3. Identify client by name; check identaband.
4. Explain procedure to client.
5. Provide privacy.
6. Wash your hands.

9. Instruct the client to lie quietly for 15 minutes until the suppository is absorbed.
10. Discard equipment, wash applicator, and return to appropriate place in client's room.
11. Wash your hands.
12. Return after 15 minutes to check on client.
13. Chart medication and any evidence of discharge or odor from vagina.

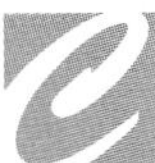

CHARTING for Suppository Medications

Client's Medical Record

- Appropriate medication form for facility
- Name of drug
- Dosage
- Times ordered
- Time administered
- Method of administration
- Initials of nurses administering drug

Nurses' Notes

- Comments made on perineal skin condition or anal area
- Results from rectal suppository

CRITICAL THINKING APPLICATION

CLINICAL PROBLEMS	CRITICAL THINKING OPTIONS
■ Client unable to retain suppositories.	• Observe if sphincter is competent. • Instruct client to maintain position for at least 15 minutes in order to allow absorption to occur. • Position on abdomen, and hold buttocks closed. • Notify physician so that an alternative route or a different medication can be tried.
■ Suppository fails to dissolve.	• Check expiration date on package and, if necessary, obtain new supply. • Instruct client to maintain appropriate position so that drug is absorbed. • Ensure that suppository has been placed in appropriate area.

unit 10 IRRIGATIONS

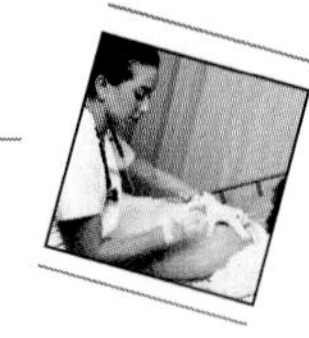

NURSING PROCESS DATA

ASSESSMENT Data Base

Identify purpose of irrigation.

Assess the area surrounding part being irrigated for signs of irritation, sloughing of tissue, and edema.

Assess area being irrigated for itching, burning, and pain.

Assess client's response to irrigating solution and irrigation.

PLANNING Objectives

To administer an irrigation using appropriate technique

To cleanse an area of excess drainage, debris, or irritating substances

To administer an antiseptic solution

To apply heat or cold

To remove foreign objects

IMPLEMENTATION Procedures

Irrigating the Eye

Irrigating the Ear

Irrigating the Throat

EVALUATION Expected Outcomes

Area being irrigated is cleansed of debris or irritating substances.

Foreign objects are removed.

Heat or cold treatments are provided.

IRRIGATING THE EYE

Equipment

2 sterile containers: 1 round bowl, 1 curved basin

Irrigating solution, 60–200 mL

Sterile 10-mL syringe or eye irrigating syringe

Sterile 4×4 gauze pad

Absorbent pad

Clean gloves

Preparation

1. Check physician's orders or client care plan.
2. Wash hands.
3. Gather equipment.
4. Warm irrigating solution to about 100°F.
5. Explain procedure to client.
6. Provide privacy if appropriate.
7. Place in Fowler's position, turned slightly to affected eye side.
8. Place absorbent pad over chest. **Rationale:** This action protects clothing from becoming wet.

Procedure

1. Open two sterile containers as with any sterile package. Place on table close to bed.
2. Pour 60–200 mL of irrigating solution into round bowl.
3. Draw up irrigating solution into syringe.
4. Have client hold curved basin on cheek under eye. **Rationale:** Basin is used to catch solution.
5. Don gloves.
6. Clean eyelids and eyelashes with moistened 4×4 gauze pad. Wipe from inner to outer canthus. **Rationale:** This method prevents contamination of opposite eye.

7. Using your thumb and forefinger, open the eye and expose lower conjunctival sac by pulling the sac down toward cheek.
8. Place the syringe over area of inner canthus pointing toward the outer canthus. Push the barrel of the syringe slowly, allowing irrigating solution to flow into the conjunctival sac.
9. Continue irrigating until eye is cleansed completely or ordered amount of solution is used. Client needs to close eyes between irrigating when large amounts of solution are used.
10. Wipe eyelid with 4×4 gauze from inner to outer canthus.
11. Place client in position of comfort.
12. Dispose of equipment in appropriate area.
13. Wash your hands.

IRRIGATING THE EAR

Equipment

Ear syringe or asepto syringe
2 sterile containers: 1 round basin, 1 curved basin
Sterile solution
Absorbent pad
Sterile cotton-tipped swabs
Sterile 4×4 gauze pad
Clean gloves

Preparation

1. Check physician's order or client care plan.
2. Wash your hands and don gloves.
3. Gather equipment.
4. Explain procedure to client.
5. Warm irrigating solution to body temperature.
6. Provide privacy if appropriate.
7. Place client in Fowler's position.
8. Place absorbent pad over shoulder. **Rationale:** This procedure protects clothing and bed linen from becoming wet.
9. Pour irrigating solution into round basin.

Procedure

1. Place curved basin under ear to catch irrigating solution.
2. Moisten cotton-tipped applicator swab with irrigating solution.
3. Clean the external structures of the ear and meatus with the moistened cotton-tipped applicator swab. Do not insert applicator into canal.
4. Fill the syringe with irrigating solution.
5. Open and straighten the canal by pulling the pinna up and backward in adults or down for infants. **Rationale:** This action allows the solution to flow into the canal.
6. Insert the irrigating syringe tip into the meatus, and as you push the plunger, direct the flow of solution toward the top of the canal. **Rationale:** This action allows the flow to reach the entire length of the canal.
7. After the solution has ceased to flow, dry the outside of the ear with a 4×4 gauze pad.
8. Position the client for comfort or on the affected side. **Rationale:** Positioning on the affected side increases the drainage of residual irrigation solution.
9. Discard equipment in appropriate area.
10. Wash your hands.

IRRIGATING THE THROAT

Equipment

Irrigation bag, tubing, catheter
Irrigation solution
Absorbent pad
Curved basin
Clean gloves

Preparation

1. Check physician's orders or client care plan.
2. Wash your hands and don gloves.
3. Gather equipment.
4. Warm irrigating solution to 100°F.
5. Explain procedure to client.
6. Provide privacy if appropriate.

7. Place in Fowler's position or position in front of the sink.
8. Place absorbent pad over chest.

Procedure

1. Establish communication system for halting the irrigation. The client can be instructed to bend the tubing to stop the flow of solution or tap you on the hand. If client can perform the irrigation him or herself, it is advisable.
2. Unclamp the tubing.
3. Direct the irrigating tip toward the throat. Move the tip slowly back and forth in the mouth to reach all areas of the throat.
4. Continue to irrigate, with interruptions as directed by the client.
5. Clamp tubing, and remove the irrigation catheter.
6. Remove equipment, and place client in bed or in position of comfort.
7. Clean equipment if to be reused or dispose of equipment in appropriate place.
8. Wash your hands.

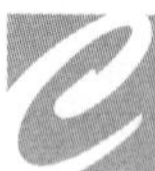

CHARTING for Irrigations

- Irrigating solution
- Amount of solution utilized
- Presence of exudate, color, odor
- Presence of edema, erythema of surrounding area
- Client's reaction to procedure

CRITICAL THINKING APPLICATION

CLINICAL PROBLEMS	CRITICAL THINKING OPTIONS
Irrigating solution runs out of ear without first reaching the canal.	• Reposition the ear to ensure the canal is open. • Point the syringe toward the top of the canal when irrigating. • Slow down the speed of the irrigation to prevent the solution from running in too quickly.
Difficulty is experienced in keeping eye open during irrigation.	• Obtain assistance from another nurse as two hands may be needed to keep eye open.
Client cannot tolerate throat irrigations.	• Allow client to do own irrigations if you have been performing them. He or she may be less apt to gag when he or she can control the flow.

GERIATRIC CONSIDERATIONS

The elderly suffer 50% of all drug side effects (estimated 17 per 100,000 population).

The elderly are at increased risk for drug toxicity.

- Renal excretion is altered—kidneys cannot process drugs as well.
- Liver enzymes are altered.
- Liver has diminished blood circulation.
- Client may be receiving multiple drugs that compete for binding and interact with one another.
- CNS is more sensitive to drugs—drugs may interfere with neurotransmitters that regulate brain function.
- Altered body mass and ratio of fat to muscle affects assimilation.

The most commonly abused drugs by the elderly

- Tranquilizers—most frequently abused
- Sleeping pills
- Medications to control pain
- Laxatives

The major problems with prescriptive drugs in the elderly

- Drug interactions—many seniors use multiple physicians and pharmacies, creating risk of drugs that interact thereby causing adverse reactions.
- Medication errors—the more medications a person takes the greater risk of medication error (people over age 75 take an average of 17 prescriptions annually).
- Noncompliance—not taking right dose at right time or discontinuing drug without consultation; common due to lack of understanding about reason to take drug and general knowledge base of drug action.
- Unpredictable drug action—physiologic changes in the elderly associated with age and disease may alter effects of the drugs.
- Drug side effects not recognized—elderly not aware or do not understand potential dangerous side effects of drugs.
- Inadequate monitoring—elderly often alone or not monitored consistently, so drug problems are not identified.
- Cost of drugs—multiple medications are costly for many elderly, so they stop taking drugs.

DRUG SUPPLEMENT

CALCULATIONS OF SOLUTIONS

Types of Solutions

1. Volume to volume (vol/vol): a given volume of solute is added to a given volume of solvent.
2. Weight to weight (wt/wt): a stated weight of solute is dissolved in a stated weight of solvent.
3. Weight to volume (wt/vol): a given weight of solute is dissolved in a given volume of solvent, which results in the proper amount of solution.

Preparing Solutions

- Liquid to Drug Solutions

  Determine the strength of the solution, the strength of the drug on hand, and the quantity of solution required.

  Use this formula for preparing solutions:

$$\frac{D}{H} \times Q = X$$

where D = desired strength; H = strength on hand; Q = quantity of solution desired; and X = amount of solute.

Example: You have a 100% solution of hydrogen peroxide on hand. You need a liter of 50% solution.

$$\frac{50}{100} \times 1000 \text{ mL} = 500 \text{ mL}$$

If the strength desired and strength on hand are not in like terms, you need to change one of the terms.

Example: You have 1 L of 50% solution on hand. You need a liter of 1:10 solution. 1:10 solution is the same as 10%.

$$\frac{10\%}{50\%} \times 1000 \text{ mL} = 200 \text{ mL}$$

Add 200 mL of the drug to 800 mL of the solvent to make a liter of 10% solution.

- Volume to Volume Solutions

  Use the formula:

$$\frac{D}{H} \times Q = X$$

Example: Prepare a liter of 5% solution from a stock solution of 50%.

$$\frac{5\%}{50\%} \times 1000 \text{ mL} = 100 \text{ mL}$$

Add 100 mL to 900 mL of diluent to make 1 L of 5% solution.

- Solutions from Tablets

  Use the formula:

$$\frac{D}{H} \times Q = X$$

where X = amount per number of tablets used.

Example: Prepare 1 L of a 1:1000 solution, using 10-gr tablets.

$$\frac{1/1000}{10 \text{ gr}} \times 1000 \text{ mL} = X$$

First convert 10 gr to grams so the numerator and denominator are in the same unit of measure. 1 g = 15 gr; therefore 10 gr = $\frac{2}{3}$ g. Now substitute the new numbers in the formula and solve for X.

$$\frac{1/1000}{2/3} \times \frac{1000}{1} \text{ mL} = X$$

$$\frac{3}{2000} \times \frac{1000}{1} = X$$

$$X = \tfrac{3}{2}, \text{ or } 1\tfrac{1}{2} \text{ tablets}$$

Place $1\frac{1}{2}$ tablets into the liter of solution and dissolve.

APPENDIX 16–1. Abbreviations and Symbols for Orders, Prescriptions, and Labels

aa	of each	p.c.	after meals
a.c.	before meals	per	by, through
ad lib.	freely, as desired	p.r.n.	whenever necessary
b.i.d.	twice each day	q.d.	every day
$\bar{c}$	with	q.h.	every hour
C	carbon	q.i.d.	four times each day
Ca	calcium	q.s.	as much as required, quantity sufficient
Cl	chlorine		
dr *or* ʒ	dram	q2h	every 2 hours
et	and	q3h	every 3 hours
GI	gastrointestinal	q4h	every 4 hours
gt *or* gtt	drop(s)	R_x	treatment, "take thou"
H_2O	water	$\bar{s}$	without
H_2O_2	hydrogen peroxide	$\overline{ss}$	one-half
IM	intramuscular	stat	immediately
in.	inch	t.i.d.	three times each day
K	potassium	tsp	teaspoon
lb *or* #	pound	WBC	white blood count
m	minimum (a minimum)	°	degree
Mg	magnesium	−	minus, negative, alkaline reaction
N	nitrogen, normal	+	plus, positive, acid reaction
Na	sodium	%	percent
n.p.o.	nothing by mouth	v	Roman numeral 5
oob	out of bed	vii	Roman numeral 7
os	mouth	ix	Roman numeral 9
oz *or* ℥	ounce	xiii	Roman numeral 13

APPENDIX 16–2. Conversion Tables

TABLE A. Household Equivalents (Volume)

Metric	Apothecary	Household
0.06 mL	1 minim	1 drop
5(4) mL	1 fluid dram	1 teaspoonful
15 mL	4 fluid drams	1 tablespoonful
30 mL	1 fluid ounce	2 tablespoonfuls
180 mL	6 fluid ounces	1 teacupful
240 mL	8 fluid ounces	1 glassful

TABLE B. Apothecary Equivalent (Volume)

Metric		Apothecary
1 mL	=	15 minims
1 cc	=	15 minims
0.06 mL	=	1 minim
4 mL	=	1 fluid dram
30 mL	=	1 fluid ounce
500 mL	=	1 pint
1000 mL (1 L)	=	1 quart

TABLE C. Apothecary Equivalents (Weight)

Metric		Apothecary		
1.0 g	*or*	1000 mg	=	gr xv
0.6 g	*or*	600 mg	=	gr x
0.5 g	*or*	500 mg	=	gr viiss
0.3 g	*or*	300 mg	=	gr v
0.2 g	*or*	200 mg	=	gr iii
0.1 g	*or*	100 mg	=	gr $1\frac{1}{2}$
0.06 g	*or*	60 mg	=	gr 1
0.05 g	*or*	50 mg	=	gr $\frac{3}{4}$
0.03 g	*or*	30 mg	=	gr $\frac{1}{2}$
0.015 g	*or*	15 mg	=	gr $\frac{1}{4}$
0.010 g	*or*	10 mg	=	gr $\frac{1}{6}$
0.008 g	*or*	8 mg	=	gr $\frac{1}{8}$
4 g			=	1 dr
30 g			=	1 oz
1 kg			=	2.2 lbs

17

Pain Management

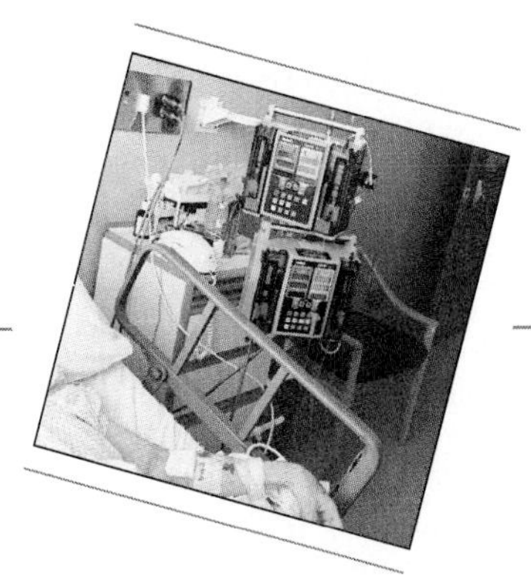

LEARNING OBJECTIVES

- Discuss what is meant by the experience of pain.
- Explain the use of endorphins for pain control.
- Describe the body's physiologic response to pain.
- Identify the most important information elicited from the client regarding pain.
- Discuss what it means for the nurse to be the client's advocate in relation to pain control.
- Discuss the gate control theory.
- Outline the main points of one noninvasive method of relieving pain.
- Describe a pain scale.
- Describe the pain relief method known as TENS.
- Discuss two advantages of epidural narcotic analgesia.
- List three criteria for client selection for PCA.
- Explain what is meant by establishing the client control mode.
- Describe the steps of teaching PCA to a client.

TERMINOLOGY

Acupressure: Chinese method of treatment that involves compression of certain areas of the body by following a system of meridians or energy flow.

Adaptive reaction: a response by which the person attempts to improve or alter his or her condition in relation to the environment.

Alleviate: to make more bearable; reduce (pain, grief, or suffering).

Angina: a sense of suffocation with symptoms of severe, steady pain and feeling of pressure in region of the heart.

Arrhythmia: irregular rhythm.

Arthritis: inflammation of a joint, usually accompanied by pain and frequently, deformity.

Autogenic training: a method of deep muscle relaxation that enables one to reduce the stress response, regain homeostasis, and prepare to handle additional stress.

Autoimmunization: immunity produced by an attack of the disease or by processes occurring within the body.

Autonomic nervous system: the part of the nervous system that regulates the functioning of internal organs and glands; it controls such functions as digestion, respiration, and cardiovascular activity.

Behavior: the manner in which one acts.

Biofeedback: a training technique that uses monitoring instruments to assist people to control stress-related disorders through self-regulation of internal functions.

Booster dose: an additional dose given to a client on a p.r.n. basis. Ordered by physician, administered by RN.

Brady: prefix indicating slow.

Bradycardia: slowed heart action, below 60 BPM.

Cardio: prefix pertaining to the heart.

Cardiovascular: pertaining to the heart and blood vessels.

Cerebral cortex: the extensive outer layer of gray tissue of the cerebral hemispheres (brain), responsible for higher nervous functions.

Coping mechanisms: means by which an individual adjusts or adapts to a threat or a challenge; actions that assist in maintaining homeostasis.

Diaphoresis: profuse sweating.

Dynamics of homeostasis: danger or its symbols, whether internal or external, resulting in the activation of the sympathetic nervous system and the adrenal medulla. The organism prepares for fight or flight.

Emotional: affected by strong feelings, as of joy and sorrow.

Endorphins: a naturally occurring body chemical similar to morphine but many times stronger.

Fight or flight: one's immediate response to stress that is, although archaic and often inappropriate, part of our central nervous system biologic heritage.

Four (4)-hour limit (mL): the maximum amount of drug that can be administered to client during a 4-hour period.

Gastro: term that denotes the stomach.

Gastrointestinal: pertaining to the stomach and the intestine.

General adaptation syndrome: a general theory of stress response formulated by Dr. Hans Selye; describes the action of stress response in three stages: the alarm reaction, the stage of resistance, and the stage of exhaustion.

-Genic: suffix indicating generation or production.

Health: the state of physical, psychologic, and sociologic well-being.

Hypertension: a condition in which the client has a higher blood pressure than judged to be normal.

Illness: a state characterized by the malfunction of the biopsychosocial organism.

Insomnia: inability to sleep.

Ischemic: local and temporary anemia due to obstruction of the circulation to a part.

Loading dose (optional): initial dose given to client as ordered by physician.

Lockout interval: period during which the PCA cannot be activated and no analgesic can be delivered by client. (A booster dose can be given during lockout interval if ordered.)

Meditation: the act of reflecting on or pondering; contemplation.

Musculo: pertaining to the muscles.

Musculoskeletal: pertaining to the muscles and the skeleton.

Nausea: inclination to vomit, usually preceding emesis.

Neuro: prefix pertaining to nerves.

Pain: a sensation in which a person experiences discomfort, distress, or suffering.

Parasympathetic nervous system: a division of the autonomic nervous system that regulates acetylcholine and conserves energy expenditure; it slows down the system.

PCA—Patient-Controlled Analgesia: a method of delivering pain medication via IV pump. Within physician-ordered parameters, the client can control the medication amount necessary to manage his or her pain level.

Physiologic: concerning body function.

Psychogenic: of mental origin.

Referred pain: pain felt in a part removed from its point of origin.

Regression: a turning back or return to a former state.

Relaxation: a lessening of tension or activity in a part.

Resistance: opposition to or the ability to oppose.

Rheumatism: a term applied to conditions of acute and chronic, characterized by soreness and stiffness of muscles and pain in joints.

Stamina: constitutional energy; strength; endurance.

Stress: a nonspecific response of the body to any internal or external event or change that impinges on a person's system and creates a demand.

Stressor: a specific demand that gives rise to a coping response.

Sympathetic nervous system: a division of the autonomic nervous system that controls energy expenditure and mobilizes for action when confronted with a threat.

Tachy: prefix meaning fast.

Tachycardia: abnormal rapidity of heart action; above 100 BPM.

TENS—Transcutaneous Electrical Nerve Stimulator: a noninvasive method to relieve pain that involves stimulation to the skin via a mild electric current.

Touch: a tactile sense.

Visceral: pertaining to internal organs.

Wellness: a state of physical, psychologic, and sociologic well-being of a whole person.

COPING WITH PAIN

The experience of pain is direct and personal. In this culture we tend to view pain as a negative condition and often go to any lengths to avoid the sensation. The positive aspect of pain is that it is an early warning system; its presence triggers an awareness that something is wrong in the body. Without the sensation of pain we could not survive, because pain provides the cues that allow us to modify our reactions and direct our behavior. One perspective of pain is that it is a message to our conscious self to check out any pain sensation before it gets worse, for that is the nature of pain. Without intervention the condition may well get worse.

Margo McCaffery, a nurse–author who writes about caring for the client in pain, defines pain as "whatever the patient experiencing pain says it is, existing whenever he says it does." The nurse is totally dependent on the client to describe the sensation of pain, identify the location, and tell about what kind of pain is being experienced.

The most important information in pain assessment, then, is the client's report. The pain experience is totally subjective. The onset of acute pain stimulates the sympathetic nervous system "fight or flight" response that results in certain signs or symptoms. While observation of these symptoms provides objective data, it cannot be considered conclusive evidence to the identification of pain—that must come from the client.

The sensation of physical pain arouses some specific responses in the client. The sympathetic nervous system response is usually stimulated by superficial pain, and the parasympathetic nervous system response is usually stimulated by deeper pain and results in the slowing down of all the systems to conserve energy.

Theories of Pain

The neurophysiologic basis of pain can be explained by several theories, none of which is mutually exclusive nor totally comprehensive.

Specificity Theory. This theory suggests that certain pain receptors are stimulated by a specific type of sensory stimuli that sends impulses to the brain. This theory dealt with the physiologic basis for pain but did not take into account the psychologic components of pain, nor the degree of pain tolerance.

Pattern Theory. This theory attempts to include factors that were not adequately explained by the specificity theory. This theory suggests that pain originates in the dorsal horn of the spinal cord. A certain pattern of nerve impulses is produced and results in intense receptor stimulation that is coded in the CNS and signifies pain. Like the specificity theory, the pattern theory does not explain the psychologic factors of pain.

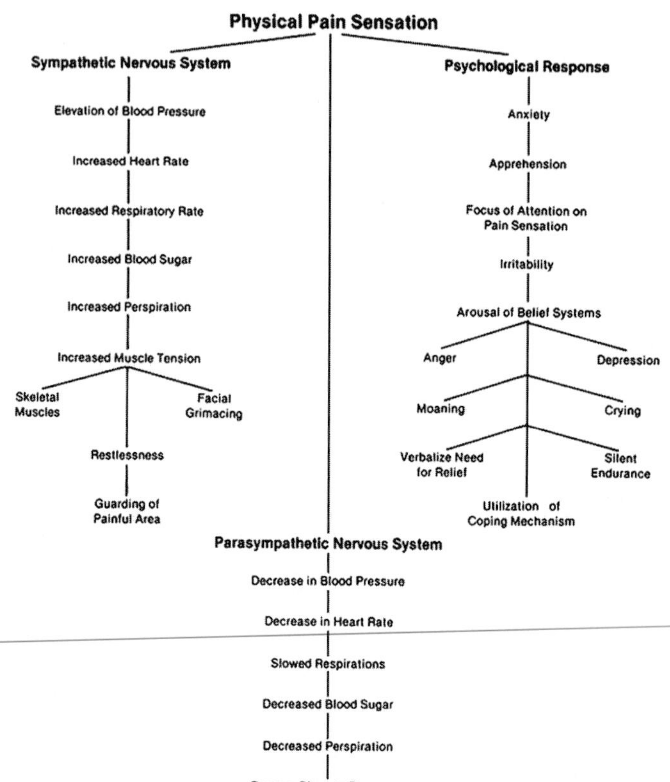

Physical Pain Sensation.

Gate Control Theory. One of the most popular and credible concepts is the gate control theory. The first premise of the gate control theory is that the actual existence and intensity of the pain experience depends on the particular transmission of neurologic impulses. Secondly, gate mechanisms along the nervous system control the transmission of pain. Finally, if the gate is open, the impulses that result in the sensation of pain are able to reach the conscious level. If the gate is closed, the impulses do not reach the level of consciousness and the sensation of pain is not experienced.

Three primary types of neurologic involvement affect whether the gate is open or closed. The first type involves activity in the large and small nerve fibers that affect the sensation of pain. Pain impulses travel along small-diameter fibers. The large-diameter nerve fibers close the gate to the impulses that travel along the small fibers. The technique of using cutaneous stimulation on the skin, which has many large-diameter fibers, may help to close the gate to the transmission of painful impulses, thereby relieving the sensation of pain. Interventions that apply this theory to practice include massage, hot and cold applications, touch, acupressure, and transcutaneous electric nerve stimulation. These interventions are described in detail later in this chapter.

The second form of neurologic involvement is the impulses from the brainstem that affect the sensation of pain. The reticular formation monitors in the brainstem regulate sensory input. If the person receives adequate or excessive amounts of sensory stimulation, the brainstem transmits impulses that close the gate and inhibit pain impulses from being transmitted. If on the other hand, the client experiences a lack of sensory input, the brainstem does not inhibit the pain impulses, the gate is open, and the pain impulses are transmitted. Interventions that apply to this part of the gate control theory are those related in some way to sensory input, such as techniques of distraction, guided imagery, and visualization.

The third type of neurologic involvement is the neurologic activities or impulses in the cerebral cortex and thalamus. A person's thoughts, emotions, and memories may activate certain impulses in the cortex that trigger pain impulses, which are transmitted to the conscious level. Past experiences relating to pain affect how the client responds to current pain. For this reason, it is important to explore the client's previous experiences and teach the client what to expect from the present situation. Interventions that apply to this part of the gate control theory include using and teaching various relaxation techniques, teaching the client about what expectations to have about pain as related to a specific illness, allowing the client to feel he or she has some control over the taking of medication for pain relief, and giving medications properly (i.e., preventively, before the pain is so severe that the client fears he or she will receive no relief).

The Discovery of Endorphins

A relatively recent theory of pain relief was developed when Avron Goldstein, looking for morphine and heroin receptors, discovered that receptors in the brain fit only morphine or morphine-like molecules. He asked himself why these receptors were located in the brain, when opiates are not naturally found in this area. The answer, learned through diligent research, is that the brain produces natural brain opiates. These substances are hormones, chemicals produced by different parts of the body to regulate certain biologic processes. At present, five of these natural opiates have been found. Three are called endorphins, one dynorphin, and one enkephalin. Endorphins fit into special cells, called receptors, and thereby activate their regulating powers. In addition to endorphin "keys" and receptor "locks," researchers have found antilocks, called antagonists, that keep endorphins from working. Endorphin receptors and antilocks have been found throughout the body—in the stomach, intestines, pancreas, spinal cord, and bloodstream, as well as the brain.

A beta-endorphin is 50 times stronger than morphine, and a dynorphin is 190 times stronger than morphine. In one test, 14 men and women suffering from extreme pain from cancer were given tiny injections of an endorphin. *All* felt relief within minutes, and the relief lasted for 1 to 3 days.

Endorphins are now being produced synthetically, but they are very expensive and at this time are used only for research. Researchers must discover how the body makes and releases endorphins before a method is developed to encourage the body to produce more of its own endorphins to control pain.

The Pain Experience

The pain experience is a mixture of physical sensations, physiologic changes, and psychosocial factors. The client's interpretation of the physical sensation is influenced by the client's culture, previous experiences with and without pain, beliefs about self, interpretation of the future, present environment, and the persons in that environment. The intensity of pain is influenced by

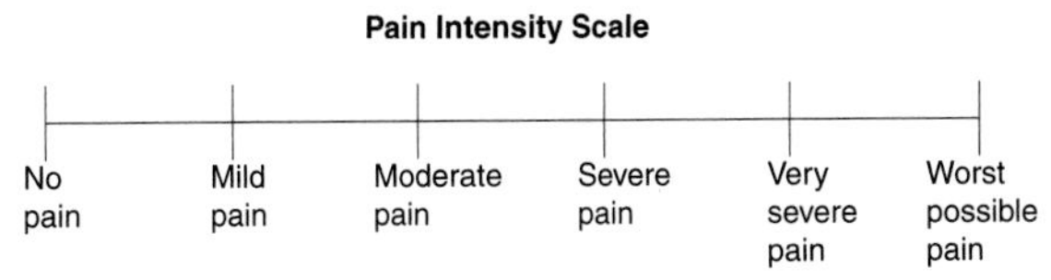

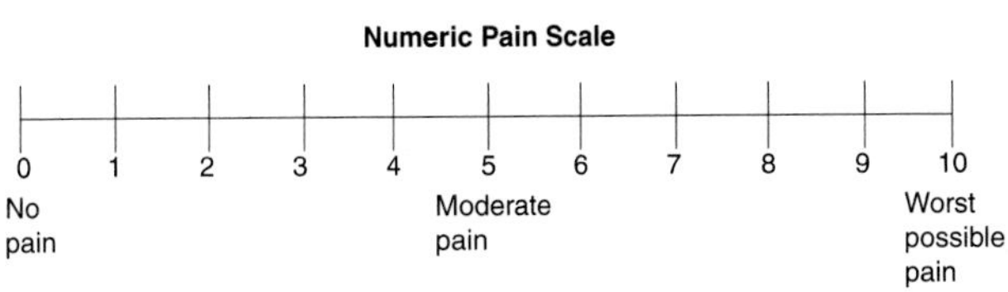

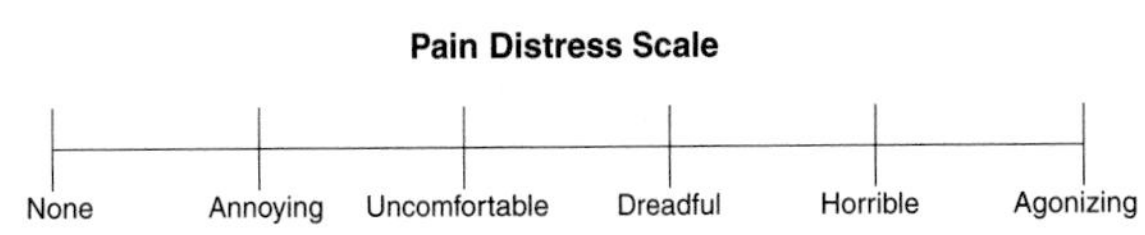

Examples of pain scales. Acute Pain Management: *Operative or medical procedures and trauma.* US Department of Health and Human Services, Public Health Service, pp. 116–117.

what the sensation means to the client, the client's level of anxiety, degree of fatigue, and the number of stressors in the client's environment.

There are several methods of assessing the degree or level of pain a client may be experiencing. Following are examples of scales you may use to assess your client's pain. After explaining the scale you are using, ask your client what level of pain he or she is experiencing at the moment. You may use a scale of 1 to 10, an intensity scale, or a pain distress scale. Whichever scale is chosen, maintain its use throughout the course of pain control.

CHARACTERISTICS OF PAIN

Location

- Area of the body
- Diffuse or localized
- Radiates and area involved

Quality

- Stabbing, knife-like
- Throbbing
- Cramping
- Vise-like, suffocating
- Searing, burning
- Superficial, deep

Intensity

- Rate on scale: 0–10 (0 = no pain, 10 = most pain ever experienced)

Factors Associated with Pain

- Nausea
- Vomiting
- Bradycardia, tachycardia
- Hypotension, hypertension
- Profuse perspiration
- Apprehension or anxiety

Precipitating Factors

- Motion affecting incision area (e.g., coughing, turning, deep breathing)
- Fear and emotional distress
- Inflammation or infection
- Trauma
- Disease state

Aggravating Factors

- Position changes
- Environmental stressors
- Fatigue
- Inadequate pain relief measures

Alleviating Factors

- Position change
- Medications
- Biofeedback
- Visualization
- Relaxation techniques
- TENS
- Massage

Pain Pathways

The pathway to pain is a complicated, fascinating expression of how our amazing bodies work. First there is the source of pain, a direct causative factor. Stimulation of a pain receptor may be mechanical, chemical, thermal, electric, or ischemic. The sensation travels along the sensory pathways and ascends the spinal cord to the thalamus. The autonomic nervous system is activated, and sensations travel to the sensory area of the cerebral cortex. Pain reception occurs in the thalamus, where awareness and integration take place, and pain interpretation occurs in the cerebral cortex. Once awareness of pain takes place and it has been interpreted by the cerebral cortex, the person becomes aware and the response patterns are activated.

NONINVASIVE PAIN RELIEF

When a method to relieve pain is noninvasive, it is both safer and results in less potential side effects for the client. Such measures will probably become the pain control choice of the future.

Current practice for controlling pain is to use both drugs and nondrug options because both, separately or combined, meet the objectives of relieving pain and making the client more comfortable.

Nondrug options may include the use of specific cognitive–behavioral techniques—deep breathing, visualization, imagery; physical agents—electric stimulators, massage-vibration, and biofeedback systems; and various adjunct therapies—cold therapy, heat therapy, or counterirritants.

The nonpharmacologic approach (Table 17–1) is appropriate for clients who are receptive to alternative methods; who have a high level of anxiety around the issue of pain; who would benefit from reducing dependence on drug therapy; who anticipate long-term or have chronic pain; or who receive inadequate pain relief from pharmacologic interventions.

The Nurse's Role

Pain reduction methods include a wide range of techniques and medications. Rarely is pain relief successfully achieved with only one method. Even massive doses of narcotics do not always control pain effectively—especially when it has been allowed to escalate.

One of the most important influences on pain relief is the relationship that exists between nurse and client. With most methods (the exception is PCA), the nurse has the power to relieve pain or to withhold pain relief. This knowledge creates anticipatory anxiety for the client. The client may request less medication when the nurse is supportive, caring, and assists with pain management.

The single most critical factor in achieving pain relief is for the nurse to be the client's advocate. This means that the nurse

- Listens to and believes clients when they describe the level of pain they are experiencing.
- Intervenes or administers the pain medication when it is needed.
- Does not allow the pain to escalate but anticipates when it is needed.
- Works with the client to control the pain and requests different medications or dosages from the physician when needed.
- Is not concerned about addiction when administering pain medication. (The incidence of opioid addiction in hospitalized clients is less than 1%.)

Nursing interventions that provide effective pain relief, in addition to pain medication, are those that encourage behaviors that assist the client not to focus on pain. For example, when the client is talking about something of great interest or pleasure, he or she is not thinking about pain. Teaching the client techniques,

TABLE 17–1. Nonpharmacologic Approaches to Pain

Physical Methods	Advantages
TENS—stimulating skin with mild electric current	Noninvasive method Higher level of activity Studies show more effective for postoperative pain Gives staff confidence they can assist client with pain Choice for chronic pain
Acupuncture—ancient Chinese form of treating diseases through insertion and manipulation of needles at specific points on the body	Insertion of thin needles is not painful to the client Pain relieving capacity extends beyond actual procedure Method may provide relief when no other method works
Biofeedback—electric monitoring device that feeds back effect of behavior so client can control internal processes (e.g., heartbeat)	Noninvasive method Completely controlled by client Promotes stress reduction as well as pain relief After mastery, instruments are not needed to achieve result
Vibration or massage—hands-on manipulation of muscles or electrical from of massage (vibration)	Noninvasive method—electrically alleviates pain by numbness or paresthesia or through touch Increases circulation and endorphins to area Relaxes muscles and reduces tension on nerves and promotes relaxation Useful only for light to moderate pain
Cold therapy—cold wraps, gel packs, cold therapy, ice massage	Relieves pain faster than heat therapy Numbs nerves and decreases inflammation and spasms Effective for nerve, abdominal, and lower back pain Alters pain threshold Decreases tissue injury response
Heat therapy—hot wraps, dry heat, moist heat	Noninvasive method Decreases pain by reducing inflammation Promotes relaxation of muscles Increases vasodilation and blood flow to area Facilitates clearance of tissue toxins and fluids
Counterirritants—mentholated ointments or lotions (Ben-Gay or Icy Hot)	May contain salicylates (reduces inflammation) but dangerous if client has potential bleeding problems May be irritating to the skin—potential skin breakdown
Acupressure application—based on the ancient Chinese method of acupuncture, this method involves using specific points located on meridians at various places on the body	Noninvasive method Redirection of energy flow through pressure on meridian points Reduces pain and increases endorphins
Cognitive–Behavioral Methods	**Advantage**
Relaxation—body relaxation of muscles used with imagery, music, or breathing. Techniques from books, tapes, and therapist instruction	Relaxes tense muscles and reduces stress Effective in reducing pain Easy to learn and implement techniques for self-mastery Reduces fear and anxiety connected to pain
Imagery—visualization technique of forming sensory images, or seeing in the "mind's eye" an image that distracts from the sensation of pain	Effective in reducing pain Client can control use and timing of technique Reduces high-level anxiety connected to pain
Deep breathing—techniques using breath to control pain	Effective in reinforcing body relaxation and visualization Reduces pain through breath control; increases oxygen utilization
Hypnosis—creating a state of altered consciousness so that client is susceptible to instruction	Effective with a client who is suggestive and who experiences tension and anxiety accompanying pain

such as deep, slow breathing and relaxation, lessens pain, whereas muscle tension and anxiety increase it. If the nurse teaches pain relief techniques before surgery, the client can more easily implement them when the pain is intense. The nurse may also encourage the client to use techniques that he or she has already found effective, no matter how "unscientific" they may be. Whatever method or technique the nurse uses to assist the client with relieving pain, the single most critical intervention is a caring and supportive attitude.

TECHNIQUES FOR PAIN CONTROL

Patient-Controlled Analgesia (PCA)

One of the most successful methods of pain relief to be introduced in the last few years is patient-controlled analgesia (PCA). The primary purpose of PCA is to allow the client to self-administer an analgesic dose of medication predetermined by the physician. PCA enables the client to assess and control his or her own pain level. This method of pain control has been found to be very efficacious because the client feels in more control of his or her life situation, there is no significant difference in the amount of analgesic medication used (if anything, it is usually less), and this method of pain control is less time-consuming for the nurse.

Epidural Pain Control

A new technique for controlling pain with the use of an epidural catheter is rapidly becoming the method of choice for controlling pain following surgery. The advantage of epidural pain control is that the narcotic moves directly from the epidural space into the spinal fluid and binds with opiate receptors in the spinal cord, blocking reception of pain. Administered by this method, the required drug dose is considerably lower because it is not metabolized in the liver.

Direct IV Pain Control

In addition to the new methods of pain control, a client may receive a continuous infusion via direct IV. The dosage may be titrated to achieve pain relief with the lowest dose (10 mg or $\frac{1}{6}$ gr of morphine sulfate). The dose is individualized according to the client's needs, tolerance, and response. When pain relief is not achieved, increments of at least 25% of the previous dose should be implemented. When morphine is administered IV, a dark bag should be placed over the narcotic bag because the medication is light-sensitive.

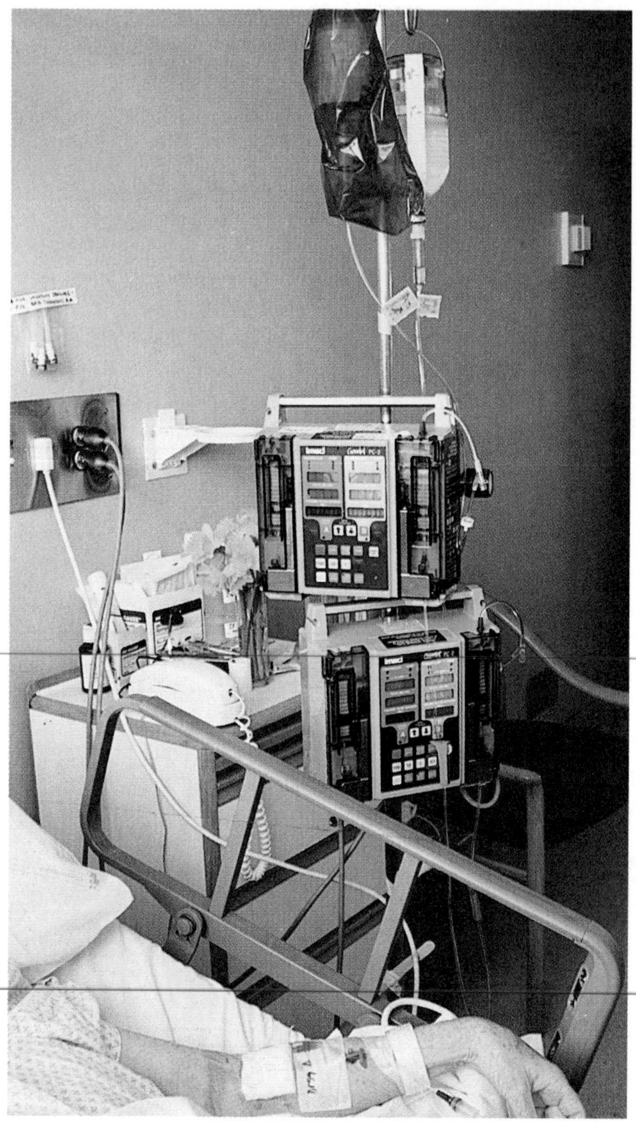

Continuous IV narcotic drip for pain control.

NURSING DIAGNOSES

The following nursing diagnoses may be appropriate to include in a client care plan when the components are related to alleviating pain in a client.

NURSING DIAGNOSIS	RELATED FACTORS
Anxiety	Anticipation of discomfort, fear, helplessness, inability to relax
Fear	Long-term disability, terminal disease, hospitalization, invasive procedures, lack of knowledge, surgery and its outcome
Pain	Trauma, immobility, surgery, chronic illness

unit 1

PAIN RELIEF

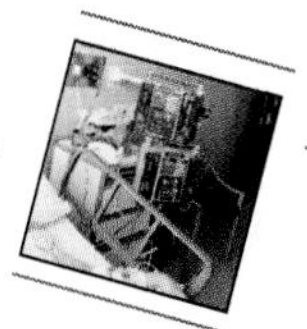

NURSING PROCESS DATA

ASSESSMENT **Data Base**

Assess type of pain.

Acute pain: short duration of a few seconds to 6 months

Chronic pain: longer duration of 6 months to years

Intractable pain: severe and constant and resistant to relief measures

Assess nonverbal indications of pain.

Assess client's behavioral responses to pain.

Depression, withdrawal, or crying

Stoicism or expressive

Assess location, quality, intensity, onset, aggravating factors, associated factors, and alleviating factors. (See Physical Pain Sensation chart)

PLANNING **Objectives**

To prevent pain from retarding recovery

To prevent pain from causing nausea and vomiting, a decrease in fluid intake which results in fluid and electrolyte imbalance

To prevent pain from causing undue fatigue

To prevent pain from inhibiting moving, ambulating, turning, and coughing; pain increases the possibilities of secondary problems from inactivity (e.g., pneumonia, emboli)

To relieve pain or prevent pain from escalating by relaxing muscles; muscle tension increases the pain

To decrease client's anxiety that present and future pain relief will not be achieved

To bring pain relief to a level acceptable to the client

To educate clients to communicate their pain level

IMPLEMENTATION **Procedures**

Alleviating Pain through Touch

Using Relaxation Techniques

Using Transcutaneous Electric Nerve Stimulation (TENS)

Administering Epidural Narcotic Analgesia

for Bolus Injection

for Continuous Infusion

EVALUATION **Expected Outcomes**

Pain is controlled to the client's satisfaction.

Pain is relieved and does not interfere with ambulation or sitting in a chair.

Client is free from nausea and vomiting due to pain.

Client's anxiety level is low.

ALLEVIATING PAIN THROUGH TOUCH

Equipment

Cream or talcum powder
Massage oil

Procedure

1. Determine whether client achieves more relief from pain with massage over painful area, near painful area, or from foot rub, back rub, or hand rub.
2. Warm your hands by rubbing them together or rinsing in warm water.
3. Warm lotion to be used by holding closed bottle under warm running water.
4. Massage area of client's choice with slow and steady motion.
5. Use deep pressure or light stroking motion, whichever is more comfortable for the client. **Rationale:** Relaxed muscles result in a decreased pain level.

USING RELAXATION TECHNIQUES

Equipment

A printed relaxation technique (the nurse can read slowly until client learns technique)
A cassette recorder and tape

Procedure

1. Help client assume a comfortable position.
   a. If lying, place support under knees, lower legs, and under head. Be sure body is in good alignment.
   b. If sitting, sit comfortably positioned with both feet on the floor, hands on knees, back straight, and head balanced comfortably straight.
2. Instruct client to inhale deeply, hold breath for a moment, then exhale deeply. Repeat several times.
3. Give the following instructions to client, using a slow, soothing voice.
   a. Continue to breathe in and out slowly. Concentrate on my voice and follow my words.
   b. Find a point of tension in your body.
   c. As you identify the tension, tense the area up even more.
   d. Then relax the area, letting all the tension drain out.
4. Continue with these instructions until the client has had time to relax all points of tension.
5. To end the process, instruct the client to open eyes slowly and say, "I feel relaxed and awake."

USING TRANSCUTANEOUS ELECTRIC NERVE STIMULATION (TENS)

Equipment

Cutaneous stimulator with lead wires and leads
Cream for lead placement

Procedure

1. Obtain physician's order (may be intermittent or continuous).
2. Follow directions for electrode placement. (Check electrode placement chart provided by manufacturer of TENS unit.)
   a. Place electrode on skin over or near the area of pain.
   b. Identify trigger points (specific points that are extremely sensitive when stimulated), and place electrode.
   c. Identify acupressure point, and place electrode.
   d. Place electrode on peripheral nerves, enervating area of pain. (Client adjusts each pair of electrodes to produce a sensation that is pleasant and to relieve pain.)
3. Apply electrodes.
   a. Some electrodes are water conductive: moisten with water.

b. Some electrodes require a conductive gel: place gel on electrode before attaching to skin.

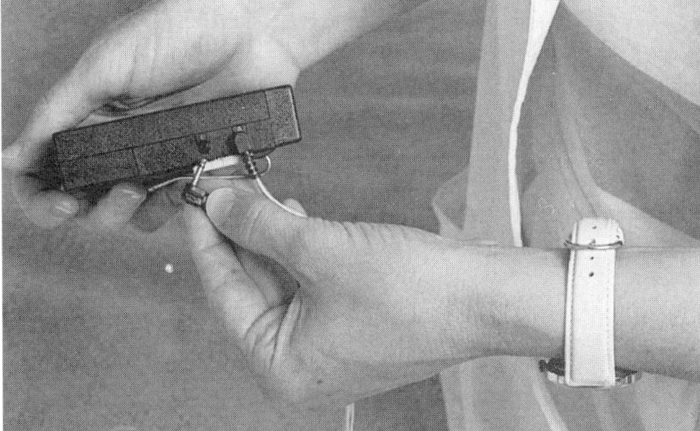

Plug TENS electrodes into unit, following directions.

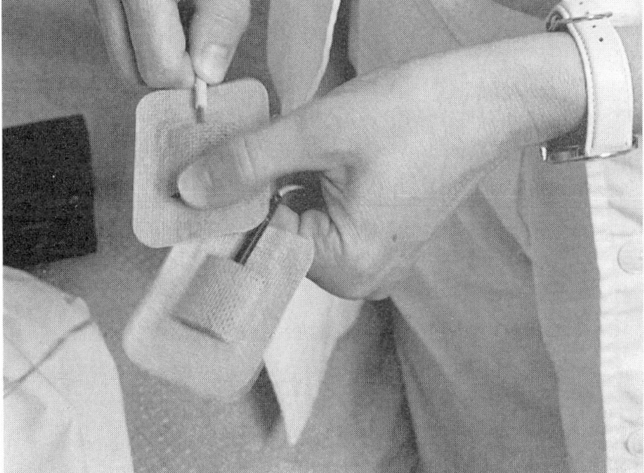

Insert TENS probe into pad before placing pad on skin.

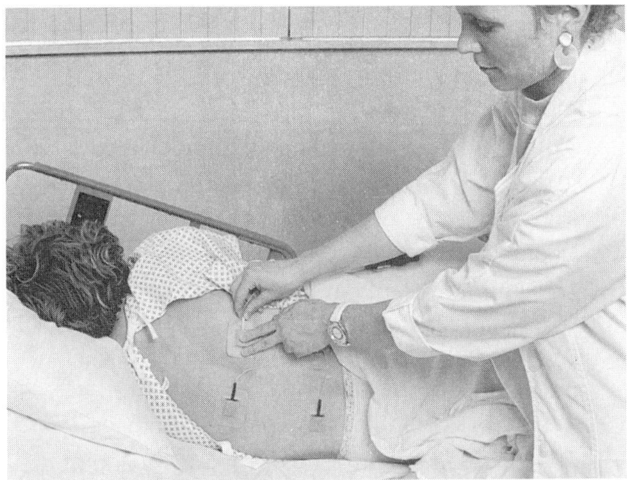

Position pads on skin around painful areas.

4. Instruct client to adjust intensity of skin stimulation until it creates a pleasant sensation that relieves the pain.

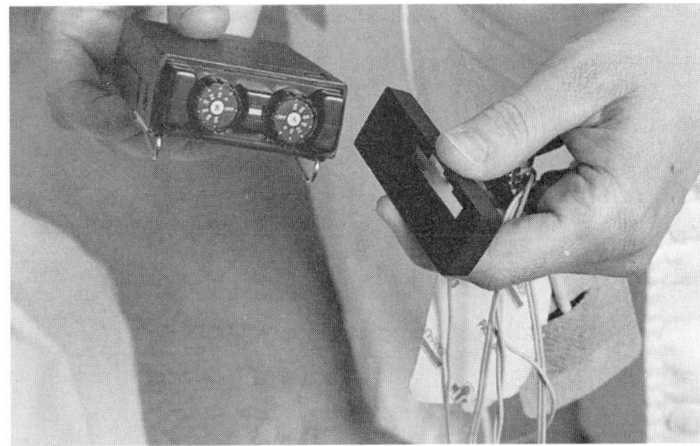

Set dials on top of unit to control pulse rate and width.

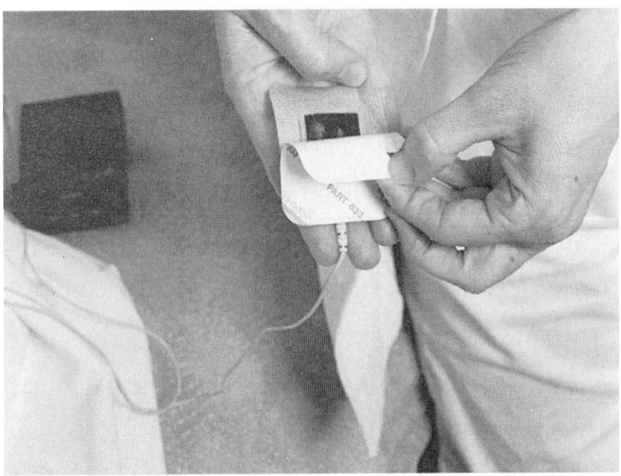

Peel backing from pad so that pad will adhere to skin.

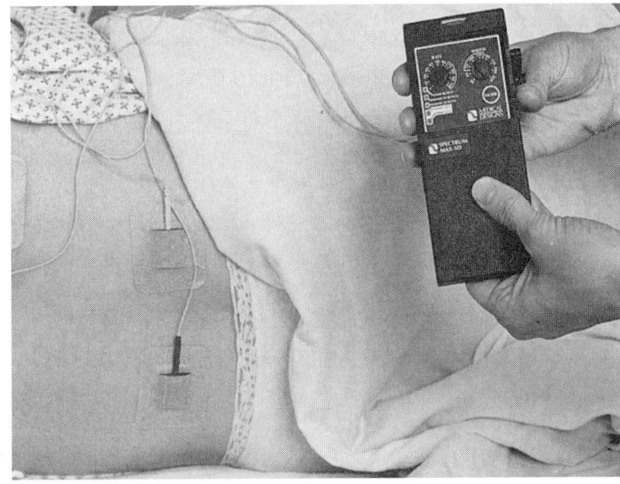

Turn on machine and instruct client to adjust level.

ADMINISTERING EPIDURAL NARCOTIC ANALGESIA*

*Many hospitals require specific certification before the RN can administer narcotics via an indwelling epidural catheter. A student nurse *should not* administer solutions via epidural catheter.

Equipment

Labels for safety precautions:
- At head of bed: "Epidural Protocol Client"
- At end of catheter: "Epidural Catheter"

3-mL syringe and ampule of naloxone hydrochloride (Narcan: 0.4 mg) as ordered at bedside
Ambu bag at bedside
Respiratory record, apnea monitor, or pulse oximeter
Sterile gloves
Tape

for Bolus Injection
- Prediluted preservative-free narcotic as ordered
- 12-mL syringe with filter needle
- 20-gauge 1-inch needle
- Povidone-iodine swabs
- Sterile 2 × 2 gauze

for Continuous Infusion
- Infusion pump
- IV tubing
- Prediluted preservative-free narcotic container

Preparation

1. Check physician's orders for epidural narcotic indicating minimum and maximum dosage.
   a. Preservative-free narcotic and dose; preservative-free saline and amount
   b. Interval between doses
   c. Infusion rate and concentration, if appropriate
2. Check that safety sign is over bed "Epidural Protocol Client." **Rationale:** Identifies client to all staff as having epidural tubing.
3. Check that catheter is labeled "Epidural catheter." **Rationale:** Identifies catheter and avoids confusing epidural catheter with IV tubing.
4. Check that a Narcan ampule and 3-mL syringe are at bedside. **Rationale:** Respiratory depression can be treated with IV Narcan, a narcotic antagonist.

> **■ CLINICAL ALERT**
>
> Place IV line as far as possible from an epidural catheter and label epidural catheter to avoid mistaking it for IV catheter—this could be a *fatal* mistake. Some catheters are specifically labeled. For example, the DuPen permanent epidural catheter has a yellow band near the Luer-Lok tip that has a sign "Epidural catheter–not an IV access."

5. Check that there is IV access for administration of Narcan. **Rationale:** Necessary to quickly administer a narcotic antagonist if respiratory depression occurs.
6. Check that Ambu bag is available on unit. **Rationale:** Necessary for complication of respiratory depression.
7. Check if an apnea monitor or pulse oximeter is ordered. **Rationale:** It is important that clients are monitored closely (at least for the first 12 hours) because of dangerous side effects, especially respiratory depression.
8. Assemble equipment.
9. Wash your hands, and maintain strict aseptic technique. **Rationale:** Maintaining sterility of insertion site, administered solutions, and infusion lines decreases potential for complications.
10. Check client's identaband.

Procedure

for Bolus Injection
1. Put on sterile gloves, and maintain sterile technique.
2. Wipe narcotic vial with povidone-iodine swab.
3. Draw up ordered dose of prediluted preservative-free narcotic in 12-mL syringe with filter needle.
4. Change filter needle to 20-gauge needle.
5. Expel air from syringe.
6. Verify narcotic with a second nurse before administering. **Rationale:** It is important to take every precaution to prevent inadvertent administration of a drug that could cause spinal cord damage.
7. Disinfect catheter injection port (Luer-Lok port or the injection cap) with nonalcohol antiseptic iodine wipe. **Rationale:** Alcohol must *never* be

used because it is extremely toxic to the spinal cord.

8. Dry injection cap or port with sterile 2×2 gauze.
9. Insert needle into injection cap or port, and attempt to aspirate for 30 seconds. **Rationale:** See Clinical Alert below.

■ CLINICAL ALERT

If more than 1 mL of fluid or blood is returned during aspiration of the catheter, the procedure *must be terminated* and physician notified.

10. Inject medication slowly.
11. Remove needle from injection cap or port.
12. Dispose of uncapped needle in appropriate safety container.
13. Check that a sterile, occlusive dressing is over catheter. Dressing is changed every 72 hours (certified RN or MD to change dressing).
14. Document dose in appropriate record.
15. Closely monitor respirations every 1 hour for 24 hours or use apnea monitor or pulse oximeter. **Rationale:** Due to risk of respiratory depression, close monitoring after administration of an epidural narcotic is essential.
16. Monitor vital signs: BP and pulse every 30 minutes for 1 hour after initial epidural dose, then every 8 hours.
17. Monitor for possible side effects of narcotic administration: respiratory depression, urinary retention, nausea and vomiting, and pruritus.

for Continuous Infusion

1. Check physician's orders for epidural narcotic.
2. Check that safety signs are near bed and label is on catheter.
3. Wash hands and don gloves.
4. Attach container of narcotic to infusion pump tubing.
5. Prime tubing (see Chapter 27 for step-by-step instruction).
6. Attach proximal end of tubing to pump and distal end to epidural catheter.
7. Tape all connections securely.
8. Set infusion pump to ordered calibration.
9. Observe for side effects of narcotic or client response and pain level.
10. Dispose of gloves and wash hands.
11. Chart pump reading every hour for 12–24 hours or as dictated by institutional policy.
12. Record narcotic on appropriate sign-out sheet.

Narcotics commonly administered via epidural continuous infusion:

- Hydromorphone hydrochloride (Dilaudid: 0.05–0.3 mg/hr)
- Fentanyl (Duragesic: 50–150 μg/hr)
- Morphine sulfate (Duramorph: 0.2–1.0 mg/hr)

Narcotics commonly administered via epidural bolus technique:

- Hydromorphone hydrochloride (Dilaudid: 0.5–2.0 mg)
- Fentanyl (Duragesic: 50–100 μg)
- Morphine sulfate (Duramorph: 5–10 mg)
- Meperidine (Demerol: 25–75 mg)

} administered in prediluted preservative-free form

CHARTING for Pain Relief

- Record drug, dose, and time given and client's response to medication
- Describe the client's pain, including location, quality, intensity, precipitating factors, associated factors, and aggravating factors
- Describe alleviating factors, including what the client does to relieve pain as well as nursing assistance
- Describe behavioral changes due to pain relief or the absence of objective changes in response to the medication or nursing interventions
- If there is a poor response to therapy, state what other measures will be attempted, and chart results
- Continue to document attempts to relieve pain until relief occurs and the client is satisfied
- Placement of epidural catheter
- Site assessment for catheter insertion

CRITICAL THINKING APPLICATION

CLINICAL PROBLEMS	CRITICAL THINKING OPTIONS
Client achieves no relief from relaxation, visualization, or massage.	• Try combining methods with use of medications (i.e., use these methods while waiting for the medication to take effect). • Client has to trust the technique before it can be effective. Have client talk to another person who has found technique helpful.
Client achieves little or no relief from TENS.	• Use another brand or type of stimulator as ordered. • If using continuous cutaneous stimulation, try using intermittent stimulation and vice versa.
Client develops skin irritation at electrode sites.	• Use hypoallergic tape to secure electrodes. • Discontinue tape. Use Velcro or elastic bandage to hold electrodes in place. • If rash appears to be caused by gel, mix cortisone gel with the electrode cream. Change gel. Cleanse skin and electrodes with soap and water frequently.
Client develops constipation from regularly administered narcotic preparations.	• Obtain order for and administer stool softener and peristaltic stimulant. • Encourage intake of high-fiber diet, if not contraindicated. • Encourage adequate fluid intake.
Client develops respiratory depression and appears to be sedated.	• Check that drug has been absorbed by systemic vasculature and epidural veins and ended up in high concentrations in the brain. • Check on other drugs the client is taking—there may be a synergistic effect. • Nursing assessment: respirations, ability to cough and deep breathe, auscultate chest, arterial blood gases. • Check that Narcan is at the bedside and may be ordered if respirations are too slow (this drug reverses analgesia so monitor for high pain level returning).
Client develops nausea and vomits.	• Assess cause of problem—consider pain, ileus, as well as reaction to drug. • Administer antiemetics as ordered, and protect client from aspiration. • Keep client n.p.o. until cause of problem is discovered.

unit 2

PATIENT-CONTROLLED ANALGESIA (PCA)

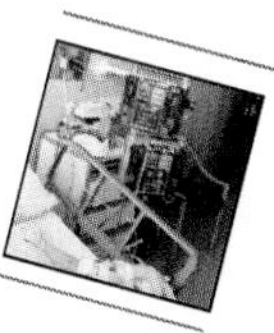

NURSING PROCESS DATA

ASSESSMENT Data Base

Assess potential use of PCA as method of pain control.

Assess reliability of candidate for PCA.

Assess which PCA model is most appropriate for client.

Assess client throughout PCA therapy (every 2 hours during first 24 hours, then every 4 hours).

Assess patency of IV lines.

Assess allergy to pain medication—morphine or meperidine.

Assess respiratory system for baseline comparison.

Assess client's type and level of pain.

PLANNING Objectives

To provide a consistent level of pain control

To allow the client, according to needs for pain control, to self-administer pain medication via PCA

To enable the client to feel in control of his or her pain management

To decrease the client's anxiety around the pain control issue

IMPLEMENTATION Procedures

Qualifying the Client for PCA

Administering PCA

Changing Dose Volume

Changing Lockout Interval

Changing 4-Hour Limit

Terminating a PCA Infusion

Teaching PCA to a Client

EVALUATION Expected Outcomes

Client feels competent to self-administer pain medication via PCA.

PCA infuser works efficiently to administer medication.

IV site used to administer PCA remains free of complications.

Pain is controlled to client's satisfaction.

Client's anxiety level remains low or manageable around issue of pain control.

QUALIFYING THE CLIENT FOR PCA

Procedure

1. Determine whether physician wishes to use PCA for pain control.
2. Determine if client is a candidate for PCA.
   a. Check criteria for client selection.
   b. After explaining PCA, determine if client wishes to use this method of pain control.
3. Determine which type—electronic or mechanical—PCA unit is appropriate.
   a. A mechanical device is fed by gravity rather than electricity; it is simple, inexpensive, disposable, and does not interfere with the client's mobility.
   b. A pump or electronic device has a computer for dosage monitoring, is more flexible, and can be reset as necessary.

4. Assess any allergy to prescribed pain medication.

> **CLINICAL ALERT**
>
> Determine if client is allergic to pain medication prescribed—usually morphine or meperidine.

5. Perform basic physical assessment before initiating PCA.
   a. Establish baseline vital sign chart.
   b. Specifically assess client's respiratory system for ongoing evaluation during PCA therapy.

Criteria for Client Selection for PCA

- Clients requiring parenteral analgesic treatment.
- Clients requiring postoperative pain relief.
- Trauma clients who have clear sensorium.
- Clients suffering from chronic pain (terminal cancer).
- Clients who are mentally alert and able to understand and comply with procedure instructions.
- Clients without a handicap that impairs ability to use PCA.
- Clients with no prior addiction to drugs or alcohol.
- Eighteen years of age is the usual minimum age for PCA use, but it has been used in children as young as 7 years of age.

ADMINISTERING PCA

Equipment

This skill applies to the Abbott Lifecare PCA Plus II pump. Specific steps of administering PCA vary with different manufacturer's equipment.

PCA Infuser Pump

PCA infuser pumps are made for home or hospital use. These special pumps allow the client to control three parameters of medication delivery:

- Stopping and starting a continuous infusion.
- Titrating the hourly dose within a preset range of milligrams per hour.
- Administering a bolus dose within preset parameters.

Specific physician's orders for PCA
PCA infuser pump
IV administration set
IV pole
IV narcotic as ordered
IV tubing for drug cartridge (PCA microbore)
Minibore extension tube with one injection site, if needed
Extension set with Leur-Lok

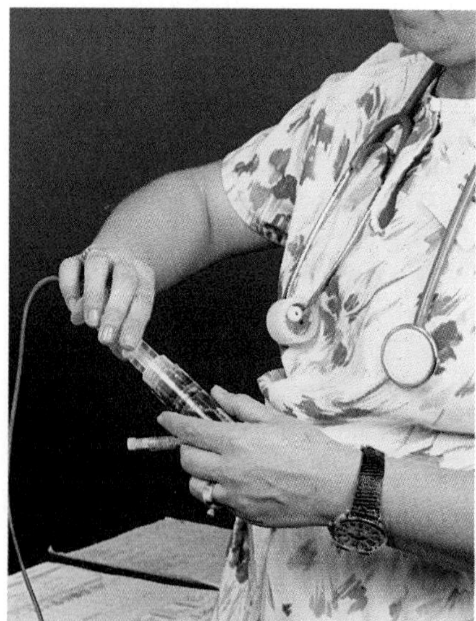
Connect plunger to vial.

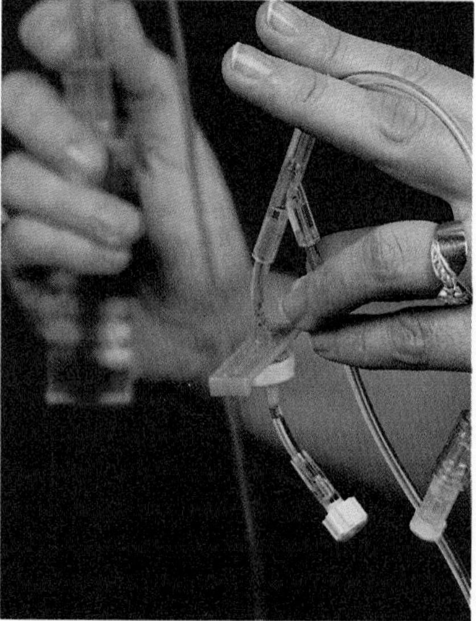
Prime PCA tubing to Y connector.

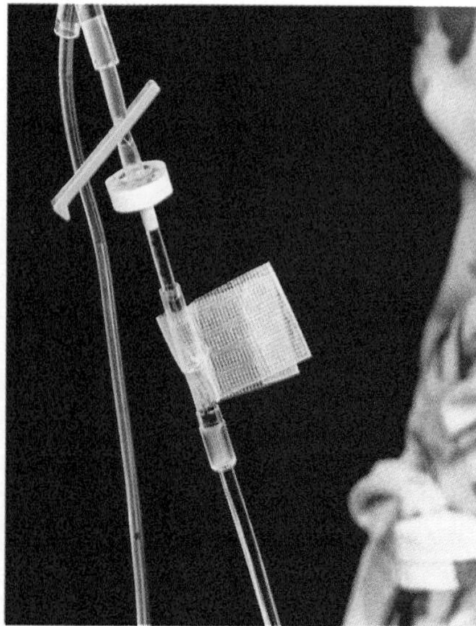
Tape maintenance IV securely.

Analgesic medication cartridge and injector (vial injector)

PCA administration record

Preparation

1. Check that physician's orders, including medication orders for PCA, are complete.
   Morphine is available in 30-mL vial injectors (concentration of 1 mg/mL or 5 mg/mL) and meperidine (Demerol) in 30-mL vial injectors (concentration of 10 mg/mL).
2. Assemble IV administration set (refer to Chapter 27, "Preparing IV System Using Plastic Bag").
3. Check client's identaband.
4. Wash your hands before preparing PCA equipment.
5. Assemble PCA vial injector following instructions on vial carton.
   a. Snap caps from injector (plunger) and vial.
   b. Connect plunger to vial by twisting them together.
   c. Prime unit by pushing down on injector to release air.
6. Secure backcheck valve on vial injector, and tighten PCA set to backvalve before proceeding. **Rationale:** Backcheck valve must be attached to prevent accidental overdosage due to a cracked or malpositioned PCA vial injector.
7. Prime PCA tubing to the "Y."
8. Attach maintenance IV to unprimed portion of the Y.
9. Tape maintenance IV securely to Y of PCA tubing. **Rationale:** This is necessary if there is no Luer-Lok on PCA tubing (Abbott).
10. Prime lower tubing of PCA set with IV solution from the gravity administration set.
11. Close slide clamps of gravity IV set after lower portion of PCA set has been primed.
12. Close slide clamp on PCA tubing. **Rationale:** Closing slide clamp maintains prime and prevents air entry.
13. Open flow control clamp on IV. **Rationale:** This clears medication already primed with maintenance IV.
14. Explain ongoing procedure to client. (You have already completed client teaching regarding pain management with use of PCA infuser.)
15. Leave PCA booklet with client for referral during pain control time.
16. Prepare IV site and start IV if not already established (refer to Chapter 27, skills "Preparing IV Site" and "Inserting a Wing-Tipped Needle").

■ CLINICAL ALERT

To administer blood or any other medication incompatible with pain medication, you must establish a second IV site.

Procedure

1. Unlock by turning key, and open door of infuser.
2. Activate drive release mechanism by pinching spring-loaded lever, and move drive assembly to uppermost position.
3. Load vial injector into vial injector holder by moving drive assembly downward. (Be sure calibrations are visible.)
4. Clamp securely, and listen for "click" sound. **Rationale:** Click lets you know vial injector is properly inserted and locked into position.
5. Rotate vial injector in holder, and inspect for leakage or cracks. **Rationale:** Improper loading may cause vial injector to crack. Vial injector may not leak until delivery pressure is applied. Cracked vial injector may cause overdelivery of medication to client.

■ CLINICAL ALERT

If vial injector is cracked and unusable, discard contents in presence of another licensed RN and sign off on narcotic record or follow hospital protocol for disposal of narcotic. Replace with new vial injector.

6. Validate drug and dose by responding to PCA screen (e.g., "Drug—morphine 1 mg? Yes or no.")
7. Continue to activate PCA by responding to screen (e.g., "Administer loading dose now? Yes or no.")
8. Deliver loading dose as ordered by physician. (Loading dose may be taken from separate vial.) **Rationale:** Loading dose is initial dose given to client, initiating pain management.
   a. Press on–off button to turn on infuser. **Rationale:** When machine is turned on, DOOR OPEN and VOLUME DELIVERED message appear.
   b. Set LOCKOUT INTERVAL at 20 (period during which PCA infuser cannot be activated). Do not close door when giving loading dose.

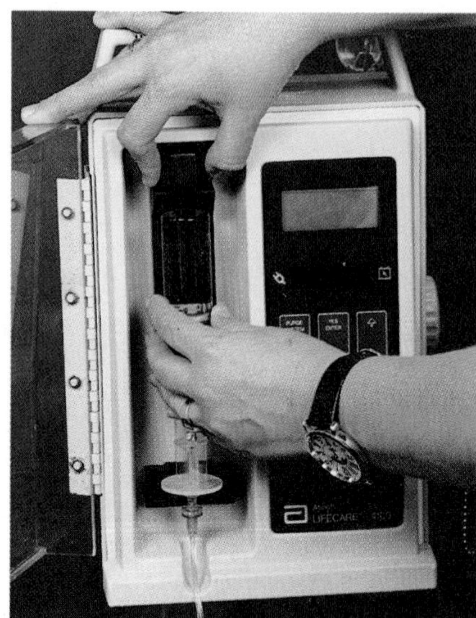

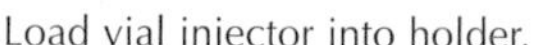

Load vial injector into holder.

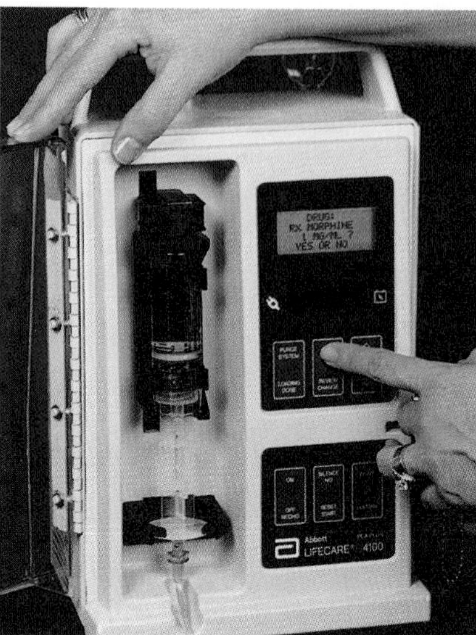

Validate drug dose on screen.

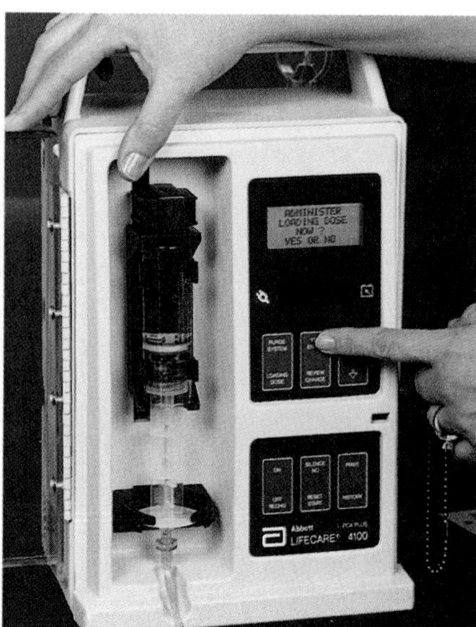

Administer loading dose.

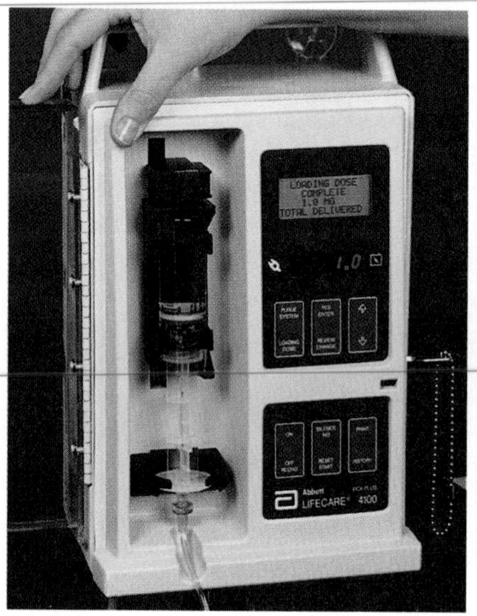

Read screen for loading dose.

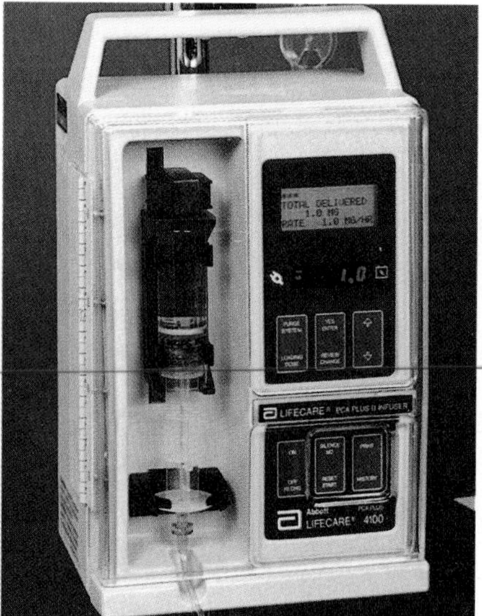

Read screen for delivered dose.

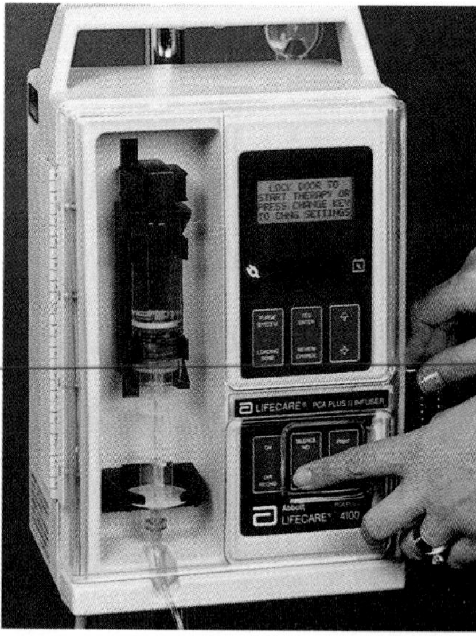

Lock door to begin therapy.

c. Use dose volume control to set DOSE VOLUME to be delivered.

d. Check that slide clamps on PCA infuser are open.

e. Calculate number of milliliters needed for the correct milligram dose.

Dose Calculation

- The PCA infuser delivers in milliliters. The nurse must calculate the number of milliliters needed for the correct milligram dose. Examples: 10 mg (1 mL) every 10 minutes; 40 mg (4 mL) every 10 minutes.
- The maximum rate of administration is 20 mL/hour.

f. Press and release LOADING DOSE.

g. Check that display screen shows volume delivered.

h. Monitor respirations every 15 minutes after loading dose until stable.

9. Set 4 HOUR LIMIT by calculating maximum dose client may receive in a 4-hour period. Control ranges from 5 to 30 mL in 5-mL increments.

Rationale: This allows 30 mL to be the maximum amount that can be delivered in 4 hours.

10. Set DOSE VOLUME according to written orders.
11. Close and lock security door to initiate client control. Remove key and place with narcotic keys or follow hospital protocol. **Rationale:** Door must be locked to read READY message. This indicates infuser is now in client control mode and that first dose is available to client.
12. Hand control button to client.
13. Review client instructions.

P.R.N. Booster Dose via PCA

If physician so orders, a booster dose may be given to a client on a p.r.n. basis. All booster doses must be administered by an RN.

- Open door.
- Set DOSE VOLUME to dose ordered.
- Set LOCKOUT INTERVAL to 00.
- Administer dose.
- Set dose back to original order.
- Set LOCKOUT INTERVAL to original order.
- Close and lock door.

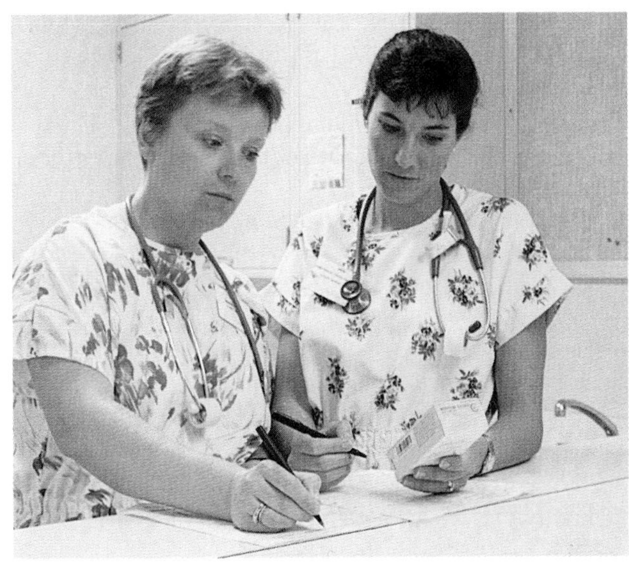

Check narcotic dose with a second nurse.

14. Evaluate how client is responding to medication schedule and revise parameters with physician, if necessary.

CHANGING DOSE VOLUME

Procedure

1. Unlock and open security door.
2. Note message. DOOR OPEN status appears.
3. Enter new DOSE VOLUME.
4. Close security door, checking that it is securely locked. **Rationale:** PCA infuser will not return to client control mode if door is not securely locked.
5. Check that READY or LOCKOUT INTERVAL message has appeared. **Rationale:** This indicates infuser is back in client control mode.

CHANGING LOCKOUT INTERVAL

Procedure

1. Unlock and open security door.
2. Read DOOR OPEN status message.
3. Enter new LOCKOUT INTERVAL.
4. Close security door making sure it is locked.
5. Read READY or LOCKOUT INTERVAL message. **Rationale:** This indicates PCA infuser is back in client control mode.

CHANGING 4-HOUR LIMIT

Procedure

1. Unlock and open security door.
2. Note DOOR OPEN status message on display. **Rationale:** This indicates infuser is ready for resetting 4-HOUR LIMIT.
3. Press and release 4-HOUR LIMIT. **Rationale:** 4-hour maximum dose is automatically set at 10 mL. It can be set at 5, 10, 20, 25, or 30 mL.

4. Redepress 4-HOUR LIMIT to change setting (while existing 4-HOUR LIMIT is displayed). Hold until desired limit appears.
5. Release when new limit appears. Note that setting a new 4-HOUR LIMIT does not erase previous 4-hour dose history.
6. Close security door, checking that it is securely locked.
7. Note READY or LOCKOUT INTERVAL message appearing. **Rationale:** This message indicates that PCA infuser is back in client control mode.

■ CLINICAL ALERT

To Discontinue an Ongoing Infusion

1. Close slide clamp proximal to Luer-Lok connector on vial injector.
2. Unlock and open security door.
3. Press OFF button to turn PCA infuser off.
4. Record amount of medication administered.

Infusion immediately ceases with these interventions.

TERMINATING A PCA INFUSION

Procedure

1. Close manual slide clamp proximal to Luer-Lok connector on vial injector.
2. Unlock and open security door.
3. Remove vial injector from PCA infuser, and disconnect from set.
4. Press OFF button to turn off PCA infuser.
5. Continue or discontinue IV as required.
6. Record and dispose of PCA narcotic vial injector per hospital policy for disposal of narcotic drugs.
7. Dispose of narcotic that remains in vial injector per protocol. **Rationale:** Narcotics must be accounted for by cosignature on controlled narcotic record or per individual hospital protocol.

TEACHING PCA TO A CLIENT

Preparation

1. Determine if client is a candidate for PCA (see skill in this chapter "Qualifying Client for PCA").
2. Allow client to directly handle equipment. **Rationale:** This reduces fear of technology and teaches basic steps of PCA before surgery.

Procedure

1. Explain how PCA device works.
   a. Set the pump's controls to deliver pain medication.
   b. Tell client that if amount of medication is not sufficient to control pain, he or she may press a button to deliver an additional bolus.
   c. After each bolus, client must wait a minimum amount of time (usually 5–10 minutes) before delivering another dose. **Rationale:** This protects client from receiving too much medication.
   d. Dose may be adjusted to maintain pain control. **Rationale:** When clients control their own medication dose, studies indicate usage is not excessive.
   e. Have client explain and demonstrate PCA use before initiating therapy.

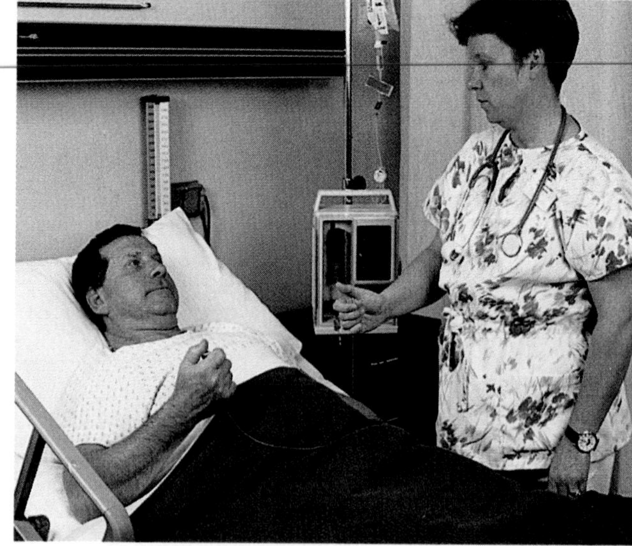

Teach PCA procedure to client.

2. Clarify with client how he or she administers medication dose when pain is felt. **Rationale:** Self-control of pain medication has been found to be very successful with clients and less time-consuming for the nurse. There is no significant difference in amount of medication used.
3. Program PCA infuser for continuous infusion plus a bolus dose.
   a. Establish amount of narcotic needed to control client's pain (i.e., give 1–5 mg morphine every 10 minutes until pain is relieved).
   b. Set pump's hourly infusion rate to equal total milligrams per hour needed to control pain.
4. Reassure client that PCA will control, but not totally abolish, pain. **Rationale:** Continuous infusion supplemented by small boluses provides steady relief (more so than IM injections) but does not eliminate pain.
5. Teach client how to evaluate pain level on a five-point scale. If client's pain is not sufficiently relieved, medication dose is increased. **Rationale:** When clients know they can control their pain level, they feel less helpless and more empowered.
   1 = Pain relieved
   2 = Occasional discomfort
   3 = Decreased pain intensity, e.g., able to walk, cough
   4 = Minimal pain relief
   5 = No pain relief
6. Evaluate client's response to medication schedule. **Rationale:** It is important to check for adverse effects of sedation to avoid complications or necessity of revising dose parameters.
7. Reassess client's ability to control pain level and effectiveness of medication dosage to control pain.
8. Instruct client to notify staff if machine malfunctions (alarm sounds or message display indicates a problem), pain is not controlled or changes in severity, or if he or she has any questions.

PATIENT CONTROLLED ANALGESIA (PCA)—USING THE PCA INFUSION PUMP

DATE:	TIME:	DRUG ALLERGIES:

A. DRUG/CONCENTRATION: Check One

Morphine = 1 mg/mL .... ☐
Meperidine = 10 mg/mL........ ☐
Other ________ ________ = mg/mL .... ☐

B. PCA/BASAL (Patient Controlled with Background Continuous Infusion)
Please specify doses in mL rather than mg when ordering.

1. Specify **DOSE** (patient controlled): ________ mL
   Pump range is 0.1–9.9 mL
   Suggested dose: Morphine **0.5–1.5 mL** (0.5–1.5 mg)
   Meperidine **0.5–1.0mL** (5-10mg)
2. Specify **DELAY** (PCA dose lockout interval): ________ min
   Pump range is 3–60 min
   Suggested interval: **10–15 min**
3. Specify **BASAL RATE** (continuous infusion): ________ mL/hr
   Pump range is 0.0-10.0 mL/hr
   Suggested continuous rate: Morphine **1.0–2.5 mL/hr** (1.0–2.5 mg/hr)
   Meperidine **1.0–1.5 mL/hr** (10–15 mg/hr)
4. Specify **1 HOUR LIMIT** (maximum combined PCA + basal rate): ________ mL
   Pump range is 1.0–30 mL
   Suggested limit: Morphine **5–10 mL/hr** (5–10 mg)
   Meperidine **4.0–5.5 mL/hr** (40–50 mg)
5. Specify **BOLUS** dose (initial loading dose) if desired: ________ mL
   Specify if bolus dose may be repeated and frequency/interval:
   ____
   Pump range is 0.0–9.9 mL
   Suggested bolus dose: Morphine **3–5 mL** (3–5 mg)
   Meperidine **2.0–2.5 mL** (20–25 mg)

C. Additional PCA orders: ________

____

D. If patient persistently complains of inadequate analgesia, notify Physician.

Physician's Signature: ________

PCA Calculation.

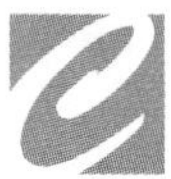

CHARTING for PCA

- Assess and chart on client using PCA infuser every 4 hours (after initial 24 hours), unless otherwise ordered.
- Describe respirations every 2 hours, and compare to baseline assessment sheet.
- Record sedation and pain legend every 4 hours. Include degree of pain relief obtained from PCA.
  - 1 = Wide awake
  - 2 = Drowsy
  - 3 = Dosing intermittently
  - 4 = Mostly sleeping
  - 5 = Only awakens when disturbed
- Initiate new PCA administration record for each narcotic vial injector used.

On PCA Record

- Chart appropriate entries throughout your shift. To determine amount of medication administered, press TOTAL DOSES and multiply by number of milliliters prescribed.
- Chart LOADING DOSE and time administered separately on medication record.
- Chart wasted narcotic—cosigned per hospital policy.
- Verify and document that calculated volume remaining and actual volume remaining in syringe are the same. Report any discrepancy and follow hospital procedure for incorrect narcotic count.

CRITICAL THINKING APPLICATION

CLINICAL PROBLEMS	CRITICAL THINKING OPTIONS
■ Vial injector is incorrectly positioned or empty.	• Close slide clamp. • Press SILENCE. • Check vial injector for contents and position. Properly install it or replace with new vial injector. • Open slide clamp.
■ Alarm signal flashes.	• Press SILENCE to mute alarm temporarily.
■ Security door is closed and locked and a. Dose volume and lockout interval controls combined allow more than 20 mL/hr, *or* b. Dose volume is greater than 5 mL or at 0.0 mL/hr, or c. Lockout interval is less than 5 minutes.	• Unlock and open security door. • Reset DOSE VOLUME and/or LOCKOUT INTERVAL to proper values. • Close and lock security door and remove key. • READY message appears.
■ Alarm signal flashes and fluid delivery stops.	• Close slide clamp.
■ Check whether a. Manual flow clamp is closed, *or* b. Administration tubing kinked or occluded, *or* c. Venipuncture is occluded.	• Press SILENCE to mute alarm. • Pinch spring-loaded lever, and move drive assembly up to relieve pressure. • Identify and correct cause of occlusion. • Reposition vial injector correctly.

CLINICAL PROBLEMS	CRITICAL THINKING OPTIONS
Audible alarm sounds.	• Press SILENCE (mutes alarm for 1–5 minutes). • Plug into AC outlet as soon as possible to recharge battery. (With a discharged battery, there is a blank message panel, loss of cumulative volume and total dose information, and nonoperation of PCA infuser.)
Alarm bar flashes because door has been open 10 minutes.	• Press SILENCE to mute for an additional 10 minutes, *or* • Close and lock security door.
Client exhibits bradypnea, hypotension, nausea, vomiting, or dizziness.	• Monitor sedation level—remember the goal of PCA is to control pain without sedation. • Report to physician that medication parameters are resulting in oversedation.
Client is insecure and anxious about using PCA mode of pain control.	• Determine which steps client feels insecure about completing, and reteach procedure while demonstrating steps.
Medication, either type or dose, is not sufficiently controlling client's level of pain.	• Reevaluate medication and dose parameters with physician.

GERIATRIC CONSIDERATIONS

The incidence of pain in the elderly has not been well studied and this population presents several pain management problems.

- Elderly people often suffer acute and chronic painful diseases or have multiple diseases, thus they often have more than one source of pain.
- Elderly are at increased risk for drug–drug as well as drug–disease interactions.
- Studies show the incidence of pain is twofold higher in those over 60. Acutely painful conditions affect the elderly disproportionately (herpes zoster, arthritis, polymyalgia rheumatica, peripheral vascular disease).
- Elderly may have impaired senses (vision, hearing) and an impaired ability to express themselves.

Pain assessment is more complex and difficult with the elderly.

- The elderly may report pain differently (not as clearly) as younger clients due to physiologic, psychologic, and cultural changes associated with aging.
- Clinicians often hold the mistaken belief that the elderly have increased pain thresholds; they may be more stoic about experiencing, thus reporting pain.
- Cognitive impairment (which may occur in as many as 50% of the institutionalized elderly) may interfere greatly with the assessment of pain. Even though behavior may be assessed (restlessness, groaning, agitation) it is nonspecific and subject to interpretation.
- See Geriatric Considerations for Medications in Chapter 16 for specific guidelines for drug use with the elderly.

Traditional approaches to pain control may not work with the elderly.

- Universal use of pain scales may not be possible with visual, hearing and motor impairments.
- Clients may report pain initially, but recall (due to cognitive impairment) may not be possible.
- Pain assessment may require frequent monitoring. Monitoring may have major implications for quality of care and quality of life, so facilities with limited staff may result in poor pain control in the elderly.
- The elderly are at risk for over- and under treatment. Adverse drug reactions are more prevalent with the elderly.
- Attitudes among health care professionals may also impede appropriate care (partially due to belief that acute and chronic pain are a normal component of aging).

18

Nutritional Management

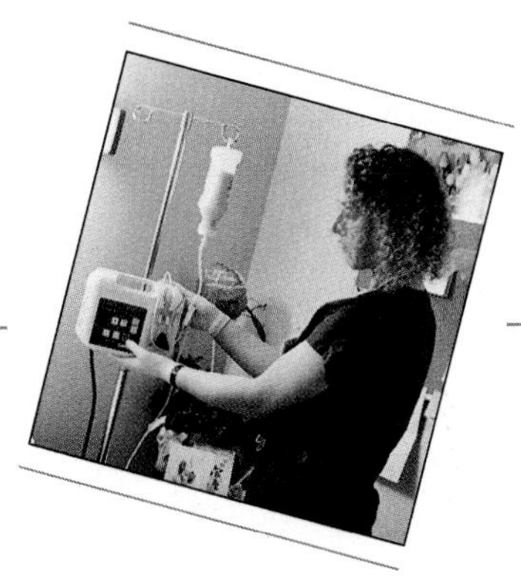

LEARNING OBJECTIVES

- List the six essential nutrients necessary to sustain life.
- Outline the primary differences between vitamins and minerals.
- Describe the primary functions of the gastrointestinal system and accessory organs.
- Identify the assessment categories important for a total nutritional assessment.
- Define the term "therapeutic diet."
- Describe a sodium-restricted diet and list at least three foods high in sodium.
- Name and discuss the purpose of at least four therapeutic diets.
- List what foods should be included in a postoperative surgical diet.
- Explain what is meant by a postoperative diet protocol.
- Outline the steps for inserting a nasogastric tube.
- Identify the primary steps of administering a tube feeding.
- Discuss at least two potential problems that may occur with a tube feeding and the suggested solutions.

TERMINOLOGY

Alimentary: of or pertaining to nutrition.

Anorexia: loss of appetite for food.

Aspirate: to remove fluids or gases by suction.

Calorie: the amount of heat necessary to raise the temperature of 1 kilogram of water 1°C. This is the "small" calorie. The dietary, or large, Calorie represents 1000 of these calories, or 1 kilocalorie.

Carbohydrates: a group of chemical substances, including sugars, glycogen, starches, dextrins, and celluloses, that contain only carbon, oxygen, and hydrogen.

Cardio: prefix pertaining to the heart.

Cardiovascular: term that pertains to the heart and blood vessels as cardiovascular system.

Diabetic: one who has inadequate production and use of insulin.

Diet: liquid and solid food substances regularly consumed.

Digestion: the process by which food is broken down mechanically and chemically in the gastrointestinal tract.

Diverticula: a sac or pouch in the walls of a canal.

Diverticulosis: diverticula of the colon without inflammation or symptoms.

Emaciation: a condition characterized by extreme leanness or thinness.

Emesis: the act of vomiting.

Erythema: redness of the skin produced by capillary congestion as in a sunburn.

Fat: substance made up of carbon, hydrogen, and oxygen, occurring naturally in most foods but especially in meat and dairy products.

Food supplement: a preparation added to the regular diet that aids nourishment.

Gastric gavage: introduction of nourishment into the stomach by mechanical means.

Gastrointestinal: term that pertains to the stomach and intestines.

Hematemesis: vomitus containing blood.

Hyperalimentation: the process of nourishing the body through parenteral means.

Hyperglycemia: condition characterized by an increase in blood sugar.

Hypertonic: solution having a higher osmotic pressure or tonicity than a solution to which it is compared.

Hypoglycemia: condition characterized by a deficiency of sugar or glucose in the blood.

Infuse: introduce a liquid into a vein.

Ingest: the process of taking material into the gastrointestinal tract or the process by which a cell takes in foreign particles.

Jejunostomy: surgical creation of a permanent opening into the jejunum.

Kwashiorkor: a state of extreme malnutrition due to severe protein insufficiency.

Lumen: the inner open space of a tube.

Malnutrition: a condition characterized by a lack of necessary food substances or improper absorption and distribution of food substances in the body.

Minerals: inorganic elements or compounds.

Nasogastric tube: a tube that is passed through the nose and into the stomach.

Nausea: a feeling of sickness accompanied with the urge to vomit.

Nutrient: nourishing; food item that supplies the body with necessary elements.

Obstruction: blocking of a structure that prevents it from functioning normally; obstacle.

Polyunsaturated: term usually referring to a fat, indicating that the carbon chain has more than one double bond. These fats tend to have higher densities (HDL) than saturated fats.

Projectile vomiting: the expulsion of vomitus with great force.

Proteins: substances that contain amino acids essential for growth and repair of tissues.

Protocol: description of steps taken.

Renal: term that pertains to the kidney.

Sepsis: pathologic state usually febrile, resulting from the presence of microorganisms or their poisonous products in the bloodstream.

Thrombo: a clot of blood; a thrombus.

Thrombophlebitis: inflammation of a vein before the development of a thrombus.

Trauma: an injury or wound.

Uremia: toxic condition associated with renal insufficiency and the retention of nitrogenous substances in the blood.

Vitamins: a group of organic substances essential for life.

Xiphoid: the lowest portion of the sternum.

ESSENTIAL NUTRIENTS

Nutrition comprises essential nutrients—carbohydrates, fats, proteins, vitamins, minerals, and water (Table 18–1)—all of which are necessary for growth and development through the life cycle. When these are supplied to the body in proper balance, the body uses them for energy, growth and development, tissue repair, and regulation and maintenance of body processes.

A useful method of organizing food intake to ensure a balance of the appropriate foods and nutrients is the food guide pyramid, a revised guide published by the nutrition section of the U.S. Department of Agriculture.

TABLE 18–1. Essential Body Nutrients

Carbohydrates	Monosaccharides Glucose, fructose, galactose Disaccharides Sucrose, lactose, maltose Polysaccharides Starch, dextrin, glycogen, cellulose, hemicellulose
Fats	Linoleic acid, linolenic acid, arachidonic acid
Proteins	Amino acids Phenylalanine, lysine, isoleucine, leucine, methionine, valine, tryptophan, threonine
Vitamins	Fat-soluble Vitamins A, D, E, and K Water soluble Vitamins B_1, B_2, B_6, B_{12}, niacin, pantothenic acid, folacin, biotin, choline, *meso*-inositol, *para*-aminobenzoic acid, and vitamin C
Minerals	Major elements Calcium, chloride, iron, magnesium, phosphorous, potassium, sodium, sulfur
Water	Trace elements

Carbohydrates

Carbohydrates are the chief source of energy and contain carbon, hydrogen, and oxygen. Carbohydrates include sugars, starches, and cellulose. Simple sugars, such as fruit sugar, are easily digested. Starches, which are more complex, require more sophisticated enzyme processes to be reduced to glucose, the end product of carbohydrate metabolism. Glucose, which is converted sugars and starches, appears in the body as blood sugar and is "burned" as fuel by the tissues. Some glucose is processed by the liver, converted to glycogen, and stored by the liver for later use.

Ingesting too many carbohydrates crowds out other important foods and prevents the body from receiving the necessary nutrients for healthy maintenance. Too few carbohydrates may lead to loss of energy, depression, ketosis, and a breakdown of body protein. Although differences in individual body structure, energy expenditure, basal metabolism, and general health status determine the amount and kind of carbohydrates that should be consumed for optimal health, there are general guidelines. The Select Committee on Nutrition and Human Needs of the U.S. Senate recom-

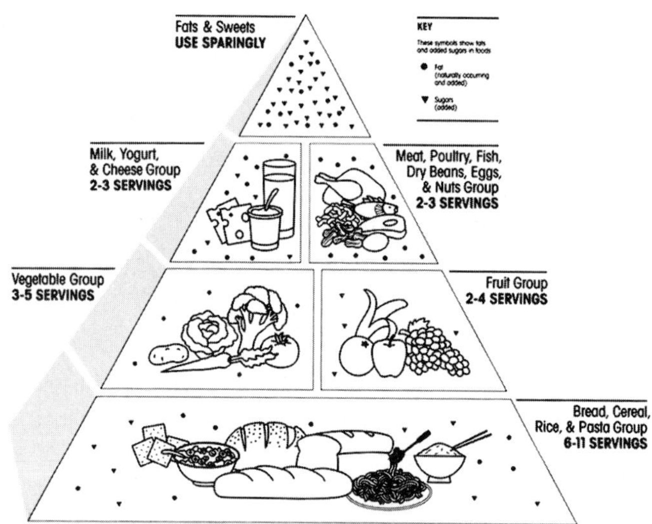

Food Guide Pyramid (US Department of Agriculture).

mends 55–60% of calories come from complex carbohydrates.

Fats

Fats or lipids are the second important group of nutrients. Fats also provide energy. In fact, when oxidized, they are the most concentrated sources of energy and, as such, furnish the calories necessary for survival. Fats also act as carriers for the fat-soluble vitamins, A, D, E, and K. Consuming too much fat can lead to weight problems and poor metabolism of food products. The optimal percentage of fat in the diet is 25–30%.

Fatty acids are the basic components of fat and comprise two main groups. Saturated fatty acids usually come from animal sources. Unsaturated fatty acids primarily come from vegetables, nuts, or seed sources. In the unsaturated group are three essential fatty acids. These acids are called "essential" because they are necessary to ensure health and growth and the body cannot manufacture them. They must therefore be obtained from the diet. These three acids are linoleic acid, arachidonic acid, and linolenic acid. They are necessary for healthy blood, arteries, nerves, and skin. A deficiency in this group leads to skin problems and illness.

Proteins

Proteins, the third essential group of nutrients, are complex organic compounds that contain amino acids. Proteins are critical to all aspects of growth and development of body tissues. They are necessary for the building of muscles, blood, skin, internal organs, hormones, and enzymes and are also a source of energy when there is insufficient carbohydrate or fat in the diet. When protein is spared, it is either used for tissue repair and maintenance or converted by the liver and stored as fat.

When digested and broken down, proteins form 22 amino acids. These amino acids are then absorbed from the intestine into the bloodstream and carried to the liver for synthesis into the tissues and organs of the body. They are the chemical basis for life, and if just one is missing, protein synthesis decreases or even stops. All but eight of the amino acids can be produced by the body. These eight must be obtained from the diet. If all eight are present in a particular food, the food is a "complete protein." Foods that lack one or more of these essential amino acids are called "incomplete proteins." Most meat and dairy products are complete proteins, and most vegetables and fruits are incomplete. When several incomplete proteins form the major portion of a person's diet, they should be combined carefully so that the result is a balance yielding complete protein. For example, the combination of beans and rice is perfectly balanced to give a complete protein food.

It is difficult to determine the exact amount of protein needed to supply all of the essential amino acids because there are many variables. Height and weight, level of activity, and nutritional and health status all influence the amount of protein necessary for a healthy body. The National Research Council recommends that 0.42 g of protein be consumed per day per pound of body weight. Previously, it was advocated that a person weighing 150 pounds should consume 75 g of protein; however, recent research shows that this amount can be decreased by about one-third without negative results. The optimal healthy diet should be 12% protein, or 40–50 g, for a person weighing 150 pounds. It appears that as long as the essential amino acids are included in the diet, the total grams of protein can be reduced.

Protein deficiency can affect the entire body—organs, tissues, skin, and muscles—as well as certain body processes. If a child is deficient in protein, he or she may suffer from kwashiorkor, a disease resulting in physical and mental impairment and, if severe enough, death. If an adult is deficient in protein, his or her stamina, mental state, and ability to withstand stress and infection is affected. Protein deficiency also interferes with recovery from diseases or surgery.

Protein is very plentiful in the body. It is an integral part of all cells and essential for growth and development. Just like fats and carbohydrates, adequate protein must be consumed in balance with other nutrients for human survival.

Water

Although not specifically a nutrient, water is essential for survival. Water is involved in every body process from digestion and absorption to excretion. It is a major portion of circulation and is the transporter of nutrients throughout the body.

Body water performs three major functions: it gives form to the body, constituting 50–75% of the body mass; it provides the necessary environment for cell metabolism; and it maintains a stable body temperature.

Almost all foods contain water that is absorbed by the body. The average adult body contains 56 quarts of water and loses about 3 quarts a day. If a person suffers severe water depletion, dehydration and salt depletion can result and can eventually lead to death. A person can survive several weeks without food but only days without water.

Vitamins

Vitamins are organic food substances and are essential in small amounts for growth, maintenance, and the functioning of body processes. Vitamins are found only in living things—plants and animals—and usually cannot be synthesized by the human body.

Vitamins can be grouped according to the substance in which they are soluble. The fat-soluble group includes vitamins A, D, E, and K. These vitamins are measured in international units. Each unit generally refers to the amount of the vitamin needed to produce a change in the nutritional health of a laboratory animal. The water-soluble vitamins include the B complex vitamins, vitamin C, and the bioflavonoids. These are usually measured in milligrams.

Vitamins have no calorie value, but they are as necessary to the body as any other basic nutrient. Currently, there are about 20 substances identified as vitamins, but recent research is concerned with identifying even more of these substances since they are so essential to survival.

For many years research groups have attempted to determine basic vitamin requirements for various age groups. The most commonly used are the listings of the Recommended Dietary Allowances (RDA), based on standards established by the National Academy of Sciences.

Minerals

Minerals are inorganic substances, widely prevalent in nature, and essential for metabolic processes. Minerals are grouped according to the amount found in the body. Major minerals include calcium, magnesium, sodium, potassium, phosphorus, sulfur, and chlorine, all of which have a known function in the body. Major minerals are measured in milligrams. A second group—trace minerals—are iron, copper, iodine, manganese, cobalt, zinc, and molybdenum. These minerals are measured in micrograms, and their function in the body remains unclear. There remains another group of trace minerals (such as boron, silica, barium, strontium, etc.) found in scanty amounts in the body and whose function is also unclear. Minerals form 60–90% of all inorganic material in the body and are found in bones, teeth, soft tissue, muscle, blood, and nerve cells.

Minerals act on organs and in metabolic processes. They act as catalysts for many reactions, such as controlling muscle responses, maintaining the nervous system and acid–base balance, transmitting messages, maintaining cardiac stability, and regulating the metabolism and absorption of other nutrients. Even though they are considered separately, all minerals work synergistically with other minerals, and their actions are interrelated. A deficiency in one mineral, therefore, affects the action of others in the body. It is essential that adequate minerals be ingested because a mineral deficiency can result in severe illness. Likewise, excessive amounts of minerals can throw the body out of balance.

Sufficient minerals can be supplied by adequate diet. Even though RDAs have not been established on all minerals, a diet that contains all the other nutrients usually supplies the necessary amount of minerals for the body. Many nutritionists and biochemists, however, recommend a daily basic vitamin–mineral supplement to ensure adequate levels.

ASSIMILATION OF NUTRIENTS

Following the discussion of the essential body nutrients, it is now important to identify how these elements are broken down, absorbed, and used in the body. Nutrients, in most cases, are ingested through the mouth, and must be broken down by the body. This process is called digestion. It takes place in the mouth, pharynx, esophagus, stomach, and the small and large intestines.

The total daily energy requirement of an individual is the number of calories needed to replace the energy loss from the metabolic rate, plus loss from a person's physical, emotional, and mental output. The number of calories ingested should be directly related to maintaining an adequate energy level and supporting the body's metabolic processes.

Gastrointestinal Tract

The main functions of the gastrointestinal system are the secretion of enzymes and electrolytes to break down raw materials that are ingested; the movement of the ingested products through the system; the complete digestion of nutrients and their absorption into the blood; and the storage or excretion of the end products of digestion.

Chewing food is the first stage of digestion. When nutrients reach the stomach, both mechanical and chemical digestive processes occur. Nutrients are churned, and peristaltic waves move the material through the stomach and, at intervals with relaxation of the pyloric sphincter, into the duodenum. The parietel cells in the gastric glands that line the stomach produce hydrochloric acid, which provides the proper medium for pepsin to split protein into proteoses and peptones. Other chemical actions produce lipase, a fat-splitting enzyme, rennin, which coagulates the protein of milk, and the intrinsic factor, which acts on certain food components to form the antianemic factor.

As nutrients move into the duodenum and the jejunum, intestinal juices provide a large number of enzymes that break down protein into amino acids, form and convert maltase to glucose, and split nucleic acids into nucleotides. The small intestine provides for the absorption of nutrients and the large intestine for the elimination of waste products. It is here that the formation of vitamins K and B_{12}, riboflavin, and thiamin occurs. Also, water is absorbed from the fecal mass as it passes through the small intestine.

The Accessory Organs

The accessory organs of the gastrointestinal tract also play an important role in the use of nutrients. These organs include the tongue, salivary glands, teeth, liver, gallbladder, and pancreas.

The liver is especially important because it has a major role in the metabolism of carbohydrates, fats, and proteins. In the metabolism of carbohydrates, the liver converts glucose to glycogen and stores it. The liver then can reconvert glycogen to glucose when the body requires higher blood sugar. The process of releasing carbohydrates (end products) into the bloodstream is called glycogenolysis.

The liver metabolizes fats through the process of oxidation of fatty acids and the formation of acetoacetic acid. Also, the liver forms lipoproteins, cholesterol, and phospholipids and converts carbohydrates and protein to fats.

Proteins are metabolized in the liver, where deamination of amino acids takes place. Also in this process, the formation of urea and plasma proteins is completed. Finally, the interconversions of amino acids and other compounds occurs in the liver.

The gallbladder's primary function is to act as a reservoir for bile. When fatty materials are in the duodenum, liberation of cholecystokinin is stimulated and the gallbladder contracts causing the relaxation of the sphincter of Oddi. Bile emulsifies fats through constant secretion (500–1000 mL in 24 hours).

The pancreas secretes pancreatic juices that contain enzymes for the digestion of carbohydrates, fats, and proteins. Enzymes are secreted as inactive precursors that do not become active until secreted into the small intestine. In the intestine, the enzyme trypsin acts on proteins to produce peptones, peptides, and amino acids; pancreatic amylase acts on carbohydrates to produce disaccharides; and pancreatic lipase acts on fats to produce glycerol and fatty acids.

In summary, the alimentary tract's primary function is to provide the body with a continuous supply of nutrients by ingestion and moving food and fluids, secreting digestive juices for breaking down the food, and absorbing the resulting nutrients, water, and electrolytes. Nutrients are essential for life, but their simple ingestion into the body is not sufficient for survival. They must be broken down, absorbed, and used efficiently if the body is to remain in proper balance or homeostasis.

NORMAL AND THERAPEUTIC NUTRITION

Normal nutrition is based on recommended daily dietary allowances. These standards are scientifically designed for the maintenance of nearly all healthy people in the United States.

Therapeutic nutrition is a modification of nutritional needs based on the disease condition or the excess or deficit of a nutrition state. Combination diets, which include alterations in minerals, vitamins, proteins, carbohydrates, fats, as well as fluid and texture, are prescribed in therapeutic nutrition.

Whether a normal or a therapeutic diet is being considered, a person's cultural, socioeconomic, and psychologic influences, as well as the physiologic requirements, must be taken into account for effective nutrition; thus, in any given situation, the nutritional requirements must be considered within the context of the total needs of an individual (Table 18–2).

TABLE 18–2. Basic Nutritional Assessment

Assessment	Normal	Abnormal
Appetite	Remains unchanged	Increased or decreased recently Particular cravings
Weight	Previous weight maintained Normal for client Appropriate for age and body build	Changed—increased or decreased recently Rapid or slow changes in weight
Nutritional intake	Adequate foods and fluids to supply body nutrients Nonallergic response to major food groups No pattern of fad diets Absence of drugs, chemicals, or other substances that influence appetite or metabolism	Elimination of certain food categories that results in limited nutrients Emphasis on some food groups (sugar) to the exclusion of others (vegetables) Allergic response to certain foods Constant use of fad diets to lose weight Use of drugs or chemicals that interfere with appetite or nutrient assimilation Presence of emotional disorder (depression, anorexia, manic response) that interferes with food ingestion
Meal patterns	3–6 home-prepared meals/day Adequate time and calm atmosphere for meals	Fast-food or packaged foods Missed meals, constant snacking, or overeating Eating "on the run" or hurried
Physical factors	Adequate chewing and swallowing capability Mouth and gums healthy so food can be ingested Physical exercise adequate for calorie intake	Teeth or gums in poor condition or ill-fitting dentures Swallowing impairs ingestion Inadequate physical exercise to burn calories
Presence of disease	No disease process that interferes with nutrient assimilation No congenital condition or postsurgery condition that interferes with nutrient assimilation	Disease present that interferes with ingestion, digestion, assimilation, or excretion Congenital condition, rehabilitation phase, or postsurgery that interferes with food assimilation
Sociocultural–religious factors	Ability to afford adequate foods in all food categories Cultural beliefs that do not eliminate whole food groups Religious beliefs that do not eliminate whole food groups Food does not lose all nutrient value in preparation	Economic position that precludes purchase of adequate food Religious or cultural beliefs that interfere with receiving balanced diet (macrobiotic diets) Inadequate knowledge, experience, or intelligence to prepare healthy meals
Elimination schedule	Regular, adequate elimination of foods Absence of constant flatus, discharge, or mucus	Irregular or painful elimination Presence of constant flatus Presence of discharge, blood, or mucus

Nutritional Problems in the Hospital

In a hospital, nutrition is frequently neglected as a viable component of client care. Studies conducted at various medical centers support the claim that clients become more malnourished the longer they remain in a hospital.

For clients who seem to be stable on admission and give no history of nutritionally related food problems, the usual hospital diet is adequate; however, these clients must be reassessed periodically to prevent nutritional problems from developing. A periodic assessment is especially important for clients hospitalized for a long time. In many long-term care facilities, clients are weighed monthly.

For clients identified as having a nutritional problem, a nursing care plan must be developed. To treat these clients correctly, the cause of depletion must first be determined. Research indicates that poor food intake is the leading cause of malnutrition. Reasons for poor food intake include fear, anxiety, or depression prior to or during hospitalization. Some clients may not be capable of feeding themselves or may have poorly fitting dentures. Treatment and therapy may limit a client's ability to eat or interfere with his or her appetite. Also, some clients may have the desire to eat and a good appetite, but shortly after eating a certain food, have cramps, pain, gas, or diarrhea or feel nauseous or vomit. This eventually leads to less food intake. Whatever the source, the cause of depletion must be determined to prevent further malnutrition. As clients become more and more malnourished, they lose the ability to handle foodstuffs metabolically. As their intake decreases below their nutritional requirements, their body cannot regenerate the epithelium of the gastrointestinal tract from the crypt cells. The villi and microvilli, needed to metabolize and absorb food, flatten and become ineffective. This leads to malabsorption, resulting in further malnutrition.

Therapeutic Management

After determining the cause and the extent of depletion, the next step is to institute therapeutic procedures that meet the needs of the client. In selecting nutrients, the clinician needs to evaluate the status of the client's gastrointestinal tract to determine if modifications in nutrients are necessary. For example, can the client split intact protein into the peptides and amino acids needed for absorption? Can the client tolerate the osmotic load of monosaccharides or disaccharides? Is the client fat-intolerant, or does he or she need special fat? Is the client lactose-intolerant? Can the client eat normally?

Most of us consider that eating and meal time is a social time. Frequently, however, nurses place clients in uncomfortable and even unsocial positions so that eating is not a pleasure. In preparing the client's environment for eating, try to make him or her as comfortable as possible. For example, it is important to plan painful or uncomfortable procedures so that they are not immediately before or after meals. Position the client as near to normal as possible; that is, sitting in a chair, dangling on the side of the bed, or with the bed elevated 90°. Provide a bright, nonodorous environment. If possible, position roommates so they can converse while eating if they so desire. Check the client care plan for client preferences: cultural or religious limitations as well as allergies and personal likes or dislikes. Food trays should be checked for compliance with orders and client preferences. If the client is n.p.o., be sure that a sign is posted on the unit door and that the client does *not* receive a tray.

When you are preparing to assist the client to eat, lower the side rail and place the tray table over the client's lap low enough so that he or she can see what is on it. If the tray is not neatly arranged, rearrange it. Food appearance and presentation influence appetite. Assist the client with whatever is needed, such as cutting meat. If the client is unable to drink from a glass, provide a straw or special cup.

Be sensitive to the client's response to food, and continually attempt to orient feeding to meet the client's needs. If the client has diminished sight or is blind but able to feed him or herself, tell the client what is on the tray and the position of each item. Often, it is clearer to describe position of foods by a clock; for example, chicken at 12, green beans at 3 o'clock.

After therapeutic diets have been ordered, it is critical that the nurse be aware of compliance by the client. The nurse is most closely involved with the client and is the one who can best determine the client's actual intake. The nurse should ensure that the client is not receiving inappropriate foods from other sources and that the client is actually eating the foods prescribed. If the prescribed diet is not meeting the client's needs, an alternative method of feeding might be considered. For example, if oral feedings prove inadequate, then alternative methods, such as feeding by nasogastric, nasoduodenal, or nasojejunal tube, should be considered. A variety of delivery systems and methods of enteral feeding are now available for adequate care of the client. The particular choice should be based on the individual client's needs and requirements.

When other methods have failed, parenteral nutrition may be the management of choice. This can be administered peripherally, using isotonic concentrations of glucose, crystalline amino acids, and fats. It can also be administered through a central, high-flow vein in which hypertonic glucose, along with crystalline amino acids, fats, electrolytes, vitamins, and trace elements, may be given. This technique requires special handling and client care and is the most expensive method of feeding. It should be used only if the intestines do not work adequately, if the client is obstructed or has a fistula, if bowel rest is required, or if the client is so debilitated that the gastrointestinal tract is nonfunctional.

In this era of sophisticated medical and nursing management, no client should become or remain malnourished or develop any kind of nutritional problem. As a nurse, you are responsible for meeting the client's needs. Among these needs are adequate nutritional requirements to maintain status and to be able to successfully deal with or overcome the medical problems for which the client is being treated.

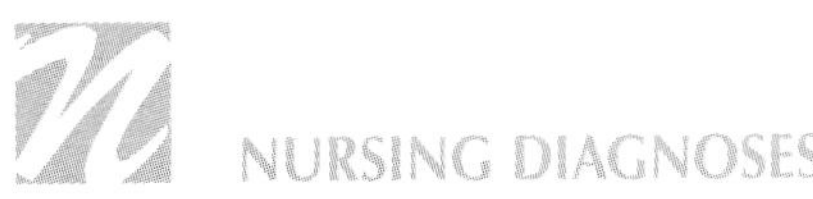

NURSING DIAGNOSES

The following nursing diagnoses may be appropriate to include in a client care plan when the components of the plan are related to nutritional problems or nutritional health maintenance.

NURSING DIAGNOSIS	RELATED FACTORS
Knowledge Deficit	Lack of appropriate dietary information, misinterpretation of information, cognitive limitation, inadequate motivation
Noncompliance	Chronic illness, disease-related symptoms, side effects of therapy, poor self-esteem
Altered Nutrition: Less than Body Requirements	Impaired swallowing, faulty metabolism, dysphagia, altered level of consciousness, inadequate absorption, eating disorders
Altered Nutrition: More than Body Requirements	Lack of basic nutritional knowledge, excessive intake in relation to metabolic requirements, decreased activity patterns, decreased metabolic needs, eating disorders

unit 1

NUTRITION MAINTENANCE

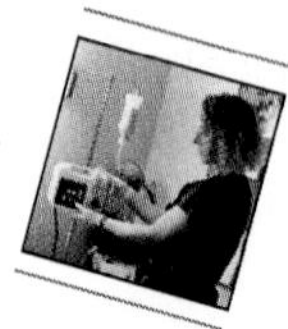

NURSING PROCESS DATA

ASSESSMENT Data Base

Check appropriate dietary order.
Assess client's nutritional needs.
Determine client's sociocultural orientation.
Obtain client's diet history, and determine eating habits and food preferences.
Assess client's ability to comply with diet regimen.
Assess client's fluid intake needs.
Check recommended daily dietary allowances and essential body nutrients.
Evaluate results of the following data:
  Analysis of appropriate diagnostic tests.
  Alterations in health status that indicate need for therapeutic vs. regular diet.
Status of GI tract, including digestion or absorption.
Client's ability to split intact protein into peptides and amino acids needed for absorption.
Client's ability to tolerate osmotic load of monosaccharides or disaccharides.
Client's ability to tolerate lactose.

PLANNING Objectives

To provide a nutritional diet based on individual needs
To identify the client who exhibits nutritional deficits and to determine an appropriate diet
To provide nutritional requirements for clients unable to consume oral feedings
To provide a diet that is tolerated physiologically and emotionally by the client

IMPLEMENTATION Procedures

Serving a Food Tray
Feeding a Client

EVALUATION Expected Outcomes

Client receives adequate diet, fluids, electrolytes, vitamins, minerals, and trace elements.
Reasonable compliance to diet is maintained.
Diet is tolerated physiologically and emotionally by client.

SERVING A FOOD TRAY

Equipment

Diet slip completed
Diet tray
Over-bed table
Utensils
Protective covering

Preparation

1. Assist physician in determining a diet appropriate for the client's needs.
2. Elicit food preferences of the client.
3. Send request to the diet kitchen for the specific diet, and keep diet sheets or diet rands up-to-date.
4. Check client care plan for changes in diet.
5. Medicate client for pain 20 minutes before eating.

6. Check all diet trays before serving to ensure the diet provided is the one ordered.
7. Ensure that hot food is hot and cold food is cold.
8. Keep food trays attractive. Avoid spilling liquids on tray.
9. Assist client to empty bladder if needed and wash hands.
10. Remove unpleasant objects from area, such as a bedpan.

Procedure

1. Wash your hands.
2. Raise bed to HIGH position, and lower side rail.
3. Assist client to sitting position if possible.
4. Place protective covering over gown if desired.
5. Place tray on tray table. Position table so client can see food.
6. Assist client as needed (e.g. cut meat, open milk carton).
7. Check on client during meal to determine if assistance is necessary.
8. Reposition tray table at bedside when completed.
9. Provide hand cleaning and oral care if desired.
10. Offer bedpan or assistance to commode or bathroom.
11. Raise side rail.
12. Position bed for comfort.
13. Note amount of food eaten.
14. Remove food tray from room.
15. Wash your hands.
16. Chart amount eaten. If necessary, record I&O.

FEEDING A CLIENT

Procedure

1. Check client care plan for current changes in diet.
2. Wash your hands.
3. Raise bed to HIGH, and lower side rail.
4. Assist client to wash hands and face, if desired.
5. Place client in sitting position if possible.
6. Place protective covering over gown if desired.
7. Place tray on tray table. Position table so client can see food.
8. Stand or sit facing the client. Bed is in low position if you are sitting.
9. Ask client the order in which he or she wants to be fed.
10. Feed a blind client using the following technique:
    a. Use the clock system by describing food arrangement on the plate.
    b. Tell the client the time on the clock at which food is placed, for example, "The corn is at 4 o'clock and the chicken is at 8 o'clock."
    c. Encourage the client to feed him or herself, but remain with client if possible.
11. Encourage the client to hold glass, bread, finger foods.
12. Allow client time to chew and swallow.
13. Provide fluids throughout meal.
14. Alternate foods; don't feed all meat then all vegetable.
15. Allow client to rest at intervals during the feeding.
16. Talk with client during meal. **Rationale:** Talking with the client makes mealtime more pleasant and encourages client not to hurry.
17. Reposition tray table at bedside when completed.
18. Provide hand cleaning and oral care if desired.
19. Raise side rail.
20. Position bed for comfort. Lower bed if it is raised.
21. Note amount of food eaten.
22. Remove food tray from room.
23. Wash your hands.
24. Chart amount eaten. If necessary, record I&O.

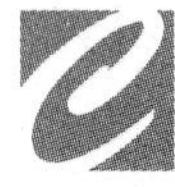

CHARTING for Nutrition Maintenance

- Appetite
- Food intake
- Tolerance to diet
- Weight
- I&O fluid status

CRITICAL THINKING APPLICATION

CLINICAL PROBLEMS	CRITICAL THINKING OPTIONS
■ Client is unable to assimilate foods metabolically.	• Document on client care plan, and make staff report of abnormal results of diagnostic tests which identify assimilation problems. Assist the physician in altering the method of feeding (enteral or parenteral).
■ Client vomits or has diarrhea.	• Evaluate allergic responses to food. Review history and physical to determine any existing food allergies. • Obtain order for clear liquid diet, gradually progressing back to regular diet. • Assess overall health status (e.g., temperature, obstruction).
■ Psychosocial behavior interferes with eating.	• Modify diet to conform to client's desires. • Request consultation with dietician.

unit 2

THERAPEUTIC DIETS

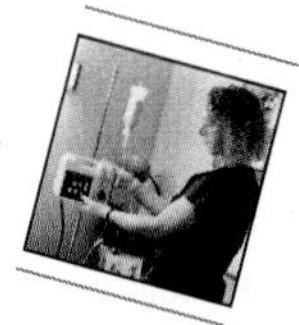

NURSING PROCESS DATA

ASSESSMENT Data Base

Assess total condition of client—physical, emotional, and mental status.

Determine appropriateness of prescribed therapeutic diet as related to altered state of health.

Evaluate ability of client to tolerate diet.

Assess client's mental state in regard to compliance with diet regimen.

Refer to general assessment steps in maintaining normal nutritional status.

PLANNING Objectives

To maintain balanced status

To meet nutritional needs based on alterations in client's health status

To allow client to tolerate foods and nutrients more efficiently

To design a therapeutic diet with which client will comply

IMPLEMENTATION Procedures

Providing Therapeutic Diets

Carbohydrate Control	*Fiber Control*
Protein Control	*Bland Food Diets*
Fat Control	*Calorie Control*
Renal Disease	*Pre- and Postoperative Diets*
Vitamin Control	*Mechanical Soft Diet*
Mineral Control	*Pureed Diet*

EVALUATION Expected Outcomes

Client complies with prescribed therapeutic diet.

Client tolerates diet well.

Disease symptoms diminish.

Client verbalizes knowledge of therapeutic diet.

Therapeutic diet conforms to ethnic preferences.

Therapeutic diet can be implemented in home setting.

PROVIDING THERAPEUTIC DIETS

Procedures

Carbohydrate Control

1. Hypoglycemia occurs when the supply of insulin is so high that most of the glucose moves from blood into the cells and leaves inadequate supply for the brain.
   a. Foods prescribed are high in protein and high in fat, and have only moderate amounts of complex carbohydrates.
   b. Foods not allowed are simple carbohydrates; for example, sugar, syrup, candy.
2. A diabetic diet modifies the insulin disorder and controls sugar intake.
   a. Foods included on the diet are balanced and provide protein, fat, and carbohydrates in relation to an individual's needs.
   b. Foods not allowed are refined sugars.

Protein Control

1. A low-protein diet is used in case of renal impair-

ment (uremia), hepatic coma, and cirrhosis (according to individual requirements).
   a. Control end products of protein metabolism by limiting protein intake.
   b. Evaluate the number of grams of protein allowed.
   c. Eliminate high-protein foods, such as eggs, meat, milk, and milk products.
2. A high-protein diet is necessary for tissue building, correction of protein deficiencies, burns, liver diseases, malabsorption syndromes, undernutrition, and maternity.
   a. Correct protein loss or maintain and rebuild tissues by increasing intake of high-quality protein food sources.
   b. Encourage the eating of high-protein foods, such as fish, fowl, organs and meats, and dairy products.
   c. Suggest protein supplements (usually ordered by physician), such as Sustagen, Meritene, and Proteinum.
3. An amino acid metabolism abnormality diet is used for phenylketonuria (PKU), galactosemia, and lactose intolerance.
   a. Reduce or eliminate the offending enzyme in the food intake of protein, and use substitute nutrient foods.
   b. Avoid milk and milk products as they constitute the main source of enzymes for the three diseases.
   c. Employ substitutes to meet daily allowances.

Fat Control

1. A restricted cholesterol diet is used to manage cardiovascular diseases, diabetes mellitus, and high-serum cholesterol levels.
   a. Control the blood cholesterol level or maintain blood cholesterol at a normal level by restricting foods high in cholesterol.
   b. Limit high-cholesterol foods, such as egg yolk, shellfish, organ meats, bacon, pork, avocado, and olives.
   c. Encourage low-cholesterol foods, such as vegetable oils, raw or cooked vegetables, fruits, lean meats, and fowl.
2. A modified fat diet is used according to individual tolerance in malabsorption syndromes, cystic fibrosis, gallbladder disease, obstructive jaundice, and liver disease.
   a. Attempt to lower fat content in diet to reduce irritation of diseased organs and to reduce fat content where there is inadequate absorption of fat.
   b. Low-fat diet: Avoid such foods as gravies, fatty meat and fish, cream, fried foods, rich pastries, whole-milk products, cream soups, salad and cooking oils, nuts, and chocolate. Allow eggs (2–3 per week), lean meat, and small amount of butter or margarine.
   c. Fat-free diet: Allow vegetables, fruits, lean meats, fowl, fish, bread, and cereal and restrict all fatty meats and fat.
3. A high-polyunsaturated-fat diet is used to manage cardiovascular diseases.
   a. Reduce intake of saturated fats, and increase intake of foods rich in polyunsaturated fats. (Physician usually prescribes caloric level as well as restrictions.)
   b. Avoid foods originating from animal sources, selected peanuts, olives, avocado, coconuts, chocolate, and cashew nuts.
   c. Allow foods originating from vegetable sources (except for those named above), margarine; corn, soybean, and safflower oils; fresh ground peanut butter; and nuts (except cashews).

Renal Disease

1. A low-protein diet and essential amino acid diet (modified Giovannetti diet) comprises 20 g of protein and 1500 mg of potassium.
   a. Prevent electrolytes and byproducts of metabolism from accumulating to a fatal level between artificial kidney treatments.
   b. Allow foods such as one egg daily, 6 ounces of milk, low-protein bread, fruit, vegetables, butter, oil, jelly, candy, tea, and coffee.
   c. Restrict foods such as meat, chicken, fish, peanuts, and high-protein bread.
2. A low-calcium diet is used to prevent formation of renal calculi.
   a. Decrease the total daily intake of calcium to prevent further stone formation. Total calcium intake is 400 mg per day instead of 800 mg (normal).
   b. Allow foods such as milk (1 cup daily), juices, tea, coffee, eggs, and fresh fruits and vegetables.
   c. Restrict foods such as rye and whole-grain breads and cereals, dried fruits and vegetables, fish, shellfish, cheese, chocolate, and nuts.
3. An acid ash diet is used to prevent precipitation of stone elements.

TABLE 18–3. Foods Rich in Vitamins

Foods Rich in Fat-Soluble Vitamins	Foods Rich in Water-Soluble Vitamins
Vitamin A—liver, egg yolk, whole milk, butter, fortified margarine, green and yellow vegetables, fruits Vitamin D—fortified milk and margarines, sunshine, fish oils Vitamin E—vegetable oils and green vegetables Vitamin K—egg yolk, leafy green vegetables, liver, cheese	Vitamin C—citrus fruits, tomatoes, broccoli, cabbage Thiamine (B_1)—lean meat, such as beef, pork, liver; whole-grain cereals and legumes Riboflavin (B_2)—milk, organ meats, enriched grains Niacin—meat, beans, peas, peanuts, enriched grains Pyridoxine (B_6)—yeast, wheat, corn, meats, liver, and kidney Cobalamin (B_{12})—lean meat, liver, kidney Folic acid—leafy green vegetables, eggs, liver

a. Establish a well-balanced diet in which the total acid ash is greater than the total alkaline ash daily.
b. Allow foods such as breads and cereals of any type, fats, fruits (one serving), vegetables, meat, eggs, cheese, fish, fowl (two servings), and spices.
c. Restrict foods such as carbonated beverages, dried fruits, bananas, figs, raisins, dried beans, carrots, chocolate, nuts, olives, and pickles.

4. A low-purine diet is used to prevent uric acid stones; also used to treat gout.
   a. Restrict purine, which is the precursor of uric acid; 4% of urinary stones are composed of uric acid.
   b. Allow foods such as milk, tea, fruit juices, carbonated beverages, breads, cereals, cheese, eggs, fat, and most vegetables.
   c. Restrict foods such as glandular meats, gravies, fowl, fish, and high meat quantities.

Vitamin Control

1. An increased vitamin diet is necessary for treatment of specific vitamin deficiencies (Table 18–3).
   a. Provide high-vitamin diet for clients with burns, healing wounds, raised temperatures, and infections. Also used for pregnant clients.
   b. Evaluate diseases, such as cystic fibrosis and liver disease, that require water-soluble vitamins.
2. Total low-vitamin diets are not generally prescribed—although specific vitamins might be decreased for periods of illness.

Mineral Control

1. A restricted sodium diet is used to manage hypertension, hepatitis, congestive heart failure, renal deficiencies, cirrhosis of liver, and adrenal corticoid treatment (Table 18–4).
   a. Correct or control the retention of sodium and water in the body by limiting sodium intake. May be done by restriction of salt in the diet or in combination with medications.
   b. Restrict salt in cooking or at the table. In clients requiring dietary modification in salt intake any product containing sodium, such as soda bicarbonate, may be prohibited.
   c. Explain sodium restrictions in diet.
      Mild: 2–3 g sodium

TABLE 18–4. Foods High in Sodium and Potassium

Foods High in Sodium
Table salt and all prepared salts, such as celery salt
Smoked meats and salted meats
Most frozen vegetables or canned vegetables with added salt
Butter, margarines, and cheese
Quick-cooking cereals
Shellfish, and frozen or salted fish
Seasonings and sauces
Canned soups
Chocolates and cocoa
Beets, celery, and selected greens (spinach)
Anything with salt added, such as potato chips, popcorn
Foods High in Potassium
Fruit juices, such as orange, grapefruit, banana, raw apple
Instant, dry coffee powder
Egg, legumes, whole grains
Fish, fresh halibut, codfish
Pork, beef, lamb, veal, chicken
Milk, skim and whole
Dried dates, prunes
Bouillon and meat broths

Moderate: 1000 mg sodium
Strict: 500 mg sodium
Severe: 250 mg sodium

2. An increased potassium diet is used to manage diabetic acidosis, extended use of certain diuretic drugs, burns (after first 48 hours), vomiting, and fevers (Table 18–4).
   a. Replace potassium loss from the body with specific foods high in potassium or a potassium supplement. (Severe loss is managed with intravenous therapy.)
   b. Avoid no specific foods unless there is a sodium restriction because some foods high in potassium are also high in sodium.
3. A high-iron diet is used to manage anemias (hemorrhage, nutritional, pernicious), postgastrectomy syndrome, and malabsorption syndrome.
   a. Replace a deficit of iron caused by inadequate intake or chronic blood loss.
   b. Include foods high in iron content, such as organ meats (especially liver), meat, egg yolks, whole-wheat products, seafood, leafy vegetables, nuts, dried fruit, and legumes.

Fiber Control

1. A high-residue (roughage) diet is prescribed to treat constipation and diverticulosis.
   a. Suggest foods high in residue, such as any meat or fish, cheese, fat, milk, whole-wheat breads, cereals, and especially unrefined bran.
   b. Instruct client that foods low in carbohydrates are usually high in residue.
2. A low-residue diet is used to manage ulcerative colitis, postoperative colon and rectal surgery, diverticulitis (when inflammation decreases, diet may revert to high residue), rheumatic fever, diarrhea, and enteritis.
   a. Inform client that low-residue foods are ground meat, fish, broiled chicken without skin, creamed cheeses, limited fat, warm drinks, refined strained cereals, and white bread.
   b. Instruct client that foods high in carbohydrates are usually low in residue.

Bland Food Diets

1. A bland diet is used to promote the healing of the gastric mucosa by eliminating food sources that are chemically and mechanically irritating (Table 18–5). Bland diets are used to manage duodenal ulcers, gastric ulcers, and postoperative stomach surgery.

TABLE 18–5. Bland Diet Allowances

1. Foods allowed
   Milk, butter, eggs (not fried), custard, vanilla ice cream, cottage cheese
   Cooked refined or strained cereal, enriched white bread
   Gelatin; homemade creamed, pureed soups
   Baked or broiled potatoes
2. Examples of foods that are eliminated
   Spicy and highly seasoned foods
   Raw foods
   Very hot and very cold foods
   Gas-forming foods (varies with individuals)
   Coffee, alcoholic beverages, carbonated drinks
   High-fat contents (some butter and margarine allowed)

   a. Instruct client that bland diets are presented in stages with the gradual addition of certain foods.
   b. Provide frequent, small feedings during active stress periods.
2. Establish regular meals and food patterns when condition permits.

Calorie Control

1. A restricted calorie diet reduces the caloric intake of food below the energy demands of the body so weight loss occurs.
   a. Provide psychologic support and exercise.
   b. Restrict such foods as refined sugars and fats.
2. An increased calorie diet is used to meet the increased metabolic needs of the body. There is usually an increase in protein and vitamins when increased calories are ordered.

Pre- and Postoperative Diets

1. A high-protein preoperative diet is essential for the maintenance of normal serum protein levels during and following surgery. This diet also restores nitrogen balance for protein-depleted clients (e.g., burn victims, the elderly, and severely debilitated).
   a. Provide adequate carbohydrates to maintain liver glycogen and adequate amino acids to promote wound healing.
   b. Provide a 2500-calorie diet that is high in carbohydrates, moderate in protein with high-protein supplements.
   c. Instruct client that an elemental diet is low in residue and contains a synthetic mixture of carbon, hydrogen, and oxygen; amino acids; and

TABLE 18–6. Recommended Nutrient Requirements

Total calories per day:
2800 for tissue repair
6000 for extensive repair
Protein:
40–50 g/day average person
50–75 g/day early in postoperative period
100–200 g/day if needed for new tissue synthesis
Carbohydrates:
55–60% of calories—sufficient in quantity to meet calorie needs and allow protein to be used for tissue repair
Fat:
25–30%—not excessive as it leads to poor tissue healing and susceptibility to infection
Vitamins:
Vitamin C—up to 1 g/day for tissue repair
Vitamin B—increased above normal for stress management
Vitamin A—adjuncts autoimmune system
Vitamin E—increases O_2 to tissues
Minerals:
Zinc—tissue repair
Selenium—cell repair
Calcium/magnesium—relaxes nerves and maintains electric stimulation

essential fatty acids with added minerals and vitamins. It is bulk-free and easily assimilated and absorbed.

2. A special postoperative surgical diet is necessary to promote wound healing, avoid shock from decreased plasma proteins and circulating red blood cells, prevent edema, and promote bone healing (Table 18–6).
   a. Provide 2800 total calories for tissue repair and 6000 calories for extensive repair.
   b. Fluid intake is 2000–3000 mL/day for uncomplicated surgery and 3000–4000 mL/day for sepsis or renal damage. Seriously ill clients with drainage can require up to 7000 mL/day.
3. A postoperative diet protocol progresses from nothing by mouth the day of surgery to a general diet within a few days following surgery. Foods allowed in each phase of the progressive diet include those listed here.
   a. A clear-liquid diet is 1000–1500 mL/day and comprises water, tea, broth, gelatin, and juices (apple, cranberry), or clear soda pop. Avoid juices with pulp.
   b. A full-liquid diet is clear liquids, milk and milk products, custard, puddings, creamed soups, sherbet, ice cream, and any fruit juice.
   c. A surgical soft diet is full liquid and pureed vegetables, eggs (not fried), milk, cheese, fish, fowl, tender beef, veal, potatoes, and cooked fruit. Do not include gas-formers.
   d. General diet: Take into consideration specific alterations necessary for client's health status.

Mechanical Soft Diet

1. A mechanical soft diet is used when clients
   a. Are edentulous.
   b. Have poorly fitted dentures.
   c. Have difficulty chewing.
   d. Do not chew food thoroughly.
2. Any food that can be easily broken down can be included in this diet. It allows clients variations in tastes that are not allowed on a soft diet (chili beans).

Pureed Diet

1. A pureed diet provides food that has been blenderized to a smooth consistency.
   a. Mainly used for clients with dysphagia or those who are unable to chew
   b. Often used with small babies
   c. Some hospitals provide this type of diet for gastrostomy feedings.
2. When assisting clients with this type of diet, talk with them about the meal, describing the different foods. **Rationale:** When the texture is all the same, distinguishing between foods is difficult.
3. Do not mix all pureed food together or feed out of one bowl or dish. Try to keep foods separate and feed alternately, with dessert last.

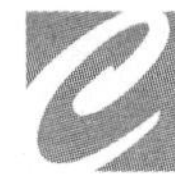

CHARTING for Therapeutic Diets

- Daily weight
- Appetite
- Client's response to diet
- Client's compliance
- Reasons for noncompliance

CRITICAL THINKING APPLICATION

CLINICAL PROBLEMS	CRITICAL THINKING OPTIONS
Client is noncompliant to diet.	• Elicit client's feelings to determine exactly what is behind the noncompliance. • Check method of diet preparation and administration to see if it is attractive and appealing. • Ensure that environment is conducive to eating. • Notify dietician to discuss diet with client.
Diet is not appropriate to disease status.	• Notify physician to change diet. • Meet with dietician to modify diet. • Modify diet within prescribed limits to enhance tolerance.

unit 3 NUTRIENTS VIA TUBE FEEDING

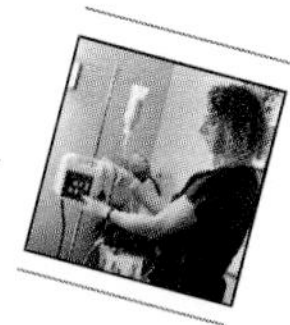

NURSING PROCESS DATA

ASSESSMENT Data Base

Assess overall status:
- Weight change
- Temperature
- Presence of sepsis
- Trauma
- Mental state
- Other medically related nutritional problems (e.g., diabetes, hyperlipidemia, alcoholism)

Evaluate oral intake and diet history. Is it adequate, moderate, or altered?

Assess nutritional requirements. Are they being met or not being met? Does the client have special needs?

Assess status of GI tract. Is it normal, limited, or obstructed? Is there a fistula or ostomy present?

Assess capacity to chew and swallow.

Assess patency of nares.

Check for presence of gag reflex.

Evaluate respiratory or thoracic conditions.

Check for renal complications.

Check for vomiting or diarrhea.

With high-protein diets, assess for fluid and electrolyte imbalance.

PLANNING Objectives

To provide alternative means of ingesting nutrients for clients with functional gastrointestinal tract

To intervene in preexisting or impending nutritional depletion from debilitation

To provide aggressive management for certain disease conditions (anorexia)

To provide means of nutrition if there is an inability to swallow or an existing obstruction in upper alimentary canal

To provide nutrients for client in comatose or semiconscious state

To provide increased nutrient requirements above oral consumption

To provide nutrients for postoperative clients with bowel sounds present

To maintain fluid and electrolyte balance

IMPLEMENTATION Procedures

Inserting a Nasogastric Tube

Irrigating a Nasogastric Tube

Collecting a Gastric Specimen from Nasogastric Tube

Removing a Nasogastric Tube

Giving an Intermittent Nasogastric Feeding

Feeding via Continuous Nasogastric Method

Giving a Gastrostomy Feeding

Inserting a Small-Bore Feeding Tube (Keofeed, Dobbhuff, Moss)

EVALUATION Expected Outcomes

Client tolerates feeding well, and weight is maintained or increased.

Appropriate residual is obtained from aspiration of stomach contents.

Client complies with feeding procedure.

Intake and output balance is maintained.

Nasogastric tube functions efficiently and remains patent.

INSERTING A NASOGASTRIC TUBE

Equipment

Portable suction equipment available
Number 6, 8, 12 Levin tube
Water-soluble lubricant
Hypoallergenic tape
pH chemstrip
Towel
Flashlight
Emesis basin
Stethoscope
Tongue blade
Glass of water
20-mL syringe or asepto syringe
Disposable irrigation set (optional)
Clean gloves

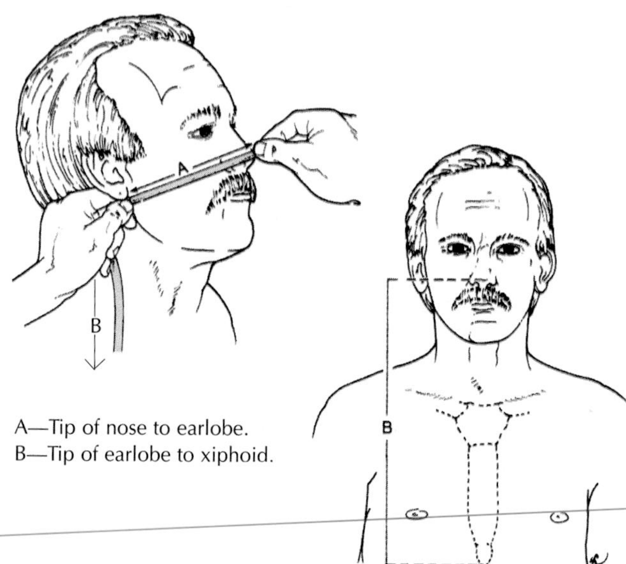

A—Tip of nose to earlobe.
B—Tip of earlobe to xiphoid.

Measure NG tube from tip of nose to earlobe to xiphoid process.

Preparation

1. Check order and client care plan for inserting a nasogastric tube.
2. Determine size of catheter based on length of time it will remain in place, client size, and viscosity of feeding solution.
3. Discuss procedure with client. **Rationale:** Demonstration and display of items to be used helps to allay client's fear and to gain cooperation.
4. Provide privacy.

Procedure

1. Wash hands. Don clean gloves.
2. Position client at 45° angle or higher with head elevated.
3. Examine nostrils, and select the most patent nostril by having client breathe through each one.
4. Measure from tip of nose to earlobe to xiphoid process of sternum to determine appropriate length for tube insertion. If tube is to go below stomach, add an additional 15–25 cm. Mark point on tube with tape.

> **CLINICAL ALERT**
>
> Nurses never insert or withdraw a nasogastric tube for clients with gastric resections. The suture line could easily be interrupted, and hemorrhage could occur.

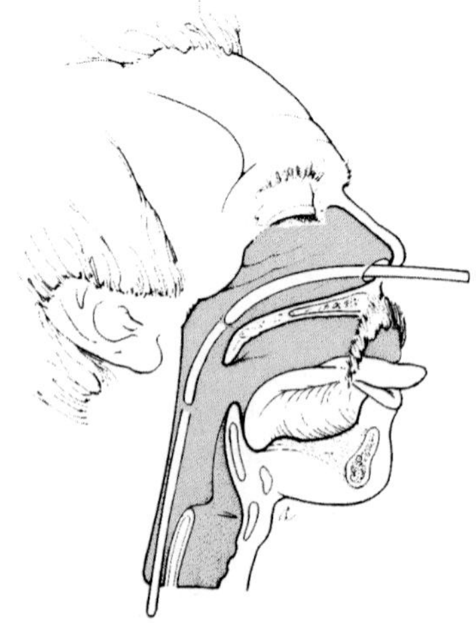

Use flashlight to check NG placement.

5. Lubricate first 4 inches of tube with water-soluble lubricant.
6. Insert tube through nostril to back of throat. Aim the tube toward back of throat and down. Suggest client swallow to assist tube insertion. **Rationale:** Sips of water may aid in pushing tube past oropharynx.
7. Instruct client to flex head toward chest. **Rationale:** This position assists in tube insertion after tube has passed through nasopharynx and reduces risk of tube entering trachea.
8. Use flash- or penlight to locate tip of tube at back of throat.
9. Continue advancing tube, giving the client sips of water, until taped mark is reached.

■ CLINICAL ALERT

It is no longer considered safe practice to hold the proximal end of the NG tube in a glass of water while asking the client to breathe. This was done to observe if bubbling occurred indicating that the tube was in the lung. Air can be trapped in the stomach and cause bubbling to occur when the nasogastric tube is inserted.

10. Check position of tube. **Rationale:** This ensures tube has not gone into the lungs.
    a. Aspirate gastric contents and check pH. If below 3, tube is in stomach. (Intestinal sites indicate a pH range of 6–7.) *Note:* This is the preferred method of safety for determining tube position.
    b. Inject 10 mL of air through nasogastric tube, and listen with the stethoscope over stomach for a rush of air.
    c. X-ray confirmation. **Rationale:** If nasoduodenal or nasojejunal feedings are required, client should have an x-ray to confirm correct placement. Passage through the pylorus may require several days.
11. Tape tube securely to nose. **Rationale:** When tube is taped securely, no tissue trauma will be caused by pull on sides of nostril.
    a. Cut tape about 4 inches long.
    b. Split one end of tape lengthwise (about 2 inches).
    c. Place unsplit end of tape over bridge of nose with bifurcated ends hanging free.

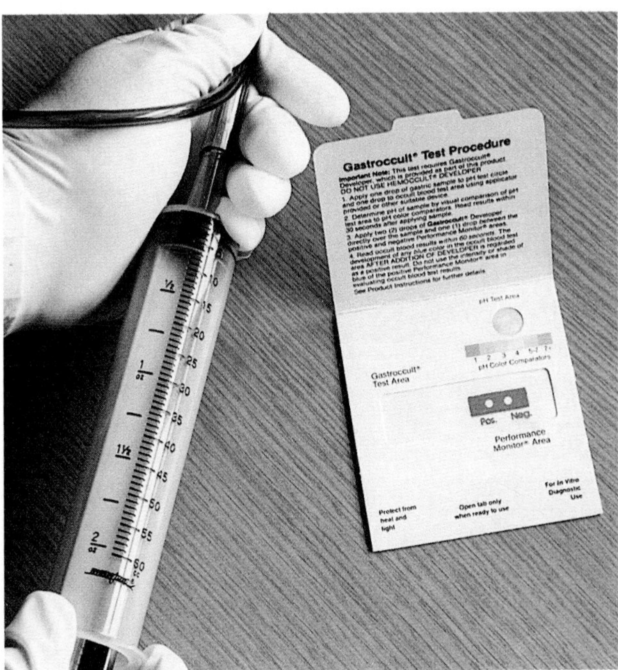

Check pH of gastric contents to validate placement.

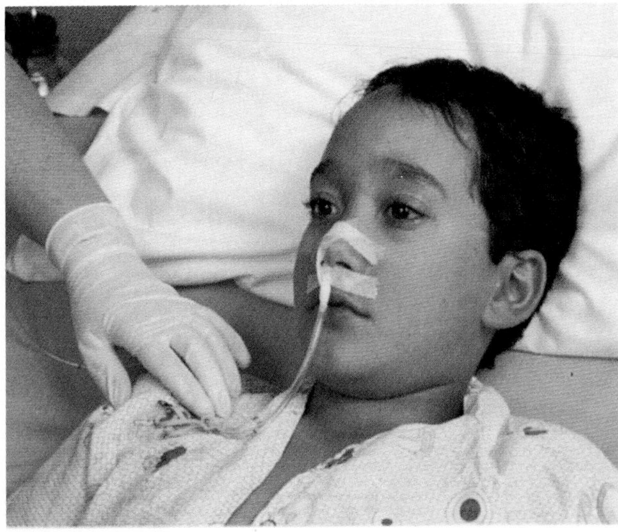
Tape NG tube securely to nose.

    d. Wrap each end of tape around the tube as it exits from the nose.
12. Secure tube with clamp or pin to client's gown or bed linen, leaving some degree of slack for head movement.
13. Remove gloves.
14. Position client for comfort.

IRRIGATING A NASOGASTRIC TUBE

Equipment

Disposable irrigation set
Emesis basin
Clean towel
20–50 mL syringe
Normal saline irrigation solution
I&O record sheet
Clean gloves

Preparation

1. Check orders and client care plan.
2. Wash hands.
3. Provide privacy.
4. Explain procedure to client.

Procedure

1. Place client in semi-Fowler's position.
2. Don clean gloves.
3. Place towel under NG tube to protect sheets.
4. Check for nasogastric tube placement by following step 10 in previous skill. **Rationale:** Solution could be instilled in lungs if NG tube is not in the stomach.
5. Draw up 20 mL normal saline into irrigating syringe (amount varies with physician's orders).
6. Gently instill the normal saline into the nasogastric tube or allow solution to flow in by gravity. Do not force the solution.
7. Withdraw the 20-mL irrigation solution and empty into basin.
8. Repeat the procedure twice. **Rationale:** Irrigating the tube once is not sufficient to clear the tube.
9. Record on I&O sheet the irrigation solution that has not been returned.
10. Remove gloves, and position client.

■ CLINICAL ALERT

If NG tube is connected to suction, disconnect tube from suction before beginning irrigation procedure, then reconnect to suction machine following irrigation.

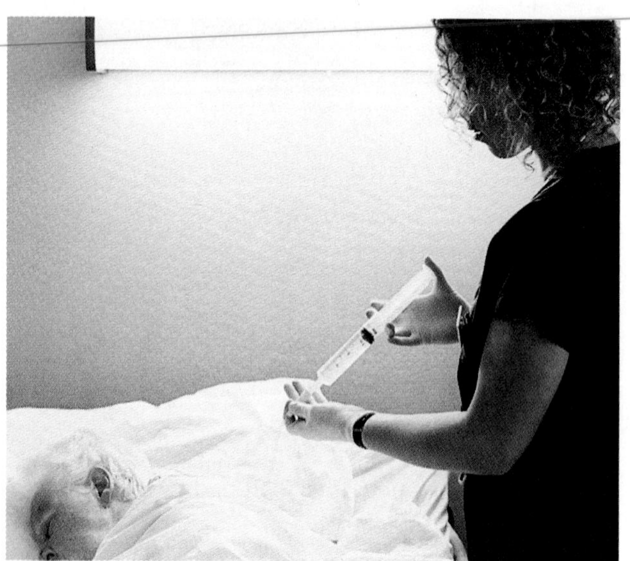

Irrigate NG tube using 20 mL of normal saline.

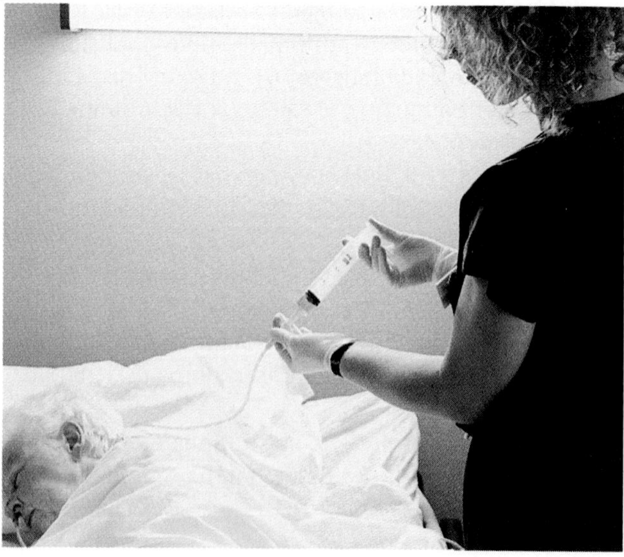

Repeat irrigation procedure twice to clear tube.

COLLECTING A GASTRIC SPECIMEN FROM NASOGASTRIC TUBE

Equipment

20-mL syringe
Specimen container
Requisition slip
Label
Clean gloves

Procedure

1. Check physician's orders or client care plan.
2. Wash your hands, and don clean gloves.
3. Place client in supine or left lateral side-lying position. **Rationale:** These positions allow secretions to "pool" near cardiac sphincter.
4. Unclamp or unplug nasogastric tube. Stand plug with flat end down on over-bed table.
5. Attach 20-mL syringe to tube.
6. Pull back on plunger of syringe to aspirate gastric contents.
7. Pinch tube, and remove syringe.
8. Reclamp or replug tube.
9. Expel aspirated contents into specimen container.
10. Reposition client for comfort.
11. Dispose of equipment from bedside.
12. Remove gloves and wash your hands.
13. Label specimen container, affix requisition, and send container to lab.

REMOVING A NASOGASTRIC TUBE

Equipment

Tube plug or clamp
Towel
Wash cloth
Paper towel
Clean gloves

Procedure

1. Check physician's orders and client care plan.
2. Wash your hands, and don clean gloves.
3. Place towel over client's chest.
4. Clamp or plug tube.
5. Unpin tube from gown.
6. Loosen tape securing tube.
7. Take paper towel in nondominant hand, and place under chin.
8. Pinch tube near nostril, and remove with a continuous steady pull. As tube is being removed, hold tube in paper towel. **Rationale:** This action prevents secretions from falling on linen.
9. Clean client's face, especially nares.
10. Offer oral hygiene.
11. Assist client to a comfortable position.
12. Dispose of equipment in trash.
13. Remove gloves, and wash your hands.

GIVING AN INTERMITTENT NASOGASTRIC FEEDING

Equipment

20–50 mL syringe
Tray
Feeding bag if used or Graduate
Formula
Water to follow feeding
Clean gloves

Preparation

1. Obtain order from physician for appropriate formula (calories or amount or both).
2. Send requisition for formula to diet kitchen.
3. Check early in shift to ensure adequate formula is available.
4. Warm formula to room temperature by placing formula in basin of hot water.
5. Assemble feeding equipment. If using bag, fill with ordered amount of formula.

6. Wash hands, and explain procedure to client. Ensure privacy.

Procedure

1. Don clean gloves.
2. Place client on right side in high-Fowler's position. Assess for abdominal distention and bowel sounds.
3. Aspirate stomach contents to determine amount of residual. **Rationale:** If residual is over 50–100 mL (or according to hospital policy), hold feeding until residual diminishes.
4. Return aspirated contents to stomach. **Rationale:** This prevents electrolyte imbalance.
5. Pinch the tubing. **Rationale:** This procedure prevents air from entering stomach.
6. Remove plunger from barrel of syringe, and attach barrel to nasogastric tube.
7. Fill syringe with formula. (If using feeding bag, adjust drip rate to infuse over 30 minutes. Usually drop factor on feeding bags is 20 drops/mL. Most bags do not give a calculated drip factor).
8. Hold container no more than 18 inches above client. **Rationale:** Holding container too high increases flow rate.
9. Allow formula to infuse slowly (between 20 and 35 minutes) through the tubing. Do not allow syringe to "run dry." **Rationale:** If syringe runs dry before the addition of more formula, it may cause gas.
10. Follow tube feeding with water in amount ordered. **Rationale:** Water cleans tube and prevents obstruction with formula.
11. Clamp end of the tube.
12. Wash, rinse, and dry equipment after each feeding.
13. Return equipment to client's bedside.
14. Give water between feedings, p.o. or per tube, if tube feeding is sole source of nutrition.
15. Provide oral hygiene.

FEEDING VIA CONTINUOUS NASOGASTRIC METHOD

Equipment

Feeding bag
Pump
Formula

Preparation

Follow steps 1 through 6 of the previous skill, *Giving an Intermittent Nasogastric Feeding.*

> **■ CLINICAL ALERT**
>
> Pour only enough formula for 4-hour infusion. Formula provides a positive medium for bacterial growth and is easily contaminated.

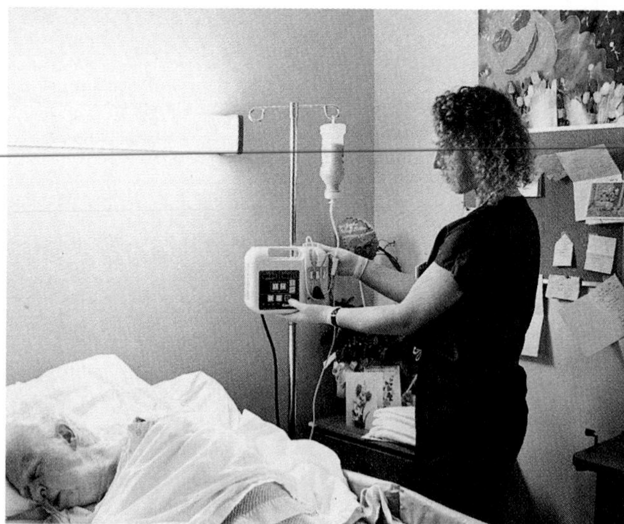
Monitor continuous NG feeding frequently.

Procedure

1. Identify client, and explain procedure.
2. Elevate head of bed 30° and keep it elevated at least 30° while tube feeding is infusing. **Rationale:** This position assists formula to go down and prevents regurgitation.
3. Check bowel sounds by listening for 1 minute. **Rationale:** Sounds indicate functioning bowel, necessary for feeding to be administered to avoid distention.
4. Check for tube placement at least every 4 hours

using procedure described in *Inserting a Nasogastric Tube.* **Rationale:** To ensure feeding tube remains in stomach.

5. Check residual at least every shift—aspirate should contain no more than 50–100 mL formula. If residual is above 100 mL, stop the feeding.
6. Return aspirate to stomach. **Rationale:** This prevents loss of electrolytes and HCl.
7. Attach feeding bag or bottle and tubing to IV pole.
8. Prime delivery tubing, and thread through feeding pump, if pump is used.
9. Attach tubing to proximal end of nasogastric tube.
10. Start feeding at prescribed rate (usually 10 mL/minute). Rate is slower than the first 4 hours.
11. Ensure infusion rate is kept at ordered rate throughout shift.
12. Monitor for signs of respiratory distress or diarrhea. **Rationale:** These are two complications associated with tube feedings: respiratory distress is an indication the tube is not in the sto[illegible] occurs as a result of infusing form[illegible]
13. Flush tubing with 30–60 mL, or pre[illegible] amount, of tap water every 4 hours. **R**[illegible] This prevents clogging of feeding tube.
14. Replace disposable feeding bag or bottle a[illegible] ing at least every 24 hours. Reusable bags a[illegible] ing are washed with soap and hot water every [illegible] hours. **Rationale:** Microorganisms accumulate i[illegible] pouch and tubing. It is best to use disposable equipment. If cost is an issue, washing equipment thoroughly decreases risk of multiplication of microorganisms.
15. Turn client every 2 hours. **Rationale:** This promotes digestion and prevents skin breakdown.
16. Provide oral hygiene frequently.
17. Record total amount of formula and water client has ingested.

GIVING A GASTROSTOMY FEEDING

Equipment

20–50 mL syringe
Graduate or feeding bag
Formula
Clean dressing

Preparation

1. Obtain order from physician for appropriate formula (calories or amount or both).
2. Send requisition for formula to diet kitchen.
3. Check early in shift to ensure adequate formula is available.
4. Warm formula to room temperature in basin of hot water.
5. Assemble feeding equipment. If using bag, fill with ordered amount of formula.

Procedure

1. Explain procedure to client and ensure privacy.
2. Place client on right side in high-Fowler's position. Assess for abdominal distention and bowel sounds.
3. Attach a syringe to gastrostomy tube, and release clamp.
4. Aspirate stomach contents to determine amount of residual. **Rationale:** If residual is over 50–100 mL (according to hospital policy), hold feeding until residual diminishes.
5. Return aspirated contents to stomach to prevent electrolyte imbalance. Flush tube with 2 ounces of water.
6. Pinch the tubing. **Rationale:** This procedure prevents air from entering stomach.
7. Remove plunger from barrel of syringe, and attach barrel to nasogastric tube.
8. Fill syringe with formula. (If using feeding bag, attach bag instead of barrel of syringe, adjust drip rate to infuse over 30 minutes.) Usually drop factor on feeding bags is 20 drops/mL. Most bags do not give a calculated drip factor.
9. Hold gastrostomy tubing straight up from insertion. **Rationale:** This position puts less stress on tube.
10. Allow formula to infuse slowly (20–35 minutes) through the tubing.
11. Clamp end of the tube, and remove syringe or feeding bag.
12. Remove dressing around gastrostomy opening.

condition.

ch feed-

16. Return equipment to client's bedside.
17. Give water between feedings if tube feeding is sole source of nutrition.

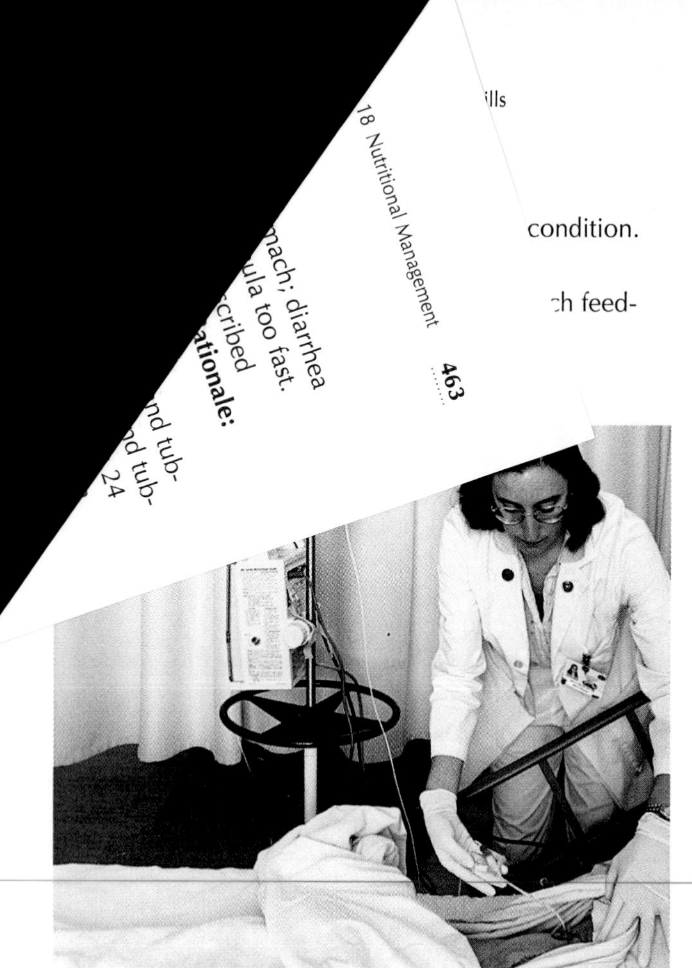

Gastrostomy feeding tube.

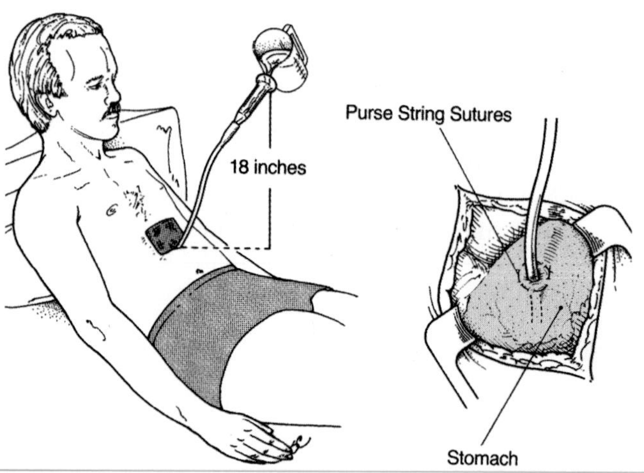

Hold gastrostomy tubing straight up from insertion and administer formula.

INSERTING A SMALL-BORE FEEDING TUBE (KEOFEED, DUBBHOFF, MOSS)

Equipment

Feeding tube package
Administration set with pump or controller
Clean gloves
Water-soluble lubricant
Micropore or adhesive tape
Glass with water and straw, if appropriate
Stethoscope
Flashlight

Procedure

1. Wash hands, and don gloves.
2. Explain procedure to client.
3. Elevate head of bed at least 45°. If possible, Fowler's position is best.
4. Determine length of tube for insertion into stomach. Use distal end of feeding tube, and measure from tip of nose to earlobe to xiphoid process. Place tape on tube to mark position.
5. Open adapter cap, snap off end of water vial, and inject water into feeding tube adapter. **Rationale:** This action activates Keolube lubricant in the tube lumen. Ensure that you have tight fit so water doesn't spill out of adapter site.
6. Close adapter cap over guide to hold in place.
7. Check that guide does not protrude through holes in feeding tube. Reposition guide as necessary.
8. Lubricate tip of feeding tube with water-soluble lubricant.
9. Assess nares to determine which nostril is most appropriate.
10. Instruct client to hyperextend neck.
11. Insert feeding tube through patent nostril. Ask client to swallow when tube reaches pharynx. (Stimulation of gag reflex is normal with tube insertion.)
12. Pull back on tube if client begins to cough or show signs of respiratory distress. **Rationale:** Tube has entered trachea not esophagus.

13. Wait several seconds, reinsert tube asking client to swallow when tube reaches pharynx.
14. Use flashlight to check position of tube at back of throat.
15. Advance tube to premeasured position.
16. Hold tube in place, open adapter cap, and slowly remove guide.
17. Tape tube in place.
18. Verify tube placement by x-ray if necessary. **Rationale:** When instilling formula, x-ray is a safety intervention to check placement.
19. Insert syringe into adapter, and gently pull back on plunger to aspirate stomach contents according to hospital policy.
20. Connect feeding tube to feeding administration set and pump.
21. Flush feeding tube with water every 4 hours as ordered or following administration of formula or medication. **Rationale:** This maintains patency of tube; small-bore tubes may become obstructed.
22. Check tape daily that secures tube to nostril. Keep clean.
23. Replace small-bore tube every 3–4 weeks or as ordered.
24. Administer daily mouth care to client.
25. Clean equipment, and replace after each feeding.
26. Remove gloves, and make client comfortable.

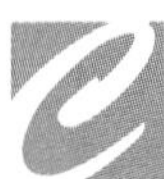

CHARTING for Tube Feeding

- Weight as ordered
- Residual obtained
- Nasogastric tube size if inserted
- Amount and type of irrigating solution used and results of nasogastric tube irrigation
- Rate and volume of feeding
- I&O
- Client's response, behavior, attitude toward feeding
- Client teaching given to encourage self-care

CRITICAL THINKING APPLICATION

CLINICAL PROBLEMS	CRITICAL THINKING OPTIONS
Client aspirates formula.	• Suction client. Evaluate respiratory status until normal breathing pattern resumes. • In future feedings, ensure that client is kept at a 30° angle or higher for at least 30 minutes following feeding.
Vomiting occurs.	• Position client quickly in high-Fowler's position (if not already) to prevent aspiration. • Suction immediately. • Assess concentration, amount, and rate with which formula was given. • Reduce rate or amount of formula infusion in future feedings.
Diarrhea	• Dilute feeding to half strength or change feeding formula (Client may be lactose-intolerant or have an allergy to formula). • Slow feeding time.

CLINICAL PROBLEMS	CRITICAL THINKING OPTIONS
■ Fluid and electrolyte imbalance occurs.	• Reevaluate procedure to make sure stomach contents were replaced after residual was checked. • Reassess formula concentration and amount of water given.
■ Stress ulcer develops in the GI tract from permanent tube placement.	• Check to see if the tube can be intermittently placed to avoid constant irritation. • Give antacids 1 hour after feeding. • Obtain gastric aspirant to test for blood before each feeding and monitor results.

GERIATRIC CONSIDERATIONS

Nutritional requirements of the elderly differ from those of younger adults.

Physical changes associated with aging affect nutritional status.

- Changes in the gastrointestinal tract, digestive enzymes, and metabolism affect nutritional status.
- Constipation is often a problem with the elderly so increased dietary fiber is important.
- As a person ages, the digestive enzymes in both the stomach (HCl) and intestines diminish. This condition affects the digestion and especially, the assimilation of nutrients, in addition to causing heartburn (a frequent complaint with the elderly).

Changes in the lifestyle of the elderly contribute to changes in the nutritional status.

- The sense of taste and smell decrease, thus the elderly are often less conscious of hunger and do not enjoy eating as much.
- Teeth are often in poor condition or dentures don't work properly, so certain foods must be eliminated from the diet.
- Physical disabilities or lack of mobility may hinder the elderly from purchasing or preparing groceries necessary for a balanced diet.
- Limited income may affect the buying of nutritious food.
- There may be a loss of interest in eating or lack of motivation when a person is living alone.
- Social isolation of loneliness may affect nutritional status.
- Health status of the elderly may affect nutritional status.

Considering nutritional needs of the elderly is essential because many are malnourished.

- Calories should be reduced by about 5% per decade.
- Fiber (fruits, vegetables, whole grains, cereals) should be increased to counter constipation.
- Sufficient water should be ingested (minimum 1500–2000 mL/day) for body function and temperature regulation. (Many of the elderly have poor thirst sensation, so they tend to drink less water than is necessary for bodily functioning.)
- Many elderly are deficient in nutrients, especially protein, B vitamins, vitamins A and C, iron, and calcium, thus nutrient supplements are important.

Assessment parameters for the nutritional status of an elderly client.

- Hydration status, body weight, edema
- Anemia
- Appetite
- Ability to feed self—physical and mental
  - Dentition
  - Mastication
  - Swallowing
  - Desire to eat
- Fatigue, energy reserve
- Constipation
- Compliance to special diets
- Effects of drugs on nutrition
  - Gastrointestinal irritation
  - Food–drug interactions
  - Some drug side effects are nausea and vomiting
- Skin and mucous membrane condition

19

Specimen Collection

LEARNING OBJECTIVES

- Discuss the nursing responsibilities for reporting abnormal laboratory values.
- Describe the major client instructions that ensure an uncontaminated midstream urine specimen.
- State two objectives for obtaining a stool specimen.
- List four precautions that must be carried out when obtaining a stool specimen for parasite identification.
- Demonstrate the procedure for testing for occult blood.
- Write charting information necessary to include in a client's record when collecting a stool specimen.
- Explain the objectives for collecting a sputum specimen.
- Outline the steps of collecting a sputum specimen from a suction trap.
- Compare and contrast obtaining an aerobic and anaerobic culture.
- State the purpose for using an autolet.
- Demonstrate the use of the autolet to obtain a capillary blood specimen.
- Write two nursing diagnoses which are relevant for specimen collection.
- Demonstrate the removal of blood using a vacutainer.
- State two critical-thinking solutions for the problem of blood not flowing into the syringe when withdrawing blood.
- State the nursing action when a hematoma occurs at the puncture site.

TERMINOLOGY

Aerobe: a microorganism that lives and grows in the presence of free oxygen.

Albuminuria: the presence of albumin in the urine.

Anaerobe: an organism that lives and grows in the absence of molecular oxygen.

Antimicrobial: an agent that prevents the multiplication of microorganisms.

Antimicrobic: preventing the development or pathogenic action of microbes.

Asepsis: prevention of contact with microorganisms.

Aspiration: the removal of fluids or gases from a cavity by the application of suction.

Autolet: a small instrument with lancet used to obtain a capillary blood specimen; usually used to measure blood glucose level.

Bacteria: unicellular plant-like microorganisms lacking chlorophyll.

Cannula: a tube for insertion into a duct or cavity.

Culture: to grow microorganisms or living tissue cells in a special medium.

Dermis: synonym for corium; the skin layer beneath the epidermis; contains vascular connective tissue.

Excoriation: a breakdown of the epidermis.

Expectorant: an agent that facilitates the removal of the secretions of the bronchopulmonary mucous membrane.

Exudate: material obtained from a wound as the result of the inflammatory process.

Genitourinary: pertaining to the genital and urinary systems.

Glucose: a monosaccharide, the end product of carbohydrate metabolism; also known as dextrose; found in the normal blood.

Glycosuria: the presence of sugar in the urine.

Granulocytes: a granular leukocyte.

Hematuria: blood in the urine.

Hemo-: prefix meaning blood.

Hypovolemia: diminished circulating fluid volume.

Inflammatory process: localized response when injury or destruction of tissue has occurred; destroys, wards off, or dilutes the causative agent or the injured tissue.

Intracellular: inside the cell.

Micturition: the process of emptying the urinary bladder; voiding.

Parasite: an organism that lives within, on, or at the expense of another organism, known as the host.

Patency: the state of being freely open.

Pathogen: disease-producing organism.

Peri: prefix meaning around or about.

Pinworm: oxyurid parasite of the intestine, usually *Enterobrus vermicularis.* Commonly found in children. Piperazine is drug of choice.

Polyuria: the excessive production and elimination of urine.

Purulent: containing pus, or caused by pus.

Pus: an inflammation product containing leukocytes and exudate.

Septic: pertinent to pathologic organisms or their toxins.

Septicemia: presence of pathologic bacteria in the blood.

Skin turgor: the tension or fullness of the cells.

Specific gravity: weight of a substance compared with an equal volume of water. Water is 1.000.

Specimen: a sample taken to show or to determine the character of the whole, as a specimen of urine.

Sputum: substance expelled by coughing or clearing the throat.

Stool: waste matter discharged from the bowels.

Transtracheal: passage of a tube or needle through the wall of the trachea.

Urinary tract infection (UTI): an infection of the urinary tract, including all or part of the organs and ducts participating in the secretion and elimination of urine.

Vacutainer: a plastic adapter that fits onto a double-ended needle for obtaining a venous blood sample.

Venipuncture: puncture of a vein with a needle or catheter.

Venous: pertaining to the veins; unoxygenated blood.

Viscosity: resistance offered by a fluid; property of a substance that is dependent on the friction of its component molecules as they slide by each other.

LABORATORY TESTS

Laboratory tests are an adjunct for diagnosing health care problems and assessing the health status of clients. Test findings can reveal occult problems, determine the stage of disease, estimate the activity of the disease process, and measure the effect of therapy. Multiple laboratory tests are usually ordered not only to assist in diagnosing problems but also to rule out certain disease states.

Laboratory tests can be analyzed individually or as a part of a screening panel. For example, a routine urinalysis screens for the chemical makeup of the urine as well as color, clarity, and presence of abnormal cells. Blood chemistry components can be tested individually as well as in combination through a multiparameter test. These tests provide data on 8, 12, or 16 different elements of blood, depending on the laboratory equipment. It is more cost-effective when all the tests are run simultaneously with one blood specimen. For example, a "panel 12" analyzes the following tests: total protein, albumin, calcium, inorganic phosphorous, cholesterol, glucose, BUN, uric acid, creatinine, total bilirubin, alkaline phosphatase, SGOT.

Every laboratory establishes its own normal values for each test. The normal values are generally printed on each laboratory slip to facilitate comparisons with the client's findings. Healthy clients do not always fall within the calculated laboratory norms. The physician, considering other variables, must judge the value and diagnostic implications of these tests.

Nursing Responsibility

Nursing responsibilities associated with the collection of specimens range from client education to reporting abnormal laboratory findings to the appropriate health team member. When specimens are ordered, it is essential that the client understands the full importance of "how" and "why" the specimen is to be obtained. If sterile or clean technique is required, client teaching can provide an understanding of the process. If the client is involved with obtaining the specimen, precise instructions should be given.

To prevent unnecessary lost time and cost to the client, the nurse must be well informed of the correct procedure for obtaining, handling, and processing each specimen. If the nurse is unfamiliar with the procedure, he or she should refer to the nursing procedure or laboratory manual for the health care facility. Specific directions are written for most tests performed by the laboratory. If there is any question about the procedure, the laboratory should be called for directions before obtaining the specimen.

The physician should be notified immediately of any abnormal laboratory findings which could be potentially life-threatening. Verbal communication is the most appropriate and efficacious method. When the nurse leaves written messages on the chart, several hours may elapse before the physician sees the findings.

All clients admitted to a health care facility have at least one laboratory specimen collected during their hospitalization. The most frequent laboratory tests ordered are those involving the urine and blood.

Urine Tests

Nursing responsibilities include collecting, temporarily storing, and performing tests on the urine specimen. Timed urine specimens are usually left in the nursing unit until completion of the test. When urine specimens are retained in the nursing unit, the nurse must take special care in the storing and handling of the specimen to ensure reliable results. Generally, urine specimens collected over a period of hours must be refrigerated or have preservatives added to the specimen to ensure accurate results. Preservatives, such as hydrochloric acid or thymol, prevent deterioration of the specimen.

Most urine specimens are collected as clean-catch, or midstream, specimens and sent directly to the laboratory. Single urine specimens are obtained through random sampling. It is best to obtain the first voided specimen in the morning for routine urine tests. This specimen is more concentrated, and the pH is more acidic. The midstream method of urine collection necessitates that proper instructions be given to the client in cleansing the genitalia and obtaining the specimen.

When timed specimens are ordered, the nursing role encompasses not only the handling of the urine specimen but also precise instructions to the client for collecting the specimen. The collection of urine needs to start and finish at the designated time. Timed tests vary from 2 hours to 24 hours. Assessment for amylase and bilirubin can be done on a 2-hour collection. Creatinine clearance and estriol determination require a 24-hour specimen. A 24-hour urine specimen that is started at 9 AM must be finished at 9 AM the next day in order to obtain accurate results. Instructions to the client include voiding at 9 AM, discarding that urine specimen, and collecting the rest of the urine at 9 AM the next morning.

Clinitest, Acetest and the test for specific gravity are usually performed by the nurse and are not done by the laboratory. Nurses should follow the specific procedures for each test to obtain accurate results.

Blood Tests

Even though blood studies are carried out on venous, capillary, or arterial blood, the usual sample is obtained from venous blood. Capillary blood specimens are usually used to obtain specimens from infants and neonates. In adult clients blood glucose and hemoglobin levels can be determined from capillary blood. Arterial samples are obtained for blood gas determination and cultures.

Blood specimens are placed in specific blood tubes according to the type of test ordered and sent to the laboratory for analysis. Each health care facility has a list of blood tests that are analyzed from blood in a specific color-top test tube. The colored top on the test tube indicates whether or not the tube contains a preservative. When whole blood is required for the test, an anticoagulant, such as heparin or trisodium citrate, is placed in the test tube to keep the blood from clotting. When serum is needed for the laboratory test, no preservative is added to the blood as the clot is used for the test. If the test tube contains a preservative, the tube should be gently agitated to prevent the blood from clotting.

Some blood tests require that the client fast for several hours prior to obtaining the specimens. Other blood tests have no special requirements for collection. Blood studies requiring a fasting specimen for accuracy include fasting blood sugar, lipid panels, glucose tolerance tests, and insulin levels.

If a needle and syringe are used for drawing blood, the top should be removed from the blood tube. After removing the top, slowly inject the blood into the test tube. When blood is ejected through both the needle and the rubber stopper, hemolysis occurs and the specimen is destroyed.

Cultures

Specimens from the throat, eyes, nose, vagina, wounds, sputum, stool, urine, and blood are often ordered to culture for pathogens. Special tubes or containers with

TEST TUBE IDENTIFICATION

Color of Top	Blood Test
Red or striped with preservative	Chemical panels, drug assays, serology, cold agglutins, isoenzymes
Small red	Blood type and cross-match
Blue top	Coagulation studies
Lavender	White blood cells, red blood cells
Purple	Hemoglobin, hematocrit
Green	Ammonia
Large red	Electrolytes
Gray	Glucose

culture media are used for organism growth. The culture is prepared in the laboratory according to the type of test ordered. It is essential that the proper technique be used to place the specimen in the appropriate container to ensure accurate results. Specimens obtained for culture and sensitivity require immediate processing and must be sent directly to the laboratory after they are obtained. If a time lapse occurs, the specimen may need to be discarded and a new one obtained. If the specimen is allowed to dry before the examination, the organism cannot be transferred to the slide and, thus, to the culture medium.

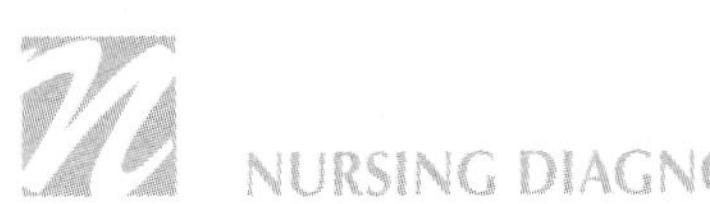

NURSING DIAGNOSES

The following nursing diagnoses may be appropriate to include in a client care plan when the components are related to collecting specimens.

NURSING DIAGNOSIS	RELATED FACTORS
Anxiety	Dread of unknown outcome, results of specimen tests
Ineffective Individual Coping	Fear, external stress, situational crisis
Knowledge deficit	Inaccurate collection of specimen (e.g., instruction not clear, unable to hear or see well enough to complete collection)
Noncompliance	Inadequate understanding of the purpose or value of diagnostic test (e.g., language and cultural barriers)
Pain	Invasive procedure, altered body function, recent surgery
Risk for infection	Invasive procedure, contamination from poor technique of specimen collection

unit 1

URINE SPECIMENS

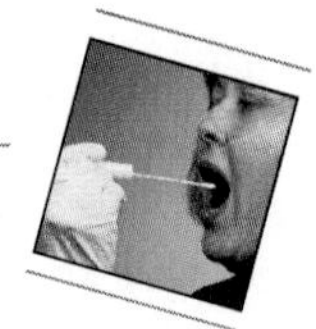

NURSING PROCESS DATA

ASSESSMENT Data Base

Assess client's ability to understand instructions and to obtain specimens properly.

Identify if signs and symptoms of urinary tract infections are present: frequency, urgency, dysuria, hematuria, flank pain, fever, and cloudy urine with sediment.

PLANNING Objectives

To instruct the client in the method for obtaining a specimen

To obtain an uncontaminated urine specimen for culture and sensitivity

To maintain the collection of urine for 24 hours

IMPLEMENTATION Procedures

Collecting Midstream Urine

Collecting 24-Hour Urine Specimen

EVALUATION Expected Outcomes

Client is able to obtain urine specimen.

Uncontaminated urine specimen is obtained.

24-hour urine specimen is completed appropriately.

COLLECTING MIDSTREAM URINE

Equipment

Soap and water
Cleaning swab or bactericidal soap
Sterile specimen container
Label for container
Clean gloves

■ CLINICAL ALERT

Clean gloves must be used when nurse assists with obtaining specimen.

Procedure

1. Gather equipment.
2. Wash your hands.
3. Identify client by checking identaband.
4. Explain procedure to client.
5. Provide perineal care as needed.
6. Instruct client to collect specimen in bathroom or place on bedpan.
7. Instruct client to clean the urinary meatus and obtain urine specimen.

   For a male:

   a. Wash hands and open container.
   b. Cleanse end of penis with cleansing swab using circular motion and moving from middle toward outside. **Rationale:** Always swab from clean to dirty area to decrease bacteria levels.

■ CLINICAL ALERT

A contaminated specimen is the single most common reason for inaccurate reporting on urinary cultures and sensitivities. To prevent contamination, place cap of container with sterile side up while collecting specimen and do not touch inside of container.

c. Initiate urine stream.

d. After single stream achieved, pass specimen bottle into stream and obtain urine sample. At least 30 mL must be obtained for adequate specimen. **Rationale:** The microorganisms which accumulate at the urinary meatus have been flushed out with the original stream of urine and are not collected in the specimen.

For a female:

a. Wash hands, and open container.

b. Spread labia minora with nondominant hand.

c. Cleanse area with disinfectant swab, beginning above the urethral orifice and moving posteriorly.

d. Initiate urine stream. Hold labia open throughout the voiding process.

e. After single stream achieved, pass specimen bottle into the stream and obtain sample.

8. To prevent contamination of specimen with skin flora, instruct the client to remove the bottle *before* the flow of urine stops and *before* releasing the labia or penis.
9. Instruct client to completely empty bladder.

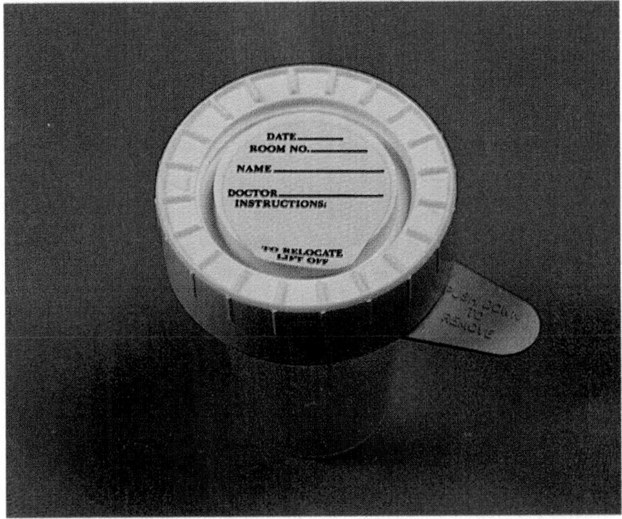

Sterile urine specimen container.

10. Wipe off outside of container after replacing cap.
11. Wash your hands.
12. Label the specimen, and take it to the laboratory within 15 minutes. If this is not possible, refrigerate the specimen.

COLLECTING 24-HOUR URINE SPECIMEN

Equipment

Urine specimen container
Preservative, if required
Requisition slip
Label for specimen
Sign that urine collection is in progress
Container with ice, if needed

24-hour urine specimens must be collected for the entire time ordered. To obtain accurate finding, the laboratory needs the entire urine specimen.

Procedure

1. Explain procedure to client. Stress the importance of saving all urine for 24 hours.
2. Place sign in client's bathroom stating that 24-hour urine specimen is in progress with date and time.
3. Collect urine specimen and discard it. **Rationale:** The first specimen is considered "old urine" or urine that was in the bladder before test began.
4. Record date and time of first specimen on label, and place bottle in appropriate area. Depending on hospital protocol, specimens may be refrigerated, placed on ice, or left in the client's bathroom.
5. Add preservative, if required.
6. Post sign in appropriate place.
7. Place all urine voided in specimen container.
8. Request client to void exactly 24 hours after first specimen was obtained. Place voided urine in container.
9. After the last voided specimen is placed in the container, cover and send entire specimen to the lab with the proper requisition.
10. Remove sign, and remind client that the test is completed.
11. If a specimen is accidentally discarded, obtain a new container, note the new date and time, and restart the procedure.

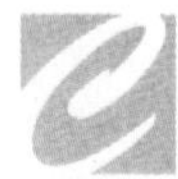

CHARTING for Urine Specimens

- Method used to obtain specimen
- Color, consistency, and odor of urine
- Amount of urine obtained (record this amount on the intake and output record also)
- Time specimen sent to laboratory
- Refrigeration, if required
- Exact time for 24-hour specimen

CRITICAL THINKING APPLICATION

CLINICAL PROBLEMS	CRITICAL THINKING OPTIONS
Client is unable to assist with obtaining a sterile specimen.	• Place female client in bed and, after cleaning perineum thoroughly, place on sterile or clean bedpan. Cleanse perineal area with swab and obtain specimen according to procedure. • Assist client into bathroom. Assist client to cleanse perineum, instruct to start urine stream, and place the sterile specimen container under the stream to collect specimen. • For male clients, cleanse the penis, and place a sterile or clean urinal under the client. Instruct to start stream of urine and then place sterile container under stream.
Urine specimen contaminated with feces or toilet paper.	• Instruct client on need for accuracy and compliance to urine collection.
Client cannot void on command at completion of test.	• Instruct client to void as close to time as possible. • Chart exact time when last specimen collected on both urine bottle and lab slip. Notify lab of findings.
Urine specimen discarded before 24-hour sample collected.	• If time period is close to 24 hours, call laboratory to determine if test can be completed on sample collected. • If 24-hour sample must be started again, instruct client of necessity to save all urine. • Place signs indicating 24-hour test collection in progress on bathroom door and client's bedside stand. • Mark in bold or underlined print in Kardex indicating 24-hour urine collection in progress.

unit 2

INFANT URINE SPECIMEN

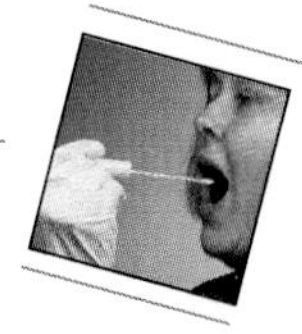

NURSING PROCESS DATA

ASSESSMENT Data Base

Determine the purpose for which the specimen is being obtained.

Determine how the collection is to be obtained.

Assess parents' understanding of the purpose for the procedure.

PLANNING Objectives

To obtain a clean urine specimen for urinary system diagnosis tests

To obtain urine specimen for routine hospital admission or as a preoperative urine sample

To provide a method for ensuring collection of all urine when a 24-hour urine collection is ordered

IMPLEMENTATION Procedure

Collecting a Specimen from an Infant

EVALUATION Expected Outcomes

An uncontaminated urine specimen is obtained.

Family is able to assist in collecting urine from small children.

COLLECTING A SPECIMEN FROM AN INFANT

Equipment

Cleansing solution
Towel
Restraints
Pediatric urine collector
Diaper
Appropriate specimen containers
Clean gloves
Clean specimen container

Procedure

1. Gather equipment.
2. Wash your hands. Don clean gloves.
3. Identify correct child by checking identaband.
4. Cleanse and dry child's perineum.
5. Remove paper backing from the adhesive on the urine collector.
6. Apply urine collector to child's perineum, avoiding extension over anus to prevent contamination.

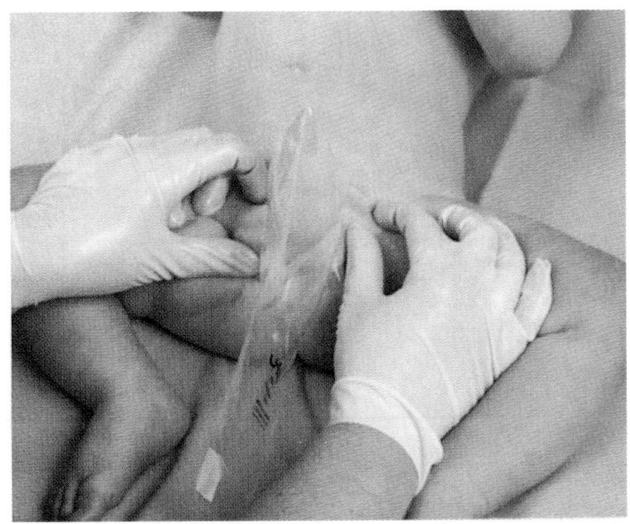

Remove adhesive backing from urine collection bag and place securely over penis.

   a. *Male*: Place child's penis through the opening of the collector.
   b. *Female*: Place the opening of the collection bag over the child's urinary meatus.

7. Remove gloves.
8. Place a diaper on the child to help hold the collector in place.
9. Restrain an active child, if necessary.
10. Wash your hands.
11. Check the collector every 15 minutes until a specimen is obtained.
12. Don clean gloves.
13. Remove the collector and place in a urine specimen container.
14. Place clean diaper on child.
15. Remove gloves and wash your hands.
16. Send the urine specimen to the lab either by placing the urine collection bag in a urine container or pouring amine from collection bag into the urine container.

CHARTING for Collecting a Specimen from an Infant

- Amount, color, character, and odor of urine
- Time specimen obtained and sent to laboratory
- Condition of perineum

CRITICAL THINKING APPLICATION

CLINICAL PROBLEMS	CRITICAL THINKING OPTIONS
Specimen is lost because collector does not adhere.	• Obtain a new collection bag, and repeat the procedure. • Tape bag in place with nonallergenic paper tape if necessary.
Specimen is lost because collection bag is the wrong size.	• Obtain appropriate size bag, and repeat the procedure.
Specimen cannot be obtained with a collection bag.	• Notify the physician that you are unable to obtain urine specimen. • If possible keep diapers off and observe when infant urinates; attempt to obtain specimen.

unit 3

STOOL SPECIMENS

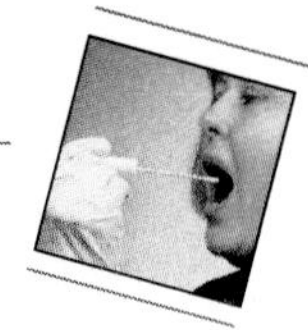

NURSING PROCESS DATA

ASSESSMENT Data Base

Determine the purpose for the test.

Check whether the specimen must be sent to the laboratory immediately.

Determine the eliminatory status of the client (i.e., liquid vs. formed stools).

Assess gastrointestinal tract dysfunction.

PLANNING Objectives

To obtain stool specimens for diagnosing dysfunction in bowel elimination

To assess for perforation or bleeding from a gastric ulcer

To detect presence of parasites

To determine presence of pinworms

IMPLEMENTATION Procedures

Collecting Adult Stool Specimen

Collecting Stool for Parasites

Collecting Infant Stool Specimen

Testing for Occult Blood

Gamma Fe-Cult Plus

Hemoccult

Collecting Stool for Bacterial Culture

Testing for Pinworms

EVALUATION Expected Outcomes

Specimen meets laboratory requirements for diagnostic testing.

Client does not experience undue discomfort or embarrassment during procedure.

Cellophane tape test completed.

COLLECTING ADULT STOOL SPECIMEN

Equipment

Waxed cardboard or plastic container with cover

Tongue blade

Label for container

Clean bedpan or bedside commode

Clean gloves

Procedure

1. Check the client's identaband, and explain the procedure to the client.
2. Before collecting stool specimen, ask the client to void. Tell client not to void on the specimen. **Rationale:** This prevents contamination of specimen with urine, which could result in inaccurate test results.
3. Don gloves.
4. Clean out all urine from the bedpan or bedside commode.
5. Raise the head of the bed so that client can assume a squatting position on the bedpan, or help client sit on the bedside commode.
6. Provide privacy until client has passed a stool.
7. Remove the bedpan or bedside commode. If necessary, help the client clean perineum.
8. Use tongue blade to obtain and place a small por-

tion (2 teaspoons) of the formed stool in a waxed cardboard or plastic container. (For some tests you may need to collect the entire specimen.) Do not contaminate the outside of container.

9. Discard remaining stool, clean bedpan or bedside commode.
10. Remove gloves, and wash your hands.
11. Label container with client's name.
12. Fill out laboratory request for appropriate test.
13. Take specimen to laboratory immediately. **Rationale:** Specimen may need to be refrigerated or examined immediately after collection.

COLLECTING STOOL FOR PARASITES

Equipment

Waxed cardboard or plastic container with cover
Tongue blade
Label for container
Clean bedpan or bedside commode
Clean gloves

Procedure

1. Follow the steps for *Collecting Adult Stool Specimen*. Don clean gloves to collect stool specimen.
2. Collect exudate, mucus, and blood with all specimens. **Rationale:** Parasites thrive in this type of medium.
3. Keep specimens at body temperature to be examined within 30 minutes. **Rationale:** Organisms must be seen in their active stages, as loose, fluid stools are likely to contain trophozoites or intestinal amoebas and flagellates.
4. There is usually no need to maintain well-formed or semiformed stool specimens at body temperature or to examine them quickly even though they may contain ova or cystic form of parasites.
5. Collect complete stools after purgative medications are administered.
6. When the presence of tapeworms is suspected, all stools must be examined in their entirety in order to find the head of the parasite.
7. Do not give barium, oil, and laxatives containing heavy metals that interfere with the extraction process for 7 days prior to stool examination. **Rationale:** Ova or cysts are not revealed.
8. Use only normal saline solution or tap water if an enema must be administered to collect specimens. Do not use soap suds or other substances.
9. Do not contaminate the specimen with urine as it kills amoeba.
10. Collect three random, normally passed stool specimens to ensure accurate test results.

COLLECTING INFANT STOOL SPECIMEN

Equipment

Diaper
Plastic diaper liner
Waxed cardboard or plastic container with cover
Cotton swabs
Label for container
Clean gloves

Procedure

1. Place a clean, disposable diaper on the child or infant.
2. Check diaper frequently so that you obtain a specimen that is not contaminated with urine.
3. If child is passing liquid stools, place a plastic liner inside the diaper.
4. Don clean gloves before taking diaper off child and collecting specimen.
5. Use cotton swabs to procure the specimen.
6. Place specimen in stool container.
7. Remove gloves, wash hands, label, and send to lab immediately.

TESTING FOR OCCULT BLOOD

Equipment

Clean bedpan or bedside commode
Tongue blade
Guaiac test (Hemoccult) or gamma Fe-Cult packet
Guaiac solution
Glacial acetic acid
Hydrogen peroxide
Clean gloves

■ CLINICAL ALERT

Overt bleeding from hemorrhoids or menstrual bleeding renders the test inaccurate.

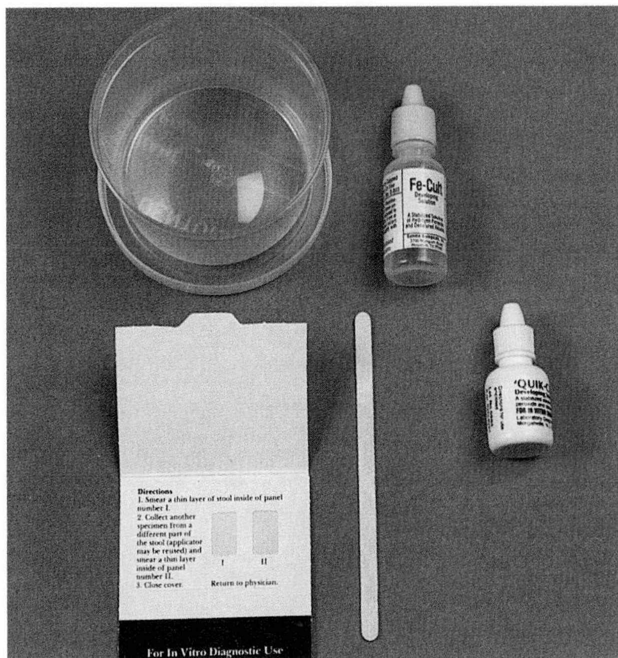

Supplies needed for testing stool for occult blood.

Procedure

1. Explain need for stool specimen to client.
2. Provide privacy.
3. Position client on bedpan or commode.
4. Don clean gloves.
5. Take stool specimen to bathroom or utility room.
6. Prepare slide for testing according to packet instructions:

   gamma Fe-Cult Plus

   a. Smear thick layer of stool on panel number 1.
   b. Obtain second specimen from a different part of stool specimen and smear thin layer on panel number 2.
   c. Turn packet over, and remove perforated flap (marked Not To Be Opened by Patient).
   d. Add 2 drops of Fe-Cult developing solution to test area over smear of stool.
   e. Read and record test results within 30 seconds. **Rationale:** Color reaction fades within 2–3 minutes. Any trace of blue indicates a positive result. No trace of blue indicates a negative result

   Hemoccult

   a. Follow steps 1 and 2 for Fe-Cult Plus test.
   b. Wait 3–5 minutes before processing text.
   c. Turn packet over, and lift flap.
   d. Apply 2 drops of Hemoccult developer over each smear.
   e. Read and record test results within 60 seconds.
   f. Apply 1 drop of Hemoccult between the + and – performance monitor test strip (orange section at bottom of packet)
   g. Interpret results within 10 seconds. If the positive side turns blue, the test slide is accurate.
7. Discard filter paper or packet.
8. Remove gloves and wash your hands.
9. Check facility policy for testing. Some laboratories conduct studies.
10. Document findings in nurses' notes.

■ CLINICAL ALERT

Bleeding from a gastric ulcer or the intestinal tract may be a slow process. If you suspect gastrointestinal bleeding, a guaiac test for occult blood is indicated. Steps for testing occult blood must be followed in sequence.

COLLECTING STOOL FOR BACTERIAL CULTURE

Equipment

Waxed cardboard container with cover
Tongue blade
Label for container
Clean bedpan or bedside commode
Clean gloves

Procedure

1. Follow steps for *Collecting Adult Stool Specimen.* Don clean gloves before collecting stool specimen.
2. Collect exudate, mucus, and blood with all specimens.
3. Place a small amount of feces in a waxed cardboard container (if entire specimen is not needed). Remove gloves, wash hands, and send entire specimen to the laboratory immediately after collection. If there is any delay, the specimen must be iced.
4. Report and calculate on the basis of daily output any stool specimens that are to undergo chemical analysis.

TESTING FOR PINWORMS

Equipment

Clear cellophane tape
Tongue depressor
Glass slide
Clean gloves

Procedure

1. Explain procedure to child and parent.
2. Obtain equipment.
3. Provide privacy.
4. Don clean gloves.
5. Place sticky side of clear cellophane tape over the end of tongue depressor. **Rationale:** Other types of tape interfere with observation.
6. Place sticky side of cellophane tape over perineal region. **Rationale:** The pinworms are expelled through the anus and adhere to the tape.
7. Leave in place for several seconds.
8. Remove tape from perineal region, and place sticky side of tape onto a glass slide for microscopic examination.
9. Wash and dry the perineal region.
10. Remove gloves, and wash your hands.
11. Label specimen, and transport to lab immediately.

CLINICAL ALERT

For better results the tape test should be done in the morning, before the client has defecated or bathed. Pinworms usually migrate to anus during the night.

CHARTING for Stool Specimens

- Time specimens collected
- Time specimens sent to laboratory
- Number of specimens sent to laboratory
- Description of stool: color, amount, odor, and any purulent patches or blood noted
- Condition of perianal skin, if client is having diarrhea
- If serial stool specimens are needed, record each specimen on the Kardex card as well as the chart

CRITICAL THINKING APPLICATION

CLINICAL PROBLEMS	CRITICAL THINKING OPTIONS
Client is embarrassed by having to give stool specimen.	• Place a bedpan or other collection device under the toilet seat in bathroom to obtain specimen. • If client is confined to bed, pull sheets over client's legs and draw curtains around the bed until procedure is completed. • If odor occurs from passage of stool, spray room with air freshener.
Client is unable to pass adequate stool for specimen collection.	• Notify physician to obtain order to give a normal saline or tap water enema.
Client passes liquid stools.	• Determine if part or entire specimen is required for test. • Obtain a plastic container with a cover and several large cotton swabs. Dip cotton swabs into the liquid stool. Place swabs in plastic container. After procedure, pay close attention to skin care. A protective ointment may be necessary to protect skin from liquid stools.

unit 4 VENOUS BLOOD SPECIMENS

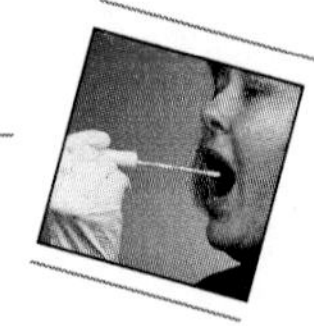

NURSING PROCESS DATA

ASSESSMENT Data Base

Check order for blood withdrawal in client's chart.

Note specific requirements for the test (e.g., fasting or administration of medications prior to the test).

Check to see if the test is routine or urgent.

Assess veins for venipuncture site.

PLANNING Objectives

To obtain an uncontaminated blood specimen

To obtain a blood sample without complications, such as hematoma formation or excessive oozing at the site

To obtain specimens of blood that can be used to diagnose the client's illness

To obtain and transfer specimens without destroying red blood cells

To ensure accurate test results by making sure the client follows all requirements for the test (e.g., fasting)

To ensure accurate test results by selecting the right tube for the right test

To ensure that uncontaminated blood specimen for culture is obtained

To obtain an accurate blood glucose level

IMPLEMENTATION Procedures

Withdrawing Blood

Using Vacutainer System

Collecting a Specimen for Culture

Obtaining Blood Specimen for Glucose Testing

Measuring Blood Glucose Using Chemstrip

Measuring Blood Glucose Using Accu-Chek—Glucometer

Measuring Blood Glucose Using Lifescan One-Touch II

EVALUATION Expected Outcomes

Blood sample is obtained without complications, such as hematoma formation or excessive oozing at the site.

Uncontaminated blood specimen is obtained.

Blood samples are sent to the laboratory in the proper tubes.

Blood glucose level obtained.

WITHDRAWING BLOOD

Equipment

5-mL or 10-mL syringe

20-gauge 1-inch needle(s)

70% alcohol wipe (with blood alcohol specimen, solution of benzalkonium is needed)

Appropriate laboratory tubes

Dry, sterile sponges

Tourniquet

Absorbent pad or towel

Clean gloves

Preparation

1. Check physician's orders for tests to be obtained.
2. Wash your hands.
3. Gather equipment.

Procedure

1. Identify client by checking identaband; introduce yourself and explain the procedure.
2. Don clean gloves.
3. Place a tourniquet 4–6 inches above the client's elbow. (If client has an IV in place, place the tourniquet on the other arm.) Tighten the tourniquet and tell the client to open and close fist.
4. Place absorbent pad or towel under arm. **Rationale:** This prevents soiling the linen with blood.
5. Cleanse the antecubital fossa (inner aspect of elbow) with an alcohol swab starting at the vein site and moving in a circular motion about 2 inches away from vein. Allow area to dry. An alternative site may be selected if appropriate.
6. With needle affixed to the syringe, hold skin taut with nondominant hand. Perform a venipuncture with bevel of needle pointed up at a 30° angle.
7. Lower needle toward skin after needle has entered vein. **Rationale:** This decreases risk of accidentally penetrating the other side of vein.
8. Thread needle along path of vein. Watch for backflow of blood in syringe.
9. Pull the syringe plunger back gently, and check for placement of the needle in the vein. If placement is correct, release the tourniquet, wait a few seconds to allow fresh blood to flow into the vein, and then pull back gently on the plunger.
10. Fill the syringe to the desired amount.
11. Remove the needle from the vein, cover the venipuncture site with a sterile sponge, and press the sponge firmly on the site. (Client may be able to hold sponge in place.)
12. Remove the top from the laboratory tube. Do not touch the inside of the tube or spill its contents.
13. Remove the needle from the blood-filled syringe, and gently eject the blood down the side of the tube. Do not allow the blood to foam or splash. **Rationale:** Red blood cells can be destroyed if the blood sample is not handled carefully.
14. Replace the tube top, and rotate the blood gently to mix the blood with the tube contents. *Alternative method*: Needle can be inserted through rubber stopper of test tube if 20-gauge needle is used. Inject blood slowly into test tube to prevent hemolysis of cells.
15. Label the tube promptly. Write the client's name, date, and the time. You may also need to write the initials of the person who drew the specimen if this information is required by hospital policy.
16. Check the client's venipuncture site for oozing. Continue to press the sponge firmly over the site if clots have not begun to form at the site.
17. Remove gloves, wash hands.
18. Take the blood specimens to a designated station or laboratory according to hospital procedure.

USING VACUTAINER SYSTEM

Equipment

5-mL or 10-mL syringe
20-gauge 1-inch needle(s)
70% alcohol wipe (with blood alcohol specimen, solution of benzalkonium is needed)
Appropriate laboratory tubes
Dry, sterile sponges
Plastic adapter (Vacutainer)
Double-ended needle that screws into the adapter
Clean gloves

Preparation

1. Check physician's orders for tests to be obtained.
2. Wash your hands.
3. Don clean gloves.
4. Obtain plastic adapter, double-ended needle that screws into the adapter, and appropriate vacuum specimen tubes.
5. Screw the double-ended needle into the plastic adapter, with the shorter needle facing the plastic adapter.
6. Explain procedure to client.

Procedure

1. Tighten the tourniquet 4–6 inches above the elbow, and cleanse the venipuncture site. An alternative site may be selected.
2. Place the vacuum tube inside the plastic adapter, with the top of the tube resting against the short needle.
3. Proceed with the venipuncture. Once the needle is positioned inside the vein and blood return is visualized, hold the plastic adapter steady and press the vacuum tube firmly into the short needle so that it pierces the top of the tube. Blood should begin to spurt quickly into the tube until the tube is filled.
4. Release the tube, and set it aside. Attach another tube to vacutainer, or prepare to remove needle.
5. Place sponge over needle site, and remove needle while applying gentle pressure to site.
6. Hold sponge on site for 1–2 minutes. Do not have client bend elbow. **Rationale:** Bending the elbow can facilitate formation of a hematoma.
7. Remove gloves, and wash your hands.

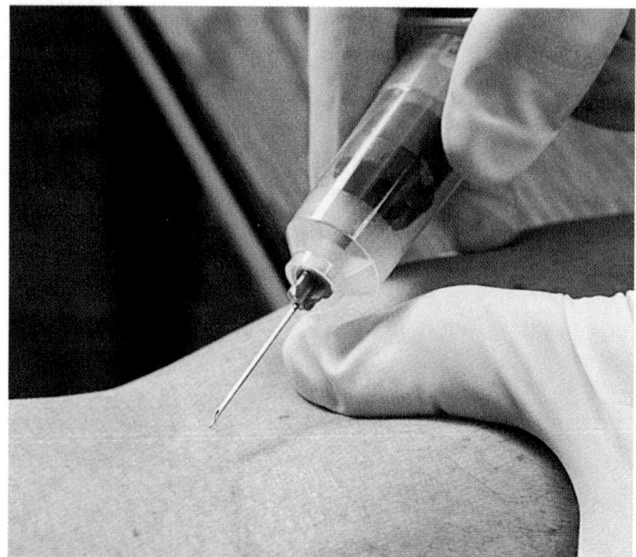

Hold skin taut, and with bevel of vacutainer needle pointed up and at a 30° angle, insert needle into vein.

8. Complete laboratory slip, and take specimen to designated station or laboratory.

COLLECTING A SPECIMEN FOR CULTURE

Equipment

2 sets of paired culture media bottles (aerobic and anaerobic)

Blood withdrawal equipment (e.g., 2 needles and syringe with attached needle)

Povidone-iodine (Betadine) swab

2 70% alcohol swabs

Additional needles

Clean gloves

Preparation

1. Check physician's orders.
2. Wash your hands.
3. Gather equipment.
4. Don clean gloves.
5. Explain procedure to client.

Procedure

1. Cleanse skin with alcohol wipe. Allow skin to dry.

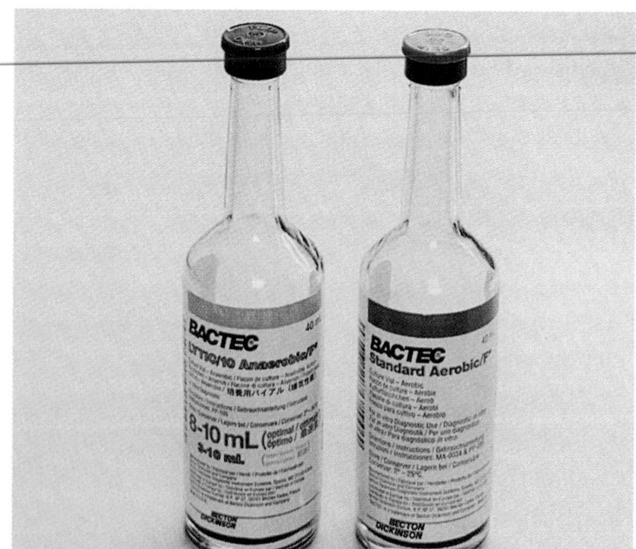

Inject blood into both aerobic and anaerobic culture bottles.

2. Prepare skin with povidone-iodine. Cleanse starting at vein site and moving in circular motion outward 2 inches.
3. Allow skin to dry.

4. Remove povidone-iodine with alcohol wipe.
5. Perform venipuncture.
6. Withdraw 20 mL of blood from vein without IV. Do not draw specimen through catheter. **Rationale:** Fluid from IV alters results.
7. Remove needle used for venipuncture and replace with new sterile needle. **Rationale:** Contamination may result if needle used to puncture skin is reused.
8. Swab top of paired blood culture bottles with povidone-iodine swab, and then alcohol swab and inject 8–10 mL blood into each bottle according to hospital policy. Change needle each time so new sterile needle used for each bottle.
9. Draw a second sample of blood after 15 minutes or according to hospital policy. Use percutaneous stick if required by hospital policy. (Prepare skin with povidone-iodine solution again.)
10. Place in second set of paired blood culture bottles, using single sterile needle technique.
11. Label bottles, and transport to lab immediately. Include site where blood specimens were obtained.

OBTAINING BLOOD SPECIMEN FOR GLUCOSE TESTING

Equipment

Automatic lancet (i.e., Autolet or Glucolet)
Penlet
Soap and water
Cotton ball, sterile sponges
Clean gloves

Preparation

1. Gather equipment—automatic lancet or Autolet wallet—and take to bedside.
2. Wash your hands.
3. Don gloves.

Procedure

1. Wash client's finger tip, especially side of finger where lancet will puncture (or heel for infant), with soap and water. **Rationale:** Use soap and water if repeated sticks are to be done, as alcohol toughens skin and may change reading.
2. Gently manipulate finger or heel to determine if good blood supply is available.
3. Take cover off Penlet.
4. Place lancet in Penlet, push and twist in place.
5. Twist cover of lancet pen to remove.

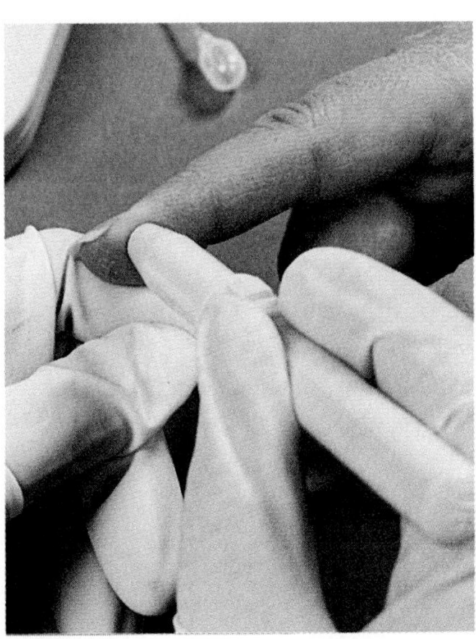

Use automatic lancet to pierce skin for blood collection.

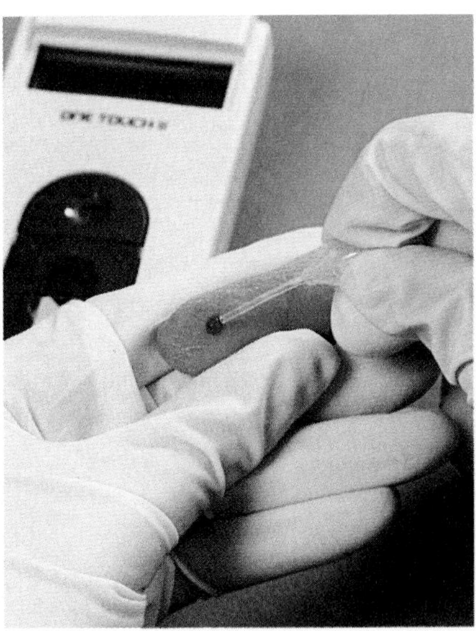

Fill tubing of capillary bulb when obtaining blood specimen.

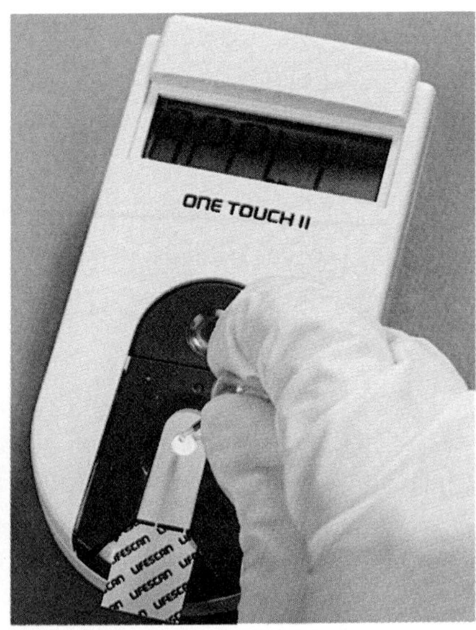

Place blood specimen in designated center of reagent strip.

6. Replace cover of Penlet.
7. Cock Penlet to pull lancet back into Penlet.
8. Place tip of sampling pen against side of finger or heel.
9. Activate to force the lancet downward by pressing gently on the activating button. The lancet punctures the skin immediately.
10. Gently massage the base of the finger, stroking toward the puncture site. Do not squeeze or apply pressure to site. **Rationale:** Massaging increases blood flow to the finger tip.
11. Wait a few seconds to allow blood to collect at puncture site.
12. Place a large drop of blood onto both zones of the reagent area on Chemstrip. May use capillary suction bulb to obtain blood specimen.
13. Wipe puncture site with cotton ball to seal.
14. Discard used equipment.
15. Wash hands.
16. Document results.

■ CLINICAL ALERT

Place tip of capillary bulb at base of blood drop. *Do not* fill bulb with blood. Fill only tubing with blood.

MEASURING BLOOD GLUCOSE USING CHEMSTRIP

Equipment

Reagent strips (Chemstrips)
Color chart
Blood specimen
Cotton ball
Clean gloves

Preparation

1. Follow steps in *Obtaining Blood Specimen for Glucose Testing.*
2. Don gloves.

Procedure

1. Place blood specimen on reagent area of Chemstrip.
2. Start the timer simultaneously with dropping blood on strip.
3. Wait 60 seconds, wipe blood from Chemstrip using dry cotton ball.
4. Wait additional 60 seconds and match color chart for results.
5. If color chart indicates reading is darker than 240 mg/dL, wait additional 60 seconds and compare Chemstrip with color scale.
6. Check Kardex or physician's orders for insulin, and administer prescribed dose.
7. Document results of blood glucose and insulin dosage on diabetic record and medication sheet.

MEASURING BLOOD GLUCOSE USING ACCU-CHEK—GLUCOMETER

Equipment

Accu-Chek or Glucometer blood glucose monitor
Chemstrips including calibration strip
Dry cotton ball

Preparation

1. Remove calibration strip from bottle of chemstrips.
2. Compare lot numbers on calibration strip to lot number on side of Chemstrip bottle. These must match.
3. Place calibration strip in meter by opening door and inserting top of strip into slot on right side of meter.
4. Insert strip until you hear a "click."
5. Close door.
6. Push ON/OFF button. Numbers 888 should appear on screen.
7. Open door of monitor.

8. Push back button on the left side of door, and slide Chemstrip under strip guide with test pads facing up.
9. Close door quickly. Numbers 000 should be displayed on screen indicator. If not, open and close door again.
10. Open door and remove strip. Leave door open.

Procedures

for Accu-Chek Machine

1. Obtain blood specimen according to steps 1 through 7 in skill *Obtaining Blood Specimen for Glucose Testing.*
2. Place blood droplet on test pad covering both the yellow and white sections of the pad. Do not touch blood on pad.
3. Press timer button.
4. Listen for "buzzer" (60 seconds later) and remove all blood from pad by wiping with cotton ball.
5. Face pad upward, depress black button door and insert chemstrip under strip guide. *Do not close door.*
6. Listen for "buzzer" (about 120 seconds), close door and read blood glucose level on display screen.
7. Observe for LLL to appear on display screen; if this occurs, remove strip and check with color chart on side of Chemstrip bottle. Blood glucose is less than 40 mg/dL.
8. Observe for HHH to appear on display screen; if this occurs, the blood glucose is over 400 mg/dL. Repeat step above to check reading.
9. Document findings on appropriate record.

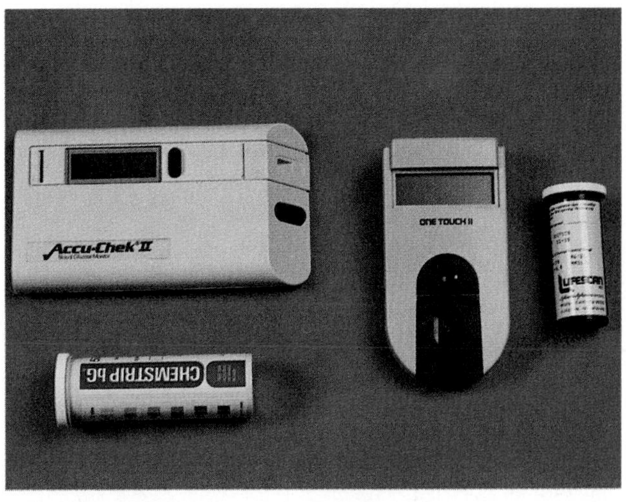

Glucose monitoring equipment and reagent strips.

for Glucometer Machine

1. Obtain blood specimen according to steps 1 through 7 in skill *Obtaining Blood Specimen for Glucose Testing.*
2. Insert Dextrose Stix into Glucometer according to manufacturer's instructions.
3. Wait 30 seconds or time noted by manufacturer. **Rationale:** Time necessary for blood to penetrate Dextrose Stix.
4. Start timer.
5. Read digital display when alarm sounds. **Rationale:** Alarm indicates glucose reading is ready.
6. Dispose of Dextrose Stix.
7. Turn off Glucometer.
8. Document findings on appropriate record.

MEASURING BLOOD GLUCOSE USING LIFESCAN ONE-TOUCH II

Equipment

Penlet II automatic blood sampler
Sterile lancet
One-Touch II meter
Test strip
Soap and water
Clean gloves

Preparation

1. Check physician's orders for specific times.
2. Wash your hands.
3. Gather equipment.
4. Check that code number on test strip matches code number on meter. **Rationale:** If code number is not same, incorrect blood glucose readings occur. Turn meter to ON. The word "Code" and the number appear on the display for several seconds. Code numbers range from 1 to 16.
5. Explain procedure to client.
6. Don clean gloves.

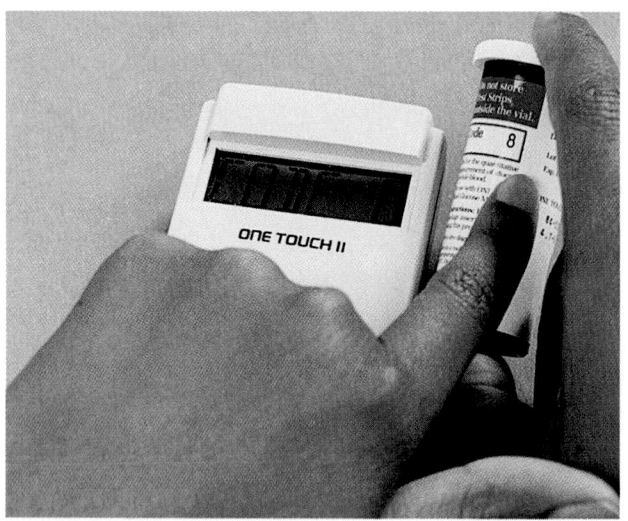

Ensure code number on test strip matches code number on meter.

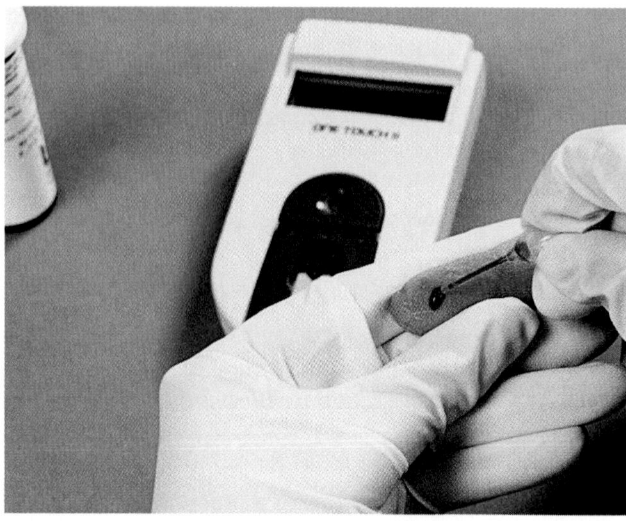
Obtain blood specimen after piercing skin with Penlet II sampler.

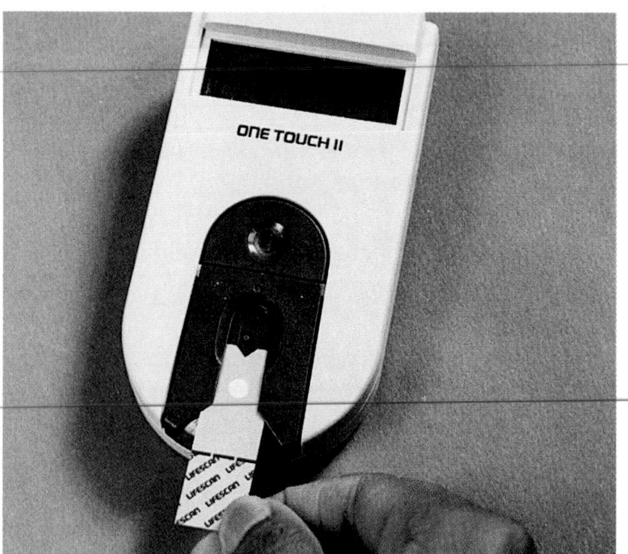

Insert strip, test spot up, into meter until it stops.

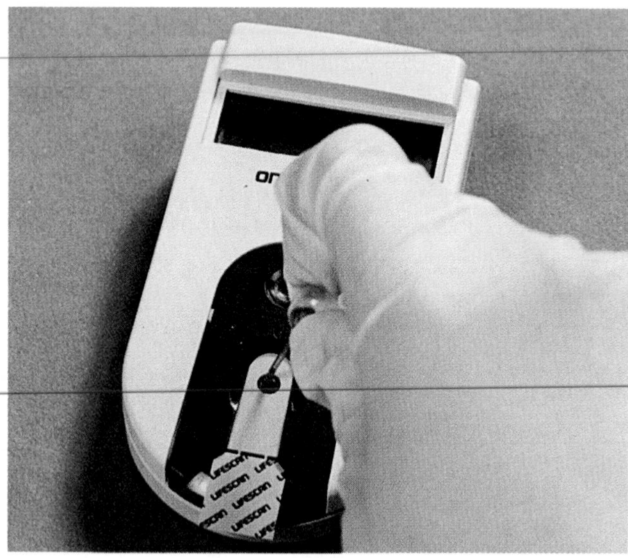
Do not smear blood when dropping on test spot.

Procedure

1. Instruct client to wash hands with soap and warm water. **Rationale:** Warm water stimulates the flow of blood to the fingers.
2. Instruct client to place arm at side of body for 10–15 seconds. **Rationale:** Blood is brought to finger tips for ease in obtaining sample.
3. Remove Penlet II cap by pulling it straight out.
4. Insert sterile lancet into lancet holder. Do not line up ridges on the lancet with the slots in the lancet holder.
5. Hold lancet firmly, and gently twist off the lancet protective disk.
6. Replace Penlet II cap.
7. Hold lower portion of Penlet II sampler, pull out gray sliding barrel until it clicks.
8. Choose a lateral surface of a finger tip. Rotate sites for sticks. **Rationale:** Rotating sites decrease callous formation and bruising of finger tips.
9. Hold Penlet II sampler firmly against side of finger, and place cap on finger.
10. Press release button. Place Penlet II sampler on firm surface while completing procedure.
11. Squeeze finger gently to obtain drop of blood.
12. Turn meter ON.
13. Remove test strip from bottle taking care not to touch white test spot. Close bottle immediately.

14. Insert test strip into meter until it stops, notched end first and test spot side up.
15. Place large drop of blood on test strip. Do not smear blood on test spot or add additional blood after test begins.
16. Wait for the beeping sound (45 seconds) to obtain reading.
17. Remove lancet by removing Penlet II cap. Grasp dark gray T-shaped prongs. Point lancet down and away from you. Pull back on dark gray sliding barrel until lancet drops out into sharps container. Clean Penlet II sampler and cap with soap and water.
18. Remove test strip, and place in disposal bag.
19. Remove gloves and wash your hands.
20. Document findings, and administer Insulin as needed.

CHARTING for Venous Specimens

- Time of blood withdrawal
- Date and name(s) of test(s) for which blood was drawn
- Any unusual conditions in either the patient or specimen
- Site where blood cultures were obtained for capillary specimen
- Results of blood glucose reading
- Insulin administered: type, amount, location of injection.

CRITICAL THINKING APPLICATION

CLINICAL PROBLEMS	CRITICAL THINKING OPTIONS
■ Blood does not flow into the syringe.	• Check the position of the needle in the vein. • Pull needle back slightly away from the wall of the vein. Rotate needle gently. Do not pull excessively on the plunger, especially if the vein is small, since this movement may cause the vein to collapse.
■ Blood does not flow into the vacuum tube.	• Check the position of the needle in the vein. If vacuum in the tube is lost or if the vein is not large enough, discard the tube and get another. • If there is pressure on the vein for vacuum pull, select a larger vein or use a syringe and needle instead of the Vacutainer method.
■ Unable to get blood sample with Autolet.	• Check that fingertip or heel not toughened with overuse of alcohol sponges. Should use soap and water to clean area. • Choose an alternative site and repeat the stick. • Stroke gently from base of finger toward the tip. Do not apply firm massage as it can interfere with blood flow.
■ One-Touch II meter shows not enough blood.	• Remove test strip, and insert new strip. • Obtain new blood drop. • Ensure blood drop is sufficient to form a round, shiny drop that covers entire strip. • Complete procedure.

unit 5

SPUTUM COLLECTION

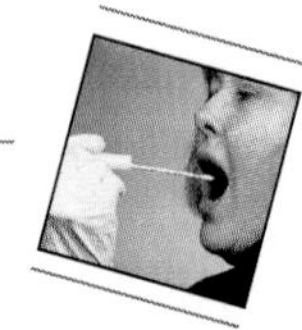

NURSING PROCESS DATA

ASSESSMENT Data Base

Check diagnosis for indication of need for specimen.

Observe client's ability to cough up specimen. You may need to assist the client while obtaining a specimen, or suction equipment may be necessary.

Determine the degree of pain the client can tolerate.

Check client's understanding of procedure so sputum and not saliva is obtained.

PLANNING Objectives

To obtain adequate sputum specimen for laboratory examination

To identify predominant organisms, if respiratory disease is present

To maintain client's respiratory status during and after procedure

IMPLEMENTATION Procedures

EVALUATION Expected Outcomes

Adequate sputum specimen is obtained for laboratory examination.

Client's respiratory status is maintained during and after procedure.

OBTAINING SPUTUM SPECIMEN

Equipment

Container and cover for specimen

Label for specimen

Small plastic bag for delivery of specimen to laboratory

Tissues

Laboratory requisition slip

Clean gloves

Gown, mask, goggles, if needed

Preparation

1. Check orders and client care plan.
2. Gather equipment.
3. Wash your hands.
4. Provide privacy.

Procedure

1. Explain procedure and rationale to client.
2. Have client rinse mouth before coughing to remove any oral contaminants.

> **CLINICAL ALERT**
>
> Strict asepsis is necessary to obtain an accurate laboratory report.

3. Don clean gloves. Don mask, gown, goggles if client requires assistance with procedure.
4. Tell client to take several deep breaths and to cough up sputum (not saliva) directly into sterile container.
5. Obtain 1–2 tablespoons of sputum in container; close and seal lid.
6. If client is unable to produce sputum specimen, assist client by placing the palms of your hands or a rolled pillow around the incision area if client is inhibited by pain. **Rationale:** Wrapping a sheet around chest or abdomen also provides support for body walls during coughing.
7. Remove gloves, gown, mask, and goggles.

8. Evaluate client's status after procedure.
9. Deliver sputum to the laboratory within 30 minutes after collection. Obtain specimen during treatment if client is receiving any respiratory treatment (IPPB or PVD).

USING SUCTION TRAP

Equipment

Suction machine
Sterile catheter and glove
Sterile saline
Sterile sputum trap
Culture tube
Plastic disposal bag
Clean gloves
Gown, mask, goggles

Preparation

1. Check physician's orders and client care plan for type of equipment needed.
2. Wash your hands.
3. Gather equipment.
4. Explain procedure to client.
5. Provide privacy.
6. Don clean gloves, goggles, gown, mask as appropriate.

Procedure

1. Set up suction equipment.
2. Attach sputum trap between suction catheter and tubing.
3. Complete suctioning as for nasooropharyngeal suctioning.
4. Place your thumb on top of sputum trap to monitor; remove your thumb and provide intermittent suction, lifting thumb at intervals until specimen is collected.

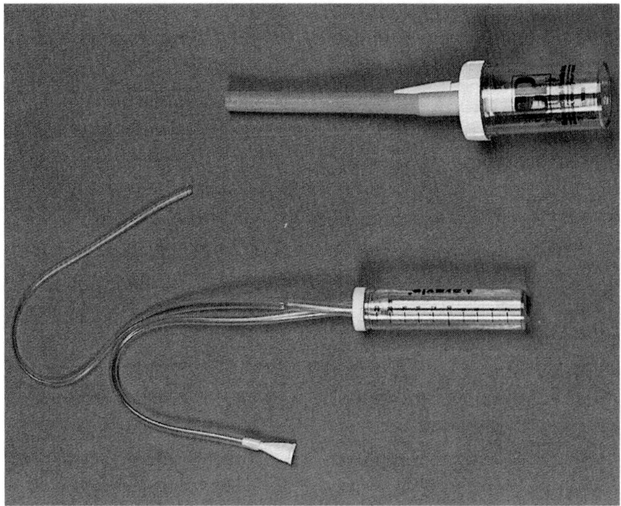

Two common types of suction traps used in client care.

5. Suction no more than 15 seconds at a time. **Rationale:** This prevents removal of too much oxygen.
6. Turn off wall suction.
7. Place suction trap in plastic bag. Follow agency protocol for double-bagging specimens before transporting to laboratory.
8. Remove gloves and other equipment; mask, gown, and goggles if used, and dispose of in appropriate receptacle.
9. Send specimen that was collected in trap to laboratory. (In many hospitals suction tube is also sent to the lab with specimen.)
10. Place client in a comfortable position.
11. Wash your hands.

COLLECTING SPECIMEN BY TRANSTRACHEAL ASPIRATION

Equipment

No. 14 needle with polyethylene tubing or small intracatheter (IV catheter)
Sterile saline and 3–5 mL syringe
Povidone-iodine (Betadine) or skin-cleansing solution dictated by hospital policy
Xylocaine injection

Procedure

1. Explain procedure to client.
2. Collect equipment.

3. Wash your hands.
4. Provide privacy for client.
5. Position by hyperextending client's neck and placing a pillow under shoulders.
6. Cleanse cricothyroid area of neck with Betadine solution.
7. Physician will anesthetize area with Xylocaine.
8. Physician will insert 14-gauge needle into cricothyroid area, thread polyethylene tubing through needle, withdraw needle, and leave tubing in place.
9. Attach syringe (3–5 mL) with 1–2 mL sterile saline into polyethylene tubing.
10. Inject saline into polyethylene tubing to initiate coughing response.
11. To obtain specimen, immediately pull back on barrel of syringe.
12. Withdraw catheter and apply pressure over puncture site.
13. Place sputum secretions in sterile container, label container, and send it to laboratory.
14. Position client for comfort.
15. Wash your hands.

CHARTING for Sputum Collection

- Amount, color, and consistency of sputum
- Mechanical sputum trap used for collection
- Client's tolerance of procedure

CRITICAL THINKING APPLICATION

CLINICAL PROBLEMS	CRITICAL THINKING OPTIONS
Pain inhibits client from coughing.	• If diagnosis permits, support painful area with rolled pillows or tight sheets so that external pressure equals internal pressure, thus minimizing pain and discomfort. • Before beginning procedure, ask client to take several deep breaths. These breaths may trigger the cough reflex and aerate the lungs. • Give client pain medication as ordered 15–30 minutes before obtaining the specimen.
Client develops coughing spasms during procedure.	• Press your third finger lightly over the client's trachea in the cricoid hollow. This pressure releases the nerve that innervates the coughing reflex. • Report to physician to obtain an order for nebulization.
Unable to obtain sputum specimen.	• Notify physician for orders: bronchodilator drugs, nebulization treatment. • Perform PVD to mobilize secretions for expectoration. • Attempt procedure early in the morning when mucus has collected during the night and is more easily expectorated.

unit 6

THROAT AND WOUND SPECIMENS FOR CULTURE

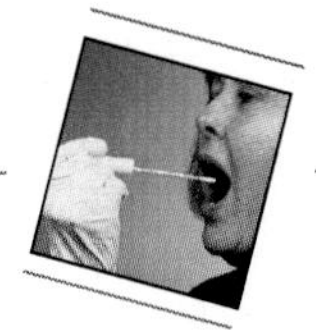

NURSING PROCESS DATA

ASSESSMENT Data Base

Identify appropriate container for specimen swabs or material.

Determine time frame for expediting specimen to lab.

Assess exact area for specimen.

Assess client's ability to cooperate with procedure.

Assess wound and drainage.

PLANNING Objectives

To obtain an uncontaminated specimen for study

To place specimen swab or material in container using appropriate techniques

To send specimen to laboratory within specified time frame

IMPLEMENTATION Procedures

Obtaining a Throat Specimen

Obtaining Aerobic Specimen

Obtaining Anaerobic Specimen

EVALUATION Expected Outcomes

Uncontaminated specimens obtained.

Specimens placed in appropriate culture medium container.

Specimens sent to laboratory in timely manner.

OBTAINING A THROAT SPECIMEN

Equipment

Tongue depressor
Culture tube with applicator stick
Light source

Preparation

1. Check physician's orders.
2. Wash your hands.
3. Gather equipment.
4. Explain procedure to client.
5. Position client in Fowler's position.
6. Place treatment light or face client toward natural light source to provide good lighting.

Procedure

1. Remove the sterile applicator from the culture tube by rotating cap to break seal.
2. Ask the client to open mouth.
3. Use tongue depressor if desired to depress tongue. **Rationale:** Prevents tongue from contaminating the swab.
4. Swab the back of the throat along the tonsillar area. **Rationale:** Swab only one side of the throat. A second specimen of the other side may be taken, check hospital protocol.

■ CLINICAL ALERT

Obtain wound specimen for both aerobic and anaerobic organisms during scheduled dressing change before any medication or antimicrobial agents have been applied.

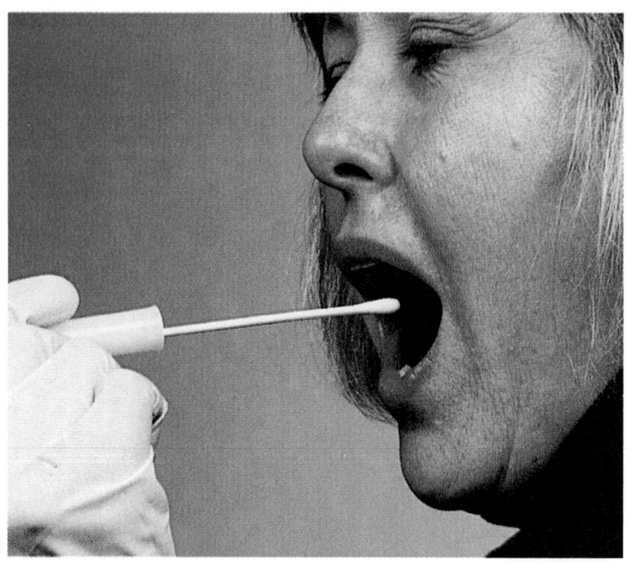

Ask client to open mouth and obtain specimen from back of throat along tonsillar area.

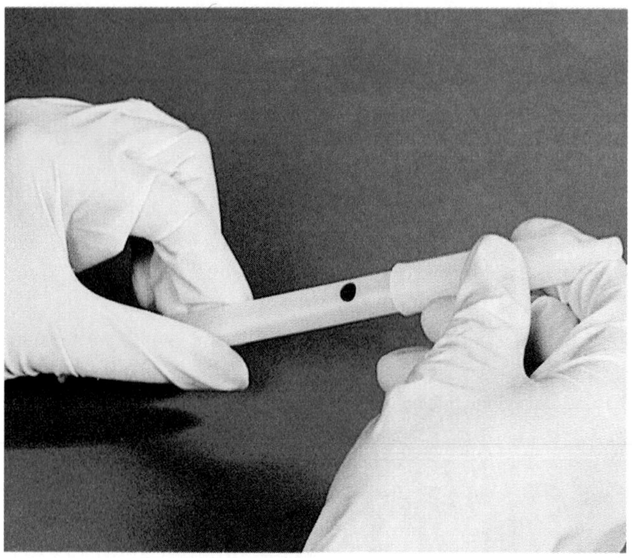

Push applicator stick in specimen tube being careful to not contaminate stick.

5. Remove the applicator stick, and place in the specimen tube.
6. Push the stick into the tube until the swab is saturated with culture medium and cap reaches black dot. **Rationale:** This places the applicator tip into the culture medium to preserve bacteria until laboratory can complete test.
7. Position client for comfort.
8. Wash your hands.
9. Label specimen tube, and send to laboratory immediately. **Rationale:** To ensure accurate identification of microorganisms.

OBTAINING AEROBIC CULTURE

Equipment

Culture transport swab with transport medium
Laboratory slip
Clean gloves
Sterile gloves
Dressing material
Disposal bag

Preparation

1. Check physician's orders and client care plan.
2. Wash your hands.
3. Gather equipment.
4. Explain procedure to client.
5. Open all sterile dressing material, and arrange for easy access during dressing change.

Procedure

1. Don clean gloves.
2. Remove and discard soiled dressing from wound into disposal bag.
3. Remove gloves and don clean gloves.
4. Remove swab, and wipe swab in wound. Obtain culture from active drainage area.
5. Avoid touching skin edges or other surfaces that will contaminate the swab.
6. Return swab to container.
7. Crush transport medium vial, and push swab tip into contact with transport medium.
8. Close container.
9. Remove clean gloves, wash hands.
10. Don sterile gloves, and replace dressing.
11. Remove gloves, and wash your hands.
12. Transport specimen to laboratory within 30 minutes. **Rationale:** This ensures organisms are still viable.

OBTAINING ANAEROBIC CULTURE

Equipment

Anaerobic transport medium kit with swab
Laboratory slip
Clean gloves
Sterile gloves
Dressing material
Disposal bag

Preparation

1. Check physician's orders and client care plan.
2. Wash your hands.
3. Gather equipment.
4. Explain procedure to client.
5. Open all sterile dressing material, and arrange for easy access during dressing change.

Procedure

1. Don clean gloves.
2. Take off dressing from wound, and discard in disposal bag.
3. Remove specimen swab, and wipe in wound as you did with aerobic culturing. Be sure you do not tip anaerobic transport medium tube because it contains carbon dioxide. **Rationale:** Tipping "spills" the gas out, making it useless to transport anaerobic organisms.
4. Return swab to container. *Do not* touch sides of container with applicator.
5. Fill out or affix label to specimen.
6. Transport specimen to laboratory *immediately.*
7. Alternative method:
   a. Draw up exudate in syringe with all air expelled or have a physician aspirate the wound.
   b. Inject drainage into anaerobic culture tube.
   c. Transport specimens to laboratory *immediately.* **Rationale:** Anaerobic organisms may appear on Gram stain even though they are not grown in the culture.
8. Remove clean gloves, wash hands, don sterile gloves.
9. Replace sterile dressing following protocol.
10. Remove sterile gloves.
11. Wash your hands.

CHARTING for Obtaining Culture

- Assessment of wound and drainage.
- Exact area where culture obtained
- Type of culture obtained
- Characteristics of material sent for culture
- Time specimen sent to lab

CRITICAL THINKING APPLICATION

CLINICAL PROBLEMS	CRITICAL THINKING OPTIONS
■ Inner surface of collection container contaminated while inserting swab into the culture medium container.	• Obtain new specimen and send to laboratory.
■ Anaerobic specimen not sent to laboratory immediately.	• Obtain new specimen and send to laboratory.
■ Anaerobic specimen not sent in appropriate container with hydrogen gas.	• Obtain appropriate container and send new specimen to laboratory.

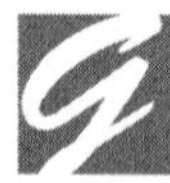

GERIATRIC CONSIDERATIONS

- Elderly clients may not clearly hear and understand the directions given regarding specimen collection. Ask specific questions to ensure compliance.
- Determine client's ability to follow directions for obtaining specimens such as urine and stool. Hearing and vision may be impaired, thereby interfering with their ability to follow through on specimen collection.
- Assess client's ability to accurately use blood glucose-monitoring equipment. Finger dexterity may be altered due to stroke, arthritis, or other chronic conditions, thus preventing them from being able to use the equipment or obtain the blood specimen.
- Residual urine may increase as a result of changes in the bladder tone, leading to urinary stasis and potential bacterial proliferation. This leads to bladder infections, necessitating accurate identification of bacteria. This is accomplished through analysis of urine obtained from specimens free of contamination. Ensure client understands the procedure for obtaining an uncontaminated urine specimen. The nurse may need to obtain the specimen if the client is unable to do so without contaminating it.
- Avoid using arms with neurological or vascular alterations when obtaining blood specimens.
- Client's receiving heparin or Coumadin require a longer pressure time over the venipuncture site to prevent bleeding.
- Elderly clients have large rolling veins that make it appear easier to perform a venipuncture. In fact, they tend to collapse and rupture quite easily.

20

Diagnostic Tests

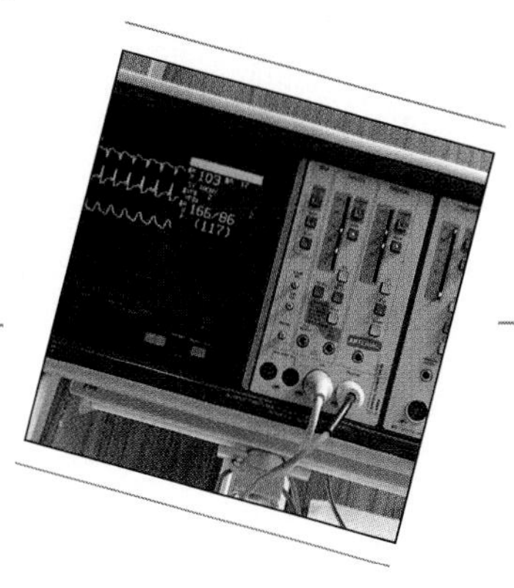

LEARNING OBJECTIVES

- Describe the major components of client teaching for diagnostic studies.
- List at least three preparatory functions for clients undergoing diagnostic studies.
- Explain the importance of determining allergic responses to shellfish before clients undergo contrast media studies.
- List the signs and symptoms that occur when the client experiences an allergic reaction.
- Explain the reason for giving blocking agents before administering radioisotopes to clients.
- Outline the nursing care responsibilities when a client returns from a myelogram.
- Discuss the nursing care responsibilities when a client returns from an arteriogram.
- Describe the care necessary after cardiac catheterization care to prevent postprocedure complications.
- Explain the steps you would take if a client is given medication prior to a GI series.
- Describe client positions for at least four diagnostic procedures commonly performed at the bedside.
- Compare and contrast postprocedure nursing observations for clients undergoing liver biopsy, paracentesis, and thoracentesis.
- Explain the nurse's role during procedures that use fiberoptic scopes.
- Describe the data that should be included in the charting for clients undergoing diagnostic procedures.

TERMINOLOGY

Abscess: a localized collection of pus in any part of the body.

Allergy: an altered reaction of body tissues to a specific substance; essentially an antibody–antigen reaction and may be due to the release of histamine.

Amniocentesis: puncturing the amniotic sac, usually by using a needle and syringe, to remove amniotic fluid for assessment of fetal maturity.

Antiemetic: an agent that prevents or arrests vomiting.

Arteriogram: study using radiopaque dye injected into an artery to assess arteries.

Barium: a radiopaque compound used in roentgenography of the gastrointestinal tract.

Bronchoscopy: a visualization of the larynx, trachea, and bronchi through a flexible scope.

Catheterization: use or passage of a catheter, a tube for evacuating or injecting fluids.

Centesis: perforation or puncture through the skin to obtain fluid.

Cholangiography: x-ray examination of the bile ducts.

Cholecystogram: x-ray picture of the gallbladder.

Cinecystourethrogram: motion picture record of radiologic investigation of the urethra and urinary bladder when they are filled and during emptying.

Computerized Tomography (CT Scan): a scanning technique that provides a series of detailed visualizations.

Contrast medium: a radiopaque substance used during x-ray examination to provide a contrast in density between the tissue being filmed and the medium.

Contusion: an injury in which the skin is not broken.

Cranio: prefix pertaining to the skull.

Craniotomy: incision involving the skull.

Diagnosis: method or art of identifying the disease or condition a person has or is believed to have.

Diaphoresis: profuse sweating.

Dissipate: to scatter, disperse, dispel, disintegrate.

Dyspnea: shortness of breath.

Enema: introduction of a solution through a tube into the rectum or colon.

Fiberoptic scope: flexible scope that uses fiberoptic materials for visualization. These materials transmit light along its course by reflecting it from the side or wall of the fiber. Devices using fiberoptic materials are used in endoscopic examinations.

Fluoroscopy: type of examination using a screen to view shadows with the aid of x-rays.

Lithotomy: incision into the bladder for removing a stone.

Lumbar: pertaining to the loins and lower vertebrae in the back.

Magnetic Resonance Imaging (MRI): is a noninvasive test that uses a magnetic field with radio frequency waves to produce cross-sectional images of the body.

Myelogram: x-ray inspection of the spinal cord by the use of radiopaque medium

Neoplasm: a new and abnormal formation of tissue, as a tumor or growth.

n.p.o.: nothing by mouth.

Oliguria: diminished amount of urine formation.

Paracentesis: puncture of the abdominal cavity for the removal of fluid.

Peripheral: outer part or surface of a body.

Pneumo: pertaining to air, gas, and respiration.

Pyelo: pertaining to the pelvis of the kidney

Pyelogram: x-ray study of the renal pelvis and ureter.

Scintillation: the emissions from radiographic substances; a subjective sensation of seeing sparks.

Septicemia: blood poisoning; septic products in blood and tissue.

Tachycardia: fast pulse above 100 BPM.

Thoracentesis: surgical puncture of the chest wall for the removal of fluid.

Tumor: uncontrolled new growth or tissue forming an abnormal mass that performs no physiologic function.

Urticaria: a vascular reaction of the skin characterized by the eruption of pale elevated wheals, which are associated with severe itching.

Ventro: denoting the abdomen or ventral (anterior) surface of the body.

Vertigo: sensation of moving or having objects move when they are actually still.

PREPARATION

The responsibility of the nurse begins with the initial scheduling of the test and continues after the results of the test are explained to the client. The physician explains the results of the test, but the nurse answers questions, interprets terminology, and listens to the client express his or her feelings or apprehensions.

The preparation of clients for diagnostic tests must be done on an individual basis. Some clients are well informed about the test they are scheduled to take. They know about diet and fluid restrictions, what to expect during the procedure, whether or not there is any discomfort with the test, and how long the procedure takes. Others need a great deal of explanation. Also, some clients prefer not to be given any explanation about the test. Nurses need to respect the client's preferences and provide only information requested, unless it in some way is a danger to the client.

Many clients who are frightened are unable to communicate. Communication involves an active, verbal interchange of ideas as well as paying attention to the client's nonverbal cues. One effective way to allow clients time to think about questions is to provide a printed form explaining the diagnostic test. The form may cover such information as how long a test takes, equipment used for the test, and any sensations experienced during the test. Leaving the form at the bedside can stimulate interest and prompt the shy, reserved client to ask questions when you return later.

Many diagnostic procedures are done on an outpatient basis. This makes it imperative that the nurse provides the necessary information about the procedure. Instructions are sent home with the client that include preprocedural preparation. When the client arrives for the diagnostic test, time should be allotted to answer questions, reassure the client, and determine if the preprocedure preparation was followed.

Another important aspect of teaching involves the way in which the nurse approaches the client. Avoid giving the impression that you are in a hurry and that you have no time to answer any questions. On the other hand, be aware of the client's ability to pay attention to what you have to say. If the client seems distracted, he or she may be worried about finances, about who is watching the children, or whether or not their job will be waiting after discharge from the hospital. This preoccupation may prevent assimilation of knowledge and the client may be unprepared for the events that follow.

Remember, the client probably does not know medical jargon; therefore, explain procedures in terms the client can understand. If the client looks puzzled and does not ask any questions, evaluate how you presented the information.

Feedback is the only way in which you can evaluate the learner's knowledge. Feedback can be in the form of direct questioning about certain aspects of the test. Feedback can also be determined through direct observation of facial expressions, posturing, and activities.

Contrast Media Studies

Many x-rays use the normal contrasts of the body, such as air, water in soft tissues, and bone; however, for some tests a contrast medium is required. Several types of contrast media are used routinely, including barium sulfate, helium, carbon dioxide, and organic iodides.

One of the major problems with the use of some contrast media is the adverse reaction or sensitivity that can occur. This is more common when iodine preparations are used. The degree of reaction varies from mild (such as nausea) to severe (such as cardiovascular collapse). The usual symptoms include urticaria, hives, nausea, vomiting, and decreased blood pressure.

Clients allergic to food, especially shellfish, or drugs are often allergic to some dyes used in diagnostic studies, particularly those that are iodine-based. Following injections of iodine dye, many tests are abnormal for varying lengths of time. Urine sodium, specific gravity, protein, and osmolality are abnormal for 16 hours. Urine catecholamines are abnormal for 16 hours.

Barium can cause some uncomfortable feelings and problems with the gastrointestinal tract, but with proper postprocedure care this condition can be greatly reduced.

Ultrasound Studies

Ultrasound is a relatively new procedure used to study alterations in soft tissue images. Many organs are now studied through this procedure, among them the gallbladder, reproductive organs, liver, spleen, and thyroid gland. Ultrasound uses a high-frequency sound wave to display an echo pattern on an oscilloscope.

Ultrasound is painless, requiring only that the client lie quietly during the 15- or 30-minute procedure. These procedures need to precede barium studies because barium impedes the transmission of sound waves.

When ultrasound is used to study the pelvic organs, the client is instructed to drink four glasses of water to promote a full bladder. The full bladder enhances the transmission of sound waves and thus improves visualization of the organs.

Echocardiography and echoencephalography procedures are similar to those for ultrasound. They are painless, noninvasive techniques that use transducers and oscilloscopes similar to those in ultrasound procedures. The echocardiogram records heart motion, not heart outline. The echoencephalogram measures, by spikes produced from the echo, the midline structures of the brain. There is no preparation or postprocedure alteration in activity for these procedures.

Nuclear Imaging Studies

Radioisotopes distribute uniformly through normal tissue but unevenly in pathologically involved or diseased tissue. The radioisotopes emit radiation and gamma rays and can be picked up by scanning devices. A scanning procedure involves less radiation exposure than a chest x-ray.

Radioisotopes tend to concentrate in specific organ tissues and thus are more effective when administered for scanning a particular organ. For example, hippuran (^{131}I) is specifically used for thyroid scanning while thallium-201 (^{201}Tl) is used to evaluate blood flow through vessels that are too small to visualize with a cardiac catheterization procedure. The newer thallium imagery is three-dimensional, the camera moves around the client in a 180–360° arc. The three-dimensional view is more precise in identifying abnormalities. Scanning allows visualization of organs that are unobservable by x-ray alone. Tumors present as areas of reduced radioisotopic activity. Radioisotope studies are contraindicated with pregnancy, breast-feeding mothers, or persons who are allergic to the radioisotopes.

The radioactive isotopes are administered intravenously or orally to the client. A specified time elapses before the scanning is done. This allows time for the radioactive material to reach the specific tissue under study. Then, a scanning device is used to record the concentration of radiation that emerges from the radioisotope.

Some clients are given blocking agents before the administration of the radioisotope. This prevents the radioactive material from entering organs other than those being studied. A common blocking agent is Lugol's solution, which is given to a client who is having a study done on an organ other than the thyroid gland.

Magnetic Resonance Imaging (MRI)

The MRI procedure has revolutionized diagnostic medicine. The procedure identifies the distribution of hydrogen molecules in the body using a three-dimensional process. The images are translated by computer and differentiate normal from abnormal tissue. The MRI detects and describes soft tissue abnormalities and yields information about the chemical nature of the cells. Gray and white brain matter can be differentiated and brain tumors and vascular abnormalities identified. Cardiac abnormalities and multiple sclerosis can also be identified through the MRI procedure. The procedure is noninvasive and does not involve harmful exposure to radiation.

Assisting the Physician during Tests

Nurses are frequently called on to assist the physician with procedures at the bedside as well as in the treatment room. The procedures presented in this chapter are the most common ones performed in the hospital unit. It is important that the nurse be aware of the correct client positioning in order to facilitate the procedure, decrease complications, and decrease the time it takes to complete the procedure.

Some diagnostic tests frequently used in the past are of limited use today. One such procedure is the lumbar puncture. Removal of fluid from the spinal tract may cause the brain, because of edema, to herniate down through the tentorium. Because of this complication, a lumbar puncture is not done on a client with head trauma or potential increased intracranial pressure. The CAT scan is now frequently used to determine intracranial bleeding.

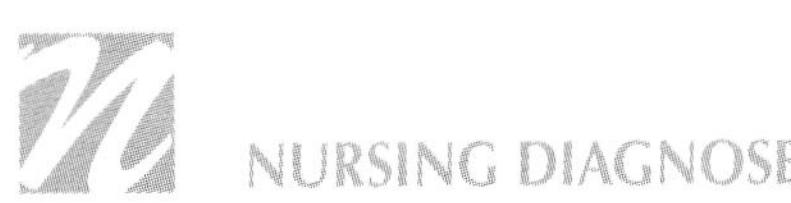

NURSING DIAGNOSES

The following nursing diagnoses may be appropriate to include in a client care plan when the components are related to clients undergoing diagnostic procedures.

NURSING DIAGNOSIS	RELATED FACTORS
Anxiety	Apprehension regarding test or procedure outcome
Fear	Results of diagnostic test, change in health status, threat to self-concept
Fluid Volume Deficit	Reaction to contrast media, n.p.o. status, side effects of medication
Knowledge Deficit	Misunderstanding of instructions or information, inadequate data or explanation of procedure (maintaining position after spinal tap, liver biopsy)
Noncompliance	Inability to follow directions as a result of poor health status

unit 1

CONTRAST MEDIA STUDIES

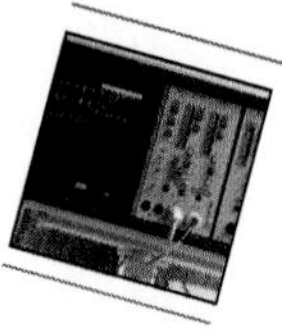

NURSING PROCESS DATA

ASSESSMENT Data Base

Assess client's knowledge of procedure to be done.
Identify any history of drug or food allergies.
Evaluate client's ability to follow directions before and during the test.
Assess vital signs and document for baseline data.

PLANNING Objectives

To determine if the client is physically prepared for the test
To determine if the client is psychologically prepared for the test
To determine if the client is at risk for an allergic reaction
To determine if the client is able to cooperate with the preparation and completion of the test

IMPLEMENTATION Procedures

Preparing for Contrast Media Studies

Procedure for Oral Cholecystogram
Procedure for Intravenous Cholangiogram
Procedure for Intravenous Pyelogram
Procedure for Myelogram
Procedure for Arteriogram
Procedure for Computerized Tomography (CT Scan)
Procedure for Cardiac Catheterization

EVALUATION Expected Outcomes

Client is able to complete the test without untoward effects.
Client understands procedure and has anxiety level under control.
Client is properly prepared for diagnostic test.

TABLE 20–1. Contrast Media Studies

Diagnostic Test	Rationale
Oral Cholecystogram	To visualize shape and position of the gallbladder and to identify the presence of stones
Intravenous Cholangiogram	To visualize the biliary tract
Intravenous Pyelogram	To visualize structures of the urinary tract
Myelogram	To visualize the subarrachnoid space to identify abnormalities
Arteriogram	To visualize abnormalities or obstructions to specific blood vessels
Computerized Axial Tomography	To visualize a cross-section of the brain to precisely localize intracranial lesions
Cardiac Catheterization	To measure oxygen concentration, provide blood samples, determine cardiac output, and visualize coronary arteries

PREPARING FOR CONTRAST MEDIA STUDIES

Equipment

Signed consent form
Pajama bottoms and hospital gown
Allergy identaband, if needed
Wheelchair

Preparation

■ CLINICAL ALERT

Symptoms of contrast media reactions
- Urticaria, hives
- Nausea, vomiting
- Respiratory distress
- Decreased blood pressure

Clients allergic to food or drugs generally are allergic to some contrast media used for diagnostic studies.

1. Identify the specific diagnostic test to be performed (Table 20–1).
2. Determine if any tests must precede others in order to schedule test appropriately.
3. Obtain client's history to determine allergies to food or drugs, and note these on the chart. Notify physician of findings.
4. Identify specific preparations that need to be carried out before the studies.
5. Monitor food and fluid restrictions that need to be altered for the studies.
6. Obtain special consent forms for all invasive diagnostic studies after the physician has explained the study to the client.
7. Provide client teaching regarding the purpose of the study, including any special preparation required and restrictions imposed by the study.
8. Provide psychologic support and reassurance to the client.
9. Obtain orders regarding medications or nutrition for clients with special problems, such as diabetes or seizure disorders.
10. Carry out safety precautions immediately prior to the study:
    a. Check identaband for accuracy.
    b. Have client void if necessary.
    c. Remove client's hairpins, jewelry, and dentures if necessary.
    d. Chart premedication given.
    e. Monitor safe transfer from the bed to gurney or wheelchair.
    f. Accompany client to x-ray department if needed. (Usually nurses accompany critically ill clients.)

Procedure *for Oral Cholecystogram*

1. Explain purpose for procedure to client.
2. Identify allergies to shellfish or iodine. Notify physician if allergy is noted.
3. Administer iodine radiopaque medication after dinner—no later than 5 PM. Usual drugs include iopanoic acid (Telepaque), iodipamide (Cholografin), and (Oragrafin).
    a. Number of tablets administered is based on client's weight.
    b. Tablets are given 5–30 minutes apart with 8 oz. of water for each tablet.
    c. Inform client that diarrhea is a common side effect.
4. Keep client n.p.o. after administration of contrast medium. **Rationale:** This prevents contraction of gallbladder and expulsion of radiopaque dye.
5. Take client to x-ray department.
6. Explain details of procedure to client.
    a. X-ray client in standing and lying positions for good visualization of gallbladder and common bile duct.
    b. Feed client a fatty meal to test ability of the gallbladder to contract.
    c. If visualization does not occur, additional medications may be given and the test repeated the following day, or an IV cholangiogram may be done.

■ CLINICAL ALERT

After injection of iodine dye the following tests are abnormal for at least 16 hours:
- Urine sodium, specific gravity, protein, and osmolality
- 24-hour urine collection for 17-hydroxyketosteroids, 17-hydroxycorticoids, and catecholamines
- Protein-bound iodine (PBI) (may be affected for 3–6 months

> **CLINICAL ALERT**
>
> Ultrasound has replaced the oral cholecystogram test in most cases. It may still be used, however, if ultrasound results are inconclusive.

Procedure *for Intravenous Cholangiogram*

1. Follow steps as appropriate in *Preparation for Contrast Media Studies.*
   a. Give client a clear liquid lunch, two glasses of water, and clear liquid dinner on day before test. **Rationale:** To clear out GI tract so duct x-rays are clearer.
   b. Keep client n.p.o. for at least 3 hours pretest.
   c. Identify allergies to shellfish or iodine.
   d. Obtain consent.
2. Explain procedure to client.
   a. Procedure involves dye injection directly into the biliary tree. The dye is given over a 15- to 30-minute period.
   b. Injection site is usually at the midclavicular line beneath the right costal margin.
   c. Tell client he or she will be strapped to tilting x-ray table and x-rays will be taken every 15–30 minutes until the common bile duct tree is visualized.
   d. The procedure may take 1–3 hours.
   e. Warn client he or she may feel nauseated and warm when dye is injected.
   f. Instruct client to inform technician immediately of any abnormal reactions.
3. Client is returned to room.
4. Encourage fluids and offer diet.
5. Have client resume previous activity orders.
6. Monitor client for allergic response to contrast media.
7. Monitor vital signs, and check for symptoms of septicemia and bleeding. Report unusual findings to physician.
8. Report any pain to physician. **Rationale:** Pain is not associated with this test, this may indicate a complication is occurring.

Procedure *for Intravenous Pyelogram (IVP)*

1. Follow steps as appropriate in *Preparation for Contrast Media Studies.*
   a. Give client clear liquids the evening before the IVP. Place client on n.p.o. after 12 midnight.
   b. Give laxative or enema as ordered. **Rationale:** To eliminate feces and gas to provide better contrast.
   c. Identify allergies to shellfish or iodine.
   d. Obtain consent.
   e. Take client to x-ray department when notified.
2. Explain details of procedure to client.
   a. Test dose of contrast medium may be injected intradermally for clients with a history of allergies. The contrast material is administered if there is no reaction within 15 minutes of test dose.
   b. Contrast medium is injected as a large single dose.
   c. X-rays are taken over period of 1 hour to determine extent to which dye is filtered through the kidneys.
3. Warn client that contrast medium can cause feelings of nausea, shortness of breath, and a hot, flushed effect.
4. Return client to room and have client resume ordered activity level.
5. Encourage fluids, and offer diet.
6. Observe signs and symptoms for reactions to contrast medium such as oliguria, nausea, and vomiting.

Procedure *for Myelogram*

1. Follow steps as appropriate in *Preparation for Contrast Media Studies.*
   a. Identify allergies to shellfish, iodine, or other contrast media.
   b. Keep client n.p.o. for 3–4 hours before test.
   c. Obtain baseline levels of motor and sensory function.
   d. Obtain consent.
   e. Medicate with sedative if ordered. **Rationale:** This provides client comfort.
   f. Take client on gurney to x-ray department.
2. Explain details of procedure to client.
   a. Client is placed in prone position with pillow under abdomen. **Rationale:** This position allows physician to visualize ruptured disc or neoplasms.
   b. A lumbar puncture needle is inserted between the vertebrae into the subarachnoid space.
   c. A small amount of cerebrospinal fluid is sent to lab for study.

d. Contrast medium is injected, and client is tilted on table to allow flow of dye to designated areas of spine to visualize it by x-rays.
e. Oil-based contrast medium, Pantopaque, is removed through aspiration. Explain to client that sudden sharp pain in legs may occur.
f. Water-based contrast medium, metrizamide, is absorbed and excreted through kidneys. It is not removed by aspiration.
g. Procedure lasts about 1 hour.
h. Client is returned on gurney to room.

3. After the test.
   a. Keep client in prone position or supine position for 12–24 hours. May turn side to side. **Rationale:** This position prevents a headache and CSF leaks.
   b. Keep head of bed elevated 15–30° if procedure has included water-soluble dye medium. Client may be ambulatory or on bed rest. **Rationale:** This position reduces rate of upward displacement of dye.
4. Monitor vital signs and motor and sensory function.
   a. Cervical myelogram: Check upper and lower extremities and bladder function.
   b. Lumbar myelogram: Check lower extremities and bladder function.
5. Medicate for pain as ordered.
6. Increase fluids to at least 2500 mL per day. **Rationale:** Fluids rehydrate and replace cerebrospinal fluid and may prevent headache following procedure. Offer diet.
7. Monitor output, and observe for distention.
8. Observe for complication of chemical or bacterial meningitis: fever, stiff neck, photophobia.
9. Use comfort measures and relaxation techniques when needed.

■ CLINICAL ALERT

A myelogram is performed less frequently today because of the wide use of the MRI and CT scanning.

Procedure *for Arteriogram*

1. Explain purpose of procedure to client.
2. Identify allergies to shellfish, iodine, or any contras' media.
3. Obtain consent.
4. Shave and scrub puncture site when ordered.
5. Place client on n.p.o. if ordered.
6. Have client void before procedure.
7. Obtain vital signs. **Rationale:** To provide comparison data following procedure.
8. Administer preprocedure medications if ordered, and transport client to x-ray department.
9. Explain details of procedure to client.
   a. Puncture site will be scrubbed and a local anesthetic administered.
   b. Contrast medium will be injected to visualize abnormalities or obstruction to specific vessels.
   c. Client may be instructed to hold breath for x-rays. Procedure takes about 1 hour if an automatic film changer is used.
10. Client is returned on gurney to room.
11. Monitor vital signs, pulses, and puncture site, as with surgical clients. **Rationale:** To identify potential complications.
12. Observe for signs of shock and presence of pain, which indicate hemorrhage or thrombosis.
13. Observe for symptoms of delayed allergic reaction to dye, such as nausea, vomiting, tachycardia, and sweating. **Rationale:** Delayed reactions can occur up to several hours following the procedure.
14. Notify physician immediately if unusual symptoms are present. **Rationale:** Immediate medical intervention is necessary to prevent anaphylaxis.
15. Apply ice pack to puncture site if ordered. Do not flex the involved extremity.
16. Maintain bed rest with head elevated slightly for required time. Check hospital policy for time.
17. Offer fluids and diet as ordered and tolerated.
18. Provide comfort measures as needed.

Procedure *for Computerized Tomography (CT Scan)*

1. Explain purpose of procedure to client.
2. Identify allergies to shellfish or iodine if contrast medium is used.
3. Obtain consent if contrast medium is used.
4. Place client on n.p.o. if contrast medium is used. **Rationale:** Dye can cause nausea, n.p.o. prevents emesis and potential aspiration.
5. Administer preprocedure medication if ordered.
6. Remove all metal objects, such as hair clips, necklace, and jewelry. **Rationale:** Metal objects block bony structures on the film.
7. Take client on gurney to x-ray department.

8. Explain equipment and procedure to client.
9. Explain client will have IV injection of contrast material if enhanced study is to be done. Explain that a warm, flushed feeling or nausea can occur.
10. Instruct client to lie very still during the procedure. **Rationale:** Movement causes artifact on the image.
11. Return client to room.
12. Provide diet and force fluids to 3000 mL or as ordered. **Rationale:** Increasing fluids assists in eliminating the contrast medium more quickly.
13. Observe for signs of delayed allergic reaction if contrast study is done.

Procedure *for Cardiac Catheterization*

1. Explain purpose for procedure to client.
2. Obtain consent.
3. Identify allergies to drugs, iodine, shellfish, or any other contrast media.
4. Complete prep and shave of groin or brachial area (or both).
5. Establish baseline data for vital signs, peripheral pulses, coagulation studies (PTT, PT), ECG pattern.
6. Place client on n.p.o. after midnight.
7. In morning, obtain vital signs, take weight, have the client void.
8. Administer preprocedure medication, usually Valium and atropine.
9. Take client on gurney to cardiac catheterization lab.
10. Explain equipment and details of procedure to client.
    a. Client is strapped onto a table. ECG leads and blood pressure equipment are applied.
    b. Groin or brachial area is scrubbed and injected with Xylocaine.
    c. Catheter is placed in femoral artery and advanced to cardiac chambers.
    d. When contrast medium is injected for coronary artery visualization, explain to client that a warm, flushed feeling, shortness of breath, or nausea can occur.
    e. Client is asked to hold breath about 10 seconds during contrast medium injection.
    f. Reinforce that client will not fall off table as he or she may be turned on side for cineangiography. Total procedure takes 1–1½ hours.
    g. Following catheterization, pressure is applied to puncture site for 10–15 minutes.
11. Transport client on gurney to room.
12. Provide postcardiac catheterization care.
    a. Monitor vital signs, puncture site, heart and lung sounds, and peripheral pulses as with a surgical client.
    b. Elevate extremity used for catheterization site. Keep extremity extended. **Rationale:** Position promotes blood supply back to heart and prevents thrombus formation.
    c. Apply pressure dressing or sandbags to puncture site if bleeding continues.
    d. Encourage fluids and diet when vital signs are stable and no evidence of nausea or drowsiness is present.
    e. Monitor for signs and symptoms of allergic response.
13. Position client for comfort. Place on back for several hours after the procedure, then turn from side to side.

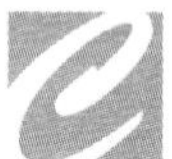

CHARTING for Contrast Media Studies

- Preparation completed (e.g., n.p.o., clear liquid dinner)
- Client teaching completed
- Medication administered
- Allergies noted
- Unusual anxiety or fears of client
- How client transported to test
- Time sent and returned from test
- Postprocedure care
- Appearance of dressing or puncture sites

CRITICAL THINKING APPLICATION

CLINICAL PROBLEMS	CRITICAL THINKING OPTIONS
Client has allergic reaction.	• Follow protocol or standing orders for allergic reactions. • Start O_2 at 6 L/min unless otherwise contraindicated. Use nasal cannula. • Place in semi- or high-Fowler's position if not contraindicated. • Administer medications as outlined in protocol or according to physician's orders. • Provide reassurance and encouragement. • Have client take slow, deep breaths. • If nausea or vomiting occur, obtain an order for an antiemetic from the physician.
Client is given meal when on n.p.o. status.	• Call x-ray and change time of test. If possible, arrange for test to be done later in the day to avoid additional hospitalization. • Instruct client on what n.p.o. means.
Client very apprehensive and refuses test at last minute.	• Identify reasons for anxiety and attempt to allay fears. • Notify physician and ask if he or she wants to cancel or postpone test to later time. Do not attempt to "talk client into it."
Bleeding or hemorrhage occurs from arteriogram puncture site.	• Notify physician. • Apply direct pressure until pressure dressing can be applied. • Monitor amount of blood loss and possible signs and symptoms of shock. • Elevate and keep extremity in extension position.
Client develops irregular pulse following cardiac catheterization.	• Notify physician immediately. • Prepare for possible code status and IV administration. • Monitor vital signs frequently.
Bleeding occurs at catheter insertion site following cardiac catheterization.	• Apply pressure dressing. • Elevate extremity. • Monitor peripheral pulse and vital signs. • If bleeding does not subside, notify physician.

unit 2

NUCLEAR IMAGING

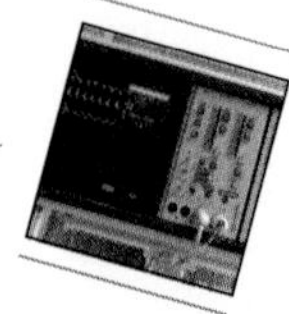

NURSING PROCESS DATA

ASSESSMENT Data Base

Assess client's understanding of nuclear imaging and the specific diagnostic test he or she is to receive.

Assess client's ability to tolerate procedure (e.g., swallowing iodine solution, fasting).

Determine client's psychologic needs in relation to the nuclear scan.

Identify any allergies the client may have to radioactive materials.

Assess need to remain with client during procedure.

Assess vital signs and document for baseline data.

PLANNING Objectives

To diagnose tumors, metastatic disease, abnormal conditions, cardiac and other organ abnormalities via noninvasive method

To prepare the client physically for the nuclear diagnostic test

To prepare the client psychologically to prevent undue stress

To complete client teaching to ensure the client understands the procedure

IMPLEMENTATION Procedures

Preparing for Nuclear Scan

Procedure for Bone Scan

Procedure for Lung Scan

Procedure for Brain Scan

Procedure for Nuclear Cardiography

Procedure for Adrenal Scan

Procedure for Thyroid Scan

Teaching for Nuclear Scans

EVALUATION Expected Outcomes

Client is physically prepared for the diagnostic study.

Client is psychologically prepared for the diagnostic study.

Client expresses an understanding of the diagnostic test.

TABLE 20–2. Nuclear Studies

Diagnostic Test	Rationale
Bone Scan	To diagnose metastatic bone disease, osteomyelitis, or fractures
Lung Scan	To diagnose pulmonary embolism, pneumothorax, or assess pulmonary status before lung surgery
Brain Scan	To determine presence of cerebral infarction, abscess, neoplasm, or contusions
Cardiology Scan	To diagnose coronary artery disease, cardiomyopathy, valvular heart disease, or to assess cardiac status and analyze ventricular function
Adrenal Scan	To diagnose adrenal gland tumors
Thyroid Scan	To diagnose thyroid nodules, abnormal function, or thyroid cancer

PREPARING FOR NUCLEAR SCAN

Equipment

Signed permit
IV equipment (for most scans)
Hospital gown and pajama bottoms

Preparation

1. Identify the specific diagnostic test that is to be performed (Table 20–2).
2. Determine if any tests must precede others in order to schedule test appropriately.
3. Identify specific preparations that need to be carried out before the studies.
4. Monitor fluid alterations that need to precede the studies.
5. Obtain special consent forms if required by facility after the physician has explained the study to the client.
6. Provide client teaching regarding the study, including any special preparation required for the study.
7. Provide psychologic support and reassurance to the client.
8. Carry out safety precautions immediately prior to the study:
   a. Check identaband for accuracy.
   b. Chart premedication if given.
   c. Monitor safe transfer from the bed to gurney or wheelchair.
   d. Accompany client to nuclear medicine department if needed. (Usually nurses accompany critically ill clients.)

Procedure *for Bone Scan*

1. Follow steps as appropriate for *Preparing for Nuclear Scan.*
   a. Explain purpose for procedure to client.
      Rationale: If client is of child-bearing age, determine whether she is pregnant. If so, test cannot be done.
   b. Have client ready for injection of tracer amount of radioactive material 2 hours before scan.
   c. Force fluids for 1 hour.
   d. Take client to nuclear medicine department.
2. Explain procedure.
   a. Client is positioned under scintillation camera.
   b. Instruct client to remain very still for 20 minutes to ensure observation of bone abnormalities.
   c. Return client to room.
3. Instruct client to resume activities.

Procedure *for Lung Scan*

1. Follow steps as appropriate in *Preparing for Nuclear Scan.*
   a. Explain purpose for procedure.
   b. Obtain consent if required.
   c. Transport client to nuclear medicine department.
2. Explain details of procedure.
   a. Explain equipment to client.
      Closed-breathing system.
      Scintillation camera.
   b. Client is injected intravenously with a tracer amount of radioactive material.
   c. Client is positioned in several ways to obtain clear images.
   d. Client is instructed to breathe through a closed system until all radioactive gas is cleared from the system.
   e. Instruct in use of mouthpiece or nose clips if used.
   f. Client is instructed to lie quietly for 30 minutes as radiography is completed.
3. Transport client on gurney to room.
4. Instruct client to resume prestudy activities.

Procedure *for Brain Scan*

1. Follow steps as appropriate in *Preparing for Nuclear Scan.*
   a. Explain purpose for procedure.
   b. Obtain consent, if required.
   c. Transport client to nuclear medicine department.
2. Explain details of procedure.
   a. IV injection of radioactive material is administered.
   b. Client's head is placed under scintillation camera and client is to remain still for 5 minutes.
   c. Client is kept comfortable and monitored carefully for 90 minutes.
   d. Client is placed in several different positions to assist distribution of radioisotopes.
   e. Client is instructed to remain still for 20 minutes.
3. Return client to room.
4. Instruct client to resume prestudy activities.

Procedure *for Nuclear Cardiography*

1. Follow steps as appropriate in *Preparing for Nuclear Scan.*
   a. Instruct client that radioactive tracer substances are used to detect and evaluate cardiovascular abnormalities.
   b. Instruct client in specific activities related to the test (i.e., exercise on a treadmill, holding certain medications, fasting). See step 2 for specific cardiology test.
2. Common tests in nuclear cardiology:
   a. *Technetium pyrophosphate scan.* The client receives an injection into the antecubital vein. He or she then waits 2 hours while the renal system clears the drug. A special camera scans the heart to identify areas of increased uptake of the radioisotope. The radioisotope accumulates in damaged areas of the heart and shows any evidence a recent MI.
   b. *Thallium scan.* A medication (^{201}Tl) is injected into the antecubital vein and scanning is done within 4–10 minutes. Necrotic or ischemic tissue does not reflect the radioisotope as tissue with normal blood supply and healthy cells does. To detect myocardial scarring and perfusion, an acute or chronic MI, or the evaluation of prior cardiac surgery are the primary purposes for this test.
   c. *Thallium scan with exercise.* When this test involves exercise, it takes 1 hour and 15 minutes; 3 hours later, a 30-minute resting scan is performed. Imaging with exercise may demonstrate perfusion problems not apparent when the client is at rest.
   d. *Gated cardiac blood pool scan.* The client receives an intravenous injection of a red blood cell tagging agent and ECG leads are positioned on him or her. The computer is then synchronized with the ECG reading. This test evaluates left ventricular function.
3. Evaluate client's status following the scan.

Procedure *for Adrenal Scan*

1. Follow steps as appropriate in *Preparing for Nuclear Scan.*
2. Purpose of scan is to diagnose adrenal gland problems.
3. Explain procedure to client.
   a. Client will have taken a strong iodine solution (Lugol's solution) for 2 days before isotope is injected. **Rationale:** This prevents isotope from being picked up by the thyroid gland.
   b. Client continues Lugol's solution for 2 weeks.
   c. Explain that the drug dexamethasone may be administered before and during the scan. **Rationale:** This is given when checking for aldosterone or androgenic tumors.
   d. Tell client scan takes 30–60 minutes to complete.

Procedure *for Thyroid Scan*

1. Follow steps as appropriate in *Preparing for Nuclear Scan.*
2. Purpose of scan is to diagnose thyroid nodules, abnormal thyroid function, or thyroid cancer.
3. Explain procedure to client.
   a. Instruct client not to consume any iodine compounds (vitamin or mineral supplements that may contain iodine or iodized table salt) or eat any foods that contain iodine—especially seafood, which has a high iodine content. **Rationale:** Consuming iodine products interferes with the test.
   b. Instruct client not to take thyroid or antithyroid drugs or x-ray contrast medium before the test. **Rationale:** These materials interfere with the thyroid scan.
   c. Tell client that after the initial iodine scan or uptake is completed, he or she must return to the lab 24 hours later.

TEACHING FOR NUCLEAR SCAN

Procedure

1. Inform client that test is to be performed in the nuclear medicine department.
   a. The department name alone may be frightening to the client.
   b. Taking the client to the department ahead of time may help to decrease anxiety.
2. Explain to the client that he or she will be receiving an injection of a radioisotope through a vein. The exceptions to this procedure are a lung scan in which the isotope is administered through an oxygen mask and a gastric-emptying scan in which the isotope is given orally with food.

a. Inform client that this isotope emits a harmless amount of radiation.
b. Also inform client that the camera used for scanning does not emit radiation. The camera detects a small and harmless amount of radiation from the isotope as it is lodged in the part of the body being imaged.

3. Explain to the client that he or she will be lying on a table (he or she will not be confined in an enclosed space) while the camera is positioned above or below the table.
4. Assure the client that someone will be with him or her throughout the test, contrasting this procedure with x-rays for which the technician must leave the room or with the MRI for which the client enters a tube-like structure.
5. Tell the client that if he or she is in pain, he or she may receive an analgesic during the procedure, as he or she must remain still while the camera is scanning the body.

CHARTING for Nuclear Imaging

- Client teaching completed
- Client's emotional state
- Any radioisotopes given on the unit
- Preprocedural preparation completed (i.e., enema or laxative)
- Means by which client transported to nuclear medicine department
- Time sent and returned from scan

CRITICAL THINKING APPLICATION

CLINICAL PROBLEMS	CRITICAL THINKING OPTIONS
Client appears not to understand purpose of diagnostic test.	• Observe for nonverbal cues or misunderstandings in order to clarify. • Provide alternative teaching aids. • Show client the equipment if necessary. • Ask client to repeat explanation to you.
Client is unable to cooperate during the procedure.	• If not contraindicated by condition, ask physician for sedation order. • Nursing staff members may be asked to help client remain quiet. If so, wear lead apron shield.
Client is uncomfortable during procedure.	• Reposition client for comfort if possible. (It may not be possible depending on area of body to be scanned.) • Provide support by propping client in position needed for scanning. • Assist client to focus on other things (e.g., the ball game, weather, or something pleasant).

unit 3

BARIUM STUDIES

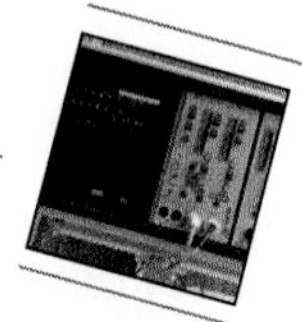

NURSING PROCESS DATA

ASSESSMENT Data Base

Assess results of laxative and enema administration to ensure a clean colon for the study. Notify physician if client is unable to "hold" enema solution.

Evaluate client's ability to cooperate with test.

Evaluate client's knowledge of test.

PLANNING Objectives

To determine the client's ability to understand the preparatory process

To clean out colon in order to ensure visualization of colon

To prepare the client psychologically for the test

IMPLEMENTATION Procedures

Preparing for Barium Studies

Procedure for Barium Enema

Procedure for Upper Gastrointestinal Study

EVALUATION Expected Outcomes

Client is able to cooperate with test.

Client's colon is clear of stool.

Barium is expelled following test.

TABLE 20–3. Barium Studies

Diagnostic Test	Rationale
Barium Enema	To visualize the lower GI tract for presence of lesions or obstructions
Upper Gastrointestinal Study	To visualize the upper GI tract for presence of lesions or obstructions

PREPARING FOR BARIUM STUDIES

Equipment

Signed consent
Enema tube and bag
Ordered solution for enema
Laxative
Wheelchair

Preparation *for Barium Enema*

1. Identify the specific diagnostic test that will be performed (Table 20–3).
2. Explain purpose for procedure to client.
3. Instruct client on low-residue diet 1–3 days before procedure.
4. Instruct client to take only clear liquid meal the evening before the procedure.

5. Administer laxative as ordered in early evening before procedure.
6. Place on n.p.o. after midnight.
7. Carry out safety precautions immediately prior to the procedure:
   a. Check identaband for accuracy.
   b. Monitor safe transfer from bed to gurney or wheelchair.

CLINICAL ALERT

Barium studies should follow IVPs, ultrasound examinations, and arteriograms because barium interferes with visualization of other structures.

Procedure *for Barium Enema*

1. Transport client to radiology department usually via wheelchair.
2. Explain details of procedure to client.
   a. An enema tube is inserted and barium solution is administered into the large bowel in order to detect lesions, obstructions, or abnormalities.
   b. X-rays are taken as the client is positioned several ways.
   c. Client is asked to retain barium while x-ray is processed.
   d. Client is allowed to expel barium in x-ray department.
   e. Entire procedure takes 15 minutes to 1 hour.
3. Transport client to room.
4. Force fluids unless contraindicated.
5. Administer laxative or enema as ordered. **Rationale:** To facilitate bowel evacuation.
6. Ensure client has bowel movement within 2–3 days.

Preparation *for Upper Gastrointestinal Study*

1. Explain purpose of procedure to client.
2. Instruct on low-residue diet 1–3 days before procedure.
3. Administer laxative or enema evening before procedure, particularly if this test follows barium enema study.
4. Place client on n.p.o. after midnight.
5. Instruct client not to smoke. **Rationale:** Smoking causes an increase in flow of digestive juices.

Procedure *for Upper Gastrointestinal Study*

1. Transport to radiology department.
2. Explain details of procedure to client.
   a. Client is instructed to drink a cup of flavored barium.
   b. Client is instructed to turn to several positions while x-rays are obtained.
   c. X-rays are taken every 30 minutes until barium advances through small bowel. This usually takes about 2 hours.
   d. Films can be taken as long as 24 hours later.
3. Transport client to room.
4. Force fluids unless contraindicated.
5. Administer laxative.
6. Ensure bowel movement within 2–3 days. Enema may need to be administered.

CLINICAL ALERT

Obtain specific orders for enemas when client has severe abdominal pain, ulcerative colitis, or history of megacolon. Do not follow general preprocedural orders.

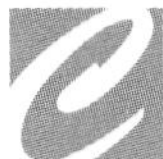

CHARTING for Barium Studies

- Laxative administered
- Type, amount of fluid, number of enemas administered
- Enema results, consistency of stool, color of returning enema solution
- Unusual symptoms such as pain, bleeding, or nausea associated with enemas
- Color of stool following test

CRITICAL THINKING APPLICATION

CLINICAL PROBLEMS	CRITICAL THINKING OPTIONS
■ Barium is unable to be expelled even following administrations of laxatives and enemas.	• Obtain order for and administer oil-retention enema. • Administer tap water enema following oil-retention enema. • Continue to administer laxatives until barium is expelled.
■ Laxatives or enemas (or both) are ordered for clients with ulcerative colitis or severe abdominal pain.	• Do not administer either the laxative or enema without checking with the physician. • If physician confirms order, administer small amount of enema fluid carefully, and observe and document effects on client. • Chart the type of pain if any, characteristics of stool, and any symptoms noted while enema is administered. • If client complains of excruciating pain, stop procedure and notify the physician.
■ Client's medications are administered in error.	• Notify x-ray department, and ask for specific orders as to what action needs to be taken regarding the test. • Inform physician, complete a medication error form and send to nursing office. An incident form may need to be completed as well. • If this is a frequent problem on the unit or in the hospital, an in-service education program should be given that includes a discussion of when medications should be given and when held.

unit 4

DIAGNOSTIC PROCEDURES

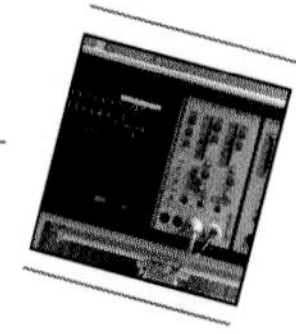

NURSING PROCESS DATA

ASSESSMENT **Data Base**

Assess vital signs prior to, during, and following the procedure.

Assess client's ability to maintain position necessary for procedure.

Assess client's knowledge of the procedure to be performed.

Review pertinent laboratory tests prior to procedure.

Evaluate signs and symptoms that indicate a potential problem could exist if test performed.

PLANNING **Objectives**

To provide reassurance for clients undergoing diagnostic tests

To position the client in a manner that facilitates the introduction of a needle through the skin surface to obtain a tissue sample

To position client in a manner for ease in passing an instrument in order to visualize a body cavity

To position the client in as comfortable a position as possible

IMPLEMENTATION **Procedures**

Assisting with Lumbar Puncture

Assisting with Liver Biopsy

Assisting with Thoracentesis

Assisting with Paracentesis

Assisting with Bone Marrow Aspiration

Assisting with Vaginal Examination and Papanicolaou (Pap) Smear

Assisting with Proctoscopy

Assisting with Fiberoptic Colonoscopy

Assisting with Gastroscopy–Endoscopy

Assisting with Cystoscopy

Assisting with Bronchoscopy

Assisting with Amniocentesis

Assisting with Magnetic Resonance Imaging (MRI)

EVALUATION **Expected Outcomes**

Client is prepared psychologically and physically for procedure.

Diagnostic tests performed with minimal discomfort.

Vital signs remain within normal range.

Specimens sent to lab in appropriate container and in a timely manner.

TABLE 20–4. Diagnostic Procedures

Diagnostic Test	Rationale
Lumbar Puncture	To obtain a cerebral spinal fluid specimen to determine presence of microorganisms, RBCs, or WBCs
Liver Biopsy	To obtain a specimen to determine presence of tumor or disease
Thoracentesis	To remove fluid from the thoracic cavity; to obtain a specimen cell study
Paracentesis	To remove fluid from the abdominal cavity; to obtain a specimen for cell study
Bone Marrow Aspiration	To study cells obtained from the specimen
Vaginal Examination and Papanicolaou Smear	To determine cell changes through a smear; to obtain a specimen for venereal disease identification
Proctoscopy	To determine alterations in tissue; to determine if active bleeding is present
Fiberoptic Colonoscopy	To obtain tissue for biopsy, remove foreign bodies and polyps
Gastroscopy–Endoscopy	To visualize areas of bleeding in upper GI tract; to obtain specimen for cell studies
Cystoscopy	To visualize the bladder and lower urinary tract
Bronchoscopy	To visualize larynx, trachea, bronchi, to obtain tissue for biopsy, and to diagnose bleeding sites
Amniocentesis	To remove amniotic fluid for studies of fetal maturity and genetic abnormalities

ASSISTING WITH LUMBAR PUNCTURE

Equipment

Diagnostic tray or equipment specific for procedure
Bath blanket
Sterile collection bottles or test tubes if indicated and not on tray
Sterile gloves
Xylocaine injection, if not on tray
Examining light
Clean gloves

Procedure

1. Explain purpose.
2. Explain procedure.
3. Obtain consent.
4. Instruct client to empty bowel and bladder.
5. Wash your hands.
6. Obtain tray and any additional equipment needed, such as sterile gloves, bath blanket.
7. Position client in lateral recumbent position with back at the edge of the examining table. Cover with bath blanket, exposing only client's back.
8. Open sterile tray if requested by physician. Pour antiseptic solution into sterile medicine cup if needed.
9. Pull client's knees up to abdomen and flex chin on chest. **Rationale:** This position widens the space between the spinous processes of the lower lumbar vertebrae for ease of needle insertion.
10. Place pillows between knees. **Rationale:** This prevents upper legs from sliding off lower legs.
11. Assist client in relaxation exercises or instruct in deep, slow breathing through the mouth.

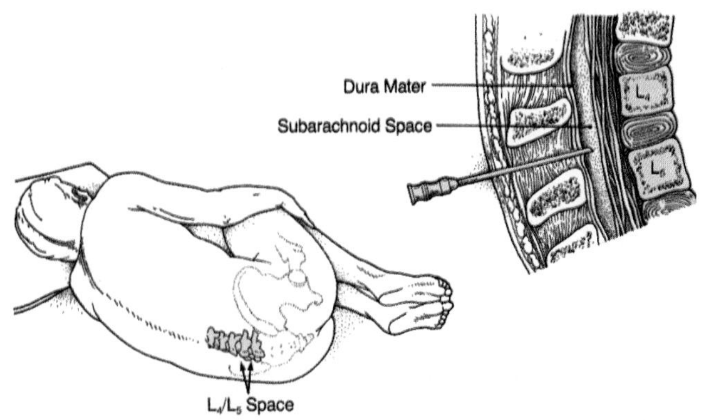

Place client in Sims' position to facilitate needle insertion for lumbar puncture.

12. Assist physician with the Queckenstedt's test when requested. After opening pressure is obtained, apply compression to neck veins with your fingers.

> **■ CLINICAL ALERT**
>
> Queckenstedt's test is used to identify blockage of CSF flow in the spinal subarachnoid space. Generally when neck pressure is applied, there is a rapid rise in pressure level on the manometer with a return to normal within seconds when pressure is released.

13. Don clean gloves.
14. Label cerebral spinal fluid samples with number on each specimen container.
15. After removal of needle, apply Band-Aid to puncture site.
16. Remove gloves, and wash hands.
17. Fill out lab slips for appropriate test (i.e., cell count, serology).
18. Instruct client to lie flat for 4–24 hours, depending on hospital policy. Head is to remain flat and even with position of body. **Rationale:** To reduce CSF leakage.
19. Encourage fluids if not contraindicated by client's condition. **Rationale:** To reduce chance of headache.
20. Observe for spinal fluid leak from puncture site.
21. Check for headaches or alterations in neurologic status.

ASSISTING WITH LIVER BIOPSY

Equipment

Same as for *Assisting with Lumbar Puncture*

Preparation

1. Obtain lab values, such as prothrombin time, bleeding time, and platelet count if ordered.
2. Determine if a blood typing and cross-matching is needed.
3. Determine if client is to be n.p.o.
4. Explain purpose of biopsy to client.
5. Explain procedure.
6. Obtain consent.
7. Assess if client has any allergies to topical anesthetic agents.

Procedure

1. Wash your hands.
2. Take vital signs. **Rationale:** This provides baseline data to compare with postprocedure data.
3. Administer sedative as ordered.
4. Obtain tray and any additional equipment needed, such as sterile gloves, sandbag, bath blanket.
5. Place client in supine position at the right edge of the bed. Raise right arm and extend it over the left shoulder behind the head. If possible, turn head to left side. **Rationale:** This position provides maximal exposure of right intercostal space.
6. Open sterile tray if requested by physician.
7. Instruct client to inhale and exhale deeply several times and then exhale and hold breath while physician inserts the biopsy needle. **Rationale:** Holding the breath prevents the needle from tearing the diaphragm or lacerating the liver.
8. Instruct the client to breathe normally after the physician removes the needle.
9. Don clean gloves, and place Band-Aid over puncture site.

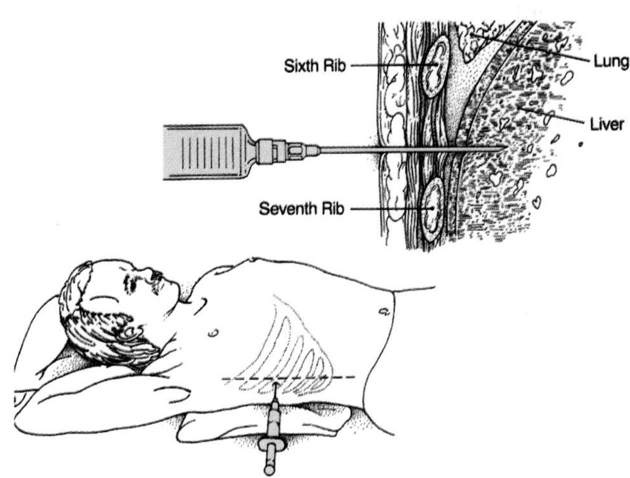

Instruct client to raise arm over head to facilitate needle insertion for liver biopsy.

10. Position client on right side for 2 to 4 hours. Sandbags may be placed under client's right side to provide hemostasis.
11. Instruct client to remain on bed rest for 24 hours.
12. Assess for signs of hemorrhage at least every hour for 12 hours.
13. Monitor vital signs as you would for a surgical client (e.g., every 15 minutes for 1 hour).

ASSISTING WITH THORACENTESIS

Equipment

Same as for *Assisting with Lumbar Puncture*

Preparation

1. Explain purpose of procedure to client.
2. Explain procedure.
3. Obtain consent.
4. Ensure chest x-ray film has been taken. **Rationale:** This film is used to compare with the film taken after the procedure.
5. Assess if client has any allergies to topical anesthetic agents.

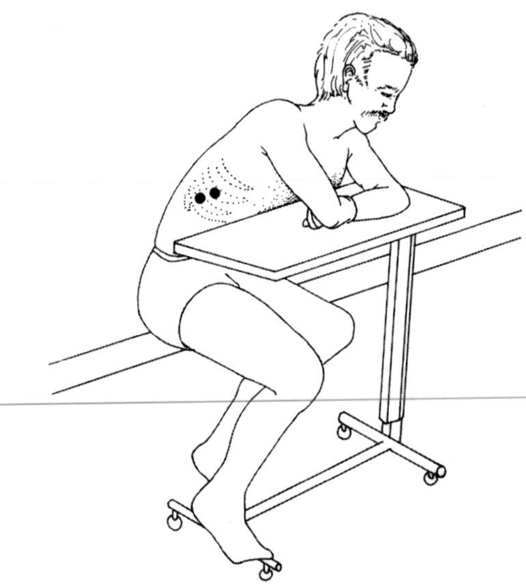

Place client in a leaning forward position to expose intercostal space for thoracentesis.

Procedure

1. Wash your hands.
2. Take vital signs, and complete a respiratory assessment. **Rationale:** This information provides post-procedure comparisons and early identification of potential complications.
3. Administer sedative as ordered.
4. Position client on edge of bed with arms crossed and resting on the overbed table. **Rationale:** This position provides good access to the intercostal spaces and facilitates fluid removal.
5. Provide adequate warmth and covering for client using bath blanket.
6. Place unwrapped sterile tray on bedside stand.
7. Open sterile gloves as indicated.
8. Assist physician as needed with skin prep.
9. Instruct client not to cough during placement of needle by the physician. **Rationale:** Pleural perforations can occur.
10. Following insertion of needle, observe client for pallor, dyspnea, tachycardia, chest pain, or vertigo. Report these findings immediately to the physician. **Rationale:** These symptoms occur with a pneumothorax.
11. Apply Band-Aid or pressure dressing (as determined by policy) after fluid is removed. Don clean gloves before applying dressing.
12. Observe client for pulmonary edema (blood-tinged sputum), cardiac distress (changes in respirations, pulse, or color), or a shift in the mediastinum.
13. Place client on unaffected side with head elevated 30° for at least 1 hour.
14. Monitor vital signs and breath sounds as with post-operative clients for 2 hours.
15. Obtain chest x-ray following procedure to check for pneumothorax.
16. Record color, amount, consistency, and samples of fluid obtained.
17. Complete lab slips, and send specimen to lab.

ASSISTING WITH PARACENTESIS

Equipment

Same as for *Assisting with Lumbar Puncture*
- Chair
- Drape
- Sterile tray
- Sterile gloves
- Bucket

Dressing—elastic adhesive patch
Blood pressure equipment
Clean gloves

Preparation

1. Explain purpose of procedure to client.
2. Explain procedure.
3. Obtain consent.
4. Assess if client has any allergies to topical anesthetic agents.
5. Wash your hands.
6. Assess client's abdominal girth and bowel sounds. **Rationale:** This information provides postprocedure comparisons and early identification of potential complications.
7. Weigh client. **Rationale:** This information can be used to assess fluid loss following the procedure.
8. Have client empty bladder. **Rationale:** This prevents accidental puncture of the bladder during the procedure.

Procedure

1. Place client in Fowler's position on chair or on edge of bed with legs spread apart.
2. Drape client, and provide adequate warmth and covering with a bath blanket.
3. Obtain vital signs, and observe client for pallor and vertigo during procedure. **Rationale:** These symptoms are indicative of shock.
4. Position and open tray on over-bed table.
5. Open sterile gloves if needed.
6. Assist physician in preparing skin with antiseptic solution or as needed.
7. Don clean gloves.

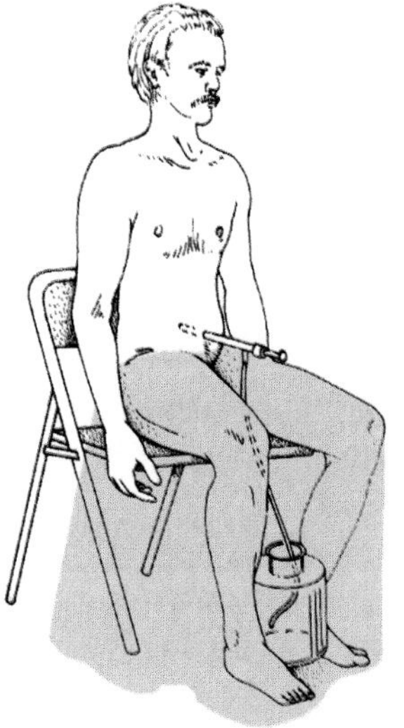

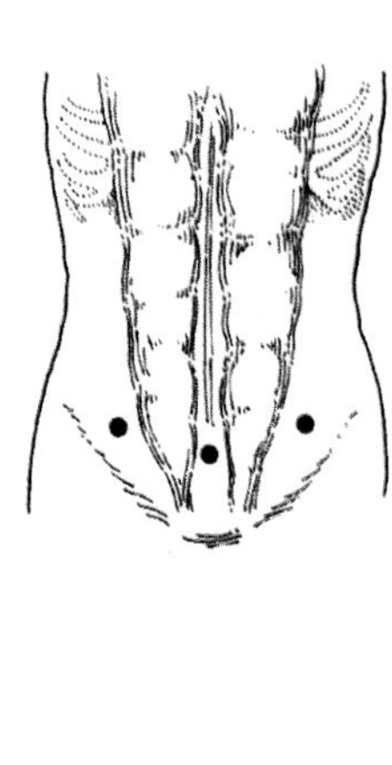

Place client in chair to facilitate trocar insertion and drainage for paracentesis.

8. Observe total amount of fluid aspirated. **Rationale:** Removing larger amounts of fluid can lead to hypotension and hyponatremia.
9. Apply pressure dressing following removal of 20-gauge needle. **Rationale:** This prevents bleeding from puncture site.
10. Remove gloves, and place in appropriate receptacle.
11. Wash your hands.
12. Return client to bed and place in semi- to high-Fowler's position. **Rationale:** These positions usually are most comfortable for client and promote lung expansion.
13. Observe for leakage at puncture site or scrotal edema in male client.
14. Monitor vital signs, urine output, and dressing every 15 minutes for at least 2 hours; every hour for 4 hours; every 4 hours for 24 hours.
15. Assess bowel sounds, and measure abdominal girth.
16. Weigh client when vital signs are stable. **Rationale:** This prevents hypotension.
17. Reinforce or change dressings as needed.
18. Record color, amount, consistency, and samples obtained from paracentesis, and send to laboratory.

ASSISTING WITH BONE MARROW ASPIRATION

Equipment

Same as for *Assisting with Lumbar Puncture*

Procedure

1. Explain purpose.
2. Explain procedure. **Rationale:** Client will experience discomfort of pressure when needle is inserted.
3. Obtain consent.
4. Obtain tray and provide any additional equipment needed, such as specimen container or gloves.
5. Premedicate with prescribed drugs.
6. Position client in supine position if sternum or anterior iliac crest is the biopsy site, or prone if posterior iliac crest is the biopsy site. Place a sandbag under iliac crest area if physician requires.
7. Open tray on over-bed table.
8. Assist physician as needed.
9. Apply direct pressure for 5–15 minutes following removal of needle. **Rationale:** To prevent bleeding.
10. Cover puncture site with small dressing or Band-Aid.
11. Monitor vital signs, and observe puncture site for drainage, edema, or pain, as with surgical client.
12. Position the client for comfort.
13. Properly label specimens, and send to laboratory.

ASSISTING WITH VAGINAL EXAMINATION AND PAPANICOLAOU (PAP) SMEAR

Equipment

Two slides
Cytology container
Vaginal speculum, several sizes
Gloves
Water-soluble lubricant jelly
Examining light

Preparation

1. Explain purpose of procedure.
2. Explain procedure.
3. Instruct client not to douche before exam.

Procedure

1. Assist client to examination room. Client may walk if not contraindicated.
2. Position in lithotomy position using stirrups.
3. Provide adequate coverings to preserve modesty and prevent chilling.
4. Open speculum package, gloves, and lubricant. Place on tray. Place cytology slides and container on tray.
5. Label two slides with client's name and area from where specimen is obtained.
6. Position light for good exposure.
7. Stay with client if she is a child or physician is a male.
8. Assist physician as needed.
9. Place slides in cytology container, and send to the lab. Complete all cytology forms.
10. Assist client in perineal care.
11. Assist client to room.

ASSISTING WITH PROCTOSCOPY

Equipment

Rigid or flexible endoscope with light source, anoscope, and obturator
Suction set up
Air insufflator
Biopsy forceps

Preparation

1. Explain purpose of procedure to client.
2. Explain procedure.

3. Administer tap water or disposable (e.g., Fleets) enema as ordered the evening before the procedure.
4. Allow clear liquids after midnight as ordered.
5. Give tap water enema morning of examination.
6. Obtain consent if necessary.
7. Have client void before procedure.

Procedure

1. Transport client by wheelchair or gurney to treatment or special procedure room. Place on proctoscopy or examination table.
2. Position in a knee–chest position if using examination table and rigid scope. Place on left side with right leg bent and placed over left leg if using flexible scope.
3. Drape client to provide for modesty and warmth.
4. Position light for good exposure. Open tray and gloves and place lubricant on tray.
5. Explain equipment and details of procedure to client.
   a. Physician examines the rectum digitally first.
   b. Lubricated proctoscope is advanced through anus into the rectum to visualize any abnormality of rectum, sigmoid colon, and large bowel.
   c. Client may feel pressure and need to have a bowel movement. Assure client this is usual feeling.
   d. Air may be introduced to increase visualization of bowel wall.
   e. Suction equipment passed through the scope may be used to remove secretions for better visualization of colon.
   f. Biopsy may be obtained by passing a snare through scope.
   g. Scope is removed, and client's rectal area is cleaned and dried.
6. Return client in wheelchair or on gurney to room, and instruct to resume preexamination activities.
7. Monitor stools for bleeding.
8. Don gloves to clean and dispose of equipment. Follow universal precautions when disposing of equipment. Return cleaned, nondisposable equipment to central supply area.

ASSISTING WITH FIBEROPTIC COLONOSCOPY

Equipment

Flexible fiberoptic colonoscope
Biopsy forceps
Cytology brush
Gloves
Specimen containers, if necessary

Preparation

1. Explain purpose of procedure to client.
2. Explain procedure.
3. Place client on liquid diet 1 day before procedure.
4. Instruct client to drink electrolyte laxative solution (Golytely or Colyte) the day before procedure. Take according to directions, usually 8 ounces every 15 minutes until 1 gallon taken. Solution should be chilled (more palatable) and swallowed quickly. **Rationale:** This osmotic solution works quickly and produces a clear colon in about 4 hours if directions are followed accurately. Watery diarrhea usually begins 30–60 minutes after first glass taken.
5. Explain side effects of nausea and fluid and electrolyte imbalance to client, especially elderly clients.
6. Instruct client to not take any routine or p.r.n. medications when drinking electrolyte solution. **Rationale:** The medications will not be digested.

> **CLINICAL ALERT**
>
> An alternative bowel preparation includes n.p.o. for 1–3 days, laxatives for 1–2 days, and enemas until the bowel is clear the morning of the procedure.

Procedure

1. Medicate client with a narcotic analgesic, usually (Demerol).
2. Transport client to special procedure room. This procedure may be done at the bedside if client cannot be moved.
3. Position client on left side with legs drawn up.
4. Explain details of procedure to client.
   a. Scope is inserted through rectum and advanced

through the sigmoid, descending, transverse, and ascending colon.

b. Client may experience discomfort when air is instilled into colon to open colon and advance scope.
c. (Valium) may be administered if client is anxious.
d. Biopsy forceps or brush is inserted through scope to obtain specimens for study.
e. Tissue or secretions obtained are placed in specimen container.
f. Scope is removed, and rectal area cleaned and dried.

5. Transport client to room.
6. Instruct client to report any rectal bleeding, abdominal pain, or distention. **Rationale:** These symptoms indicate possible bowel perforation or hemorrhage.
7. Monitor vital signs as with any client. **Rationale:** Vital signs changes indicate complications especially increased temperature and pulse and decreased blood pressure.
8. Complete laboratory slips, and send specimens to laboratory.

ASSISTING WITH GASTROSCOPY–ENDOSCOPY

Equipment

Fiberoptic endoscope for specific area to be studied or universal endoscope
Light source
Local anesthetic preparation (lidocaine spray)
Specimen containers

Procedure

1. Explain purpose.
2. Obtain consent.
3. Keep n.p.o. for 6–12 hours.
4. Remove dentures.
5. Transport to special procedures room on gurney. (May be done at bedside for critically ill clients.)
6. Explain details of procedure:
   a. Client is awake during procedure.
   b. Cardiac monitoring and pulse oximetry are done.
   c. Throat is anesthetized by swabbing with local anesthetic.
   d. Client is sedated with intravenous medication (usually [Valium] or [Versed]). Atropine may be administered to decrease secretions.
   e. Client is placed in left lateral recumbent position. **Rationale:** This facilitates drainage of saliva.
   f. Endoscope passed through esophagus to the duodenum.
   g. Specimens may be taken and sent to lab.
7. Transport client to room on gurney.
8. Monitor vital signs as for surgical client.
9. Check for signs and symptoms of bleeding or perforation. **Rationale:** Sharp, intense pain in stomach or chest and cool, pale skin indicate perforation.
10. Check gag reflex. **Rationale:** May take 2–3 hours before gag reflex returns.
11. Keep side rails up until effects of medications have subsided.
12. Provide ice chips or throat lozenges for sore throat.

ASSISTING WITH CYSTOSCOPY

Procedure

1. Explain purpose of procedure to client.
2. Obtain consent.
3. Premedicate as for surgical client.
4. Keep client n.p.o.
5. Transport client on gurney to cystoscopy room.
6. Place client in lithotomy position. Provide covering to preserve modesty and prevent chilling.
7. Prepare external genitalia with povidone-iodine solution.
8. Explain equipment and details of procedure to client.
   a. Local anesthetic may be instilled into urethra before scope is inserted.

b. Cystoscope is inserted through the urethra to inspect bladder and urethral wall and facilitate a biopsy.
c. Bladder is filled with sterile irrigating solution to assist in distending the bladder and irrigating bladder of clots. **Rationale:** Irrigation allows for better visualization of bladder.
d. Biopsy forcep may be passed through cystoscope to obtain tissue.
e. Bladder is emptied, and scope removed.

9. Return client on gurney to room.
10. Observe closely for signs of septicemia (i.e., chills, fever, flushed feeling).
11. Force fluids unless contraindicated.
12. Monitor urine for persistent bright red color.
13. Assess client for severe pain (colicky pain is normal with urethral catheterization), continual burning, and frequency.
14. Monitor vital signs.

ASSISTING WITH BRONCHOSCOPY

Equipment

Bronchoscopy tray
Flexible fiberoptic bronchoscope
Local anesthetic preparation (lidocaine spray)
Sterile water-soluble lubricant
Suction equipment
Sterile suction catheters
Oxygen equipment
Emesis basin
Gloves

Preparation

1. Explain purpose of procedure to client.
2. Explain procedure.
3. Place client on n.p.o. for 6–8 hours before procedure. **Rationale:** This decreases risk of aspiration while gag reflex is blocked during the procedure.
4. Obtain consent.
5. Obtain baseline data: vital signs and respiratory assessment. **Rationale:** This provides comparison data after procedure.

Procedure

1. Remove dentures. **Rationale:** This prevents damage or lodging of dentures in the throat during procedure.
2. Premedicate client with sedative and atropine if ordered. **Rationale:** These medications inhibit vagal stimulation, suppress gag reflex, and decrease the client's anxiety.
3. Transport client on gurney to special procedure room or operating room. Place client on table.
4. Wash hands, and don gloves.
5. Assist physician as necessary.
   a. Attach bronchoscope to machine for light source.
   b. Suction client if necessary.
   c. Attach oxygen source if client is hypoxic. **Rationale:** Hypoxia can occur as airway is partially obstructed when scope is inserted.
6. Explain procedure to client.
   a. Physician sprays nasopharynx and oropharynx with topical anesthetic. **Rationale:** This prevents laryngospasm, depresses gag reflex, and prevents discomfort when scope is inserted.
   b. Client is instructed to avoid swallowing anesthetic agent. Instruct client to expectorate into emesis basin.
   c. Bronchoscope is inserted into mouth and advanced to trachea and bronchi.
   d. Tissue specimens or secretions are collected and sent to laboratory for study.
   e. Bronchoscope is removed.
7. Cleanse client's nose of lubricant following removal of scope.
8. Assist with cleaning tray, and send to central supply. Follow universal precautions when disposing of equipment.
9. Remove gloves, and wash your hands.
10. Monitor vital signs and respiratory status as with a surgical client. **Rationale:** This determines possible complications, such as bleeding or hypoxia.
11. Monitor for bloody sputum. **Rationale:** Bleeding can occur as a result of the bronchoscopy. Notify physician immediately if this occurs.
12. Instruct client not to eat or drink until gag reflex returns, usually 1–2 hours. **Rationale:** Aspiratic can occur when gag reflex is absent.

ASSISTING WITH AN AMNIOCENTESIS

Procedure

1. Explain purpose for procedure to client.
2. Obtain consent.
3. Have client void prior to test. **Rationale:** This prevents injury to the bladder.
4. Transport client to treatment room.
5. Instruct client to lie quietly in supine position for 30 minutes.
6. Obtain fetal heart tones.
7. Open amniocentesis tray and gloves. Place Xylocaine nearby if not included on tray. **Rationale:** Procedure is performed under sterile conditions to prevent infection.
8. Explain details of procedure to client.
   a. Physician prepares abdomen with povidone-iodine (Betadine) or alcohol.
   b. Xylocaine injection provides local anesthesia for needle insertion area.
   c. Needle is inserted, and amniotic fluid is withdrawn.
   d. Amniotic fluid is placed in specimen container and labeled with client's name. Appropriate lab slips are completed.
   e. Procedure takes about 10 minutes.
9. Place small dressing or Band-Aid over needle site.
10. Monitor fetal heart tones, and observe for signs of labor.
11. Instruct client to notify physician of any unusual occurrences, signs of labor, or signs of infection.

ASSISTING WITH MAGNETIC RESONANCE IMAGING (MRI)

Preparation

1. Evaluate client for following conditions. **Rationale:** These conditions exempt clients from having MRI because the magnet can move and displace metal, such as clips, staples.
   a. Clients with pacemakers
   b. Clients with hip prostheses, cardiac surgery, or metal implants
   c. Clients with vascular clips and staples from recent surgery
2. Clients with cardiac or respiratory complications may be excluded.
3. Check for allergies if contrast medium is to be used.
4. Obtain consent.

Procedure

1. Instruct client to remove all metal or magnetically sensitive objects: jewelry, watches, hair clips, credit cards.
2. Describe MRI machine and procedure to client.
   a. Client needs to lie flat, still, and relax inside the tube magnet. **Rationale:** Movement can produce artifact on image.
   b. Procedure lasts 60–90 minutes.
   c. Entire body is encased in machine.
   d. Inform client he or she will feel nothing but may hear noises. **Rationale:** Noises are caused by changing magnetic fields.
   e. Inform client he or she will have ear plugs in place but will be able to communicate with MRI staff through microphone. **Rationale:** This allays feelings of claustrophobia.
3. Instruct client to void before procedure. **Rationale:** This prevents the need for client to void while undergoing procedure.
4. Administer premedication as ordered, usually Valium.
5. Place client in a comfortable position on table.
6. Instruct client on feelings of warmth or shortness of breath if contrast medium is used during procedure.
7. Transport client to room following procedure.
8. Observe for symptoms of delayed reaction to dye if used during procedure.

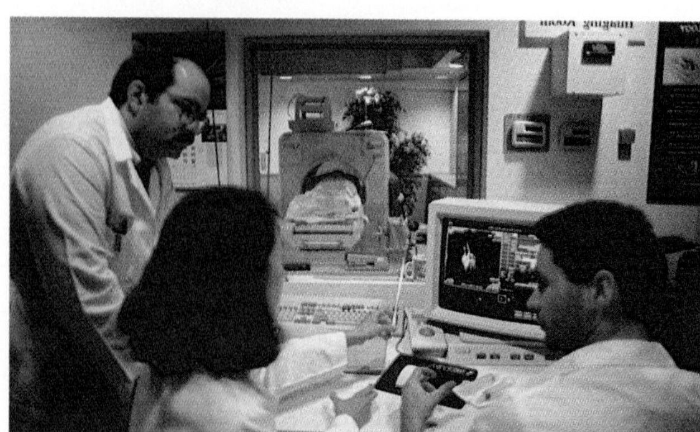

Magnetic Resonance Imaging machine (MRI).

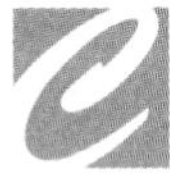

CHARTING for Diagnostic Procedures

- Preparation completed for test
- Client teaching completed
- Client's tolerance of procedure
- Fluid or specimens sent to laboratory for analysis
- Preprocedure and postprocedure vital signs if required
- Record color and amount of fluid withdrawn from paracentesis, thoracentesis, or lumbar puncture
- Type of dressing applied
- Specific position assumed after procedure
- Abnormal findings following procedure

CRITICAL THINKING APPLICATION

CLINICAL PROBLEMS	CRITICAL THINKING OPTIONS
Client has spinal fluid leak following lumbar puncture.	• Keep client in supine position. • Notify physician. • Keep sterile dressing over puncture site. Do not allow dressing to become wet. • If leak persists, physician may place client in Trendelenburg's position to prevent headache. This position is contraindicated in clients with increased intracranial pressure or following a craniotomy.
Client complains of shortness of breath or expectorates blood-tinged sputum following a thoracentesis.	• Place client in Fowler's position. • Assess vital signs. • Administer oxygen. • Monitor breath sounds. • Notify physician and check on order for chest x-ray. • Have chest tube insertion tray available. • Allay client's fears, and provide emotional support.
Urine output is blood-tinged following paracentesis.	• Notify physician at once; bladder may have been punctured during procedure. • Monitor vital signs for shock. • Maintain client on bed rest. • Observe for urine output.
Lower gastrointestinal tract not clear and proctoscopy not completed.	• Repeat laxative and enemas per physician orders. • Observe results of enema; if solution not clear, notify physician.
Vertigo occurs while maintaining knee–chest position during proctoscopy.	• Have client lie in supine position for few minutes. • Have client assume standing position slowly.
Upper gastrointestinal bleeding begins when scope inserted.	• Insert nasogastric tube, and apply suction. • Monitor vital signs for evidence of shock.

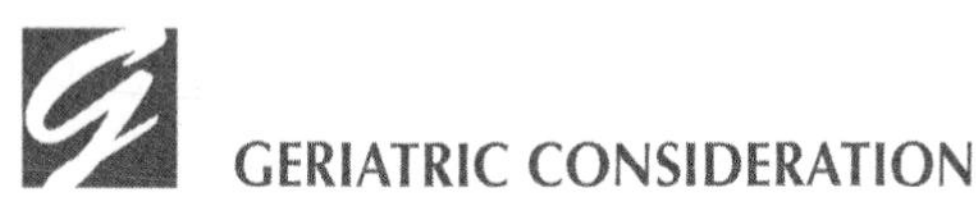

GERIATRIC CONSIDERATIONS

Elderly clients requiring diagnostic tests are at risk for the following problems:

- Dehydration can result from fluid restriction, use of contrast agents for the tests, and bowel preparation using enemas. Osmolar imbalances and hypovolemia can result from the dehydration.
- Extracellular fluid volume excess can occur if large volumes of fluid are required for the test. Renal studies, which usually require the use of large volumes of fluid, should not be considered if the client is at risk for circulatory overload. Elderly clients may have a compromised cardiorespiratory status. A secondary choice of tests may need to be considered such as a CT scan.
- Renal dysfunction resulting from multiple tests using contrast agents should be avoided. Acute renal failure can result from multiple tests with contrast agents in elderly clients who already have a compromised renal system. Spacing tests over time helps prevent this problem.

Nursing responsibilities for elderly clients requiring diagnostic tests should include the following:

- Carefully monitor fluid and electrolyte balance.
- Adequately hydrate client prior to and following tests unless contraindicated.
- Monitor laboratory tests, such as electrolytes and osmolarity.
- Monitor intake and output frequently.
- Monitor vital signs
- Weigh clients who are at risk for fluid volume disturbances.
- Complete physical assessment, including mental status, each shift, and report unusual findings to physician.

21

Urine Elimination

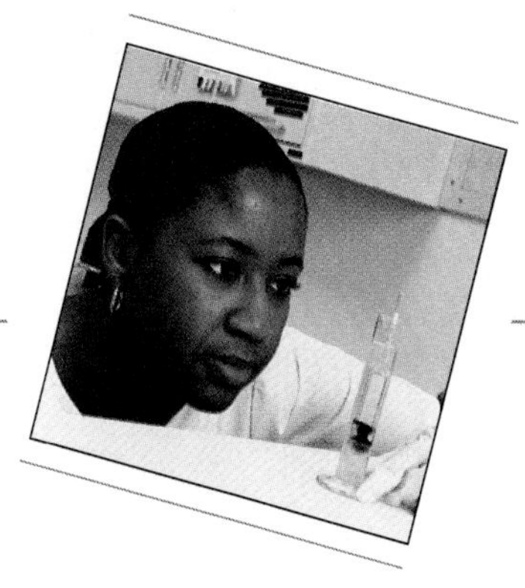

LEARNING OBJECTIVES

- Describe the process of forming urine as the filtrate passes through the renal tubules.
- List four alterations that result in urinary elimination problems.
- State two nursing diagnoses that relate to urine elimination.
- Complete an intake and output bedside record.
- Outline the steps of monitoring specific gravity.
- Describe a ketone test, and discuss its purpose.
- Compare and contrast the steps of inserting a straight catheter in a male and female client.
- Describe the major parameters needed to preserve a sterile environment when inserting a Foley catheter.
- Explain the cleansing procedure for both a male and female client when inserting a Foley catheter.
- Demonstrate the clamping protocol used for clients with suprapubic catheters.
- Explain how a catheter is attached to a leg bag.
- Identify the most important steps to take if infection occurs with a suprapubic catheter.
- List the major steps of irrigating by opening a closed urinary system.
- Discuss how medications are instilled through a closed urinary system.
- Outline the steps necessary to obtain a urine specimen from a closed urinary drainage system.
- Outline the steps in applying a urinary diversion pouch.
- Compare and contrast nursing interventions for clients on peritoneal dialysis and hemodialysis.

TERMINOLOGY

Albuminuria: the presence of albumin in the urine.

Anemia: a condition in which the number of circulating red blood cells, or hemoglobin, is reduced.

Antibiotic: a substance that has the power to inhibit or destroy other organisms, especially bacteria.

Antidiuretic: decreasing the rate of urine secretion; an agent having such an action.

Anuria: a total suppression or lack of production of urine.

Bactericidal: able to destroy bacteria.

Calyx: any cuplike division of the kidney pelvis.

Catheterization: a sterile tube insertion for the injection of or removal of fluids from a vessel or body cavity.

Dehydration: the process of losing water as in depriving the body tissues of water.

Distention: stretching out or inflating of an organ such as the bladder.

Diuresis: the excessive production and elimination of urine.

Dorsal: pertaining to the back.

Dysuria: difficult or painful urination.

Edema: a condition in which body tissues contain an excessive amount of fluid.

Electrolyte: composed of acids, bases, and salts; a compound that dissociates into ions when placed into solution and becomes a conductor of electricity.

Excoriation: a breakdown of the epidermis.

Extracorporeal circuit: blood is circulated outside the body through a system for removal of substances, such as excess urea and electrolytes from the urine.

Foley catheter: a type of indwelling tube that is inserted through the urethra into the bladder to provide continuous urinary drainage.

Genitourinary: pertaining to the genital and urinary systems.

Glycosuria: the presence of sugar in the urine.

Hematuria: the presence of blood in the urine.

Hemorrhage: abnormal internal or external escape of blood from the vessels.

Hydrometer: instrument used to determine the specific gravity of urine.

Incontinence: inability to retain urine, semen, or feces through loss of sphincter control.

Indwelling urethral catheter: a retention, or Foley, catheter.

Infection: condition in which the body or a part is invaded by a pathogenic agent.

Irrigation: the flushing of a tube, canal, or area with solution.

Malpighian corpuscle: a spheric body consisting of a glomerulus and Bowman's capsule found in the cortex of a kidney.

Micturition: the process of emptying the urinary bladder; voiding.

Nocturia: excessive urination during the night.

Oliguria: the diminished production of urine by the kidneys.

Patency: the state of being freely open.

Peri: prefix meaning around or about.

Peristalsis: a progressive wavelike movement that occurs involuntarily in hollow tubes in the body, especially the alimentary tract.

Polyuria: the excessive production and elimination of urine.

Pyuria: the presence of pus in the urine.

Renal: pertaining to the kidney.

Sediment: a substance settling at the bottom of a liquid.

Septic: pertinent to pathologic organisms or their toxins.

Septicemia: presence of pathologic bacteria in the blood.

Shock: a state of collapse resulting from acute peripheral circulatory failure.

Specific gravity: weight of a substance compared with an equal volume of water. Water is 1.000.

Stoma: artificially created opening in the abdominal wall.

Suction: the act of sucking up by reduction of air pressure over part of the surface of a substance.

Urethra: a canal for the discharge of urine from the bladder to the outside.

Urinary diversion: an interruption in normal flow or urine through the urinary system by surgical intervention.

Urinary tract infection (UTI): an infection of the urinary tract, including all or part of the organs and ducts participating in the secretion and elimination of urine.

URINARY SYSTEM

The primary structures of the urinary system are the kidneys, ureters, bladder, and urethra. Each kidney produces urine, which is carried to the bladder by a ureter that is about 25 cm (10 inches) long and 0.6 cm in diameter. Peristaltic waves, pressure, and gravity propel urine through the ureters so that it can be discharged into the bladder.

The bladder serves as a reservoir for urine until the urge to void takes place. When the act of micturition, or urination, occurs, urine passes through two sphincters and is transported from the bladder to the external environment by the urethra.

The anatomic position of the bladder and the structure of the urethra differ in males and females. The bladder in both sexes is posterior to the symphysis pubis. In a female, however, the bladder is anterior to the vagina and the neck of the uterus. In a male the bladder is anterior to the rectum. The urethra of the female is about 4 cm (1.5 inches) long, and the male urethra is 20 cm (8 inches) long.

The urethra, bladder, ureters, and kidney pelves are lined with a continuous layer of mucous membrane. Because there is no break in the continuity of the lining, bacteria introduced into the normally sterile system can spread rapidly throughout the tract. When the bladder is empty, the lining falls into folds which provide pockets where bacteria can multiply. Since the membrane is highly vascular, bacteria can easily enter the bloodstream and septicemia can result.

Urine Production

Nephrons, the functional units of the kidneys, produce urine. Each nephron consists of a renal corpuscle and a renal tubule, which is surrounded by a capillary bed. Each kidney has approximately a million nephrons.

Urine formed in the renal tubule enters a collecting duct. The collecting ducts from a number of nephrons attach to a single, larger collecting duct, which empties urine into the kidney calyx. The urine collects in the renal pelvis until enough accumulates to flow to the bladder. If movement of urine from the pelvis is interrupted, infection or formation of calculi may occur.

Filtration of blood plasma occurs within the renal corpuscle. Two arterioles circulate blood to and from a capillary network called the glomerulus. Because the inlet to the glomerulus is larger than the outlet, hydrostatic pressure in the capillary network is higher than the pressure in other capillaries of the body. This high pressure causes filtration to occur.

Alterations in pressure change the rate of filtration. The afferent and efferent arterioles control the flow of blood and maintain the appropriate pressure in the glomerulus by constricting and dilating. Other factors that influence the rate of filtration from the glomerulus are the plasma colloidal osmotic pressure and the pressure in the Bowman's capsule into which the filtrate passes.

Due to the pressure in the glomerulus, certain substances are filtered from the blood through the capillary walls into the Bowman's capsule, which surrounds

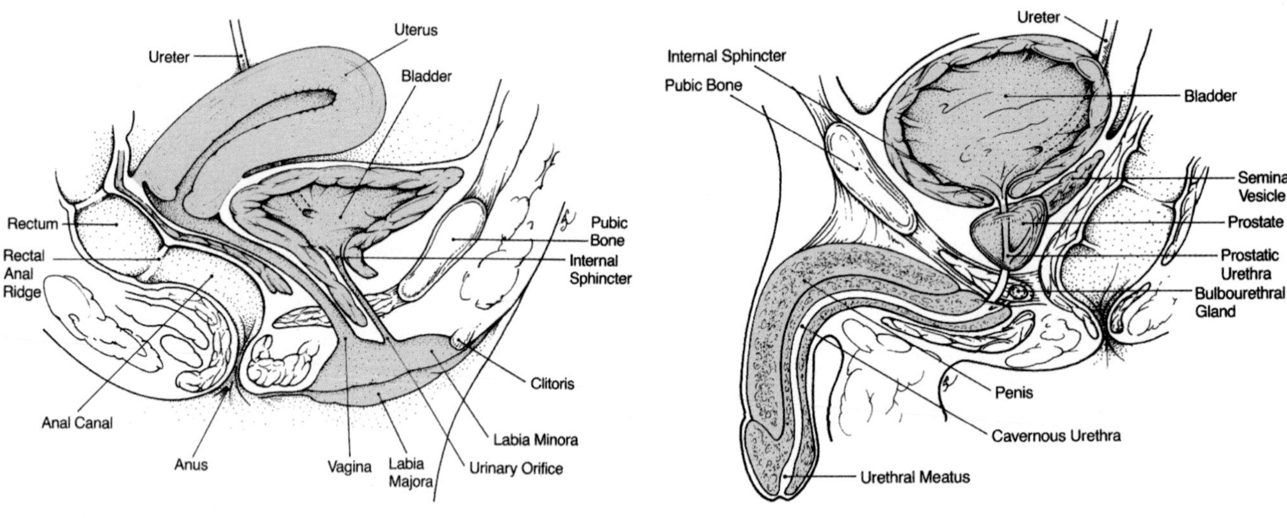

Female genitourinary system.

Male genitourinary system.

the glomerulus. These substances, which include water, amino acids, electrolytes, glucose, and waste products, form a filtrate that closely resembles blood plasma. This filtrate leaves the Bowman's capsule through the renal tubule.

The renal tubule comprises three parts: the proximal convoluted tubule, the loop of Henle, and the distal convoluted tubule. As the filtrate travels through the tubule, some substances are removed through mechanisms, such as active transport and osmosis. Other substances are added to the filtrate through excretion (a summary of the functions of the segments of a tubule appears in Table 21–1).

The process of urine formation in all the nephrons of both kidneys reduces 120 mL of filtrate produced each minute to 1 mL of urine. The average daily urine output is, therefore, about 1500 mL. Alterations in the rate of filtration, the filtrate, or functions of the tubule may result in changes in the volume of urine or its constituents.

Micturition

Micturition (urination) is a reflex act that occurs in response to pressure changes within the bladder. When urine begins to collect, the muscular walls of the bladder are relaxed, with little change in pressure. After about 300 mL of urine accumulates, the bladder walls tighten, and pressure increases. This rising pressure stimulates receptors in the bladder wall, which send impulses to the spinal cord. After 400–500 mL of urine is collected, the bladder walls contract and the internal

TABLE 21–1. Tubular Alterations of Filtrate

Proximal tubule and descending limb	Obligatory water reabsorption, which accounts for about 80% of the absorption of water, occurs in the proximal tube and descending limb. Glucose, amino acids, vitamins, and sodium are actively reabsorbed. Chloride, sulfate, phosphate ions, and urea are passively reabsorbed. Bicarbonate is actively reabsorbed in relation to systemic pH. Water is reabsorbed with these substances, leaving the filtrate osmotic pressure unchanged.
Loop of Henle	Sodium is actively transported from the filtrate in the ascending limb into the medullary interstitial fluid, thus raising its osmotic pressure. This rising pressure causes more water to be reabsorbed from the descending limb and the collecting duct and results in the concentration of the urine.
Distal tubule and collecting ducts	Facultative or optional reabsorption of water, which accounts for about 10–15% of the absorption of water, occurs in the distal tubule and collecting ducts. Sodium is actively reabsorbed in exchange for secreted potassium or hydrogen. As water continues to be reabsorbed, the filtrate becomes more concentrated and its volume is greatly reduced.

sphincter relaxes, causing a sense of urgency to void. When urine enters the urethra, the external sphincter relaxes and voiding occurs.

Micturition can occur sooner if the tone of the bladder is increased because of such factors as emotional stress or infection. Micturition can be delayed by voluntary contraction of the external sphincter or contraction of the abdominal muscle. Once the volume of urine reaches about 700 mL, however, most individuals lose their ability to delay micturition.

If an individual is unable to void, as much as 1000 mL of urine can accumulate in the bladder. When a large volume of urine is retained, the bladder's lining and blood vessels can be damaged by the increased stretching and pressure. When this happens, an individual experiences pain, restlessness, chilling, flushing, headache, diaphoresis, and a rise in blood pressure.

TABLE 21–2. Average Daily Urine Output

Age (years)	Amount (mL)
<1	400–500
1–5	500–700
5–8	700–1000
8–14	800–1400
14–older adult	1500
Older Adult	<1500

ALTERATIONS IN URINARY ELIMINATION

Alterations in urinary elimination can result from changes in the intake and output of fluids, obstructions to the flow of urine, changes in the secretion of the antidiuretic hormone (ADH), and changes in blood volume.

Alterations Related to Fluids

The average person takes in approximately 2600 mL of fluid each day: 1200 mL from drinking, 1100 mL from the water content of food, and 300 mL from changes in metabolism. An increase or decrease in fluid intake results in a parallel increase or decrease in urine output.

Healthy individuals rarely experience decreases in urine output because they take in more fluids whenever they are thirsty. Individuals who are ill, however, often experience decreases in urine output because they are unable to respond to the thirst response, their intake is limited due to testing that requires n.p.o. preparations, or their IV fluid intake is not properly maintained.

Fluid is lost from the body not only from urine, but also through respiration, perspiration, and feces. On a daily basis, most individuals lose approximately 2400 mL of fluid: 1500 mL through urine output, 200 mL through respiration, 600 mL through perspiration, and 100 mL through the elimination of feces. Individuals who are ill may also lose fluids through vomiting, bleeding, wound drainage, and suctioning.

Alterations Related to Obstructions

A decrease in the output of urine may also be caused by an obstruction to the flow of urine from the bladder. If the obstruction is large enough, the bladder does not empty completely. Instead, it retains fluid and, over time, becomes distended. Individuals who have obstructions in the urinary tract experience the need to void more frequently. When they do void, however, they eliminate only very small amounts of urine.

Alterations Related to Secretion of the Antidiuretic Hormone

Changes in the rate of secretion of ADH also alter urine output since this hormone controls the amount of water that is reabsorbed in the distal renal tubules and collecting ducts. Common factors that increase the secretion of ADH and reduce urine output include emotional stress, accidental or surgical trauma, pain, hemorrhage, anesthesia, and drugs, such as morphine and barbiturates. Factors that reduce the secretion of ADH and thus increase urine output include alcohol, caffeine, cold, and increased carbon dioxide in the blood.

Alterations Related to Changes in Blood Volume

Because the production of urine is influenced by the volume of blood filtrate, decreases in this filtrate lead to reductions in the output of urine. Hemorrhage, severe dehydration, and shock reduce the flow of blood through the glomeruli and cause decreases in the filtrate. If the volume of the filtrate is reduced substantially, severe oliguria, or even anuria, may occur.

Other factors that may increase or decrease the output of urine include pathophysiologic states of the kidneys or other body systems, drugs, treatment modalities, diet, and metabolic rate.

NURSING INTERVENTIONS

The primary purpose for performing nursing interventions associated with urinary elimination is to maintain the integrity of the urinary system, which allows the body to eliminate fluid waste, and thereby promote homeostasis.

Aseptic technique is essential whenever performing procedures that could introduce bacteria into the urinary tract. Handwashing, using sterile gloves, and maintaining a closed urinary collection system decrease the incidence of ascending bladder contamination. Securing catheters to the skin minimizes to-and-fro motion, thus reducing infections of the urinary tract. Retrograde flow of urine must be prevented in order to prevent bladder contamination. Keeping urine collection bags below the level of the bladder helps prevent retrograde flow.

NURSING DIAGNOSES

The following nursing diagnoses may be appropriate to include in a client care plan when the components are related to promoting urine elimination.

NURSING DIAGNOSIS	RELATED FACTORS
Body Image Disturbance	Alteration in body appearance, urinary diversion stoma
Fluid Volume Excess	Decreased urine output, renal system dysfunction, decreased cardiac output
Ineffective Individual Coping	Poor adjustment to illness or treatment, chronic disease state
Noncompliance	Inadequate knowledge base, denial of health status, cultural or spiritual beliefs
Altered Urinary Elimination	Incontinence, lack of muscle tone, urinary tract infection, motor or sensory impairment, abdominal surgery
Urinary Retention	Inability to void, bladder distention or atony, surgical repair

unit 1

INTAKE AND OUTPUT

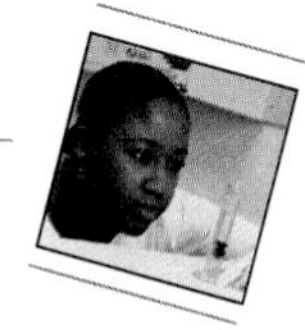

NURSING PROCESS DATA

ASSESSMENT Data Base

Assess if strict measurement of intake and output is ordered.

Assess client's ability to assist in keeping I&O record.

Assess all potential sources of intake (e.g., IVs, oral fluids) and output (e.g., urine, drainage from tubes).

Observe color, clarity, and odor of urine.

Determine all forms where documentation of I&O must occur.

Assess for signs of dehydration or overhydration.

Evaluate weight changes.

PLANNING Objectives

To accurately measure all sources of fluid intake

To accurately measure all sources of fluid output

To identify alterations in fluid balance based on urine and weight assessment

To record data on appropriate records

IMPLEMENTATION Procedure

Measuring Intake and Output

EVALUATION Expected Outcomes

All sources of intake and output are identified.

Intake and output measurements are accurately maintained.

Signs of fluid imbalance are identified.

Intake and output records are current and accurate.

MEASURING INTAKE AND OUTPUT

Equipment

Glass or cup

I&O bedside form with fluid conversions

I&O chart record

Graduate for urine and other output measurement

Bedpan or urinal

Clean gloves

Preparation

1. Explain purpose of keeping I&O record to client.
2. Instruct client to keep record of all fluids taken orally. Keep an I&O record at the bedside for the client to document intake.
3. Instruct client to void into bedpan or urinal, not into toilet.
4. Instruct client not to place toilet tissue in bedpan or defecate in bedpan.

Procedure

Oral Intake

1. Measure all fluids taken orally according to hospital values (e.g., cup = 150 mL, glass = 240 mL).
2. Record time and amount of oral fluids in the appropriate space on bedside form. Record all IV fluids and NG feedings on record.
3. Check hospital procedure manual or the bedside I&O record for approximate amounts of oral fluid containers.
4. Transfer 8-hour total fluid intake from bedside I&O record to graphic sheet for 24-hour intake and output record on chart.
5. Record all forms of fluid intake except blood and blood products in the total amount column of the

24-hour record (IVs and oral fluid). These are recorded separately.

6. Complete 24-hour intake record by adding together all three 8-hour totals.

Output

1. Don clean gloves.
2. Empty urinal, bedpan, or Foley drainage bag into graduate or commode "hat." For accurate record, empty urine into graduate. **Rationale:** Measurement is only approximate from Foley drainage bag or "hat."

BEDSIDE INTAKE AND OUTPUT RECORD

Name ________________ Date __________

Room # ________

Intake			Output			
	Oral	IV		Urine	Emesis	Drainage
7 am – 3 pm			7 am – 3 pm			
Total			Total			
3 pm – 11 pm			3 pm – 11 pm			
Total			Total			
11 pm – 7 am			11 pm – 7 am			
Total			Total			
24hr Total			24hr Total			

Measurements

Glass 240cc	Ice Cream 100cc
Cup 150cc	Jello 100cc
Bowl 150cc	Ice Chips 5cc/Cube
Juice Glass 100cc	
Coffee Pot 240cc	

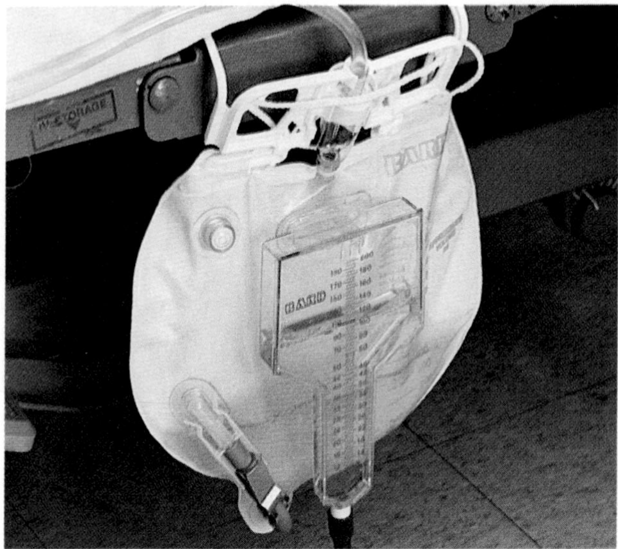

Close monitoring of urine output is accomplished when calibrated drainage bag is used.

3. Remove gloves, and wash hands.
4. Record time and amount of output on bedside I&O record. Record all urine, drainage from NG tubes, drainage tubes.
5. Transfer 8-hour output totals to graphic sheet or 24-hour I&O record.
6. Complete 24-hour output record by adding together all three output totals, and place total on graphic sheet.

METHODS TO STIMULATE VOIDING

- Run water in sink.
- Massage the lower abdomen.
- Place a hot washcloth on the abdomen.
- Pour warm water over the perineum with client positioned on toilet or bedpan.
- Give client a sitz bath after obtaining an order.
- Put oil of wintergreen on a cotton ball in the bedpan or urinal.

CHARTING for Intake and Output

- Time and amount of all oral fluid intake
- 8-hour totals of all IV and enteral fluids
- 24-hour total of all fluid intake
- Time and amount of all urinary output
- Time and amount of all drainage (e.g., NG or T tube)
- 8-hour total of all fluid output
- 24-hour total of all fluid output

CRITICAL THINKING APPLICATION

CLINICAL PROBLEMS	CRITICAL THINKING OPTIONS
Fluid balance is not correct as stated on intake and output record.	• Report to charge nurse so he or she can determine if all nurses are keeping accurate records. • Check if client or family can help with keeping the I&O record. • Check the addition on the I&O record to see if an error was made.
Client does not maintain an intake of at least 1500 mL.	• Ensure that the diagnosis allows a 1500-mL intake. • Check if the client is able to drink fluids by him or herself, or if he or she needs assistance. • Ensure that adequate fluids are available for the client. • Determine client's preferences for fluid (i.e., juice, jello, etc.)

unit 2

URINE STUDIES

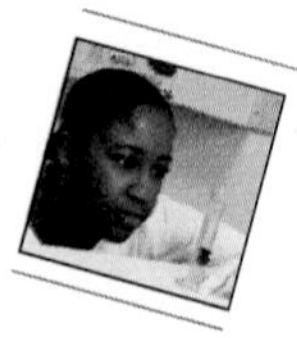

NURSING PROCESS DATA

ASSESSMENT Data Base

Assess client's ability to void when specimens are needed.

Assess color, clarity, and odor of urine.

Assess appropriate time when testing should be done.

Review diagnostic tests and drugs that interfere with test results.

PLANNING Objectives

To assist the client to void to obtain urine specimen

To obtain a nonsterile urine specimen for testing

To monitor the client's sugar and acetone levels

To measure urine specific gravity

IMPLEMENTATION Procedures

Monitoring Specific Gravity with Urinometer

Monitoring Specific Gravity with Spectrometer

Determining Urine Glucose with Tape

Measuring Urine Glucose

Measuring Urine Ketone Bodies

EVALUATION Expected Outcomes

Client able to void when test required.

Accurate specific gravity measured.

Sugar and acetone urine levels monitored.

MONITORING SPECIFIC GRAVITY WITH URINOMETER

Equipment

Clean gloves

Cylinder

Urinometer

Procedure

1. Don clean gloves.
2. Fill a cylinder with 20–30 mL of urine (about three-fourths full).
3. Place cylinder on a flat surface.
4. Place urinometer into cylinder, and spin with your fingers so the urinometer floats freely and does not touch the side of the cylinder. **Rationale:** If urinometer stays against side of cylinder, a false reading occurs.

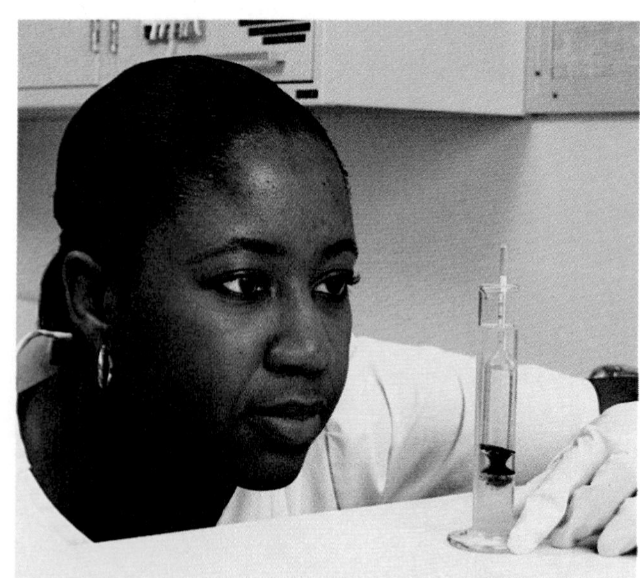

Specific gravity can be measured using the cylinder and urinometer.

5. Take the reading just before the spinning stops by checking the curved portion of the urine level to the scale on the urinometer. Urinometer scale is 1.000–1.060. Normal specific gravity is 1.003–1.030.
6. Empty and wash the cylinder, and rinse the urinometer with cool water. **Rationale:** Cool water prevents coagulation of urinary proteins and adherence to side of cylinder.
7. Put cylinder and urinometer in appropriate place.
8. Remove gloves, and wash your hands.

MONITORING SPECIFIC GRAVITY WITH SPECTROMETER

Equipment

Spectrometer
Urine specimen
Clean gloves
Paper towel
Medicine dropper

Procedure

1. Don clean gloves.
2. Obtain urine specimen.
3. Place 1–2 drops of urine on slide.
4. Turn instrument light on and look through scope. Specific gravity results will be present.
5. Clean urine off slide with damp paper towel.
6. Turn off spectrometer light.
7. Discard urine specimen.
8. Remove gloves, and wash hands.
9. Document findings.

DETERMINING URINE GLUCOSE WITH TAPE

Equipment

Clean gloves
Urine and specimen container
Reagent strips (Testape, Urostix, or Clinistix)

Procedure

1. Don clean gloves before handling urine specimen.
2. Have client void, and take urine specimen to bathroom. Test it, and keep results if unable to obtain second urine specimen. **Rationale:** In case second voided specimen cannot be obtained the first specimen gives data and assists in determining actions for care.
3. Obtain second voided specimen approximately 10–20 minutes after first specimen.
4. Take urine specimen to bathroom (from bedpan or urinal).
5. Pour small amount of urine into specimen container.
6. Dip test strip into urine.
7. Compare color change with color chart on test strip container after waiting prescribed amount of time identified on container. Results are read as percent, 1/10–2% or as a plus, one plus (+ or 1+) to four plus (++++ or 4+).
8. Replace tape dispenser, away from sink area. **Rationale:** If tape becomes wet it is ineffective.
9. Return bedpan or urinal to bedside stand or bathroom.
10. Remove gloves, and wash hands.

MEASURING URINE GLUCOSE

Equipment

Clean gloves
Urinal or bedpan
Test tube
Reagent (Clinitest) tablets
Urine testing kit (test tube, dropper)
Color charts
Paper towel
Watch for timing

Procedure

1. Wash hands, and don clean gloves.
2. Ask client to void in urinal or bedpan 30 minutes before urine specimen for testing glucose is needed. **Rationale:** Urine collected overnight does not accurately reveal present concentration of glucose in urine.

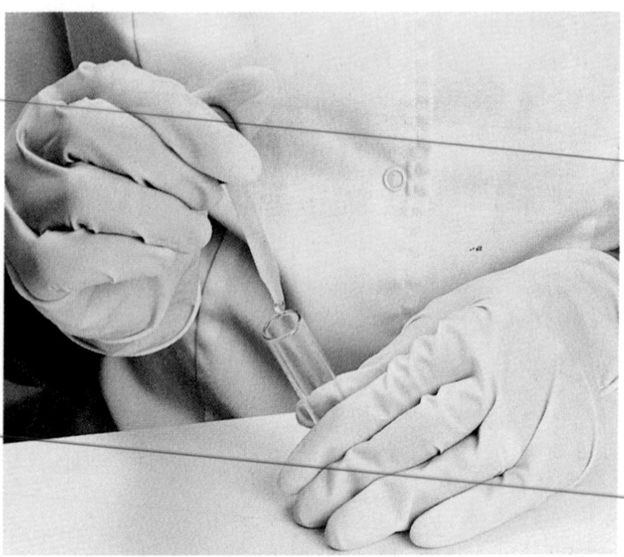

Place 5 drops of urine and 10 drops of water into test tube.

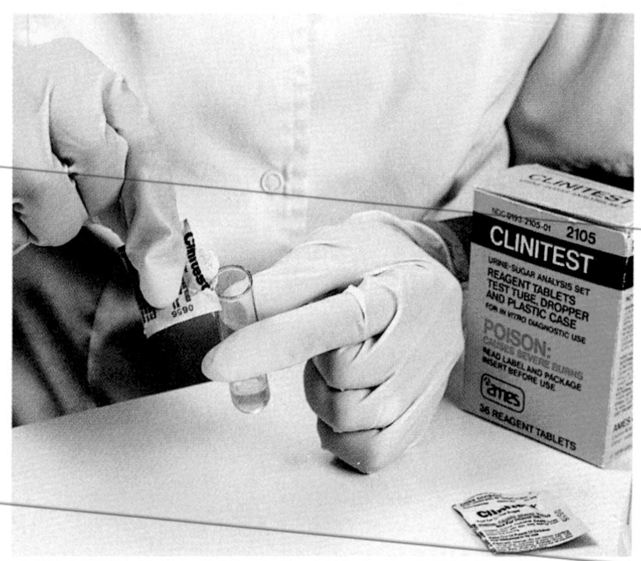

Drop Clinitest tablet into test tube without touching tablet.

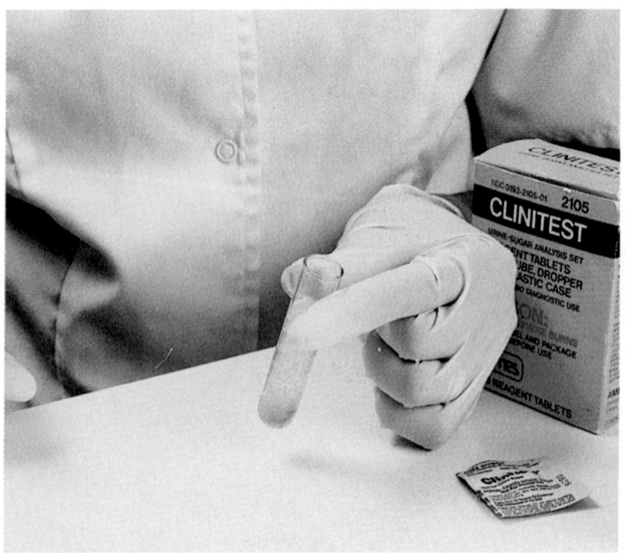

After bubbling stops, wait 15 seconds and shake gently.

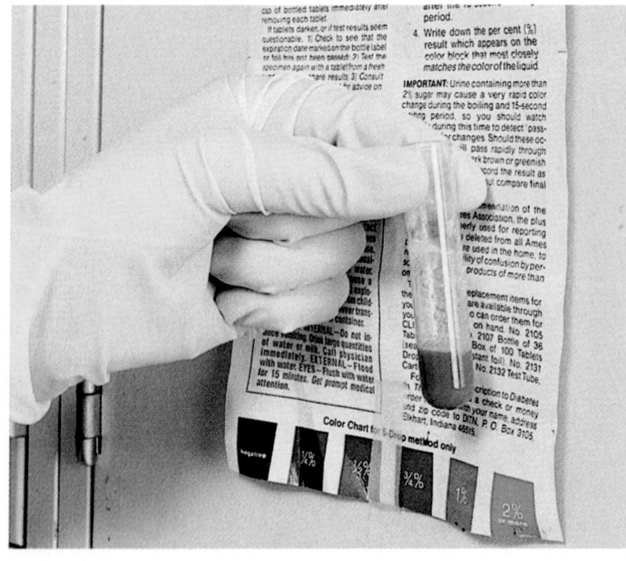

Compare color of test tube mixture with color chart.

3. Take first voided specimen to utility or bathroom. Empty small amount of urine from bedpan or urinal into test tube.
4. Test first voided specimen and record findings if required to do so by facility. **Rationale:** Some facilities require two tests, even though second voided specimen is more accurate.
5. Obtain second voided specimen and take to utility or bathroom. **Rationale:** Second voided specimen is a more accurate measure of present condition of the body.

■ CLINICAL ALERT

Place test tube in holder or grasp by top of tube as it gets very hot when bubbling occurs. Reagent tablet contains sodium hydroxide which, when added to water, boils.

for Clinitest—5-drop method

a. Place 5 drops of urine and 10 drops of water into test tube.
b. Drop one reagent (Clinitest) tablet into test tube.
c. Allow reaction to bubble until it stops.
d. Wait 15 seconds, shake gently, and compare results with chart:

   Blue indicates negative test.

   Orange indicates highly positive test.

   Dark greenish-brown preceded by rapid change in color from green to orange indicates urine glucose level about 2%.

COMMUNITY HOSPITAL

DIABETIC RECORD

DIRECTION: Test second voiding whenever possible. Place "U" in 2nd void column twice.

DATE												
TIME	1st void / 2nd void											
VOLUME	1st void / 2nd void											
SUGAR												
ACETONE												
INSULIN	TYPE											
	DOSE											
	TIME											
	ROUTE											
	SITE											
SIGNATURE												

for Clinitest—2-drop method

a. Place 2 drops of urine and 10 drops of water into test tube.
b. Drop reagent (Clinitest) tablet into test tube.
c. Allow reaction to bubble until it stops. (Do not shake tube.)
d. Wait 15 seconds, shake test tube, and compare results with chart:

   Seven colors are contained on chart.

   Scale ranges from 0–5%.

6. Rinse out test tube and return to container.
7. Discard gloves and wash hands.
8. Discuss results with client.
9. Document findings as negative or positive, and determine if insulin is needed.

MEASURING URINE KETONE BODIES

Equipment

Same as for *Measuring Urine Glucose* except add (Acetest tablets or Keto-Diastix strips)

Procedure

1. Ask client to void in urinal or bedpan 30 minutes before urine specimen for testing acetone is needed. **Rationale:** Urine collected overnight does not accurately reveal present concentration of acetone in urine.
2. Don clean gloves.
3. Take first voided specimen to utility or bathroom. Empty small amount of urine from bedpan or urinal into test tube or dip Keto-Diastix strip into urine.
4. Test first voided specimen and record findings if required to do so by facility. **Rationale:** Some facilities require two tests, even though second voided specimen is more accurate.

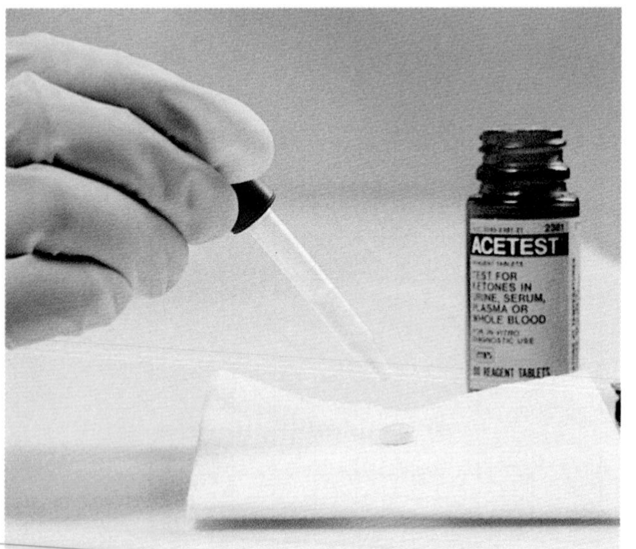

Place one drop of urine on acetest tablet to check for ketone bodies.

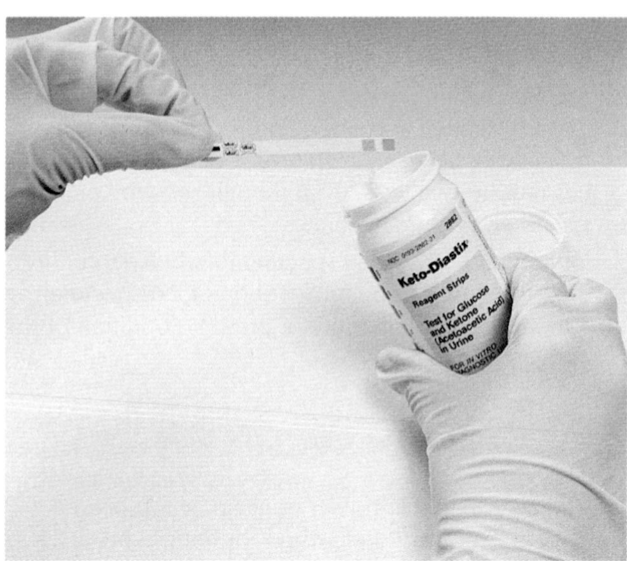

Keto-Diastix strips are used to check urine for ketone bodies.

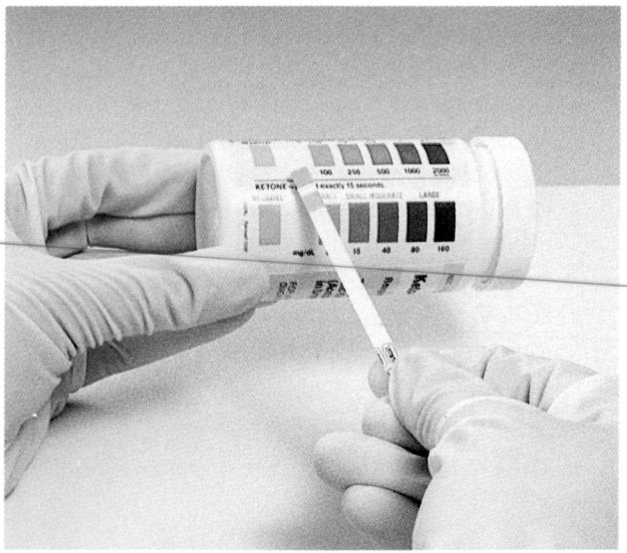

Reagent strips are checked against the chart found on bottle.

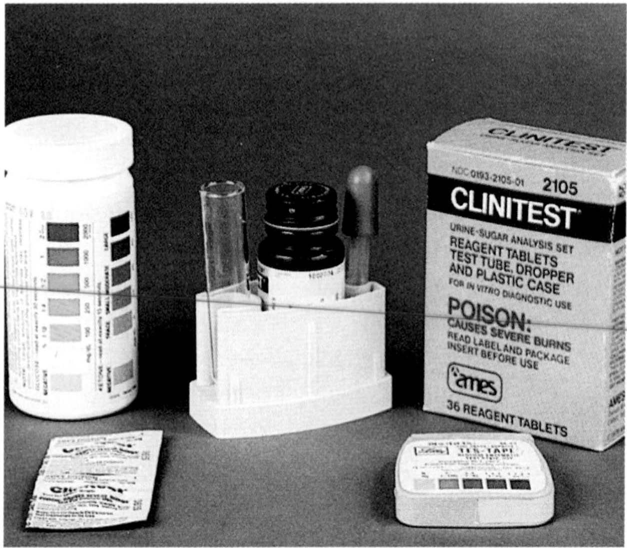

Equipment used to check urine for glucose and ketone bodies.

5. Obtain second voided specimen and take to utility or bathroom. **Rationale:** Second voided specimen is a more accurate measure of present condition of the body.
6. Place ketone (Acetest) tablet on piece of paper towel. **Rationale:** White towel reflects color and absorbs more efficiently.
7. Place one or two drops of urine on Acetest tablet. Wait 1 minute.
8. Compare color of tablet and chart. Dark purple indicates positive results. (Results range from negative to positive to strongly positive.)
9. Alternative method: Dip Keo-Diastix strip into urine and compare results on color chart found on bottle.
10. Clean and replace equipment to proper storage area.
11. Discard gloves.
12. Wash your hands.
13. Document findings, and determine if insulin is needed.
14. Discuss results with client. **Rationale:** It is important to reinforce the need for compliance.

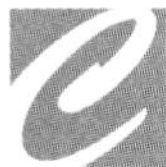

CHARTING for Specific Gravity and Glucose

- Amount, color, appearance, and odor of urine
- Techniques effective in stimulating voiding
- Type of urine testing equipment used (e.g., test tape)
- Percentage and "plus" readings from urine test
- First or second voided specimen used for testing
- Specific gravity reading
- Actions taken based on results
- Physician notified, if appropriate

CRITICAL THINKING APPLICATION

CLINICAL PROBLEMS	CRITICAL THINKING OPTIONS
Urine glucose level positive for unknown reason.	• Check if new medication contains sugar (e.g., elixirs, cough syrups). • Assess if client is taking large quantities of ascorbic acid and aspirin. The urine tests positive even though glucose is not present. • Check if client is taking medications that cause false-positive results, e.g., Benemid, levodopa, NegGram, Keflin.
Strips or tablets are discolored or moist.	• Sensitivity is lost. They need to be disposed of and new strips or tablets used. • Keep tablets and strips away from moisture by keeping them in tightly covered container (original bottle for tablets and baby food jar for tape). • Always check tablet before using to ensure accurate results.

unit 3

CATHETERIZATION

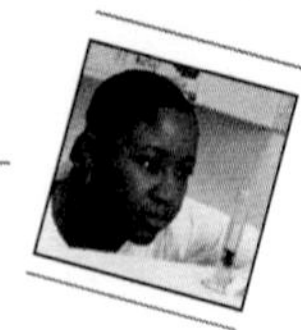

NURSING PROCESS DATA

ASSESSMENT Data Base

Assess the client's bladder for distention.

Assess purpose of catheterization.

Check physician's orders for method of catheterization to be done.

Assess the client's physical ability to cooperate with positioning.

Assess urinary meatus and catheter for exudate, edema, inflammation, and general cleanliness.

Assess need for perineal care before catheterization procedure.

PLANNING Objectives

To prevent or relieve discomfort due to bladder distention

To promote urinary elimination

To obtain a sterile urine specimen

To obtain accurate measurements of bladder function

To provide continual urinary bladder drainage

To instill medication

To measure the amount of residual urine

To monitor the output of a critically ill client

To facilitate studies of the urinary system

To prevent skin breakdown in incontinent bedridden clients

To prevent urinary tract infections through catheter care

IMPLEMENTATION Procedures

Draping a Client

Inserting a Straight Catheter (Female)

Inserting a Straight Catheter (Male)

Inserting a Retention Catheter (Female)

Inserting a Retention Catheter (Male)

Providing Catheter Care

Removing a Retention Catheter

EVALUATION Expected Outcomes

Residual urine measured.

Sterile urine specimen obtained.

Catheterization performed using sterile technique.

Retention catheter inserted without difficulty.

Bladder emptied when client unable to void.

Urinary tract infections prevented through aseptic catheter care.

Urinary medications instilled using sterile technique.

DRAPING A FEMALE CLIENT

Equipment

Bath blanket

Procedure

1. Bring bath blanket to bedside.
2. Identify client, and explain procedure.
3. Provide privacy.
4. Wash your hands.
5. Place bed in HIGH position, and lower side rail nearest you.
6. Place bath blanket over client's top linen so that one corner of the blanket is pointed toward the client's head to form a diamond shape over the client.
7. Instruct client to hold onto bath blanket. Fanfold linen to foot of bed and place on chair.
8. Request that client flex knees and keep them apart with feet firmly on bed.
9. Wrap lateral corners of bath blanket around feet in a spiral fashion until they are completely covered.
10. The corner of the blanket between knees and extending over perineum can later be folded back over the abdomen.

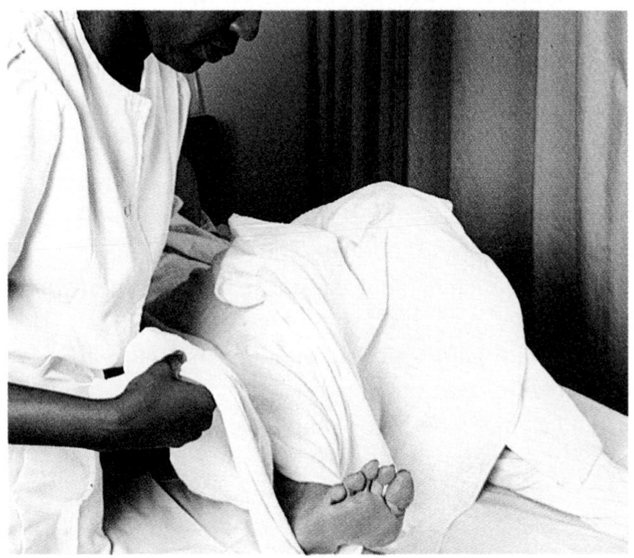

Use bath blanket to drape client before catheterization.

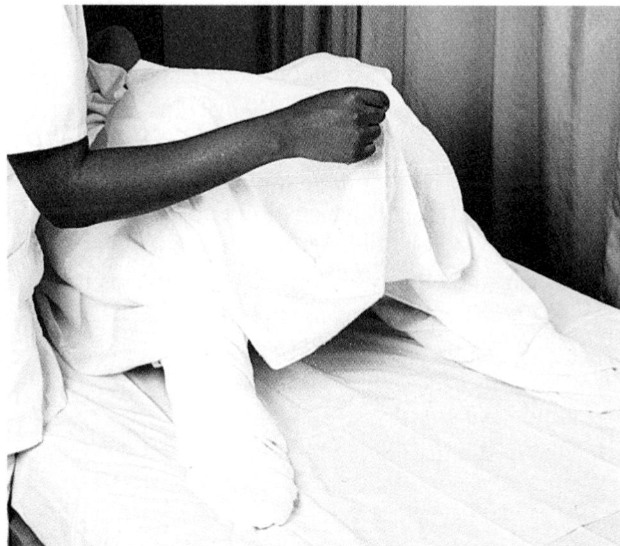

Corner of blanket is folded back over abdomen to expose perineum.

INSERTING A STRAIGHT CATHETER (FEMALE)

Equipment

Disposable catheterization tray with straight catheter
Bath blanket
Additional light source, if needed
Towel, washcloth
Basin with warm water and soap
Clean gloves

Preparation

1. Bring equipment to bedside table.
2. Check lighting source.
3. Identify client, and explain procedure and need for client to keep knees positioned during procedure.
4. Provide privacy.
5. Wash your hands.
6. Place bed in HIGH position, and lower side rail on working side.
7. Drape the client (see *Draping a Female Client*).
8. Have client bring knees up and out. May need assistance to keep knees in this position.
   Rationale: This position provides for good visualization of urinary meatus.

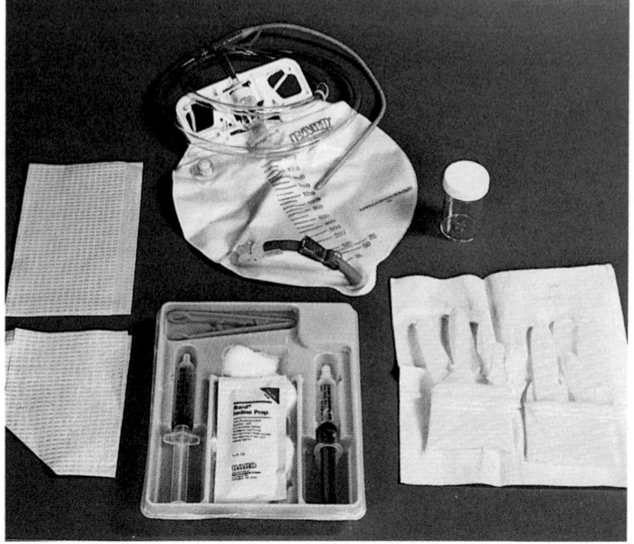

Disposable kit includes equipment necessary for performing a catheterization.

9. Adjust light source to ensure that exposure is adequate.
10. Fold up bath blanket corner to expose perineum.
11. Provide perineal care if necessary with soap and water using clean gloves.
12. Dry perineum thoroughly. Fold bath blanket corner over perineum for privacy.
13. Discard towels, water, and replace basin.
14. Dispose of gloves, and wash your hands.

Procedure

1. Open sterile package by tearing the package on the lined edge of plastic wrap. Place plastic wrap at foot of bed for waste disposal.
2. Place cath tray on bed between client's legs.
3. Fold back bath blanket to expose perineum.
4. Open white outer wrap away from sterile package with last turn toward client.
5. Position white wrap under client's buttocks. **Rationale:** Used for added protection of the bed.
6. Remove sterile absorbent pad, and position under client's buttocks. Have client lift buttocks if able. Position pad by holding on to corners of pad only.
7. Put on sterile gloves, remove sterile articles from tray, and arrange conveniently on sterile field or place tray up close on field.
8. Open package, and pour antiseptic solution over cotton balls.
9. Uncap syringe filled with lubricant, or tear open package, pick up catheter tip, and lubricate the tip of the catheter generously. Place catheter back on tray. (May place lubricant on sterile field and put catheter tip on lubricant and leave in place.)
10. If specimen is required, uncap the specimen container.
11. Move the urine collection receptacle close to client.
12. Place the fenestrated drape over the perineum exposing meatus.

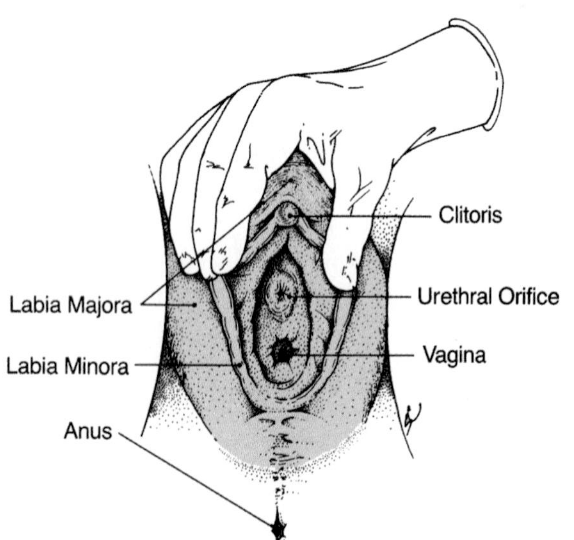

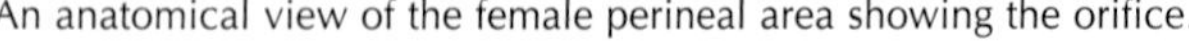

An anatomical view of the female perineal area showing the orifice.

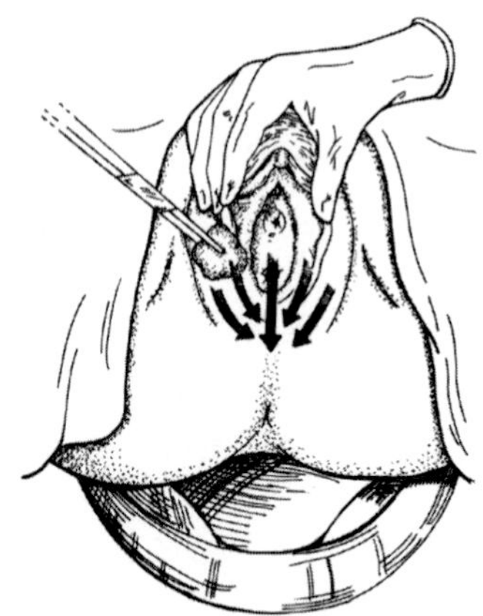

Cleanse meatus with saturated cotton ball in one downward stroke.

13. Cleanse the client's meatus:
    a. Separate the client's labia minora with your nondominant hand.
    b. With your dominant hand, *use forceps* to pick up an absorbent ball that has been saturated with antiseptic solution.
    c. Cleanse the client's meatus with one downward stroke of the forceps. **Rationale:** Using a downward stroke cleans from least contaminated to most contaminated area. Discard the absorbent ball in the plastic cover at foot of bed. **Rationale:** Using a new cotton ball with each downward stroke prevents transfer of microorganisms.
    d. Repeat step c at least three to four times.
    e. Continue to hold the client's labia apart until you insert the catheter. **Rationale:** This prevents contamination of urinary meatus.
14. Discard the forceps in the plastic bag at the foot of the bed. Using sterile gloved hand, pick up lubricated catheter keeping drainage end in collection container, and insert 2–3 inches or until urine begins to flow.
15. Move nondominant hand from holding labia open to hold catheter in place.
16. Place the sterile specimen container under the drainage end of the catheter if specimen is needed, and fill the container with approximately 30 mL of urine.
17. Replace catheter drainage end in collection container, and allow urine to flow until it ceases.

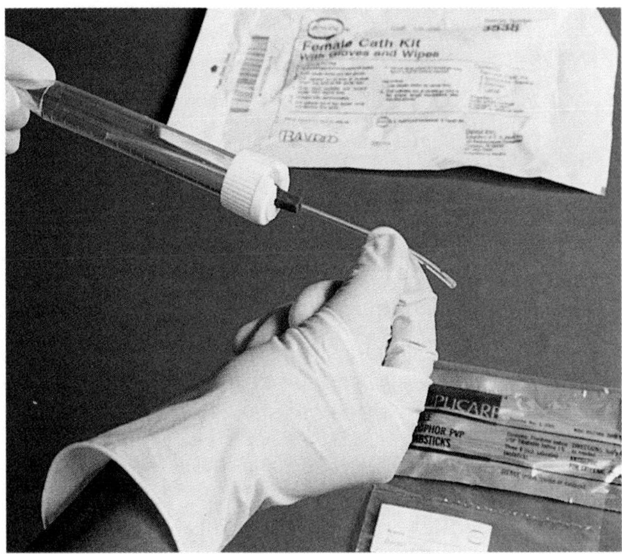

Female catherter kit can be used to obtain sterile urine specimen.

18. Pinch catheter closed when urine ceases to flow, and remove gently and slowly.
19. Remove the drapes, wash and dry the perineum.
20. Position the client for comfort, put the bed in LOW position with the side rails up.
21. Measure and record urine output on the I&O bedside record.
22. Discard gloves and the equipment in the utility room.
23. Wash your hands.

INSERTING A STRAIGHT CATHETER (MALE)

Equipment

Same as for *Inserting a Straight Catheter (Female)*

Preparation

1. Follow steps 1 through 6 in *Inserting a Straight Catheter (Female).*
2. Place client in a supine position with knees slightly apart. **Rationale:** This position relaxes abdominal and perineal muscles.
3. Drape client by placing a bath blanket over chest area and fanfold top linen down to cover lower extremities, exposing only genital area.

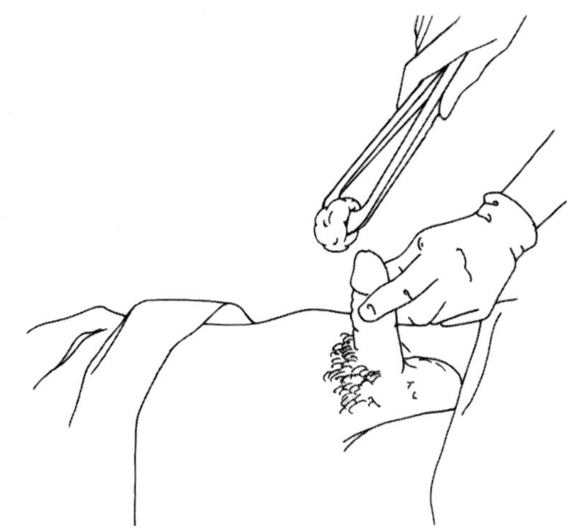
Cleanse tip of penis with forceps holding saturated cotton ball.

4. Don clean gloves, and wash genital area if necessary.
5. Remove gloves, and prepare for catheterization.

Procedure

1. Open sterile package by tearing the package on the lined edge of plastic wrap. Place plastic wrap at foot of bed for waste disposal.
2. Place sterile kit on client's thighs if client is cooperative, or at client's side near thigh.
3. Open outer white wrap away from sterile package with last turn toward penis.
4. Place first drape over penis.
5. Don sterile gloves.
6. Place fenestrated drape over penis.
7. Open antiseptic package, and pour solution over cotton balls.
8. Uncap syringe filled with lubricant, or tear open package, pick up catheter tip, lubricate generously, 5–7 cm (2–3 inches). Place catheter back on tray.
9. Hold penis upright with your nondominant hand. Hold sides of penis to prevent closing of urethra.
10. With your dominant hand, use forceps to pick up cotton ball saturated with antiseptic solution.
11. Cleanse meatus first with one circular stroke of the forceps. Discard cotton ball into plastic bag at foot of bed.
12. Repeat circular cleansing motion around tip of penis. Cleanse three times using a new cotton ball each time.
13. Continue to hold penis with your nondominant hand.
14. Discard forceps into plastic bag. Place end of catheter in specimen container or urine collection container. **Rationale:** This allows specimen to be collected or urine to drain into container without urine leaking over sterile field.
15. Pick up catheter with sterile hand about 8–10 cm (3–4 inches) from tip of catheter.
16. Lift penis to a 90° angle (perpendicular to body) and exert slight traction by pulling upward. **Rationale:** This movement straightens the urethra for easier insertion of catheter.
17. Insert catheter about 20 cm (8 inches) until urine begins to flow.
18. If catheter meets resistance at sphincter, twist catheter and ask client to take deep breath. **Rationale:** Taking a deep breath helps relax external sphincter. If persistent resistance is felt and catheter is unable to be inserted without difficulty, remove catheter and notify physician.
19. Obtain urine specimen if needed. Place 30 mL urine in specimen container. Pinch tubing, and transfer end of catheter into collection container.
20. Allow urine to drain into collection container until flow stops.
21. Remove catheter, place lid on specimen bottle.
22. Dry penis, and remove drapes.
23. Make client comfortable.
24. Discard equipment in appropriate container.
25. Remove gloves, and wash hands.
26. Send specimen to lab and document findings.

INSERTING A RETENTION CATHETER (FEMALE)

Equipment

Disposable catheter kit with appropriate size catheter (size 8–10 for child, size 14–16 for adult female, and size 18–20 for adult male)
Closed drainage set, if not included in kit
Additional lighting, if needed
Bath blanket
Towels, washcloth
Basin with warm water
Soap
Tape

Preparation

Same as for *Inserting a Straight Catheter (Female).*

Procedure

1. Open sterile package by tearing the package on the lined edge of plastic wrap. Place plastic wrap at foot of bed for waste disposal.
2. Place catheter tray on bed between client's legs.
3. Fold back corner of bath blanket to expose perineum.
4. Open white outer wrap away from package with last turn toward client.
5. Bring white wrap under client's buttocks.

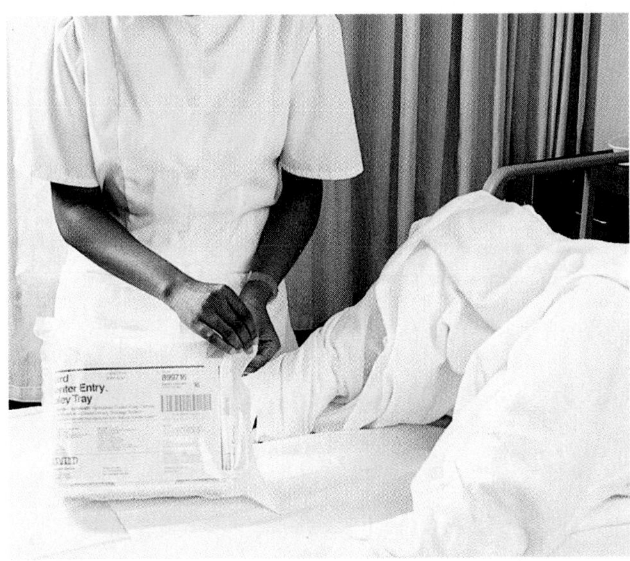

Open sterile package by tearing it along lined edge of plastic wrap.

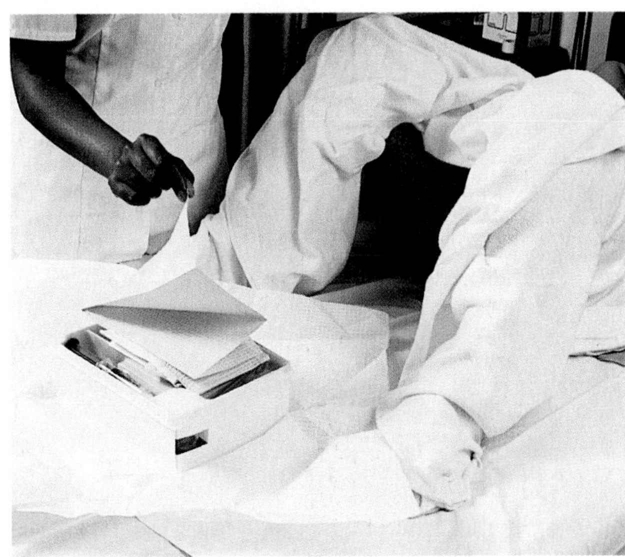

Remove sterile absorbent pad and place it under client's buttocks.

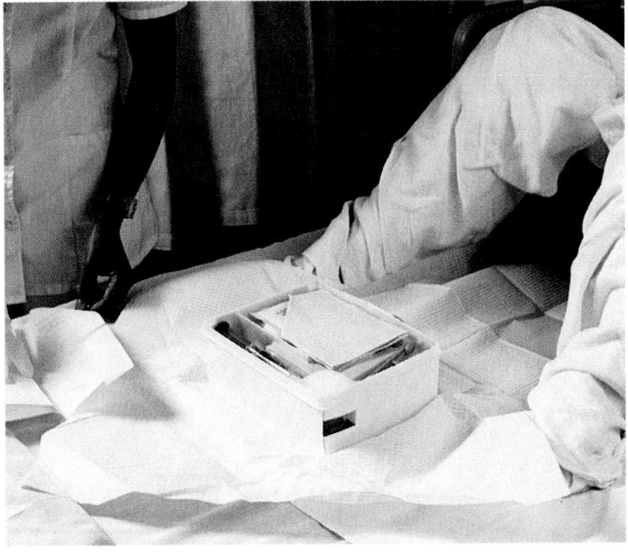

Put on sterile gloves being careful not to contaminate sterile field.

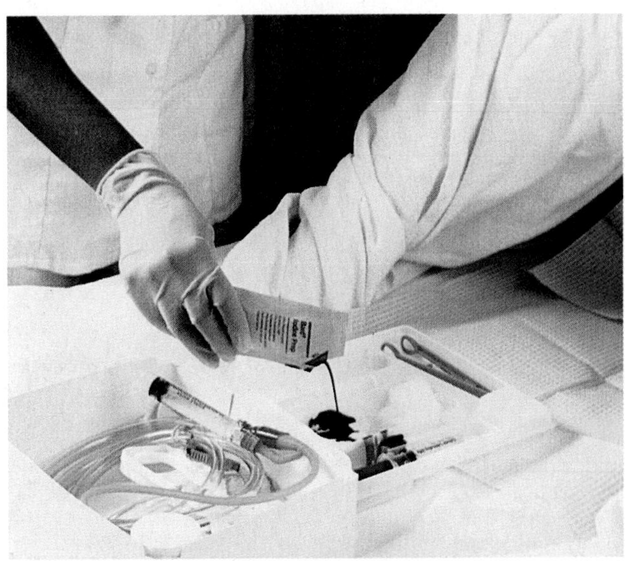

Open package and pour antiseptic solution completely over cotton balls.

6. Remove sterile absorbent pad, and position under client's buttocks. Have client lift buttocks if able. Position pad by holding on to corners of pad only. **Rationale:** Holding onto the edges keeps the center sterile.
7. Put on sterile gloves, and separate the two containers. Place container with cotton balls and lubricant toward client. Place container with catheter and bag toward foot of bed (next to first container).
8. Open package, and pour antiseptic solution over cotton balls.
9. To test catheter bag, remove rubber protector and insert tip of the prefilled syringe into catheter side arm to inflate balloon. Standard catheters have 5-mL balloons. Omit pretesting step for catheters with prefilled balloons on drainage end of catheter. **Rationale:** Once prefilled balloons are opened and fluid forced into balloon at tip of catheter, the fluid cannot be aspirated back into drainage end.
10. After testing balloon, pull back on syringe to remove fluid. **Rationale:** Testing is done to ensure that balloon is able to be inflated without leaking.
11. Lubricate catheter by uncapping syringe filled with lubricant or open package, and generously lubricate tip in lubricant. Keep catheter on tray.

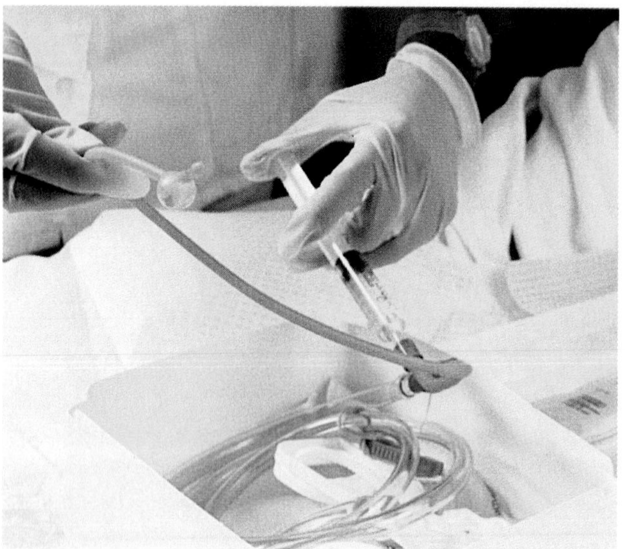
Test catheter balloon by inserting pre-filled syringe into side arm of catheter.

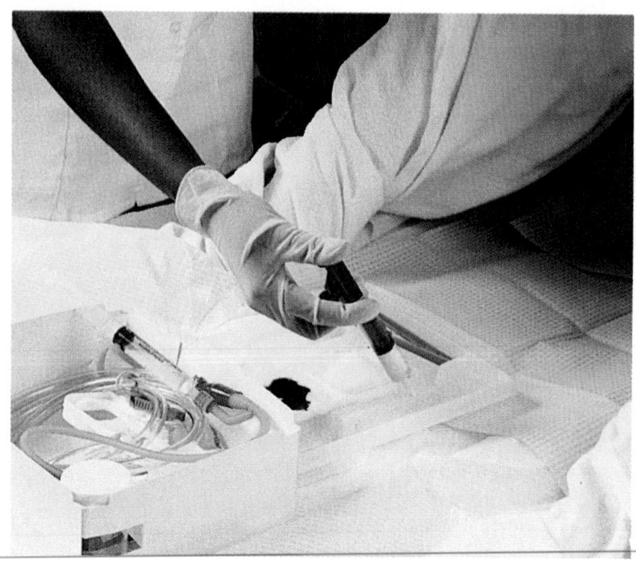
Uncap lubricant syringe and squeeze lubricant onto tray.

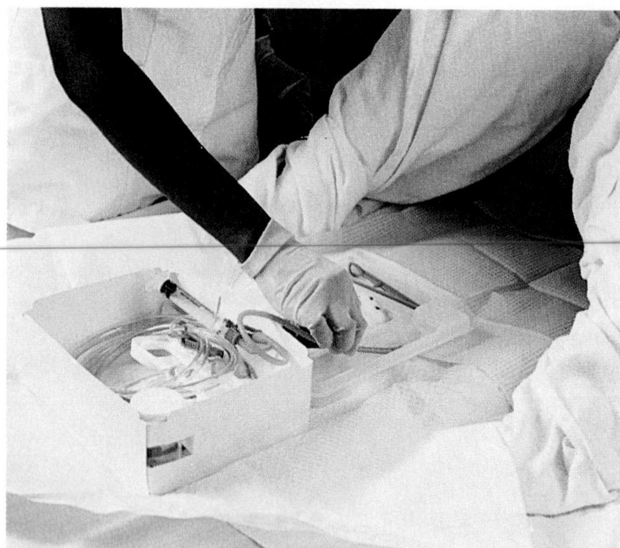
Generously lubricate tip of catheter to facilitate insertion without trauma.

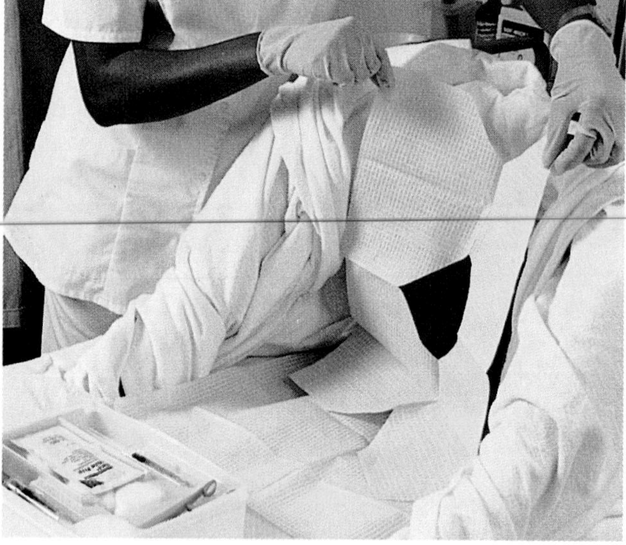
Position sterile fenestrated drape over client to expose genitalia.

Rationale: Lubricating the catheter prevents friction and trauma to the meatus.

12. Position fenestrated drape over the client to expose the genitalia.
13. Cleanse the client's meatus:
    a. Separate the client's labia minora with your nondominant hand.
    b. With your dominant hand, *use forceps* to pick up an absorbent ball that has been saturated with antiseptic solution.
    c. Cleanse the client's meatus with one downward stroke of the forceps. Discard the absorbent ball in plastic bag at foot of bed.
    d. Repeat step c at least three to four times.
    e. Continue to hold the client's labia apart until you insert the catheter.
14. Discard forceps in plastic bag at foot of bed.
15. With uncontaminated hand, take catheter from tray, and insert gently into meatus 2–3 inches or until urine starts to flow.
16. Guide the catheter gently 1–2 inches beyond the point at which urine begins to flow. **Rationale:** Inserting the catheter further into bladder ensures it is beyond the neck of the bladder.

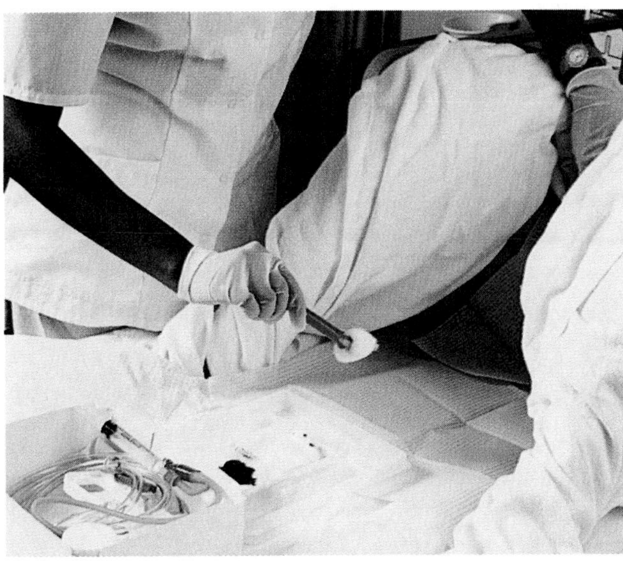
Cleanse meatus by using downward strokes with antiseptic soaked cotton balls.

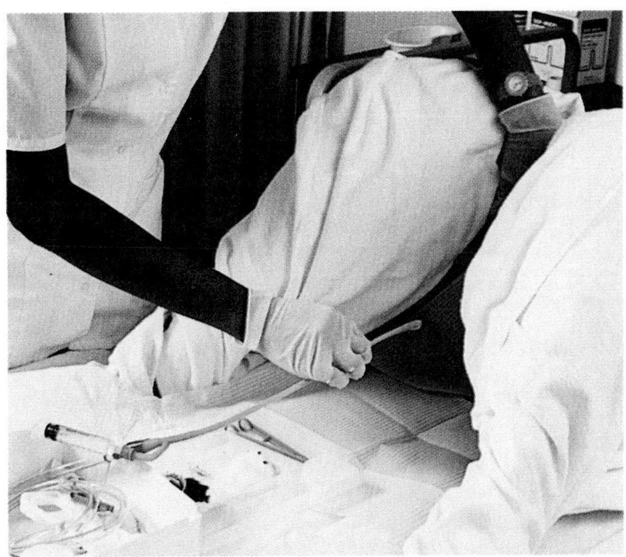
Insert catheter while holding labia apart to prevent contamination of catheter.

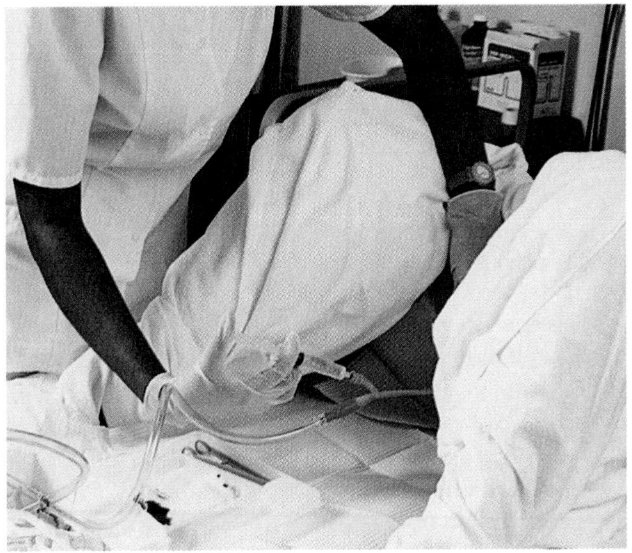
Inject water from prefilled syringe after inserting catheter into bladder.

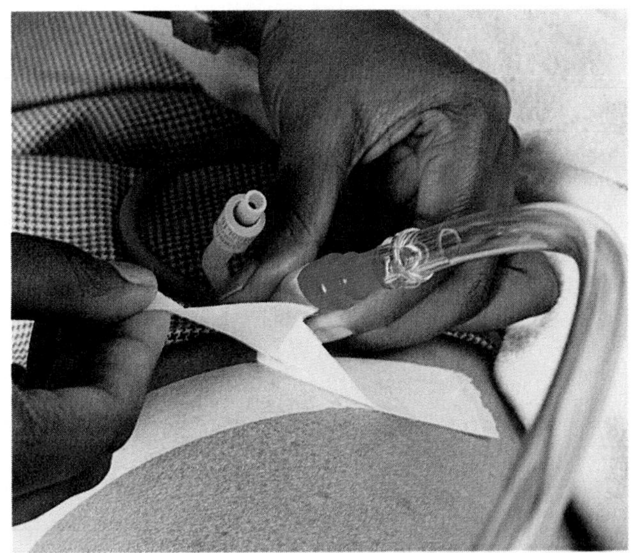
Tape catheter to leg using non allergenic tape to prevent pulling on catheter.

17. Inject the entire contents of the prefilled syringe into the side arm of the catheter used for balloon inflation. If the catheter has a prefilled balloon at the drainage end of catheter, inflate the retention balloon by releasing the clamp on the prefilled balloon.
18. Retract the catheter until you feel resistance.
19. Tape the catheter to the side of the leg with 1-inch tape.
20. Attach drainage bag to bed frame (not side rails).
21. Cleanse the client's perineum of the antiseptic solution. Remove drapes.

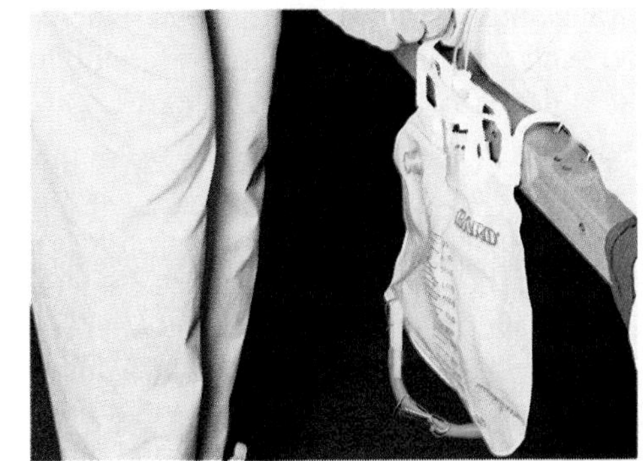
Attach drainage bag to bed frame to ensure it does not come in contact with floor.

22. Reposition the client for comfort; put bed in LOW position with side rails up.
23. Remove all equipment, including gloves, and discard disposable trash in the appropriate container.
24. Measure and record urine output on I&O bedside record.
25. Wash your hands.

INSERTING A RETENTION CATHETER (MALE)

Equipment

Same as for *Inserting a Retention Catheter (Female)*

Preparation

1. Follow steps 1 through 6 in *Inserting a Straight Catheter (Female).*
2. Place client in a supine position with knees slightly apart. **Rationale:** This position relaxes abdominal and perineal muscles.
3. Drape client by placing a bath blanket over chest area and fanfold top linen down to cover lower extremities, exposing only perineal area.
4. Don clean gloves, and wash client's perineal area if necessary.
5. Remove gloves, and prepare for catheterization.

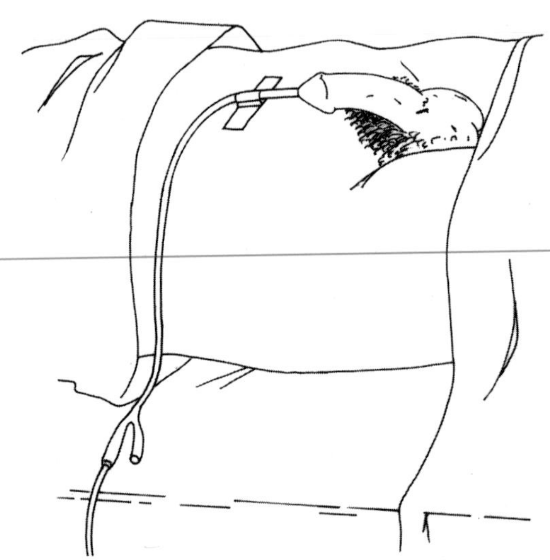

Tape catheter to abdomen to prevent pressure on penoscrotal angle.

Procedure

1. Open sterile package by tearing the package on the lined edge of plastic wrap. Place plastic wrap at foot of bed for waste disposal.
2. Place sterile kit on client's thighs if client is cooperative, or at client's side near thigh.
3. Open outer white wrap away from sterile package with last turn toward penis.
4. Place first drape under penis.
5. Don sterile gloves.
6. Separate two containers. Place container with cotton balls and lubricant toward client. Place container with catheter and bag toward foot of bed (next to first container).
7. Open package and pour antiseptic over cotton balls.
8. To test catheter bag, remove rubber protector, and insert tip of the prefilled syringe into catheter side arm to inflate balloon. Standard catheters have 5-mL balloons. Omit pretesting step for catheters with prefilled balloons on drainage end of catheter. **Rationale:** Once prefilled balloons are opened and fluid forced into balloon at tip of catheter, the fluid cannot be aspirated back into drainage end.
9. After testing balloon, pull back on syringe to remove fluid. **Rationale:** Testing is done to ensure that balloon is able to be inflated without leaking.
10. Lubricate catheter by uncapping syringe filled with lubricant or open package, and generously lubricate tip for 5–7 cm (2–3 inches). Keep catheter on tray. **Rationale:** Lubricating the catheter prevents friction and trauma to the meatus.
11. Position fenestrated drape over the penis.
12. Hold penis upright with your nondominant hand. Hold sides of penis to prevent closing of urethra.
13. With your dominant hand, use forceps to pick up cotton ball saturated with antiseptic solution.
14. Cleanse meatus first with one circular stroke of the forceps.
15. Discard cotton ball into plastic bag at foot of bed.
16. Repeat circular cleansing motion around tip of penis. Cleanse three times using a new cotton ball each time.
17. Continue to hold penis with your nondominant hand.
18. Discard forceps into plastic bag.

19. Pick up catheter with sterile hand about 8–10 cm. (3–4 inches) from tip of catheter.
20. Lift penis to a 90° angle (perpendicular to body) and exert slight traction by pulling upward. **Rationale:** This movement straightens the urethra for easier insertion of catheter.
21. Insert catheter about 20 cm. (8 inches) until urine begins to flow.
22. If resistance is met at sphincter, twist catheter and ask client to take deep breath. **Rationale:** Taking a deep breath helps relax external sphincter. If persistent resistance is felt and catheter is unable to be inserted without difficulty, remove catheter and notify physician.
23. Guide the catheter gently 1–2 inches beyond the point at which urine begins to flow. **Rationale:** Inserting the catheter further into bladder ensures it is beyond the neck of the bladder.
24. Inject the entire contents of the prefilled syringe into the side arm of the catheter used for balloon inflation. If the catheter has a prefilled balloon at the drainage end of catheter, inflate the retention balloon by releasing the clamp on the prefilled balloon.
25. Retract the catheter until you feel resistance.
26. Tape the catheter to abdomen with 1-inch tape. **Rationale:** This prevents pressure on the penoscrotal angle. Alternative taping to upper thigh.

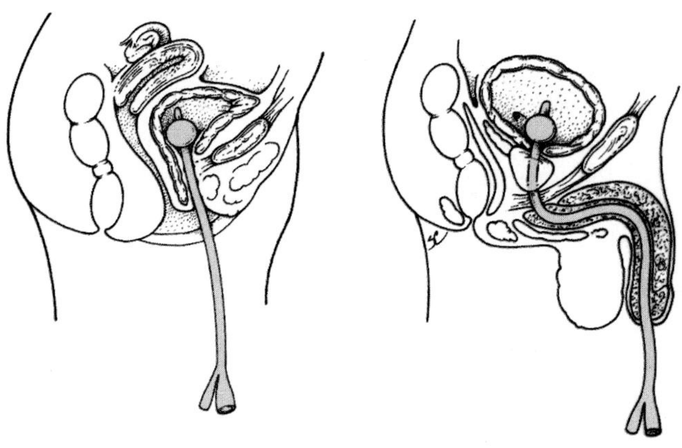

Foley catheter placement is maintained with inflated retention balloon

27. Attach drainage bag to bed frame (not side rails).
28. Cleanse the client's perineum of the antiseptic solution. Remove drapes.
29. Reposition the client for comfort; put bed in LOW position with side rails up.
30. Remove all equipment, including gloves, and discard disposable trash in the appropriate container.
31. Measure and record urine output in I&O bedside record.
32. Wash your hands.
33. Document findings.

PROVIDING CATHETER CARE

Equipment

Commercially prepared kit *or*
Antiseptic solution
Sterile swabs or sterile cotton balls
Clean gloves
Sterile bowl
Paper bag

Procedure

1. Check physician's orders and client care plan.
2. Gather equipment.
3. Identify client by checking identaband.
4. Provide privacy.
5. Wash hands.
6. Explain procedure to client.
7. Raise bed, and lower side rail on working side.
8. Place client in supine position, and expose perineal area to easily visualize the meatus.
9. Open sterile catheter care kit or assemble equipment on over-bed table within easy reach.
10. Pour antiseptic solution over cotton balls or open package of cleansing swabs.
11. Place paper bag near working area.
12. Remove tape.
13. Put on clean gloves.
14. Cleanse urinary meatus using circular motion moving from middle toward outside with antiseptic soaked cotton ball or swab. Dispose of cotton ball into paper bag. **Rationale:** This motion prevents bacteria from entering the urinary meatus.
15. Gently pull catheter taut and cleanse with new

swab or cotton ball from catheter insertion site down catheter tubing approximately 4–5 inches toward drainage bag. Dispose of cotton ball into paper bag.

16. Remove gloves and discard. Retape catheter.
17. Position client for comfort.
18. Lower bed, and raise side rail.
19. Discard equipment.
20. Wash hands.

REMOVING A RETENTION CATHETER

Equipment

10-mL syringe
Paper towel
Catheter clamp
Soap, water, towel
Clean gloves

Preparation

1. Check physician's orders.
2. Wash your hands.
3. Gather equipment.
4. Explain procedure to client.
5. Provide privacy.
6. Don clean gloves.

Procedure

1. Clamp catheter. Remove tape attaching catheter to client.
2. Insert syringe into balloon port of catheter. Do not cut the catheter with a scissors. **Rationale:** Balloon may not totally deflate if cut.
3. Withdraw fluid from balloon (usually 5–10 mL water in balloon).
4. Pull gently on catheter to ensure balloon is deflated before attempting to remove. **Rationale:** Damage to the urethra can occur if balloon is not totally deflated.
5. Hold a paper towel under the catheter with your nondominant hand.
6. If resistance is not met, slowly withdraw the catheter allowing it to fall into paper towel.
7. Disconnect catheter bag from bed frame.
8. Empty catheter bag into graduate and measure output.
9. Record output on I&O bedside record.
10. Dispose of catheter in trash.
11. Wash perineum with soap and water. Dry thoroughly. Remove gloves.
12. Position client for comfort.
13. Wash your hands.
14. Instruct client to drink oral fluids as tolerated and observe for signs and symptoms of urinary tract infections (burning, frequency, urgency).
15. Offer bedpan or urinal at least every 2–4 hours after removing catheter, until voiding occurs. Keep accurate I&O record.

CHARTING for Catheterizations

- Type of catheterization
- Amount, color, and odor of urine obtained
- Size of catheter used
- Client's tolerance of procedure
- Specimen sent to lab (if ordered)
- Catheter care provided
- Condition of urinary meatus
- Catheter removed
- Voiding: time and amount after catheter removal
- Intake and output

CRITICAL THINKING APPLICATION

CLINICAL PROBLEMS	CRITICAL THINKING OPTIONS
■ Catheter is inserted in the vagina of a female client.	• Leave the catheter in place and follow these actions: a. Reposition your fingers to assist in visualizing the urethral meatus. b. Have someone obtain a new catheter and new gloves. You may need a whole new kit if contamination of the sterile field has occurred. c. Locate the client's urinary meatus before inserting the catheter. d. Repeat the catheterization procedure.
■ Catheter is contaminated when attempting to insert.	• Obtain a new catheter and repeat the catheterization. • If the sterile field has been contaminated, obtain a new catheter kit. Repeat the catheterization procedure.
■ Unable to insert catheter into a female client.	• Repeat the procedure following these actions: a. Ask client to hold her legs apart or ask for assistance from another health team member so you have better access to the urethral meatus. b. Before cleansing the client, identify the area of the urethral meatus. c. When cleansing with antiseptic solution, observe the urethral opening for movement when pressure is applied to meatus. d. Repeat the catheterization procedure using a new catheter kit or new gloves and a new catheter if the kit has not been contaminated.
■ Unable to insert catheter into male client.	• Obtain a new catheter kit and follow these actions: a. Hold penis vertical to client's body. b. Insert catheter while applying slight traction by gently pulling upward on the shaft of the penis. c. If you encounter resistance, rotate the catheter, increase the traction, and change the angle of the penis slightly. d. When urine begins to flow, lower the client's penis.

CLINICAL PROBLEMS	CRITICAL THINKING OPTIONS
■ Urine exceeds 1000 mL with catheterization.	• If Foley catheter is inserted, clamp catheter for 20–30 minutes and then unclamp. • If bladder appears to be grossly distended when palpated, insert Foley catheter instead of straight catheter. a. If urine exceeds 1000 mL, inflate balloon and clamp for 30 minutes. b. Open clamp and drain remaining urine, then deflate balloon. c. Remove catheter after urine flow ceases or notify physician of results and ask if Foley should be left in place.
■ Catheter comes out with balloon still inflated.	• Assess client for signs of urethral trauma (e.g., bleeding, pain). • Obtain a new catheter and repeat the catheterization procedure, making sure that the balloon is inflated with at least 10 mL water. • Monitor urine output for bleeding. • Notify physician to determine if a Foley with a 30-mL balloon should be inserted.

unit 4

EXTERNAL CATHETER SYSTEM

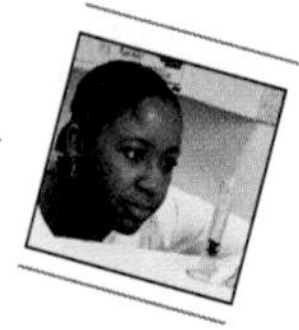

NURSING PROCESS DATA

ASSESSMENT Data Base

Assess the genital area for signs of irritation and edema during the use of condom catheter.

Assess activity level of client to determine when a leg bag or a continuous drainage system is necessary.

PLANNING Objectives

To provide a means for preventing incontinency

To provide a means of collecting urine in a system which allows client ambulation

To prevent urinary tract infections in clients who are at risk but require a method of urine collection to maintain continency

IMPLEMENTATION Procedures

Applying a Condom Catheter

Attaching Catheter to Leg Bag

EVALUATION Expected Outcomes

Urinary tract infection is prevented.

Client remains continent.

Genital area remains free of inflammation.

Client is able to ambulate without a catheter drainage bag.

APPLYING A CONDOM CATHETER

Equipment

Soap, water, towel

Commercial condom catheter

Leg bag or continuous drainage system

Alcohol wipes

Clean gloves

Preparation

1. Check physician's orders and client care plan.
2. Gather equipment, condom catheter, soap, towel, and basin with warm water.
3. Explain procedure to client.
4. Wash your hands, and provide privacy.
5. Raise bed, and lower side rail on working side of bed.
6. Don clean gloves.
7. Wash genital area with soap and water, and dry area thoroughly.

Procedure

1. When commercial condom catheters are used, apply protective coating to skin on penile shaft and allow to dry completely (30 seconds).
2. Peel off paper from both sides of the adhesive liner that accompanies the commercial product.
3. Spirally wrap the adhesive liner around the penile shaft behind the glans.
4. Take the latex condom catheter and place the prerolled latex sheath so the funnel is against the glans.
5. Unroll the latex sheath up the penis until it is completely over the adhesive liner.
6. Gently squeeze the condom against the liner to seal it after the sheath is completely rolled over the penis. Do not wrinkle the latex as wrinkles cause urine to leak through the catheter.
7. Attach the condom to a drainage system. The drainage system can be a leg bag or a continuous drainage system depending on the activity level and condition of the client.
8. Lower bed, and raise side rail or assist client out of

bed if he is to be ambulated.
9. Remove gloves, and wash your hands.
10. Observe penis 30 minutes after condom applied to check for edema, discoloration, and urine flow. **Rationale:** This detects complication with application.

ATTACHING CATHETER TO LEG BAG

Equipment

Leg bag
Alcohol swab
Clean gloves

Procedure

1. Obtain order for leg bag from physician.
2. Gather leg bag and alcohol wipe.
3. Wash your hands, and provide privacy.
4. Raise bed, and lower side rail on working side of bed.
5. Don clean gloves.
6. Disconnect drainage tubing from indwelling or condom catheter.
7. Wipe the leg bag and catheter connectors with alcohol.
8. Connect the tip of the leg bag into the catheter.
9. Place the cap from the leg bag tip on the collection tubing.
10. Secure the leg bag to the lower leg by placing the rubber strap through the bag and around the leg. Secure the strap by placing the button through the opening in the strap.
11. When removing leg bag, disconnect the catheter from the leg bag and wipe each connection end with alcohol wipes.

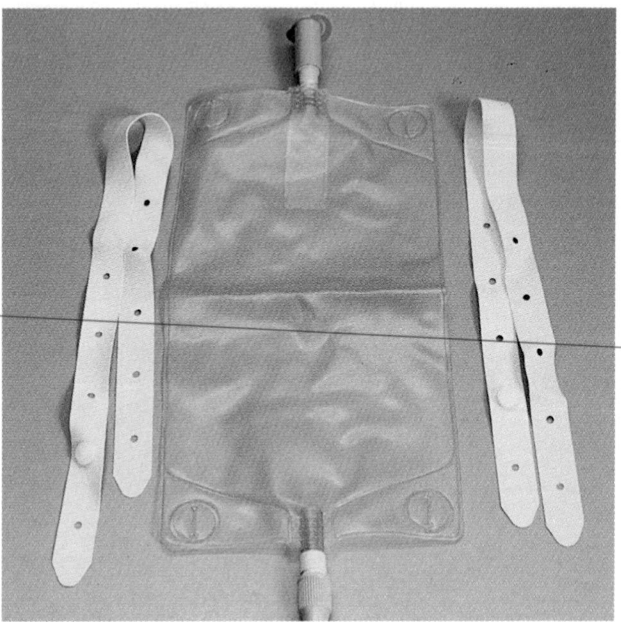

Leg bag is secured to leg by placing rubber strip through bag and around leg.

12. Take leg bag cap off the drainage tubing and replace it on the leg bag.
13. Connect the catheter to the drainage tubing.
14. Lower bed, and raise side rail.
15. Rinse the leg bag in warm soap and water, and place in bathroom to dry.
16. Remove gloves, and wash your hands.

CHARTING for External Catheter

- Condom catheter applied
- Size of catheter used
- Condition of genital area
- Type of protective coating applied to skin
- Whether catheter connected to leg bag or continuous drainage
- Amount, color, and odor of urine obtained
- Client's tolerance of procedure

CRITICAL THINKING APPLICATION

CLINICAL PROBLEMS	CRITICAL THINKING OPTIONS
■ Incontinence continues with use of condom catheter.	• Use smaller condom to provide wrinkle-free application.
■ Penis becomes reddened and excoriated.	• Remove condom catheter as much as possible to allow air to reach penile shaft. • Notify physician for topical medication order. • Diaper the client, and change frequently. Keep condom off penis until area is healed. • Wash perineal area frequently.

unit 5 SUPRAPUBIC CATHETER CARE

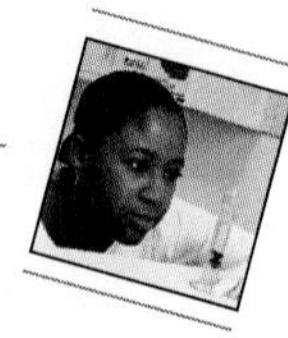

NURSING PROCESS DATA

ASSESSMENT Data Base

Observe for urine flow through catheter.

Observe for excessive bleeding through catheter or at insertion site.

Check that suture site is clean, dry, and intact.

Check that straight drainage is maintained.

Assess that fluid intake is at least 2000 mL daily.

Assess client for pain, bladder distention, or spasms.

Assess client's ability to assist with clamping procedure.

Assess client's ability to tolerate catheter being clamped.

PLANNING Objectives

To prevent urinary tract infection when a suprapubic catheter is inserted

To maintain a patent suprapubic catheter

To monitor the suprapubic clamping procedure

To prevent infection at catheter insertion site

To provide discharge teaching if catheter is to remain in place when client is discharged

IMPLEMENTATION Procedure

Providing Suprapubic Catheter Care

EVALUATION Expected Outcomes

Catheter remains patent; bladder drains completely.

Client voids spontaneously after routine clamping.

Client remains free of urinary tract infections.

Insertion site is clean and dry.

PROVIDING SUPRAPUBIC CATHETER CARE

Equipment

Closed drainage system, including Foley catheter tubing and bag

Catheter clamp

Dry sterile dressing and tape if ordered

Clean gloves

Sterile gloves

Preparation

1. Check physician's orders and client care plan.
2. Explain purpose of catheter.
3. Describe procedure for monitoring and clamping suprapubic catheter.
4. Wash your hands.
5. Provide privacy.

Procedure

1. Observe catheter for patency. **Rationale:** The most common problem with suprapubic catheters is occlusion with sediment or clots.
   a. First 24 hours: check the catheter every hour to detect possible obstruction. Urine output should be in excess of 30 mL/hour.
   b. Second day: check the catheter every 8 hours.
   c. Third day: check the catheter when the catheter is unclamped.

2. Maintain a closed drainage system. Do not open system to irrigate or obtain urine sample.
3. Observe for signs and symptoms of urinary tract infection (color, odor, presence of sediment).
4. Keep the dressing dry around site of insertion. Apply a new dressing, maintaining sterile technique, every morning and as necessary at other times.
5. Perform clamping protocol after the third postoperative day. Use this protocol or clamp according to physician's orders.
   a. Explain the clamping procedure and ask client to help you monitor the clamping.
   b. Instruct client to notify you if he or she feels fullness in the bladder during clamping.
   c. Don gloves.
   d. Clamp the catheter.
   e. Empty the drainage bag. Remove gloves. Record urine output on I&O bedside record.
   f. Leave the catheter clamped for 3–4 hours depending on client's level of comfort and physician's orders.
   g. At 3- to 4-hour intervals, or when client feels fullness in bladder, ask client to void normally. Don gloves to measure the urine and record output on I&O bedside record.
   h. Immediately after client voids, unclamp catheter and leave unclamped for 5 minutes, collecting the residual urine.
   i. Don gloves to measure the residual urine following unclamping of the catheter.
   j. Reclamp catheter.
   k. Send a urine specimen to laboratory after the first clamping. **Rationale:** This checks for the presence of microorganisms.
6. Repeat clamping protocol every 3–4 hours. (For the first few days of the clamping procedure the catheter may be open to drainage from bedtime until 6 in the morning.)

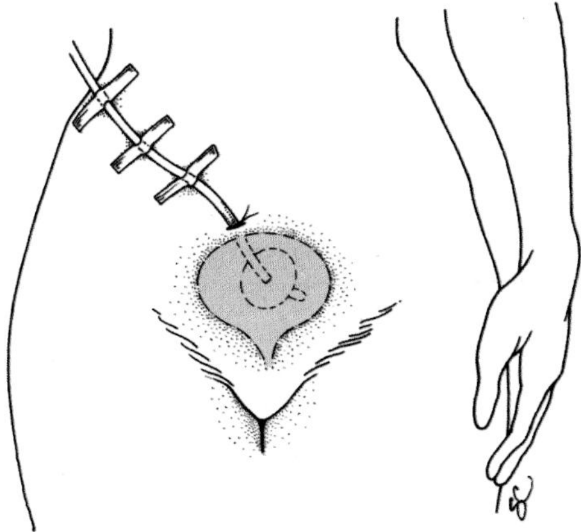

Tape catheter and connect to a closed system.

7. When the client is voiding normally, clamp the catheter throughout the night in preparation for its removal.
8. When the client's residual urine output is less than 100 mL on two successive checks, notify the physician for removal of the catheter.
9. Apply a Band-Aid or small 2×2 sterile dressing over the insertion site.
10. Dispose of the catheter in biohazard bag.
11. If the client is discharged from the hospital with the catheter, provide the following teaching for home care:
    a. Instruct the client to drink one glass of fluid every hour while awake.
    b. Instruct client to follow clamping procedure when awake or as instructed by physician.
    c. Instruct the client to leave the catheter open to the drainage system at night. (Drainage system may be urinary tubing and bag or leg bag.)
    d. Tell client to notify physician if dysuria occurs when voiding or if urine becomes cloudy, odorous, or full of sediment.

CHARTING for Catheter Care

- Time catheter clamped
- Length of time clamped
- Client's ability to void spontaneously
- Client's feelings of fullness
- Time specimen sent to laboratory
- Color, amount, and odor of urine obtained
- Color, amount, and odor of residual urine

CRITICAL THINKING APPLICATION

CLINICAL PROBLEMS	CRITICAL THINKING OPTIONS
■ Suprapubic catheter was not sutured in place and becomes dislodged.	• Place sterile dressing over puncture site. Do not attempt to replace the catheter. • Notify physician immediately. • Have new suprapubic catheter ready for insertion by physician.
■ Client develops urinary tract infection.	• Observe client for signs and symptoms of urinary tract infection: temperature; cloudy, foul-smelling urine with sediment present; bladder spasms. • Inform physician of possible urinary tract infection and obtain order for urinary antibiotic. • Force fluids to at least 2000 mL per day unless contraindicated by diagnosis. Give cranberry juice or fluids that acidify urine. • Clarify physician's order for protocol regarding clamping catheter or keeping the catheter open to straight drainage while evidence of infection is present.
■ Client unable to void spontaneously through urethra.	• Notify physician for orders.

unit 6

BLADDER IRRIGATION AND INSTILLATION

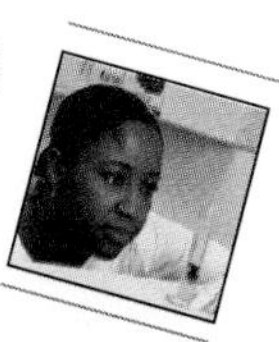

NURSING PROCESS DATA

ASSESSMENT Data Base

Determine presence of active bleeding (i.e., dense, dark red drainage).

Note rate of urine flow from bladder.

Assess for distended bladder.

Assess for bladder discomfort.

PLANNING Objectives

To remove blood clots from client's bladder

To instill medications into client's bladder

To ensure patency of drainage system

To relieve bladder spasms

IMPLEMENTATION Procedures

Irrigating by Opening a Closed System

Irrigating a Closed System

Instilling Medications

Maintaining Continuous Irrigation

EVALUATION Expected Outcomes

Blood clots are removed from client's bladder.

Medications are instilled easily into client's bladder.

Continuous flow of antibacterial solution is instilled into client's bladder to prevent or treat a urinary tract infection.

Continuous flow of solution is maintained to evacuate clots and prevent catheter obstruction.

Catheter remains patent and unobstructed by sediment.

IRRIGATING BY OPENING A CLOSED SYSTEM

Equipment

Sterile irrigation set (new set for each irrigation)

Clean gloves, sterile gloves

Sterile normal saline irrigant (or solution as ordered)

Catch basin

Antiseptic swab

Absorbent pad

Procedure

1. Check physician's order and client care plan.
2. Gather equipment.
3. Check client's identaband.
4. Explain procedure and rationale to client.
5. Wash your hands.
6. Provide privacy, and place the client in a comfortable position. The dorsal-recumbent position is the most convenient if client can tolerate this position. Raise bed, and lower side rails if needed. Fanfold linen to expose catheter.
7. Palpate client's bladder to check for distention.
8. Open sterile container on bed or on the over-bed table. Maintain sterility of the inside of the container. Don clean gloves.
9. Place an absorbent pad under the connection of tubing and catheter to form a working field.

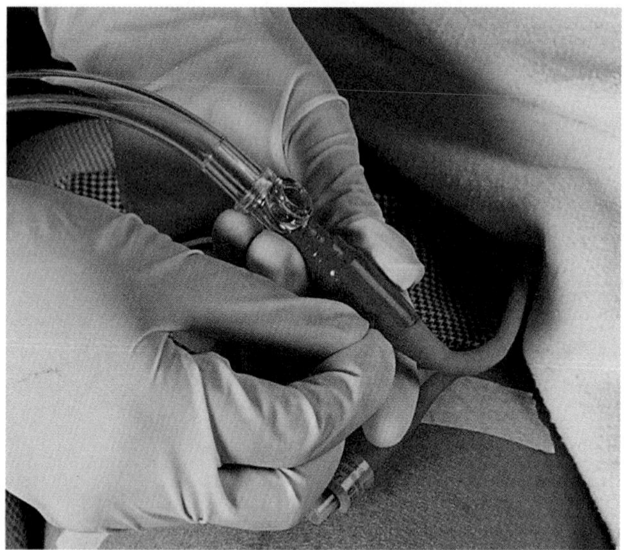
After cleaning injection port of catheter insert solution-filled needle and syringe and irrigate closed system.

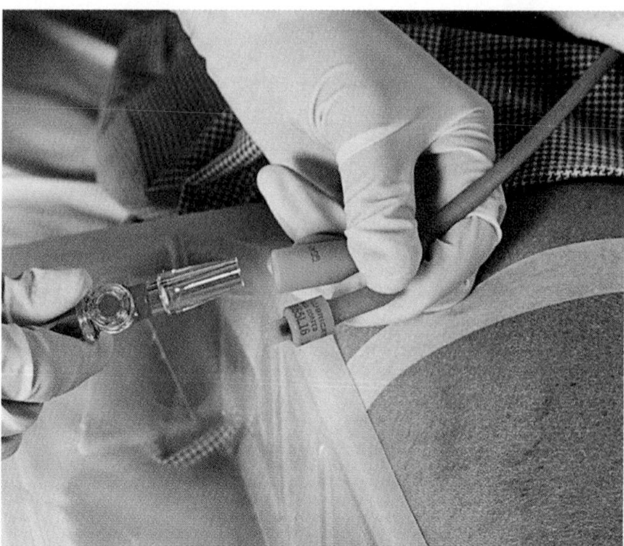
Carefully disconnect catheter from drainage tubing and place protective cap over end of drainage tubing to maintain sterility.

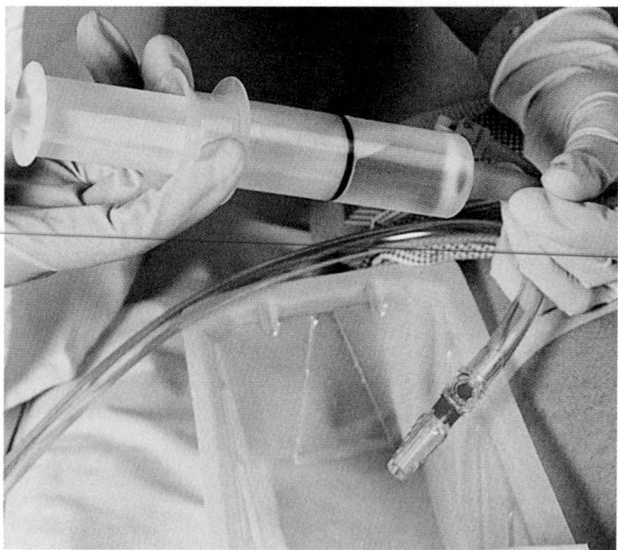
Instill 30-50 mL of irrigant into catheter with a gentle but firm pressure to irrigate an open system.

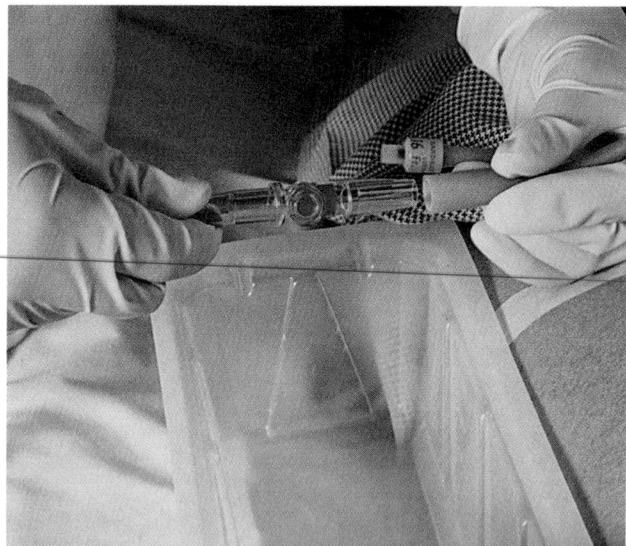
Wipe end of catheter with alcohol swab before reconnecting catheter to drainage tubing.

10. Pour irrigant into solution container.
11. Place syringe in container. Do not contaminate the syringe tip.
12. Place catch basin on pad to form the working field. (Always keep syringe tip and irrigant uncontaminated.)
13. Disconnect catheter from drainage tube. Place the sterile protective cap over the end of the drainage tube or hold in nondominant hand being careful not to contaminate tip of tubing.
14. Coil tubing on bed.
15. Place catheter over the edge of the catch basin. Do not allow end of catheter to touch covers, underpad, exposed skin surfaces, or drainage tube.
16. Don sterile gloves after removing clean gloves.
17. Instill 30–50 mL of irrigant into catheter with a gentle but firm pressure.
    a. Remove syringe and allow solution to drain.
    b. Lower the catch basin to facilitate solution return via gravity.
    c. Continue to irrigate client's bladder with 30–50 mL of irrigant until fluid returns are clear or clots removed.

18. Remove the protective top from the drainage tube and wipe it with an antiseptic swab.
19. Wipe the end of the catheter with an alcohol sponge, and connect the catheter to the drainage tube.
20. Ensure straight line from tubing to drainage bag. Curl excess tubing loosely on the bed and secure the tubing to the linen.
21. Tape catheter to the inner thigh for a female and to the abdomen for a male.
22. Lower bed, and raise side rails.
23. Remove gloves, and discard equipment.
24. Make sure the client is clean and comfortable. Place the call light within easy reach.
25. Wash your hands.
26. Subtract any irrigating solution still remaining in the urinary drainage system from the client's intake and output record.

IRRIGATING A CLOSED SYSTEM

Equipment

Irrigation set
30-mL syringe and 21- or 25-gauge 1-inch needle
Alcohol or povidone-iodine (Betadine) swab
Irrigating solution
Catheter clamp
Clean gloves

Procedure

1. Check physician's order and client care plan.
2. Gather equipment.
3. Check client's identaband. Explain procedure and rationale to client.
4. Wash hands.
5. Provide privacy, and place client in dorsal-recumbent position, if tolerated.
6. Raise bed, and lower side rail on working side of bed.
7. Open sterile container. Maintain sterility on the inside of the container.
8. Place absorbent pad under the end of the catheter to form a working field.
9. Pour irrigant into solution container.
10. Fill large 30-mL syringe with the amount of irrigating solution ordered.
11. Place the needle onto the syringe.
12. Don clean gloves.
13. Clamp tubing just distal to injection port.
14. Swab the injection port of catheter with alcohol or Betadine solution.
15. Insert the needle into the injection port.
16. Inject solution slowly to prevent back pressure in urinary drainage system.
17. Remove syringe and needle from the injection port.
18. Unclamp drainage tube, and lower catheter. **Rationale:** This facilitates drainage.
19. Repeat irrigation steps until return is free of clots and debris.
20. Lower bed, and raise side rail.
21. Remove gloves, and dispose of equipment.
22. Wash your hands.
23. Subtract the irrigating solution from the client's intake and output record.

INSTILLING MEDICATIONS

Equipment

Syringe (size depends on amount of solution to be instilled) and 25-gauge needle
Alcohol or povidone-iodine (Betadine) solution and swabs
Appropriate medication for irrigation or instillation
Clamp for catheter
Clean gloves

Procedure

1. Check physician's orders and client care plan.
2. Explain procedure to client.
3. Provide privacy.

4. Assemble equipment, and draw up ordered medication in syringe.
5. Wash your hands, and don gloves.
6. Scrub port site on Foley catheter tubing with alcohol or Betadine solution.
7. Clamp drainage tubing so that medication is retained in the client's bladder.
8. Insert the needle at an angle into the injection port.
9. Instill medication slowly.
10. Withdraw the needle, and cleanse the port site with an alcohol or Betadine swab.
11. Keep tubing clamped for 15–20 minutes.
12. Remove gloves, and wash your hands.
13. Observe for bladder distention or spasms while catheter is clamped.
14. Unclamp tube after 15–20 minutes.

MAINTAINING CONTINUOUS IRRIGATION

Equipment

Irrigating solution and container
Tubing
IV pole
Alcohol or povidone-iodine (Betadine) swab
Clean gloves

PURPOSE OF CONTINUOUS IRRIGATION

Rinse bladder of clots and debris following prostatic surgery
Provide hemostasis
Instill medication

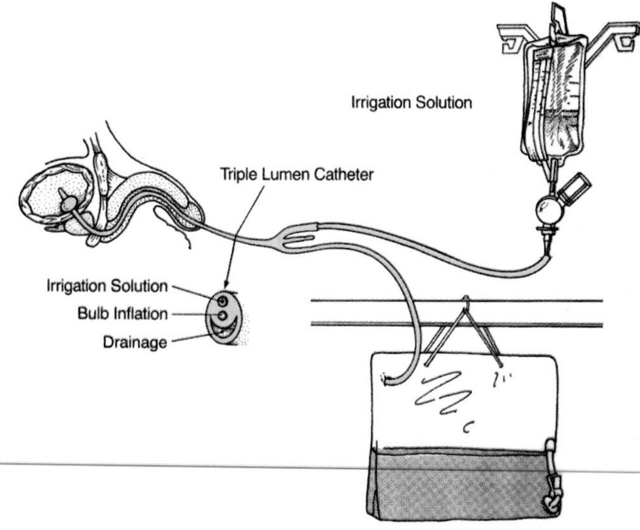

Maintain continuous bladder irrigation by using a triple lumen catherter for procedure.

Procedure

1. Check physician's orders and client care plan.
2. Obtain irrigating solution from pharmacy or central supply.
3. Place label on irrigating bag if not labeled. Include client's name, date, room number, type of solution, and additives.
4. Check client's identaband.
5. Explain procedure to client and provide privacy.
6. Wash your hands, and don clean gloves.
7. Remove protective covering from spike on tubing, and insert spike into insertion port of solution container. Use aseptic technique.
8. Place irrigating solution container on IV pole and prime tubing. Height of pole is usually 24–36 inches above bladder.
   a. Fill drip chamber by pinching fluid chamber until half full.
   b. Remove protective cover from end of tubing using aseptic technique.
   c. Open roller clamp, and allow irrigating solution to run through tubing until all air is expelled. **Rationale:** This prevents air from entering bladder and causing discomfort.
   d. Close roller clamp, and replace protective cover on end of tubing.
9. Connect tubing to third lumen using aseptic technique.
10. Remove gloves.
11. Adjust drip rate of the solution by adjusting the clamp on the tubing to deliver prescribed hourly rate of irrigant.
    a. With clear drainage, drip rate should be approximately 40–60 drops per minute.
    b. When drainage is bright red or contains blood clots, increase drip rate. **Rationale:** Increased

drip rate will clear the drainage and flush out clots.

c. Change irrigation solution bottle using aseptic technique.
d. Tubing should be changed at a minimum of every 24 hours.

12. Monitor urine output at least every hour to observe patency of system.
13. Empty drainage bag at least every 4 hours. Subtract amount of irrigant infused from total output to obtain urine output.
14. Wash hands.

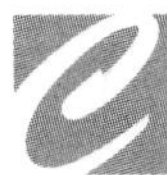

CHARTING for Irrigation and Instillation

- Type and amount of medications administered
- Type and amount of solution administered for irrigation
- Rate of administration of irrigating solution
- Description of urinary output, including color and presence of clots
- Any signs of discomfort or cramping
- Amount of actual urine output (total urine output minus amount of irrigant instilled)
- Signs and symptoms indicative of potential infection.

CRITICAL THINKING APPLICATION

CLINICAL PROBLEMS	CRITICAL THINKING OPTIONS
■ Irrigation flow is not infusing at prescribed rate.	• May need to raise or lower IV standard with attached irrigation bag to assist in regulating flow using gravity. • Move the flow adjuster clamp to a new site on the tubing if flow is slower than ordered. Tubing may be collapsed due to constant pressure from clamp. • If infusion rate slows, may indicate clots are blocking flow. Irrigate catheter following physician's orders.
■ Irrigation solution is not returned because of an obstruction in the system.	• Follow these steps to obtain irrigation solution: a. Aspirate the solution from the catheter, using moderate "pull back" pressure. b. If the irrigant does not return, palpate the client's bladder and instill 30–50 mL of irrigating solution to agitate and clear any clots. c. If irrigant does not return, reconnect urinary system and observe for 30 minutes. Bladder spasms can block the flow of urine through the system.

CLINICAL PROBLEMS	CRITICAL THINKING OPTIONS
	d. If irrigant does not return, cleanse client's urinary meatus and the catheter tubing with povidone-iodine (Betadine) solution. Gently insert the Foley catheter further into the client's bladder. If the lumen opening of the catheter is against the wall of the bladder, it obstructs the flow of urine. e. If irrigant still does not return after performing the above procedures, notify physician for further orders.
■ Client's pain and anxiety causes "clamping down" and creates an obstruction in the outflow opening to the catheter thus irrigation solution is not returned.	• Help client practice relaxation techniques. • Place a warm towel over client's abdomen to ease bladder spasms. • Reposition client to reduce pressure on the catheter. • If client is unable to expel the irrigant, administer medications to relieve client's pain or bladder spasms.
■ Client experiences excessive bladder spasms.	• Notify physician of bladder spasms in order to obtain an order to place a heating pad on the client's abdomen. • Follow physician's order and administer urinary antispasmodic.
■ Bright red drainage continues even when solution flow rate is increased.	• Notify physician. • Continue to infuse solution at a rapid rate to cleanse client's bladder until you obtain physician's orders. • Assess client for signs of anemia or significant blood loss. Take vital signs, observe capillary filling pressure, and observe mucous membranes for signs of anemia.

unit 7

SPECIMENS FROM CLOSED SYSTEMS

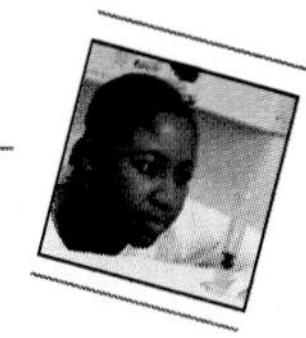

NURSING PROCESS DATA

ASSESSMENT Data Base

Assess the type of specimen needed: Sterile specimens for culture and sensitivity tests; clean specimens for urinalysis.

Check to see if the closed urinary system has a port for obtaining a specimen or catheter is made of self-sealing material (not silastic or silicone).

Identify amount of urine needed for specimen.

PLANNING Objectives

To prevent urinary infection by obtaining a urine specimen without interrupting a closed urinary drainage system

To determine the specific microorganism causing a urinary tract infection

To obtain a urine specimen for use in a diagnostic urinary work-up

IMPLEMENTATION Procedure

Collecting Specimen from a Closed System

EVALUATION Expected Outcomes

Noncontaminated urine specimen is obtained from the closed urinary drainage system.

Catheter does not develop a leak from improper puncture for urine specimen.

COLLECTING SPECIMEN FROM A CLOSED SYSTEM

Equipment

Catheter clamp

Syringe with 25-gauge needle

Sterile specimen container

Antimicrobial or alcohol swab

Clean gloves

Procedure

1. Gather equipment.
2. Identify client by checking identaband.
3. Explain the procedure and rationale to the client. Clamp catheter tubing for 15 minutes. **Rationale:** This ensures urine specimen is adequate.
4. Wash your hands, and don gloves.
5. Wipe the aspiration port of the drainage tubing with the antimicrobial or alcohol swab.
6. Insert the needle at a 30–45° angle into the aspiration port. **Rationale:** This facilitates sealing of the rubber in the port following removal of needle. Allow urine to accumulate in the tubing. (2 mL urine is sufficient for a specimen.)
7. Aspirate the urine sample by gently pulling back on the syringe plunger, and then remove the needle.
8. Wipe the aspiration port with the antimicrobial swab. Remove clamp.
9. Empty the syringe into the sterile urine container, ensuring needle does not touch inside of sterile container. (Sometimes the urine is sent to the laboratory in the syringe.)
10. Remove and discard gloves.
11. Wash your hands.
12. Label the container, and take it to the laboratory within 15 minutes. If this is not possible, refrigerate specimen.

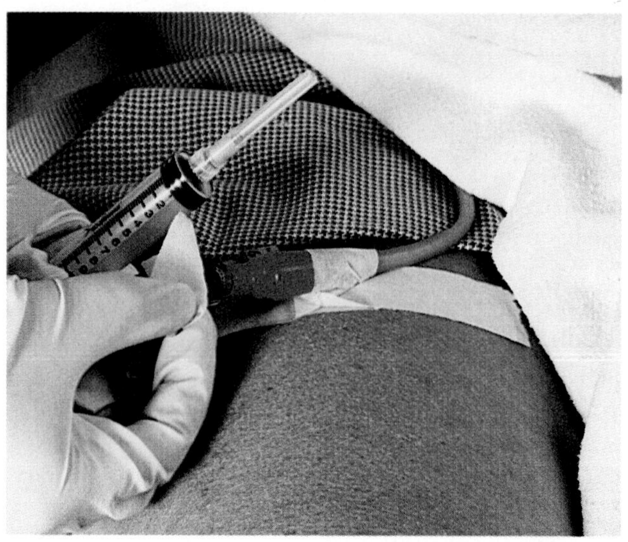
Wipe aspiration port of drainage tubing before inserting sterile syringe and needle.

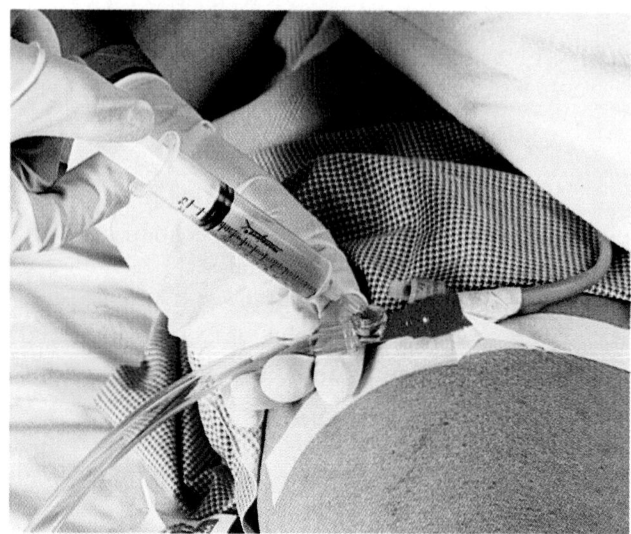
Insert needle at 30-45 degree angle into aspiration port and gently pull back on barrel of syringe.

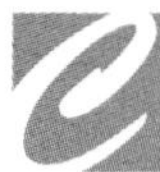

CHARTING for Collecting Specimen

- Type of specimen obtained
- Mode of obtaining specimen from port
- Color, consistency, and odor of urine
- Time of urine collection
- Time specimen sent to laboratory

CRITICAL THINKING APPLICATION

CLINICAL PROBLEMS	CRITICAL THINKING OPTIONS
Insufficient amount of urine available when specimen collection is attempted.	• Clamp catheter tubing for 30 minutes. • Reposition client. • Check for kinking of catheter.
Signs and symptoms of urinary tract infection occur.	• Notify the physician of client's signs and symptoms. • Make sure there are no kinks in urinary system tubing or that the system is not clamped off. This ensures that the urine drains into the catheter bag and does not stagnate in bladder. • Give ordered antibiotics on correct time schedule. • Do not interrupt the closed urinary drainage system.
Bacteremia develops secondary to urinary tract infection.	• Administer antibiotics as ordered. • Encourage client to force fluids to flush out bladder. • Use cranberry juice or other acid-producing (noncitric) juices. • Obtain frequent vital signs and assessment data. • Observe color and clarity of urine for further infectious problems.

unit 8

URINARY DIVERSION

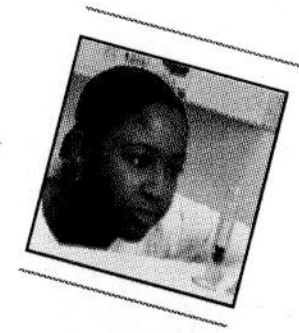

NURSING PROCESS DATA

ASSESSMENT Data Base

Assess location of stoma on client's abdomen.

Check abdomen for folds, contour, incision line.

Observe stoma color (same color as mucous membrane lining the mouth).

Assess skin for erythema and excoriation.

Ascultate bowel sounds.

Assess most appropriate pouching system for client. (System depends on client's age, manual dexterity, and size of stoma.)

Assess client's ability to manage self-care.

PLANNING Objectives

To provide a pouching system that prevents skin irritation

To instruct the client in self-care

To monitor stoma for viability

To obtain a sterile urine specimen

IMPLEMENTATION Procedures

Applying a Urinary Diversion Pouch

Obtaining Specimen from an Ileal Conduit

Emptying Continent Ileostomy

EVALUATION Expected Outcomes

Client demonstrates self-care skills.

Pouching system fits tightly, and skin remains free of irritation.

Sterile urine specimen is obtained.

Stoma remains viable.

APPLYING A URINARY DIVERSION POUCH

Equipment

Two-piece urinary pouch with skin barrier, flange, and spigot at bottom of pouch to empty urine

Items to clean stoma (e.g., soft cloth or gauze sponges)

Plastic bag for disposal of used equipment

Tissue for drying skin

Tissue or tampon for wicking stoma

Underpad to protect bedding

Scissors with sharp point

Protective barriers such as skin prep, skin gel, or protective barrier film

Stoma measuring guide

Clean gloves

Preparation

1. Check physician's order and client care plan.
2. Gather equipment.
3. Wash your hands.
4. Explain procedure to client.
5. Provide privacy.
6. Place client in supine position.
7. Place bath blanket over client's chest and position top covers over lower abdomen.

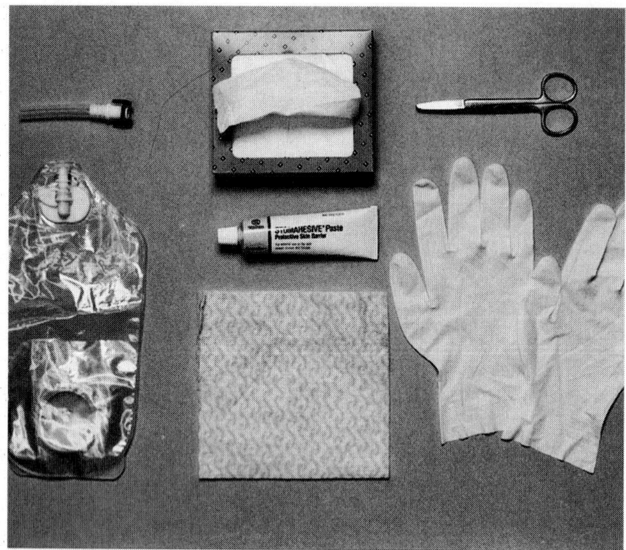
Equipment for urinary diversion pouching.

Procedure

1. Place protective pad under client.
2. Don clean gloves.
3. Prepare new urinary pouch. First measure stoma site with measuring guide.
4. Trace size of stoma on wafer and cut $\frac{1}{8}$-inch larger than size.
5. Snap pouch onto flange.
6. Remove old pouch, and discard in plastic bag.
7. Wash skin with warm water. Check stoma for healing.
8. Remove paper from adhesive on wafer.
9. Wick stoma with tissue or tampon. **Rationale:** To keep urine from contact with skin during pouch change.
10. Apply protective barrier to healthy skin surrounding stoma. **Rationale:** Protective barriers placed on excoriated skin contain alcohol and cause burning and pain.
11. Let dry thoroughly.

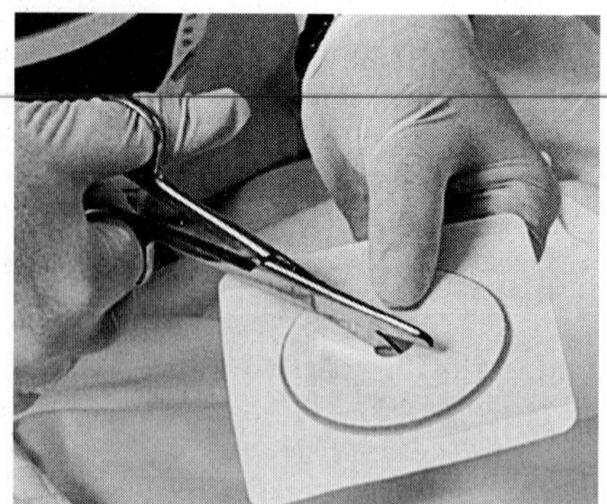
Cut panel to fit stoma.

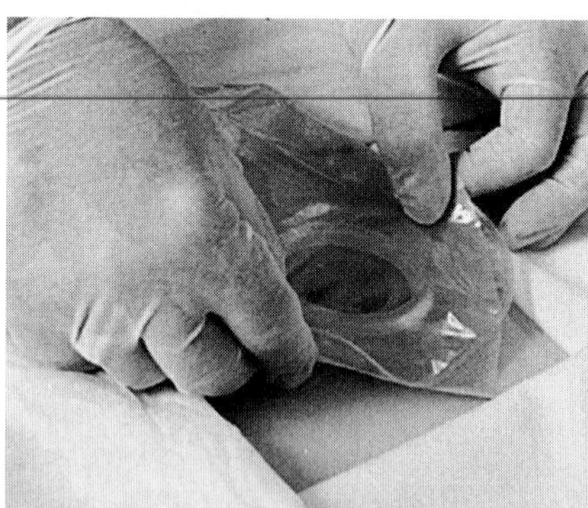
Remove old pouch.

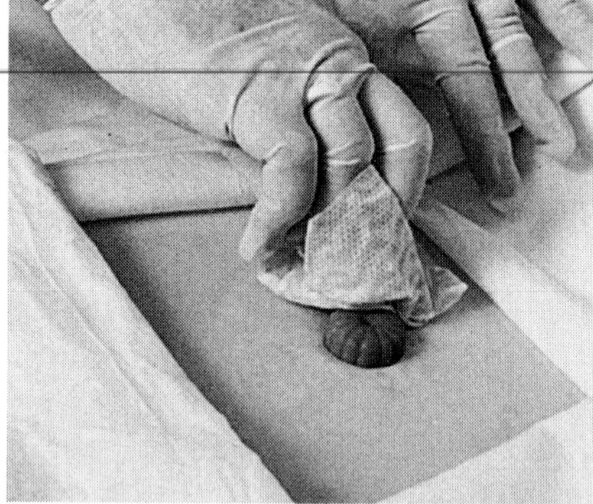
Clean skin around stoma before wicking.

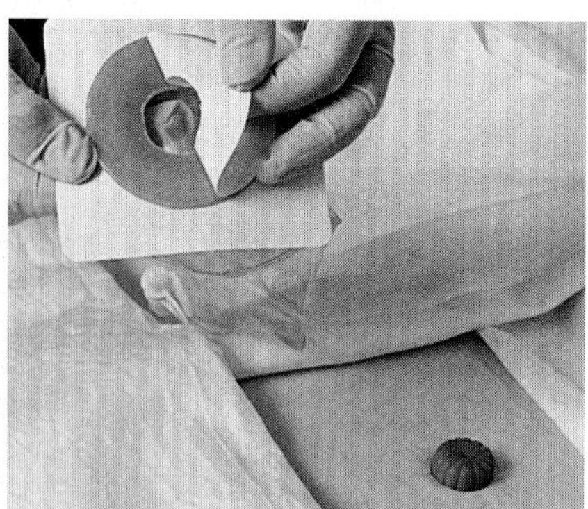
Remove paper from backing.

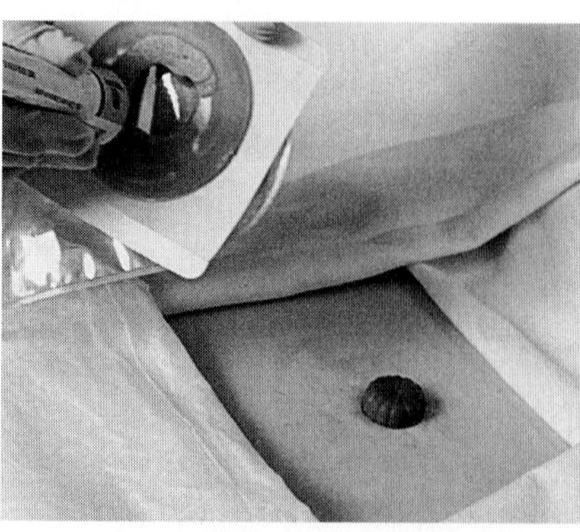
Apply protective barrier to ring.

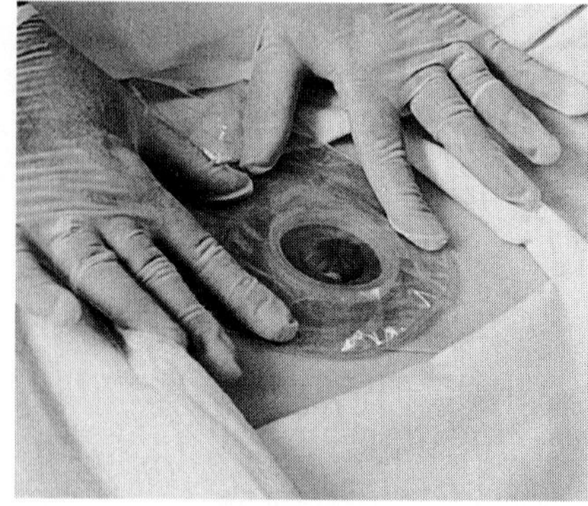
Apply pouch and press firmly.

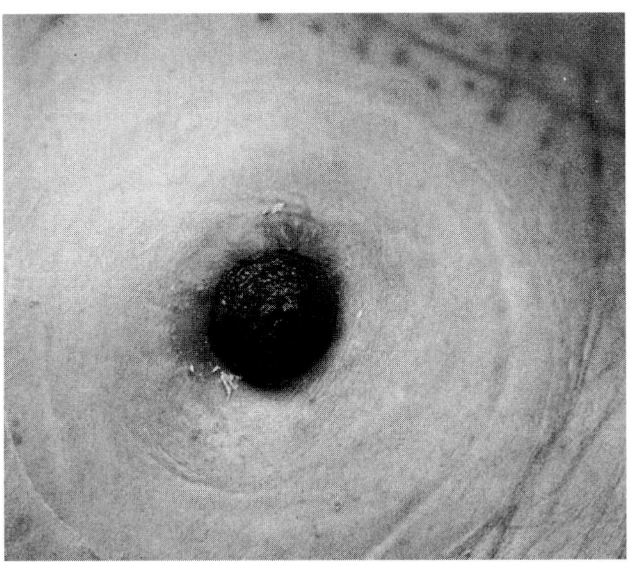
Well-healed urinary diversion stoma.

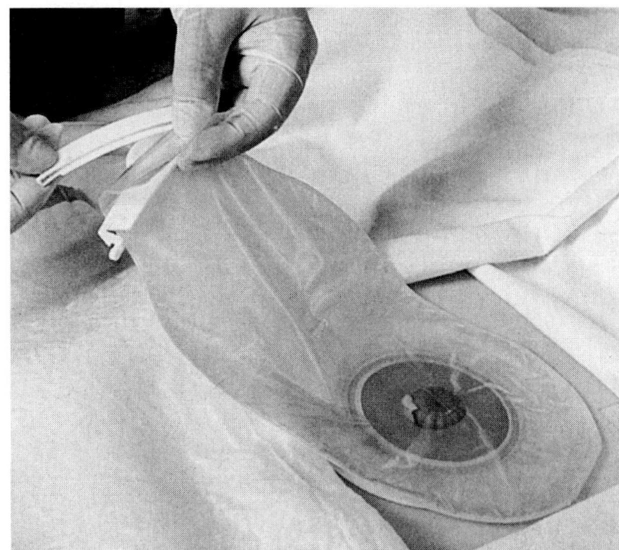
Pouch attached to well-healed stoma.

THREE TYPES OF URINARY DIVERSIONS

Cutaneous Ureterostomy

- Opening from ureters to abdominal surface—one or both ureters are attached to abdominal wall or flank.
- Stoma is smaller than colostomy or ileostomy.

Ileal Conduit

- Ureterostomy constructed from portion of bowel—ileum is resected and a pouch formed and attached to abdominal wall.
- Ureters are connected to internal pouch.
- An external pouch collects urine output.
- Stoma is larger than ureterostomy.

Continent Urostomy (Koch's Pouch)

- Pouch is constructed from ileum and two nipple valves are created by pulling ileum back onto itself.
- Ureters are implanted near internal nipple valve.
- Outlet valve is attached to abdominal wall and stoma.
- Catheters are inserted to drain urine.

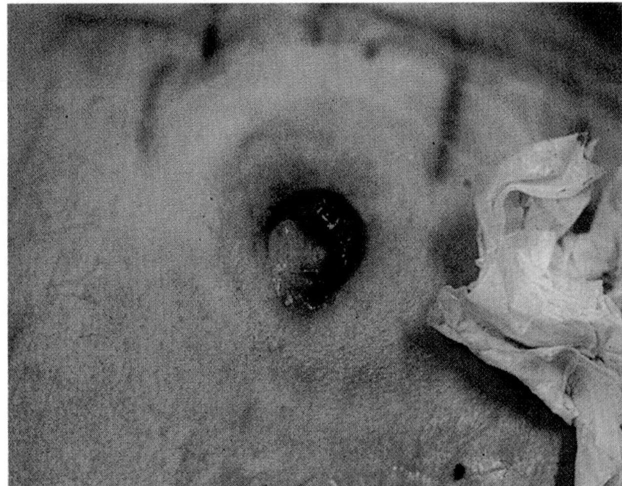
Ureterostomy.

12. Remove wick and center pouch over stoma; apply pouch to dry skin.
13. Smooth tape onto skin.
14. Attach pouch to gravity drainage bag.
15. Remove gloves, and discard in appropriate receptacle.
16. Wash your hands.

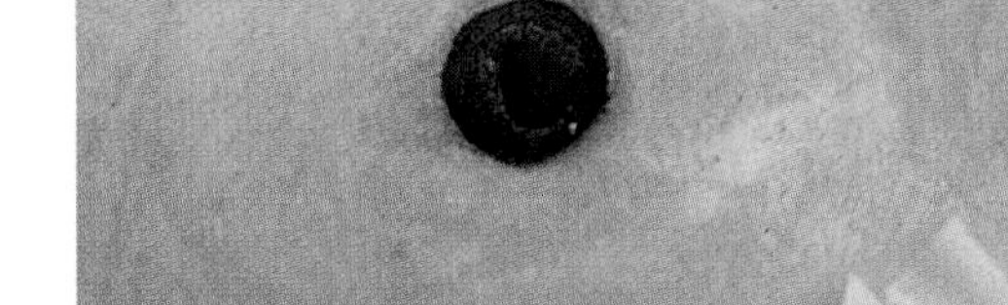
Urinary diversion.

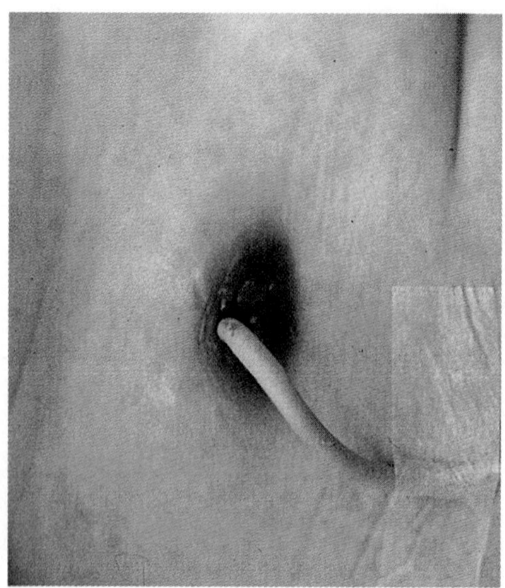

Ureterostomy with catheter.

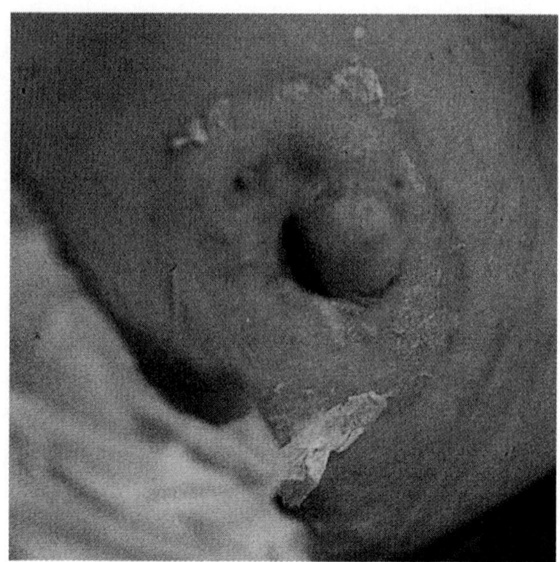

Ureterostomy.

OBTAINING SPECIMEN FROM AN ILEAL CONDUIT

Equipment

Sterile catheter kit
Prep solution
Sterile saline or water
Underpad
New urinary pouch
Supplies to apply new pouch
Bath blanket
Clean gloves

Preparation

1. Check physician's orders and client care plan.
2. Gather equipment.
3. Wash your hands.
4. Explain procedure to client.
5. Provide privacy.
6. Place bath blanket over client's chest and position top covers over lower abdomen.

Procedure

1. Open sterile packages.
2. Remove pouch.
3. Put on gloves.
4. Place sterile drape over stoma.
5. Remove top from specimen container, and place end of catheter into container.
6. Apply lubricant to catheter.
7. Use forceps to pick up cotton ball and prep stoma with solution and rinse with sterile saline or water.
8. Insert tip of catheter into stoma. When abdominal musculature relaxes, slide catheter into conduit.
9. When flow of urine completed (usually not more than 5–25 mL), clamp catheter with fingers and remove.
10. Return lid to specimen container, apply label, and send to lab.
11. Remove completely any residual prep solution and lubricant.
12. Continue with pouching procedure.
13. Remove gloves, and wash hands.

CLIENT TEACHING FOR EVACUATION OF POUCH

Instruct client to

- Use bathroom if possible.
- Place distal end of pouch between thighs into toilet.
- Unclamp pouch or open drainage port to allow effluent to drain.
- Clean end of pouch or port with soapy warm water.
- Reclamp pouch or close drainage port.
- Wash hands.

EMPTYING CONTINENT ILEOSTOMY

Equipment

Clean catheter
Water-soluble lubricant
Clean gloves
Bedpan (if client unable to use toilet)
Plastic zip-lok bag
Warm water and soap
Washcloth, towel

Preparation

1. Check physician's orders and client care plan.
2. Gather equipment.
3. Explain procedure to client.
4. Wash hands.
5. Assist client to bathroom or position in bed, and provide privacy.
6. Don clean gloves.
7. Remove appliance or dressing if present.

Procedure

1. Position client on chair facing toilet or place bedpan next to client if on bedrest.
2. Remove clean catheter from zip-lok bag.
3. Lubricate tip of catheter.
4. Insert catheter $1\frac{1}{2}$–2 inches into stoma. Place distal end of catheter into toilet or bedpan.
5. Instruct client to take deep breath as you gently insert catheter through nipple valve until effluent returns. **Rationale:** When the abdominal muscles are relaxed it is easier to advance catheter through nipple valve.
6. Leave catheter in place until effluent stops draining.
7. Pinch catheter, and remove gently.
8. Wash and dry peristomal area with soap and water.
9. Replace pouch or dressing if needed. Assist client back to bed, or position for comfort.
10. Clean catheter with warm soap and water, allow to dry, and place in clean zip-lok bag. Return to storage area in client's bathroom.
11. Remove gloves, and wash hands.

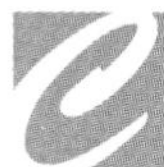

CHARTING for Urinary Diversion Care

- Color and amount of urine obtained from catheterization or emptying continent ileostomy
- Amount of residual urine
- Catheter size used for catheterization
- Peristomal skin and stoma condition
- Client's acceptance of stoma
- Type and method of drainage pouch applied

CRITICAL THINKING APPLICATION

CLINICAL PROBLEMS	CRITICAL THINKING OPTIONS
■ Urinary tract infection is suspected.	• Ensure that catheterized specimen is not contaminated before sending to lab. • Force fluid to eight glasses per day. Encourage use of cranberry juice to acidify urine.

CLINICAL PROBLEMS	CRITICAL THINKING OPTIONS
Excess of 50 mL urine present in ileal conduit when catheterized.	• Notify physician as stasis of urine could be caused by urine remaining in conduit.
Pouch does not keep client dry.	• Check area for crease or dip in skin which allows urine to pool and leak out. • Fill in area with skin barrier to prevent pooling. • Belt may be applied to minimize leak if it appears on one side only. • If leak due to dissolving of skin barrier, change more frequently or change to different barrier.
Client unable to manage own urinary diversion.	• Simplify pouch procedure if possible. Provide detailed instruction in a more simplified manner if possible. • Include family in teaching to enable them to support and assist the client. • May need referral to home health care facility for follow-up care.
Unable to insert catheter into conduit.	• Insert catheter into stoma but do not force it. Wait for a few seconds to see if abdominal muscles relax enough to allow catheter to slide in. If not, notify physician.
No urine obtained from conduit.	• Rotate catheter, or position client on side to allow urine to flow into catheter. As little as 1–3 mL is needed for culture and sensitivity.
Odor in pouch.	• Odor usually due to alkaline urine in pouch turning to ammonia. Keep urine acidic by taking vitamin C, 500 mg b.i.d. to t.i.d., and drinking cranberry juice. Other citrus juices should be avoided because they form an alkaline ash. • Wash urinary equipment clean with mild soap and water and rinse in vinegar weekly. • Inform client that certain foods and drugs, such as asparagus and vitamin B complex, give an odor to the urine. The pouch should be emptied frequently if these substances are ingested. • Cloudy and strong odor to urine may be due to urinary tract infection. Advise physician, and collect sterile urine specimen.
Unable to insert catheter into continent ileostomy.	• Instruct client to take in deep breath as you gently push catheter into nipple valve. • Notify physician if intubation unsuccessful; nipple valve may be malfunctioning.

unit 9

PERITONEAL DIALYSIS

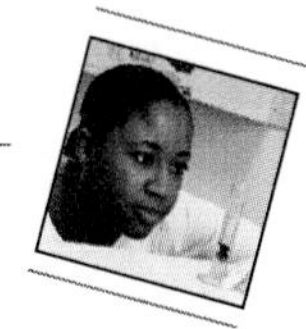

NURSING PROCESS DATA

ASSESSMENT Data Base

Obtain baseline measurements of vital signs (especially blood pressure).

Assess for edema; measure abdominal girth.

Check client's weight.

Review renal function tests.

Examine dietary regimen: Prior to dialysis, a low-protein diet is prescribed to reduce end products of protein metabolism. During dialysis, protein restriction may not be necessary. Provide diet that is high calorie, with limited sodium and potassium.

Evaluate client's abdomen for signs of infection or distention. Report any abnormalities to the physician.

Assess for signs of shock.

Auscultate breath sounds for rales and possible atelectasis.

Assess results of stool analysis for occult blood.

Assess condition of skin.

Review orders for solution to be used; number of exchanges; and inflow, diffusion, and outflow times.

Verify signed consent form.

PLANNING Objectives

To remove end products of metabolism when the kidneys are nonfunctional

To provide an effective method of reducing symptoms of renal failure

To remove excess fluid and reestablish fluid balance

To remove toxic substances that kidneys are unable to process from clients who have taken an overdose of drugs

To control blood pressure, creatinine, and BUN levels

To manage peritoneal dialysis procedure and provide catheter care

INTERVENTION Procedures

Assisting with Catheter Insertion

Managing Peritoneal Dialysis

Maintaining Peritoneal Dialysis

Providing Catheter Site Care

EVALUATION Expected Outcomes

Specific symptoms decrease, and complications of renal failure diminish.

Excessive fluid is reduced through use of peritoneal dialysis, and fluid balance is regulated.

Creatinine and BUN levels are reduced.

Asepsis is maintained throughout the procedure.

Complications are detected early, and treatment initiated promptly.

Catheter site remains free of infection.

ASSISTING WITH CATHETER INSERTION

Equipment

Sterile gowns, caps, masks, and gloves
Razor and blade
Povidone-iodine (Betadine) solution, alcohol swabs
Catheter insertion tray, with sterile drapes, catheter, trocar, connector, syringes, needles, sterile dressings, and sutures
Local anesthetic, usually 1% Xylocaine without epinephrine
Scalpel and blade
Clean gloves
4×4 gauze pads
Antimicrobial ointment
Tape
Dialysis inflow tubing
Dialysate solution with admixtures, as ordered

Preparation

1. Explain procedure to client, reinforcing physician's explanation and correcting any misconceptions.
2. Have client empty bladder or insert Foley catheter. **Rationale:** To lessen the risk of bladder perforation.
3. Weigh client to establish baseline weight.
4. Prime dialysate delivery system.
   a. Check bag labels and compare with orders.
   b. Check bag for signs of contamination.
   c. Add admixtures to dialysate solution bag, if ordered.
   d. Connect dialysate bag to administration set.
   e. Clear air from inflow tubing, and clamp line. If using an automated delivery system, set controls according to manufacturer's directions.

Procedure

1. Wash your hands.
2. Provide privacy.
3. Remove top linens, and place bath blanket over client's lower extremities.
4. Place client in supine position.
5. Don clean gloves.
6. Shave abdomen between umbilicus and symphysis pubis.
7. Perform surgical scrub of shaved area.
8. Remove gloves.
9. Don sterile attire.
10. Hold bottle of local anesthetic so that physician can withdraw desired amount.

Physician's Actions

   a. Physician dons sterile gown and gloves.
   b. Abdomen is draped with sterile towels.
   c. Local anesthetic is withdrawn and administered.
   d. Insertion area is infiltrated and catheter inserted.
   e. Trocar is removed.
   f. Catheter is sutured in place.

11. Assess client's level of comfort during procedure, and relieve client's anxiety as necessary.
12. After physician has removed the trocar, connect the inflow tubing to the catheter.
13. Apply Betadine to insertion site.
14. Apply a sterile occlusive dressing around the catheter site following suturing of catheter.
15. Tape securely.

MANAGING PERITONEAL DIALYSIS

Equipment

Dialysis administration set
Sterile, prewarmed dialysis solution, 1.5% or 4.25% dextrose concentration
Heparin IV
Potassium chloride IV
Dialysis flow sheet
Mask and sterile gloves

Procedure

1. Inject admixtures to dialysate solution bag as ordered (e.g., potassium, heparin), and connect inflow tubing to dialysate bag.
2. Don mask and sterile gloves according to hospital policy.
3. Infuse dialysate solution by following protocol for inflow phase.
   a. Open all clamps between bag(s) of dialysate and catheter.

b. Check that all clamps between catheter and drainage bag are closed.
c. Make sure tubing is not kinked.
d. Infuse amount of solution as quickly as possible. Usually it takes 5–10 minutes to infuse 1500–2000 mL.
e. Observe client's breathing pattern and level of comfort.
f. Inspect catheter insertion site for leakage or bleeding.

4. Shut off the inflow line. Allow dialysate to dwell in abdomen 20 minutes (diffusion or dwell period).
5. Complete dialysis cycle by following protocol for outflow phase:
   a. Place the client in semi-Fowler's position.
   b. Place bed in HIGH position.
   c. Open clamps between catheter and outflow bottle.
   d. Provide an airway in bag by inserting needle into air vent if required. **Rationale:** This assists in drainage of fluid into bag.
   e. Allow dialysate to drain by gravity for 30–35 minutes.
   f. Observe appearance of outflow fluid.
   g. Send dialysis fluid sample to lab as ordered.
   h. When drainage slows to a drip rate, clamp off drainage tubing, and begin next exchange.
6. Calculate fluid balance at end of cycle:
   a. Subtract the amount drained from the amount infused.
   b. Describe the results as positive or negative in relation to the peritoneal cavity.
   c. If the number is positive, fluid was retained in the cavity. If the number is negative, more fluid was drained out than instilled.
   d. Document findings on peritoneal dialysis flow sheet.
7. Throughout the cycle, monitor client status by assessing:
   a. Vital signs
   b. Abdominal distention
   c. Mental status
   d. Blood pressure and pulse every 15 minutes during the first cycle and every hour thereafter
   e. Temperature every 4 hours
   f. Color of dialysate solution
   g. Area surrounding catheter site
8. Culture the outflow fluid from the first cycle and one cycle a day thereafter.
9. Weigh client daily with abdomen empty.

MAINTAINING PERITONEAL DIALYSIS

Procedure

1. Monitor hydration status.
   a. Check intake and output daily.
   b. Record daily weight.
   c. Check for edema.
   d. Auscultate lungs for rales.
2. Evaluate electrolyte balance.
   a. Check for muscle weakness and diarrhea (signs of hyperkalemia).
   b. Monitor ECG for tall, peaked T waves and widening QRS segment (evidence of hyperkalemia).
   c. Check potassium levels frequently. **Rationale:** Potassium levels are frequently decreased in chronic dialysis clients.
3. Evaluate lung status at least every shift.
   a. Perform deep breathing and coughing to prevent pulmonary complications.
   b. Check for signs of pulmonary edema (dyspnea, restlessness, rales).
   c. Assess need for nasal cannula.
4. Examine site for possible infection (high temperature, leukocytosis, lethargy).
5. Monitor for seizure activity: padded side rails and tongue blade at bedside, if indicated.
6. Check Chvostek's and Trousseau's signs frequently for indications of low calcium level.
7. Monitor diet: low potassium and sodium, high calorie, high bulk, and adjusted protein to complete amino acids (necessary to maintain positive nitrogen balance and replace protein lost through dialysis).
8. Maintain good skin care to prevent skin breakdown and pruritus.
9. Evaluate for signs of bleeding at catheter site, in stools, and in urine; check hemoglobin and hematocrit frequently.
10. Monitor any medications. If iron is given as a supplement, have client take iron with meals.

PROVIDING CATHETER SITE CARE

Equipment

4×4 gauze pads
ABD pad
Tape
Povidone-iodine (Betadine) swab or solution
Applicator sticks
Sterile saline
Mask
Sterile gloves (two pairs)
Forceps (optional)

Procedure

1. Explain procedure to client.
2. Wash hands.
3. Provide privacy.
4. Put on mask and gloves.
5. Remove old dressing with forceps or sterile gloves.
6. Inspect site for infection or bleeding.
7. Use normal saline to remove any dried blood or drainage.
8. Dry area thoroughly.
9. Change gloves.
10. Cleanse area surrounding catheter with povidone-iodine swab or applicator sticks. Allow to dry.
11. Apply sterile pads around catheter at exit site and on top of catheter.
12. Remove gloves.
13. Tape dressing nonocclusively.

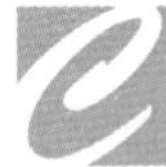

CHARTING for Peritoneal Dialysis

- Predialysis weight and baseline assessment
- Time of catheter insertion
- Composition of dialysis solution
- Time of onset and termination of each cycle
- Number of cycles
- Amount of solution infused for each cycle
- Amount of fluid recovered for each cycle
- Cumulative fluid balance
- Appearance of outflow
- Postdialysis weight and clinical status
- Signs or symptoms of complications
- Nursing interventions to prevent or treat complications

CRITICAL THINKING APPLICATION

CLINICAL PROBLEMS	CRITICAL THINKING OPTIONS
■ Pain occurs during procedure.	• Evaluate characteristics to differentiate dialysis-related pain from other types (for example, myocardial infarction). • If on inflow, reassure client that pain sometimes occurs. • Check that dialysate is at body temperature. • Promote effective fluid drainage. • Provide diversionary activities. • If persistent, consult with physician about decreasing infusion volume or instilling a local anesthetic through the catheter.

CLINICAL PROBLEMS	CRITICAL THINKING OPTIONS
	• If accompanied by signs of peritonitis (abdominal rigidity, rebound tenderness, cloudy outflow fluid or fever), alert physician immediately.
■ Dialysate return is not clear.	• If dialysate is cloudy, send specimen immediately to laboratory for culture and sensitivity. • Monitor client for signs of abdominal wall rigidity, abdominal palpation tenderness, cloudy dialysate outflow, and increased temperature. • Notify physician. • If dialysate contains blood, this is usual for the first two "runs" following catheter insertion. If condition persists, reassess catheter insertion. • Observe for signs of bleeding: petechiae, ecchymosis, or signs of blood in stool and urine. • Monitor hemoglobin and hematocrit to determine extent of bleeding.
■ The amount of fluid return is less than desired.	• Increase dialysate glucose concentration according to physician's orders. The higher glucose level "pulls" more fluid across the semipermeable membrane (peritoneal cavity). • Make sure dialysate is body temperature when infusing. Cold fluid can promote vasoconstriction and decrease fluid loss.
■ Creatinine and BUN levels are not reduced.	• Make sure each dialysis cycle is only 1 hour long. To increase diffusion of BUN and creatinine across the peritoneal membrane, make sure the dialysate is allowed to stay in the abdomen no more than 20 minutes. Longer time periods cause equilibration of the BUN and creatinine on either side of the membrane so that BUN and creatinine are not reduced as effectively. • Warm the dialysate to body temperature to increase urea clearance. • Increase glucose, as ordered, in dialysate solution to increase urea clearance.
■ During catheter insertion, client experiences sudden pressure in bladder, rectum, or epigastrium.	• Alert physician immediately, as these signs indicate malposition of catheter and require repositioning.
■ Inflow is slower than normal.	• Check inflow tubing for kinks. • Lower bed position.
■ Outflow is slow or absent.	• Check that outflow clamps are open. • Check for kinks in outflow tubing. • Check for and eliminate any air in drainage tubing. • Turn client from side to side. • Raise the head of the bed to a higher position. • Gently massage the abdomen.

CLINICAL PROBLEMS	CRITICAL THINKING OPTIONS
	• Consult physician about possible blockage of catheter. He or she may probe catheter to dislodge fibrin plugs or reposition it to release a subcutaneous kink.
■ There is positive fluid balance at end of cycle.	• Repeat outflow phase. • If positive balance is within limits specified by physician (usually 250 mL maximum), continue with next cycle.
■ Client experiences dyspnea.	• Elevate head of bed. • Institute deep breathing and coughing exercises to prevent atelectasis. • If acute respiratory distress, immediately drain the fluid and notify the physician.
■ Client appears confused or lethargic; other signs of hyperglycemia are present during dialysis; signs of hypoglycemia are present after dialysis.	• Check that dialysate glucose concentration on bottle label matches ordered concentration of glucose. • Be sure that dialysate is drained promptly at the end of the diffusion period. • Place diabetics on routine blood glucose monitoring. • Consult with physician about discontinuing dialysis slowly, giving the body time to readjust blood glucose and insulin levels.
■ Fecal-colored drainage or decreased drainage and diarrhea are present.	• Notify physician because these signs indicate possible bowel perforation. Surgical repair may be necessary.
■ Client experiences bladder fullness and increased urinary output, and there is decreased drainage.	• Notify physician because these signs indicate possible bladder perforation; surgical repair may be necessary.
■ Client on high glucose dialysate develops tachycardia or hypotension.	• Alert physician and implement changes in orders. A dialysate with lower glucose concentration usually is ordered for future cycles to minimize recurrence of these signs.
■ There is leakage around catheter site.	• Change dressing as needed. • Apply sterile plastic drape over skin. • Weigh dressings to estimate fluid loss (1 g = 1 mL).

unit 10 HEMODIALYSIS

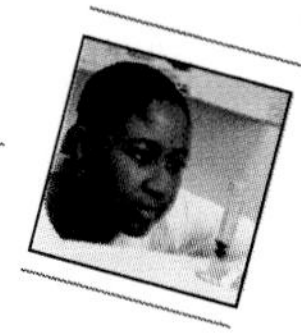

NURSING PROCESS DATA

ASSESSMENT Data Base

Review dialysis orders.

Determine type of vascular access.

a. Femoral vein catheter: dual-lumen vascular device used for immediate vascular access in life-threatening situations.
b. Central venous dual-lumen catheter (DLC): vascular device placed in superior vena cava; used for temporary access for acute or chronic hemodialysis clients.
c. Permanent dual-lumen catheter (PDLC): vascular device inserted through internal jugular vein and advanced to right atrium; used long term when access is unavailable through peripheral veins.
d. Arteriovenous fistula: surgically created internal anastomosis between an artery and vein; used for clients undergoing chronic hemodialysis.
e. Arteriovenous graft: surgically implanted synthetic material (Goretex) or biologic material (human umbilical vein) used for anastomosis between an artery and vein for clients undergoing chronic hemodialysis.

Review chart and laboratory reports for factors that may alter management of dialysis (especially potassium, sodium, calcium and phosphorus levels, albumin, hemoglobin, hematocrit levels, BUN, and creatinine).

Assess client's response to ultrafiltration.

Assess vital signs.

a. Observe for shock and hypovolemia.
b. Assess causes of hypotension: fluid loss; decreased blood volume; hypoalbuminemia; or use of antihypertensive drugs before dialysis.

Check serum electrolytes, BUN, and creatinine before and after dialysis according to physician orders.

Weigh client before and after dialysis to determine fluid loss. Complete physical examination for signs of fluid and electrolyte imbalances (e.g., periorbital, sacral, or pedal edema; asterixis; S_3 heart sounds, or adventitious lung sounds).

Establish data base for monitoring HBSag, HBSab, HIV status if client consents.

Assess for serum liver enzyme elevations.

PLANNING Objectives

To remove byproducts of protein metabolism: urea, creatinine, and uric acid

To remove excessive fluid, thereby reestablishing normal fluid status

To maintain or restore normal level of electrolytes in the body

To maintain a patent access site for hemodialysis

To maintain patent femoral or subclavian catheters

To instruct the client in self-care

INTERVENTION Procedures

Initiating Hemodialysis

Managing Hemodialysis

Terminating Hemodialysis

Maintaining Central Venous Dual-Lumen Catheter (DLC)

Flushing Permanent Dual-Lumen Catheter (PDLC) with Heparin

EVALUATION Expected Outcomes

Asepsis is maintained throughout the procedure.

Creatinine and BUN levels are reduced, and electrolyte balance remains in a satisfactory state.

Excessive fluid is reduced.

Toxic substances are removed, and client's health status is improved.

Access site remains patent.

Client is able to care for self following client teaching.

Femoral catheters remain patent.

INITIATING HEMODIALYSIS

Equipment

Dialyzer (types are hollow fiber and parallel plate)
1000-mL bag of 0.9% normal saline IV solution
Macrodrop administration set
Fistula needles, $\frac{15}{16}$ gauge, 1 – $1\frac{1}{4}$ inches in length
Sterile gauze pads, alcohol swabs, and povidone-iodine swabs
Hemostats, cannula clamps
Tape
Sterile gloves and clean gloves
Gown
Protective goggles and face mask or visor shield
Sterile bowl
30-mL syringe and needle
Infusion pump
Heparin solution 1:1000
APTT
APTT tubes
Stop watch
Hemastix
Dialysis log
Gelfoam (optional)

Preparation

1. Obtain dialysate bath composition as ordered.
2. Set up 1000-mL IV of normal saline using macrodrop tubing.
3. Fill a 30-mL syringe with heparin 1:1000 solution, and place syringe in infusion pump.
4. Connect heparin-filled syringe to heparin port in arterial limb (limb refers to tubing that connects arterial access site to dialyzer) of dialysis tubing. **Rationale:** Heparin is added to system just before blood enters dialyzer to prevent clotting. The clotting mechanism is activated when blood moves outside body and is in contact with foreign substances.
5. Check location of nearest emergency power outlet. **Rationale:** To maintain electric current if routine power fails.
6. Test dialysis machine for presence of bleach with Hemastix. **Rationale:** This detects presence of caustic agents that could result in client complications.
7. Prime dialyzer and arterial and venous blood lines with saline.
8. Hang additional IV solution of saline. **Rationale:** Saline infusions must be available immediately for

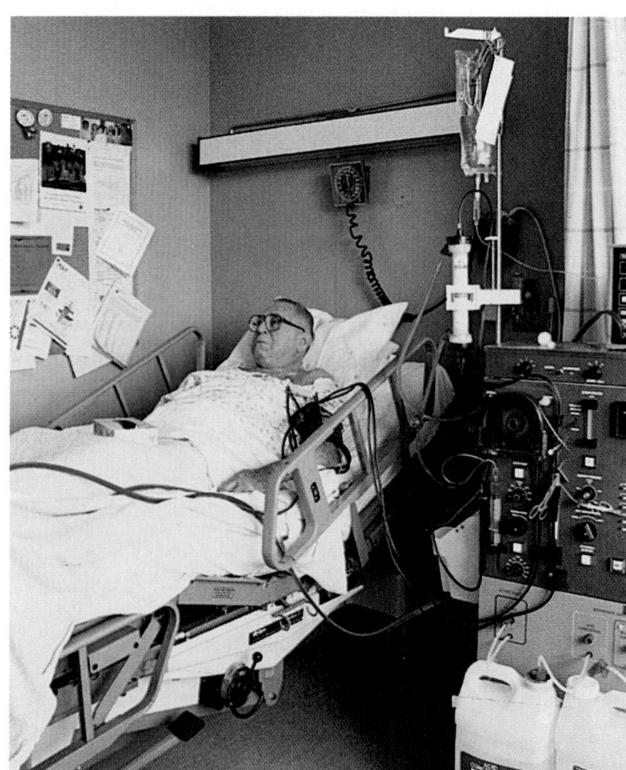

Hemodialysis unit used to treat renal failure clients.

rapid reversal of hypotension or discontinuation of dialysis.

9. Connect pressure monitor lines to both arterial and venous drip chambers. **Rationale:** This monitors the amount of hydrostatic pressure exerted on blood in the ultrafiltration process used to extract fluid throughout dialysis treatment.
10. Set the alarm pressures—high and low.
11. Connect air leak detector to venous drip chamber.
12. Test all machine alarms—venous and arterial pressure, air detector, and blood leak detector.

THE HEMODIALYSIS PROCESS

Hemodialysis works by removing blood from the client's arterial access site (shunt, fistula, or catheter) circulating it through a tubing system to a dialyzer. In the dialyzer, which acts like a semipermeable membrane, fluid, electrolytes, and toxins are removed from the blood through a process of osmosis and diffusion. The blood then flows from the dialyzer through a tubing system to the client's venous access site. Fluid is removed through the use of hydrostatic pressure applied to the blood and a negative hydrostatic pressure applied to the dialysate bath. The difference between these two pressures is termed transmembrane pressure and this results in the process of ultrafiltration.

Procedure

for Internal Shunts or Grafts

1. Place blood line at the same level as the bed.
2. Don mask and gown. Put on goggles, and wash hands.
3. Don clean gloves, and remove dressing, if used. Remove and discard gloves.
4. Don sterile gloves.
5. Clean access site using povidone-iodine swab. Using a circular motion, cleanse from needle insertion site outward. Allow to dry. Wipe site with alcohol swab according to hospital policy.
6. Insert needles into shunt. Tape securely to extremity.
7. Obtain blood for predialysis blood samples as ordered by the physician. (Usually electrolytes, hematocrit, clotting time, etc.)
8. After blood is drawn for lab work, heparin load should be given to client according to baseline ACT and client's weight. Connect to extension tubing.
9. Prime the extracorporeal circuit with blood.
   a. Connect arterial tubing of the blood line to client's arterial site.
   b. Place end of venous tubing into sterile basin to "bleed off" saline or connect to client's venous cannula—depending on client's need for saline prime. **Rationale:** Some clients require more volume to maintain vital signs when initiating hemodialysis.
   c. Remove venous blood line clamp.
   d. Remove arterial blood line clamp.
   e. Clamp saline infusion line. (Should be changed before "bleed off.")
   f. Remove arterial cannula clamp. Do not remove venous cannula clamp unless client is to receive the saline as a prime.
   g. As blood enters the arterial drip chamber on the arterial line, begin heparin infusion at prescribed rate according to specific orders.
   h. Allow blood to circulate through system until saline in venous drip chamber is pink.
   i. Clamp venous blood line if "bleeding off" saline into basin.
10. After priming extracorporeal circuit, if "bleeding off" saline, complete the circuit.
    a. Wipe venous cannula end with alcohol swab.
    b. Attach venous blood line to venous cannula.
    c. Remove venous blood line clamp.
    d. Remove venous cannula clamp.
11. Note time of dialysis initiation.

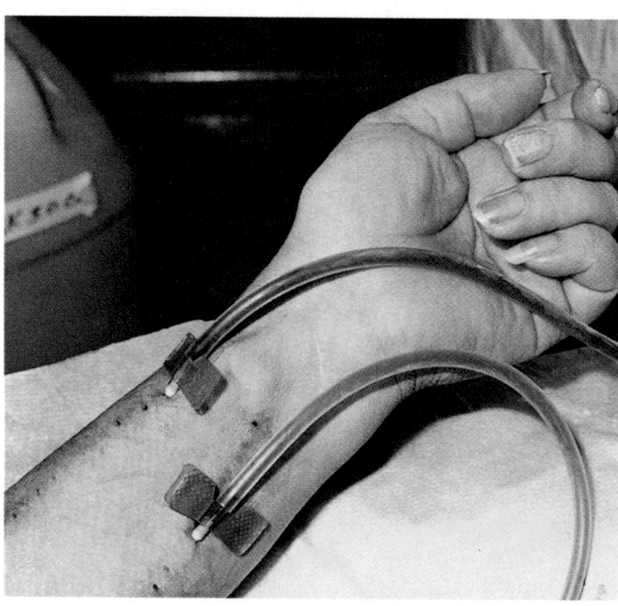

Arterial and venous needle sites used in hemodialysis.

12. Tape all connections securely; secure blood tubing to client's extremity.
13. Connect pressure monitor lines to each drip chamber.
14. Set alarm pressures—high and low.
15. Connect air leak detector to venous drip chamber. **Rationale:** Presence of air leak activates alarm—requires immediate intervention.
16. Establish blood flow rate (usually 250–450 mL/min).
17. Check client's blood pressure and pulse once dialysis has been initiated, then hourly unless otherwise indicated.
18. Maintain ordered clotting times of client and dialyzer. **Rationale:** It is necessary to keep heparin dosage at a level that maintains desired clotting time.
    a. Check ACT every 30 minutes.
    b. Turn heparin infusion off last 30–60 minutes.
19. Assess client at least hourly for vital signs and potential complications.
20. Administer any ordered medication through the venous line. **Rationale:** Medication infuses into client, not machine.
21. When dialysis treatment stabilizes, increase negative pressure, if ordered, to establish ultrafiltration. **Rationale:** This action is necessary to obtain required fluid loss.

PROTOCOL TO MAINTAIN CLOTTING TIMES WITH HEPARIN

Dosage is determined by an arbitrary formula followed by assessment of clotting time values.

- 10 units × dry weight (kg) = heparin low dosage
- 15 units × dry weight (kg) = heparin mid dosage
- 20 units × dry weight (kg) = heparin high dosage

Amount of heparin administered to keep clotting time at appropriate level.

MANAGING HEMODIALYSIS

Procedure

1. Limit fluid intake to prescribed amount.
2. Maintain diet: low sodium (20–40 g), low protein, high carbohydrate, high fat, and foods low in potassium.
3. Check vital signs for hypovolemia; check temperature for infection.
4. Auscultate heart and lung sounds for signs of pulmonary edema and pericarditis.
5. Provide shunt care.
6. Observe level of consciousness—indicative of fluid and electrolyte imbalance or thrombus.
7. Administer antihypertensive drugs between dialysis if ordered.
8. Administer diuretics if ordered.
9. Administer blood if ordered (cellular portion only is needed because of low hematocrit).
10. Weigh daily to assess fluid accumulation.
11. Use antibacterial soap and lotion to bathe. **Rationale:** This decreases risk of staphylococcal infections.
12. Provide continued emotional support.
    a. Allow for expression of feelings about change in body image.
    b. Encourage expression of fears of death especially during dialysis.
    c. Encourage family cooperation.
    d. Give support for required change in life style.

ASSESSING ARTERIOVENOUS FISTULA

- Wash your hands.
- Position client's arm so fistula is easily accessed.
- Palpate the area over the shunt to feel for the thrill (vibration). This indicates a patent fistula.
- Auscultate the area over the shunt with a stethoscope to detect a bruit (swishing noise). This indicates a patent fistula.
- Palpate distal pulses to fistula to check circulation.
- Observe capillary refill in fistula extremity.
- Assess for numbness, tingling, or alteration in sensation in digits of fistula extremity.
- Assess for signs and symptoms of infection: redness, edema, soreness, warmth, or increased temperature.

SAFETY PRECAUTIONS FOR SHUNTS

- Do not measure blood pressure on shunt extremity.
- Do not apply tourniquet on shunt extremity.
- Do not perform venipuncture above shunt site.
- Counsel client not to wear constrictive clothing on shunt extremity.

TERMINATING HEMODIALYSIS

Equipment

Clean gloves
Gown
Goggles
Mask
Sterile pads
Tubing clamps

Procedure

1. Reduce negative pressure to zero.
2. Don gloves, gown, goggles, and protective mask.
3. Remove tape and dressing to visualize needle insertion site.
4. Place sterile pads under connectors.
5. Clamp arterial cannula and arterial blood line.
6. Open IV of normal saline to return blood in extracorporeal tubing.
7. Release arterial line clamp, and infuse normal saline to rinse arterial tubing.
8. Clamp saline and arterial lines.
9. Separate venous line from venous cannula.
10. Perform site care.
11. Measure and record postdialysis vital signs and weight.

Acceptable Lab Values Following Dialysis

- Sodium 134–145 mEq/L
- Potassium less than 6.2 mEq/L
- Chlorine 94–104 mEq/L

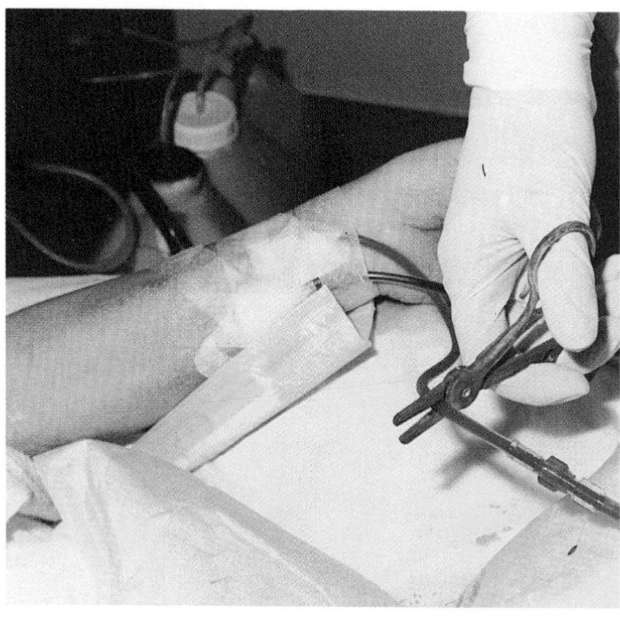

Clamp arterial cannula first when terminating dialysis.

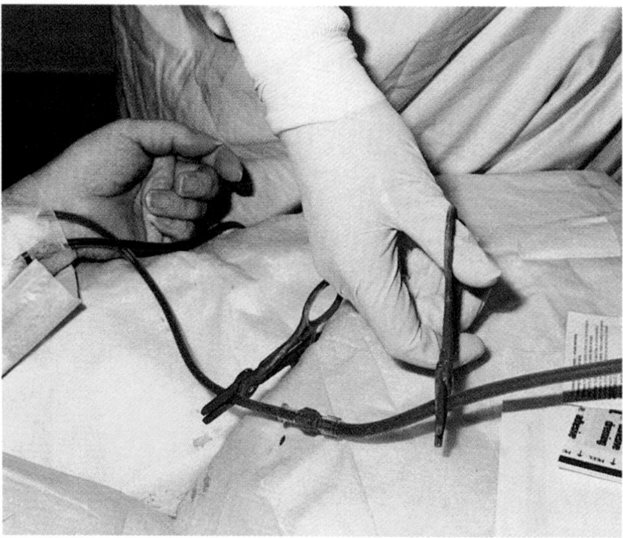

Clamp arterial blood line next.

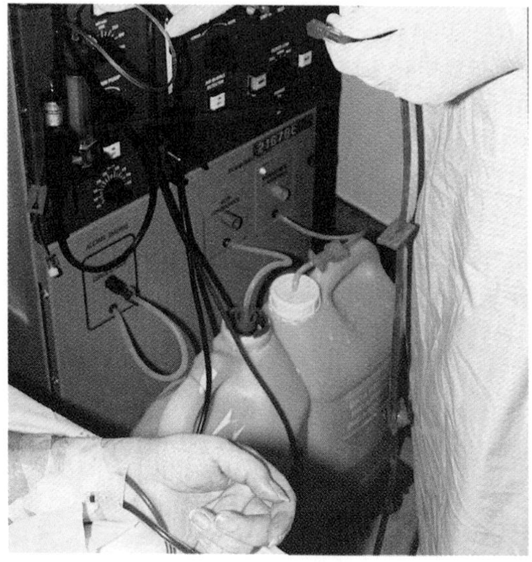

Disconnect arterial blood line from machine.

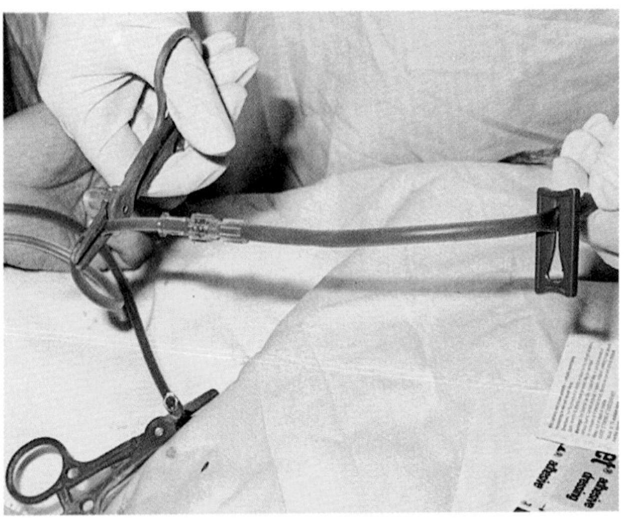
Clamp venous line after clearing first with saline.

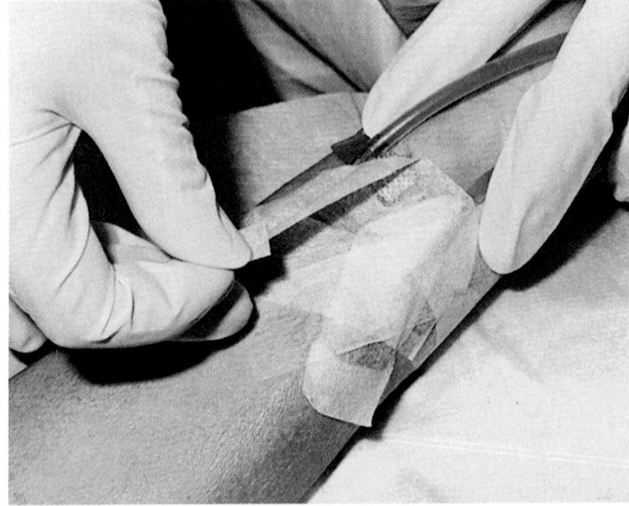
Carefully remove tape from needle site.

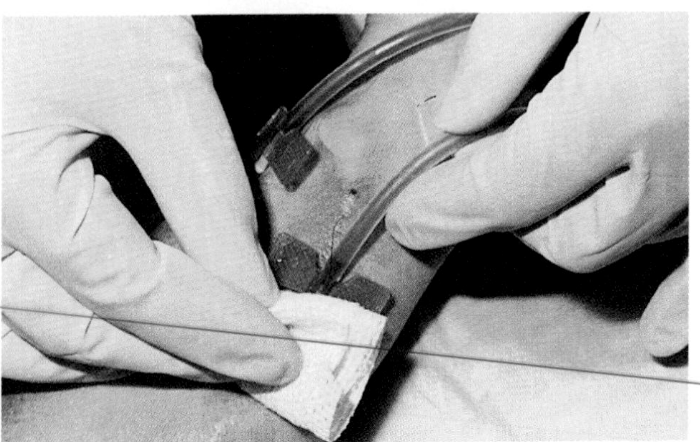
Remove arterial and venous needles.

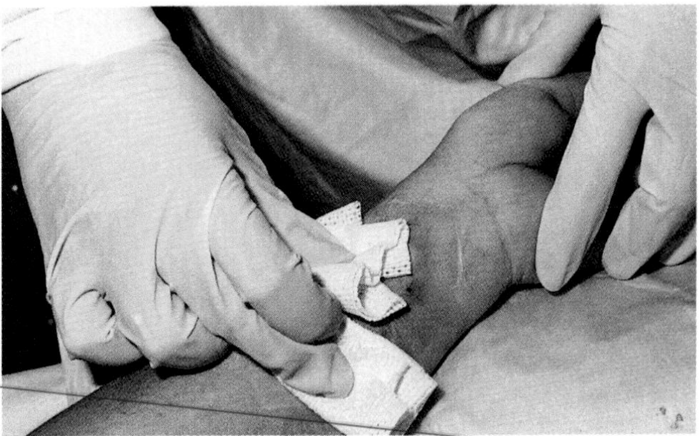
Apply pressure over needle site for five to ten minutes.

- Hydrochloric acid 18–24
- BUN greater than 60, less than 85 mg/dL
- Creatinine less than 13 mg/dL
- Uric acid less than 10 mg/dl
- Glucose 100 mg/dL
- Calcium greater than 9.5, less than 11 mg/dL
- Phosphorus 5.0–6.0 mg/dL
- Alkaline phosphorus less than 90 units/L
- Magnesium less than 3.0 mEq/L
- Albumin greater than 3.5 g/dL

MAINTAINING CENTRAL VENOUS DUAL-LUMEN CATHETER (DLC)

Equipment

Heparin 1000 units/mL
Normal saline
Two dialysis clamps
Povidone-iodine swabs, skin prep
2×2 gauze pads
4×4 sterile transparent occlusive dressings
Tape
Luer-Lok catheter caps
Two 10-mL syringes
Sterile gloves
Mask
Gown

Procedure

1. Wash your hands.
2. Fill two 10-mL syringes with 500 units heparin

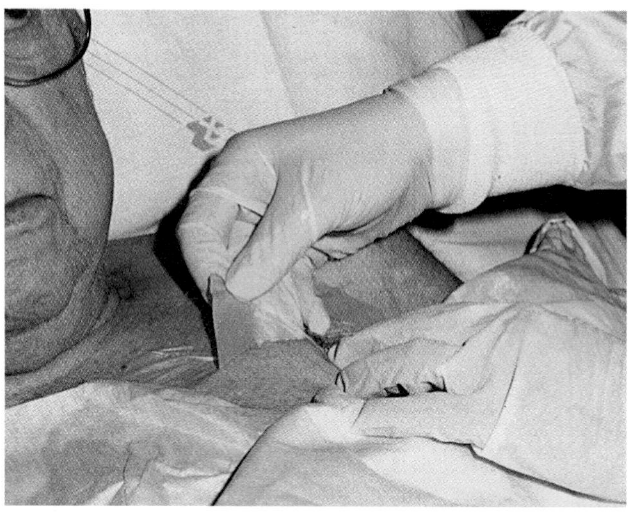
Maintaining sterility, carefully remove dressing from dual-lumen catheter.

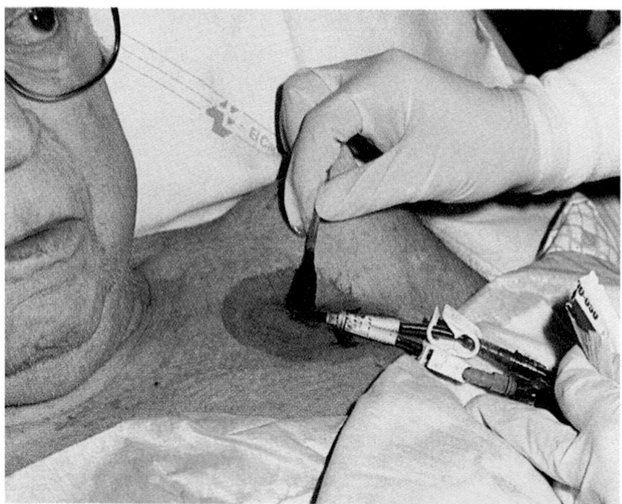
Cleanse catheter insertion site with Povidone-iodine swabs using circular motion.

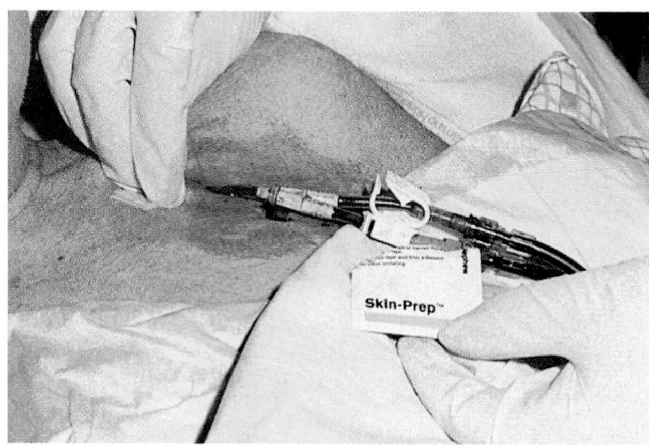

Swab area surrounding catheter site with skin prep before applying dressing.

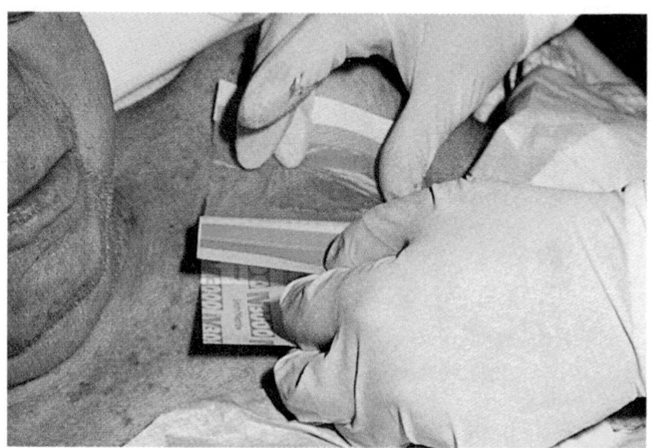
Apply transparent dressing over catheter insertion site for easy assessment.

and 2.5 mL normal saline.

3. Prime Luer-Lok caps with heparinized normal saline.
4. Don sterile gloves and mask.
5. Place caps on arterial and venous limbs of catheter; tape securely.
6. Inject remainder of heparinized saline solution into lumen.
7. Clamp catheter by placing clamp on arterial and venous lines.
8. Flush catheter with heparinized saline according to facility procedure.
9. Remove old dressing, and discard in appropriate receptacle.

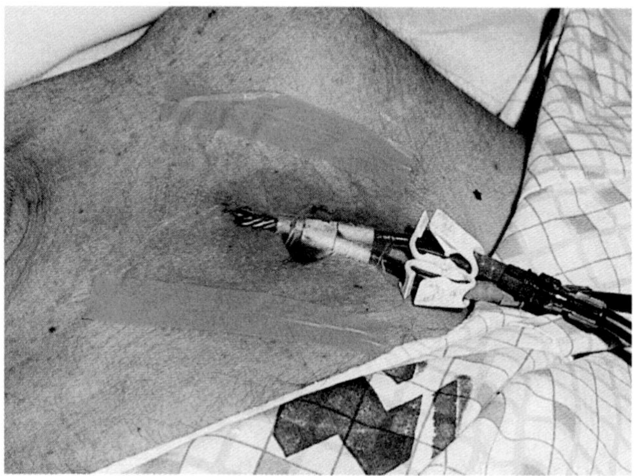
Monitor frequently for signs of infection, bleeding or catheter displacement.

10. Cleanse area surrounding catheter with povidone-iodine swabs using circular motion. Begin at catheter insertion site and work outward. Swab area with skin preparation.
11. Place 4×4 transparent dressing over catheter insertion sites.
12. Provide catheter site care daily and after each dialysis.
13. Remove gloves and mask, and discard.
14. Monitor for signs of infection, bleeding, or displacement of catheters daily.

FLUSHING PERMANENT DUAL-LUMEN CATHETER (PDLC) WITH HEPARIN

Equipment

Two 3-mL syringes filled with 2 mL heparin solution 1:1000
Two 3-mL syringes
Sterile gloves
Two catheter clamps
Two Luer-Lok caps
Two 10-mL syringes filled with normal saline
Two sterile 4×4 gauze pads
Povidone-iodine swabs
Gloves
Mask
Gown

Preparation

1. Wash your hands.
2. Gather equipment.
3. Fill 3-mL syringes with 2 mL of 1:1000 heparin solution.
4. Fill 10 mL syringes with normal saline.
5. Open sterile 4×4 gauze pads and place on overbed table.

Procedure

1. Don sterile gloves.
2. Place sterile gauze under both lumen tips.
3. Cleanse outside of hub connections with povidone-iodine swabs.
4. Open catheter ports, and discard Luer-Lok caps.
5. Connect 3-mL syringe to each port.
6. Unclamp each port and gently aspirate 3 mL of blood. **Rationale:** This removes indwelling heparin.
7. Close clamps, and remove syringes.
8. Attach 10-mL syringes filled with normal saline to each port.
9. Open clamps, and flush catheters.
10. Close clamps. Replace 10-mL syringes with 3-mL syringes filled with heparin solution.
11. Instill heparin.
12. Close clamps simultaneously with instillation of last amount of heparin solution. **Rationale:** This creates positive pressure within the catheter preventing backflow of blood into the catheter when syringe is removed.
13. Attach new Luer-Lok caps, and fasten securely.
14. Discard used equipment in appropriate receptacle.
15. Remove gloves and discard.

■ CLINICAL ALERT

If PDLC is clotted, the physician may order a urokinase injection into the catheter. Inject the fibrinolytic agent slowly, wait 5 minutes, then aspirate to check for catheter patency. After the second try, if the catheter is still clotted, notify physician.

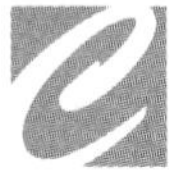

CHARTING for Hemodialysis

- Predialysis assessment, subjective and objective data
- Time dialysis initiated and scheduled termination time of dialysis
- Dialyzer type and dialysate used
- Findings of all safety checks: chloramines, total dissolved solids, bleach, conductivity, air detector, venous and arterial pressure, blood leak
- Any complications during procedure and actions taken
- Client symptoms at hourly intervals for chronic clients and 15-minute intervals for acute clients
- Vital signs
- Postdialysis assessment

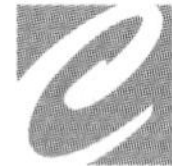

CHARTING for Maintaining Catheters

- Assessment of catheter site
- Amount of heparin solution instilled
- Any complications associated with flushing or instilling heparin

CRITICAL THINKING APPLICATION

CLINICAL PROBLEMS	CRITICAL THINKING OPTIONS
■ Decreased pulse, thrill, or bruit in shunt.	• Notify physician promptly of potential shunt clotting. Shunt needs to be aspirated or irrigated with heparin, or possibly the vessel needs to be stripped of clots. (Success of declotting depends on speed with which it is instituted.)
■ Hypotension occurs during dialysis.	• Anticipate possibility if antihypertensive or diuretic drugs were not omitted before dialysis. • Prime line with 1 unit albumin. • Administer normal saline into the extracorporeal circuit. • Reduce pressure gradient if the client is on ultrafiltration. • If hypotension is severe, place client in Trendelenburg's position if tolerated; consult physician about use of albumin, blood, or vasopressors. • Before future dialyses, consult with physician about using smaller volume dialyzer, less ultrafiltration, or intermittent normal saline doses to maintain blood pressure.
■ Bleeding occurs during dialysis.	• Administer protamine sulfate as ordered to return clotting time to desired range. • If blood leak alarm sounds, observe dialysate. If no blood is apparent, check dialysate with Hemastix since air bubbles can cause false alarms. • If bleeding or blood leak is present, discontinue dialysis.

CLINICAL PROBLEMS	CRITICAL THINKING OPTIONS
■ Alarms sound during dialysis.	• Before dialysis, thoroughly familiarize yourself with alarm sounds, functions, and troubleshooting maneuvers. • When alarms sound, quickly check for possible causes, such as obstructions or separations of tubing. • In an emergency, such as clots, air emboli in venous line, or failure of bypass mode, clamp venous blood line tubing immediately, and place client in Trendelenburg's position on left side.
■ Near the end of or following dialysis, dialysis disequilibrium syndrome develops.	• Suspect dialysis disequilibrium if client develops confusion, seizures, headache, nausea, vomiting, or hypertension. • If these signs appear during dialysis, consult physician, and implement possible orders to slow blood flow rate or discontinue dialysis. • Administer medications as ordered to control symptoms, for example, Dilantin for seizures. • For future dialyses, consult with physician about possible orders regarding prevention, such as early dialysis before BUN rises excessively, shorter dialysis, to a change or the less-efficient peritoneal dialysis.
■ Signs and symptoms of fluid overload or electrolyte imbalance occurs during dialysis.	• Increase ultrafiltration. • Check serum electrolyte values on fresh blood sample. • Consult physician about possible changes in orders.

GERIATRIC CONSIDERATIONS

- Elderly clients may have difficulty with vision and manual dexterity therefore it is imperative that a self-care evaluation is made by the nurse if the client needs to manage a urinary diversion.
- As the thirst mechanism decreases with age, elderly clients need to be encouraged to drink liquids throughout the day to prevent urinary tract infections. Make a list of the client's favorite liquids and formulate a plan for fluid intake throughout the day.
- Clients with long-term indwelling catheters must be monitored carefully for signs of infection. Aseptic catheter care and replacement must be maintained to prevent infection.
- Elderly clients who have long-term indwelling catheters and are ambulatory or in wheelchairs should be evaluated for using leg bags during the day rather than the drainage bag. This provides for more comfort and increases self-esteem.
- Urinary incontinence is a common problem among the elderly. It can lead to both altered self-esteem and body image. Assessment and planning for methods to promote continence or interventions to prevent incontinence are a high priority when caring for these clients.
- Positions, other than dorsal recumbent, may need to be considered when inserting catheters in elderly clients on bed rest. A side-lying position with the upper leg placed across the lower leg exposes the urinary meatus and provides an alternative method for catheter insertion.

22

Bowel Elimination

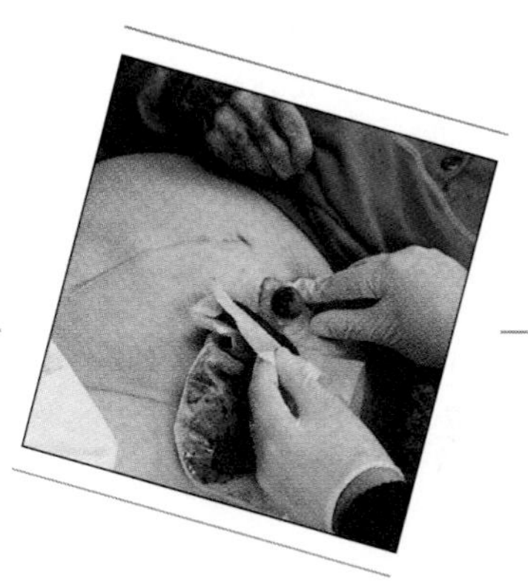

LEARNING OBJECTIVES

- Explain both the mechanical and chemical aspects of digestion.
- Compare and contrast hypermotility with hypomotility.
- Discuss what is meant by obstruction of the bowel.
- Describe the anatomic locations for an ileostomy, cecostomy, or colostomy.
- List the components of a good bowel training program.
- Outline the essential steps in administering a tap water or saline enema to an adult client.
- Describe the precautions necessary when performing digital stimulation to remove a fecal impaction.
- Compare and contrast stoma care of an ileostomy and a colostomy.
- Outline the steps for performing a colostomy irrigation.
- State the conditions under which ostomy irrigations are contraindicated.
- Describe at least three potential problems encountered when irrigating a colostomy.
- Describe at least three precautions necessary when applying a fecal ostomy pouch.
- Discuss the corking and intubation procedure for client with a continent ileostomy.

TERMINOLOGY

Anal fissure: a small linear ulcerated area in the anal area.

Bacteria: unicellular plantlike microorganisms lacking chlorophyll.

Bowel: the intestine.

Bowel movement: the emptying of the intestinal tract.

Carminative: an agent that removes gases from the gastrointestinal tract.

Cathartic: a drug to induce emptying of the intestinal tract; a laxative.

Colitis: inflammation of the colon.

Colon: the large intestine, which extends from the cecum to the anus.

Colostomy: an artificially created opening from the colon to the abdominal surface for the elimination of waste.

Constipation: difficult defecation; the passage of dry, hard fecal material.

Defecation: emptying of the intestinal tract; bowel movement.

Diarrhea: the passage of unformed liquid stools.

Digestion: the process by which food is broken down, mechanically and chemically, in the gastrointestinal tract.

Diverticulitis: inflammation of diverticuli in the intestinal tract causing stagnation of feces in the small distended sacs (diverticula).

Diverticulum: an outpouching of the mucous membrane of the intestine.

Emulsification: the breaking down of large fat globules in the intestine to smaller, uniformly distributed particles.

Enema: the introduction of fluid through a tube into the lower intestinal tract.

Feces: intestinal waste products consisting of bacteria and secretions of the liver, in addition to a small amount of food residue.

Fistula: an abnormal tubelike passage from a normal cavity or tube to a free surface or another cavity.

Flaccid: relaxed, flabby; having defective or absent muscle tone.

Flatulence: excessive gas in the stomach and intestines.

Gastro: pertaining to the stomach.

Gastrointestinal: having to do with the stomach and intestines.

Guaiac: test for blood in stool.

Hemorrhoids: abnormally distended rectal veins due to a constant increase in venous pressure.

Hypermotility: unusually quick motility in the gastrointestinal tract.

Hyperreflexia: increased action of reflexes.

Hypertonic: having a higher osmotic pressure than normal body fluid.

Hypomotility: unusually slow motility of the gastrointestinal tract.

Ileostomy: an artificially created opening from the ileum to the abdominal surface for the elimination of wastes.

Impaction: condition of being tightly wedged into a place, as of feces in the bowel.

Integumentary: relative to a covering, as the skin.

Laxative: a mild-acting drug to induce emptying of the intestinal tract.

Mucosa: mucous membrane.

Necrosis: death of areas of tissue or bone caused by enzymatic action or lack of circulation.

Obstipation: the act or condition of obstructing; extreme constipation due to obstruction.

Occlude: to block off, obstruct.

Occult blood: blood in such minute quantities that it can only be detected by a microscope or chemical means.

Ostomy: a surgically formed artificial opening that serves as an exit site for the bowel or intestine.

Parasite: an organism that lives within, on, or at the expense of another organism, known as the host.

Perforation: the act or process of making a hole, such as that caused by an ulcer.

Peristalsis: a progressive wave-like movement that occurs involuntarily as in the gastrointestinal tract.

Reflux: a return of or backward flow.

Sphincter: circular band of muscle fiber constricting a natural orifice.

Stoma: an artificially created opening between two passages or between a passage and the body surface.

Stool: waste matter discharged from the bowels.

Suppositories: semisolid substances for introduction into the rectum, vagina, or urethra where they dissolve; serves as a vehicle for medicines to be absorbed.

Villi: short filamentous processes found on certain membraneous surfaces.

ANATOMY AND PHYSIOLOGY

The gastrointestinal system converts food into products that can be used as nutrients on the cellular level and disposes of wastes incurred in the process. The primary structures in this system include the mouth, esophagus, stomach, small intestine, and large intestine.

The mouth, esophagus, and stomach are the structures of the upper gastrointestinal tract, where the process of digestion begins. The small intestine, where digestion is completed and most absorption takes place, is a 12-foot tube composed of the duodenum, jejunum, and ileum. The large intestine is made up of the cecum, colon, and rectum. The cecum contains the ileocecal valve and the appendix. The colon is divided into the ascending, transverse, descending, and sigmoid colon. The rectum extends from the sigmoid colon to the anus. The terminal end of the rectum is called the anal canal and is guarded by the internal and external sphincter muscles. The chief functions of the colon are to reabsorb water and sodium and to store wastes.

Digestion is accomplished mechanically and chemically. Food is mechanically churned through the intestinal tract by sharp contractions, or peristaltic waves, of the circular and longitudinal muscles of the intestinal wall. Muscular sphincters and valves are located at strategic points throughout the intestinal tract. These structures help propel the food bolus or feces at appropriately timed intervals in a process called rhythmic segmentation. The sphincters and valves, when functioning properly, prevent reflux of contents. Peristaltic waves, coupled with rhythmic segmentation, allow maximal contact between food and the bowel wall so that chemical reactions can accomplish digestion and absorption can take place.

The chemical aspects of digestion in the small intestine begin in the duodenum with the introduction of pancreatic juices and bile. Pancreatic juices are rich in enzymes, which work to break down proteins and fats

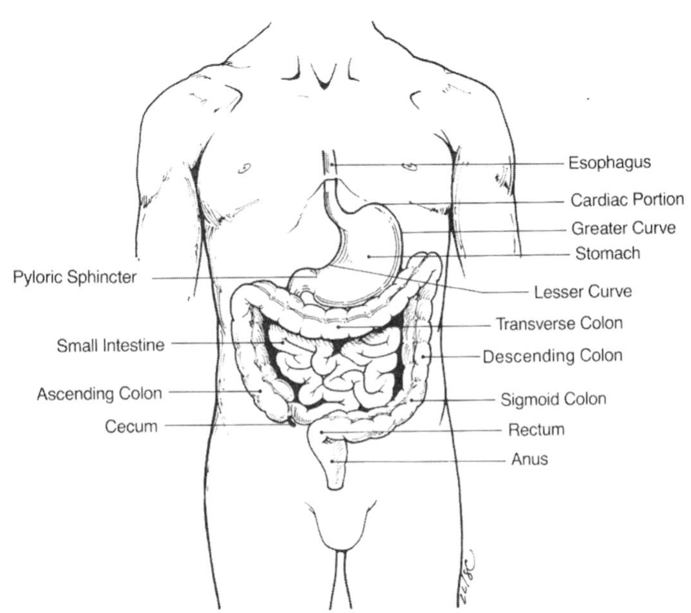

Anatomy of the gastrointestinal tract.

and to complete the transformation of starch to sugar. Bile, secreted by the liver, aids in the emulsification and absorption of fats. These substances work in an alkaline medium that combines with the acidity of chyme to provide a neutral pH in the duodenum, thereby protecting the duodenal mucosa.

In the 20 feet of jejunum and ileum, approximately 3000 mL of digestive enzymes are secreted. These enzymes, which are secreted by the mucus glands of the intestines, complete the digestive processing of food prior to absorption. Again, the alkaline nature of these secretions works to protect the mucous membrane of the intestinal tract.

The peristaltic activity of the gastrointestinal tract, as well as its secretory functions, is governed, to a large degree, by parasympathetic and sympathetic nerve fibers. Stimulation of the parasympathetic system increases the activity of the intestinal tract, while stimulation of the sympathetic nervous system inhibits activity in the tract. The internal anal sphincter, however, is activated by sympathetic stimulation, whereas the external anal sphincter is under voluntary control.

Absorption, another primary function of the small bowel, is the passage of prepared materials from the gastrointestinal lumen to the blood and cells. Most absorption in the small intestine results from the churning action of the bowel. Chyme is continually exposed to the circular folds of the mucosal surface, which is lined with thread-like projections called villi. Villi serve as the sites of absorption of fluid and nutrients. The duration of contact between chyme and the mucosal surface of the bowel is very important in absorption. Hypermotility in the small intestine can result in decreased contact with the mucosal wall and deficient absorption; hypomotility can result in increased absorption of fluids as well as problems with elimination.

The circulatory system delivers nutrients to tissue cells and transports the waste products of metabolism. The small bowel and colon are supplied by the superior and inferior mesenteric arteries. Blood that contains absorbed nutrients is carried from the gastrointestinal tract by the superior and inferior mesenteric veins, which become a part of the portal system delivering blood to the liver. Each villus on the intestinal wall contains a network of small capillaries, which absorb sugar and amino acids, and a central lymph channel, which absorbs fatty acids and glycerol. When circulation is compromised, absorption is decreased and cells are lost.

By the time chyme reaches the ileocecal valve—the junction between the small and large intestines—most nutrients have been absorbed. Whereas 3 L of fluid pass through the small bowel, only 500 mL actually pass through the ileocecal valve. The semiliquid material received by the large intestine consists of living and dead bacteria, undigested food and residue, and cell debris. As residue is slowly passed along the colon by peristaltic-like mass movements, fluid is absorbed. These movements occur relatively infrequently (perhaps two or three times per day) and are stimulated by the entrance of food into the stomach by the gastrocolic reflex.

Absorption of fluid in the colon takes place primarily in the ascending and transverse colon. Fecal masses are stored in the sigmoid colon and move into the rectum with mass peristaltic movement. When the rectum fills and becomes sufficiently distended, centers in the sacral area of the spinal cord facilitate a defecation reflex, which contracts the rectum and relaxes the internal and external anal sphincters. The resulting urge, facilitated by higher centers, leads to contraction of the abdominal, perineal, and diaphragmatic muscles. Willful defecation is a coordinated, learned habit. Voluntary inhibition of the act returns the stool to the sigmoid colon.

DEFECATION

Defecation is defined as evacuation of the bowels. The pattern of defecation varies with each individual. It can occur from several times each day to two to three times each week. The type and amount of stool evacuated is also individualized. It is determined by such factors as diet and normal changes in the intestinal flora. Additional factors that influence bowel patterns include age, fluid intake, exercise, psychologic factors, alterations in lifestyle, and medications.

Normal feces are composed of about 75% water and 25% solid material. The stool is soft, but formed, and the color ranges from light to dark brown. The color of the stool is due to the presence of stercobilin and urobilin, derived from bilirubin. In the absence of bile pigment the stool takes on a characteristically clay-colored or white appearance. The action of bacteria in the colon plays a role in the color of the stool. Ingestion of certain foods, drugs, and vitamins can alter the color and consistency of the stool. The nurse must complete an accurate bowel history to determine normal or abnormal findings. Conclusions should not be made on observation alone. Iron supplements, vitamins with iron, beet, red peppers, licorice, grape juice, and spinach affect the color of the stool, which could lead to an incorrect conclusion of blood in the stool. Feces that are red or black in color can be a direct result of ingestion of these foods. Medications can also affect the color and consistency of the stool. Medications, such as codeine and morphine, can cause constipation. In addition to consistency and distinct color of the feces there is an odor associated with the feces. The odor is a result of the action of microorganisms on the chyme.

Abnormal characteristics of the feces include the presence of exudate, parasites, fat, and large amounts of mucus. Large amounts of mucus are generally associated with an inflammatory process of the bowel. The stool appears slimy in this condition. Diseases, such as ulcerative colitis or Crohn's disease, produce a stool with large amounts of pus when inflammation is present. Stools with abnormally high fat content are foul-smelling and float to the top of the water. Children with cystic fibrosis commonly produce this type of stool.

ALTERATIONS IN ELIMINATION

By-products of digestion must be continually eliminated to maintain normal body function. Alterations in normal elimination can result from changes in motility, obstruction of the lumen of the bowel, circulatory deficiencies, disease process, and surgically induced alterations to the structures of the intestinal tract.

Changes in Motility

Motility in the gastrointestinal system is the ability to move spontaneously. Normal motility of the bowel provides peristaltic activity that pushes and churns food and chyme through the upper tract and feces through the lower tract at timed intervals.

Hypermotility may be caused by direct stimulation or irritation of the autonomic nervous system, as well as by inflammatory processes in the gastrointestinal tract. Stimulation of parasympathetic nerves promotes peristalsis and increases bowel muscle tone. Increased peristalsis speeds the propulsion of chyme through the upper tract, resulting in deficient absorption of nutrients. When increased peristalsis speeds the propulsion of feces through the lower tract, diarrhea occurs.

Stimulation of the autonomic nervous system may be psychic in origin. Anxiety, for example, may be mediated through either parasympathetic nerves, with resultant diarrhea, or through sympathetic nerves, with resultant constipation. The action on the parasympathetic nervous system of certain drugs may also cause hypermotility of the intestine. Antihypertensive drugs, such as reserpine, and cholinergic drugs can cause diarrhea by their stimulation of parasympathetic nerves.

Hypermotility caused by the stimulating effect of an irritant on intestinal peristalsis may arise from infectious agents, chemical agents, or inflammatory disease processes. The most common intestinal irritants are the products of certain bacteria that release toxins in the digestive tract. Chemical agents that irritate the intestinal mucosa include cytotoxic drugs, castor oil, and quinidine. Ulcerative and inflammatory disease processes include diverticulitis, tuberculous lesions, ulcerative colitis, and Crohn's disease.

Hypomotility may be caused by direct stimulation or blockage of the autonomic nervous system, intestinal muscle weakness, and chemical agents that inhibit peristalsis and induce flaccidity in the intestinal tract. Decreased peristalsis causes chyme to move sluggishly through the upper tract so that fluids are overabsorbed. Decreased peristalsis also slows the propulsion of feces through the lower tract and causes constipation, fecal impaction, and obstruction.

Stimulation or blockage of the autonomic nervous system may be congenital in origin, as is the case in Hirschsprung's disease, where the absence of parasympathetic nerve ganglia results in failure of peristalsis of the affected portion of the bowel. The effects of trauma or toxins on autonomic innervation of the intestine, which occur with paralytic (adynamic) ileus, inhibit motility to the point of obstruction.

Intestinal muscle weakness that results from disease processes, old age, or a lack of essential vitamins (notably the B group) or electrolytes (particularly potassium) may all contribute to hypomotility. Certain drugs, such as codeine and morphine, can also cause hypomotility by relaxing the smooth muscles of the digestive tract and by increasing spasms of the intestinal sphincters.

Obstruction of the Lumen of the Bowel

Obstruction of the lumen of the bowel may be partial or complete. The severity of the obstruction depends on the region of the bowel that is affected, the degree to which the lumen is occluded, and the degree to which the circulation in the bowel wall is disturbed.

A small-bowel obstruction that occurs as a consequence of persistent vomiting (reverse peristalsis) can cause severe disturbances in the electrolyte balance of the body. Large-bowel obstructions, even if complete, are not as dramatic, provided that the blood supply to the colon is not disturbed.

The causes of intestinal obstruction are varied. In rare instances, obstruction may result when a foreign body, such as a large fruit stone or a mass of parasitic worms, becomes lodged in the bowel. More frequently, intestinal obstructions are caused by strictures, adhesions, hernia, volvulus, intussusception, polyps, neoplasms, and fecal impactions.

The physiology of an obstruction in the lumen of the bowel is generally the same, regardless of cause. As the lumen of the bowel is blocked, the body attempts to overcome the obstruction by increasing peristalsis. During this process, liquid feces move past the site of obstruction and cause diarrhea and increased obstruction, which leads to constipation. Within several hours peristalsis is reduced, and the bowel becomes flaccid. As intraluminal pressure builds up, fluid is retained and absorption decreases. The increased intraluminal pressure then leads to the compression of the bowel wall and its capillaries, which causes necrosis of the bowel wall.

Circulatory Deficiencies

An adequate circulatory flow is essential for maintaining the structure of the bowel and for carrying on cellular nutrition. Any interruption of the arterial blood supply inhibits the bowel function. An occlusion of the circulatory flow, also called an intestinal infarction, results in gangrene of the bowel unless surgical intervention is carried out. A partial occlusion of the mesenteric arteries due to atherosclerosis can cause abdominal angina, a condition that occurs when the blood supply is increasingly interrupted.

Surgically Induced Alterations in the Structure of the Bowel

When alterations in bowel elimination become life-threatening and medical management fails, surgical intervention becomes necessary. Diversionary surgical procedures of the bowel include ileostomy, cecostomy, and colostomy.

An ileostomy is a surgically created opening from the ileum through the abdominal wall. The entire large intestine is bypassed or removed (or both), and the distal ileum is brought through the abdominal wall to form a stoma. The discharge from an ileostomy contains water and many digestive enzymes that have not yet been absorbed by intestinal villi. Strict attention should be paid to skin protection around the ileostomy stoma to prevent breakdown caused by the digestive enzymes.

A cecostomy is a surgically created opening from the cecum through the abdominal wall. This procedure is generally a temporary method of decompressing the bowel to relieve obstruction. Frequently a catheter is left in the opening. This catheter requires frequent irrigation to ensure a patent lumen. If a catheter is not left in the opening, the cecostomy opening should be pouched in the same manner as an ileostomy.

A colostomy is a surgically created opening from the colon through the abdominal wall. In a colostomy the diseased portion of the colon is bypassed or removed, and a portion of healthy colon is brought to the outside of the abdomen to form a stoma. Colostomies are named after the section of the colon surgically altered. The location of the colostomy dictates the type of drainage as well as the proper method of management.

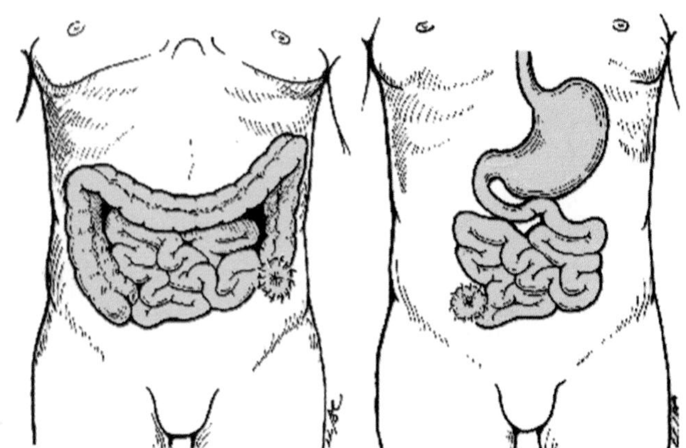

A sigmoid colostomy is permanent. An ileostomy is permanent.

An ascending colostomy has liquid to semisoft effluent, which may flow throughout the day and night. The discharge from an ascending colostomy contains some digestive enzymes caused by this portion of the colon's proximity to the small intestine. It also contains a great deal of water, since much of the water-absorbing portions of the colon are bypassed. The stoma is usually located on the right lower quadrant of the abdomen. A drainable pouch with good skin protection is required for management of an ascending colostomy.

The discharge from a descending, or sigmoid colostomy, is formed and firm, since most of the water has been absorbed by the time the feces reaches these portions of the colon. The flow of output from a descending or sigmoid colostomy may be controlled by diet, the careful use of stool softeners, or colostomy irrigations, Table 22–1.

Colostomy irrigations are not commonly used today to establish regularity of bowel elimination. Clients usually reestablish bowel habits similar to those prior to the surgery. There may still be some clients who do perform daily irrigations; however, there are situations when irrigations must not be done. Irrigations are always contraindicated in clients with unstable fluid and electrolyte balance and in those clients in whom vagal stimulation is dangerous. Irrigations are also contraindicated when clients are receiving radiation therapy or are experiencing chemotherapy-induced diarrhea. For clients who have a nonregulated descending

TABLE 22–1. Comparison Chart for Ostomies

Colostomy	Ileostomy
Etiologic Factors	
Cancer of colon—Permanent	Ulcerative colitis
Traumatic or congenital disruption of intestinal tract—Permanent or temporary	Crohn's disease (regional ileitis)
Diverticulitis (double barrel)—Can be reanastomosed after inflammatory process healed, usually 3–6 months	Birth defects Trauma Cancer
Surgical Procedure	
Portion of colon brought through abdominal wall	Portion of ileum brought through abdominal wall
Bowel Control	
Sigmoid—Yes Ascending—No	None
Stool Consistency	
Sigmoid—Formed Ascending—Semiformed	Liquid to semiliquid
Irrigation for Bowel Control	
Sigmoid—May irrigate Ascending—Not usually irrigated	No
Use of Appliance	
Sigmoid—Not usually Ascending—Yes	Yes
Nursing Care Priorities	
Control bowel evacuation a. Diet b. Irrigation (ascending)	Control not possible
Maintain skin integrity a. Wash peristomal area b. Provide skin barrier c. Ensure proper fit of appliance, if used	Maintain skin integrity a. Wash stoma area b. Provide skin barrier c. Ensure proper fit of appliance, if used
Fluid Requirement	
Sigmoid—Usual Ascending—Increased	Increased
Diet Control	
Avoid gas-forming foods, odor-forming foods, popcorn, and mushrooms	Low residue High calorie Avoid gas-forming foods
Medications	
Sigmoid—Stool softeners Ascending—Electrolyte replacement: K, Na, $NaHCO_3$ Odor control	Electrolyte replacement: K, Na, $NaHCO_3$, Mg, Ca Vitamins, especially K minerals B_{12}
Psychosocial	
Promote self-image Refer to Ostomy Club	Promote self-image Refer to Ostomy Club

or sigmoid colostomy, a drainable pouch with an appropriate skin barrier is necessary. Once bowel control is reestablished a small, closed-ended pouch or dome may be used to cover the stoma.

A loop colostomy is often performed in the transverse or ascending colon to allow the remaining portion of the colon to rest. This type of colostomy is usually temporary. The surgical procedure for a loop colostomy requires the surgeon to lift a loop of healthy bowel through the abdominal wall and to place a rod of some type behind the loop to stabilize the bowel on the abdomen. During the surgery or shortly afterward, the surgeon opens the loop to allow fecal elimination. When the bowel adheres to the abdominal wall, usually 5–7 days after the operation, the surgeon removes the rod.

A double-barrel colostomy, which may also be temporary, is one that has two stomas. The proximal stoma, which connects to the rest of the digestive tract, is the functioning part of the colostomy. The distal stoma, which connects to the rectum, is the nonfunctioning part of the colostomy. The proximal stoma discharges fecal material, while the distal stoma discharges mucus. Irrigation procedures are not usually taught to clients with a temporary colostomy.

An end colostomy has only one stoma, which originates from the proximal portion of the bowel. The distal end of the colon is either resected or is closed off with sutures and remains in the abdomen. When it remains in the abdomen it is referred to as an end colostomy and Hartmann's Pouch.

NURSING DIAGNOSES

The following nursing diagnoses may be appropriate to include in a client care plan when the components are related to alterations in bowel elimination.

NURSING DIAGNOSIS	RELATED FACTORS
Body Image Disturbance	Presence of stoma, fear of rejection, psychosocial factors
Colonic Constipation	Inadequate intake of fluid or bulk, decreased exercise, disease states, medication, personal habits
Ineffective Denial	Change in body image secondary to stoma, ostomy care, disease process
Diarrhea	Nutritional intake, medication, disease state
Anticipatory Grieving	Loss of body contiguity, operative procedure (colostomy, ileostomy)
Altered Health Maintenance	Cognitive impairment, depression, immobility, cultural beliefs, lack of social support
Impaired Skin Integrity	Skin irritation or breakdown, poor pouching techniques, incontinence or diarrhea, poor-fitting equipment, economic situation
Noncompliance	Inability to manage equipment, impaired manual dexterity, poor vision

unit 1

RECTAL TUBE INSERTION

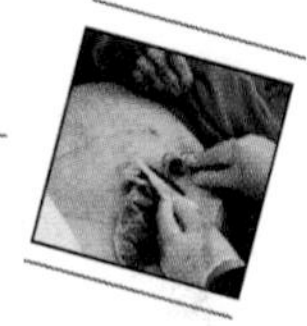

NURSING PROCESS DATA

ASSESSMENT Data Base

Palpate client's abdomen to determine the degree of abdominal distention. May need to measure abdominal girth.

Assess discomfort caused by flatulence.

Note quality and rate of respirations and pulse.

Note the presence or absence of hemorrhoids.

Assess condition of perianal skin.

PLANNING Objectives

To promote removal of flatulence in the digestive tract following abdominal surgery

To promote removal of flatulence that occurs with excessive swallowing of air

To stimulate expulsion of flatus in the lower digestive tract

To prevent abdominal distention caused by flatulence, which can interfere with diaphragmatic muscle contraction and cause dyspnea

To manage continuous diarrhea

IMPLEMENTATION Procedure

Inserting a Rectal Tube

EVALUATION Expected Outcomes

Abdominal distention is relieved, and comfort increased.

Dyspnea is relieved if flatulence has caused respiratory distress.

Flatus is removed from lower gastrointestinal tract.

Stool contained; skin and wound are not contaminated.

INSERTING A RECTAL TUBE

Equipment

Rectal tube: size 22–24 straight (French) for adults and size 12–18 French for children

Small plastic bag or stool specimen container

Hypoallergenic paper tape

Water-soluble lubricant

Bed protector

Clean gloves

Procedure

1. Check physician's orders and client care plan.
2. Wash your hands.
3. Gather equipment.
4. Identify the correct client, and explain the procedure.
5. Provide privacy. Place client on left side in a recumbent position and drape. **Rationale:** This position facilitates insertion of tube following the normal curve of rectum and sigmoid colon.
6. Place bed protector under client.
7. Tape the plastic bag around the distal end of the rectal tube or insert the tube into the stool specimen container.
8. Vent the upper side of the plastic bag to prevent inflation.
9. Don gloves.
10. Lubricate the proximal end of the rectal tube with water-soluble lubricant.
11. Gently separate buttocks, and ask client to take in

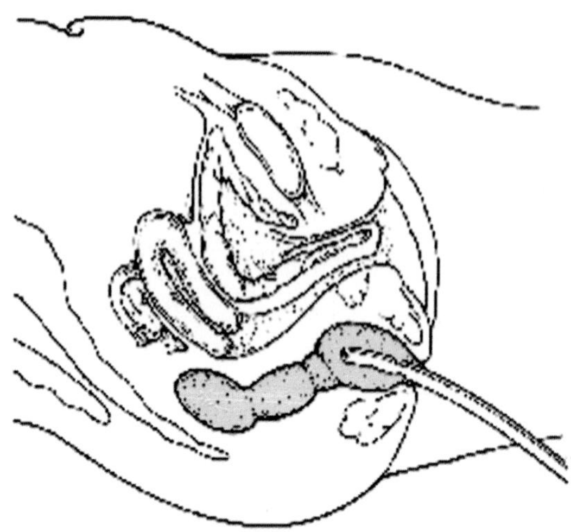
Insert rectal tube past the external and internal anal sphincters.

a deep breath. Gently insert the tube into the client's rectum, past the external and internal anal sphincters (2–4 inches in adults, 1–3 inches in children). **Rationale:** Taking a deep breath relaxes the anal sphincter and prevents tissue trauma during tube insertion.

12. With adults, gently tape the tube in place, using hypoallergenic paper tape. With children, hold the tube in place manually.
13. Take client's pulse. **Rationale:** Alterations in pulse rate can indicate a vagal stimulation and the rectal tube may need to be removed. This can occur particularly in a client with a cardiac condition.
14. Leave the tube in place no longer than 20 minutes. **Rationale:** Prolonged stimulation of the anal sphincter may result in a loss of the neuromuscular response. The prolonged presence of a catheter may cause pressure necrosis of the mucosal surface.
15. Remove the tube, and provide perianal care as needed.
16. Help the client assume a comfortable position.
17. Clean the tubing, and replace in bathroom if to be reused. Remove and discard the plastic bag.
18. Instruct client that chewing gum, sucking on candy, drinking liquids through a straw, carbonated beverages, and smoking tend to promote the swallowing of air and increase abdominal distention.
19. Remove gloves, and wash your hands.

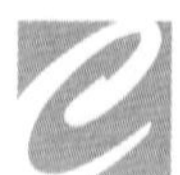

CHARTING for Rectal Tube Insertion

- Time rectal tube inserted, size of tube
- Amount, color, and consistency of feces collected
- Time rectal tube removed
- Presence, absence, or change in abdominal distention
- Client's reaction to procedure
- Any unexpected outcomes and measures taken to treat these outcomes
- Pulse rate before and during procedure

CRITICAL THINKING APPLICATION

CLINICAL PROBLEMS	CRITICAL THINKING OPTIONS
■ No relief of abdominal distention.	• Reposition client at an angle that raises the lower part of the body (e.g., in a prone position with the foot of the bed raised). • Instruct client to circle, raise, and lower his or her legs. • Reinsert the tube after 2–3 hours. • Remove the tube and check for feces that may be clogging the outlet. Clean tube, and reinsert.
■ Fecal impaction lower in rectum prevents insertion of rectal tube.	• Perform digital examination with gloved finger and water-soluble lubricant. Break up impaction if present. • Position client on left side in Fowler's position. • Reinsert the rectal tube.

unit 2

BOWEL EVACUATION

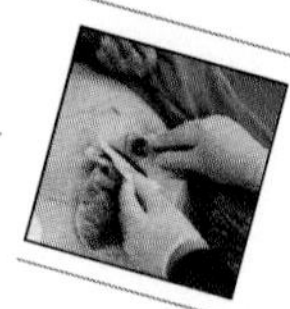

NURSING PROCESS DATA

ASSESSMENT Data Base

Evaluate client's diet.

- Amount of high-bulk foods.
- Amount of fluid intake daily.

Evaluate client's physical status.

- Ability to ambulate (i.e., spinal cord injury, CVA).
- Ability to perform bed exercises, abdominal exercises.
- Extent of disease process.

Assess effectiveness of drugs, such as stool softeners, bulk formers, suppositories.
Assess time of day client usually evacuates bowels.
Identify client's ability to adapt and psychologic readiness for the above program.
Identify position most effective for bowel evacuation.
Assess consistency and amount of stool for abnormal findings (diarrhea or fecal impaction).
Assess when client had last bowel movement.
Assess for abdominal distention.
Assess perianal area for tears, ulcerations, or excoriation.

PLANNING Objectives

To promote regular bowel evacuation
To prevent constipation
To remove a fecal impaction
To establish a bowel program to which the client can easily adapt
To develop a bowel program that the client can perform him or herself
To relieve pain and discomfort

IMPLEMENTATION Procedures

Removing a Fecal Impaction
Providing Digital Stimulation
Developing a Regular Bowel Routine
Administering a Suppository

EVALUATION Expected Outcomes

Client establishes regular bowel evacuation program.
Fecal impaction is removed.
Client is able to evacuate bowels at a convenient time.
Client is free of pain, flatus and discomfort.

REMOVING A FECAL IMPACTION

Equipment

Clean gloves, 2 or 3 pair
Water-soluble lubricant
Absorbent pad
Washcloth and towel
Bedpan
Basin of warm water

Preparation

1. Check physician's order for impaction removal if the client is at risk for possible complications from vagal stimulation (i.e., cardiac or spinal cord injured patient). **Rationale:** Vagal stimulation can result from manual removal of feces. It should be used only as a last resort and with specific physician's order. It causes a decreased pulse rate by decreasing conductivity at the sinoatrial (S-A) node and decreasing the rate of impulse firing at the node.
2. Gather equipment.
3. Identify the correct client, and explain procedure.
4. Provide privacy.
5. Wash your hands.

> ■ CLINICAL ALERT
>
> Some hypertonic tube feedings predispose clients to constipation and fecal impaction. Review formula ingredients if this occurs.

Procedure

1. Obtain baseline pulse and blood pressure.
2. Place client on left side with knees flexed.
3. Place absorbent pad on bed.
4. Place bedpan next to client's buttocks.
5. Don gloves, and lubricate fingers of dominant hand. You may want to double-glove dominant hand to prevent contamination if glove tears.
6. Ask client to take a deep breath and exhale slowly through the mouth as your index finger is gently inserted into rectum. **Rationale:** Encouraging breathing assists in relaxing the sphincter.
7. Gently remove the hardened stool.
8. Allow client to rest between digital removal if any untoward effects, such as palpitations or faintness, are exhibited.
9. Obtain vital signs if client complains of any discomfort.
10. When stool is removed, change gloves; wash and dry buttocks thoroughly.
11. Dispose of stool in toilet or send stool specimen to laboratory.
12. Clean bedpan, and replace in appropriate area.
13. Remove gloves, and wash your hands.
14. Position client for comfort.
15. Wash your hands.

PROVIDING DIGITAL STIMULATION

Equipment

Clean gloves, 1 or 2 pair
Lubricant
Bedpan or commode
Absorbent pad
Washcloth and towel
Medication if ordered

> ■ CLINICAL ALERT
>
> Digital stimulation, given ½ hour after dinner or breakfast, is usually required for spinal cord-injured clients.

Procedure

1. Check physician's orders and client care plan.
2. Gather equipment.
3. Identify the correct client, and explain procedure.
4. Provide privacy.
5. Place client in position for bowel evacuation (bedpan, commode, toilet).
6. Don gloves, and lubricate fingers of nondominant hand. You may want to double-glove to prevent contamination if gloves tear.
7. Insert finger into rectum 1½–2 inches.
8. Move your finger from side to side in a circular motion to slightly stretch the rectal wall. Move toward the spine and not the bladder to prevent injury to the bladder.
9. Continue stretching the rectal wall for 1–3 minutes until the internal sphincter muscle relaxes.
10. Work with client to discover an associated stimulus to help establish a good bowel routine. **Rationale:** Abdominal massage, coughing, deep inhalations, and tightening of abdominal muscles, in conjunction with digital stimulation, assist in bowel evacuation.
11. Repeat digital stimulation for 1–3 minutes at 5-

minute intervals up to 20 minutes if a bowel movement does not occur.

12. After bowel evacuation occurs, assist the client with cleaning and drying perineum.
13. Remove equipment from room.
14. Wash equipment, and return to storage area.
15. Discard gloves, and wash hands.
16. Position the client for comfort.

DEVELOPING A REGULAR BOWEL ROUTINE

Equipment

Clean gloves, 1 or 2 pair
Lubricant
Bedpan or commode
Absorbent pad
Specific enema if ordered
Washcloth and towel

Preparation

1. Check physician's orders and client care plan.
2. Identify the correct client, and explain procedure.
3. Identify time of day client usually evacuates bowels.
4. Evaluate diet, exercise, former use of medications for bowel evacuation.
5. Administer the following drugs as ordered:
   a. Stool softener—(Colace or Parlax)—daily.
   b. Bulk former—(Metamucil)—q.d. to t.i.d.
   c. Mild laxative (Senokot, Doxidan)—8 hours before program.
   d. Suppository (glycerin or Dulcolax) just before digital stimulation.
6. Wash your hands.

Procedure

1. Don gloves. You may want to double-glove to prevent contamination if glove tears.
2. Perform digital stimulation $\frac{1}{2}$ hour after dinner or breakfast (see previous intervention).
3. Place client on toilet or commode. (Use bedpan if client is on bed rest.)
4. Remove gloves.
5. Wash your hands.
6. Provide privacy and sufficient time for evacuation.
7. Don gloves.
8. Wash and dry perineal area if client is unable to do so.
9. Remove gloves.
10. Place client in wheelchair or bed and position for comfort.
11. Wash your hands.
12. Wean client away from suppositories and laxatives when spontaneous bowel movements occur with digital stimulation.

BOWEL TRAINING

Good bowel training programs include

- Initiation of defecation on demand with digital stimulation and abdominal massage
- Evacuation at same time each day
- Proper diet
- Daily physical exercise regimen
- Client and family education

ADMINISTERING A SUPPOSITORY

Equipment

Clean gloves
Lubricant
Bedpan or commode
Absorbent pad (optional)
Suppository as ordered
Washcloth and towel
Paper towel

Procedure

1. Check physician's orders and client care plan.
2. Wash your hands.
3. Gather equipment.
4. Identify the correct client, and explain procedure.

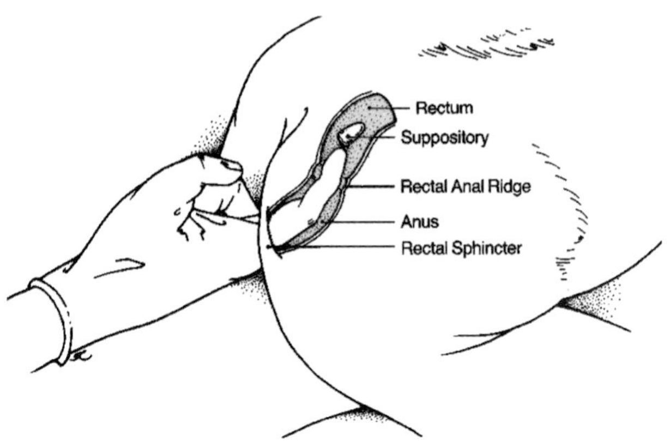

Insert rectal suppositories beyond the rectal–anal ridge for retention.

5. Provide privacy. Place client in Sims' position.
6. Place bed protector on bed if necessary.
7. Don gloves, lubricate fingers of nondominant hand.
8. Place small amount of lubricant on paper towel.
9. Open suppository foil; lubricate tip of suppository.
10. Insert suppository (usually glycerin) with pointed end first, and place high in rectum beyond external and internal sphincters. **Rationale:** This prevents expulsion of suppository.
11. Push the suppository against the side of the rectal wall. Ensure it is not placed into fecal mass. **Rationale:** It is ineffective if placed in feces as it cannot be absorbed.
12. Place client on toilet or commode.
13. If bowel movement does not occur in 20 minutes, perform digital stimulation.
14. Repeat with stronger suppository if ordered (Dulcolax) after 20 minutes if there are no results.
15. Allow client to retain Dulcolax suppository for 20 minutes. If no results, do digital stimulation again.
16. Following bowel evacuation, cleanse and dry perineal area.
17. Remove gloves, and wash your hands.
18. Position client in wheelchair or bed.

■ CLINICAL ALERT

If client has a spinal cord injury, observe for signs of autonomic hyperreflexia (goose pimples, pounding headache, hypertension, perspiration above level of spinal cord injury).

If signs and symptoms of autonomic hyperreflexia occur, discontinue digital stimulation, apply Nupercainal and Xylocaine ointment around anus and rectum as ordered. This anesthetizes the area and decreases the stimulation that caused the response. Wait 10 minutes for symptoms to decrease, and then gently remove the feces.

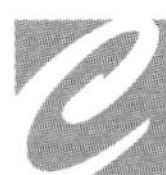

CHARTING for Regular Bowel Evacuation

- Type and number of suppositories used
- Digital stimulation used
- Approximate time used for digital stimulation
- Amount, consistency, characteristics of stool
- Protocol for bowel evacuation for client
- Untoward complications of bowel training
- Nursing interventions needed to correct complications

CRITICAL THINKING APPLICATION

CLINICAL PROBLEMS	CRITICAL THINKING OPTIONS
When digital stimulation is performed, client exhibits reflex spasm that prevents stool expulsion.	• Apply local anesthetic around rectum and anus, if ordered. • Wait for spasm to relax, and then proceed with stimulation.
Client develops diarrhea.	• Identify possible cause of diarrhea. • Observe dietary intake for possible cause. Provide for bulk. • Hold the laxatives and stool softeners temporarily. • Instruct client to eat yogurt and drink milk if not contraindicated by condition. • Inform physician of diarrhea and obtain orders for Kaopectate. Administer 2 teaspoons after each loose stool for 24 hours. • Check with physician if medications should be readjusted for bowel training as needed.
Client exhibits signs and symptoms of vagal response during removal of fecal impaction.	• Immediately discontinue procedure. • Place client in shock position. • Monitor vital signs every 5–15 minutes until condition is stable. • Notify physician of findings and request medication order for antispasmodic such as atropine. • Be prepared for "Code" situation, even though it is not likely to occur.
Effective bowel evacuation program is not established.	• Ask dietitian for altered diet (including more fruits and vegetables). • Check if client can have fluids increased to 3000 mL daily. • Obtain order from the physician to administer stool softeners and bulk formers in greater quantity. • Have client increase physical activity, especially exercise of the abdominal muscles if not contraindicated by condition. • Ensure that client begins bowel training program ½ hour after a meal.

unit 3

ENEMA ADMINISTRATION

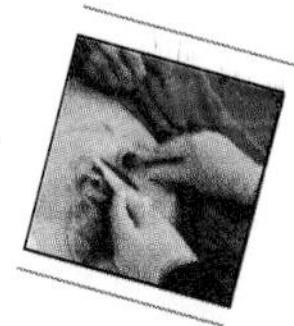

NURSING PROCESS DATA

ASSESSMENT Data Base

Review client's present and past eliminatory status.

Assess the need for an enema.

Evaluate amount of solution a client can tolerate.

Assess if fecal impaction is present.

Assess the degree of abdominal distention.

Assess degree of sphincter control.

Assess current medical regimen.

Assess dietary history.

Assess vital signs before and after procedure, as necessary.

PLANNING Objectives

To relieve constipation.

To relieve fecal impactions.

To cleanse the bowel prior to surgery, childbirth, or diagnostic examination.

To evacuate the bowel in clients with neurologic dysfunction.

To provide nutrients.

To introduce an exchange resin.

To relieve abdominal distention.

To stimulate peristalsis.

IMPLEMENTATION Procedures

Administering an Enema.

Administering an Enema to a Child.

Administering a Disposable Enema (Fleet's).

Administering a Retention Enema.

Administering a Harris Flush Enema.

EVALUATION Expected Outcomes

Client experiences increased comfort and relief from abdominal distention.

Returns are clear if preparing client for diagnostic examination or surgery.

Relief obtained from fecal impaction.

Return of solution plus formed, soft feces is complete.

ADMINISTERING AN ENEMA

Equipment

Fluid container with attached rectal tube (size 22–32, straight, or French, for adults)

Normal saline, tap water, soap solution

Water-soluble lubricant

Clean bedpan with cover; bed protector

Skin care items (e.g., soap, water, towels)

Clean gloves

Preparation

1. Check physician's orders and client care plan.
2. Gather equipment.

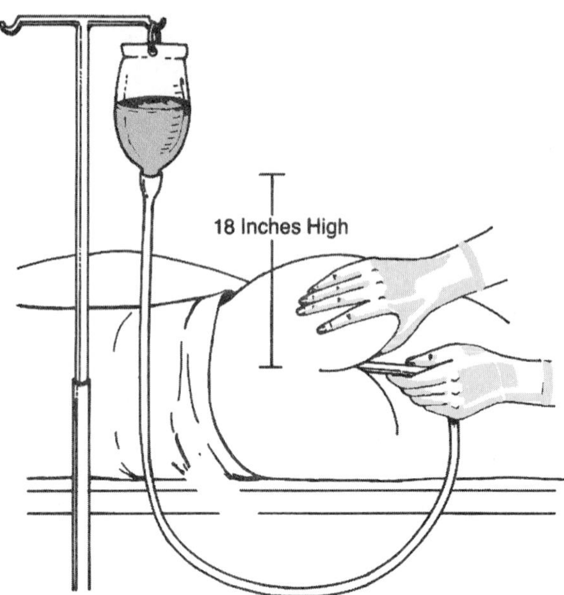

Place enema solution container no more than 18 inches above rectum for safety.

3. Identify correct client and explain the procedure. Explain the benefits of relaxing and taking periodic deep breaths.
4. Provide privacy.
5. Wash your hands, and don gloves.

Procedure

1. Fill water container with 750–1000 mL of lukewarm solution, 105–110°F. **Rationale:** Solutions that are too hot or too cold or solutions that are instilled too quickly can cause cramping, damage to rectal tissues, and extreme shock.
2. Allow solution to run through the tubing so that air is removed. Clamp tube. **Rationale:** If air is instilled during the procedure, the client experiences discomfort as a result of distension of the colon.
3. Hang container on IV pole next to bed.
4. Raise bed to HIGH position, and lower side rails on side where you will be working.
5. Don gloves.
6. Place bed protector under client.
7. Place bedpan within easy reach.
8. Place client on left side in Sims' position.
9. Provide privacy, and drape client.

TABLE 22–2. Enema Administration

Fluid Volumes (mL)

Infant	150–250
Toddler	250–350
Child	300–500
Adolescent	500–750
Adult	750–1000

Types of Enemas

Cleansing

Stimulates peristalsis through irritation of colon and rectum and by distention. Agents: Soap suds, tap water, and saline.

Soap suds: Mild soap solutions stimulate and irritate intestinal mucosa. Strong soap solutions can cause severe irritation of the mucous membrane of the colon. Dilute 5 mL of castile soap in 1000 mL of water.

Tap water: Give with caution to infants or to adults with altered cardiac and renal reserve. Tap water is a hypotonic solution.

Saline: For normal saline enemas, use a smaller volume of solution. Hypertonic solutions draw fluid into the colon from the body tissues. These solutions are mildly irritating to the mucous membrane of the colon.

Retention

Solution or nutrient is retained for specified time. Agents: mineral, olive, cottonseed oil, liquid petrolatum. Nutrient agent: dextrose solution.

Emollient (Oil): Lubricates the rectum and colon protecting the intestinal mucous membrane. Feces absorb oil and become softer and easier to expel. Client retains enema for several hours.

Nutritive: Provides nourishment in temporary or emergency situations. Enema is retained.

Distention Reduction

Provides relief from flatus causing distention. It improves ability to expel flatus. Types: carminative and return flow.

Carminative: Two common types include; 1-2-3 enema (30 gm of magnesium sulfate, 60 g of glycerin, and 90 mL warm water) and milk and molasses (180–240 mL of equal amounts).

Return flow: Harris flush most common. Mild colonic irrigation using 100–200 mL of enema solution. After instillation, enema container is lowered and solution siphoned back into container.

Medicated

Enemas containing drugs used for reducing bacteria or removing potassium. Agents: Kayexalate and neomycin.

Kayexalate: A resin is introduced into the large intestine removing the excess potassium by exchanging it for sodium ions.

Neomycin: Antibiotic solution used to reduce bacteria prior to bowel surgery.

10. Lubricate tip of tubing with generous amount of water-soluble lubricant.
11. Gently spread buttocks, instruct client to take slow breath, and insert tubing.
12. Raise the solution container to a maximum height of 18 inches.
13. Allow solution to flow slowly. **Rationale:** If the flow is slow, the client experiences fewer cramps. The client will also is able to tolerate and retain a greater volume of solution.
14. Hold the tubing in place in the client's rectum at all times. Keep a bedpan nearby.
15. Lower solution container or momentarily clamp tubing if client experiences cramping, is unable to retain solution, or exhibits anxiety. Resume infusion of solution after a few minutes.
16. After you have instilled the solution, gently remove the tubing. Instruct client to hold solution for 10–15 minutes.
17. Clean and dispose of equipment.
18. Remove gloves, and wash hands.
19. Elevate the head of the bed so that the client can assume a squatting position on the bedpan, or assist to bathroom.
20. Provide privacy until the client has expelled the total volume of the instilled solution.
21. Don clean gloves.
22. Remove bedpan, and immediately empty, clean, and replace to proper storage area.
23. Assist client with perineal care, and help client to assume a comfortable position.
24. If client is on strict I&O, measure returns to make sure total volume of the solution is expelled.
25. Remove gloves and wash your hands.

ADMINISTERING AN ENEMA TO A CHILD

Equipment

Water container with attached rectal tube (size 14–18 straight [French] for children, and size-12 French or infant enema syringe with bulb for infants)

Normal saline, tap water, soap solution

Water-soluble lubricant

Clean potty chair for children

Bed protector

Skin care items (e.g., soap, water, towels)

Clean gloves

Preparation

1. Check physician's orders and client care plan.
2. Gather equipment.
3. Provide privacy for child.
4. Wash your hands.
5. Identify correct client, and explain procedure to child or family. Take time to calm a frightened child and to answer the child's questions.

Procedure

1. Fill water container with 100°F solution (500 mL or less for child, 250 mL for an infant).
2. Allow solution to run through the tubing so that air is removed.
3. Hang solution container on IV pole.
4. Place bed protector under child.
5. Place child on left side or in knee–chest position.
6. Don clean gloves.
7. Lubricate tip of tubing or infant enema syringe with bulb.
8. Gently separate buttocks and insert catheter or syringe into child's rectum (1 - $1\frac{1}{2}$ inches for infants, 2–3 inches for children).
9. Elevate solution container no more than 12–18 inches. **Rationale:** Height increases pressure of solution entering colon—too much pressure may damage colon.
10. Allow solution to flow slowly for 10–15 minutes.
11. After you have instilled the solution, gently remove the tubing or syringe.
12. Hold child's buttocks together or tape them with hypoallergenic paper tape. If child is toilet trained, place a potty chair nearby.
13. Retain solution 10–15 minutes for cleansing enemas.
14. Place the child on a potty chair or bedpan to expel solution.
15. If there are no contraindications, you may gently

massage child's abdomen to help child expel returns.

16. If the child wants to be left alone while expelling returns, provide privacy. Child should expel the total volume of the instilled solution.
17. Remove the potty chair or bedpan.
18. Clean the child's perineal area, and help child assume a comfortable position.
19. Estimate returns to determine that the child expelled the total volume of the solution.
20. Clean all equipment, and replace in appropriate area.
21. Remove gloves, and wash your hands.

ADMINISTERING A DISPOSABLE ENEMA (FLEET'S)

Equipment

Commercially prepared enema
Water-soluble lubricant
Bedpan or commode
Clean gloves
Bed protector
Skin care items (e.g., soap, water, towels)

Preparation

1. Check physician's orders and client care plan.
2. Gather equipment.
3. Wash your hands.
4. Identify correct client and explain the procedure. Explain the benefits of relaxing and taking periodic deep breaths.
5. Place bed protector under client.
6. Place client on left side in a Sims' position.
7. Provide privacy.
8. Don clean gloves.

Procedure

1. Read directions on enema container.
2. Lubricate with water-soluble lubricant if necessary. (Usually rectal tube is self-lubricated.)
3. Expose the anal opening to assist you in inserting the tube without traumatizing the tissue.
4. After inserting rectal tube, squeeze the container, and empty entire 120 mL of hypertonic solution.
5. Instruct client to hold solution 5–7 minutes.
6. When ready to expel solution elevate the head of the bed so that the client can assume a squatting position on the bedpan. If able, client may expel solution in toilet.
7. Provide privacy until the client has expelled the total volume of the instilled solution.
8. Remove and cover bedpan.
9. Assist client with perineal care, and help client to assume a comfortable position.
10. Measure returns if on strict I&O.
11. Dispose of equipment, and remove gloves.
12. Wash your hands.

ADMINISTERING A RETENTION ENEMA

Equipment

Commercially prepared disposable oil retention enema
Oil: adult 150–200 mL, child 75–100 mL, 91°F
Water soluble lubricant
Bedpan or commode
Bed protector
Skin care items (e.g., soap, water, towels)
Clean gloves

Procedure

1. Identify and prepare client as for any enema.
2. Disposable oil retention enema is administered like a disposable Fleet's enema. Read directions on enema container.
3. Don clean gloves.
4. Expose anal opening, and gently insert rectal tube tip of container 3–4 inches. Commercially prepared enemas are prelubricated.
5. Squeeze contents slowly, and empty entire amount into rectum.

6. Remove rectal tube gently.
7. Discard equipment, following universal precautions.
8. Explain to client that oil should be retained for 1–3 hours before it is expelled. **Rationale:** Purpose of enema is to soften stool.
9. A cleansing enema may need to be given to remove oil and stimulate defecation.

ADMINISTERING A HARRIS FLUSH ENEMA

Equipment

Fluid container with attached rectal tube
Normal saline or tap water heated to 105–110°F
Water-soluble lubricant
Clean bedpan
Bed protector
Skin care items (e.g., soap, water, towels)
Clean gloves

Preparation

1. Check physician's orders and client care plan.
2. Gather equipment.
3. Provide privacy.
4. Wash your hands.
5. Check identaband.
6. Fill fluid container with 100–200 mL of ordered solution; check that temperature is between 105–110°F.
7. Allow solution to run through tubing so that air is removed. **Rationale:** If air is instilled during procedure, client experiences discomfort.
8. Hang on IV pole.

Procedure

1. Explain procedure to client. Explain the benefits of relaxing and taking periodic deep breaths during procedure.
2. Raise bed to HIGH position, and lower side rails.
3. Don gloves.
4. Place bed protector under client.
5. Place client on left side in a Sims' position. **Rationale:** This position facilitates instillation of fluid.
6. Lubricate tip of tubing with water-soluble lubricant.
7. Gently spread buttocks, and insert tubing 3–4 inches into client's rectum, past external and internal sphincters. Avoid traumatizing hemorrhoids during insertion. **Rationale:** Vagal nerve stimulation from enemas, digital examination, or rectal tube placement may cause cardiac arrhythmias.
8. Raise water container to a maximum height of 18 inches above bed.
9. Allow solution to flow slowly into rectum and sigmoid colon. If cramping occurs, clamp tube for a few minutes and then continue infusion.
10. Lower solution container below level of rectum and allow all fluid to flow back into container.
11. Raise container 18 inches above rectum and allow solution to flow back into rectum.
12. Repeat inflow–outflow process 5–6 times, changing solution when it becomes thick with feces. **Rationale:** This assists in stimulating intestinal peristalsis with expulsion of flatus.
13. Provide privacy until client has expelled total volume of instilled solution following last inflow–outflow series.
14. Assist client with perineal care, and help client assume a comfortable position.
15. If client is on strict I&O, measure returns to make sure total volume of solution is expelled.
16. Clean all equipment, and replace in bathroom or appropriate location.
17. Remove gloves, and wash your hands.

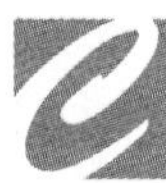

CHARTING for Administering an Enema

- Time enema given
- Volume and type of solution used
- Results obtained: amount, consistency, and color
- Any unexpected outcomes and measures taken to remedy problems
- Client's reactions to procedure
- Relief of flatus

CRITICAL THINKING APPLICATION

CLINICAL PROBLEMS	CRITICAL THINKING OPTIONS
■ Client expels solution prematurely.	• Calm and ease client's distress by reassuring him or her as you clean the equipment. • Place bedpan under client. Place client in semi-Fowler's position with knees flexed. • Hold the rectal tube in client's rectum between thighs. Slow the water flow, and continue with the enema.
■ Client complains of severe and sudden abdominal pain, nausea, and distention.	• Remove tubing, and notify physician immediately of possible perforation. • Assess vital signs. If you suspect cardiac dysrhythmias, remove bedpan and notify physician immediately. • Be prepared to administer emergency drugs, such as atropine. • If an IV is not in place, start an IV of 5% dextrose in water (D_5W) using a large-bore needle for emergency use.
■ The flow of water is impeded or an obstruction is felt.	• Open clamp on tubing. Allow a small amount of solution to flow. (The warm solution may help relax the internal sphincter.) • Withdraw tube slightly, and reinsert. • Gently perform a digital examination for the possibility of fecal impaction. Break up impaction if present. Ask physician for order to give a retention enema, followed by a cleansing enema 2–3 hours later.
■ Client cannot return enema solution.	• Gently massage client's abdomen if not contraindicated. • Replace rectal tube. Lower the enema bag below the level of the bed. • If client is not uncomfortable, do nothing. If client complains of discomfort or pain, notify physician.
■ Enema returns are not clear prior to surgery or diagnostic testing.	• Repeat enema. If, after three enemas, returns are still not clear, notify physician of findings. • May need to give an enema with a stronger solution.
■ Fecal impaction is not relieved.	• Check orders for oil retention enema. • Check catheter size needed. • Obtain order for and use digital stimulation and manual extraction of feces if not contraindicated by diagnosis of cardiac or neurologic involvement.

unit 4

COLOSTOMY IRRIGATIONS

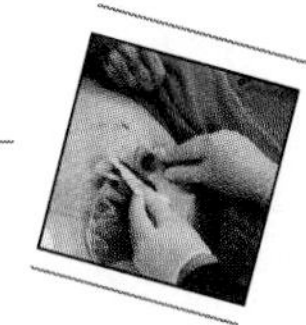

NURSING PROCESS DATA

ASSESSMENT Data Base

Assess types of colostomy, double barrel, single barrel.
Assess the permanence of the colostomy and client's prognosis.
Identify the location of the colostomy along the large intestine.
Assess bowel sounds.
Check abdomen for distention.
Assess for stomal complications (i.e., peristomal hernia, stenosed stoma, or prolapsed stoma).
Note any presence of disease in the client's bowel.
Assess the client's ability to sit for a prolonged period.
Note client's age and bowel habits prior to surgery.
Assess client's feelings about colostomy management.
Assess the client's mental alertness and ability to learn.
Assess time of bowel evacuation before surgery.
Check pulse and blood pressure before procedure.

PLANNING Objectives

To manage regular bowel elimination.
To evacuate stool from the colon.
To assist client to develop a positive attitude toward living with a colostomy.
To assist client to become proficient in colostomy care.

IMPLEMENTATION Procedures

Performing a Colostomy Irrigation.
Performing Irrigation in Bed.

EVALUATION Expected Outcomes

Complete return of solution plus soft or formed feces.
Bowel elimination is regulated.
Client develops positive attitude toward living with a colostomy.
Client becomes proficient in colostomy care.
Pulse and blood pressure remain within normal limits during procedure.

PERFORMING A COLOSTOMY IRRIGATION

Equipment

Solution container with 1000 mL warm water
Irrigating tubing with cone
Three pairs of clean gloves
Irrigating sleeve cut long enough to reach water level in toilet
Items to clean skin and stoma (e.g., wash cloths or gauze sponges)
Plastic bag for disposal of used pouch
Clean pouch and closure device
Skin barriers
Water-soluble lubricant
IV pole

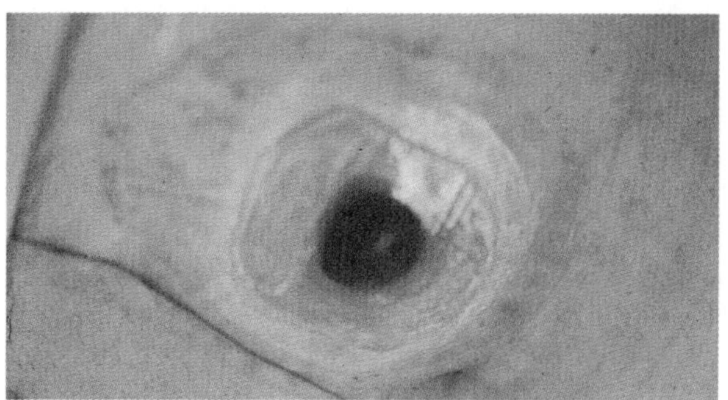

Ileostomy.

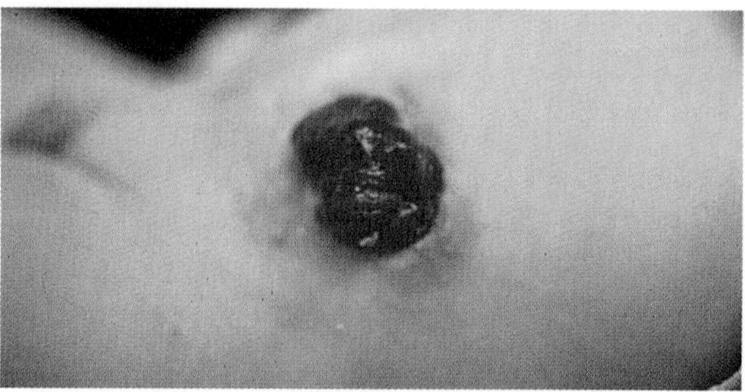

Transverse colostomy.

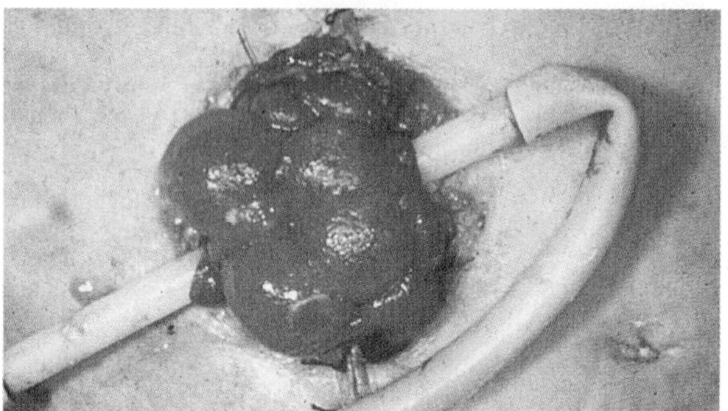

Transverse loop colostomy with rod.

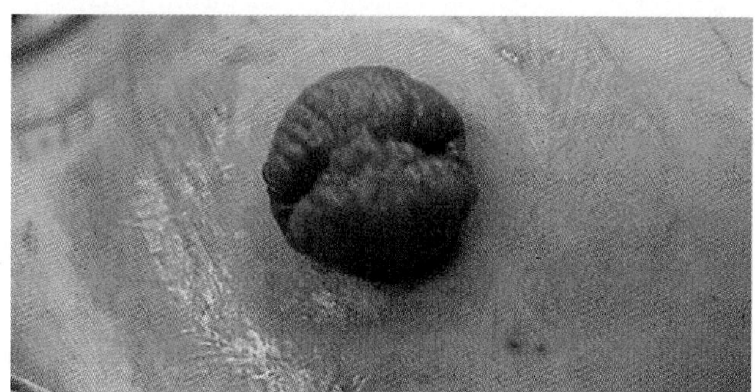

Loop colostomy.

Preparation

1. Check physician's orders and client care plan. Irrigations can be daily or every other day.
2. Wash hands.
3. Gather equipment.
4. Provide privacy.

Procedure

1. Check identaband, and explain procedure to client.
2. Explain benefits of relaxing and taking periodic deep breaths.
3. Don clean gloves.
4. Remove and dispose of used pouch in plastic bag.
5. Clean stoma and skin with warm water and soft cloth. Assess skin for signs of irrigation or breakdown.
6. Apply irrigation sleeve to peristomal skin, and place belt around waist.
7. Fill container with 1000 mL lukewarm water (500 mL for first irrigation). **Rationale:** Lukewarm water temperature is 105–110°F. This temperature prevents injury from hot solutions and cramping from cold solutions.
8. Suspend container on bathroom hook or IV pole at level of client's shoulders.
9. Open roller clamp and allow solution to run through tubing; close clamp. **Rationale:** This removes air from tubing and prevents discomfort for client.
10. Assist client to sit on toilet or on chair in front of toilet.
11. Place sleeve between client's thighs and direct end into toilet.
12. Lubricate cone tip with water-soluble lubricant.
13. Position cone in sleeve by placing through top opening. If cone cannot be inserted easily do not force it.
14. Hold cone snugly against stoma. **Rationale:** This prevents back flow of solution.
15. Open roller clamp on tubing and allow water to run through cone while inserting cone into stoma.
16. Instill solution (1000 mL) over 5–10 minutes. **Rationale:** The container height and rate of water flow affects results obtained. If client complains of feeling light-headed or has vertigo, take pulse and stop instillation. **Rationale:** These are symptoms of a vagal response.

■ CLINICAL ALERT

A distended colon can cause a vagal response resulting in hypotension, bradycardia, and even loss of consciousness.

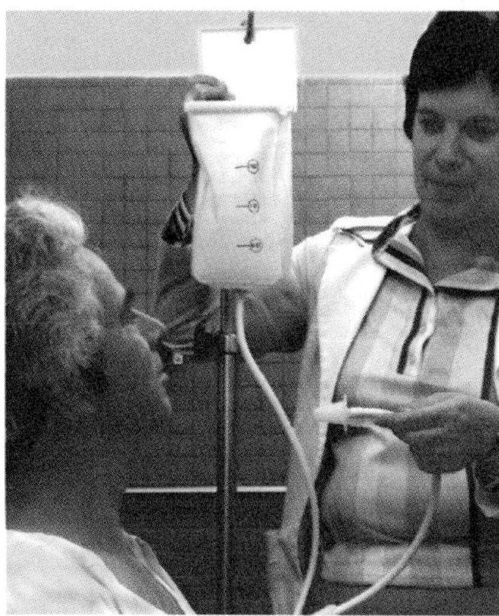

Establishing a nurse-client relationship supports client while learning colostomy care.

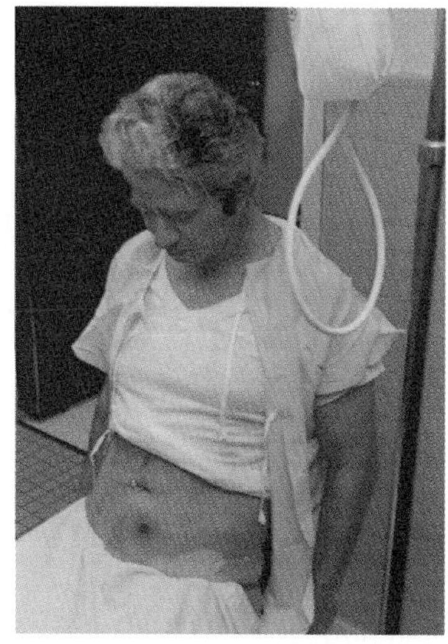

Encourage client to look at stoma and participate in care.

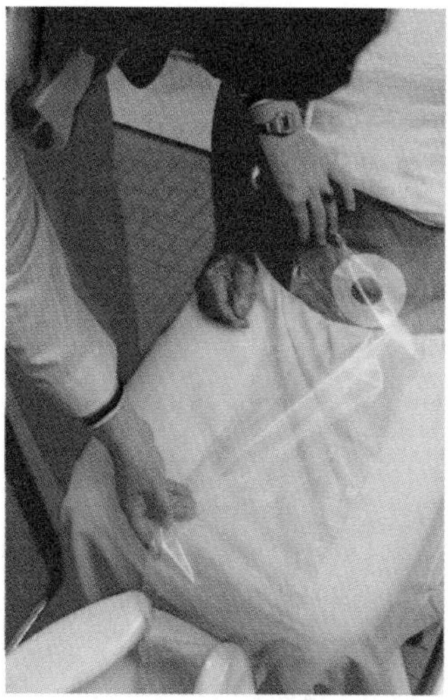

Place sleeve between client's thighs and place end in toilet.

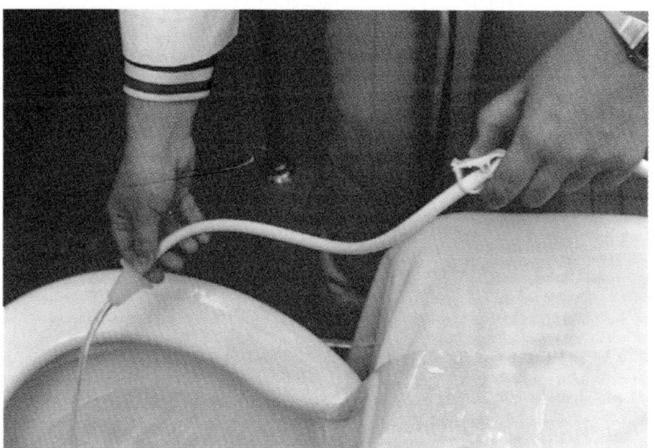

Open clamp and allow fluid to run through tubing to cone.

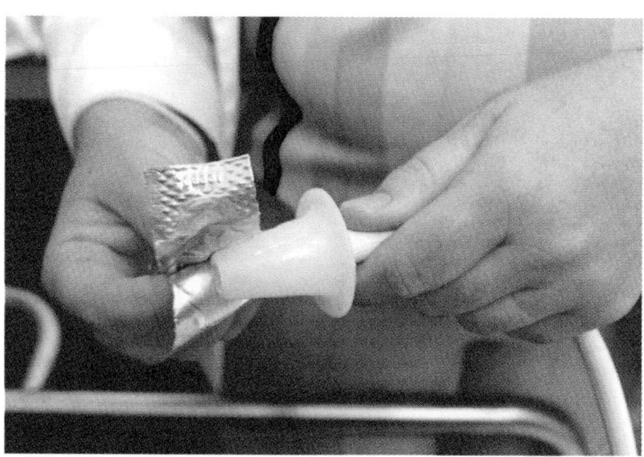

Lubricate cone tip with water-soluble lubricant.

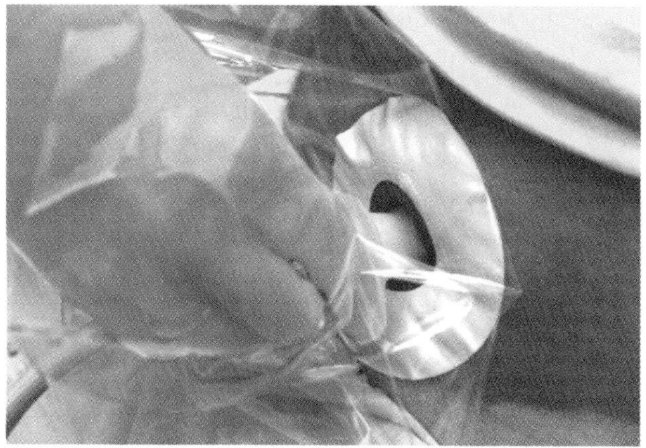

Place cone through top opening of sleeve.

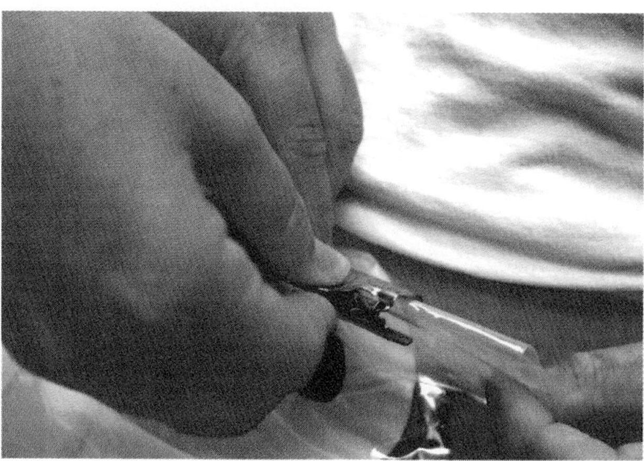

Fold sleeve over and close with clamp.

17. Clamp tubing for a few minutes if cramping occurs. Instruct client to take a deep breath when solution is instilled. **Rationale:** Deep breathing relaxes abdominal muscles.
18. Remove cone, and close off or fold over top of sleeve after solution is instilled.
19. Allow client to remain seated while the majority of stool and solution return, usually 10–15 minutes.
20. Remove gloves, and discard.
21. Don clean gloves.
22. Rinse sleeve with water. Dry bottom of sleeve and close end of sleeve.
23. Remove gloves.
24. Ask client to wear sleeve in this manner for 30–60 minutes. Client may return to bed, walk around, or proceed with other activities during this time. **Rationale:** This provides additional time for expelling solution or feces and thus prevents accidental evacuation.
25. Don clean gloves.
26. Remove sleeve, clean, and store for client's use.
27. Clean client's skin and stoma with warm water, and dry thoroughly.
28. Apply skin barriers, and clean pouch.
29. Remove gloves, and wash your hands.
30. Put away all supplies, and reorder as needed.

■ CLINICAL ALERT

The danger of perforation of the colon is much greater when irrigating a colostomy with a catheter. The use of an irrigation cone results in safer administration and better water flow.

PERFORMING IRRIGATION IN BED

Equipment

Water container with cone

Water at 105–110°F (500 mL for the first irrigation; 1000 mL thereafter)

Irrigating sleeve cut long enough to reach bedpan on chair at bedside

Items to clean skin and stoma (e.g., wash cloths or gauze sponges)

Plastic bag for disposal of old pouch

Clean pouch and closure device

Skin barriers

Water-soluble lubricant

IV pole

Bedpan

Chair

2 Bed protectors

Three pairs of clean gloves

Preparation

1. Check physician's orders and client care plan.
2. Wash hands.
3. Gather equipment.
4. Provide privacy.

Procedure

1. Identify and explain procedure to client. First irrigation is usually performed in bed.
2. Position client comfortably in bed, using side-lying position. **Rationale:** This position facilitates drainage into bedpan.
3. Place bed protector on bed.
4. Don clean gloves.
5. Close off the bottom of the irrigation sleeve and allow it to rest in a bedpan at the client's side.
6. Remove and dispose of used pouch in plastic bag.
7. Clean stoma and skin with warm water and soft cloth.
8. Apply irrigation sleeve to peristomal area.
9. Fill container with 500–1000 mL lukewarm water. **Rationale:** Water that is too hot can cause vertigo.
10. Suspend container on IV pole.
11. Remove air from tubing.
12. Place bedpan on chair by bedside. Place bed protector under bedpan to prevent soiling chair.
13. Place sleeve in bedpan.
14. Lubricate cone tip with water-soluble lubricant.
15. Follow steps 13–18 for *Performing a Colostomy Irrigation.*
16. Remove gloves, and discard.
17. Wait 55–60 minutes to allow most of the irrigation fluid to return.
18. Don clean gloves.
19. Open bottom of sleeve into bedpan.
20. Remove sleeve, clean, and return to storage place.
21. Clean client's skin and stoma with warm water, and dry thoroughly.

22. Apply appropriate pouch and skin barriers.
23. Remove and discard gloves.
24. Place client in a comfortable position.
25. Wash your hands.
26. Put away all supplies, and reorder as necessary.

CHARTING for Colostomy Irrigation

- Time irrigation administered
- Amount and type of solution used
- Results obtained; amount, color, and consistency of returns
- Place where irrigation occurred: bathroom or bed.
- Condition and color of stoma (it should be healthy red)
- Condition of peristomal skin
- Pouch application
- Extent of client participation
- Client's reaction to procedure

CRITICAL THINKING APPLICATION

CLINICAL PROBLEMS	CRITICAL THINKING OPTIONS
Stool leaks out under irrigation sleeve.	• Secure belt to sleeve. • Ensure skin is dry before applying sleeve. • Flatten abdomen before applying sleeve. • Use self-adhering irrigating pouch. • Reposition client.
Water does not flow easily into colostomy stoma.	• Change angle or position of cone slightly. • Check for kinks in tubing from container. • Check height of water container. • Remove cone, stool may be expelled. • Ask client to relax and to take deep breaths. • Instill small amounts of water to loosen stool.
Client experiences cramping, nausea, or dizziness during irrigation.	• Stop flow of water, leaving cone or catheter in place. • Do not resume until cramping has passed. • Check water temperature. Water that is too hot can cause vertigo. • Check height of water bag. Water that flows too rapidly can also cause vertigo.
Inability to run water into colostomy.	• Cone is perhaps against wall of bowel. Rotate cone to different position to start flow. • Do not force cone into stoma and attempt to instill solution.
No return of stool or water from irrigation.	• Apply drainable pouch. • Have client increase fluid intake. Client may be dehydrated. • Repeat irrigation next day.

CLINICAL PROBLEMS	CRITICAL THINKING OPTIONS
■ Continual spillage of stool between irrigations.	• Reassess type of colostomy—only those in descending or sigmoid colon are to be irrigated. • Be sure client uses and retains 1000 mL of tap water. • Assess the client's past bowel habits prior to surgery. Clients who have had very irregular bowel habits or frequent stools may not be candidates for irrigation.
■ Poor returns due to constipation or fecal impaction.	• Assess the client's diet. The dietician may need to be notified to provide more bulk foods. • Assess medications client is taking. (Drugs, such as codeine, iron, and vincristine, can be very constipating.) • Stool softeners or mild laxative may be needed. • Assess client's fluid intake. Increasing the amount of fluids may be necessary. • Perform a digital examination to check for impaction. If impaction or severe constipation persists, colostomy may be irrigated with 30 mL soap, 60 mL oil, and 500 mL water. (Warn client that this can cause severe cramping.) This procedure requires physician's order. • Obtain physician's order to add liquid Colace, milk, and molasses or mineral oil to irrigating solution to soften stool. A soft rubber catheter may be used to put the liquid medication nearer to the obstruction. • Administer low-volume (100–200 mL) solution, keep cone in place to keep fluid in place to assist with stool softening.
■ Diarrhea occurs.	• Do not irrigate colostomy. Apply drainable pouch. • If client is receiving radiation therapy, which usually causes diarrhea, check with physician about stopping irrigations until therapy is completed. • Assess client's medications. (Antibiotics or chemotherapy drugs can cause diarrhea.) • If diarrhea is excessive or prolonged, alert the physician because client may need to be monitored for potassium loss and have diet adjusted accordingly.
■ Client does not develop a positive attitude toward living with a colostomy.	• Arrange visit between ostomy visitor and client to demonstrate the rehabilitation possible following surgery. • Ask physician to refer client to health specialist skilled in teaching ostomy management. • Ask physician to refer client to ostomy club. • Ask physician if referral to psychologist for support would be advisable. • Allow client to grieve over change in body image.

unit 5

FECAL OSTOMY POUCH APPLICATION

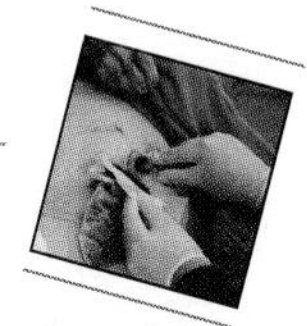

NURSING PROCESS DATA

ASSESSMENT Data Base

Observe stoma color.

Inspect client's abdomen for creasing, firmness, softness, contour, scars, folds, and incisions.

Inspect client's peristomal skin for signs of erythema, excoriation, ulceration, and fistula formation.

Assess client's learning abilities, age, manual dexterity, and visual acuity.

PLANNING Objectives

To collect effluent for accurate assessment of output in the hospital.

To collect effluent for the comfort of the client.

To contain drainage and odors so that the client feels that he or she is socially acceptable.

To protect peristomal skin from erythema, excoriation, and infection.

To protect the client's clothing.

IMPLEMENTATION Procedure

Applying a Fecal Ostomy Pouch.

EVALUATION Expected Outcomes

Pouch remains intact without leakage for 3–5 days.

Pouching system provides maximal skin protection.

Pouching system remains odorproof for 3–5 days.

Client gradually assumes an active role in applying the pouch.

Client's skin remains free of erythema or excoriation.

APPLYING A FECAL OSTOMY POUCH

Equipment

Clean drainable pouch with attached skin barrier
Skin barriers (e.g., Skin Gel or Skin Prep)
Warm water in basin
Soft cloths
Bath blanket
Plastic bag for disposal of old pouch
Tail closure for pouch
Clean gloves
Measuring guide
Deodorant (optional)
Hypoallergenic paper tape (optional)
Tissues
Scissors

Preparation

1. Check physician's orders and client care plan.
2. Determine exact supplies client uses.
3. Gather equipment.
4. Explain procedure to client.
5. Provide privacy for client.
6. Wash hands, and don clean gloves.
7. Raise bed to HIGH position, and lower side rails on working side of the bed.

■ CLINICAL ALERT

To promote the client's self-esteem and body image, be aware of your own body language. Even subtle changes in the way you look at the stoma could indicate disgust or disapproval and an altered self-esteem could result.

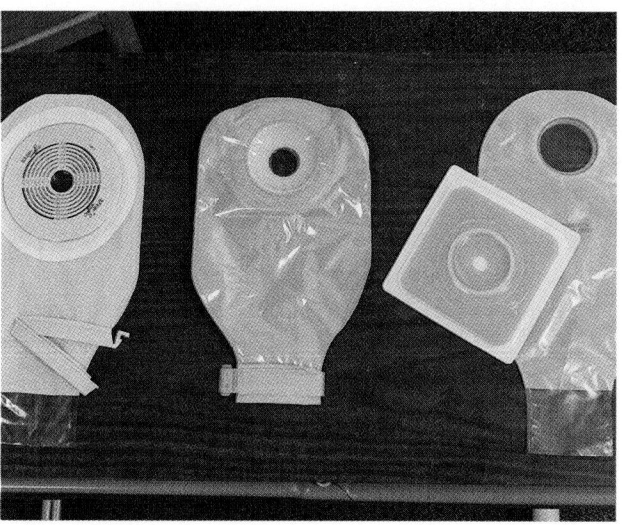
Drainable pouches for ostomies.

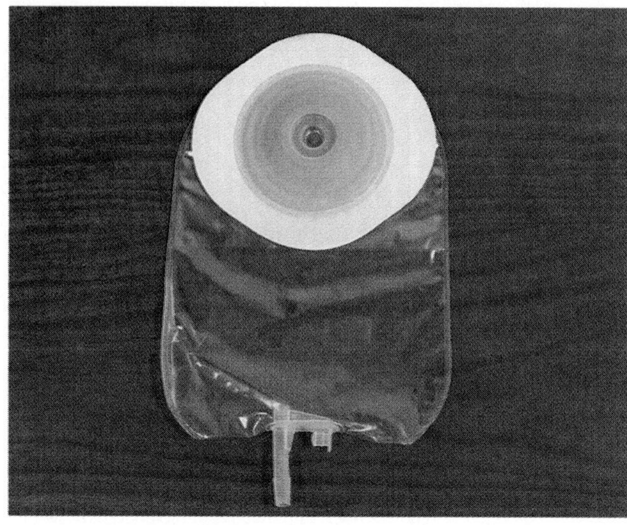
Drainable ileostomy pouch.

Procedure

1. Place bath blanket over client, and fold top linen to bottom of bed.
2. Empty old pouch. Pouches should be emptied when one-third to one-half full of feces or flatus. **Rationale:** This prevents the weight of the pouch contents from loosening the pouch.
3. Remove old pouch by pushing against skin as you pull backing from skin and discard in plastic bag. Save tail closure on bottom of pouch.
4. Clean client's skin and stoma gently with warm water and soft cloth. **Rationale:** Oily substances interfere with the pouch adhesive.
5. Dry client's skin well with a soft cloth. Keep tissues available if stoma evacuates stool while pouch is off.
6. Observe skin and stoma for changes in size, ulceration, or color—stoma should be a healthy red. **Rationale:** Breakdown of peristomal skin may be caused by improperly fitting pouch, leakage of stool on skin, hair follicle irritation, misuse of skin barriers, bacterial or fungal infections, perspiration, or allergic reactions.

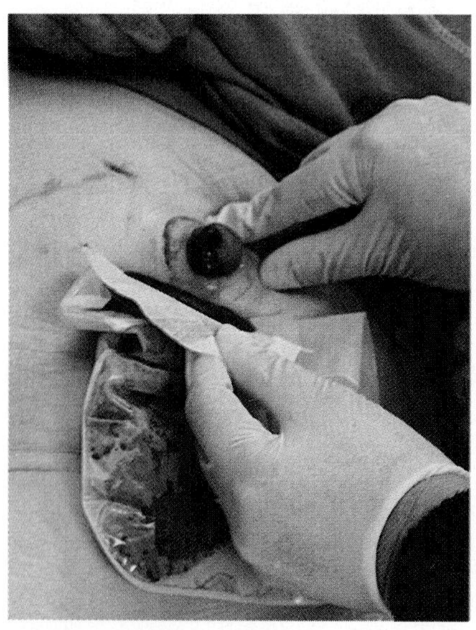
Remove old pouch.

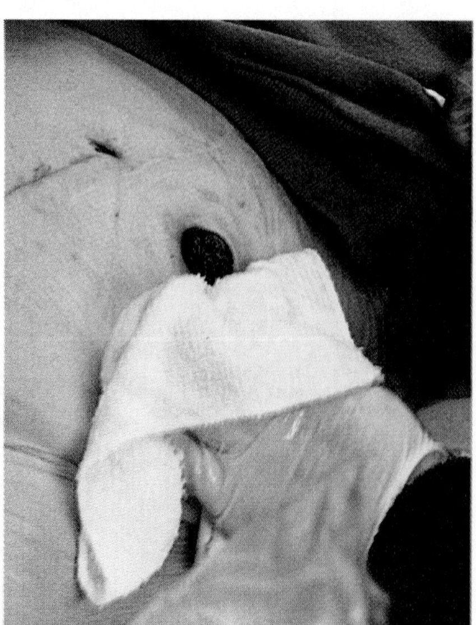
Cleanse peristomal skin.

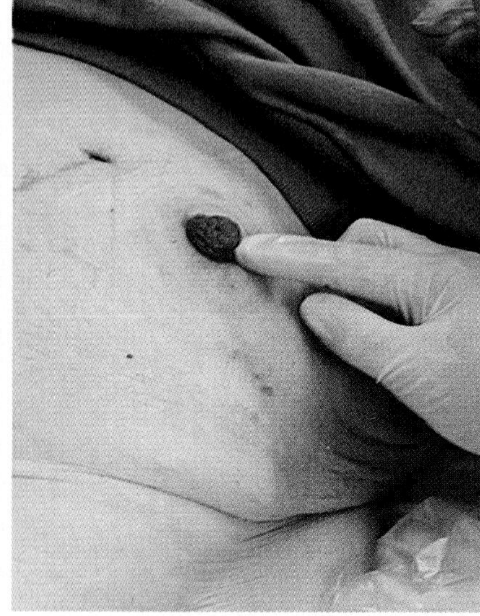
Assess stoma for change.

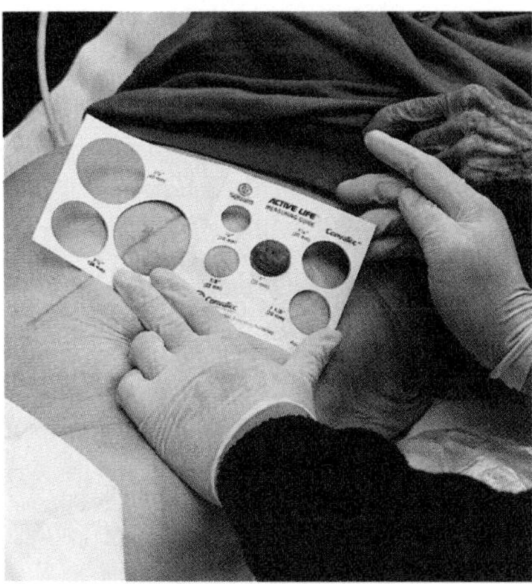
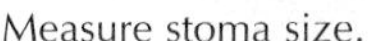
Measure stoma size.

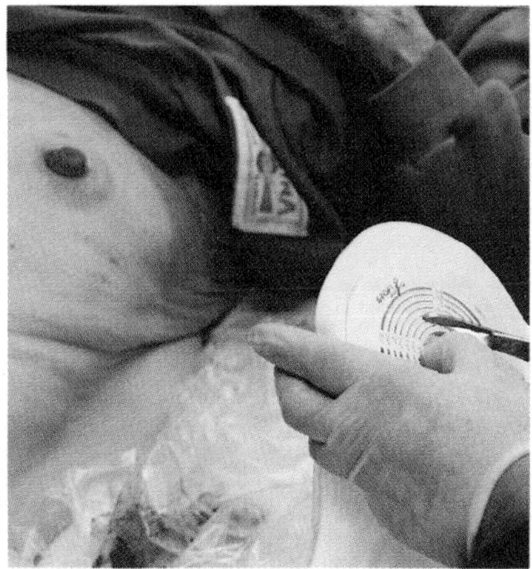
Cut pouch to fit stoma.

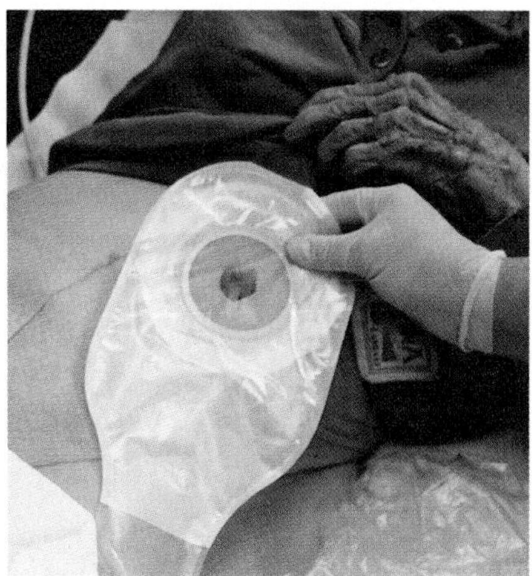
Check opening size.

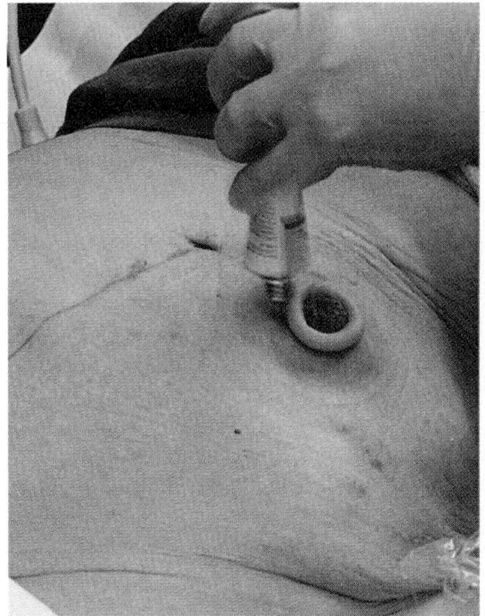
Apply skin barrier paste.

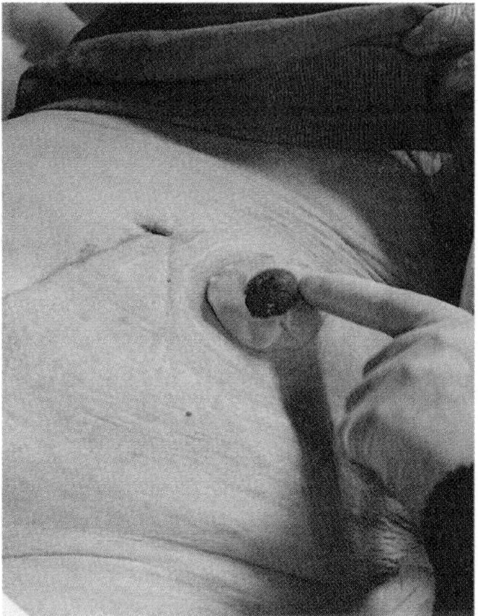
Wet fingers and spread paste.

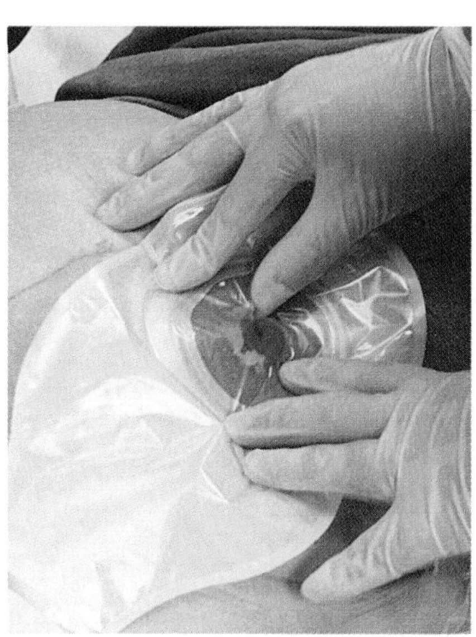
Center and apply pouch.

7. Prepare clean pouch:
   a. Measure stoma with measuring guide.
   b. Cut pouch about $\frac{1}{8}$ inch larger than measurement. **Rationale:** To prevent trauma to stoma.
   c. Check to ensure opening is large enough to encircle stoma without pushing on edges.
   d. Remove paper from skin barrier on pouch.
8. Apply skin barrier paste to peristomal area.
9. Wet fingers, and spread paste around stoma.
10. Center and apply clean pouch. Pouch may be applied over incision. **Rationale:** Incisions are sealed within 24 hours; therefore contamination from fecal material does not occur.
11. Instruct client to "puff" out stomach. **Rationale:** This prevents wrinkles from occurring when pouch is applied.
12. Press the adhesive around the stoma to form a seal. Do not allow adhesive to wrinkle. **Rationale:** This prevents leakage from pouch.

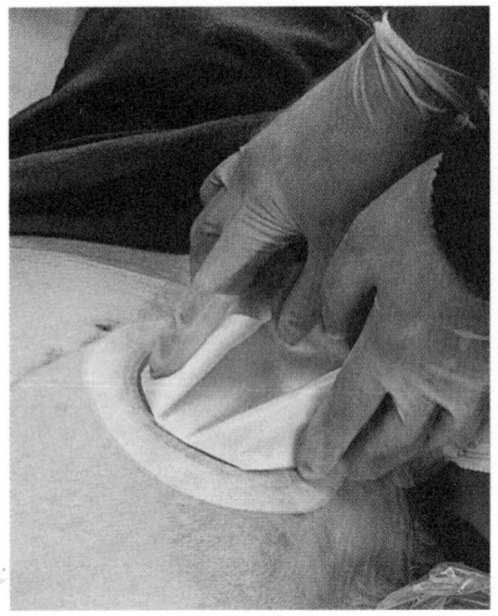
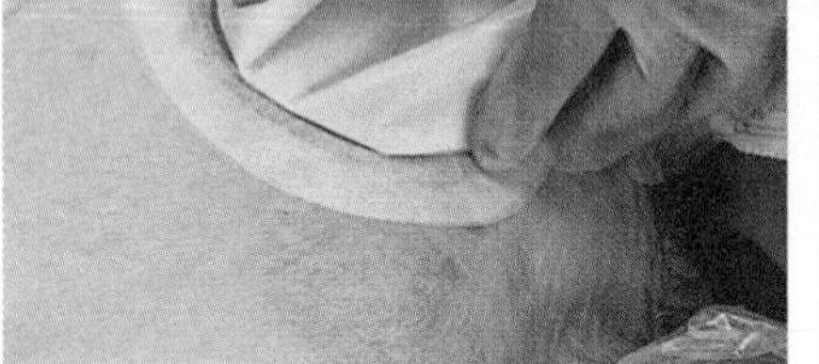

Press adhesive around stoma.

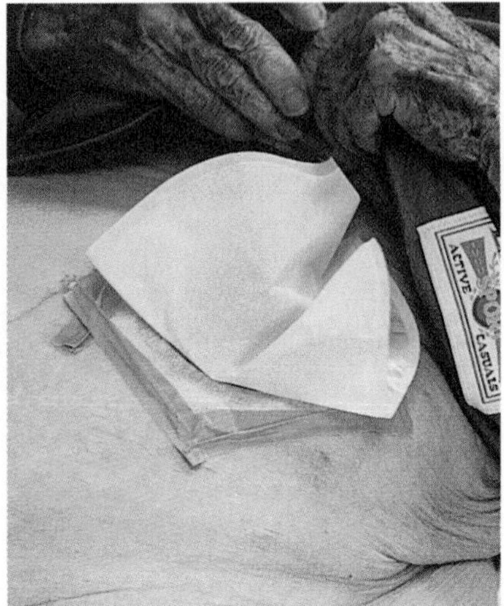
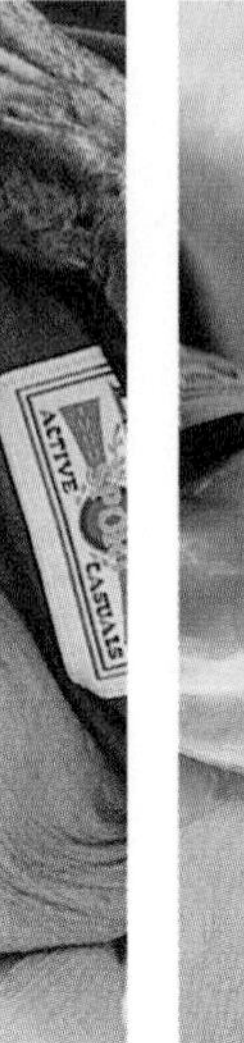

Reinforce ring with tape.

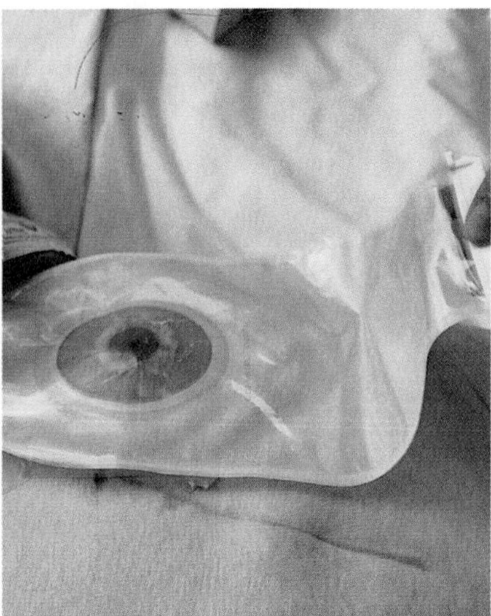

Close pouch with tail closure.

TYPES OF OSTOMY POUCHES

The surgical construction of the stoma, the contour of the abdomen, and the firmness of the abdomen dictate the types of skin barriers and pouches used.

- If stoma protrudes nicely above skin, a broader range of skin barriers and pouches may be applied.
- If stoma is flush to skin, a convex pouch or belt may be needed to prevent leakage.
- If abdomen is very soft and large, a convex pouch may be needed to prevent leakage.
- If abdomen is firm and small, a pouch without ridges may be used.

13. Check that adhesive ring is wrinkle-free. **Rationale:** Prevents seepage of effluent from pouch onto skin.
14. Reinforce ring with tape to balance weight of pouch and prevent edges from loosening when client showers.
15. Instruct client to lie quietly for 3–5 minutes to allow pouch to seal.
16. Close and secure end of pouch with tail closure.
    a. Ensure bowed end is next to body. **Rationale:** This provides a better fit to the body, and prevents outpouching of clamp through clothing.
    b. Lay hook on top of bag and fold bag 1 inch over end of pouch.
    c. Squeeze clamp together to close.
    d. Check clamp is positioned correctly; bowed end is toward body and hook is in top left-hand corner.
    e. Lift up and push clamp in to open clamp.
17. Attach belt to faceplate of pouch (optional).
18. Remove gloves, and wash hands.
19. Position client for comfort.
20. Lower bed, and raise side rails.
21. Put away supplies, and reorder as necessary.

CLINICAL ALERT

To prevent odor from being emitted from the pouch

- Fold the end of the pouch like a cuff before emptying.
- Rinse the pouch with tepid water.
- Wipe the lower 2 inches of pouch with facial tissue or 4×4 gauze pad to remove remaining effluent.
- Fold down cuff, and apply clamp.

Client Teaching

- Empty pouch when one-third full of stool or flatus.
    a. Empty into toilet
    b. Rinse pouch using peribottle filled with soapy water.
    c. Pouch should last for 3–4 days with cleaning regimen.
- Empty each morning and last thing at night even if not one-third full.
- Check seal on daily basis for tight fit, change if needed.
- Instruct client to avoid wearing tight-fitting

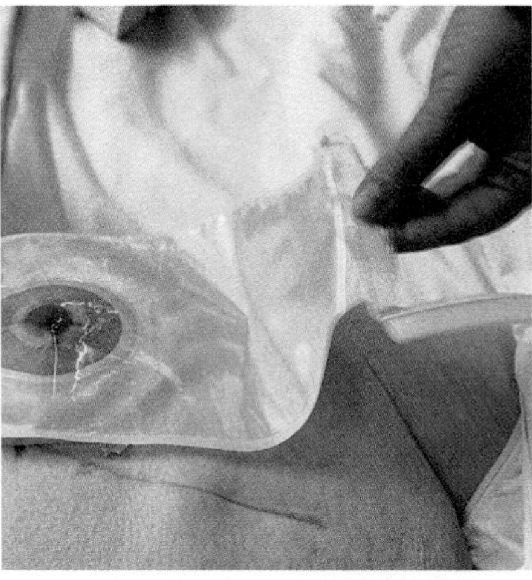

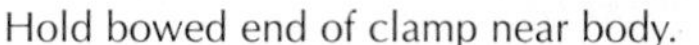

Hold bowed end of clamp near body.

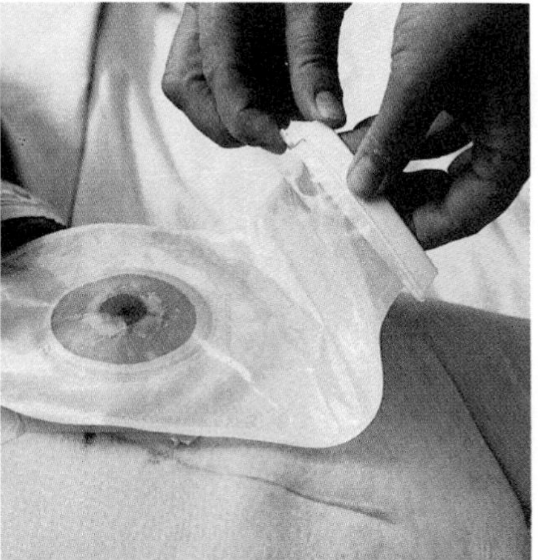

Fold colostomy bag end over clamp and close.

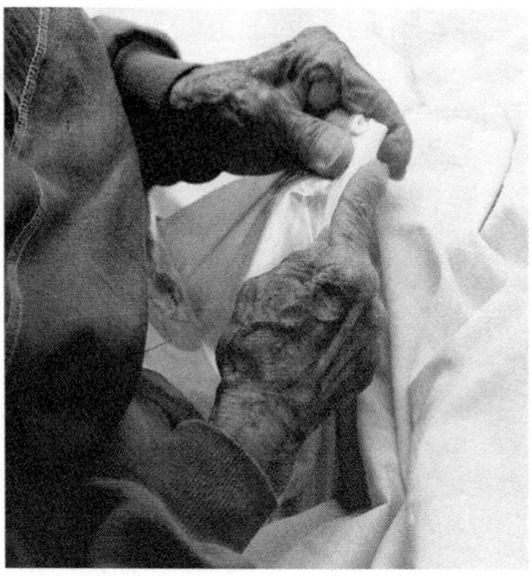

Encourage client to practice closing clamp.

clothes. it can cause stomal bleeding.

- Keep follow-up appointment with enterostomal therapist. (Stoma shrinks up to 3 months after surgery and client may need different type of pouch.)
- Instruct client to always carry a supply of ostomy equipment for emergency use.
- Instruct client on emptying and cleaning pouch, opening and closing clamp, observing and cleaning periostomal area, and changing pouch.
- Have client return demonstration until able to perform activities correctly.

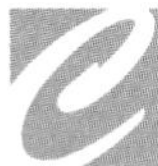

CHARTING for Applying a Fecal Ostomy Pouch

- Type of pouch and skin barrier used
- Time pouch applied
- Time pouch emptied
- Amount, color, and consistency of stool emptied from pouch
- Presence or absence of flatus through the stoma
- Client participation in pouch application
- Condition of peristomal skin and stoma
- Condition of incision line (i.e., any redness or swelling)
- Condition of abdomen (e.g., distention)

CRITICAL THINKING APPLICATION

CLINICAL PROBLEMS	CRITICAL THINKING OPTIONS
The stoma appears dark, dusky-colored, or black.	• Notify physician of findings, and document in chart.
The stoma becomes ulcerated or cut.	• Examine pouching system to see if opening of pouch may be rubbing or cutting into stoma. • Recut opening to $\frac{1}{8}$ inch larger than stoma to avoid traumatizing stoma. • Notify physician of findings. • Assess placement of client's waistband and belt.

CRITICAL THINKING APPLICATION

CLINICAL PROBLEMS	CRITICAL THINKING OPTIONS
■ The pouching system does not provide skin protection.	• Reassess the abdomen and the pouching system for weak points. Modify system to eliminate leakage. • Change the pouch a little more frequently (once per day or every other day) until the peristomal skin is healed. • Assess for allergy to products being used.
■ Client experiences itching, burning, or a feeling of irritation under ostomy appliance.	• Prepare to change pouch. This is usually a sign of periostomial skin irritation. • Remove pouch and thoroughly clean the skin with warm water and soap. Dry thoroughly. • Apply new pouch.

unit 6

INTESTINAL TUBE INSERTION

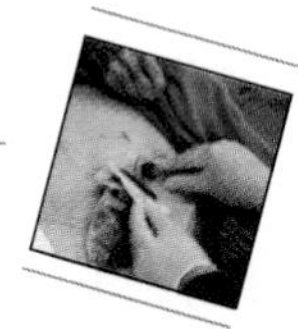

NURSING PROCESS DATA

ASSESSMENT Data Base

Determine client's level of consciousness.

Assess client's knowledge of the procedure.

Auscultate the client's abdomen for presence of bowel sounds.

Palpate abdomen for distention.

Assess amount, color, and odor of drainage.

PLANNING Objectives

To decompress the bowel proximal to an obstruction

To stimulate peristalsis

To assess gastrointestinal bleeding (infrequent)

To relieve abdominal distention through tube placement

To prevent muscosal damage on removal of the tube

IMPLEMENTATION Procedures

Assisting in Intestinal Tube Insertion

Removing an Intestinal Tube

EVALUATION Expected Outcomes

Tube is properly placed and advanced.

A clear tube lumen is maintained throughout the intubation.

Relief of abdominal distention occurs through suction.

Bowel is compressed proximal to obstruction.

Peristalsis is reestablished.

Tube is removed without trauma to the intestinal mucosa.

ASSISTING IN INTESTINAL TUBE INSERTION

Equipment

Water-soluble lubricant

Ice in basin

Miller–Abbott tube (double-lumen, 6–10 feet in length) *or*

Cantor tube (single-lumen, 10 feet in length) or

Harris tube (single-lumen, 6 feet in length)

Stethoscope

Piston syringes: 5 mL, 10 mL, 50 mL

Emesis basin

Tissues or wash cloth, towel

Clean gloves

2–5 mL mercury or tungsten

Normal saline solution

Items for oral hygiene

Clean gloves

Preparation

1. Check physician's orders and client care plan.
2. Gather necessary equipment.
3. Notify physician that you are ready to assist with insertion.
4. Wash your hands.
5. Take equipment to client's room.
6. Identify client via identaband.
7. Inform client about procedure and what can be

expected during and after insertion.

8. Explain how the client can help with tube insertion.
9. Agree on a signal that the client can use to stop the procedure for a moment or two.
10. Test the patency of the balloon, and measure the capacity by filling it with air (20–50 mL of air used). Then completely deflate the balloon.
11. Fill the balloon bag's upper portion with mercury or tungsten, and aspirate all air from bag before inserting the Cantor and Harris tubes. Do *not* place mercury or tungsten in Miller–Abbott tube before inserting. **Rationale:** The second lumen is used to insert and remove the material.
12. Label adapters of Miller–Abbott tube at proximal end. One adapter should be labeled for suction; the other should be labeled balloon.

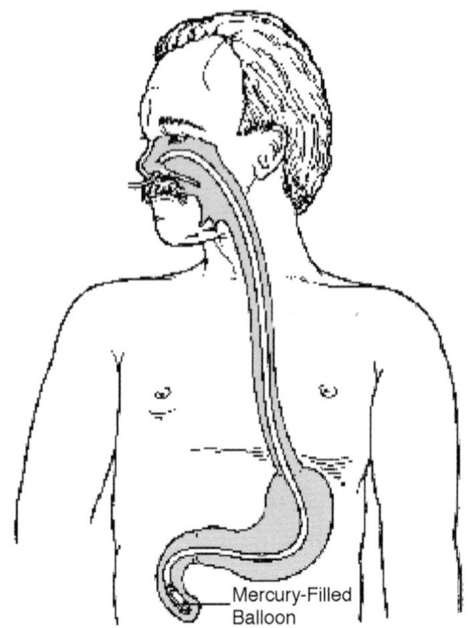

This tube is advanced in increments of 1–2 inches every hour. Suction is applied only after balloon passes pyloric valve.

The Miller–Abbott tube is a double-lumen tube. One lumen drains secretions. A balloon containing air or mercury (or tungsten) is attached to the end of the other lumen to stimulate peristalsis. The Cantor tube and Harris tube are single-lumen tubes. All three tubes progress through the duodenum, jejunum, and ileum by gravity and peristalsis. They are used to aspirate bowel contents. The Harris tube is also used for lavage.

Procedure

1. Place client in a high-Fowler's position with neck flexed.
2. Spread towel "bib fashion" over chest.
3. Measure tubing, using the distance from the tip of the nose to the earlobe to the xiphoid.

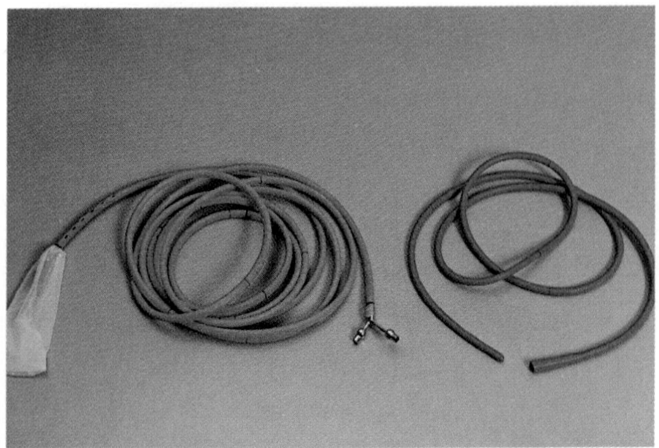

Miller-Abbott and Cantor tubes.

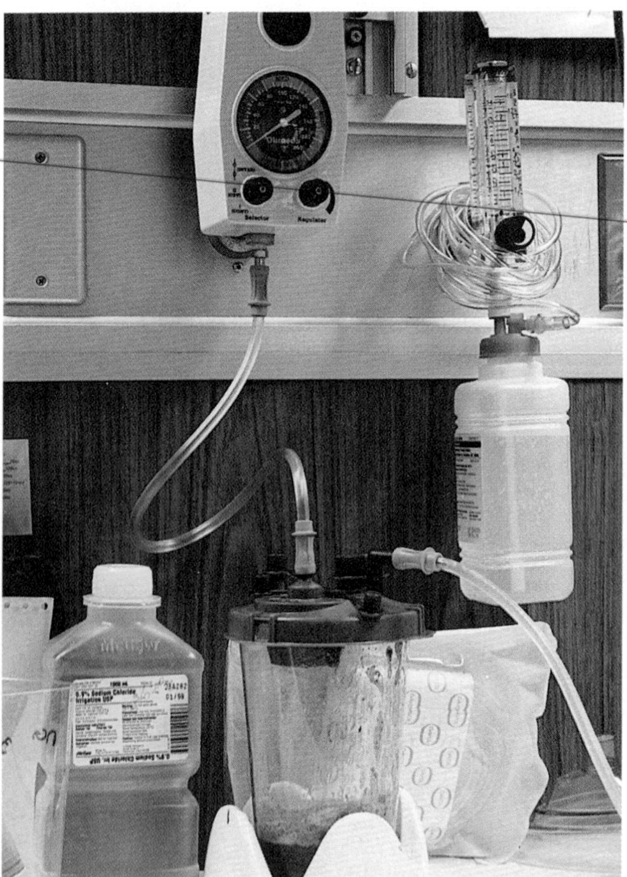

Intestinal tubes are attached to low suction.

4. Wrap a piece of tape around the tube, and mark the distance you measured.
5. Chill the tube; then lubricate the distal end sparingly.
6. Don clean gloves.
7. Remove dentures. Instruct the client to breathe through the mouth.
8. Observe as physician inserts the tube into the client's nostril. The tube is gently but firmly advanced. The client is instructed to swallow as the tubing is advanced past the pharynx. **Rationale:** The tube is not secured to the nose until tube has been advanced to the desired position. This halts the progress of the tube and may lead to bowel injury or intussusception.
9. The tube is advanced to the premarked area on the tube. Observe for aspiration of secretions. **Rationale:** Advancement of the tube more than 2–4 inches at a time can create knots and kinks in the tubing, which may prevent relief from the obstruction or cause intussusception of the bowel.

■ CLINICAL ALERT

If the client is suffering from a small-bowel obstruction, the drainage from the tube is yellow and fecal smelling. If the client is suffering from a complete bowel obstruction, the drainage is clear and may approach 3000 mL per day.

10. Assist with determining the placement of the tube in stomach using one of the following measures:
    a. Instill 5 mL of air into the suction portion of the tube while you listen with a stethoscope over the stomach area. If you hear a "whooosh" sound, the tube is in the stomach.
    b. Use a syringe to aspirate for stomach contents through the suction portion of the tube.
    c. Send client to x-ray to confirm tube placement.
11. Physician instills 2–5 mL of mercury (or tungsten) into the balloon portion of the Miller–Abbott tube. Clamp tube to prevent leakage of mercury. **Rationale:** Mercury-weighted tip helps the balloon move through the pyloric valve.
12. Reposition client on right side. **Rationale:** This position facilitates passage of the tube through the pyloric valve.
13. Remove gloves.
14. Send client for fluoroscopy to determine if the balloon has passed the pyloric valve. When the balloon has passed the pyloric valve, air is injected into the balloon portion of the tube.
15. Reposition the client every 2 hours, turning from right to left side and back to high-Fowler's position. Encourage ambulation. **Rationale:** Repositioning and ambulation move the balloon through the gastrointestinal tract.
16. Attach the tube to intermittent low suction any time after the balloon has passed the pyloric valve.
17. Advance the tube as ordered: 1–2 inches every hour, or 2–4 inches every 2 hours. When the client is in bed, coil and pin extra tubing to the bed. When the client is standing, coil and pin tubing to the gown.
18. When the tube reaches the desired position, secure it with tape to the client's nose or forehead. Make sure that the tubing is not putting pressure on the lumen of the nostril.
19. Don gloves to administer oral hygiene at least once every 4 hours. **Rationale:** Colonic bacteria travel to the client's mouth by "wick action."
20. Assess amount, color, and odor of drainage.
21. Don gloves to irrigate. Slowly instill 30–60 mL normal saline in the suction portion of the tube and then aspirate contents of the tube.
22. Advance tube according to schedule.
23. Notify physician if unable to advance or if any untoward effects occur.
24. Observe client frequently, and note relevant changes.

REMOVING AN INTESTINAL TUBE

Procedure

for Removing a Tube That Has Not Reached the Ileocecal Valve.

1. Explain what the client should expect as you remove the tube. **Rationale:** Client may experience nausea as tube is removed.
2. Insert 5-mL syringe in tube balloon port, aspirate and ensure that the mercury (or tungsten) and air are removed from balloon portion of the tube.
3. Gradually remove the tube 6 inches every hour or as ordered.

4. Give client oral hygiene immediately.

for Removing a Tube That Has Passed the Ileocecal Valve.

1. Explain what the client should expect as you remove the tube.
2. Cut the tubing at the client's nose.
3. Allow the tube to advance through the rectum.
4. Remove the remaining portion of the tube from the rectum with the aid of peristalsis.
5. Provide perineal care.

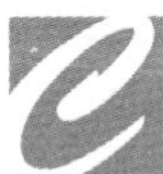

CHARTING for Intestinal Tube

- Time and date tube inserted
- Type of tube inserted
- Time intervals of advancement of tube
- Amount of mercury inserted and removed
- Amount, consistency, color, and odor of drainage obtained from suction
- Oral care given
- Records of intake and output
- Dates and times irrigated
- Amount of irrigant used
- Time intervals tubing is pulled during removal
- Number of inches tubing is pulled during removal
- Client's reactions to all phases of nursing intervention

CRITICAL THINKING APPLICATION

CLINICAL PROBLEMS	CRITICAL THINKING OPTIONS
■ Proper placement and advancement of the tube does not occur.	• Assess that tube is not kinked or coiled by pulling back on the tube and then allowing it to advance again. • Ensure that the tube is not pinned to gown or bed in such a way as to prevent advancement. • Reposition client to aid in advancement of the tube. If not contraindicated, ambulate client to assist in advancement of tube.
■ There is no relief of abdominal distention through suction.	• Irrigate the tube through the suction portion of the tube. • Insert rectal tube for 20 minutes as ordered.
■ Clear tube lumen is not maintained throughout intubation period.	• Irrigate tube. • Notify the physician for additional orders.
■ Removal of tube is traumatizing to intestinal mucosa.	• Observe stool for occult blood, and notify physician.

GERIATRIC CONSIDERATIONS

- Elderly clients frequently have concomitant cardiac problems, which can be affected by vagal stimulation during fecal removal or enema administration. Check with the physician before these skills are performed on elderly clients. Monitor the pulse carefully during the procedure.
- Fecal impaction is not uncommon with elderly clients due to decreased mobility and exercise, dietary habits, and tendency to overuse enemas and laxatives.
- Encourage clients to decrease use of laxatives and enemas, increase fluid intake and fiber in diet, and increase exercise. Dehydration resulting from inadequate fluid intake leads to constipation and fecal impaction.
- To select the proper ostomy appliance for an elderly client, the nurse must determine if the client has any physical limitations that could influence the type of appliance needed. These limitations include poor vision, use of only one hand, arthritis, and inability to perform cleaning and pouching procedure.

23

Heat and Cold Therapy

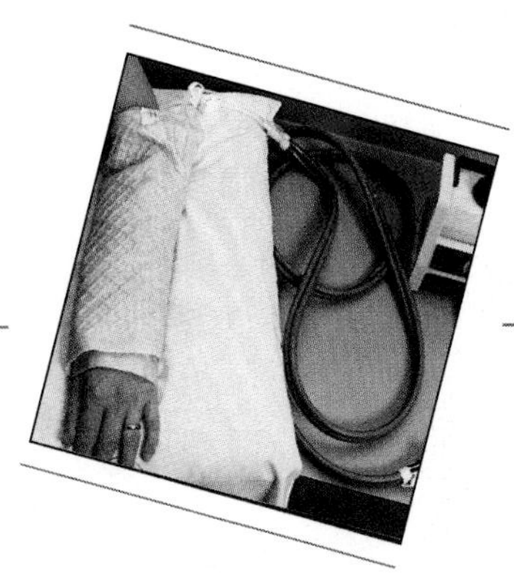

LEARNING OBJECTIVES

- Describe the mechanisms responsible for the body's heat loss and heat production.
- Discuss the role of the hypothalamus in the body.
- List at least three adaptive processes that maintain the body temperature within a normal range.
- Discuss how heat transmission occurs.
- Outline the steps necessary to prepare for the administration of hot, moist applications.
- List four safety factors to consider when applying heat and cold treatments.
- Explain the steps of providing a sitz bath.
- State at least three precautions for providing dry heat treatments.
- Compare and contrast the effects of heat and cold therapy on the body.
- List two safety factors used to prevent skin irritation for infants in a radiant warmer.
- Demonstrate preparation of the infant radiant warmer.
- Explain the use of an aquathermic pad.
- Discuss the safety factors that need to be assessed while administering a tepid sponge bath or ice application.
- List the steps in preparing a cooling blanket.
- Describe major nursing interventions performed for clients requiring a cooling blanket.
- State two nursing diagnoses related to thermic treatments.

TERMINOLOGY

Adipose: fatty; pertaining to fat.

Ambient air temperature: the temperature of the air surrounding a person.

Antipyretic: an agent that reduces febrile temperatures.

Brown adipose tissue: a special lipid cell that is capable of producing heat through chemical processes; brown fat.

Circadian biorhythms: physiologic rhythms that run a full cycle in 24 hours. The high temperature is usually experienced in late afternoon, and the low in the early morning. Temperature can vary up to 2°F.

Compress: a pad of cloth applied firmly to a part of the body; compress may be dry or wet, cold or warm.

Conduction: transfer of heat by direct contact through fluids or solids or any suitable substance.

Constriction: a narrowing or closing in.

Continuous fever: consistently elevated fever.

Convection: transfer of heat by air.

Crisis: sudden drop in fever to a normal value.

Cyanosis: bluish coloring of the skin and the mucous membrane due to decreased oxygenation.

Dermatitis: inflammation of skin evidenced by itching, redness, and skin lesions.

Diaphoresis: an excessive amount of perspiration, as when a person's skin is moist and perspiring.

Erythema: increased reddish color of the skin due to vasodilatation of capillaries.

Euthermia: a normal body temperature.

Evaporation: to convert from a liquid or solid state to a gaseous state.

Fastigium: the course of a fever wherein the body attempts to give off heat. The person feels flushed, sweaty, and lethargic.

Flush: redness of the skin, as in a blush, usually associated with an elevated temperature. The face and neck are more likely to be affected.

Hyperemia: increased blood supply to an area.

Hyperthermia: a body temperature much higher than normal.

Hypothermia: a body temperature lower than normal.

Insulator: substance that is a poor conductor or a nonconductor of heat; a substance that helps prevent the escape or entrance of radiant heat.

Intermittent fever: body temperature alternates between normal and fever.

Lysis: slow or gradual drop to normal temperature.

Mottling: blue-gray to purplish blotches seen usually peripherally; it is usually the result of peripheral vasoconstriction.

Nonshivering thermogenesis: production of body heat by chemical processes, and not involving the muscle cocontraction (shivering) process.

Onset: phase of fever during which chills and shivers are experienced.

Pallor: loss of reddish hue due to superficial vasoconstriction produced by sympathetic stimulation.

Palpitation: rapid, violent, or throbbing pulsation, as of the heart.

Periphery: outer part or surface of a body.

Physiologic: concerning body function.

Pyrexia (terminology associated with fever): a disorder of the thermoregulation where the "set point" is displaced upward and the body actively seeks to raise its temperature; "true fever" temperature.

Radiation: transfer of energy (heat) in the form of waves.

Remittent fever: body temperature alternates between pyrexia and several degrees above normal.

Resolution: period when the temperature begins to drop.

Shivering: the tremoring of the body usually in response to coolness. It is the result of reflex action coordinated by the hypothalamus.

Shivering thermogenesis: production of body heat by shivering or muscle contraction (tremors).

Sitz bath: bath to sit in with water above the hips.

Suppuration: the process of pus formation.

Thermogenesis: heat production by the body.

Vasoconstriction: a narrowing of blood vessels.

Vasomotor: pertaining to nerves having muscular control of the blood vessel walls.

TEMPERATURE CONTROL

The temperature of the human body is regulated and maintained by a group of interrelated feedback systems. When these homeostatic mechanisms are altered by disease or environmental conditions, the body may need assistance to regain its normal temperature.

Temperature control of the body is a homeostatic function that balances heat production and loss to maintain body temperature within a fairly constant range. The body uses neuronal pathways to collect, organize, and transmit temperature information. These pathways also transmit physiologic responses to produce temperature adjustments. The main integrative function is carried out by the hypothalamus.

The hypothalamus is the body's thermostat, and it functions to maintain the body as close as possible to a constant, or "set point," temperature. Information reaches the hypothalamus by indirect and direct means: indirectly through receptors and directly by circulating blood. The hypothalamus triggers body response in the tissues and vasomotor tone in the organs to produce shivering, sweating, and changes in convection, conduction, and evaporation. The body uses these physiologic processes to alter temperature.

The body continuously strives to maintain a constant optimal temperature. As heat is gained through metabolism, exercise, or environmental factors, the body throws off excess warmth through convection, conduction, or evaporation. In contrast, on sensing a loss of heat (cold), the body triggers one or more processes to produce heat (thermogenesis), conserve it, or dissipate it. Although these dynamic processes cannot be observed, their resulting effects, such as violent shivering, are readily evident. The hypothalamus continuously makes adjustments, varying in intensity, to maintain the core body temperature.

Our body works to maintain a neutral thermal environment. We consciously and unconsciously alter levels of activity in response to the physiologic stimulus from the body's thermostat, the hypothalamus. When we sense cold, we huddle or curl up to decrease heat lost from the body surface. When warm, we extend our bodies and separate our limbs. There are sensors in the hypothalamus and in the dermis that are distributed widely over the body surface. These sensors react to changes in temperature. In fact, the hypothalamus is sensitive to very minute changes, as slight as 0.01°C in the circulating blood.

Adjustment Processes

An important adjustment process is heat conservation. When the body perceives a cooling sensation, heat-conserving and heat-producing mechanisms are activated.

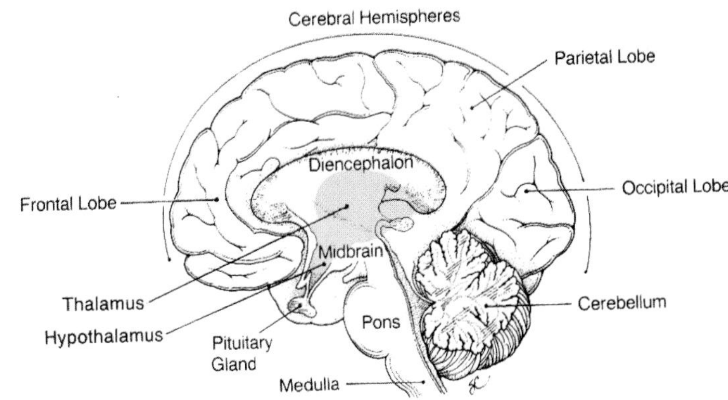

The hypothalamus is located in the diencephalon portion of the brain. It controls the body's thermostat.

Vasomotor constriction, a heat-conserving mechanism, removes warmed blood from the surface area of the skin. This reduces heat loss to the cooler exterior through conduction. Sweating removes heat from the body through the process of evaporation. The piloerector muscles contract, raising all the body hairs, to create an insulating (nonconductive) layer of air around the body. The latter reaction produces "goose flesh" and may lead to the behavioral response of huddling, curling up, or adding clothing to modify the microenvironment.

An emotional reaction can also produce a vasomotor response. Psychologic perception of danger triggers the body's alarm system causing epinephrine to be released. This results in vasoconstriction on the periphery of the body, piloerection, and increased respiratory rate.

Heat production, or thermogenesis, is a progressive adaptive process. A mild cold stimulus causes an increase in respiratory rate. This is the result of the increased oxidative process going on in muscles as they are tensing. More oxygen is consumed, shivering begins as muscle tension increases, and heat is produced. This process continues until the temperature, as sensed by the thermostat hypothalamus, is high enough or has reached the "set point."

A second kind of thermogenesis, nonshivering thermogenesis, also activates metabolic processes. Production of norepinephrine, mediated through neuroendocrine control, stimulates the metabolism of brown fat. Oxygen consumption is raised during this process, heat is produced, and body temperature increases. Brown adipose tissue has a special kind of cell structure and is normally present in newborns. Newborns, incapable of shivering, still are able to produce body heat through metabolic processes. Brown adipose tissue reserves are felt to decrease with age, which perhaps explains why we feel extremes of cold more severely as we grow older.

In contrast, when the body perceives excess heat, opposite measures are activated. Sources of excess body heat may be internal (excessive muscle activity) or external (a very warm environment). The adaptability of the multiple systems to maintain temperature within the critical range is again demonstrated when mechanisms are activated to dissipate heat. The thermostat of the hypothalamus and the peripherally situated warmth receptors provide neurologic information to set the cooling mechanisms in motion. Peripheral vasodilatation occurs, and warmed blood is brought to the surface of the body. Surface vessels dilate, promoting radiation of heat away from the body. Behavioral responses are to remove insulative layers and to extend our body to increase the surface area for greater heat conduction. Heat conservation mechanisms are reduced, muscle activity is decreased, and heat production is minimized.

When mild thermoregulatory activities are ineffective, sweating begins. Sweating is stimulated by thermal signals from circulatory and integumentary receptors. Sweat glands are innervated by the cholinergic sympathetic nervous system. Thus, emotions, such as anxiety and fear, can trigger sweating.

One of the most effective mechanisms for heat loss is evaporation. As internal temperature increases, the sweating and vasodilator responses work together. Behavioral responses to heat include a decrease in activity manifested by apathy and inertia, and decreased hunger sensations. Heat dissipation processes become more efficient as the heat load persists. Then, as the body approaches normal temperature, the activities decrease and the dynamic process for thermoregulation continues.

Some processes associated with heat production may also promote heat loss, and vice versa. For example, physical exercise produces heat, but it also allows a larger body area to be exposed for heat dissipation. Exercise also disturbs the insulative thin-air layer around the body.

All thermoregulatory activities require functional pathways for receptors and effectors. Physiologic systems must be healthy and intact to respond to the constant adjustments. The behavioral–intellectual systems must also function effectively to be able to manipulate the immediate environment to maintain body temperature. Our ability to adapt to alterations in temperature is affected by many external factors, such as pathogens; medications; physical disorders; and general health conditions related to age, circulation, physical fitness, and nutrition.

Conditions That Affect Adaptive Processes

Pathogens in the form of viruses and bacteria can trigger fever, generally a temperature of over 38.3°C, or 101°F. Fever caused by a pathogenic process is a thermoregulation disorder in which the "set point" is displaced upward. In response, the body perceives it is cold and seeks to conserve heat (i.e., shivering). The basal metabolic rate increases approximately 7–8% for every half degree Celsius of temperature elevation. Age, the duration and amount of temperature increase, and the overall disease condition are variables influencing the body's reaction.

Medications can alter the "set point" of the hypothalamus as well as affect one's ability to shiver or to exert vasomotor control. Drugs such as Thorazine, Demerol, or Phenergan may suppress the brain's temperature regulatory center.

Disorders of or damage to a major adaptive system can make it more difficult for the body to cope with even small changes. For example, the skin is a major organ in the cooling and heating of the body. A severe inflammation or skin infection may render this system unresponsive to temperature fluctuations.

Other health conditions that affect the adaptive processes are poor circulation to the skin, which makes heat dissipation difficult; dermatitis, which decreases the ability of temperature sensors and circulation to respond; and an insufficient amount of muscle mass, which decreases thermogenesis. A very thin person or one with a muscle-wasting disease may not have sufficient muscle mass to be able to shiver. Neurologic systems of elderly persons may not be able to transmit or process sensory information. Clients with a pathologic condition of the thyroid may be over or under normal levels yet not be euthermic. A person whose immune responses are deficient may not be able to adequately exhibit a febrile response. Interruptions of the hypothalamus through increased intracranial pressure grossly alter body temperature itself as well as the ability to thermoregulate. Finally, clients with decreased or absent body functions, or underdeveloped or very aged systems, also have difficulty responding to alterations.

In addition to these internal sources, the environment itself influences the body's ability to adapt to alterations in temperature. For example, a person undergoing a surgical procedure may suffer extreme exposure in a cold operating room. The client may be without covering for an extended period and have the abdomen opened to this environment, causing loss of core body heat. Other external conditions may cause cooling problems even if the cooling is mostly peripheral or surface. Peripheral cooling produces vasomotor changes or vasoconstriction. Continued cool blood from the periphery can eventually reduce the core to subnormal temperature. This cooling process causes alterations of activity in most organ systems. With extended cooling stress, the thyroid is stimulated and produces an increase in metabolic rate.

Alterations in body temperature are influenced by the body systems' integrity, age, particular disease process, and temperature stresses that a healthy person in a moderately neutral environment may experience. Many of these alterations can have temporary as well as chronic qualities. Persons may need assistance for a relatively short time or for the rest of their lives. It is apparent that assistance is often needed to maintain body temperature. Nursing attention and action can make a difference in many situations vital to the client's comfort, healing, and coping.

THERAPEUTIC EFFECTS OF HEAT

The physiologic effects of heat application to the body include vasodilation, increased metabolism leading to growth of new tissue, increased capillary permeability, activation of the autonomic nervous system, and increased muscle relaxation.

Heat dilates blood vessels and increases capillary permeability. This physiologic response increases the blood flow to a specific area of the body. Capillary permeability and increased blood supply provide a mechanism for nutrients and oxygen to reach tissues and at the same time remove toxins and wastes. Heat also decreases venous congestion and pain at an injury site. As fluid is removed through vasodilation, pain is decreased as a result of less pressure on the nerve endings.

Heat stimulates metabolism and growth of new tissue through increased blood supply to the injured area. Increased capillary permeability resulting from heat therapy assists in clearing debris from an infected area through suppuration. Heat also reduces blood viscosity, which allows leukocytes and antibiotics to reach the affected area more readily.

Heat is applied not only to reduce inflammation and relieve pain and congestion but also to relieve muscle spasm, provide comfort, and occasionally to increase body temperature. Dry heat applications, such as heat lamps and Aqua-K pads are generally used to relieve pain and support suppuration. Moist heat applications, sitz baths, and warm soaks are used to promote muscle relaxation, reduce edema and inflammation, debride wounds, and apply medications to wounds.

Supportive and preventive measures are also therapeutic. When administering thermic applications, keep in mind that heat applications produce widespread effects. Warm applications of short duration produce vasodilation of peripheral vessels, a decrease in general heat production, and an increase in mobility of leukocytes. The application of heat to one body area produces heat over other body parts, and intermittent warmth to an area allows warmth receptors to fully respond with each treatment.

THERAPEUTIC EFFECTS OF COLD

The physiologic effects of cold treatments to the body are mainly vasoconstriction and decreased metabolism. Vasoconstriction of blood vessels and decreased supply of blood to an injured area prevents edema. Decreased metabolism and decreased cellular activity reduce inflammation, available oxygen, and nutrients to the tissue. Cold therapy also blocks pain receptors and slows nerve impulse conduction, which reduces pain. Increased blood coagulation at the injury site occurs as a result of increased blood viscosity.

Cold therapy is used to reduce edema in sprains and strains, to control bleeding and pain, and to reduce fever. Cold therapy, like heat therapy, can be either moist or dry. Moist therapy is in the form of the tepid bath or cold compresses. The application of an ice pack or ice collar is considered dry therapy.

Cold therapy is effective for 15–20 minutes. If the commercial cold pack has an outer covering it can be applied directly to the skin. Ice should not be applied directly to the skin surface because it can cause tissue injury. Prolonged use of cold treatments reverse the effect of the protective mechanism.

Full-body hypothermia is used in some surgical procedures to reduce the metabolic needs of the client during prolonged surgical events. It lowers body temperature below normal range, in some cases to 78°F or below. It is also used when the client has a very high temperature that is not controlled with medication or if there is a risk of cerebral edema following head injury or cranial surgery.

The following principles of client safety are important to consider when applying heat and cold treatments.

- In most hospitals, the water temperature is controlled at a temperature not to exceed 110°F (43.3°C) to prevent client injury.
- A protective layer of petroleum jelly assists in preventing tissue damage when hot packs are applied.
- Place hot pack on client's skin for a few seconds, then remove and check condition of skin before leaving pack on the prescribed length of time.
- Monitor vital signs frequently when cold is applied.
- Observe skin for purplish color, and check client for numb feeling after cold applications are removed.

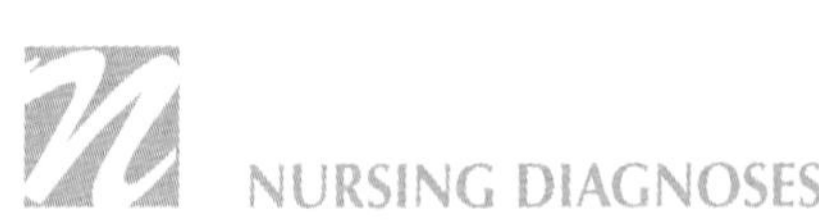

NURSING DIAGNOSES

The following nursing diagnoses are appropriate to use on patient care plans when the components are related to thermic treatments.

NURSING DIAGNOSIS	RELATED FACTORS
Risk for Injury	Heat or cold application remains on skin for prolonged time
Noncompliance	Inadequate knowledge base, misinterpretation, discomfort from treatment
Pain	Low pain threshold, tissue damage
Impaired Skin Integrity	Prolonged use of cold or hot treatment, excessive temperature of therapy, impaired sensation, impaired circulation, mechanical factors, altered tissue perfusion, extreme temperature or prolonged time of treatment

unit 1

MOIST HEAT

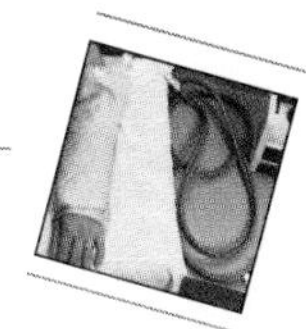

NURSING PROCESS DATA

ASSESSMENT Data Base

Assess skin condition for possible complications, such as redness, burns, and blisters related to previous applications of moist heat.

Determine if sterile technique is required.

Check for length of time heat treatment is ordered.

Assess vital signs, especially respirations on debilitated clients before applying heat.

PLANNING Objectives

To conduct heat through moist application

To produce local vasodilation

To improve tissue metabolism in an infected area

To increase circulation to the affected area

To promote comfort for an injured area

To increase mobility of leukocytes

To decrease heat loss due to evaporation by using waterproof materials (moisture barriers)

To apply medications to a specific area

To hasten suppuration and soften exudate from a wound

To assist in redistribution of heat to other body parts

IMPLEMENTATION Procedures

Applying Hot Moist Pack

Applying Hot Sterile Moist Compress

Providing a Sitz Bath

EVALUATION Expected Outcomes

Increased circulation occurs to the affected area.

Increased warmth occurs to area of application.

Suppuration progresses.

Pain is decreased with heat application.

APPLYING HOT MOIST PACK

Equipment

Terry towel or 4 × 4 gauze pads for hot packs

Plastic drape or absorbent pad for moisture barrier

Container for warming solution

Petroleum jelly for skin protection

Safety pins

Bath blanket or terry towel for securing pack

Aqua K pad (optional)

Bath thermometer

Gauze wrap (Kerlix)

Preparation

1. Check orders for type of hot moist treatment ordered, length of treatment, and time interval between treatments.
2. Gather specific equipment for type of hot moist pack ordered.
3. Place material in a warming solution (usually water).

4. Determine amount of time elapsed since last application.
5. Considering age of client, body part involved, and type of treatment, determine safe temperature of application to prevent burning. **Rationale:** Water temperature in hospitals is usually controlled at 110°F, but the individual client may require altered temperature.
6. Identify correct client and explain treatment.
7. Determine if client is able to identify alterations in sensation if they were to occur.
8. Inspect skin surface for possible complications associated with heat treatments.
9. Take baseline vital signs.
10. Bring equipment to bedside.
11. Wash your hands.
12. Provide privacy, and position client for application of moist pack.

Procedure

1. Lubricate skin with petroleum jelly.
2. Place moisture-proof pad under affected area. **Rationale:** This pad keeps bed linens dry as well as allowing the pack to totally cover body area.
3. Wring out towel or gauze pads as dry as possible.
4. Place towel or gauze pads over affected area for several seconds.
5. Remove material after 30 seconds, and check skin for redness.
6. Ask client if temperature of pack is comfortable.
7. Replace moist pack over affected area.
8. Wrap entire surface involved with plastic drape.
9. Place towel or bath blanket over plastic wrap.
10. Place Aqua K-pad over plastic drape (optional).
11. Secure blanket or towel with safety pins or kerlix.
12. Take pulse to determine response to heat treatment.
13. Assess client for possible complications of heat treatment (e.g., diaphoresis, flushed face, palpitations).
14. Remove pack after 20 minutes or as ordered by physician.
15. When treatment is completed, remove pack, inspect area for redness or tissue damage, remove petroleum jelly, dry client, and apply dressing if ordered.
16. Reposition client in comfortable position, and determine any side effects from treatment.

CLINICAL ALERT

Unless physician orders continuous heat application, treatment time is usually 20 minutes.

APPLYING HOT STERILE MOIST COMPRESS

Equipment

Terry towel or wool pieces for hot packs
Plastic drape or absorbent pad for moisture barrier
Sterile container for warming solution
Bath blanket or terry towel for securing pack
Heating pad or Aqua K-pad
Sterile solution
Sterile 4 × 4 gauze dressing
Clean gloves, 2 pair
Sterile gloves, 2 pair
Sterile towel or ABD pad for covering compress

Preparation

1. Check orders for type of hot moist treatment ordered, length of treatment, and time interval between treatments.
2. Gather specific equipment for type of hot moist pack ordered.
3. Determine amount of time elapsed since last application.
4. Considering age of client, body part involved, and type of treatment, determine safe temperature of application to prevent burning.
5. Identify correct client and explain treatment.
6. Determine if client is able to identify alterations in sensation if they were to occur.

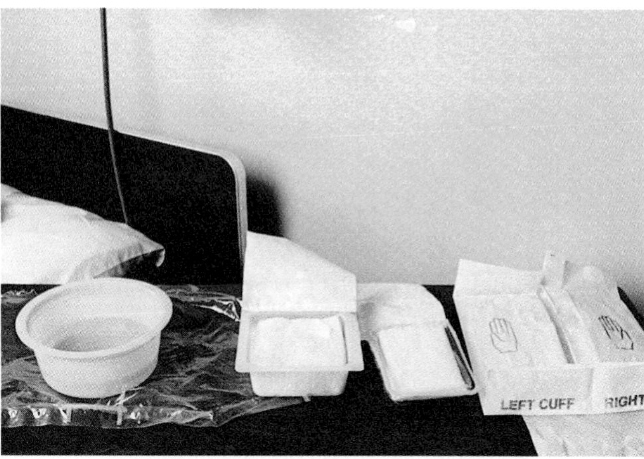

Open sterile supplies and place on overbed table in preparation for applying sterile compress.

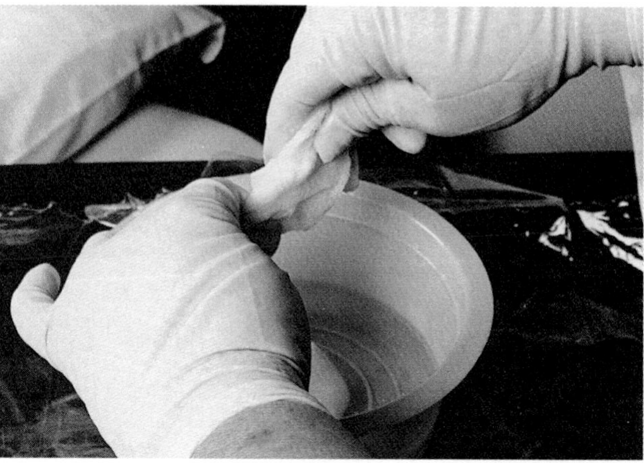

Wring out gauze pads as dry as possible, maintaining sterility, before applying to specific area.

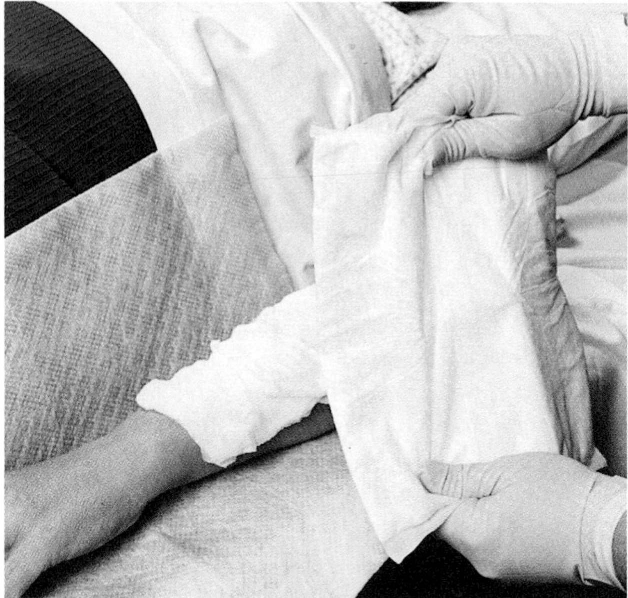

Cover gauze pads with sterile ABD pad before wrapping with sterile towel.

7. Inspect skin surface for possible complications associated with heat treatments.
8. Take baseline vital signs.
9. Bring equipment to bedside, and provide privacy.
10. Wash your hands.

Procedure

1. Warm sterile solution.
2. Place sterile gauze dressing in sterile basin maintaining sterile technique. Pour warm solution over the gauze.
3. Don clean gloves.
4. Remove old dressings, and cleanse wound of exudate.
5. Remove clean gloves, and wash your hands.
6. Don sterile gloves.
7. Wring out gauze dressing.
8. Place gauze dressing over wound (may cover with ABD pad).
9. Wrap sterile towel around dressing.
10. Remove gloves.
11. Place plastic drapes over towel.
12. Apply Aqua K-pad (105–110°F; 40.5–43.3°C) over drape.
13. Wrap towel over heating pad, and secure with tape.
14. Change compress every 1–2 hours using sterile technique.
15. Don clean gloves.
16. Remove compress, and discard gauze dressing using the double-bagged technique.
17. Remove clean gloves, and don sterile gloves.
18. Apply sterile dressing to wound between treatments of moist compresses if indicated.
19. Reposition client for comfort.

PROVIDING A SITZ BATH

Equipment

Available bathroom with appropriate size tub for client
Towels and bathmat
Inflatable tub ring
Bath blanket
Client's clean clothes
Clean gloves, if needed

Procedure

1. Check physician's orders for sitz bath.
2. Wash your hands.
3. Take linen to bathroom.
4. Fill clean bathtub or sitz bath about one-third full with warm water.
5. Check with your hand to determine that temperature of water is between 105° and 110°F, or 40.5° and 43.3°C.
6. Place towel or inflatable ring, if appropriate, on tub bottom and bathmat on floor beside tub.
7. Explain purpose and procedure to client.
8. Instruct client to undress.
9. Assist client into tub or sitz bath, supporting back with rolled towels. Put towel or bath blanket around shoulders for warmth.
10. Check with client if the water temperature and level are alright.

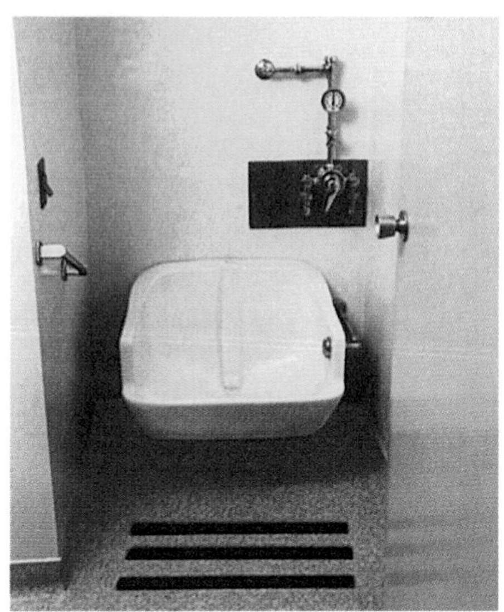

The sitz bath is used to promote healing of the perineal area, especially after surgery or childbirth.

11. Remain with client during sitz bath or check frequently. Procedure takes 20 minutes.
12. Assess client for any untoward reactions. Instruct client to ring for assistance if he or she feels dizzy, faint, or weak. Remove client immediately.
13. When sitz bath is completed, assist client from tub. If drainage present, don clean gloves.
14. Assist with drying and dressing, and accompany client to room.
15. Discard soiled linen, clean tub, using clean gloves if drainage present.

CHARTING for Applying Moist Heat

- Type of solution
- Length of time of application
- Type of heat application
- Condition and appearance of wound
- Comfort of client

CRITICAL THINKING APPLICATION

CLINICAL PROBLEMS	CRITICAL THINKING OPTIONS
Affected extremity throbs with increased circulation.	• Elevate the extremity above the level of the heart to increase venous return. • Determine if application material is too heavy and is putting too much pressure on wound. • Check for presence of peripheral pulses.
Pain in affected area is increased.	• Assess if application is too hot. • Ensure that temperature is not over 110°F (43.3°C) if a heating pad is used. • Observe surrounding skin for erythema or burning.
Client refuses to keep application intact.	• Elicit reason for uncooperative behavior. Determine if client is uncomfortable. • Explain rationale for treatment.
Pack is difficult to secure due to affected area or activity of client.	• Use a roll of kerlix (wide gauze) to wrap and mold the pack to the body. • Use a small sheet to wrap around the trunk. • Have a person (parent for child) hold the pack in place only if absolutely necessary.
Elderly client is confused.	• Assign health care team member to stay with client during treatment, or schedule treatment when client can be checked on frequently.
Vasoconstriction occurs due to heat treatment being on too long.	• Observe the treatment time carefully and remove the heat on time. • Observe the skin for possible damage due to prolonged heat. Report to physician. • Take vital signs to assess for cardiovascular changes. • Reduce temperature of heat application (i.e., decrease Aqua-K pad or sitz bath temperature) or solution temperatures for moist soaks.

unit 2

WARM DRY HEAT

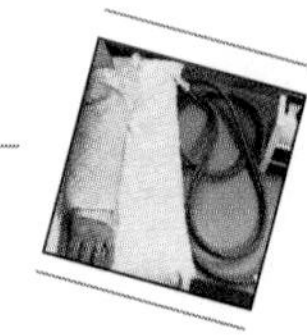

NURSING PROCESS DATA

ASSESSMENT Data Base

Observe client's skin for possible reaction to previous heat treatments.

Assess vital signs, especially temperature, to determine if overheating occurs.

Observe for and remove ointments and creams, which are nonheat-conductive materials.

Assess pain relief obtained from heat treatment.

Check cast for dampness.

PLANNING Objectives

To increase circulation to compromised area of the body

To provide comfort and relaxation

To promote drying of wound or cast

To warm a body part

To promote healing

IMPLEMENTATION Procedures

Using a Commercial Heat Pack

Using a Heat Cradle

Using the Infant Radiant Warmer

Applying an Aquathermic Pad

EVALUATION Expected Outcomes

Body part is warmed.

Drying of cast is accomplished.

Relaxation of muscle spasms occurs.

Healing is accomplished.

Circulation is increased to compromised body area.

USING A COMMERCIAL HEAT PACK

Equipment

Prepackaged heat pack

Tape

Procedure

1. Check physician's orders for type of heat treatment.
2. Wash your hands.
3. Gather equipment.
4. Explain procedure to client.
5. Provide privacy.
6. Remove heat pack from outer wrapper.
7. Break inner seal by holding pack tightly in the center and in an upright position.
8. Squeeze firmly to break seal. **Rationale:** Breaking the seal activates the chemical ingredients and produces the heat.
9. Check for leakage from the pack. Remove pack immediately if leakage occurs. **Rationale:** Chemicals from the pack may cause a burn to the skin.
10. Gently shake the pack, and then apply to treatment area.
11. Remove pack after 30 seconds, and assess skin for erythema.

12. Replace pack and secure with tape. Keep in place 15–30 minutes or as ordered by physician.
13. Remove pack, and discard in appropriate container.
14. Wash your hands.

USING A HEAT CRADLE

Equipment

Heat cradle with 25-watt bulb

Pillows to ensure client comfort and alignment during treatment

Sheet or bath blanket

Preparation

1. Review physician's orders to determine treatment area, type of application, and length of treatment.
2. Gather equipment and check it for safety factors (i.e., frayed cords, water leaks).
3. Bring equipment to client's room.
4. Explain procedure to client.
5. Wash your hands.

Procedure

1. Ensure that 25-watt bulbs are used (Table 23–1).
2. Place cradle over affected area, 18–24 inches from the client.
3. Cover client and cradle with sheet or bath blanket to prevent exposure and chilling.
4. Remove heat cradle after 10–15 minutes.
5. Observe skin for erythema, burning, or untoward effects.
6. Reposition client for comfort.
7. Return equipment to proper storage area.

TABLE 23–1. Dry Heat Application

Application	Use	Precautions
Heat lamp*	Provide heat to skin surface or mucous membrane	Use only 60-watt bulb
	May be used in drying casts	When used to dry casts, be aware that cast may be dry on outside only
Infrared lamp	Provide heat to skin surface or mucous membrane	Be aware that heat penetrates only 3 mm of body tissue
Heat cradle	Supply heat to abdomen, perineum, or chest	Use only 25-watt bulbs Ensure that temperature inside cradle does not exceed 125°F
Aquathermic pad	Supply heat to small body part or to portions of back	Ensure that temperature does not exceed 105°F Do not secure with safety pins
Heating pad*	Supply heat to any body surface	Do not secure with safety pins as could cause shock if wire were hit Set temperature control on medium

*Generally not used in hospitals due to safety problems (i.e., burns and electrical malfunctions).

USING THE INFANT RADIANT WARMER

Equipment

Radiant warmer with skin or rectal probe

Bedding appropriate for warmer

Preparation

1. Several different radiant warmers, or infant care centers, are available. Follow the manufacturer's operating instructions for safety and to determine if a manual or proportional controller is used. (General operating instructions and protocols are presented here.)
2. Check caster locks to make certain that each caster is in locked position.
3. Adjust procedure table to desired position.
4. Plug line cord into a three-wire receptacle.
5. Turn power switch ON; the red pilot light and the alarm indicator should glow. Turn alarm

switch ON to test alarm system.
6. Turn manual knob to automatic.
7. Install skin or rectal probe in controller and set switch to either rectal or skin, depending on which probe is being used.
8. Warm unit for 7 minutes.
9. Adjust temperature to degree ordered by physician; temperature is dialed on digital temperature set switch.

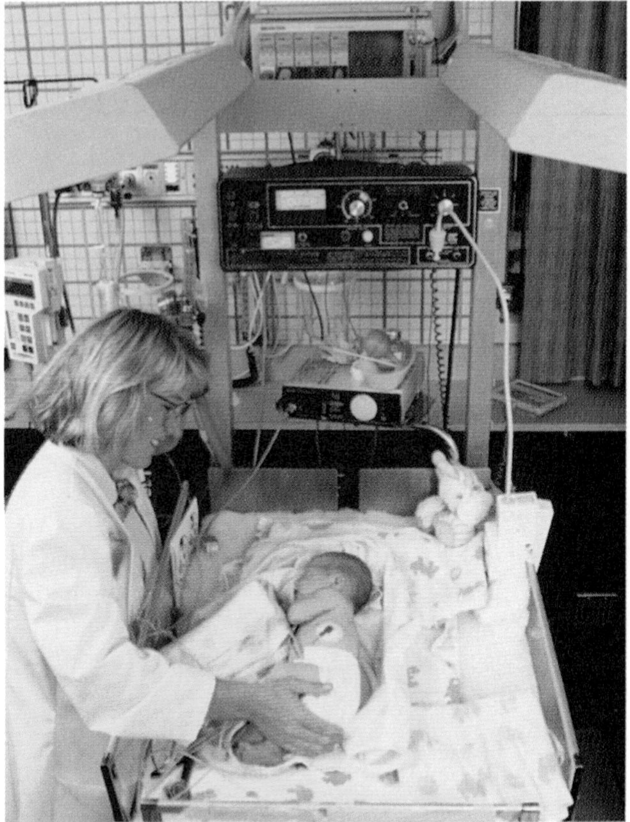

Infant overhead warmer is used to maintain body temperature.

Procedure

1. Place infant in warmer.
2. Attach skin probe.
   a. Place 1-cm skin probe with polished surface touching skin to left of the umbilicus.
   b. Use a rectal probe if hospital protocol permits.
3. Monitor placement of skin probe.
   a. Inspect infant's skin under probe at regular intervals. **Rationale:** Infant's skin is delicate and irritates easily.
   b. Change the probe location if irritation begins to appear.
   c. Do not use adhesive tape or pads. **Rationale:** These may cause skin irritation or allergic reactions. Infant's skin is very thin and fragile.
4. Allow 3–5 minutes for probe to reach infant's temperature.
5. Activate audible alarm by setting switch to ON. **Rationale:** If the infant's temperature exceeds 102°F (38.8°C), the audible alarm sounds and the visible alarm light flashes.
6. When the infant is removed from the warmer, provide preventive maintenance of warmer, such as cleaning thoroughly and inspecting all parts.

APPLYING AN AQUATHERMIC PAD

Equipment

Aquathermic reservoir container
Aquathermic pad (disposable)
Distilled water
Towel or pillow case (optional)

Preparation

1. Review physician's orders to determine treatment area, type of application, and temperature of treatment.
2. Wash hands.
3. Gather equipment, and check it for safety factors (i.e., frayed cords, water leaks).

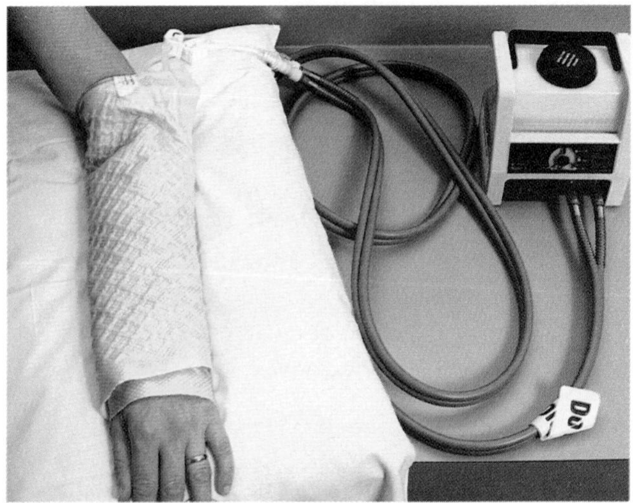

Aqua K pads serve multiple purposes in client care.

4. Bring equipment to client's room.
5. Explain procedure to client.
6. Fill reservoir container two-thirds full of distilled water and check that it is free of air bubbles.
7. Place the reservoir container on bedside stand, and plug into electric outlet. **Rationale:** If reservoir is placed below bed level the water cannot circulate through the system.
8. Place temperature control on LOW setting. **Rationale:** This prevents burning.
9. Turn on switch. Allow water to circulate through pad to warm pad. Ensure that temperature does not exceed 105°F (40.5°C).

Procedure

1. Cover pad with towel or pillow case, and place pad on affected area. (Optional: Most pads are for one use only and are discarded after use.) If arm or leg is used, pad may be tied around extremity using kerlix or towel and tape. **Rationale:** Pins should not be used to secure pad, as pins may puncture pad and cause a leak.
2. Check client's skin after 2–3 minutes. **Rationale:** This is to assess for possible skin reaction as a result of the pad temperature being too hot.
3. Instruct client to notify you if the pad seems too warm. **Rationale:** This prevents burning of skin.
4. Remove pad after 15–20 minutes. Observe area for redness, pain, or any untoward reaction.
5. When pad is used to keep dressings or soaks warm, continue treatment longer than 20 minutes if ordered. Treatment may be continuous when used for clients with back pain.
6. Place pad on bedside stand until next treatment or place in appropriate disposal area.
7. Reposition client for comfort.

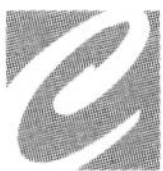

CHARTING for Warm Dry Heat

- Appearance of area before and after application
- Length of time of application
- Type of application used
- Client's response to application

CRITICAL THINKING APPLICATION

CLINICAL PROBLEMS	CRITICAL THINKING OPTIONS
■ Client experiences discomfort with heat.	• Reduce the control settings. • Remove heat application. • Examine client for burns or tissue damage. • Check for malfunctioning equipment.
■ Client's internal (core) temperature rises above normal or desired value.	• Remove the heat source. • Avoid chilling the client. • Take client's vital signs frequently, including temperature, until returned to normal.
■ Client turns up equipment control settings on own volition.	• Explain reasons why settings must not be changed (e.g., burns). • Reset, and observe settings frequently. • Assess for tissue damage. Report to physician. • Discuss reasons why client may have not been sensing the true temperature of the equipment (peripheral receptors become depressed after a time and pad may not feel hot). • Move machine out of client's reach.
■ Client is losing too much body fluid from a full body warmer (exposure to heat produces sweating and evaporative heat loss).	• Give fluids unless contraindicated. • Use fluid-retaining material between the client and ambient air (e.g., plastic Saran wrap) to allow heat to come through but retard fluid and heat loss through evaporation.
■ Client is burned by presence of creams or ointments on the skin.	• Remove creams or ointments. Notify physician. • Assess skin carefully for damage. • Obtain order for and apply cooling measures such as ice bag to area.

unit 3

COLD APPLICATIONS

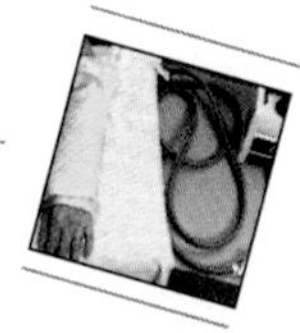

NURSING PROCESS DATA

ASSESSMENT Data Base

Check the purpose for the cool application (e.g., injury, fever).

Determine client's ability to tolerate cold application.

Assess baseline vital signs, and assess any hazards to client's vital functions with the application of cold.

Check if antipyretic medications have been administered (identify type, amount, time, and response) in addition to the cool application.

Observe fluid and electrolyte status, especially in clients with elevated temperatures.

Assess condition of skin before and after application to determine if alterations occur.

PLANNING Objectives

To promote vasoconstriction

To decrease edema

To reduce pain

To decrease temperature

To decrease or stop bleeding

IMPLEMENTATION Procedures

Providing a Tepid Bath

Using Ice Application

Using Instant Cold Pack

EVALUATION Expected Outcomes

Edema is slowed or reduced locally.

Client's internal (core) temperature is reduced.

Pain is reduced or alleviated.

Bleeding is reduced or alleviated.

PROVIDING A TEPID BATH

Equipment

Water source or source of coolant (e.g., water, or alcohol and water mixture) for equipment

Basin or tub for sponge bath

Washcloth and towels

Thermometer

Bath blanket

Lightweight linens

Preparation

1. Review order for type of bath to be given: water, or alcohol mixed with equal parts of water.
2. Note temperature of solution ordered and length of time of application.
3. Gather equipment, and bring to client's room. Identify client.
4. Provide privacy, and explain procedure.
5. Wash your hands.

Procedure

1. Remove client's clothing to allow for cooling and observation. Use bath blanket for privacy.
2. Observe skin surface before cold wrap is applied, and take vital signs, especially temperature.
3. Monitor body color and vital signs every 15–30 minutes during cooling.

4. Immerse washcloths or material for sponging in ordered solution, generally 70–80°F (21–27°C). **Rationale:** Alcohol is infrequently used due to its drying effect; however, due to efficiency of action, it should be used when the temperature needs to be decreased quickly.
5. Wring out excess solution, and place cloths on forehead, back of neck, axilla, groin, and wrists. **Rationale:** The vascularity of these areas promotes cooling.
6. Depending on type of bath, change wraps or soaks every 5 minutes. **Rationale:** This prevents wraps from holding body heat.
7. Replace warmed cloths, and continue procedure for 20–30 minutes, then stop, and reassess client's condition.
8. Do not allow shivering to occur. Stop the treatment or modify it to prevent shivering. **Rationale:** If the body senses a loss of heat, it attempts to produce it by thermogenesis, conserve it, or dissipate it.
9. Cool the air to 68–72°F (20.0–22.2°C) if possible.
10. Promote movement of air (fanning) if possible.
11. If using alcohol solution, promote ventilation of the room, and observe carefully for client's response.
12. Take temperature every 15 minutes. When temperature has decreased to desirable level, dry skin and replace light covering over client and reposition for comfort.
13. Determine client's response to cool treatment.
14. Continue to take vital signs every 1–2 hours until temperature is stabilized.
15. Provide high-calorie diet. **Rationale:** Increased temperatures cause an increased metabolic rate. Carbohydrates, proteins, and 2500–3000 mL fluid intake is essential for maintaining homeostasis.

USING ICE APPLICATION

Equipment

Ice cap, ice bag, ice collar, ice glove, freeze bag
Crushed ice
Plastic drape or absorbent pad
Face towel

Preparation

1. Review order for type and length of treatment.
2. Gather equipment for specific applications.
3. Wash your hands.
4. Fill container, if needed, two-thirds full with crushed ice, express air, and secure top shut.
5. Place absorbent covering over ice applicator.
6. Take equipment to client's room.

Procedure

1. Identify client by checking identaband.
2. Explain procedure.
3. Provide privacy as needed.
4. Take baseline vital signs, if needed, and observe the skin surface where ice is to be applied.
5. Cover ice pack with face towel. **Rationale:** This prevents direct contact with skin.
6. Place ice pack over designated area.
7. Secure with gauze strip or tape.
8. Remove ice pack after 5–10 minutes to check skin's response to cold.
9. Remove every 10 minutes, and check skin until treatment is completed.
10. Remove ice pack after 30 minutes or when absorbent cover becomes wet. Observe skin for any untoward effects, such as bluish, purple appearance or a feeling of numbness.
11. Reposition client for comfort, and provide warmth if needed.
12. Dispose of ice pack or empty ice from collar or glove for reuse.
13. Reapply ice pack in 1 hour if necessary.

USING INSTANT COLD PACK

Equipment

Packaged cold pack

Preparation

1. Review orders, and check length of treatment.
2. Gather equipment.
3. Wash your hands.
4. Identify client by checking identaband.
5. Explain procedure.
6. Provide privacy.

Procedure

1. Grasp top of cold pack, and shake contents to bottom of bag.
2. Hold package in the middle with both hands, or follow directions on package.
3. Squeeze the package firmly to break the inner pouch.
4. Shake the package gently to mix the chemicals together.

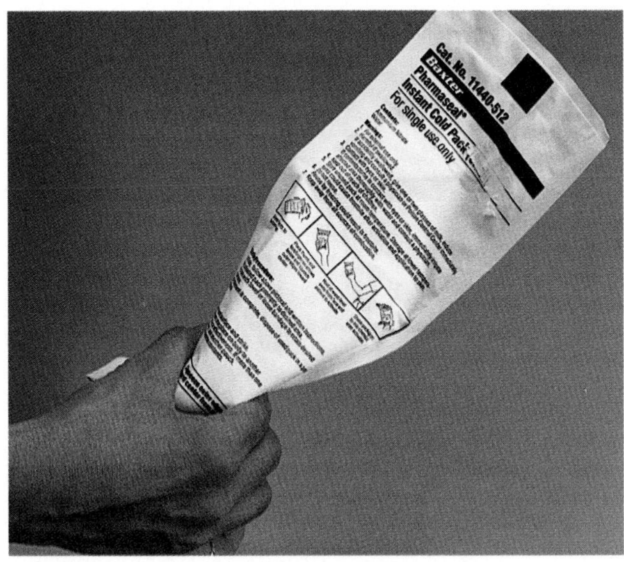

Commercially packaged, single-use cold pack.

5. Apply directly on the injured area.
6. If package is punctured or opened and the solution touches the skin, flush the area with water. **Rationale:** The chemicals can burn the skin.

CHARTING for Cold Applications

- Specific cold application used to reduce temperature
- Time of treatment
- Effectiveness of treatment
- Client's response to procedure
- Vital signs taken during application

CRITICAL THINKING APPLICATION

CLINICAL PROBLEMS	CRITICAL THINKING OPTIONS
■ Local edema is not reduced.	• Elevate extremity above level of heart. • Ensure that body surface is sufficiently covered with cold application to cause vasoconstriction. • Apply cold treatment for first 24 hours until edema has dissipated, as ordered.

CLINICAL PROBLEMS	CRITICAL THINKING OPTIONS
■ Bleeding continues even with cold applications.	• Reassess area for possible "bleeders," which may require cautery or ligation by the physician. • If bleeding continues for extended time or large blood loss is observed, notify physician immediately. • If bleeding occurs in an extremity, elevate the extremity above the level of the heart to decrease blood flow to the area. • Continue with cold application because cold constricts the arterioles and increases the viscosity of the blood, assisting in the control of bleeding.
■ Client feels cold.	• Apply warmth to soles of feet. • Place bath blanket over unaffected area.
■ Internal (core) temperature drops too low.	• Monitor the temperature frequently, every 30–60 minutes. • Warm the client slowly. • Take vital signs every 15–30 minutes.
■ Skin becomes irritated or macerated from sponging or cooling measures.	• Remove cold application from the area and use alternative surface site. • Apply petroleum jelly or oil to area when using cold applications. • Do not massage or rub the area as this action can cause tissue damage.
■ Total numbness occurs at the site of the cold application.	• Warm the area immediately by placing body surface in 110°F (43.3°C) water. Remove extremity from water when red flush appears. • Apply loose dry dressing if area appears broken down. • Observe circulation closely for any alterations. • Observe for signs of frostbite.
■ Pain occurs at the site of cold applications.	• Remove cold application. • Warm the site a few degrees. • Inspect for tissue damage.
■ Client becomes nauseated or disoriented from alcohol fumes.	• Discontinue using alcohol; remove it from area. • Provide ventilation in room. • Assess vital signs.
■ Client becomes very cyanotic or mottled.	• Discontinue cooling. • Assess vital signs. • Warm the site a few degrees. • Observe site for signs of frostbite.

unit 4

HYPOTHERMIA BLANKET

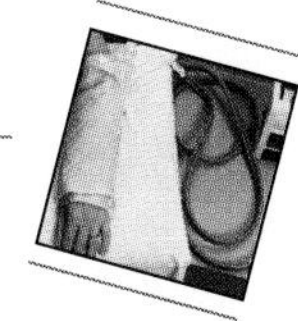

NURSING PROCESS DATA

ASSESSMENT Data Base

Evaluate if client's temperature can be reduced by less intensive measures.

Assess skin condition, especially of face, ears, hands, and feet, before, during, and following treatment.

Determine client's ability to tolerate treatment.

Assess baseline data (i.e., vital signs, neurologic signs, mental status, peripheral circulation).

Assess that the cooling blanket and machine are functioning properly.

Evaluate ECG findings throughout treatment.

Assess fluid and electrolyte balance (especially potassium level).

Evaluate fluid intake and output throughout treatment.

Assess for shivering.

PLANNING Objectives

To protect the skin from injury during use of the cooling blanket

To prevent shivering during cold applications

To ensure that the cooling blanket functions properly

To reduce body's internal (core) temperature

To provide hypothermia for operative procedures

To decrease metabolic processes, thereby preventing irreversible states

IMPLEMENTATION Procedure

Using a Cooling Blanket

EVALUATION Expected Outcomes

Skin remains free of injury during use of the cooling blanket.

Cooling blanket functions properly.

Client's internal temperature is reduced without any untoward effects.

Shivering is avoided during use of the cooling blanket.

USING A COOLING BLANKET

Equipment

Disposable cooling blanket, top or bottom (or both), machine

Thermometer

Sphygmomanometer

Stethoscope

Thermometer probe

Sheet or thin blanket (optional)

Towels, 4

Preparation

1. Check physician's orders and client care plan.
2. Gather equipment.
3. Check that electrical plugs are grounded.
4. Ensure that amount of coolant is sufficient. If not, add 20% isopropyl alcohol solution through the

reservoir cap. To mix a 20% alcohol solution:
   a. Mix 1 quart 50% alcohol with $1\frac{1}{2}$ quarts distilled water.
   b. Mix 1 quart 70% alcohol with $2\frac{1}{2}$ quarts distilled water.
5. Connect the cooling pad to the machine.
   a. Push back the collar. Insert the male tubing connector of the cooling pad into the inlet opening. Release the collar.
   b. Repeat connection using the outlet opening.
   c. If two pads are being used, connect the second pad in the same manner.
6. Turn the unit on by moving the master temperature control knob to the desired temperature. The pads from the machine reservoir fill automatically.
7. Add the alcohol mixture to the reservoir as the pads fill. Observe the reservoir sight gauge to determine the fluid level.
8. Set the master temperature control knob to either automatic or manual operation. **Rationale:** There are two separate temperature control knobs, one for automatic and one for manual operation.
9. When using automatic control, insert the thermister probe plug in the electronic control thermister probe jack.
10. When using manual control, set the master "temperature control knob" to the desired temperature.
11. Bring equipment to client's room.
12. Identify client and explain procedure.
13. Provide privacy.
14. Wash your hands.
15. Take baseline vital signs.

CLASSIFICATION OF HYPOTHERMIA

- Mild 32–37°C
- Moderate 28–32°C
- Deep 20–28°C
- Profound 0–20°C

Procedure

1. Place the cooling blanket on bed, and connect it to the machine. Precool blanket to 5–10°C.
2. Place a sheet or a thin bath blanket over the cooling blanket. (Optional: Cooling blankets are disposable and designed for one time use only.)
3. Obtain baseline client data before starting treatment.

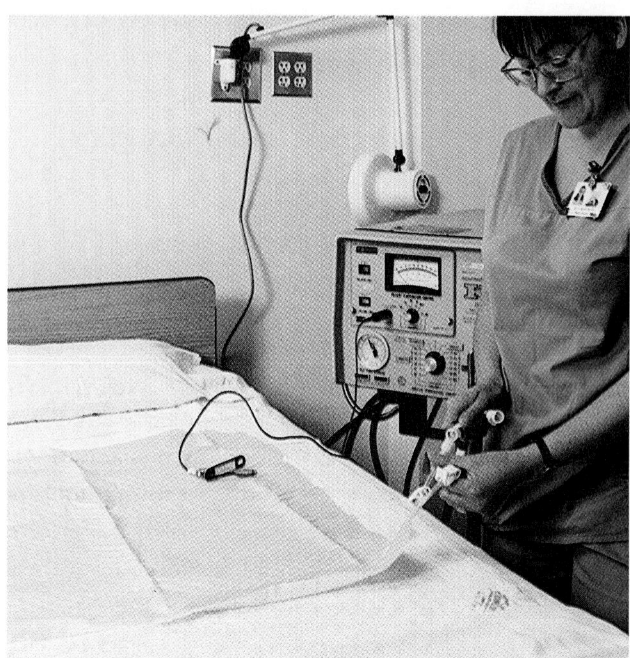

Disposable cooling blanket pad and machine.

4. Place client on the cooling blanket. Wrap client's hands and feet in towels. **Rationale:** This prevents frostbite or skin damage.

For Automatic Control

   a. Insert the probe into client's rectum.
   b. Check that temperature control knob is at the desired temperature.
   c. Observe that the automatic mode light is on.
   d. Check that the pad temperature limits are set at desired safety limits.

For Manual Control

   a. Insert the probe into client's rectum.
   b. Observe that the cool mode light is on.
   c. Watch that the cool limit warning light does not illuminate. **Rationale:** This light indicates that unit temperature is below 37°C.
   d. Monitor the fluid thermometer, which indicates temperature of pad. **Rationale:** This ensures pad temperature is maintained at desired level.
5. Set the temperature control to 37°C, and begin lowering temperature 1°C every 15 minutes until 33° or 34°C is reached.
6. Monitor client's temperature every 15 minutes.
7. Observe client for signs predicting onset of shivering: ECG muscle tremor artifact, visible facial mus-

cle twitchings, hyperventilation, and verbalized sensations.

8. If manifestations of shivering occur, obtain order for IV medications, usually chlorpromazine.
9. While client undergoes hypothermia, monitor vital signs every 30 minutes during reduction of temperature control and then every 2 hours.
10. Monitor with ECG if the client has cardiac disease or hypokalemia.
11. Observe obese clients for fluid balance alterations.
12. Remove and clean rectal probe every 4 hours.
13. Check the automatic temperature control every 4 hours for accuracy by taking temperature with an external thermometer. **Rationale:** The type of thermometer used—oral, axillary, or rectal—depends on the client's condition. Remember that oral and axillary temperatures tend to be less accurate indicators of the true internal body temperature.
14. Check physician's order for and apply thigh-high support stockings. **Rationale:** Stockings prevent venous stasis.
15. Turn, cough, and deep-breathe client every 30 minutes.
16. Monitor client's skin condition, and massage bony prominences every 2 hours.
17. When physician orders hyothermia to be discontinued, gradually increase temperature from 30–37°C over 6 hours.
18. Monitor vital signs every 15 minutes during warming.
19. Observe for edema. **Rationale:** This is caused by increased cell permeability, acidotic shock due to shivering, fluid imbalance, and hypothermia.
20. Clean and return equipment to central supply following use. Dispose of blanket.
21. Monitor client's vital signs frequently after discontinuation of treatment.
22. Make client comfortable.

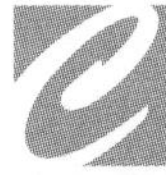

CHARTING for Cooling Blanket

- Client's temperature and method of taking temperature
- Baseline vital signs
- Any untoward effects of the treatment (i.e., shivering)
- Setting of the cooling blanket
- Whether the top blanket is used
- Skin condition
- Skin treatments done prior to use of cooling blanket
- Length of cooling blanket treatment

CRITICAL THINKING APPLICATION

CLINICAL PROBLEMS	CRITICAL THINKING OPTIONS
■ Client's core temperature decreases rapidly and falls below 37°C.	• Turn off cooling blanket. • Take top blanket off if you are using one.
■ Client begins to shiver.	• Stop the procedure or warm the solution a few degrees (or both). • Monitor temperature because shivering causes an increase in the metabolic rate leading to an increase in heat production. • Monitor temperature every 15 minutes to detect additional temperature decrease. • If temperature continues to drop, the blanket can be turned on to the warming control and the client can be warmed.
■ The rectal temperature probe does not seem to be accurate.	• Assess client's skin condition for cold, presence of peripheral pulses, and ability to feel pressure. • Take client's temperature every 2 hours with glass or electronic thermometer to evaluate the accuracy of the thermister. • Calibrate the thermister to ensure that the temperature reading of the thermister is accurate.
■ Client's core temperature is not reduced.	• Check the master temperature control to see what limits are set. May need to decrease lower limit. Do not set below 30°C without checking with physician. • Place a top cooling pad on client to provide a greater body surface area in contact with pads. • Place a blanket over the top pad to insulate and provide a more effective and rapid control of temperature. • Attach small cooling pads to the extra connections on the machine to provide cold areas to body where the arteries are close to the surface, such as groin, axilla, and neck.
■ Skin is injured during use of the cooling blanket.	• Make sure client is turned every 30 minutes. • Lubricate skin with petroleum jelly to provide protection. • Wrap client's hands and feet securely to prevent frostbite. • Massage bony prominences at least every hour. • Ensure that the master control temperature is not set too low. • Chart changes in skin condition.

CLINICAL PROBLEMS	CRITICAL THINKING OPTIONS
Cooling blanket does not function properly.	• Check that plug is not disconnected from the outlet. • Check that the alcohol level is sufficient and that unit freezing has not occurred. • Check that the thermister probe is properly connected. • Check that the cool limit on the pad is not set too high. • Check that there is no constriction through pads or tubing.

GERIATRIC CONSIDERATIONS

Elderly clients are more susceptible to injury from heat and cold therapy as a result of physiologic changes.

- There is increased epidermal replacement time and cells are replaced more slowly in the elderly.
- Skin in the elderly is thin and contains less moisture.
- The elderly have a reduced sensitivity to pain, and therefore may not feel untoward effects of heat and cold treatment.

With the high risk for injury during heat and cold therapy, the nurse must pay particular attention to skin assessment of the treatment area.

- Water temperature needs to be decreased when using heat therapy because the elderly client's skin burns more easily.
- The skin of the elderly gives less protection against trauma.

Vital signs and frequent assessment may need to be carried out during heat and cold therapy as vasodilation from heat or vasoconstriction from cold can cause changes in cardiac function and blood pressure.

24

Wound Care and Dressings

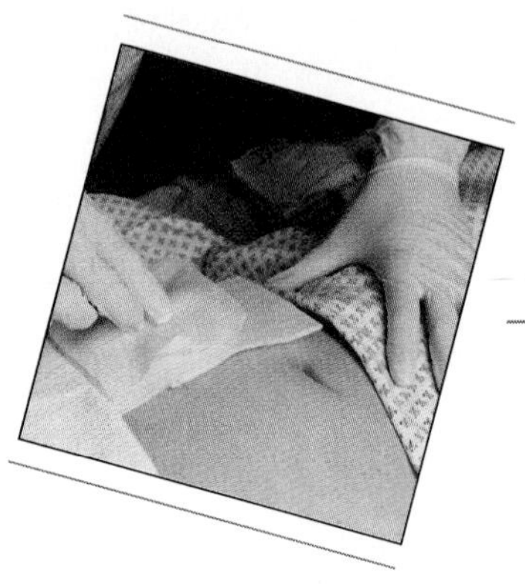

LEARNING OBJECTIVES

- Describe the three phases of wound healing.
- Define the three types of wound healing.
- Discuss three factors that affect wound healing.
- State three complications associated with wound healing.
- State criteria used to assess a wound.
- Compare and contrast the four stages of pressure ulcers.
- Write three nursing diagnoses for a client requiring wound care.
- State three goals of wound care.
- Discuss the effect of topical agents in wound healing.
- Differentiate between clean, contaminated, and infected wounds.
- Compare and contrast clean and sterile technique.
- Explain appropriate use of dressings: gauze, adhesive clear film, hydrocolloid, and hydrogel.
- Outline the steps in irrigating a wound.
- List steps to obtain a wound specimen for culture.
- Perform the steps of a surgical hand scrub.
- Prepare a sterile field for a dressing change.
- Demonstrate the steps of putting on sterile gloves.
- Describe the procedure for cleaning around a drain site.
- List steps used to maintain a Hemovac or Jackson–Pratt suction drain.
- Outline the steps for removal of staples and sutures.
- Outline the procedure for changing a wet-to-damp dressing.
- Demonstrate changing a sterile dressing.
- Complete charting on a wound assessment and wound care.

TERMINOLOGY

Adhesions: formation of fibrous scar tissue around the incision as a result of surgical intervention. Adhesions can cause obstruction or malfunction by distorting the organ.

Aerobe: a microorganism that lives and grows in the presence of free oxygen.

Anaerobe: an organism that lives and grows in the absence of molecular oxygen.

Antimicrobial: an agent that prevents the multiplication of microorganisms.

Asepsis: prevention of contact with microorganisms.

Collagen formation: formation of the protein substance of the white fibers of skin, bone, and cartilage.

Contracture: abnormal shortening of muscle tissue making the muscle resistant to stretching.

Debris: remains of damaged or broken down tissue or cells.

Decubitus ulcer: see Pressure ulcer.

Dermis: synonym for corium; the skin layer beneath the epidermis; contains vascular connective tissues.

Dehiscence: a bursting open, as a graafian follicle or wound, especially abdominal wounds.

Edematous: the presence of abnormally large amounts of fluid in the intercellular tissue spaces of the body.

Epidemiology: division of medical science concerned with defining and explaining the interrelationships of the host, agent, and environment in causing disease.

Epithelium: outer covering of the body; top layer of skin.

Erythema: redness of the skin due to congestion of capillaries.

Evisceration: protrusion of the viscera; removal of the viscera.

Exudate: material obtained from a wound as the result of the inflammatory process.

Gangrene: death and putrefaction of body tissue precipitated by poor or absent blood supply to the tissue. Occurs as a result of infection, injury, or disease processes.

Granulation: formation of granules; fleshy projections formed on the surface of a gaping wound that is not healing by the normal joining together of skin edges.

Incision: a cut made with a knife.

Infection: morbid state caused by multiplication of pathogenic microorganisms within the body.

Inflammatory process: localized response when injury or destruction of tissue has occurred; destroys, wards off, or dilutes the causative agent or the injured tissue.

Irrigate: to rinse or wash out with a fluid.

Isolation: limitation of movement and social contacts of a client; especially those having communicable diseases.

Keloid: scarlike growth of collagen that results in a rounded, hard, shiny, white benign tumor.

Macrophage: a large monocyte that has left the circulation and settled and matured in tissue and serves as scavenger of the blood, cleaning it of old cells and cellular debris.

Microorganism: minute living body not perceptible to the naked eye.

Monocyte: phagocytic white blood cell that matures into a macrophage.

Monokine: chemical mediator released by monocytes and macrophages during the immune response. They affect growth and activity of other white blood cells.

Myofibroblast: an atypical fibroblast with features of a fibroblast and a smooth muscle cell.

Necrotic: death of a portion of tissue.

Neutrophil: white blood cells responsible for body's protection against infection. Plays a large role in the inflammatory process.

Occlusion: the closure or state of being closed, of a passage.

Organism: a living thing, either plant or animal.

Pathogen: disease-producing organism.

Phagocytosis: ingestion and digestion of bacteria by phagocytes.

Pressure ulcer: a break in the skin caused by pressure and restricted blood flow to the area. The ulcer generally occurs over bony prominences of the heels, sacrum, hip, and shoulder.

Primary healing: the first stage in the wound-healing process in which the blood clot forms and the inflammatory reaction develops at a wound site.

Purulent: containing pus, or caused by pus.

Pus: an inflammation containing leukocytes and exudate.

Second intention healing: second stage in wound healing in which granulation occurs.

Tertiary healing: using open method of wound healing; allows granulation to occur.

Wound dehiscence: the separation of layers of a surgical wound.

Wound evisceration: protrusion of the internal viscera or organs through an opened incisional site.

WOUND HEALING

The three major phases of wound healing are inflammation, proliferation (or granulation), and maturation (or wound remodeling).

Inflammatory Phase

The onset of the first phase of wound healing occurs immediately after an injury and lasts 4–6 days. After the injury small blood vessels dilate and become more permeable and serous fluid leaks into the traumatized tissue. Neutrophils reach the site in about 6 hours. Through the process of phagocytosis they assist in preventing infection by ingesting and digesting bacteria. Oxygen is necessary for the neutrophils to destroy the bacteria. They survive only several hours after ingesting bacteria and necrotic tissue before releasing their intracellular contents, which forms part of the wound exudate. By the fourth day monocytes enter the wound and differentiate into macrophages, which digest necrotic tissue, remove debris, and inhibit microbial growth. They also play a role in creating collagen synthesis. If macrophages are depleted, deposition of wound collagen decreases significantly. Macrophages direct healing through the release of monokines.

Proliferative, or Granulation, Phase

This phase begins between 1 and 4 days after the injury and ends 14–21 days later. During granulation there is rapid growth of epithelial cells to produce a protective covering for the wound. The granulation tissue is formed from a rebuilding of the vascular capillary network and collagen tissue. The collagen fibers increase the tensile strength of the wound and provide wound integrity. Collagen fibers fill in the gaps and form the scar. Wound scar tissue is very fragile and susceptible to reinjury. In 6 weeks the scar is only 10% of the tensile strength of normal skin. Large wounds may take months to build enough granulation tissue to close the wound. Healthy granulation tissue has a beefy red color.

Maturation, or Wound-Remodeling, Phase

Wound contraction begins between 14 and 21 days after the injury and can last up to 2 years. During this phase the scar shrinks and thins. It becomes less red as the capillaries regress. Contraction of the wound occurs as a result of myofibroblasts, which assist in moving the wound edges toward the center of the wound. The skin and fascia of the healed wound achieve only about 70–80% of the tensile strength of normal skin.

TYPES OF WOUND HEALING

Primary Intention

This is the simplest form of healing. The skin is cleanly incised through a surgical incision or a traumatic laceration. The wound can be closed with sutures or staples, which approximates, or pulls together, the wound edges. These wounds close rapidly because there are no gaps in the tissue. The top layer of cells migrate, or epithelize, within 72 hours. The wound surface is "sealed," thus preventing bacteria from entering and fluid from escaping. The tensile strength of the wound is very weak at this stage of healing.

Secondary Intention

These wounds heal by granulation. As granulation tissue builds, it fills the gap under the skin and cells epithelize from the edge of the wound to create the closure. Burns, pressure ulcers, and wounds with large pieces of skin missing heal by this method. In these types of wounds no edges are available to be approximated and sutured. These wounds are at risk for local and systemic infection due to the destruction of the dermis and the increased time necessary for healing to occur.

Tertiary Intention

Healing by tertiary intention is a method that leaves the wound open to heal. These wounds are infected and need frequent irrigations and dressing changes to facilitate healing. Clients with peritonitis, a ruptured appendix, or diverticula frequently require this type of wound healing. After irrigations and dressing changes for approximately 10 days, the wound is sutured and allowed to heal by primary and secondary intention.

MAJOR FACTORS AFFECTING WOUND HEALING

Nutrition

The nutritional state of the client plays a major role in wound healing. Low serum albumin levels slow the diffusion of oxygen and diminish the ability of neutrophils to kill bacteria. Low oxygen at the capillary level diminishes the proliferation of healthy granulation tissue. Zinc deficiency can slow the rate of epithelialization and decrease wound and collagen strength. Adequate amounts of vitamins A and C and of iron and copper are necessary for effective collagen formation. Collagen synthesis also depends on appropriate intake of protein, carbohydrates, and fats. Wound healing requires almost double the usual protein and carbohydrate requirements for age. For the scar to develop adequate tensile strength, the client's intake of vitamin C, iron, and zinc must be increased.

General Physical Health

The major obstacle to wound healing is infection. Infected wounds have friable tissue, bleed easily, and have delayed healing. Immunosuppressed clients have more difficulty healing wounds because the inflammatory phase is impaired. When the blood glucose level is consistently over 200 mg/dL or the hemoglobin is below 10 g/dL, wounds do not follow the usual phases of healing. Any condition that reduces the formation of adequate white blood cells, especially macrophages, adversely affects healing. Such conditions include diabetes mellitus, anemia, uremia, cancer, atherosclerosis, infection, and malnutrition. Older clients, clients who smoke or are obese, and those undergoing radiation or steroid therapy are also prone to delayed wound healing.

Medications

Any medication that reduces the inflammatory response, such as steroids and nonsteroidal medications used to treat arthritis or respiratory conditions, also impairs wound healing. Antiinflammatories decrease epithelialization and wound contraction and may also affect fibroblast proliferation and collagen synthesis. Steroids decrease the tensile strength of a closed wound and cause inadequate deposits of collagen. Administration of vitamin A can reverse the processes associated with steroid use.

GOALS OF WOUND CARE

Wound assessment and measures to treat wounds have changed dramatically over the last 10 years. The major trend is to treat wounds using moisture-retentive dressing rather than drying the wound. Wound care specialists also diverge on the use of sterile versus clean technique during dressing changes.

Whatever plan is used in treating a wound, the goals remain the same.

- Remove necrotic tissue to promote wound healing.
- Prevent, eliminate, or control infection.
- Absorb drainage (exudate).
- Maintain a moist wound environment.
- Protect the wound from further injury.
- Protect the surrounding skin from infection and trauma.

To accomplish these goals a moist wound environment must be maintained to allow tissue to granulate. A

wound bed that is too moist or too dry kills healthy tissue and impairs healing. Drainage from the wound site needs to be contained to protect adjacent healthy skin from maceration. All wounds require a dressing which is dry on the air-exposed side to prevent bacterial invasion by downward capillary mobility of contaminants. The dressing should be secured over the wound and taped in place using the "window paning" method of taping. Using this method, the edges remain taped down and the dressing stays intact. Trauma to the wound is prevented by padding the wound with layers of dressing material.

Complications Associated with Wound Healing

One complication that may occur after wound healing has seemed to progress satisfactorily is adhesions. Adhesions frequently form in the peritoneal cavity after abdominal surgery and can either constrict or fold around the intestines.

Frequently clients are admitted to the hospital with incisional strangulated internal hernias that may even be gangrenous. Other complications are surgical or incisional hernias that may occur when the intraperitoneal pressure is such that it pushes against the scar tissue and causes a hernia (or outpouching) through the incision.

Contractures, formed as a result of a shortening of scar tissue, can decrease mobility and joint movement. Contractures caused by incisional scars are far less common than those caused by scar tissue from burns.

Excessive collagen formation results in the formation of a keloid, a complication that does not present a serious problem with body function; however, it generally causes an altered self-image if the keloid is large or in a prominent place on the body.

WOUND INFECTIONS

All wounds may be considered contaminated but not necessarily infected. The clinical symptoms of wound infection generally begin in 36–48 hours postoperatively or following injury. When the client's temperature and pulse rate increase, an associated tachypnea occurs. As the inflammatory process proceeds, the wound becomes progressively more tender and edematous. Erythema surrounds the edges of the wound unless the infection is in the deeper tissues. Foul-smelling, purulent drainage may occur. An absence of local signs of infection does not necessarily mean that deep wound infections are absent.

Several microorganisms are responsible for the majority of wound infections. *Staphylococcus aureus* is still a major cause of postoperative infection. *Escherichia coli, Streptococcus faecalis, Proteus vulgaris, Klebsiella, Enterobacter,* and *Pseudomonas aeruginosa* are also closely associated with wound infection. Antimicrobial agents themselves can promote infection by increasing the susceptibility of clients to colonization with nosocomial microflora; these agents also select and concentrate antibiotic-resistant organisms on or in the host.

Maintaining asepsis during dressing changes assists in preventing wound infections. Using sterile equipment, including gloves, is the first barrier against infection. A mask and gown should be worn during dressing changes to prevent the spread of microorganisms to other clients and to the health care worker.

When wounds become grossly infected or are extensive in nature, the physician may order wound irrigations. Normal saline or Ringer's solution are the usual irrigating solutions used for wounds. Most of the agents used in the past have been identified as toxic to the cells generated in the inflammatory phase of healing.

Each hospital has its own protocol for wound irrigation and you should become familiar with the institution's procedure. This chapter presents one method of wound irrigation that is helpful in most clinical situations.

Wound Specimens for Culture

Exudate, or purulent drainage, from infected wounds can contain a variety of aerobic and anaerobic microorganisms. In the majority of wound infections the causative agent is usually found in the upper respiratory tract, gastrointestinal tract, and genitourinary tract. When these organisms invade other body parts, they can cause severe infections and sometimes death.

Before a wound can be cultured, it should be irrigated with normal saline to remove the surface bacteria. The best method of obtaining a culture specimen is to rotate a swab along the wound edge. Refer to Chapter 19, Specimen Collection, for skill. For the most accurate results, the physician should take a biopsy of the tissue.

Pressure Ulcers

Pressure ulcers are defined by the National Pressure Ulcer Advisory Panel as any lesion caused by unrelieved pressure resulting in damage to underlying tissue. Four mechanical factors contribute to the development of pressure ulcers: pressure, friction, shearing, and moisture. Pressure ulcers are usually located over a bony prominence, where normal tissue is squeezed between the bone and pressure or friction caused by the bed or chair. External pressure that lasts long enough to result in decreased blood flow causes altered oxygenation and nutrition to the tissue, resulting in a pressure ulcer.

Immobility, especially associated with the elderly, is the primary cause of pressure ulcer formation. In addition to mechanical factors and immobility, aging skin and malnutrition increase the risk of skin breakdown.

Pressure ulcers affect about 9% of hospitalized clients and 23% of all nursing home clients. Elderly clients are affected most often and account for the highest number of cases. A large percentage of the clients who develop pressure ulcers in a nursing home die as a result. These statistics are appalling when one considers that ulcers are preventable and treatable.

Pressure ulcers are classified in stages by the degree of tissue damage observed. See unit four for illustration and description.

Management of pressure ulcers is best accomplished using a team of health care providers, including physicians, nurses, an enterostomal therapist, dietician, physical therapist, family members, and the client.

Client education should include

- Discussion of pressure ulcer treatment options
- Discussion of client's active participation in his or her own care
- Developing a plan of care that is consistent with the client's goals and desires

Client treatment plan should include

- Assessment of the pressure ulcer
- Managing tissue loads
- Ulcer care
- Managing bacterial colonization and infection
- Operative repair of the pressure ulcer
- Education and improvement in pressure ulcer

Management and prevention of pressure ulcers should begin on hospital admission with a thorough assessment of the client's skin, especially over bony prominences. Preventive steps for high-risk clients include the following:

- Ensure that skin is kept clean, and prevent it from getting too dry by using moisturizing lotions.
- Provide a balanced diet high in protein, vitamins, and minerals for tissue repair.
- Ensure a fluid intake of 2000 mL/day for adequate hydration.
- Place clients on a pressure-reducing mattress or chair cushion.
- Do not elevate head of the bed more than 30° for a client on bed rest.
- Reposition a bedridden client at least every 2 hours and a chair-bound client every hour—positioning remains the basic standard of ulcer prevention.
- Complete a risk assessment for the client, evaluating factors for developing pressure ulcers.

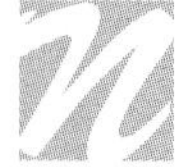

NURSING DIAGNOSES

The following diagnoses may be appropriate to include in a client care plan when the components are related to the client requiring wound care.

NURSING DIAGNOSIS	RELATED FACTORS/RISK FACTORS
Risk for Infection	Altered circulation, invasive procedures, trauma
	Exposure to nosocomial agents, surgical incision, open wound
Pain	Tissue injury, extensive dressing changes, recent surgery
Impaired Physical Mobility	Bed rest, wounds, or pressure ulcers
Impaired Skin Integrity	Mechanical factors (shearing force, pressure), altered circulation due to pressure on a bony prominence, immobility, poor nutritional intake
Altered Tissue Perfusion	Interrupted blood supply to site depleting oxygen and nutrient saturation

unit 1

MEASURES TO PREVENT INFECTION

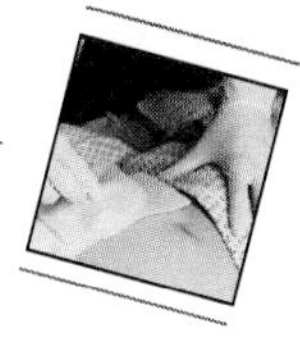

NURSING PROCESS DATA

ASSESSMENT Data Base

Identify clients at risk for infection.

Identify length of time client remained in surgery (the more hours in surgery the greater the risk for infection).

Identify the components necessary to prevent infection for individual clients.

Assess need for sterile technique compliance in client care.

PLANNING Objectives

To prevent clients with impaired resistance from becoming infected

To prevent microorganisms from entering the wound

To provide a sterile working field for dressing changes

IMPLEMENTATION Procedures

Completing a Surgical Hand Scrub

Using Sterile Gloves

Pouring from a Sterile Container

Preparing a Sterile Field

Preparing a Sterile Field Using Prepackaged Supplies

EVALUATION Expected Outcomes

Infection is prevented in clients with impaired resistance.

Sterile technique is maintained throughout wound care.

Sterile field is set up appropriately.

COMPLETING A SURGICAL HAND SCRUB

Equipment

Plastic or orangewood stick

Antimicrobial solution

Sterile towel

Procedure

1. Turn on water using foot or knee pedal or hand lever.
2. Wet your hands thoroughly.
3. With your arms held up in front of you, begin to scrub by cleaning your fingernails with a plastic or orangewood stick.
4. Scrub your hands for 4–5 minutes with an antimicrobial solution.

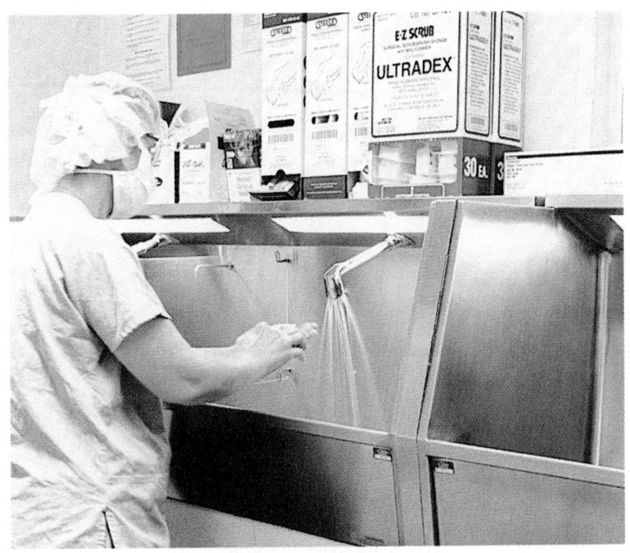

Scrub hands for 4 to 5 minutes with an antimicrobial solution.

a. Scrub may be done using brush or friction of hands.
b. Start at fingertips and with circular motion work around each finger and between each finger.
c. Move to back of hand and use circular motion with scrub.
d. Move to palm of hand, wrist, and then up arm to elbow continuing with circular scrubbing motion.
e. Placing arms under water faucet, keep fingertips pointed upward and rinse thoroughly with water flowing down toward elbows. **Rationale:** This method keeps fingers and hands free of contamination.

5. Dry your hands with a sterile towel starting at the fingertips and moving toward the elbows.
6. If hand levers are used to control water flow, turn faucets off with sterile towel used for drying hands. Do not touch faucet or sink with hands. **Rationale:** Contamination of hands occurs if objects are touched after handwashing.

USING STERILE GLOVES

Equipment

Packaged sterile gloves

Procedure

1. Wash and dry your hands.
2. Grasp two upper edges of outside wrapper and pull laterally to open. Remove gloves.
3. Open glove wrapper, keeping both package and gloves sterile. Open wrapper from the middle of the package outward, maintaining sterility.
4. With your nondominant hand, remove the first glove by grasping the section that has a folded edge. Lift the glove up and away from the wrapper. Be careful not to touch the inside of the package or any part of the glove except the inner surface of the cuff.
5. Slip your dominant hand into the glove opening. Gently pull the glove into place with your nondominant hand, touching only the folded-up cuff. **Rationale:** Don't worry if you have difficulty easing your fingers all the way into the glove. After you have placed both gloves on your hands, you can move your fingers into place.

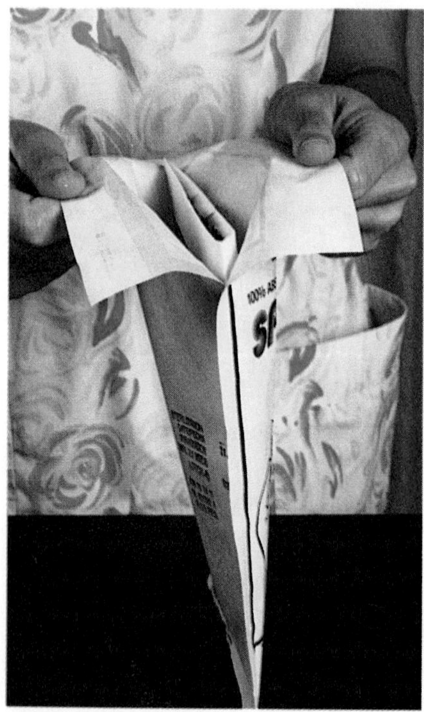

Grasp two upper edges of the glove package and pull laterally to open package.

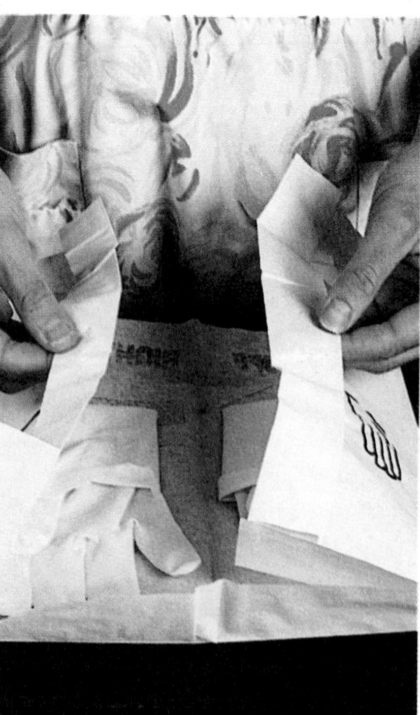

Place sterile glove wrapper on clean, flat surface and lift wrapper edges away from gloves.

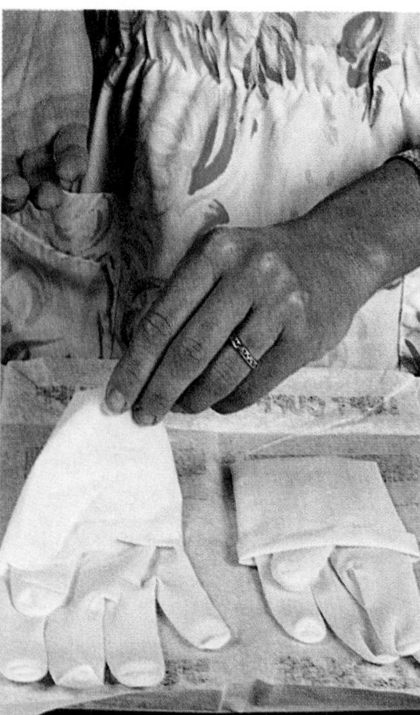

Grasp folded edge of glove with nondominant hand and lift glove away from wrapper.

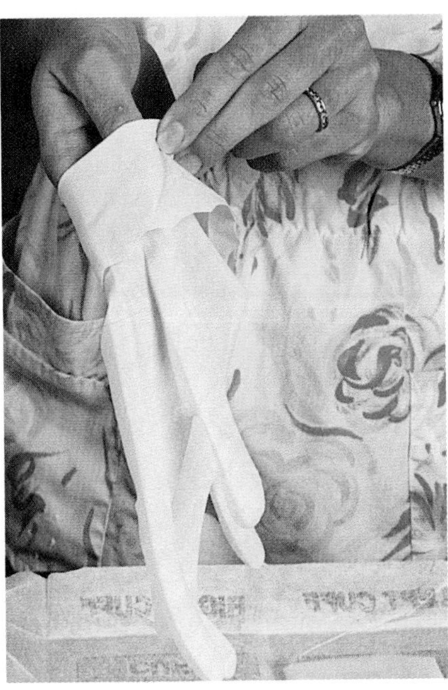

Slip dominant hand into glove opening without contaminating glove.

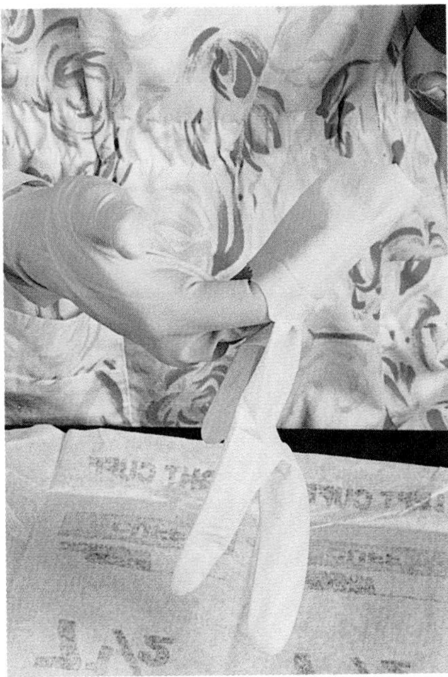

Remove second glove from wrapper by placing gloved hand under cuff.

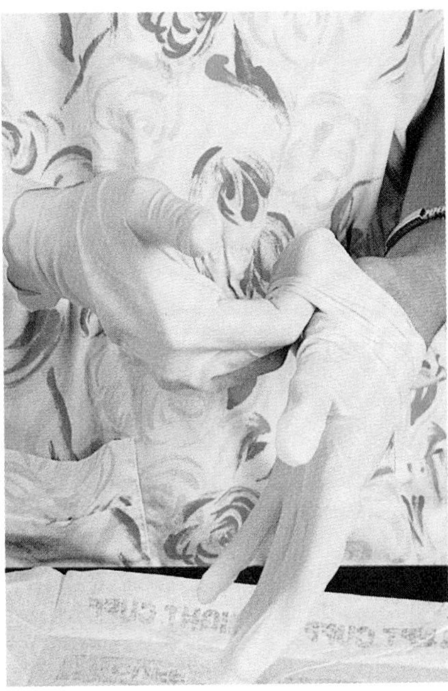

Continue to keep fingers under cuff of glove as the glove is pulled on.

6. With your dominant, gloved hand, remove the other glove from the package, making sure you touch only the inside of the folded cuff. Lift this glove up and away from the wrapper.
7. Place your ungloved fingers into the new glove opening. Gently pull the glove over your hand as before.
8. Adjust both gloves, remembering to touch sterile surfaces with sterile surfaces.
9. Keep both sterile gloves in front of you above your waist level. **Rationale:** Being able to see gloves at all times helps prevent potential contamination.

POURING FROM A STERILE CONTAINER

Equipment

Sterile container

Nonsterile container

Sterile solution

Procedure

1. Wash your hands.
2. Gather equipment.
3. Open sterile container according to procedure.
4. Place container on firm surface.
5. Take cap off the bottle and invert the cap before laying on firm surface. **Rationale:** This keeps the cap sterile.
6. Hold the bottle with the label facing up.
7. Pour a small amount of liquid into a nonsterile container. **Rationale:** This action cleans the lip of the bottle.
8. Pour the liquid into the sterile container while keeping the label facing up and not touching the container with the bottle. Do not reach over a sterile field if the container has been placed on one.
9. Replace the cap if liquid remains in the bottle. If total contents have been used, dispose of bottle in trash.
10. Replace partially filled bottle to storage area if it is to be reused.

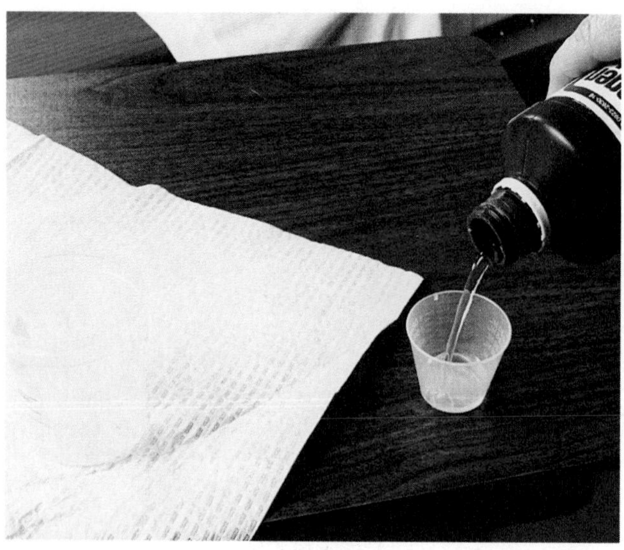

First pour a small amount of liquid into nonsterile container.

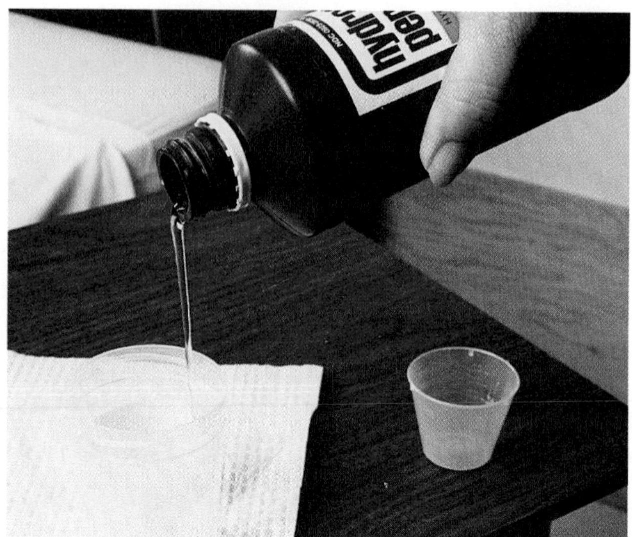

Pour liquid by placing container close to edge of sterile area.

PREPARING A STERILE FIELD

Equipment

Antiseptic cleansing solution, as ordered
Two packages of sterile towels
Number and type of dressings required for dressing change
Tape
Container for antiseptic solution
Disposable paper bag for soiled dressings
Mask
Sterile gloves

> ■ CLINICAL ALERT
>
> Preparing a sterile field is commonly used for burn dressings or large wound dressings.

Preparation

1. Check physician's orders and client care plan.
2. Gather equipment from supply area.
3. Clean off over-bed table.

Procedure

1. Wash your hands, using aseptic techniques.
2. Place sterile towel packages on over-bed table or on another surface close to the table. Place packages so that first wrapper edge can be opened away from the sterile area. **Rationale:** This prevents contamination from crossing over a sterile field.
3. Don sterile gloves and mask according to hospital policy.
4. Using both hands, pick up the two side edges of the first wrapper and open them away from the middle of the sterile field. Unfold the last edge toward you, without touching the wrapper.
5. Pick up one edge of the sterile towel, and move away from the table. Gently shake the towel away from the sterile area.
6. When the towel is open, use your other hand to pick up the two edges that are away from you. Be careful to not touch towel with clothing.
7. Lower the towel onto the tray or bedside stand so the towel is furthest away from you. Then lay the towel down on the tray by bringing it toward you, covering the entire tray.
8. Repeat the same steps with a second sterile towel.
9. If solutions for cleansing the skin are required, place sterile medicine cups near one side of the sterile towel.
10. Take the cap off the antiseptic bottle.
11. Pour a small amount of solution into a container, not on the sterile field, keeping the label in upper-

most position. **Rationale:** This action rinses contaminated particles from the lip of the bottle.

12. Pour the antiseptic solution, from the side of the sterile field, directly into the medicine cup.
13. Open sterile packages of dressings, and place on sterile surface.

Commercially Prepared Packages:

a. Open package at designated end by pulling edges apart and downward to expose contents.
b. Grasp the edges of the two sides of the package and invert the package over the edge of the sterile field. Allow the contents to drop onto the sterile field.
c. Repeat procedure for each item to be placed on sterile field.

Hospital-Wrapped Packages:

a. Hold package in your hand, and securely grasp one edge.
b. Open package wrapper by allowing edges to drop down, away from package.
c. Grasp the edges of the wrapper with your free hand and pull them toward your wrist, thus exposing the sterile contents.
d. Gently drop the contents on the sterile field. **Rationale:** Touching the sterile field with the wrapper contaminates it.
e. Repeat procedure for each item to be placed on the sterile field.

14. If sterile supplies are not to be used immediately, cover with sterile towels.
    a. Open sterile towel package by opening wrapper away from you so that you do not cross over a sterile field.
    b. Pick up one towel at the edge and open towel by moving yourself away from the sterile field and allowing towel to fall open.
    c. Grasp corner of towel opposite to one you are holding. Keep towel from touching contaminated areas.
    d. Place towel over sterile field starting at edge nearest you. Lay the towel down without touching the tray with your hand. Move the towel across the tray toward the opposite edge.
    e. Repeat procedure with second sterile towel.

GUIDELINES FOR STERILE FIELD

- Never turn your back on a sterile field.
- Avoid talking, coughing, sneezing, or reaching across a sterile field.
- Keep sterile objects above waist level.
- Do not spill solutions on the sterile field.
- Open all sterile packages away from the sterile field to prevent crossover and contamination.

PREPARING A STERILE FIELD USING PREPACKAGED SUPPLIES

Equipment

Packaged supplies

Procedures

1. Ensure working surface if clean and dry. Client's over-bed table is frequently used as preparation area. **Rationale:** This prevents contamination of sterile package.
2. Place package in center of work area and position so that you first open package flap away from you. **Rationale:** This prevents reaching across the sterile field as you continue to open package.
3. Grasp edge of the first flap of the wrapper, move it away from you, and place it on the working surface.

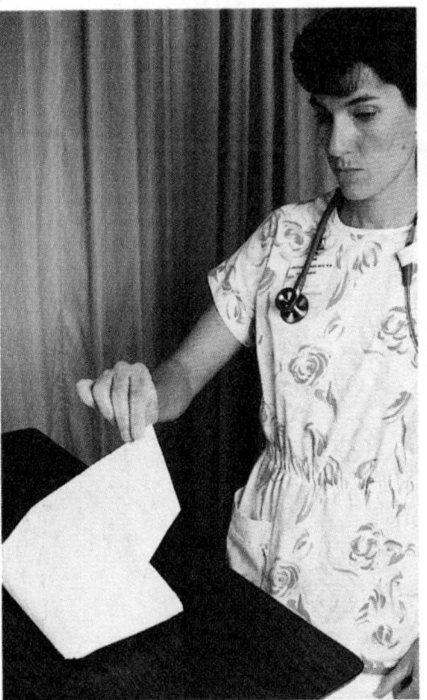

Grasp edge of the first flap of the wrapper and move it away from you.

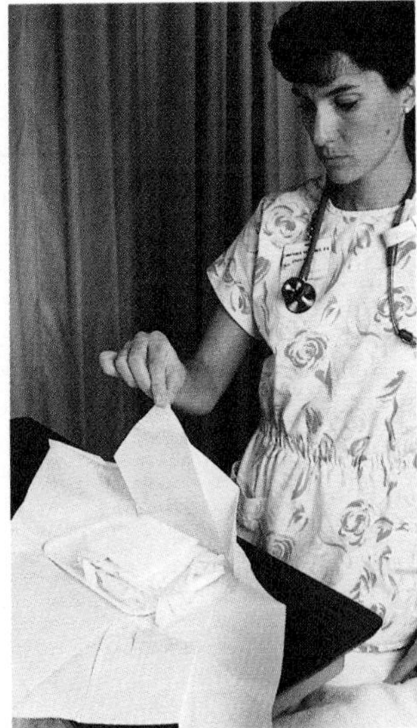

Open last flap toward you—do not cross sterile field.

4. Grasp the first side flap, lift it up; grasp the second side flap and together move both hands out toward the sides. Place the flaps down on the working surface.
5. Grasp the last flap of the wrapper and open it toward you, taking care not to touch the inside of the flap or any of the contents of the package. **Rationale:** This prevents contamination of the supplies.

CHARTING for Measures to Prevent Infection

- Type and amount of sterile dressings used
- Antiseptic solution used

CRITICAL THINKING APPLICATION

CLINICAL PROBLEMS	CRITICAL THINKING OPTIONS
Hole develops in glove while performing sterile technique.	• Discard gloves and replace with sterile gloves. • Examine hands for cuts if hole caused by sharp object. • If hands are cut, scrub hands and replace sterile gloves.
Sterile field becomes wet or damp.	• Discard supplies on sterile field. • Set up new sterile field.

unit 2

DRESSING CHANGE

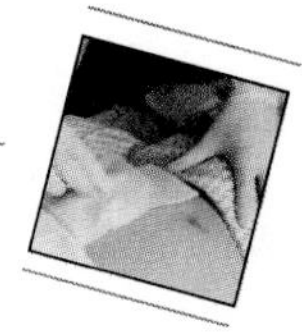

NURSING PROCESS DATA

ASSESSMENT Data Base

Identify type of dressing required.

Determine if sutures or staples need to be removed.

Assess incision for infection.

Assess extent of healing.

Assess nutritional status.

PLANNING Objectives

To promote incision healing

To prevent wound infection

To maintain sterility during dressing change

To remove sutures or staples using appropriate technique

IMPLEMENTATION Procedures

Changing a Dry Sterile Dressing

Removing Sutures

Removing Staples

EVALUATION Expected Outcomes

Incision is healing without infection.

Sterility is maintained throughout dressing change.

Sutures and staples are removed using proper technique.

CHANGING A DRY STERILE DRESSING

Equipment

Sterile gloves

Clean gloves

Mask

Gown

Disposal bag for used dressings

Dressing supplies, as needed

Micropore tape

Sterile normal saline, optional

Package sterile cotton swabs, optional

Bath blanket

Preparation

1. Check physician's orders and client care plan.
2. Wash your hands.
3. Gather equipment.
4. Identify the client, and explain procedure.
5. Provide privacy.
6. Clean off over-bed table.
7. Place sterile supplies on over-bed table.
8. Raise bed to HIGH position, and lower side rails on working side of bed.
9. Place bag for soiled dressings near incision site.
10. Fanfold linen to expose incision area.
11. Cover client with bath blanket, leaving incision area exposed.
12. Open sterile packages, and place on over-bed table. Arrange packages to ensure you don't cross over the sterile field when reaching for dressings. **Rationale:** Commercially prepared sterile packages can be opened and used for the sterile field because the inside of the package is sterile.
13. Cut tape into appropriate length strips and place on edge of over-bed table.

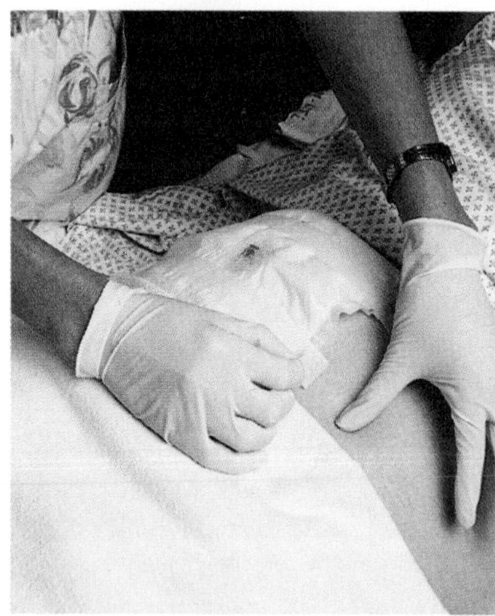
Remove tape by pulling tape toward wound.

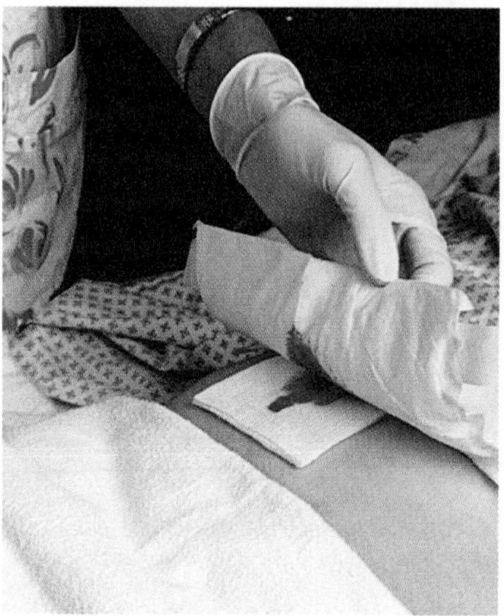
Remove soiled dressing carefully.

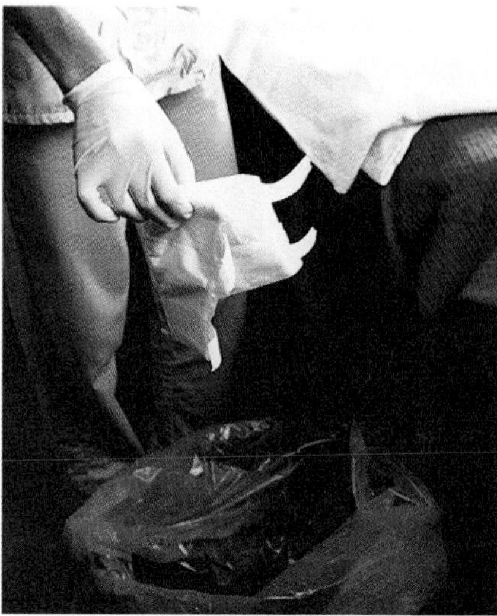
Dispose of dressing in appropriate container.

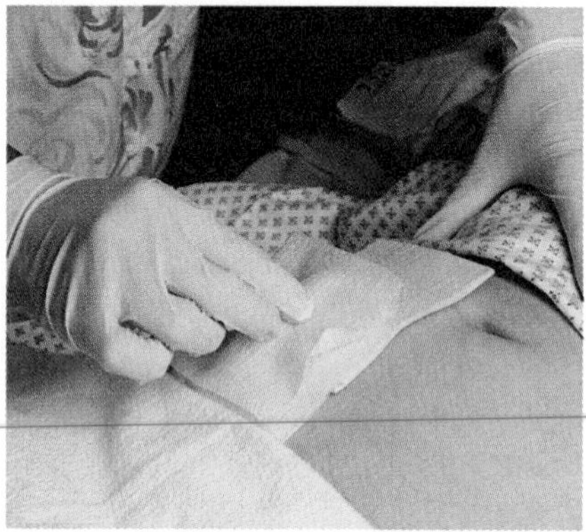
Do not touch incision when applying dressing.

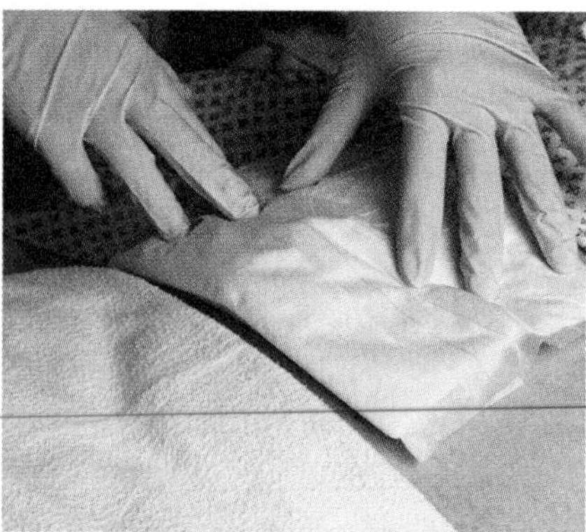
Place abdominal pad over center of incision.

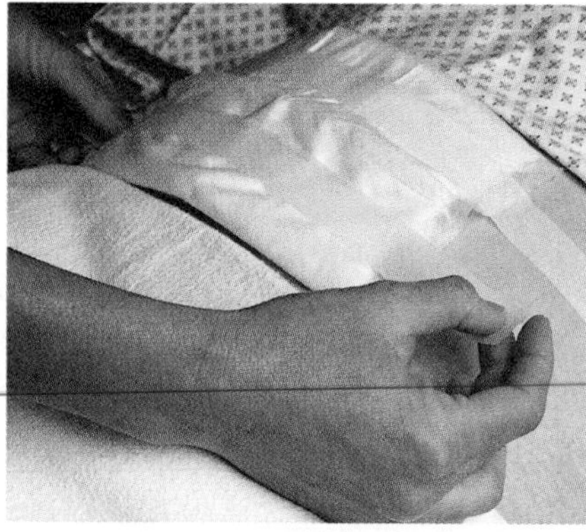
Tape dressing securely to prevent slipping.

Procedure

1. Remove tape slowly by pulling tape toward the wound. **Rationale:** Pulling toward the wound decreases the pain of tape removal by not putting pressure on the incision line.
2. Don clean gloves.
3. Remove soiled dressings, and dispose of in the proper bag. Wet dressing with sterile normal saline if it adheres to the suture line.
4. Assess incision area for erythema, edema, or drainage.
5. Remove clean gloves, and discard.
6. Move over-bed table next to working area.
7. Don sterile gloves.
8. Cleanse incision area with swabs soaked in normal saline, according to hospital policy. Cleanse from incision line outward, using swab only once. Discard swabs in disposal bag. **Rationale:** Cleaning outward from incision cleans from least to most contaminated area.
9. Place 4×4 gauze pads over incision area, being careful not to touch incision or client with your gloves. **Rationale:** Touching the incision or client contaminates the gloves. You need to reglove if this occurs.
10. Place abdominal pad over incision, being careful not to contaminate the gloves.
11. Remove gloves and discard.
12. Tape dressing securely.
13. Discard trash in appropriate receptacle.
14. Position client for comfort.
15. Wash your hands.

REMOVING SUTURES

Equipment

Sterile suture removal set
Antiseptic solution
Tape
Butterfly tape
Disposable bag for dressings
Two pairs clean gloves (1 pair optional)

Procedure

1. Gather equipment.
2. Wash hands, and don clean gloves.
3. Remove dressing and discard in disposable bag. (Discard gloves only if soiled.)
4. Open suture removal set, and don gloves if second pair needed.
5. Pick up forceps with nondominant hand.
6. Grasp suture at the knot with forceps and lift away from skin.
7. Pick up suture scissors with dominant hand.
8. Place curved tip of suture scissors under suture, next to knot.
9. Cut suture, and with forceps, pull suture through skin with one movement.
10. Discard suture into disposable bag.
11. Check that entire suture is removed.
12. Continue to remove remaining sutures according to hospital policy. Some policies state that every other suture is removed and then remaining sutures are removed at a later time. **Rationale:** This prevents wound dehiscence.
13. Cleanse suture site with antiseptic solution.
14. Take off gloves, and place in disposal bag.
15. Place dressing or butterfly tape over incision area, if ordered.
16. Discard disposal bag into contaminated waste container.
17. Wash hands.

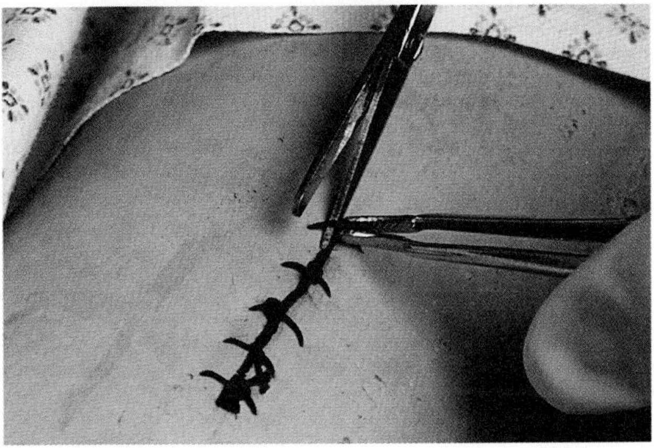

Grasp suture at the knot with forceps and lift away from skin.

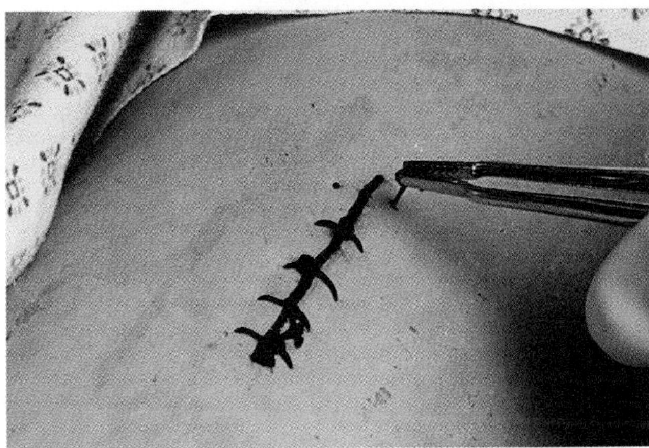

After cutting suture, grasp suture with forceps and pull through skin.

REMOVING STAPLES

Equipment

Sterile staple remover
Disposal bag
Two pairs clean gloves (1 pair optional)
Dressings
Tape or butterfly tape
Antiseptic solution

Procedure

1. Gather equipment, and open sterile staple remover.
2. Wash hands, and don clean gloves.
3. Remove dressing, and discard in disposal bag. (Discard gloves only if soiled.)
4. Don gloves if necessary.
5. Place lower tip of staple remover under staple.
6. Press handles together to depress center of staple.

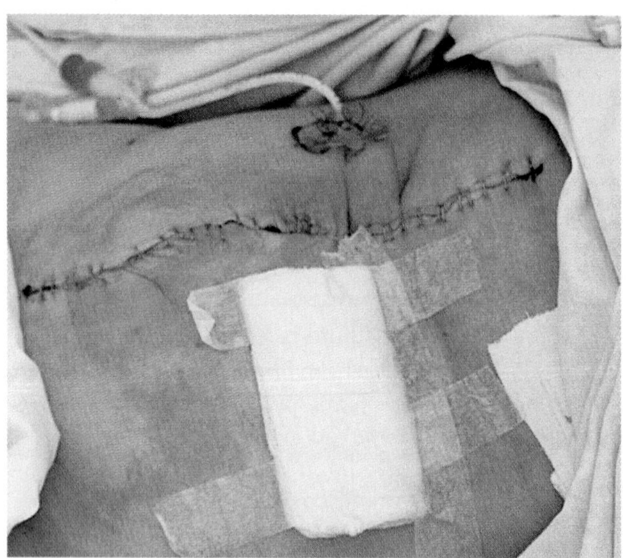
Large abdominal wound with staples closing incision.

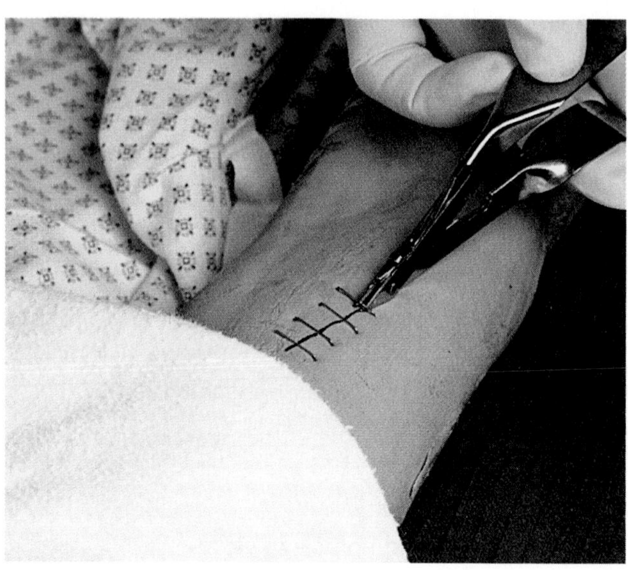
Place lower tip of staple removal device under staple.

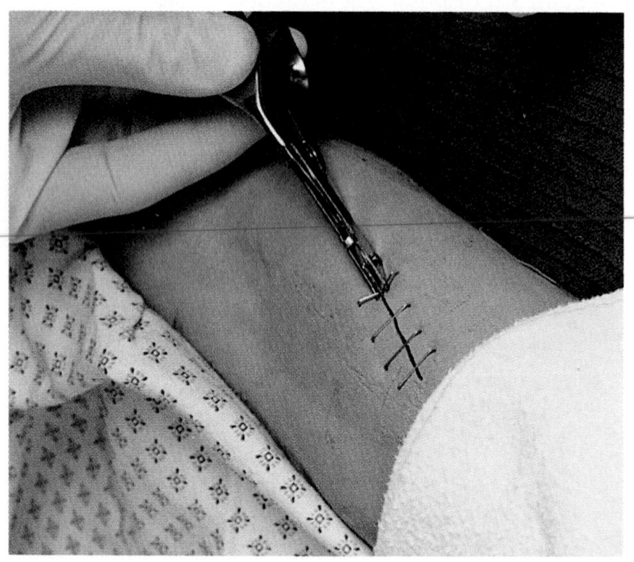
Press handle together to depress center of staple.

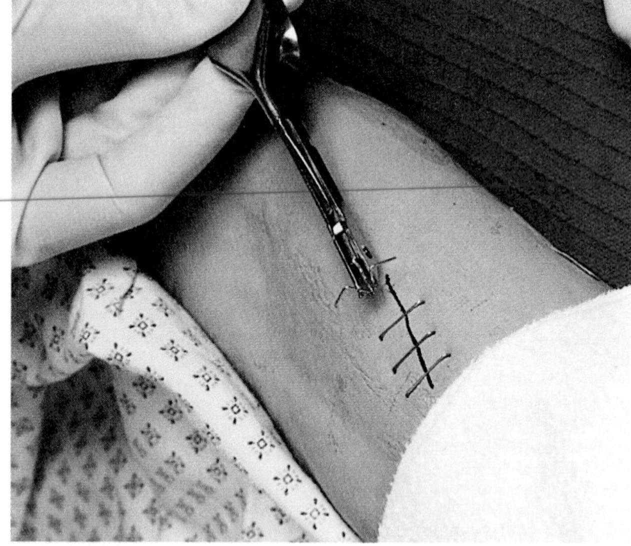
Lift staple remover device upward and away from incision.

7. Lift staple removal upward, away from incision site when both ends of staple are visible.
8. Place staple removal device over disposal bag and release handles to release staple.
9. Remove all staples or as directed by hospital policy. Some policies indicate every other staple is removed with remaining staples done at a later time.
10. Cleanse incision area with antiseptic solution if ordered.
11. Take off gloves, and place in disposal bag.
12. Place dressing over incision and secure with tape,

or place butterfly tape over incision.

13. Discard disposal bag in contaminated waste container.
14. Wash hands.

■ CLINICAL ALERT

Steristrips may be applied over incision to protect incision after staples are removed.

CHARTING for Sutures and Staples

- Conditions of suture line
- Presence of exudate or erythema
- Sutures removed
- Staples removed
- Dressing applied, if appropriate

CRITICAL THINKING APPLICATION

CLINICAL PROBLEMS	CRITICAL THINKING OPTIONS
■ Wound appears to be infected	• Obtain order for wound culture. • Obtain order for different type of dressing. • Document observations.
■ Client complains of fever, pain in incisional area	• Check incision for edema erythema, or drainage; wound could be infected.
■ Wound edges separate when suture or staple is removed	• Do not continue to remove sutures or staples. • Place steristrip over edges. • Notify physician.

unit 3 WOUND CARE

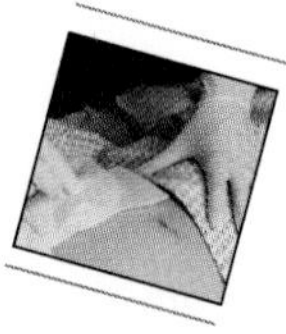

NURSING PROCESS DATA

ASSESSMENT Data Base

Identify type of dressing needed (Table 24–1)

Assess level of pain associated with wound care and dressing change.

Determine if infection is present.

Assess for function of Hemovac suction.

Assess for extent of wound healing.

Assess wound.

PLANNING Objectives

To assess wound appropriately

To promote wound healing by first or second intention

To prevent microorganisms from entering the wound

To decrease the presence of purulent wound drainage

To maintain sterility during a dressing change

To maintain patency of Hemovac suction

To immobilize and support a wound

To assist in removal of necrotic tissue

To apply medication to wound

IMPLEMENTATION Procedures

Changing a Wound Dressing

Changing a Dressing for a Peripheral Vascular Wound

Caring for a Wound with Drain

Applying an Abdominal Binder

Maintaining Wound Drainage System

Irrigating Wounds

EVALUATION Expected Outcomes

Granulation takes place, and healing occurs.

Sterility is maintained during dressing change.

Drain is advanced appropriately.

Hemovac suction remains patent.

Abdominal binder keeps dressing in place and supports abdomen.

TABLE 24–1. Moisture-Retentive Dressings

	Advantages	Disadvantages	Clinical Use
Transparent Adhesive Film	• Transparency allows wound visualization • Conforms to area of application • Can reduce friction of area • Promotes autolysis of dry eschar • Semipermeable vapor can escape and environmental oxygen can enter to reduce chance of anaerobic bacterial growth • Barrier to bacterial invasion; can aspirate fluid and patch • Does not require secondary dressing	• Does *not* absorb exudate • Exudate may macerate skin around wound • Edges will roll in friction area • May be difficult to apply • May be too tightly applied • Removal may tear underlying skin • May increase bacterial growth in infected wounds	• Pressure ulcers, stage I and II • Donor sites • Abrasions • Extend edge to minimum $1\frac{1}{4}$ inch beyond wound; skin around wound must be dry for adhesion; apply without tension • Change when fluid build-up and leaking occurs and when edges are loosening to potentially expose wound
Hydrogel	• Comes in sheets or gel to conform to the wound • May be soothing • Absorbs some exudate • Provides moist wound healing • Rehydrates dry wound beds	• Expensive • Held in place with gauze dressing or transparent film • May have transparent film on both sides (film next to wound must be removed)	• Wounds with necrosis and slough • Partial thickness (use sheets) • Gel can be used to fill wound cavity • Change every day or twice a day—based on wound exudate
Hydrocolloids	• Use on acute and chronic wounds • Absorbs exudate • Conforms to area • Prevents bacterial invasion	• Not transparent • Melts down with exudate • Characteristic drainage and odor • Edges may need to be taped to prevent rolling • Most do *not* allow environmental oxygen, so growth of anaerobic bacteria may be a problem	• Noninfected dermal ulcers • May leave in place up to 7 days • Change if leaking • Change in clinical signs of infection • Cleanse wound before application • Roll dressing over wound • Do *not* stretch; press securely

Adapted from Frommhagen.

CHANGING A WOUND DRESSING

Equipment

Sterile, prepackaged dressing(s) as needed
Tape; micropore, paper, or Montgomery tie tapes
Clean gloves
Sterile gloves
Sterile normal saline irrigation solution
Wound culture media, as needed
Plastic bag
Bath blanket
Emesis basin

Preparation

1. Check physician's orders and client care plan.
2. Wash your hands.
3. Gather equipment.
4. Identify the client, and explain procedure.
5. Provide privacy.
6. Clean off over-bed table.
7. Place sterile supplies on the over-bed table.
8. Raise bed to HIGH position, and lower side rails on working side of bed.
9. Place bag for soiled dressings near wound site.
10. Open sterile packages and place on over-bed table. Arrange packages to ensure that you don't

cross over the sterile field when using dressings. **Rationale:** Commercially prepared sterile packages can be opened and used for the sterile field; the inside of the package is sterile.

11. Fanfold linens to expose wound site.
12. Cover client with bath blanket, leaving wound area exposed.
13. Cut tape into appropriate strips, and place on over-bed table.

Procedure

1. Remove tape slowly by pulling tape toward the wound. **Rationale:** Pulling toward the wound decreases the pain of tape removal by not putting pressure on the incision line.
2. Put on clean gloves.
3. Remove soiled dressings, and dispose of in bag. Soaking dressings that are dried to skin or incision with sterile normal saline prevents tissue damage and pain when dressings are removed.
4. Obtain wound specimen for culture if ordered.

HOW TO OBTAIN A WOUND CULTURE

- Rinse wound thoroughly with sterile saline.
- Use noncotton-tipped swab.
- Rotate swab while obtaining specimen.
- Swab edges starting at top, criss-cross wound to bottom.
- Do *not* take specimen from exudate or eschar.

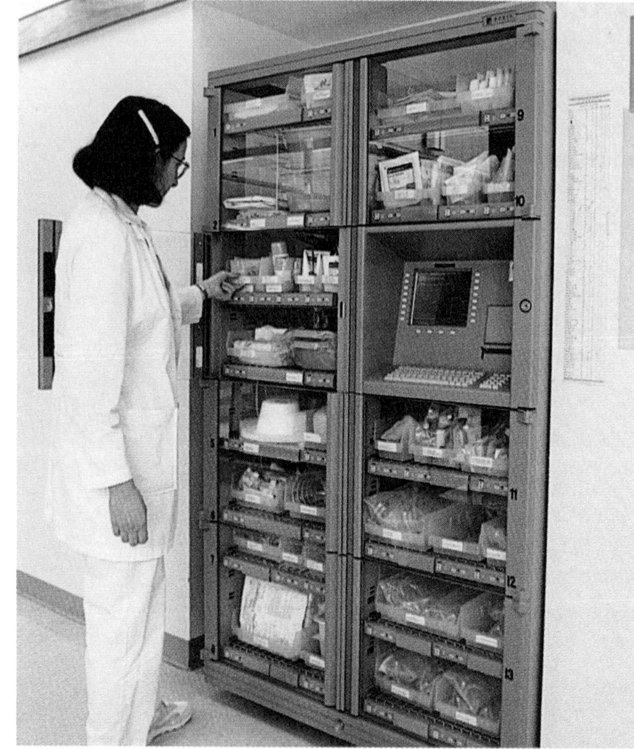

Pyxis supply station provides easy access for dressing supplies.

5. Remove clean gloves, and discard into plastic bag.
6. Bring over-bed table close to working area.
7. Open cleansing solution, and pour over wound. Place emesis basin next to skin surface to catch overflow.
8. Don sterile gloves.

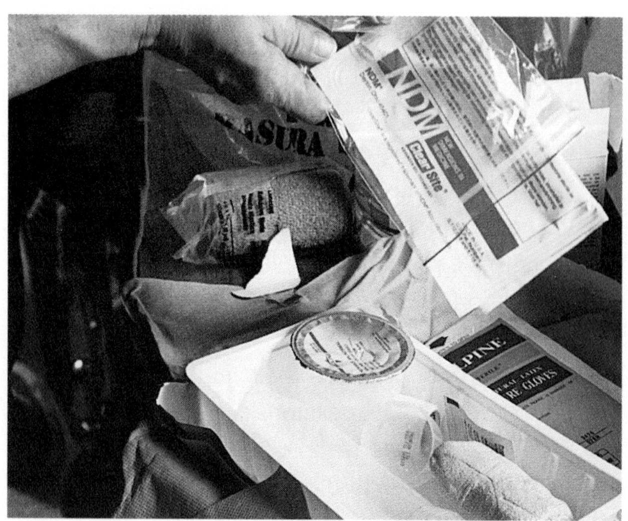

Obtain appropriate wound dressing kit, if available.

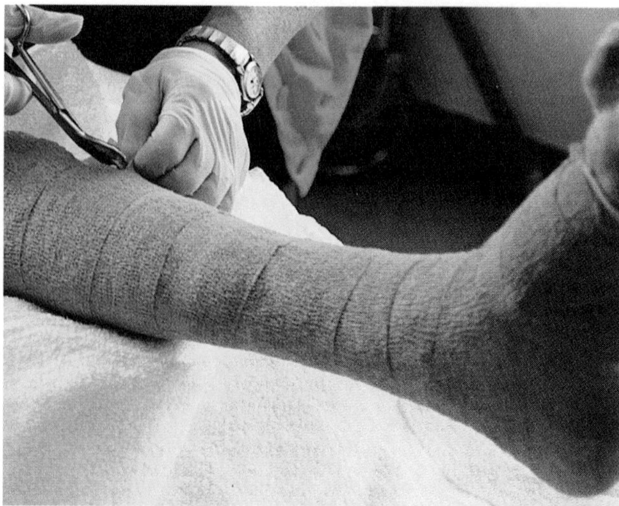

Don clean gloves and remove soiled dressing.

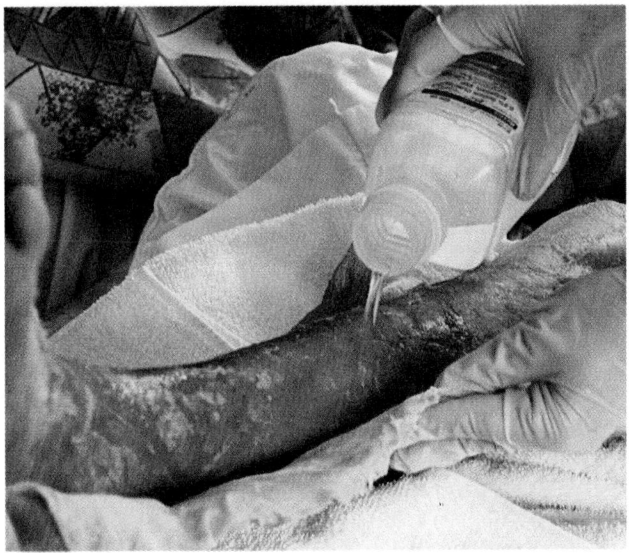

Pour cleansing solution over wound to clean off debris.

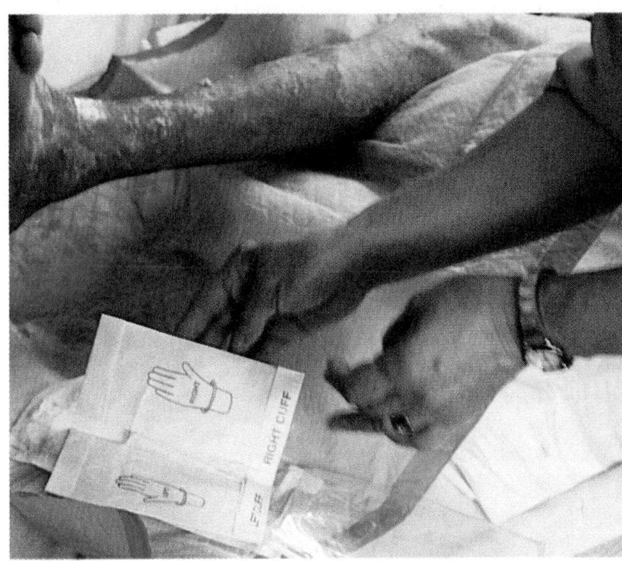

Don sterile gloves before cleaning wound with 4 × 4 gauze pads.

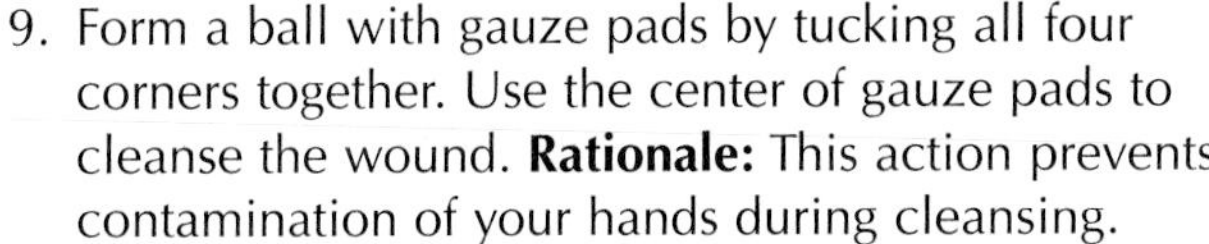

9. Form a ball with gauze pads by tucking all four corners together. Use the center of gauze pads to cleanse the wound. **Rationale:** This action prevents contamination of your hands during cleansing.
10. Cleanse wound. When cleansing an area, always start at the cleanest area and work away from that area. Never return to an area you have previously cleaned. Usually start at middle of wound and work toward periphery.
11. Cleanse under the drain and around the site with a 4 × 4 gauze pad and cleansing solution if a drain is present.
12. Place several gauze pads under the drain.
13. Place several 4 × 4 gauze pads over the wound. Cover with an ABD pad if necessary; remove gloves, and tape securely. (Montgomery straps (tie tapes) may be used if frequent dressing changes are required or the client has sensitive skin.) **Rationale:** Once a dressing has been placed over the wound it is not to be moved and readjusted, as microorganisms from the skin could be introduced into the wound.
14. A moisture-retentive dressing may be placed over 4 × 4 gauze pad and even over ABD, if used.
15. Cover client.
16. Close the plastic bag, and dispose of bag as isolation material.
17. Remove gloves, and wash your hands thoroughly.
18. Check with client to see that he or she is comfortable before leaving room.
19. Lower the bed, and raise the side rail.

CHANGING A DRESSING FOR A PERIPHERAL VASCULAR WOUND

Equipment

Cleansing solution
Normal saline
Sterile 4×4 dressings
Translucent dressing
Gel
Compression dressing
Clean gloves
Sterile gloves
Biohazard bag
Scissors
Absorbent pad

Preparation

1. Wash hands.
2. Gather equipment.
3. Explain procedure to client.
4. Provide privacy for client.
5. Raise bed to HIGH position.

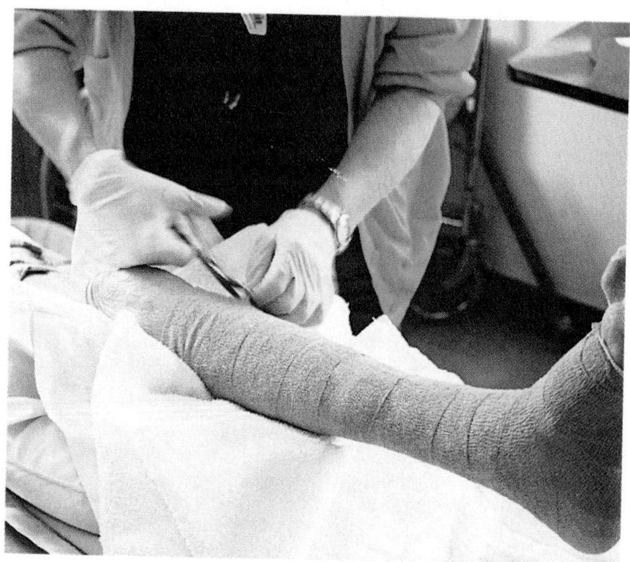
Remove compression dressing being careful not to cut skin.

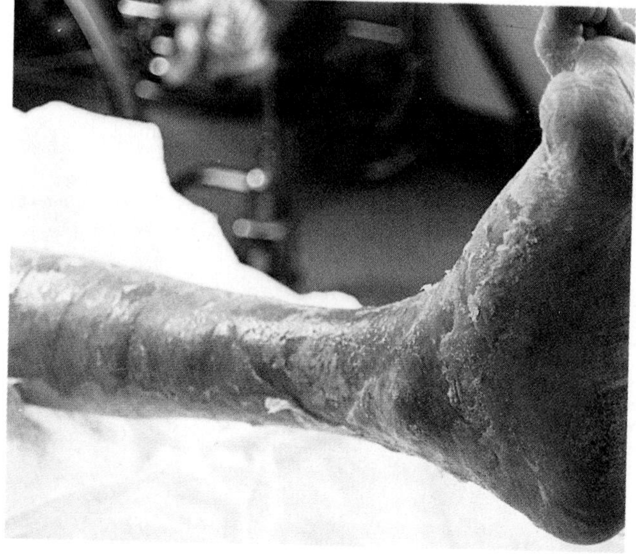
Assess wound healing and evaluate progress (Stage II).

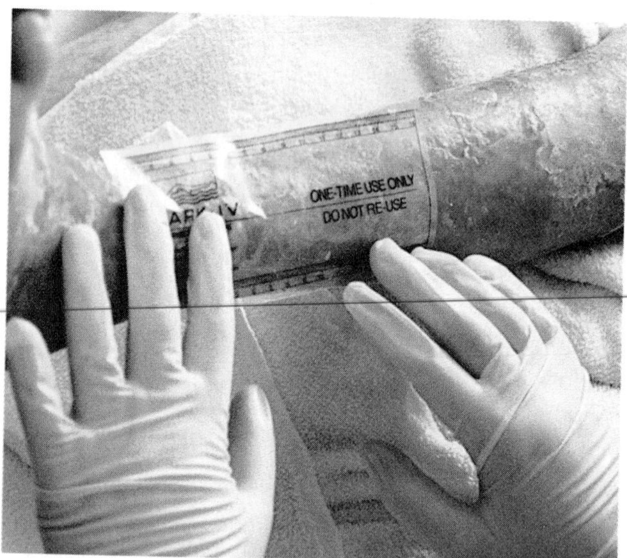

Wound is measured to evaluate effectiveness of treatment.

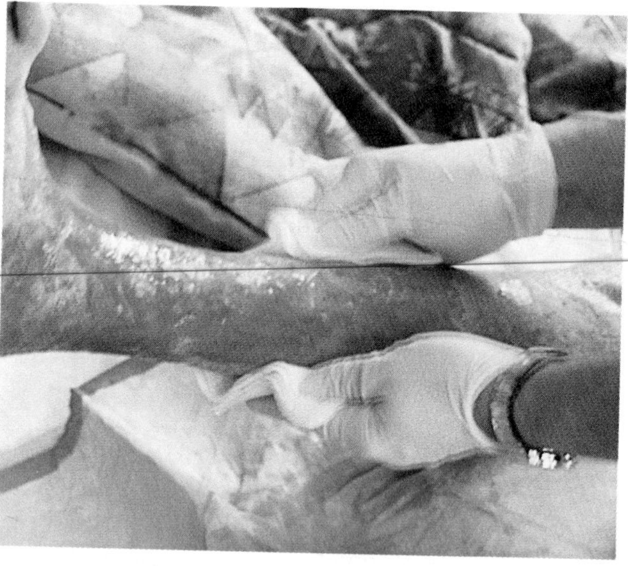
After cleansing wound, dry with 4 × 4 gauze pad.

6. Open sterile packages, and arrange on over-bed table.
7. Place absorbent pad under wound.

Procedure

1. Don clean gloves.
2. Remove old dressing, and place in biohazard bag.
3. Assess and measure wound. **Rationale:** This determines effectiveness of treatment.
4. Cleanse off debris by pouring cleansing solution over wound.
5. Rinse wound with sterile normal saline.
6. Dry wound using sterile 4×4 dressings. Place in biohazard bag.
7. Remove gloves, and don sterile gloves.
8. Apply medicated moisturizer over wound. **Rationale:** This keeps wound area moist.
9. Remove backing on transparent dressing, and place over open wound site.
10. Apply compression dressing.
11. Reposition leg in elevated position. **Rationale:** This prevents venous stasis and promotes healing.

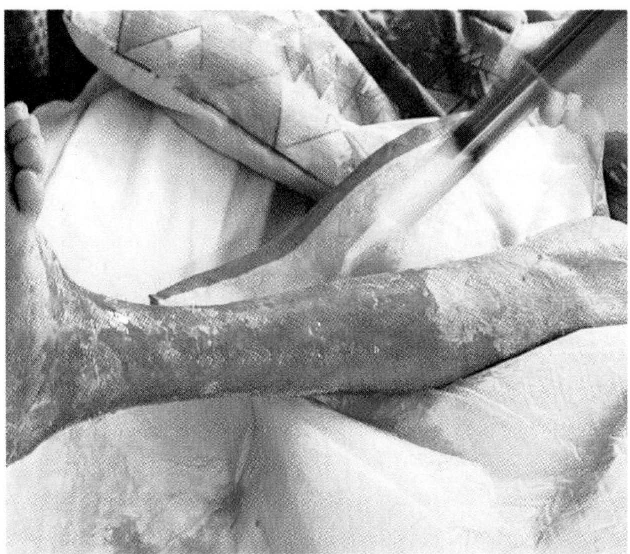
Apply medicated moisturizer on wound.

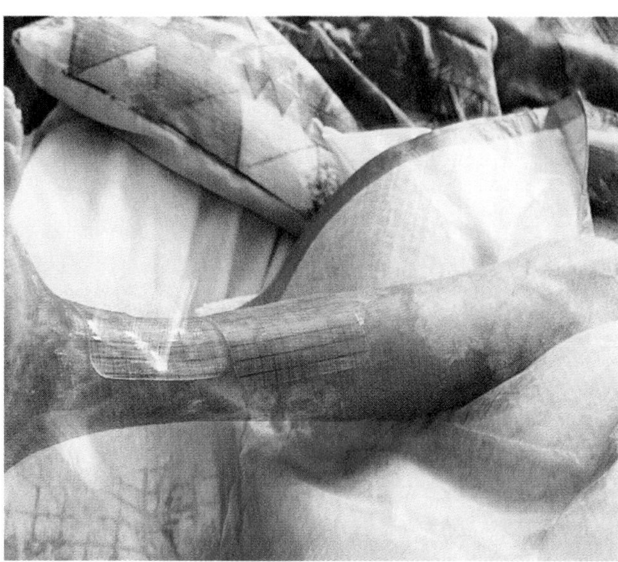
Apply transparent dressing over wound site.

12. Remove gloves, and place in biohazard bag. Place all used supplies in bag.
13. Place biohazard bag in appropriate receptacle.
14. Wash your hands.
15. Assess peripheral circulation every 4 hours. **Rationale:** This ensures compression dressing is not too tight.

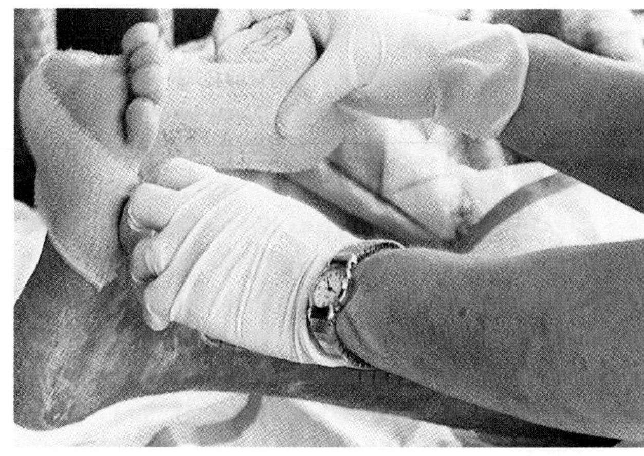
Apply compression dressing for venous or lymphatic conditions.

CARING FOR A WOUND WITH A DRAIN

Equipment

Same items as for *Changing a Wound Dressing*
Sterile cotton applicators
Sterile safety pin
ABD dressings
Sterile scissors
Sterile gloves
Clean gloves

AN ALTERNATIVE TO GAUZE DRESSING FOR DRAINING WOUNDS

Apply a pouch to

- Collect drainage
- Measure drainage
- Protect skin from drainage
- Contain drainage
- Contain microorganisms so spread is decreased
- Lessen frequency of care; dressing change is every 24–48 hours

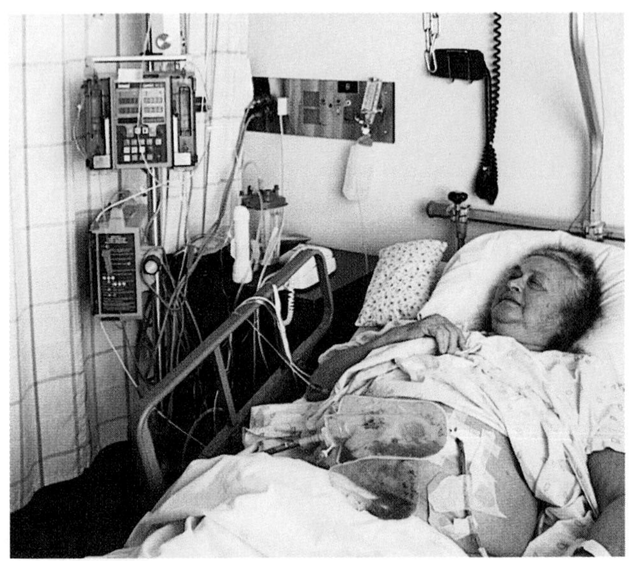
Use of drainage pouches for wounds with drains.

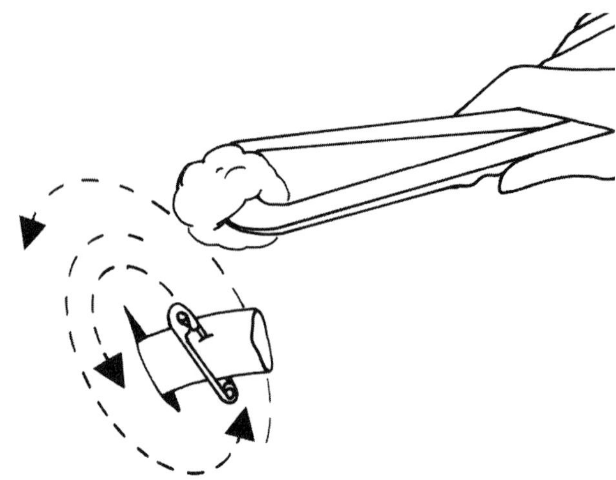
Cleanse the drain site, using a circular motion from the inside to the periphery of the wound.

Preparation

1. Check physician's orders and client care plan.
2. Wash your hands.
3. Gather equipment.
4. Provide privacy.
5. Identify client, and explain procedure.
6. Clean off over-bed table.
7. Raise bed to HIGH position, and lower side rails on working side of bed.
8. Place plastic bag for soiled dressings on bed near wound site.
9. Open sterile packages, and place on over-bed table.

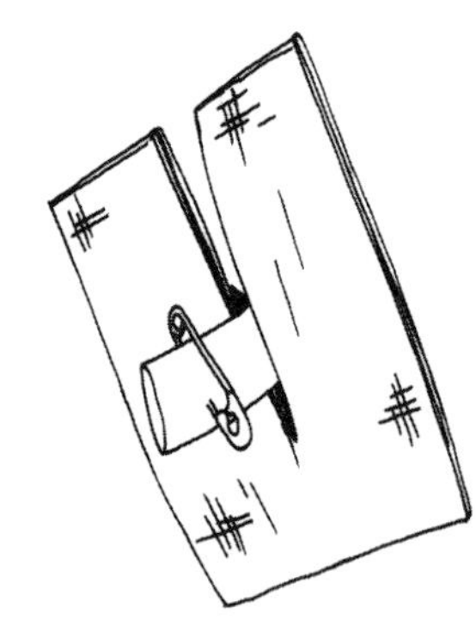
Place a pre-cut sterile 4 × 4 gauze dressing around the drain site to prevent skin excoriation.

Procedure

1. Remove tape from client's skin by pulling *toward* the incision.
2. Don clean gloves.
3. Remove soiled dressing.
4. Discard gloves and dressings into plastic bag.
5. Observe wound closely for signs of infection or healing. Don sterile gloves.
6. If pin on the Penrose drain is crusted, replace it with a sterile pin. Be careful not to dislodge drain or suction tubing.
7. Using cotton applicators or gauze pads, cleanse drain site with cleansing solution and then saline.
8. Start cleansing at drain site, moving in a circular motion toward the periphery.

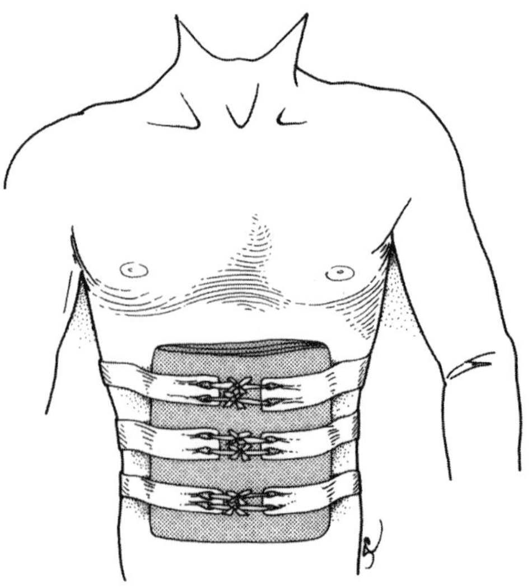
Montgomery straps are used when frequent dressing changes are needed to prevent skin irritation from tape removal.

9. Discard applicators in plastic bag.
10. Advance drain if ordered:
    a. Using sterile forceps, pull drain out of wound the ordered number of centimeters.
    b. Reposition the safety pin so it is at the level of the skin. **Rationale:** The pin prevents the drain from slipping back into the wound.
    c. Cut off the excess tubing with sterile scissors. Leave at least 2 inches of tubing on the outside.
11. Place several 4×4 dressings around the drain.
12. Apply gauze pad with a precut slit under the drain site.
13. Apply dry, sterile gauze pads over drain.
14. Apply ABD pads over sterile gauze.
15. Remove gloves, and dispose of them in refuse bag.
16. Tape dressing or retie Montgomery straps (tie tapes).
17. Remove bag with soiled dressing from room.
18. Wash your hands thoroughly.
19. Position client for comfort.
20. Lower bed, and raise side rail.

APPLYING AN ABDOMINAL BINDER

Equipment

Abdominal binder: woven-cotton, synthetic, or elasticized material

Safety pins for binders without Velcro closure

Procedure

1. Obtain binder. Most facilities use commercial Velcro binders.
2. Explain use of binder to client.
3. Place client in supine position.
4. Ask client to raise hips, and then slide the binder under client's hips at level of gluteal fold. Place top of binder at client's waist.
5. Bring ends of binder around client, and secure by pressing Velcro surfaces together. If using non-Velcro binder, secure binder with safety pins placed vertically along edges. Start pinning at bottom of binder and pin toward waist. **Rationale:** Pinning binder from bottom to waist provides uplifting support for abdominal muscles.
6. Observe for wrinkles in binder. **Rationale:** Wrinkles can cause pressure areas especially over iliac crest.
7. Assess client's ability to move freely, breathe deeply, and feel secure pressure over abdominal incision.

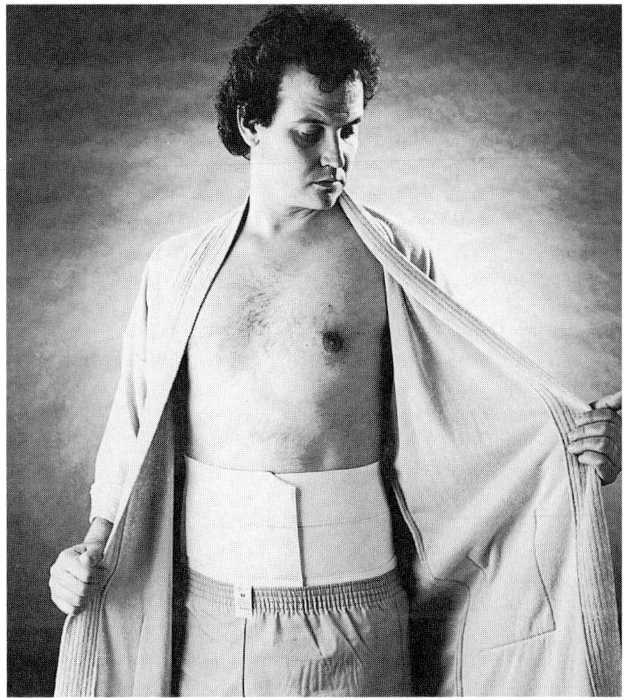

Apply abdominal binder by bringing end around client's waist and pressing velcro surfaces together.

8. Assess effectiveness of binder every 4 hours, and rewrap every 8 hours if non-Velcro binder is used. Many clients use this binder only when ambulating.

MAINTAINING WOUND DRAINAGE SYSTEMS

Equipment

Specimen cup for measuring drainage
I&O bedside record
Absorbent pad
Clean gloves
Hemovac suction or Jackson–Pratt suction drainage system

Preparation

1. Check physician's order and client care plan.
2. Bring specimen cup to bedside.
3. Identify client, and explain procedure, giving client time to ask questions.
4. Provide for comfort and privacy.
5. Wash your hands, and don gloves.
6. Elevate bed to workable height.

Procedure

1. Expose catheter insertion site while keeping client draped. Place drainage system on absorbent pad.
2. Examine pump and catheter for patency, seal, and stability. If catheter is occluded, notify physician.
3. Remove Hemovac plug, which is labeled "Pouring Spout," or disconnect tubing from Jackson–Pratt system.

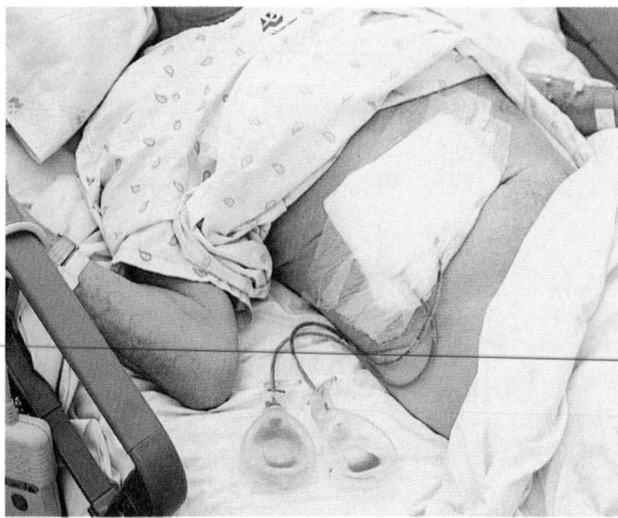

Jackson-Pratt drainage system in place.

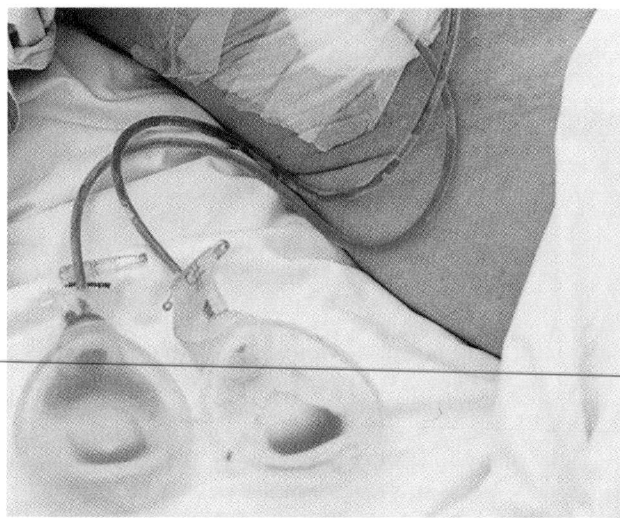

Ensure pump and catheter are patent and sealed.

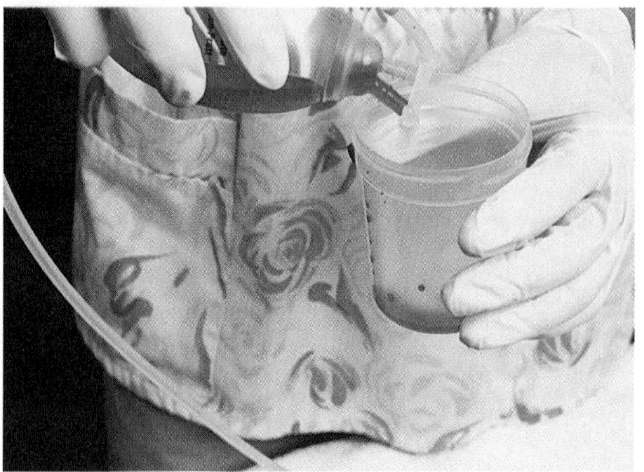

Empty, measure, and record drainage every shift.

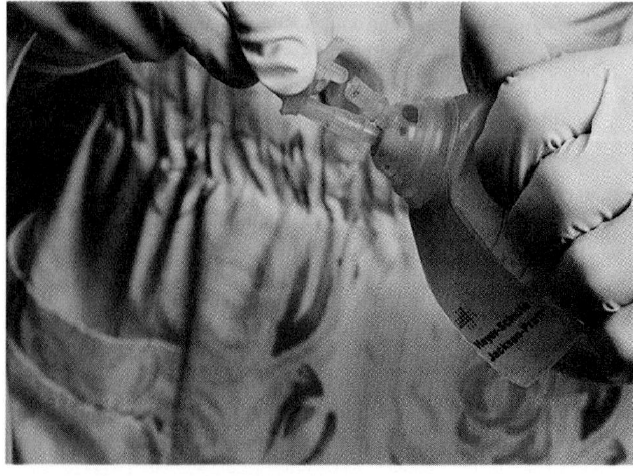

Squeeze bulb and reconnect to drainage tubing.

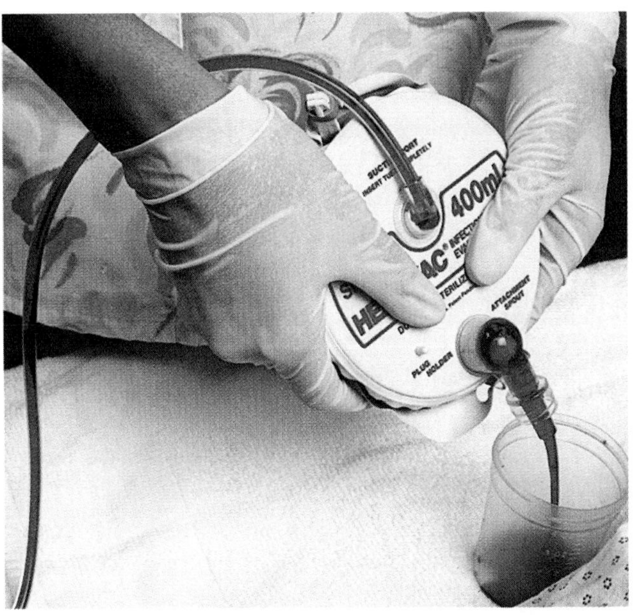

Remove Hemovac plug from "Pouring Spout" for emptying.

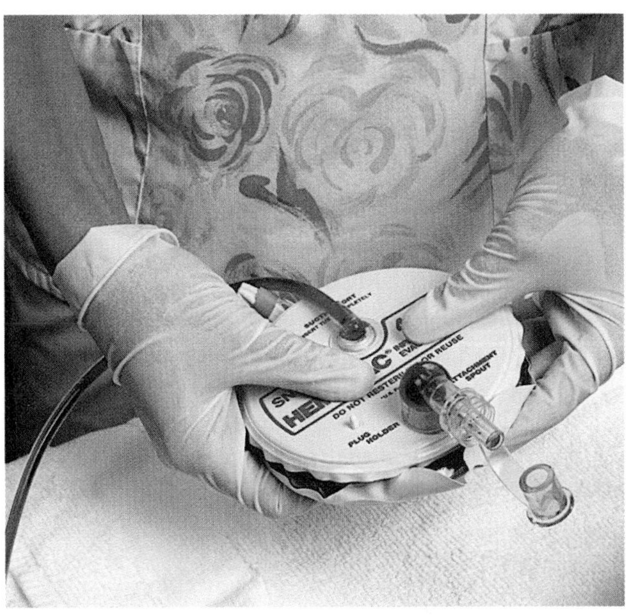

Compress Hemovac by pushing top and bottom together.

4. Pour drainage into specimen cup.
5. Compress the Hemovac by pushing the top and bottom together with your hands, or compress bulb on Jackson–Pratt.
6. Hold pump or bulb tightly compressed, and reinsert plug or connect tubing to reestablish closed drainage system.
7. Position suction devices on bed.
8. Measure and record amount of drainage.
9. Examine drainage for color, consistency, and odor.
10. Discard drainage and container; remove gloves, and wash hands.
11. Send culture specimen to laboratory if ordered.
12. Make client comfortable, and lower bed.
13. Compress evacuator at least every 4 hours to provide suction. Measure drainage at least every 8 hours.

■ CLINICAL ALERT

A Jackson–Pratt catheter or similar drainage system is connected to a drainage system or suction. This prevents the accumulation of secretions on the skin.

IRRIGATING WOUNDS

Equipment

Sterile irrigation solution
Sterile irrigating set
Absorbent pad
Sterile gloves
Equipment for dressing change

Preparation

1. Check physician's orders and client care plan.
2. Gather irrigation equipment and dressing material.
3. Check client's identaband.
4. Assemble equipment.
5. Explain procedure to client, and answer any questions.
6. Wash your hands.
7. Open sterile packages on the over-bed table as with dressing change.
8. Pour sterile irrigating solution into container.

Procedure

1. Place absorbent pads under the client. Place a bath blanket under absorbent pads when irrigating

a large wound to absorb any spilled irrigation solution.
2. Position client so that solution flows from wound to basin.
3. Put on clean gloves.
4. Remove and discard used dressing.
5. Remove gloves, and discard into plastic bag.
6. Place bedside stand near working area with all packages open.
7. Don sterile gloves.
8. Inspect area surrounding wound for redness, tissue integrity, and signs of granulating tissue.
9. Place sterile basin under wound area.
10. Draw solution from sterile container into 60-mL syringe.
11. Allow irrigating solution to flow over wound so that all organisms, tissue debris, and drainage are washed into basin. Cleanse from cleanest to dirtiest area of wound if possible.
12. Repeat until all irrigation solution has been used.
13. After the irrigation, cleanse client's skin around wound and dry.
14. Apply sterile dressing.
15. Dispose of equipment properly.
16. Remove gloves. Check to see that client is comfortable before leaving the room.
17. Lower bed, and raise side rails.
18. Wash your hands.

CHARTING for Wound Care

- Observation of wound site, including amount, color, and odor of drainage, as well as appearance of suture site
- Observation of granulating tissue and redness
- Pertinent observations concerning client's tolerance of procedure
- Observation of skin condition around incision site
- Changes in vital signs that indicate possible infection
- Type of dressing applied
- Observations on wound irrigation
- Type and amount of irrigation solutions used
- Unusual tension on sutures if present
- Amount and color of hemovac drainage

CRITICAL THINKING APPLICATION

CLINICAL PROBLEMS	CRITICAL THINKING OPTIONS
■ Wound becomes infected with different microorganisms.	• Notify physician about changes in color or odor of drainage. • Obtain culture and sensitivity if physician orders one. • Wash your hands thoroughly after caring for client to prevent the spread of infection. • Pay strict attention to changing dressings.
■ Edges of wound split open (wound dehiscence).	• Place client in supine position. Apply butterfly tape to wound edges. Cover opening with sterile dressings. • Apply binder for abdominal incisions after obtaining order. • Notify physician if signs of infection are present.

CLINICAL PROBLEMS	CRITICAL THINKING OPTIONS
	• Obtain culture of drainage if physician orders one. • Observe client for signs of shock. If client in shock, notify physician immediately. • Encourage high-protein diet.
■ Evisceration occurs (protrusion of bowel contents).	• Institute emergency measures. Place the client in supine position. Cover bowel with sterile gauze moistened with sterile saline. Have certified IV nurse insert intravenous catheter and infuse normal saline. Reassure client. Obtain vital signs, and treat for shock if present. • After above measures are completed, notify physician, and prepare client for return to surgery. • After surgical repair, notify dietician for diet change to increase protein and vitamin C in diet. • Apply abdominal binder if ordered.
■ Wound hemorrhages.	• Outline area of blood on dressing with a pen and observe outline to see how quickly the bleeding spreads. • If bleeding is excessive, notify the physician immediately. • Apply pressure dressing to site if there is excessive bleeding.
■ Skin appears red and broken.	• Clean area with sterile saline and dry thoroughly with sterile 4 × 4 pads. • Apply moisture-retentive dressing.
■ Wound is too extensive for application of drainage bag or ABD pads cannot contain drainage.	• Obtain Stomahesive or Hollihesive 8 × 8 sheets and cut on diagonal $\frac{1}{8}$–$\frac{1}{4}$ inch larger than wound. • If larger barrier needed, Stomahesive may be pieced together to form larger barrier reinforcing juncture points with Karaya paste. • A superadhesive pouch may then be applied. • If dressings are used, they may be secured with Montgomery straps (tie tapes).
■ Abdominal binder is not effective in supporting incisional area.	• Evaluate the effectiveness of the abdominal binder. • Assess if the binder is properly positioned at the hip level and waist level to provide support. • Assess if the binder is too loose.
■ Client is too large for the abdominal binder.	• Fold a drawsheet in half lengthwise and place under client. Position the edges at the waist and pubic area. • Pull tightly on the drawsheet, and secure the edges with safety pins.

unit 4

WET-TO-DAMP DRESSINGS

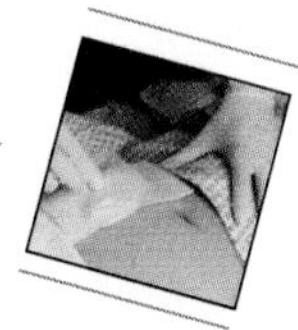

NURSING PROCESS DATA

ASSESSMENT Data Base

Assess wound edges for presence of granulation tissue.
Assess for changes in amount of drainage.
Assess if necrotic tissue is decreasing in amount.
Identify if appropriate dressing is used for wound care.

PLANNING Objectives

To promote wound healing by secondary intention
To maintain a moist environment conducive to wound healing
To provide the most appropriate treatment for wound care
To enhance local healing
To maintain sterile technique throughout procedure
To remove trapped exudate from wounds

IMPLEMENTATION Procedure

Applying Wet-to-Damp Dressings

EVALUATION Expected Outcomes

Wound heals without complications.
Sterile technique is maintained throughout procedure.

APPLYING WET-TO-DAMP DRESSINGS

Equipment

Sterile 4 × 8 noncotton gauze dressings
Sterile gloves
Clean gloves
Tape
Plastic bag for contaminated dressings
Solution for dressings
Sterile receptacle (round basin or emesis basin)
Montgomery straps, if desired

Preparation

1. Check physician's orders and client care plan.
2. Wash hands.
3. Gather equipment.
4. Explain procedure to client.
5. Provide privacy.
6. Raise bed to HIGH position, and lower side rail nearest you.
7. Remove tape by pulling it toward the wound. **Rationale:** This action prevents injury to newly formed tissue.
8. Don nonsterile gloves.
9. Moisten dressing with normal saline before removing if dressing is dry. **Rationale:** Removal of a dry dressing traumatizes granulating tissue and delays wound healing.
10. Remove wound packing by gently grasping the gauze without touching the wound. **Rationale:** Touching only the gauze prevents contamination of the wound.
11. Place soiled dressings in disposable bag.
12. Remove gloves, and dispose of them in bag.
13. Wash your hands.

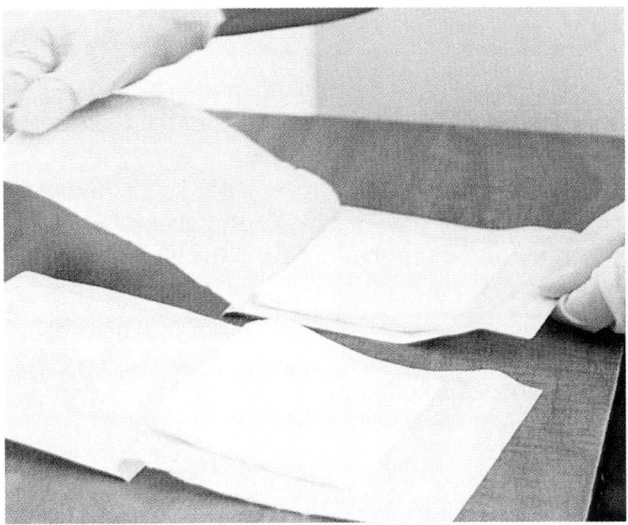
Open sterile packages before beginning dressing change.

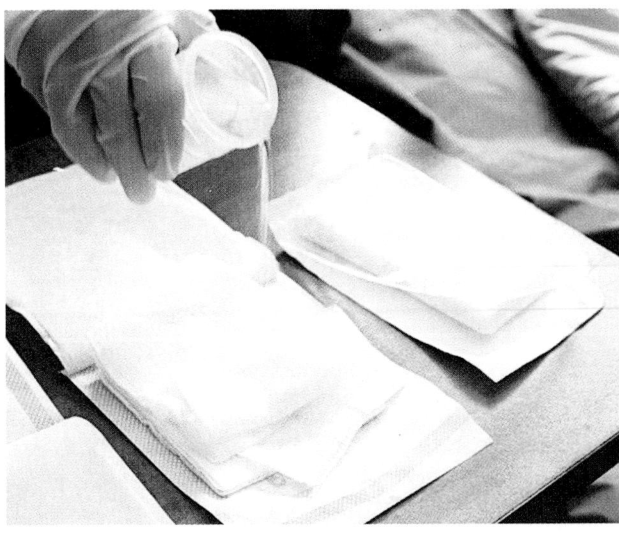
Pour sterile saline solution over dressings to moisten.

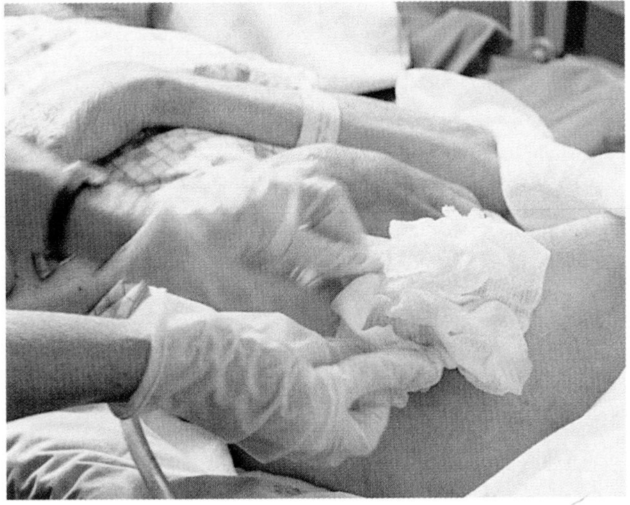
Place fluffed dressings over wound covering all exposed surface.

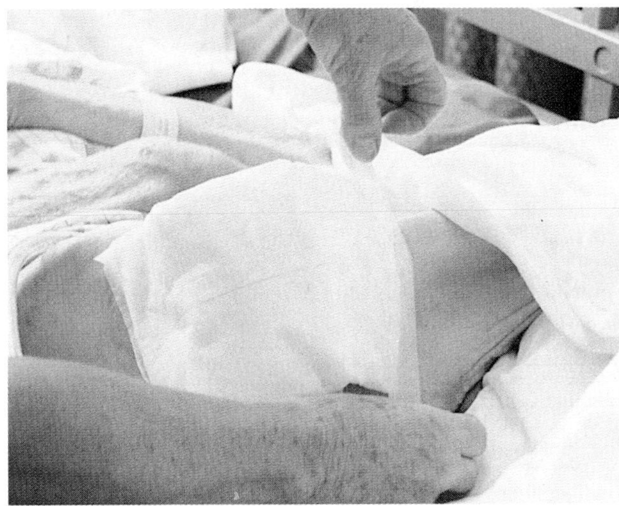
Place moist ABD pad over dressings, then cover with dry pad.

Procedure

1. Open packages of dressings making sure sterility is maintained.
2. Pour normal saline solution over dressings.
3. Don sterile gloves.
4. Pick up sterile gauze dressings one at a time.
5. Fluff each dressing, and place over wound.
6. Place gauze in the wound, covering all exposed surfaces. Press gauze into depressions or cracks. **Rationale:** Necrotic tissue is more prevalent in these areas.
7. Unfold a moist, sterile, 4 × 8 (ABD pad) dressing into a single layer and place it on top of wet dressings covering the entire area.
8. Place a dry 4 × 8 pad over the dressing to hold it in place.
9. Remove gloves, and place in plastic bag.
10. Tape only the edges of the dressing. Montgomery tapes may be used to prevent excessive skin irritation and damage due to frequent dressing changes.
11. Position client for comfort. Lower bed, and raise side rail to UP position.
12. Discard soiled material in appropriate container.
13. Wash your hands thoroughly.

14. Observe wound for excessive drainage between dressing changes. **Rationale:** Unless excessive drainage occurs, or dressing dries out, dressings are usually changed every 8 hours.
15. Provide client or family teaching regarding wound care, if appropriate.

■ CLINICAL ALERT

Normal saline is the primary irrigating solution. Other solutions previously used for these dressings are now contraindicated:

Hydrogen peroxide: Disturbs new capillaries in granulation tissue; may cause alterations in new tissue formation due to effervescent action.

Povidone-iodine: Retards collagen synthesis; can be absorbed into circulation; continuous or prolonged use can cause extreme iodine level leading to renal shutdown.

Dakin's solution: Toxic to granulation tissue and fibroblasts; retards collagen synthesis; delays epithelialization; inhibits migration of neutrophils to wound, thus inhibiting body's

CHARTING for Wet-to-Damp Dressings

- Condition of wound
- Solution used
- Number and type of dressings used
- Signs and symptoms indicative of wound infection
- Color, consistency, presence of odor, amount of drainage on soiled dressings
- Condition of skin surrounding wound
- Client's reaction to procedure

CRITICAL THINKING APPLICATION

CLINICAL PROBLEMS	CRITICAL THINKING OPTIONS
■ Wound drainage increases.	• Decrease time between dressing changes. Change every 4 hours. • Obtain order for culture and sensitivity to determine if different microorganisms are present or antibiotic medication is not sensitive to drug.
■ Dressings dry between dressing changes.	• Moisten dressing with sterile normal saline before removing to prevent debridement of granulation tissue. • Ensure that dressing is moist when applied to wound and cover with dry dressing. • Moisten and change dressing more frequently.

unit 5

PRESSURE ULCERS

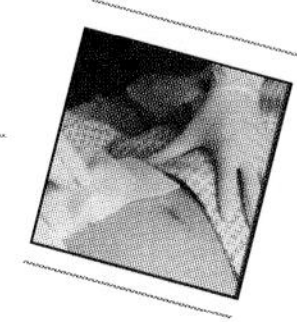

NURSING PROCESS DATA

ASSESSMENT Data Base

Assess stage of ulcer.

Identify if infection is associated with pressure ulcer.

Evaluate effectiveness of ulcer treatment.

Assess healing process of the ulcer.

Assess other bony prominences for potential formation of pressure ulcers.

Assess for presence of conditions that inhibit wound healing.

Assess wound size for changes.

PLANNING Objectives

To identify the stage of the ulcer

To provide appropriate treatment for specific ulcer stage

To promote healing of established ulcer

To prevent new ulcer formation

To prevent spread of pathogens from ulcerated area

IMPLEMENTATION Procedures

Preventing Pressure Ulcers

Applying Transparent Adhesive Film Dressing

Using Hydrocolloid Dressing

EVALUATION Expected Outcomes

Stage of pressure ulcer is accurately assessed.

Pressure ulcer is treated effectively according to stage of ulcer formation.

TABLE 24–2. Pressure Ulcer Staging and Treatment*

Stage†	Treatment Protocol for Pressure Ulcer Stages
Stage I: Nonblanchable erythema of intact skin, the heralding lesion of skin ulceration.	*Stage 1:* Apply an adhesive film dressing over the red area. These dressings are semipermeable to oxygen and prevent bacterial invasion. Healing can occur in 24 hours.
Stage II: Partial-thickness skin loss involving epidermis or dermis. The ulcer is superficial and presents clinically as an abrasion, blister, or shallow crater.	*Stage 2:* Apply a transparent adhesive film dressing if ulcer is not draining. If wound is draining, irrigate with normal saline and apply a hydrocolloid dressing. These occlusive dressings remain in place for 5–7 days, creating a moist environment that promotes epithelialization and restoration of the epidermis.
Stage III: Full-thickness skin loss involving damage or necrosis of subcutaneous tissue that may extend down to, but not through, underlying facia. The ulcer presents clinically as a deep crater with or without the undermining of adjacent tissue.	*Stage 3:* Irrigate with normal saline, cover with a hydrocolloid dressing. With excessively draining wounds, absorptive products are placed in the wound for absorption, and then the dressing is applied.
Stage IV: Full-thickness skin loss with extensive destruction, tissue necrosis, or damage to muscle, bone, or supporting structures (tendon or joint capsule are examples). Undermining and sinus tracts may be associated with this stage ulcer.	*Stage 4:* Chemical debridement, autolysis, or surgery are required for treatment of this stage. Wet-to-damp or wet-to-tacky dressing changes are used for small wounds; surgical interventions are used for larger wounds.

*Source: *Pressure Ulcers in Adults: Prediction and Prevention.* Rockville, MD: U.S. Department of Health and Human Services, Public Health Service, Agency for Health Care Policy and Research.

†Pressure ulcers are classified in stages by the degree of tissue damage observed.

Accurate staging of pressure ulcers is not possible until eschar has sloughed or wound is debrided.

Nursing Guide for Assessment of Pressure Ulcers

Identify at-risk individuals needing preventative measures:

- Bed- and chairbound individuals
- Clients with impaired ability to reposition themselves
- Clients who are immobilized
- Clients who are incontinent
- Clients with nutritional deficits, such as inadequate dietary intake, malnutrition
- Clients with altered level of consciousness
- Identification of stage I pressure ulcer may be difficult in a dark-skinned client.

A risk assessment tool should be used for all clients admitted to long-term care facilities, an acute care setting, or receiving home care (Braden scale or Norton scale). Systematic reassessments should be done at designated intervals.

Factors that contribute to development of pressure ulcers:

- Pressure
- Friction
- Shearing
- Moisture

PREVENTING PRESSURE ULCERS

Procedure

1. Inspect skin at least daily, particularly over bony prominences. Document assessment findings.
2. Individualize client's bathing schedule. Daily baths are not essential. **Rationale:** Daily cleansing can destroy the skin's natural barrier, making it more susceptible to external irritants.
   a. Avoid hot bath water. **Rationale:** Tepid water prevents injury to skin.

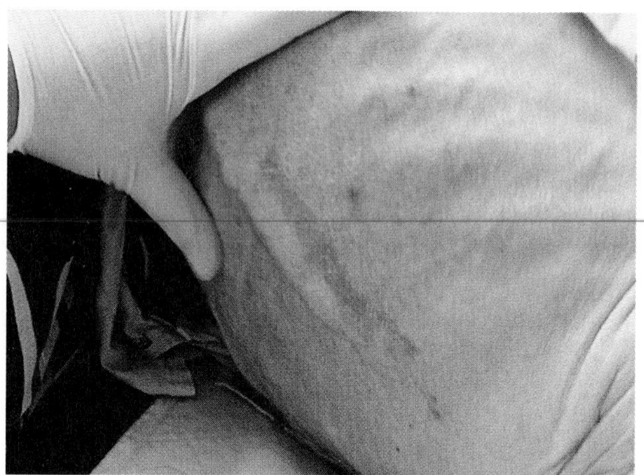

Stage I Pressure ulcer.

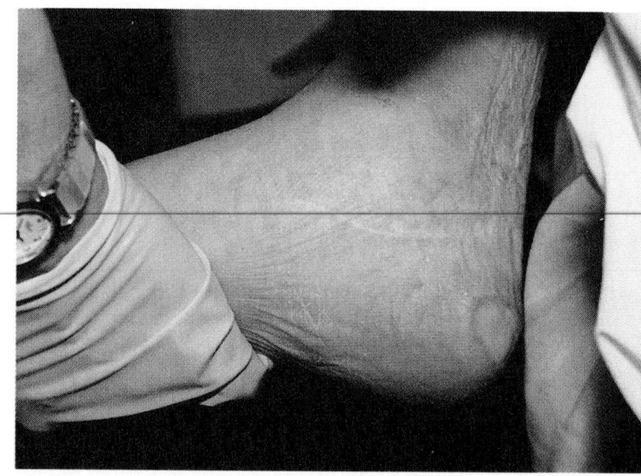

Stage II Pressure ulcer.

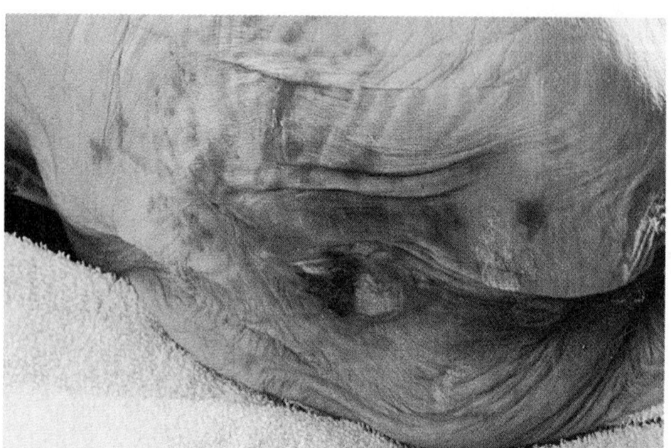

Stage III Pressure ulcer.

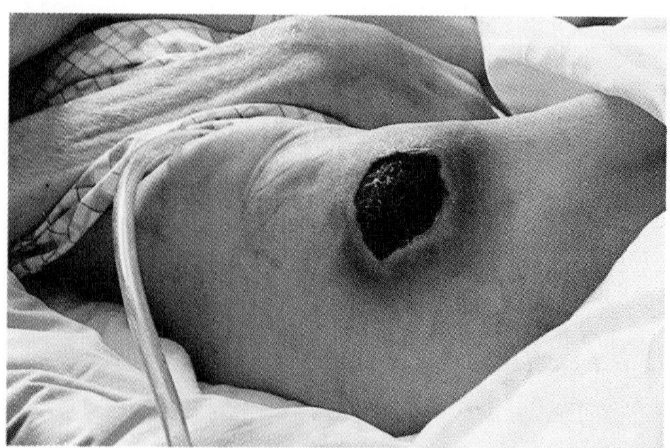

Stage IV Pressure ulcer.

b. Use mild cleansing agents to minimize dryness.
c. Cleanse skin immediately if urine, fecal incontinence, or wound drainage seeps onto skin.
d. Provide humidity to prevent drying of skin.

3. Avoid massaging bony prominences. **Rationale:** Massaging can lead to deep tissue trauma.
   a. Keep bony prominences from direct contact with one another.
   b. Use pillow, foam wedges, or other positioning devices.
4. Promote adequate dietary intake of protein, calories, and nutrients. **Rationale:** Adequate protein intake in addition to vitamins and minerals help prevent pressure ulcer formation.
5. Reposition bedridden client every 2 hours.
   a. Do not position directly on trochanter.
   b. Raise heels off bed by placing pillows under legs; allow heels to hang over edges.
   c. Use trapeze or turning sheet to reposition client.
6. Encourage mobility of range-of-motion exercises. **Rationale:** Range-of-motion exercises promote activity and reduce effects of pressure on tissue.

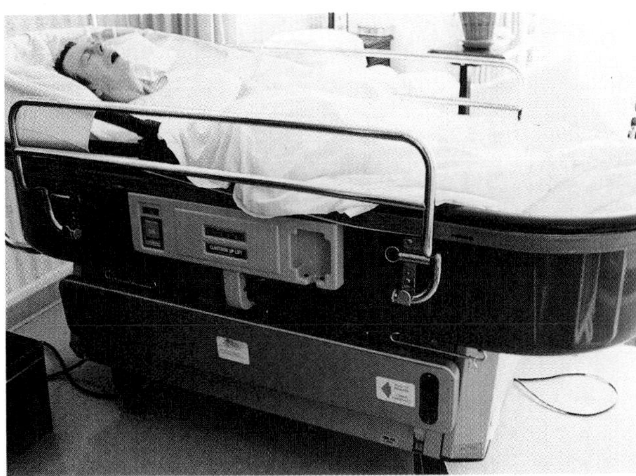

Commonly used air fluidized mattress.

7. Minimize force and friction or skin when turning, positioning, or transferring the client.
8. Maintain head of bed at lowest degree of elevation consistent with medical problem.
9. Place at-risk clients on pressure-reducing devices, such as foam, static-air, alternating gel, water mattress, or air fluidized mattress.

APPLYING TRANSPARENT ADHESIVE FILM DRESSING

Equipment

Sterile normal saline
Transparent dressing (e.g., Op-Site, Tegaderm)
Sterile 4 × 4 gauze pads
Scissors
Hypoallergenic tape
Clean gloves
Plasticizing agent (e.g., skin prep [optional])

■ CLINICAL ALERT

Adhesive transparent film dressings remain in place for 5–7 days. It is imperative to observe the ulcer area daily to determine if a large amount of secretions or serous fluid has accumulated under dressing. If fluid has increased, aspirate with a 26-gauge needle. These dressings are not used for infected areas.

Preparation

1. Check physician's orders and client care plan.
2. Gather supplies.
3. Obtain appropriately sized transparent dressing. Dressing can be applied to flat surface. (Coccyx area cannot be treated with this type of dressing.)
4. Wash your hands.
5. Explain procedure to client.
6. Provide privacy.

Procedure

1. Raise bed to HIGH position, and lower side rail on working side of bed.
2. Don clean gloves.
3. Remove old dressing, "walk off" dressing from one edge to the other, and discard in appropriate receptacle.
4. Wash pressure ulcer with sterile gauze pads moistened with sterile normal saline.
5. Dry thoroughly with sterile gauze pad.
6. Measure wound using pliable device. **Rationale:**

SAMPLE PRESSURE ULCER ASSESSMENT GUIDE

Patient Name: ______________________ Date: ____________ Time: ____________

Ulcer 1:			Ulcer 2:		
Site ____________			Site ____________		
Stage[a] ______			Stage[a] ______		
Size (cm)			Size (cm)		
Length ______			Length ______		
Width ______			Width ______		
Depth ______			Depth ______		
Sinus Tract	☐	☐	Sinus Tract	☐	☐
Tunneling	☐	☐	Tunneling	☐	☐
Undermining	☐	☐	Undermining	☐	☐
Necrotic Tissue	☐	☐	Necrotic Tissue	☐	☐
Slough	☐	☐	Slough	☐	☐
Eschar	☐	☐	Eschar	☐	☐
Exudate	☐	☐	Exudate	☐	☐
Serous	☐	☐	Serous	☐	☐
Serosanguineous	☐	☐	Serosanguineous	☐	☐
Purulent	☐	☐	Purulent	☐	☐
Granulation	☐	☐	Granulation	☐	☐
Epithelialization	☐	☐	Epithelialization	☐	☐
Pain	☐	☐	Pain	☐	☐
Surrounding Skin:					
Erythema	☐	☐	Erythema	☐	☐
Maceration	☐	☐	Maceration	☐	☐
Induration	☐	☐	Induration	☐	☐

Description of Ulcer(s):

____

____

Indicate Ulcer Sites:

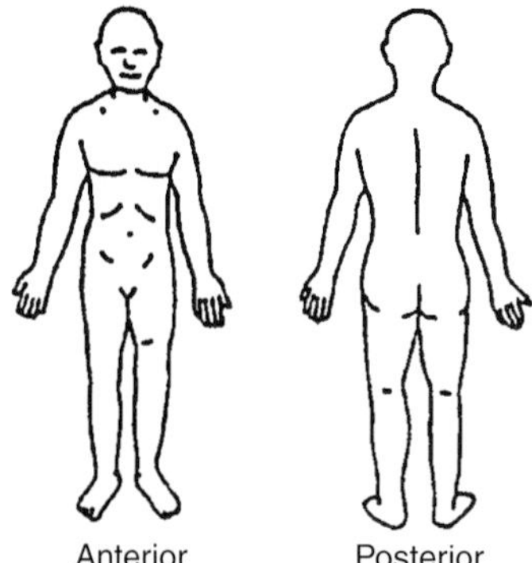

(Attach a color photo of the pressure ulcer[s] [Optional])

[a]Classification of pressure ulcers:

Stage I: Nonblanchable erythema of intact skin, the heralding lesion of skin ulceration. In individuals with darker skin, discoloration of the skin, warmth, edema, induration, or hardness may also be indicators .

Stage II: Partial thickness skin loss involving epidermis, dermis, or both.

Stage III: Full thickness skin loss involving damage to or necrosis of subcutaneous tissue that may extend down to, but not through, underlying fascia. The ulcer presents clinically as a deep crater with or without undermining adjacent tissue.

Stage IV: Full thickness skin loss with extensive destruction, tissue necrosis, or damage to muscle, bone, or supporting structures (e.g., tendon or joint capsule).

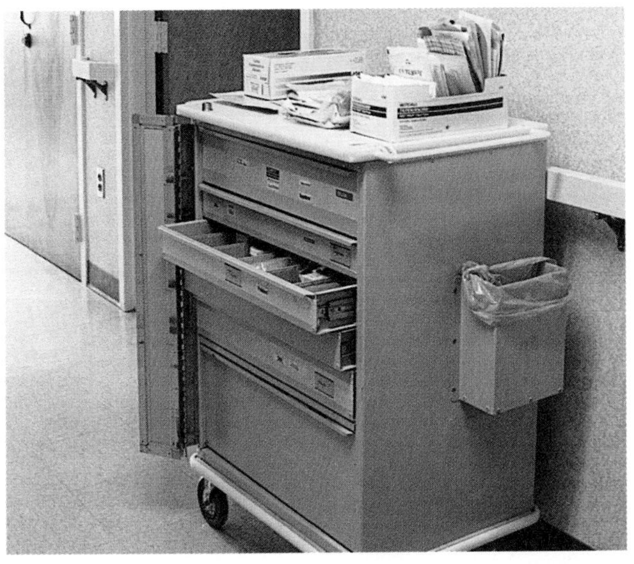

Dressing carts may be used to keep supplies closer to client area.

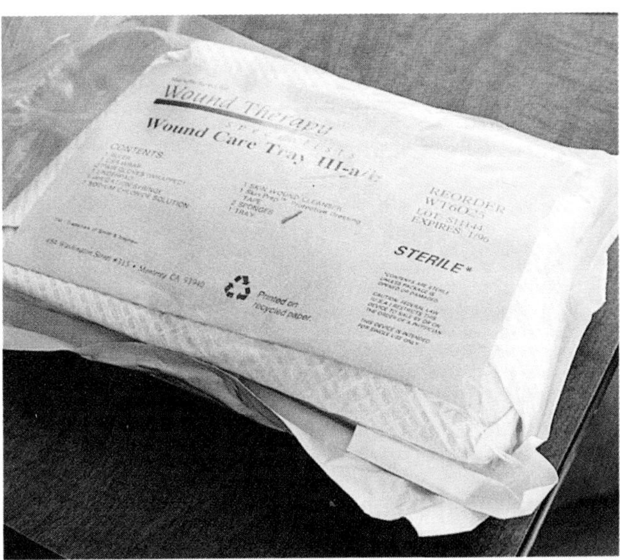

Obtain specific dressing tray for ordered treatment.

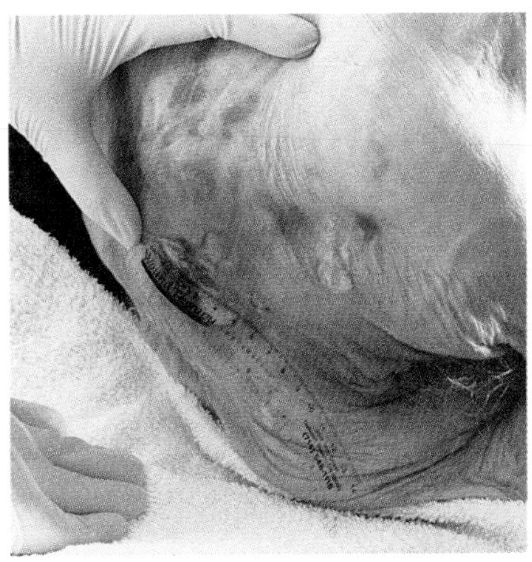

Assess size of wound to determine appropriate size of transparent dressing.

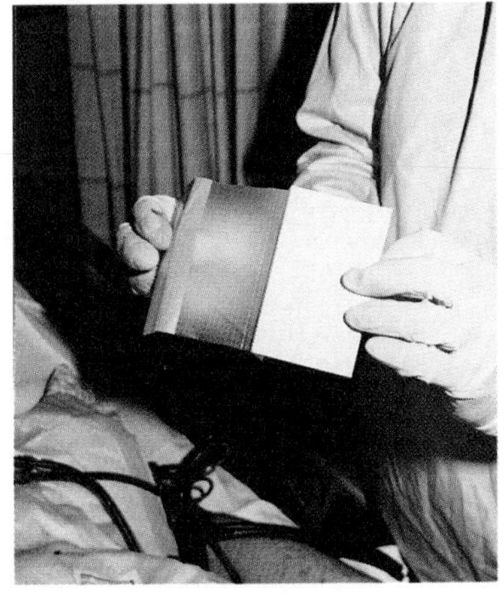

Remove backing from op-site dressing before applying.

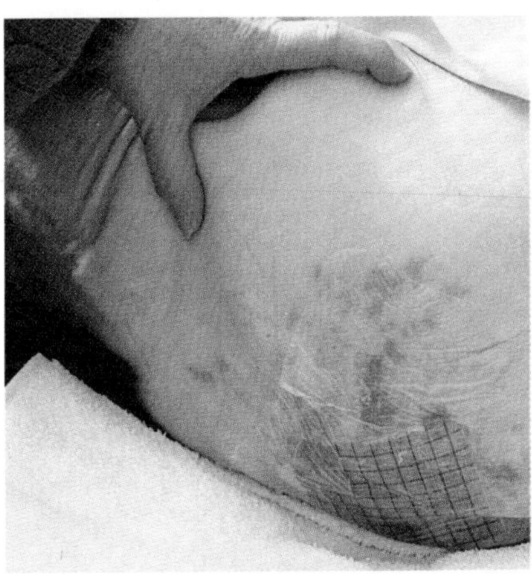

Apply transparent adhesive dressing over wound.

Comparison of measurement assists in determining effectiveness of treatment.

7. Apply plasticizing agent (skin prep, skin gel) over surrounding tissue if ordered. **Rationale:** Do not apply directly on ulcer area because the agent contains alcohol, which burns the ulcer area.
8. Loosen transparent dressing from one side of backing paper.
9. "Walk on" dressing: Start at one edge of site and gently lay the dressing down, keeping it free of wrinkles. Allow at least a $1\frac{1}{2}$-inch margin of dressing beyond ulcer margin. **Rationale:** This ensures coverage of entire wound area.
10. Cut off tabs if using Op-Site after wound is completely covered.
11. Tape edges with hypoallergenic tape. **Rationale:** This assists in preventing frequent dressing changes due to loose dressings.
12. Remove gloves, and discard in appropriate receptacle.
13. Position client for comfort.
14. Lower bed, and raise side rails.
15. Remove and discard equipment.
16. Wash your hands.

NUTRITIONAL ASSESSMENT OF CLIENT WITH PRESSURE ULCER(S)

Client Name: ______________________ **Date:** __________ **Time** __________

To be filled out for all clients at risk on initial evaluation and every 12 weeks thereafter, as indicated. Trends will document the efficacy of nutritional support therapy.

Protein Compartments

Somatic:

Current Weight (kg) ______
Previous Weight (kg) ______ (______ date)
Percent Change in Weight ______

Height (cm) ______
Height/Weight ______
Current Body Mass Index (BM) ______ [wt/(ht)^2]
Previous BMI ______ (______ date)
Percent Change in BMI ______

Visceral:

Serum Albumin ______
(Normal $\geq$ 3.5 mg/dL)
Total Lymphocyte Count (TLC) ______ (optional)
(White Blood Cell count x percent Lymphocytes/100)

Guide to TLC:

- Immune competence $\geq$ 1,800 mm^3
- Immunity partly impaired $<$ 1,800 but $\geq$ 900 mm^3
- Anergy $<$ 900 mm^3

State of Hydration

24-Hour Intake ______ mL 24-Hour Output ______ mL

Note: Thirst, tongue dryness in non-mouth-breathers, and tenting of cervical skin may indicate dehydration. Jugular vein distention may indicate overhydration.

Estimated Nutritional Requirement

Estimated Nonprotein Calories (NPC) ______ /kg Estimated Protein ______ (g/kg)
Actual NPC ______ /kg Actual Protein ______ (g/kg)

Recommendations/Plan

1.

2.

3.

4.

USING HYDROCOLLOID DRESSING

Equipment

Sterile normal saline

Hydrocolloid dressing (e.g., DuoDERM, Restore, Ultec, ClearSite)

Hydrocolloid gel if needed

Sterile 4 × 4 gauze pads

Hypoallergenic tape

Clean gloves

Procedure

1. Select dressing size to ensure coverage $1\frac{1}{4}$ inch beyond ulcer margin. (Dressing available in 4 × 4 to 8 × 8 size.)
2. Don clean gloves.
3. Cleanse skin with gauze pad moistened with sterile normal saline and pat dry with gauze pad.
4. Measure wound using pliable device.
5. Fill ulcer area with gel if ordered—usually used when exudate is present. Do not overfill with gel.
6. Remove silicone release paper backing from dressing. Minimize finger contact with adhesive surface. **Rationale:** Dressing is sterile and contamination should be avoided.
7. Center dressing over affected area. Gently roll dressing over pressure ulcer—do not stretch dressing.
8. Mold the dressing gently to skin, and hold down with hand for approximately 1 minute.
9. Apply skin prep to area that is to be covered by tape if ordered. Allow to dry. *Do not apply* skin prep under hydrocolloid dressing.
10. Picture-frame sides of hydrocolloid dressing with silk or hypoallergic tape.
11. Check dressing daily for leakage.
12. Change dressing at first sign of leakage. Dressings should not be left on longer than 7 days.
13. Remove dressing by pressing hand down on adjacent skin surface while carefully lifting edge of dressing from skin. Continue lifting dressing around periphery until all edges are released, then lift dressing carefully away from wound.
14. Record stage, size, and appearance of ulcer; date; and reason for removal of hydrocolloid dressing.

TABLE 24–3. Comparisons of Moisture-Retentive Dressings

	Transparent	Hydrocolloid
Common Brands	Tegaderm Op-Site Bioclusive	Tegasorb DuoDerm Comfeel Restore
Characteristics	Sterile Semipermeable membranes with hypoallergenic adhesive Permeable to oxygen and moisture vapor Allows oxygen exchange Impermeable to bacteria, prevents contamination	Impermeable to oxygen Dressing gel maintains moist environment that promotes autolysis Impermeable to external bacteria and contamination Minimally to moderately absorptive
Function	Provides moist environment Promotes autolysis and protects newly formed tissue Assists with debridement	Dressing contains hydroactive particles that absorb exudate to form a hydrated gel over wound When dressing removed, gel separates from dressing, which protects newly formed tissue
Use	Easy assessment of wound, dressing is transparent Nondraining or minimally draining wounds only, nonabsorbable Pressure ulcers, stage I and some stage II Minor burns, lacerations	Absorbs exudate while preserving moist environment needed for autolysis of slough Irrigate gel with saline to allow for assessing wound Pressure ulcers, some stage III and some clean stage IV Wounds with mild or moderate exudate Wounds with necrosis or slough
Contraindications	Infected wounds Wounds with fragile surrounding skin	Wounds that need frequent assessment, not transparent Wounds with heavy exudate

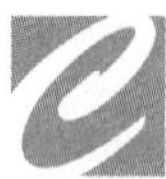

CHARTING for Pressure Ulcer

- Client's general skin condition
- Assessment of wound (i.e., drainage, evidence of tissue granulation)
- Type of ulcer care given
- Pressure ulcer record completed
- State the exact location of pressure ulcer
- *Size*: Indicate size in centimeters
- *Stage*: Write the number of the stage that corresponds to the description of the pressure ulcer (stage 1–4)
- *Treatment*: Chart treatment used (e.g., hydrocolloid dressing applied, transparent adhesive film applied, etc.)
- *Position:* Indicate time client's position was changed.

CRITICAL THINKING APPLICATION

CLINICAL PROBLEMS	CRITICAL THINKING OPTIONS
Client does not have sufficient exercise; appetite decreased.	• Encourage small, frequent feedings. • Offer high-calorie drinks like eggnog or Isocal.
Client's wound does not heal with traditional types of treatments.	• In client care conference discuss the following: Is everyone following same treatment? Are causative agents preventing healing? Should treatment be adjusted or changed? Would use of a flotation or pressure-relieving mattress be useful? Is surgical debridement and grafting necessary for healing?

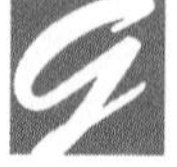

GERIATRIC CONSIDERATIONS

The inflammatory and proliferation phases of wound healing are often defective with elderly clients who have chronic diseases.

- A hemoglobin below 10 g/dL increases susceptibility.
- Uncontrolled diabetes mellitus or a blood glucose level that exceeds 200 mg/dL presents a risk.
- Hyperglycemia retards neutrophil production.
- T and B cells diminish in function and number, indicating a reduced inflammatory response. Elderly clients are at risk for cutaneous viral and fungal infections.
- Clients with rheumatoid arthritis who take steroids or nonsteroidal anti-inflammatory medications are at risk for decreased wound healing. There is a slower rate of epithelialization and severely inhibited contraction.
- Ischemia, anemia, and edema from vascular insufficiency or pressure leads to lack of blood flow to a wound area. Lower oxygen-carrying capacity results from anemia. Edema makes it difficult to transport oxygen and cellular wastes to and from cells. Ischemia leads to diminished oxygen necessary for wound healing.

Nursing actions to counteract risks against wound healing

- All at-risk elderly clients should have a pressure ulcer risk assessment completed at the time of admission and at regular intervals thereafter.
- Use of compression stockings assists in treating both the edema and ultimately the ischemia, therefore increasing blood flow to wound area.
- Turning frequently, at least every 2 hours, for clients free of pressure ulcers and every 1 hour for those at high risk, should be a priority.
- Use of pressure-relieving mattresses decreases risk potential.
- Wound care, including irrigation, use of appropriate dressings, and maintaining aseptic technique with dressing changes, should be priority care for clients with any type of wound.

25

Respiratory Care

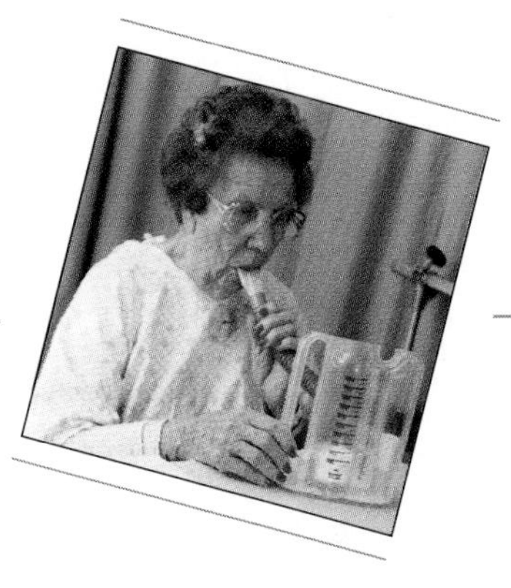

LEARNING OBJECTIVES

- Outline the three process of respiration.
- Identify three nursing diagnoses of ventilatory dysfunction.
- Describe the steps for teaching a client deep breathing and coughing exercises.
- Discuss the purpose of using an incentive spirometer.
- Describe positions used for chest percussion, vibration, and drainage.
- Describe safety measures used when suctioning clients.
- Compare and contrast the FIO_2 delivered and specific nursing interventions required by at least four of the common modes of oxygen administration.
- Describe the nursing actions included in performing tracheostomy care.
- Explain the procedure for inflating and deflating the tracheostomy cuff.
- Identify at least four interventions that promote chest tube drainage.
- List the safety measures that are carried out to promote safe, effective care for clients with chest tubes in place.
- Describe the difference between two- and three-bottle suction systems.
- Outline the steps of endotracheal intubation.

TERMINOLOGY

Acidosis: accumulation of acids (metabolic or respiratory), potentially disturbing acid–base balance and causing acidemia (low pH)

Adventitious: abnormal extra sounds (crackles, wheezes) superimposed on breath sounds

Alkalosis: condition in which the alkalinity of the body tends to increase beyond normal, potentially resulting in alkalemia (high pH)

Antiemetic: an agent that prevents or arrests vomiting

Apnea: cessation of breathing, usually of a temporary nature

Atelectasis: collapse of alveoli, which may lead to hypoxemia and increased PCO_2 and pneumonia

Auscultation: process of listening for sounds produced by body organs

Bradycardia: slow heart rate (below 60 beats/minute)

Bronchiectasis: dilation of a bronchus or bronchi with production of large amounts of malodorous secretions

Chylothorax: milky chyle that has entered pleural space from the thoracic duct

Crackles: discontinuous popping (opening) sounds indicative of hypoventilation of alveoli, usually auscultated at end of inspiration in dependent lung areas

Cyanosis: bluish or grayish discoloration of the skin resulting from reduced oxygen saturation of hemoglobin

Diaphoresis: profuse sweating

Dyspnea: a subjective feeling of having difficulty breathing

Expectorant: an agent that facilitates the removal of the secretions of the bronchopulmonary mucous membrane

Hemothorax: blood in the pleural space compressing normal lung tissue

Hyperventilation: abnormally deep breathing that results in a decrease in PCO_2 (respiratory alkalosis)

Hypoventilation: reduced rate and depth of breathing resulting in retention of carbon dioxide (respiratory acidosis)

Hypoxemia: insufficient oxygenation of the blood (decreased PO_2)

Hypoxia: lack of adequate amount of oxygen transported to the tissues

Intrapulmonic: within the lungs

Intubation: to insert a tube into a body opening, as into the trachea

Narcosis: unconscious state due to narcotics or other depressing agent

Nares: the nostrils

Nebulizer: a device for breaking a drug into small particles to produce a mist or fog for inhalation

Percussion: tapping the body lightly but sharply to determine position, size, and consistency of an underlying structure

Pneumothorax: presence of air in the intrapleural space resulting in lung collapse

Polycythemia: excess number of red blood cells

Postural Drainage: the use of gravity to drain secretions from the lungs

Spirometer: device used for measuring inhalation and exhalation volumes

Spontaneous Pneumothorax: condition developing from air leak in pulmonary alveoli or from erosion by disease process through the visceral pleura allowing positive pressure to be established in the intrapleural space

Sputum: substance expelled by coughing

Tachypnea: increased rate of breathing (over 24 breaths/minute)

Tension Pneumothorax: lung collapse and shift of contralateral mediastinal structures resulting from accumulation of air or fluid in the intrapleural space

Tracheostomy: opening into the trachea usually for insertion of a tube to provide airway patency

Ventilation: the acts of inspiration and exhalation for the exchange of oxygen and carbon dioxide between the lungs and the atmosphere

Vibration: therapeutic high-frequency shaking of a body part

Wheezes: musical adventitious sounds heard on inspiration or expiration due to airway spasm, retained secretions, or other obstruction

THE RESPIRATORY SYSTEM

The respiratory system provides for the exchange of gases between the blood and the external environment so that cellular respiration can occur. The respiratory structures involved include the nose, pharynx, larynx, trachea, bronchi, lungs, diaphragm, intercostal muscles, and ribs.

The upper respiratory tract includes the nose, pharynx, and larynx. These structures filter, warm, and humidify the air before it passes into the lower airways. When the upper respiratory tract is bypassed by intubation or tracheostomy, an artificial humidification process is often used.

The lower respiratory tract is considered a sterile environment. It begins below the larynx. The trachea is composed of smooth muscle reinforced by C-shaped rings of cartilage lined with a membranous sheath. It branches into the right and left mainstream bronchi. The right bronchus extends vertically from the trachea, whereas the left bronchus branches from the trachea at an angle.

The right and left bronchi divide further and further into terminal bronchioles and finally into respiratory bronchioles, alveolar ducts, and alveoli. The respiratory unit (respiratory bronchiole, alveolar ducts, and alveoli) is surrounded by capillaries, which allow for the exchange of oxygen and carbon dioxide. Alveoli must

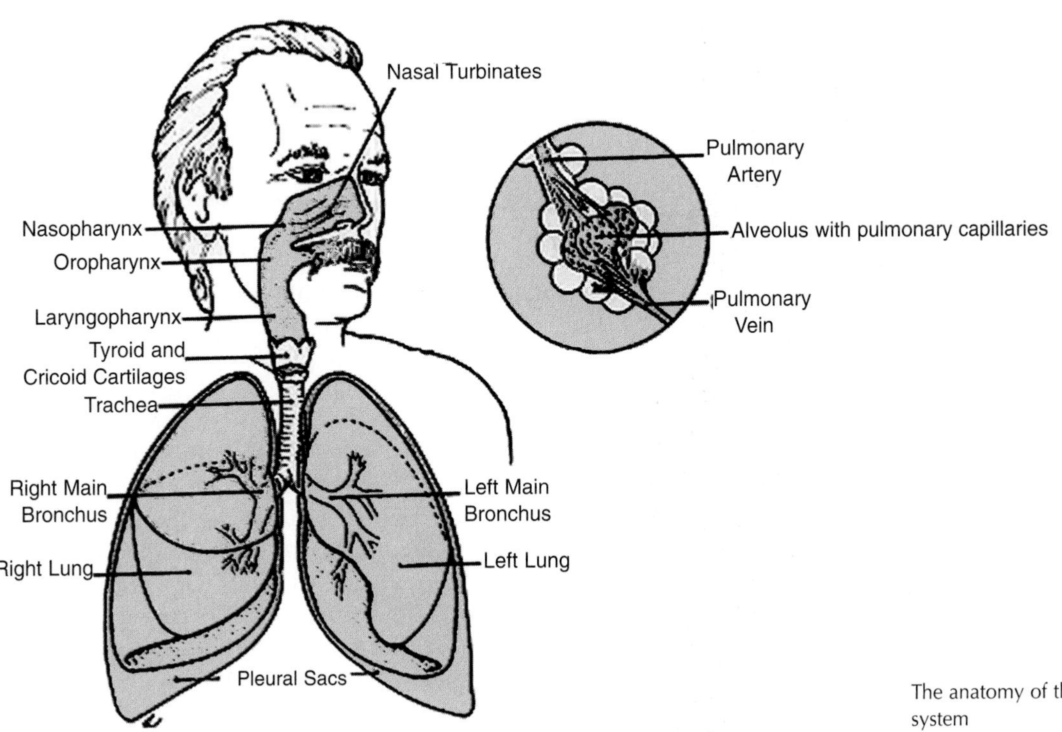

The anatomy of the respiratory system

be ventilated and must remain diffusable for gas exchange to prevent respiratory failure.

Because of the anatomical difference of the bronchi, migration of an endotracheal tube (ET) into the right bronchus is more likely. Such a migration would result in ventilation of only the right lung. Chest x-rays are taken to ensure proper placement of ET tubes in the trachea. Auscultation of *bilateral* breath sounds also helps to verify optimal ventilation of intubated clients.

THE RESPIRATORY CYCLE

Cellular respiration occurs when oxygen is transported from the atmosphere to the cell, and carbon dioxide is carried from the cells to the atmosphere. Three processes—ventilation, diffusion, and perfusion—are essential for this to occur.

Ventilation is the mechanical exchange of air between the lungs and the atmosphere. *Inspiration* is the *active* phase of ventilation. It depends on contraction of the diaphragm and external intercostal muscles to expand the thorax. When expansion occurs, intrapulmonic pressure becomes less than atmospheric pressure, and air flows into the lungs. *Exhalation* is the *passive* phase of ventilation. It occurs when alveolar pressure increases due to elastic recoils, and air flows out of the lungs back into the atmosphere.

Ventilation is controlled by the brainstem, which responds to a rise in blood carbon dioxide level (PCO_2). As breathing eliminates CO_2, there is a negative feedback to the brain. Through exhalation of carbon dioxide (which with water forms the volatile acid carbonic acid in the bloodstream) the lungs play a vital role in maintaining the normal alkaline pH of the blood (7.35–7.45). Conditions that result in metabolic acidosis (e.g., diabetic ketoacidosis) make the blood more acidic, also stimulating the brainstem to increase the rate and depth of breathing. The resultant lowering of PCO_2 (exhalation of volatile acid) helps return the blood pH to an alkaline state. This process is called respiratory compensation for metabolic acidosis.

Although CO_2 is the major stimulus for breathing, high sustained levels of carbonic acid depress the respiratory center, and respiratory arrest can occur. Individuals who have chronically elevated PCO_2 levels due to obstructive pulmonary disease (COPD) may become insensitive to PCO_2 as a stimulus for breathing. Instead, their brain responds to a lower than normal PO_2 (less than 60 mm Hg) to stimulate breathing. The administration of high flows of oxygen to such "hypoxic-dependent breathers" can eliminate their stimulus to breathe. Such individuals are at high risk for CO_2 narcosis.

Diffusion is the process of gas exchange between the alveolar air and the blood. Oxygen tension in blood flowing through alveolar capillaries is *lower* than the oxygen tension in the alveoli. This pressure gradient causes oxygen to pass from the alveoli to the blood, thus increasing the PO_2 and "arterializing" the blood. Conversely, carbon dioxide tension is *higher* in the capillary blood than it is in the alveoli, thus promoting the elimination of carbon dioxide so it can be exhaled.

Perfusion is the process of transport of oxygen and carbon dioxide between the lungs and tissue cells. Without this transport and exchange of gases at both the pulmonary and tissue capillary levels, survival is impossible.

Alterations in Respiration

Alterations in tissue respiration can result from dysfunction of any of the three essential processes previously outlined.

Alterations in Ventilation

Ventilation depends on patent airways, the ability to clear airways, chest expansion, and compliant alveoli. Many factors and disease processes can interfere with adequate ventilation, including any limitation on alveolar expansion (pneumonia, congestive heart failure, fractured ribs, pain, thoracic deformity, neurologic disease, respiratory depressants, immobility), any limitation in ability to clear airways (ineffective cough, intubation, decreased level of consciousness), and factors that interfere with surfactant activity, which is essential for alveolar inflation (narcotics, anesthetics, hypoventilation, high oxygen flow rates). Inadequate ventilation results in abnormal arterial blood gases (low PO_2 and low SaO_2, and eventually, an increase in PCO_2). Pathologic processes that cause ineffective exhalation due to loss of alveolar elastic recoil or decreased air-

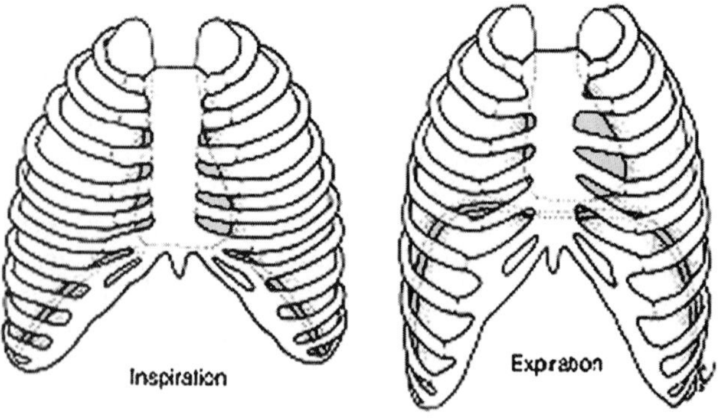

Position of diaphragm at full-end inspiration and full-end exporation.

way resistance to increased intrathoracic pressure (as with exhalation or coughing) also result in an increased Pco_2 (respiratory acidosis). Chronic obstructive pulmonary disease is an example. Two nursing diagnoses associated with alterations in ventilation are ineffective breathing patterns and ineffective airway clearance.

Alterations in Diffusion

Diffusion is dependent on a partial pressure difference in gases and an adequate amount of permeable alveolar surface area. Any disease that thickens the alveolar membrane (fibrosis, congestive heart failure) reduces alveolar permeability and leads to a reduced Po_2 (hypoxemia). Alveolar surface area can be reduced by lobectomy or pneumonectomy. A nursing diagnosis associated with alterations in diffusion is impaired gas exchange.

Alterations in Perfusion

For cells to receive oxygen and give off their wastes, blood must flow at both the pulmonary and tissue capillary levels. Adequate perfusion depends on a normal blood volume, an adequate amount of hemoglobin capable of combining with oxygen and carbon dioxide, effective cardiac function, and competent vasculature. Any pathology that interferes with blood cell production, maintenance of blood volume, cardiac function, or vascular patency can result in inadequate tissue perfusion. Likewise, any factor that prevents blood from flowing through pulmonary capillaries (pulmonary embolism) disrupts the process of gas exchange for replenishment of oxygen and the elimination of carbon dioxide. A nursing diagnosis associated with alterations in perfusion is altered tissue perfusion.

ASSESSMENT OF RESPIRATORY FUNCTION

Arterial blood gases and pulmonary function tests reflect pulmonary capacity. The pH of the blood is affected by pulmonary function. If carbon dioxide is not eliminated by the lungs due to hypoventilation for any reason, the Pco_2 rises. Since CO_2 creates an acid in the bloodstream, its accumulation (respiration acidosis) causes the blood pH to decrease (acidemia). *Hypoventilation* is the only mechanism for Pco_2 accumulation and is encountered when factors depress the respiratory center, inhibit breathing, or a client has a disease, such as COPD, that prevents efficient exhalation. *Hyperventilation* (due to anxiety, neurologic dysfunction, or iatrogenic overventilation) causes the Pco_2 to fall below normal (respiratory alkalosis) and the blood pH to rise above normal (alkalemia).

Arterial blood gas (ABG) studies also evaluate diffusion and perfusion as reflected by the Po_2 and Sao_2. Pulse oximetry is often preferred over ABGs as a cost-effective laboratory test of Sao_2.

It is essential that ventilation of alveoli is matched with blood flowing through alveolar capillaries. If alveolar ventilation occurs without matched perfusion (e.g., pulmonary embolism), the Po_2 falls, but the Pco_2 remains normal because of the great solubility of CO_2; the Pco_2 may even decrease due to hyperventilation (respiratory alkalosis). Conversely, if the alveoli are perfused but not ventilated (as in atelectasis), the blood is not adequately oxygenated. This condition results in a low Po_2 and a normal Pco_2, because carbon dioxide is highly diffusible. Continued hypoventilation, however, eventually results in an increased Pco_2 (respiratory acidosis).

Pulmonary tests of lung volume reflect the chart for normal *arterial blood gases.*

pH	7.35–7.45
Pco_2	35–45 mm Hg
HCO_3	22–26 mEq/L
Po_2	80–100 mm Hg (breathing room air)
Sao_2	96–100%

Pulmonary function (spirometry) tests measure lung volume and capacity, and help differentiate restrictive and obstructive defects of ventilation.

VC (vital capacity)	75–80% of that predicted by age, sex, and height (decreased in restrictive disease)
FEV (forced expiratory volume)	65–85% of VC in 1 second and 95% in 3 seconds (decreased in obstructive disease)
FEV_1 (forced expiratory volume in 1 sec)	normal = 75% VC (decreased in obstructive disease)

Nursing Interventions

The primary goal of nursing interventions associated with respiratory function is to improve vital capacity and pulmonary ventilation.

Nursing interventions are used routinely as preventive measures in most clinical settings. These interventions help prevent pulmonary complications for clients with known pulmonary problems, for clients who are at risk for pulmonary complications (e.g., immobility), or for surgical clients who have undergone general anesthesia and who experience pain.

To maintain maximum vital capacity with minimal effort, assist the client to a Fowler's position. It is also beneficial for the client to assume a forward-leaning position (e.g., using the over-bed table).

Other nursing interventions that support respiratory function are: maintaining adequate hydration (2–3 L of water/day unless contraindicated); humidification of inspired oxygen to help liquefy secretions for easier removal; turning to help to ventilate dependent lung areas; deep breathing to stimulate surfactant and inflate hypoventilated alveoli; coughing to remove retained secretions; and airway suctioning to assist ineffective airway clearance. Protective splinting of operative sites promotes client compliance and prevents wound strain.

The most common clinical manifestations indicative of inadequate ventilation are

- tachycardia (heart rate over 100/minute)
- tachypnea (breathing rate over 24/minute)
- restlessness
- use of accessory muscles for breathing
- change in cognition or level of response
- increased blood pressure

Early recognition of these indicators of possible hypoxemia should prompt further investigation and appropriate intervention.

NURSING DIAGNOSES

The following nursing diagnoses are appropriate to use on client care plans when the components are related to respiratory conditions.

NURSING DIAGNOSIS	RELATED FACTORS
Activity Intolerance	Fatigue, pain, inadequate oxygenation
Altered Nutrition, Less than Body Requirements	Excessive expectoration, intubation, fatigue, prolonged coughing, chronic respiratory states, nausea and vomiting
Altered Oral Mucous Membrane	Prolonged mouth breathing, bypassed airway, disease state, intubation, comatose state
Anxiety	Pulmonary congestion, chronic respiratory disorders (COPD), pain, hypoxic state
Impaired Gas Exchange	Ventilation perfusion imbalance, diminished functional lung tissue, changes in arterial blood gases
Ineffective Airway Clearance	Inability to clear secretions, excessive secretions, obstructed respiratory tract, chest trauma, surgical interventions, pain, edema
Ineffective Breathing Pattern	Inability to maintain sufficient oxygen supply to cells, neuromuscular impairment, chronic respiratory disease states
Pain	Inflammatory process, acute respiratory states (pleurisy, pneumonia), terminal states (cancer)
Self-Care Deficit Syndrome	Fatigue, hypoxic states (confusion), chronic respiratory disorders, impaired gas exchange

unit 1

DEEP BREATHING EXERCISES

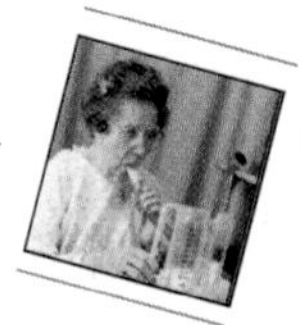

NURSING PROCESS DATA

ASSESSMENT Data Base

Observe client's physical ability to perform exercise (e.g., to assume Fowler's position, the degree of pain experienced, and the amount of medication needed to control pain).

Auscultate breath sounds.

Observe rhythm, rate, and depth of breathing.

Note presence of cough reflex.

Note proximity of incision to muscles necessary for breathing and coughing.

PLANNING Objectives

To improve vital capacity and pulmonary ventilation

To conserve energy

To loosen secretions and promote full lung expansion

To counteract effects of hypoventilation

IMPLEMENTATION Procedures

Instructing Clients to Deep Breathe

Instructing Clients to Cough

Teaching Diaphragmatic Breathing

Using Incentive Spirometers

EVALUATION Expected Outcomes

Vital capacity and pulmonary ventilation are improved.

Client reaches predetermined tidal volume level when using incentive spirometer.

Client's energy is conserved.

Secretions are loosened and lungs fully expanded.

Abdominal breathing is more automatic and respirations more efficient and relaxed.

INSTRUCTING CLIENTS TO DEEP BREATHE

Equipment

Straight chair or hospital bed in upright position

Pillows for positioning and incisional support

Preparation

1. Wash your hands.
2. Provide privacy.
3. Explain the rationale for the procedure.
4. Help client to sit up in bed as straight as possible, with head and shoulders supported by a firm surface. **Rationale:** This position promotes maximum vital capacity.

Procedure

1. Demonstrate the deep breathing steps, allowing time for client to practice each step.
2. Place your hands palm down around the sides of client's lower ribs. **Rationale:** This action supports deep breathing and assists you to evaluate depth of inspiration.

3. Tell client to breathe in slowly through nose until chest is expanded and abdomen rises visibly.
4. Check client's response to determine how often exercise should be performed—varies according to the client's condition.
(After abdominal or chest surgery, client should practice this exercise hourly. At least five breaths should be taken.)

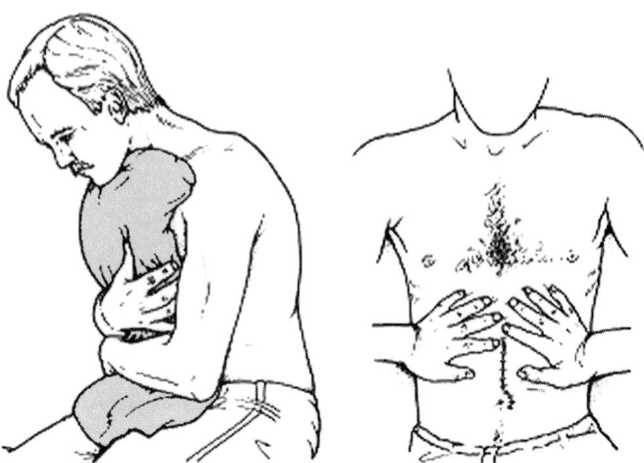

Instruct the client in deep breathing and coughing exercises preoperatively to enhance lung expansion postoperatively.

INSTRUCTING CLIENTS TO COUGH

Equipment

Straight chair or hospital bed in upright position
Pillows for positioning and incisional support
Tissues for secretions
Protective gear: gloves, gown, goggles, mask

Preparation

1. Wash your hands.
2. Provide privacy.
3. Explain procedure to client.
4. Don protective gear.

Procedure

1. Place client in upright position, upper body positioned slightly forward. **Rationale:** This position assists client to cough more effectively.
2. Ask client to slowly take two or three deep breaths through the nose and exhale passively through the mouth.
3. Instruct client to inhale deeply, hold breath for 1–2 seconds, and cough using abdominal and chest muscles. **Rationale:** This promotes a more forceful, effective cough.
4. Instruct client with pulmonary condition to exhale through pursed lips and to cough midway through exhalation (not at end of deep inspiration). **Rationale:** This helps prevent high expiratory pressures that collapse diseased airways, thus facilitating movement of secretions along the tracheobronchial tree.
5. Support any incision with the palms of your hands. You may also place a rolled pillow firmly against the incision. **Rationale:** This prevents incisional strain and encourages client to cough more effectively.
6. Encourage client to cough frequently if cough is productive. Explain why coughing is beneficial. **Rationale:** Accumulated secretions in airways promotes bacterial growth and interferes with ventilation.

TEACHING DIAPHRAGMATIC BREATHING

Equipment

Hospital bed in flat position

Preparation

1. Check physician's orders and client care plan.
2. Wash your hands.
3. Provide privacy.
4. Inform client that the purpose of this exercise is to learn how to breathe by using abdominal muscles. (Clients with COPD tend to overwork the upper chest muscles and suck in the abdomen on inspiration, making it difficult for the diaphragm to descend. This exercise improves breathing efficiency.)

Procedure

1. Place your hands on client's abdomen, below ribs.
2. Have client breathe in through the nose and try to push stomach outward against your hands.
3. Instruct client to hold his or her breath for 1–2 seconds to keep alveoli open.
4. Have client breathe out slowly through the mouth as you apply slight pressure at the base of the ribs.
5. Encourage client to practice abdominal breathing frequently, using own hands to feel the abdomen rise.

USING INCENTIVE SPIROMETERS (IS)

Equipment

Hospital bed in upright position or straight chair

Pillows for positioning

Incentive spirometer with flow rate indicator (e.g., Voldyne); save bag for storage of device

Preparation

1. Check physician's orders and client care plan.
2. Gather equipment.
3. Wash your hands.
4. Explain purpose and procedure to client.
5. If preoperative measurement was not done, use guide in Voldyne package to determine client's volume goal, and set marker at this goal.
6. Attach open end of tubing to stem on front of exerciser.

Procedure

1. Instruct client to hold exerciser, place mouth tightly around mouthpiece, and sip in a trial breath. **Rationale:** Client can see the flow floater to visualize appropriate flow rate for inhalation.
2. Explain that a slow deep breath is better than a fast breath.

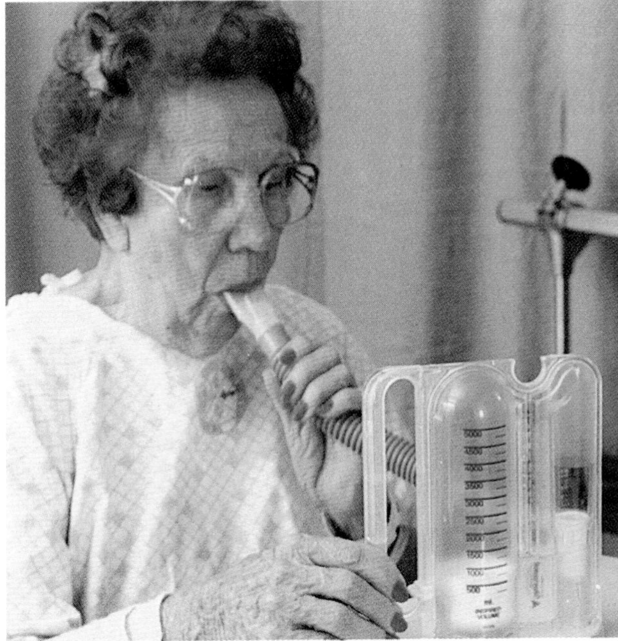

Client places mouth tightly around mouthpiece, inhales slowly and maintains piston in chamber to promote lung expansion.

3. Instruct client to exhale normally then place mouth tightly around mouthpiece.
4. Instruct client to inhale slowly to raise and maintain piston in the chamber at the "best" flow rate range,

and continue inhaling to try to raise piston to prescribed (or preoperative measured) level.

5. Instruct client to remove mouthpiece but hold breath at maximum inspiration several seconds, then exhale normally. Repeat a few times, then cough.
6. Encourage client to use spirometer hourly, coordinating use with TV program breaks, for instance, as a reminder.
7. Provide positive feedback as client uses IS to reattain preoperative inspiratory capacity using marked goal as an incentive.
8. Replace unit in bag when not in use, and keep in accessible place for client.

Note: Recent studies show that sustained inspiration (breathing in deeply through the nose, holding for 3 seconds, and exhaling) is just as effective as using a commercial incentive spirometer (and more cost-effective) in preventing pulmonary complications.

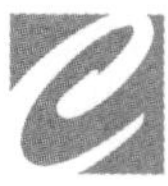

CHARTING for Deep Breathing, Coughing, and Use of IS

- Frequency of deep breathing exercises or use of IS
- Whether cough is productive or not
- Amount and character of secretions expectorated
- Changes in pulse rate or client response
- Inspiratory capacity attained on IS

CRITICAL THINKING APPLICATION

CLINICAL PROBLEMS	CRITICAL THINKING OPTIONS
■ Client is unwilling to complete exercise because of misunderstanding or fear of pain or dehiscence.	• Instruct again on rationale and necessity for procedure. • Support the incision area more fully, using the palms of your hands or a firmly rolled pillow to allay fears of dehiscence. • Medicate 30–60 minutes before using spirometer or participating in breathing exercises.
■ Nasal congestion inhibits client's breathing capability.	• Ask client to blow nose prior to the breathing exercise. • Check with physician so he or she can prescribe medications to open nasal passages.
■ Client is unable to master use of incentive breathing devices.	• Position client in Fowler's position to assist with lung expansion. • Instruct client to start slowly and increase volume over several exercise sessions. • Supervise practice with encouragement. • Provide positive reinforcement with increments in volume.

unit 2

CHEST PHYSIOTHERAPY (CPT)

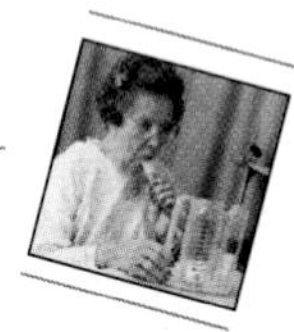

NURSING PROCESS DATA

ASSESSMENT Data Base

Auscultate breath sounds. Check for normal breath sounds and any adventitious sounds or ventilation.

Determine rhythm, rate, and depth of breathing.

Note time elapsed since eating (perform between meals to prevent regurgitation).

Observe quality of secretions. Thick, tenacious secretions may require humidification therapy prior to treatment.

Note any complicating conditions: hypertension, congestive heart failure (CHF), cerebral edema, head trauma, abdominal distention, arrhythmias, end stage COPD.

PLANNING Objectives

To facilitate clearance of retained secretions through increased coughing effort and force

To decrease adventitious lung sounds

To increase aeration of affected lung and increase air exchange

To reduce shortness of breath

To assist coughing to be more productive and effective

To decrease respiratory rate and increase ventilation and air exchange

To minimize potential complications

IMPLEMENTATION Procedure

Preparing Client for CPT

Performing Percussion

Performing Vibration

Performing Postural Drainage

EVALUATION Expected Outcomes

Lungs cleared of retained secretions.

Breath sounds clearer to auscultations.

Rales or rhonchi decreased.

Shortness of breath reduced.

Coughing is more productive and effective with reduced effort and pain.

Potential complications are minimized.

Client's sense of well-being is improved.

PREPARING CLIENT FOR CPT

Procedure

1. Validate physician's orders for CPT. (This procedure is tiring to clients and contraindicated in cases of osteoporosis, pulmonary embolism, or lung cancer.)
2. Establish the location of each lung segment. If the entire lung field is to undergo CPT, the most affected segment should be drained first. **Rationale:** Usually the lower areas are the most affected.
3. Provide privacy during procedure. (Client may be embarrassed or uncomfortable.)

4. Remain with client during initial procedure.
5. Administer treatment every 2 to 4 hours as ordered. Allow 30 minutes for draining if secretions are thick and tenacious.
6. Prepare client by discussing CPT procedures.
7. Explain importance of CPT procedures to counteract effects of hypoventilation and to prevent complications.
8. Auscultate chest for adventitious sounds prior to initiating CPT.
9. Place towel over skin when performing CPT.

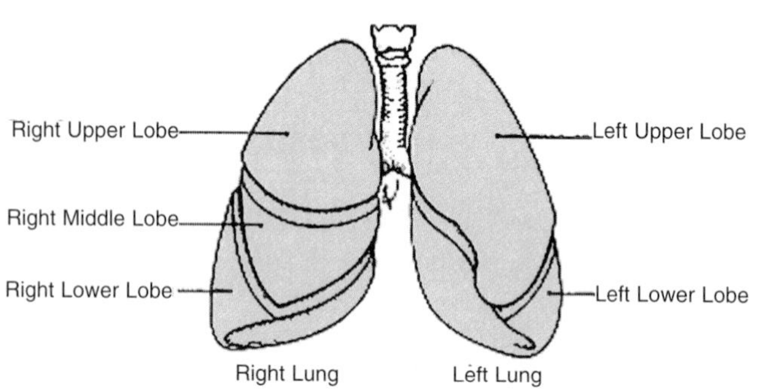

The lobes of the lungs.

PERFORMING PERCUSSION

Equipment

Pillows for positioning
Hospital bed that can be placed in Trendelenburg's position (optional)
Tissues
Container for sputum
Towel or gown for area percussed

Preparation

Same as *Preparing Client for CPT*

Procedure

1. Cover area to be percussed with gown or towel.
2. Cup your hands, keep wrists loose and relaxed, and clap rhythmically and rapidly over designated areas. **Rationale:** This motion produces vibrations that loosen secretions for easier removal with postural drainage and coughing.
3. Percuss with alternate hands and listen for hollow sound with movements.
4. Percuss each area for 3–5 minutes.
5. Do not percuss over bony prominences, such as vertebral column or scapula. **Rationale:** Vibrations are not transmitted to the chest wall through bony prominences and percussion here can cause the client discomfort.
6. Encourage client to cough after percussion of lung areas.
7. Auscultate all lung areas for changes in breath sounds.

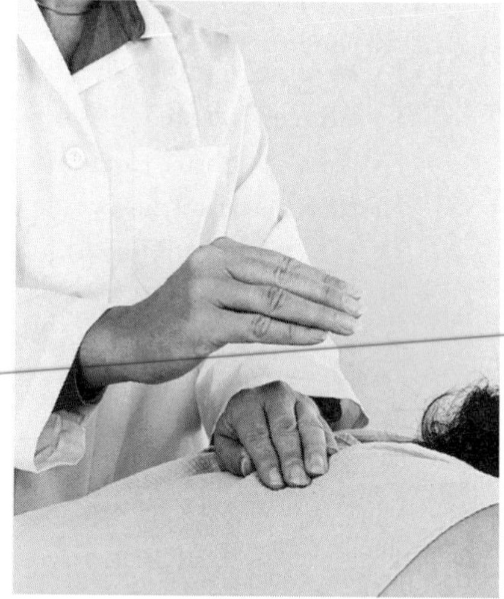

Cup your hands and use a rhythmic clapping when performing percussion.

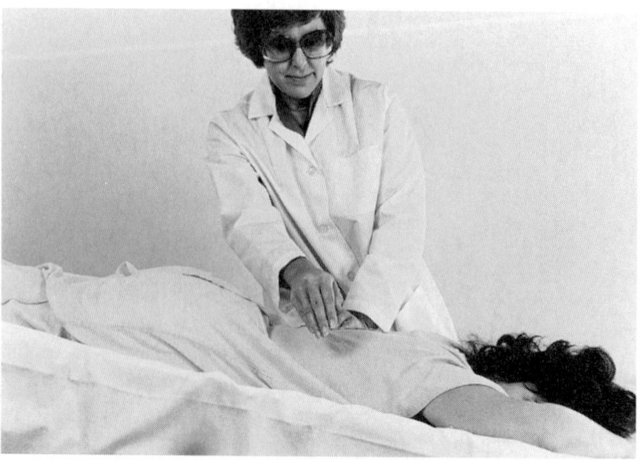

Position the client so that "most affected" area is drained first, or place client in Trendelenburg's position to drain lower areas first.

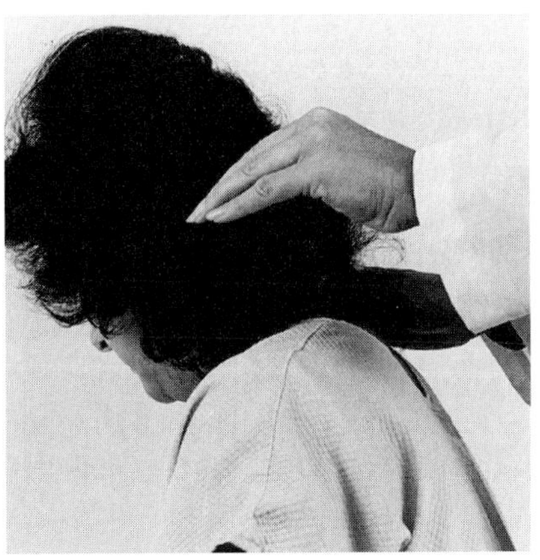

An upright, slightly forward postion allows secretions to drain from the upper lobes.

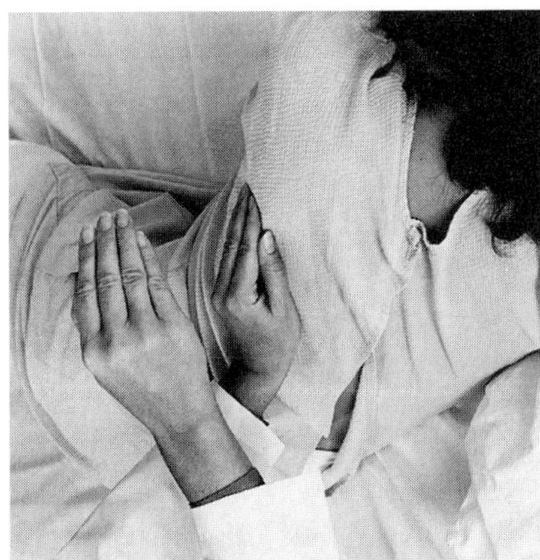

Position client on side with head of bed raised slightly to facilitate drainage.

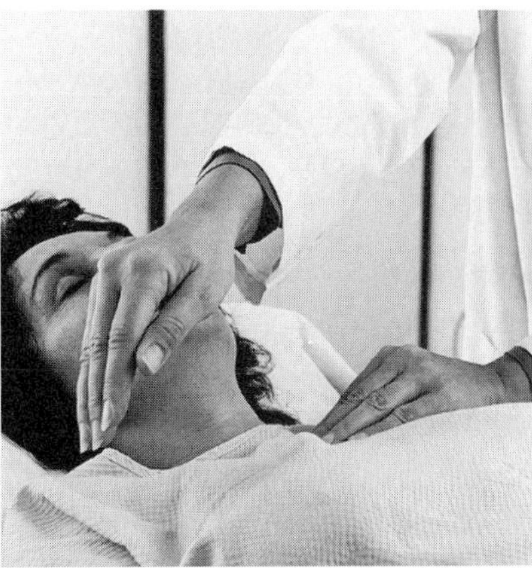

Percuss client's anterior upper lobes after lower lobes to facilitate drainage.

PERFORMING VIBRATION

Equipment

Pillows for positioning
Hospital bed or other method to place client in Trendelenburg's position to facilitate drainage of secretions
Bath towel or gown
Container for sputum
Tissue

Preparation

Same as *Preparing Client for CPT*

Procedure

1. Cover area to be percussed with gown or towel.
2. Instruct client to breathe in through nose and exhale slowly through mouth.
3. Place your hands flat over area to be vibrated, with one hand on top of the other. Keep your arms and shoulders straight. (A vibrating machine set at midrange can be used in place of manual vibration.)
4. Vibrate as client exhales by quickly contracting and relaxing your arms and shoulders for 10 seconds. **Rationale:** This loosens secretions that move into the bronchus for easier expectoration.
5. Vibrate for 5–10 minutes, depending on viscosity of secretions and client's tolerance.

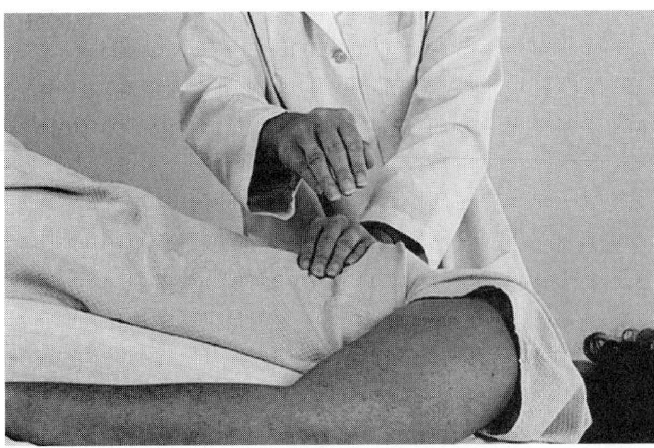

Place client in side-lying positions to drain lower lung areas.

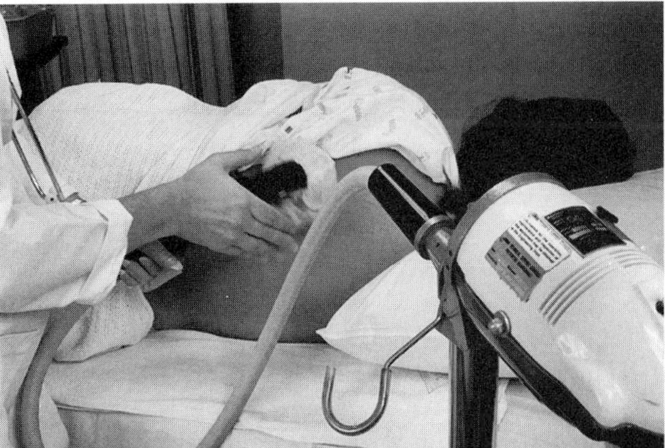

Vibrating machines can be more effective in mobilizing secretions.

6. Encourage coughing as needed.
7. Auscultate chest for changes in breath sounds.

PERFORMING POSTURAL DRAINAGE

Equipment

Hospital bed or other method to place client in Trendelenburg's position

Tissues

Container for sputum

Mouthwash and emesis basin

Preparation

Same as *Preparing Client for CPT*

Procedure

1. Loosen any binders or tight clothing.
2. Lower head of bed slowly so that client's head is positioned in a 30° downward angle if not contraindicated. (Head is lower than chest.)
3. Place sputum container and tissues within client's reach.
4. Tell client to remain in position from 5 to 15 minutes to allow secretions to drain. (Amount of time varies depending on client's need and tolerance.) **Rationale:** This allows time for drainage of secretions.
5. Instruct client to expectorate secretions.
6. Instruct client to turn to other side to facilitate drainage of other base areas. (Clients should deep breathe and cough between each position change.)
7. Assist client to slowly return to normal sitting position, after coughing in dependent position.
8. Offer oral hygiene with mouthwash.
9. Discard sputum container or send sputum specimen to laboratory, if ordered. *Note: It may take ½ - 1 hour after treatment to obtain sputum specimen.*
10. Observe client's condition.
11. Auscultate chest areas for breath sounds.

CHARTING for CPT

- Quantity and character of sputum
- Rate, and character of breath sounds, pulse
- Any unusual symptoms following procedure
- Client's physical tolerance of procedure
- Client's acceptance of and willingness to participate in procedure
- Lung sounds before and after CPT

CRITICAL THINKING APPLICATION

CLINICAL PROBLEMS	CRITICAL THINKING OPTIONS
■ Client experiences dyspnea during postural drainage.	• Change position so that client's head is not as low, especially if client is elderly or very weak. • Report to physician so that mechanical means, such as suctioning, may be used to help remove secretions.
■ Client is unable to assume head-down position for postural drainage.	• Use all positions but modify degree of Trendelenburg's position so that client's head is slightly lower than chest. • Turn client on side with pillow support to facilitate bronchial drainage.
■ Client vomits with CPT treatment.	• Perform treatments between or before meals. • Encourage use of other treatment modalities until sputum is more readily expectorated without vomiting.

unit 3

OXYGEN THERAPY

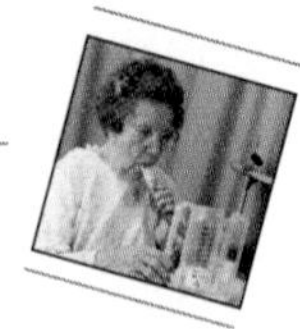

NURSING PROCESS DATA

ASSESSMENT Data Base

Review ABG results or pulse oximetry for Sa_{O_2}.

Assess client's vital signs.

Observe client for signs of hypoxia.

Assess skin under oxygen mask for irritation.

Assess for signs of carbon dioxide narcosis.

PLANNING Objectives

To return arterial P_{O_2} and Sa_{O_2} to normal range

To correct hypoxic condition so that client is adequately oxygenated

To assist breathing to return to normal rate

To increase comfort, breathing efficiency, and activity tolerance for clients with chronic lung disease

IMPLEMENTATION Procedures

Monitoring Clients Receiving Oxygen Therapy

Using an Oxygen Cylinder

Using Pulse Oximetry

Using an Oxygen Analyzer

Using a Nasal Cannula

Using an Oxygen Face Mask

Using a Pediatric Oxygen Mask

Using a Pediatric Oxygen Tent

Using an Oxygen Hood

EVALUATION Expected Outcomes

Arterial P_{O_2} and Sa_{O_2} return to normal range.

Correction of hypoxic condition results.

Comfort, breathing efficiency, and activity tolerance increased for clients with chronic lung disease.

MONITORING CLIENTS RECEIVING OXYGEN THERAPY

Equipment

Oxygen administration set

Oxygen flowmeter

SAFETY PRECAUTIONS

- Set up "No Smoking" and "Oxygen in Use" signs at the site of administration and at the door.
- Remove matches, lighters, and ashtrays from bedside (these items should only be present with physician's orders, as hospitals are smoke-free facilities.)
- Remove any friction-type toys.
- Disconnect grounded electric equipment.
- Remove all volatile materials except solutions and equipment to be used during intervention.
- Make sure that all electrical monitoring equipment is properly grounded.
- Locate fire extinguishers and oxygen meter turn-off lever.

Procedure

1. Check physician's orders for type of oxygen therapy, administration set, and prescribed oxygen liter flow.

> **■ CLINICAL ALERT**
>
> Oxygen is used conservatively on clients with chronic lung disease because high levels of oxygen may suppress breathing stimulus and lead to respiratory arrest due to CO_2 narcosis.

2. Place client in semi- or high-Fowler's position to facilitate lung expansion.
3. Turn and reposition client frequently to promote ventilation.
4. Encourage deep breathing and coughing exercises unless directed otherwise.
5. Ensure adequate fluid intake, especially if secretions are thick and tenacious.
6. If ordered, humidify oxygen when flow rate is greater than 4 L/minute.
7. Assess client's progress by frequently checking vital signs, color, and level on consciousness.
8. Assess clients with COPD frequently for signs of carbon dioxide narcosis:
   a. bounding peripheral pulses
   b. high blood pressure
   c. increased pulse pressure
   d. warm, clammy skin
9. Remain with clients who are frightened or anxious until they feel secure.

Conditions Requiring Oxygen Therapy

- Atmospheric hypoxia: oxygen therapy corrects depressed level of oxygen.
- Hypoventilation hypoxia: 100% oxygen provides five times the oxygen of room air.

Conditions for Which Oxygen Therapy Is Not Corrective

- Hypoxia caused by anemia, abnormal hemoglobin, or vascular insufficiency.
- Inadequate tissue use of oxygen (cyanide poisoning).

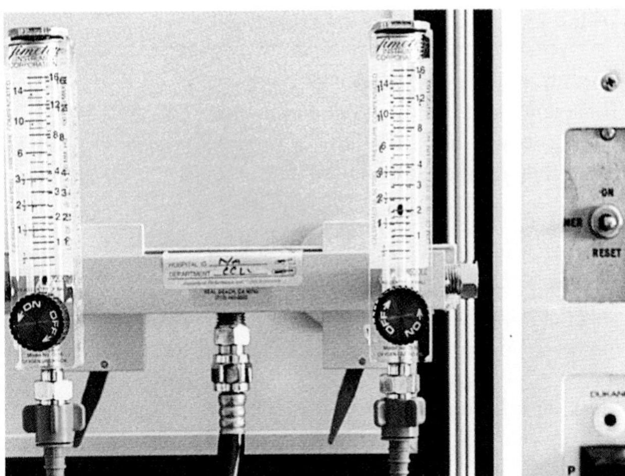

Oxygen flow meter indicates liters per minute delivered to administration set-up.

- Chronic obstructive lung disease often requires that oxygen be used with caution since oxygen can suppress respiratory drive and result in respiratory arrest.

Symptoms of Hypoxia

Early symptoms

- Restlessness
- Headache
- Visual disturbances
- Confusion or change in behavior
- Tachypnea
- Tachycardia
- Hypertension
- Dyspnea

Advanced symptoms

- Hypotension
- Bradycardia
- Metabolic acidosis (production of lactic acid)
- Cyanosis

Chronic hypoxia

- Polycythemia
- Clubbing of fingers and toes
- Thrombosis
- Right-sided heart failure

TABLE 25-1. Special Oxygen Equipment

Nasal Cannula and Prongs
This equipment is easily tolerated by most clients. It is also simpler than a mask. The flow of inspired oxygen (FIO_2) varies depending on the flow and the depth of client breathing.

FIO_2: 24–38% Flow: 1–2 L
FIO_2: 30–35% Flow: 3–4 L
FIO_2: 38–44% Flow: 5–6 L

Face mask without Reservoir Bag
This equipment requires fairly high flows to prevent rebreathing of carbon dioxide. Accurate FIO_2 is difficult to estimate.

FIO_2: 35–65% Flow: 8–12 L

Mask with Reservoir Bag
The reservoir allows higher FIO_2 to be delivered. At flows of less than 6 L/min, the risk of rebreathing carbon dioxide increases.

Two types are available:

Partial rebreathing mask: No inspiratory valve so that the beginning portion of exhaled air returns to the bag and mixes with the inspired air. Ports are present so that expired air escapes.

FIO_2: 40–60% Flow: 6–10 L

Nonrebreather: Valve in this type closes during expiration so that any exhaled air is not rebreathed, but is forced through the expiratory valve on the face piece.

FIO_2: 60–100% Flow: 6–15 L

Venturi Mask
This mask delivers a fixed or predicted FIO_2. It is used effectively on clients with COPD when accurate FIO_2 is necessary. Carbon dioxide buildup is kept at a minimum. Humidifiers are not used.

FIO_2 does not relate to liter flow; cone selector determines O_2 concentration

FIO_2: 24–50%

Face Tent
This aerosol mask is well tolerated by clients but is sometimes difficult to keep in place. It is convenient for providing humidification and oxygenation.

FIO_2: 28–100% Flow: 8–12 L

Oxygen Hood
This disposable vinyl box fits over a child's head to provide warm humidified oxygen at a controlled temperature. It is useful because it includes an oxygen limiter to prevent oxygen concentration from exceeding 40%, thus reducing the hazard of oxygen toxicity.

FIO_2: 28–40% Flow: 5–8 L
FIO_2: 40–85% Flow: 8–12 L

Less than 5 L flow may lead to carbon dioxide narcosis.

Croupette
A croupette is used to provide oxygen with cool humidification and to maintain temperature. It is also useful for a child who requires oxygen or high humidification. The unit prevents chilling in an atmosphere of aerated mist.

FIO_2: up to 50% Flow: 10–15 L

USING AN OXYGEN CYLINDER

Equipment

Source of oxygen supply: steel cylinder (oxygen tank) or portable tank
Regulator: flowmeter
Humidifier if ordered
Sterile distilled water

Procedure

1. Place oxygen cylinder in secure, upright position.
2. Check tag to determine amount of oxygen in the tank. Tag should say "Full."
3. Slowly turn hand knob on cylinder clockwise to crack tank open for a brief second to clear opening of tank; then close.
4. Attach regulator to valve outlet. **Rationale:** Regulates gas flow in liters per minute.
5. Fill humidifier, if ordered, with sterile distilled water to indicated level on bottle or use prefilled disposable humidifier bottles. **Rationale:** Humidity prevents mucous membranes from drying out.
6. Attach top of humidifier to oxygen flowmeter. Turn oxygen cylinder hand knob to open flow.
7. Slowly open handwheel and adjust flowmeter to prescribed rate in liters per minute.
8. Change sign on oxygen cylinder to read "In Use."

USING PULSE OXIMETRY

Equipment

Oximeter
Sensor, clip-on or disposable adhesive sensor

WHY PULSE OXIMETRY?

Arterial blood gas (ABG) analysis has been used for decades to determine a client's gas exchange and oxygenation transport ability. Pulse oximetry technology allows for PRN or continuous monitoring of arterial oxygen saturation (Sa_{O_2}), rather than a one-time analysis. The primary advantages of this method are

- It is cost-effective.
- It is a noninvasive evaluation tool.
- Minute-to-minute changes in saturation can be assessed and an intervention made before hypoxemia produces complications.
- The client's response to treatment can be evaluated immediately.

Preparation

1. Check physician's orders for sensor sight.
2. Determine if client has had recent tests using intravenous (IV) dyes. **Rationale:** Some dyes may make oximetry readings inaccurate.
3. Evaluate client's status before using oximetry. **Rationale:** Clients with alkalosis or with a low CO_2 level may have inadequate tissue oxygenation even with high saturation levels. Hemoglobin binds more easily with oxygen under these conditions.

Inaccurate oximetry readings can be found in clients with

- Alkalosis, acidosis
- Fever, hypothermia
- Low CO_2 levels
- Carbon monoxide poisoning
- Recent dye injection studies

4. Remove nail polish or artificial nails, if using fingers for sensor placement. **Rationale:** These substances can distort readings.
5. Obtain appropriate sensor. **Rationale:** Sensor probes are designated for specific sites, e.g., fingers, toes, earlobes.
6. Follow manufacturer's directions when selecting

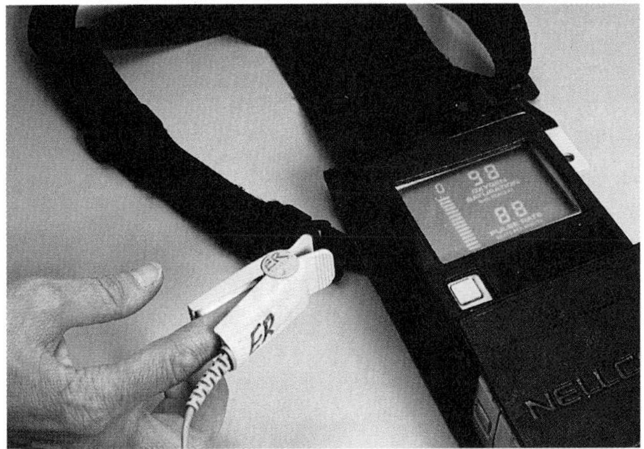

Sensor probe placed on finger for oxygen saturation analysis.

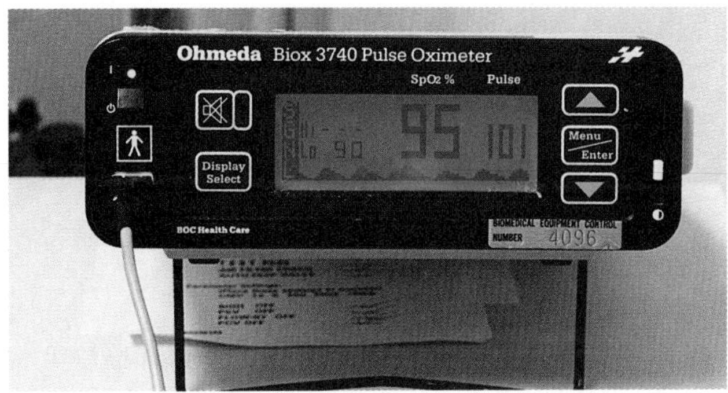

Oximeter display panel indicates percent of oxygen saturation.

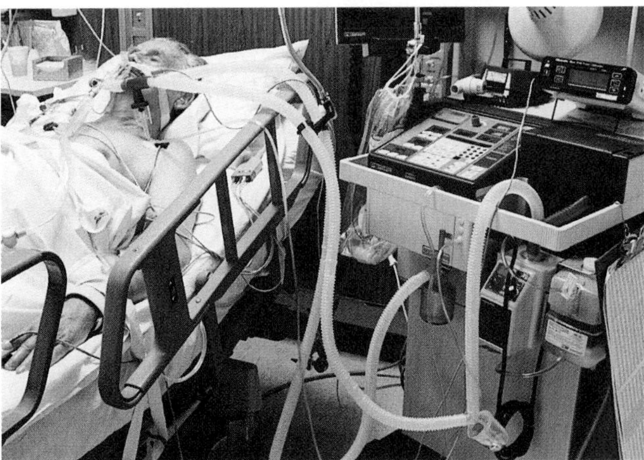
Critical care client with continuous moniter for oxygen saturation.

sensors and changing sites. **Rationale:** To prevent inaccurate readings and malfunction of equipment.

Procedure

1. Identify client and explain purpose and procedure for pulse oximetry.
2. Plug machine into electric outlet.
3. Turn on power.
4. Apply sensor probe flush with skin and secure. Make sure both sensor probes are aligned directly opposite each other. **Rationale:** Oximeter sensors contain both red and infrared light-emitting diodes (LEDs) and a photodetector. The photodetector registers light passing through vascular bed, the basis for microprocessor determination of oxygen saturation.
5. Set alarms to predetermined saturation levels or pulse rate.
6. Read oxygen saturation level on digital readout monitor.
7. Evaluate findings with previous saturation levels and changes in oxygen therapy.
8. Rotate site of clip-on probes every 4 hours and disposable probes at least every 24 hours. **Rationale:** Skin breakdown can occur with continuous usage.
9. Document findings on appropriate hospital record.

USING AN OXYGEN ANALYZER

Equipment

Analyzer

Procedure

1. Calibrate analyzer with room atmosphere prior to each reading.
2. Open tubing to the air, and compress two full times to fill analyzer.
3. Depress button. Analyzer should read 20% for room air. Adjust dial as necessary to obtain this reading.
4. Place tubing close to client's nose.
5. Compress bulb three to six times, depress button, and read findings.

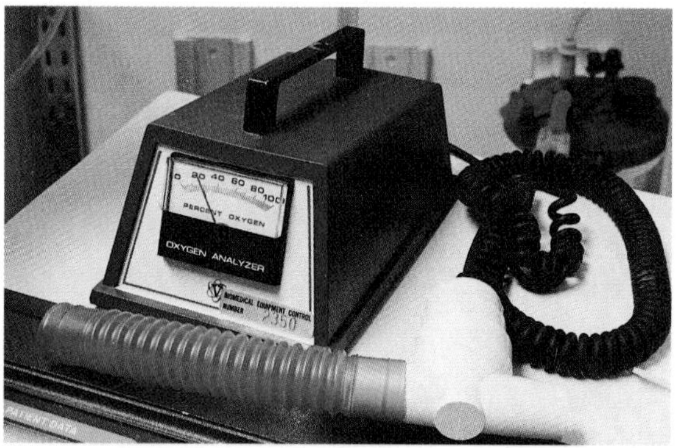

Oxygen analyzer, most often used in pediatrics.

6. Based on reading, adjust oxygen flow.
7. Check analyzer with 100% oxygen at least once a day.

USING A NASAL CANNULA

Equipment

O_2 supply
Regulator
Humidifier if ordered
Nasal cannula

Preparation

1. Check physician's orders for oxygen.
2. Gather equipment.

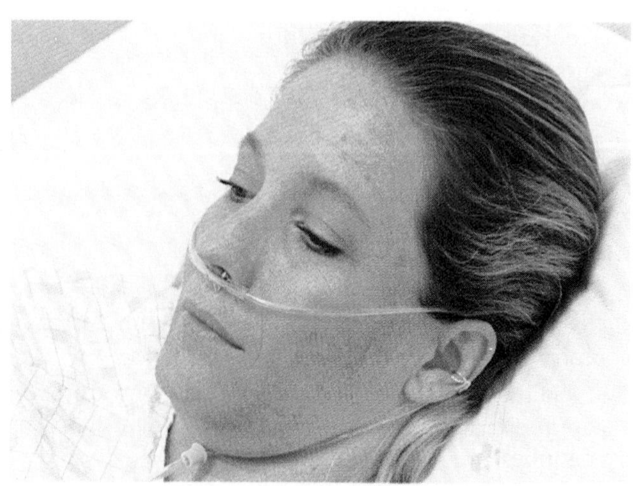
Oxygen administration by nasal cannula.

Procedure

1. Explain the purpose and procedures of oxygen therapy to client.
2. Place tips of cannula no more than ½ inch into client's nares.

> **■ CLINICAL ALERT**
>
> Humidification of low-flow O_2 through a nasal cannula is no longer considered essential and may be contraindicated because it supports bacterial growth.

3. Fasten tubing to pillow and bed sheets if bed rest is maintained.
4. Adjust flow of oxygen. Should be limited to 6 L/minute for nasal prongs. **Rationale:** Oxygen concentration varies since atmospheric air mixes with prescribed oxygen concentration as client inhales.

   The FIO_2 varies depending on the flow and nature of client's breathing. Deep breathing dilutes rather than enhances the FIO_2 because more room air is inhaled.

   FIO_2: 24–44% Flow: 1–6 L

5. Monitor vital signs and check client's condition frequently.
6. Provide nose care every 4 hours—use water-soluble products (e.g., aquaphor) and avoid petroleum products (e.g., petrolatum) since they are combustible.
7. Change equipment (tubing, cannula) according to hospital policy.

USING AN OXYGEN FACE MASK

Equipment

Oxygen mask
Oxygen source
Flowmeter
Humidifier

Preparation

1. Check physician's orders for oxygen.
2. Gather equipment.
3. Wash your hands.

Four Types of Masks

1. Oxygen mask.
2. Partial rebreathing oxygen mask with reservoir bag.
3. Nonrebreathing mask with reservoir bag.
4. Venturi mask used to specifically control oxygen concentrations.

Procedure

1. Explain procedure and rationale for administration of oxygen to client.
2. Check size of face mask to make sure it fits client.

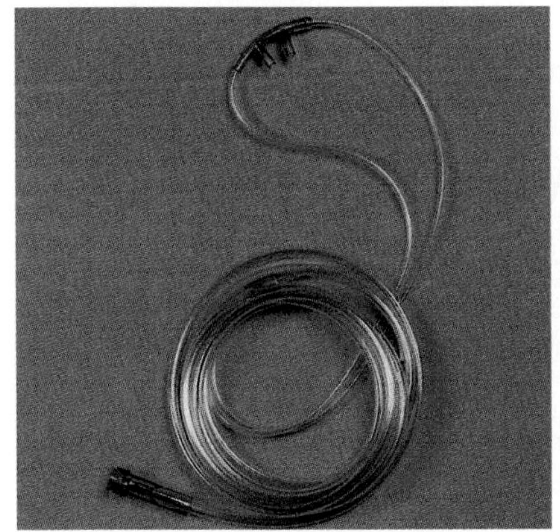

Nasal prongs, the most frequently used method, delivers up to 44% oxygen.

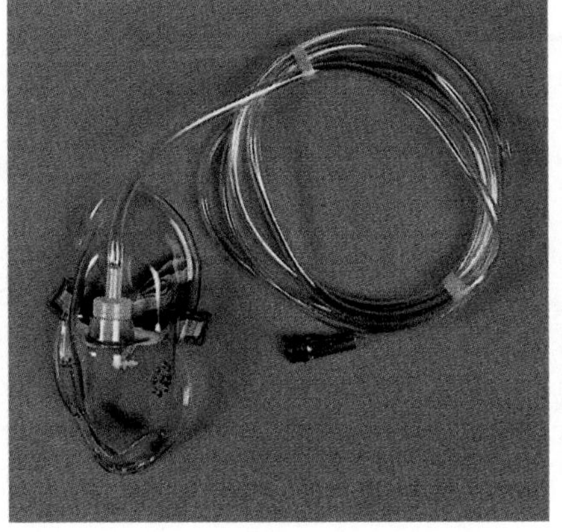

Face mask which delivers moderately high flow of oxygen.

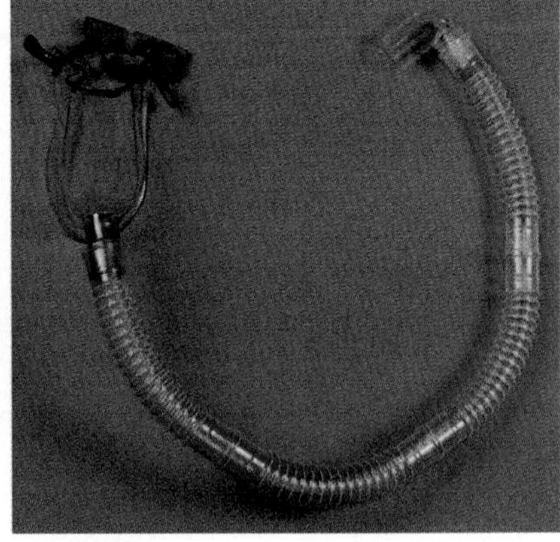

The oxygen face tent delivers unpredictable oxygen flow with high humidity.

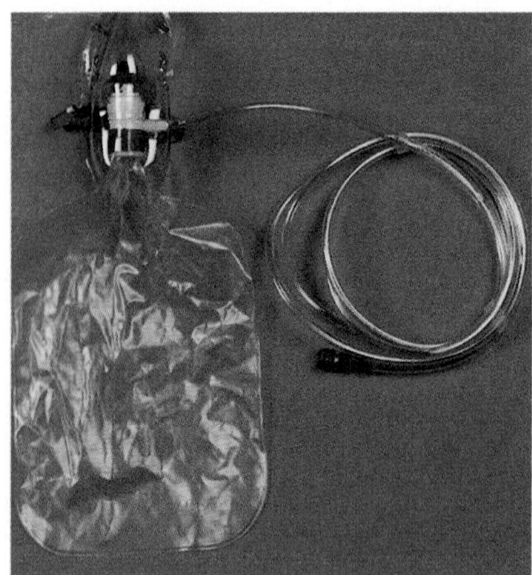

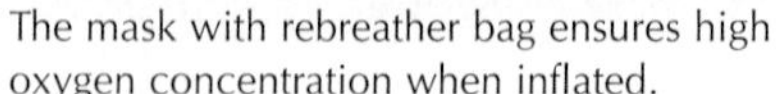

The mask with rebreather bag ensures high oxygen concentration when inflated.

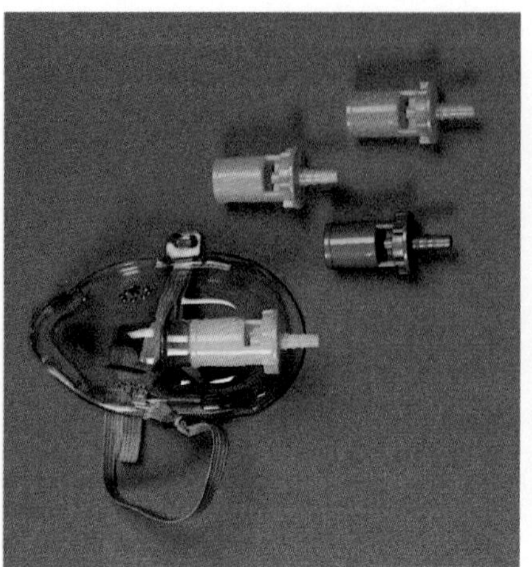

Face mask with oxygen percent control pieces.

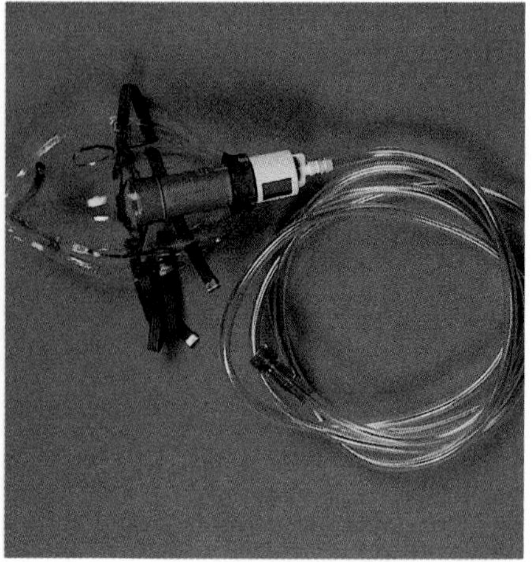

Face mask with Dial-in oxygen percent control.

3. Turn on oxygen flow to number of liters prescribed. If reservoir bag is attached, partially inflate it with oxygen.
4. Place client in semi- or high-Fowler's position.
5. Fit mask to client's face from nose downward during expiration. If reservoir bag is attached, oxygen flow must be at a level to prevent bag from collapsing. **Rationale:** A tight fit prevents oxygen from escaping around eyes or nose.
6. Place elastic band around client's head.
7. Attach tubing to pillows and bedclothes, keeping tubing free of kinks.
8. Stay with client until client feels at ease with mask. **Rationale:** Some clients may be afraid of suffocating.
9. Assess client's condition by checking vital signs and respiratory process.
10. Change mask and tubing daily, and provide skin care to face.
11. Observe for any change in client's condition.
12. Check equipment frequently. If humidifier is attached, check water level.
13. Check with physician to order a nasal cannula during meals.

USING A PEDIATRIC OXYGEN MASK

Equipment

Pediatric mask
Oxygen source
Flowmeter
Humidifier

Preparation

1. Check physician's orders for oxygen administration.
2. Gather equipment.
3. Explain purpose and rationale for mask to client and family.

Procedure

1. Choose a mask that fits the child. **Rationale:** The mask should cover child's mouth and nose but not eyes.
2. Place mask so that it fits snugly.
3. Secure mask with elastic strap.
4. Adjust oxygen concentration as ordered.
5. Remove mask at frequent intervals for skin care if the child's condition is stable and provided no ABGs are scheduled within 1 hour. **Rationale:** Taking mask off distorts ABG findings.
6. Observe child frequently for complications.
7. Spend extra time with the child as an oxygen mask may be frightening.

USING A PEDIATRIC OXYGEN TENT

Equipment

Oxygen tent
Oxygen machine
Oxygen analyzer
Bath blankets (2)

Preparation

1. Check physician's orders.
2. Gather equipment.
3. Select a tent that delivers the prescribed concentration of oxygen to the child.
4. Explain purpose of tent to child and parents.

Procedure

1. Secure tent, and place machine at head of empty bed with control knobs on opposite side where working area is required.
2. Connect regulator into oxygen source.
3. Plug in machine.
4. Set up humidifier, and check to make sure that water level (tray at back of machine) is adequate.
5. Pad the frame that supports the canopy.
6. Turn on the oxygen to desired concentration (30–50%), and maintain temperature at 17.8°–21.2°C (64°–70°F).
7. Secure the canopy by tucking in all sides and maintaining closure whenever possible. **Rationale:** To prevent oxygen leak at bottom of tent.
8. Monitor temperature regularly since overheating can occur with enclosed system.
9. Analyze and record tent oxygen concentration, and check child's vital signs every 2 hours, or as ordered.

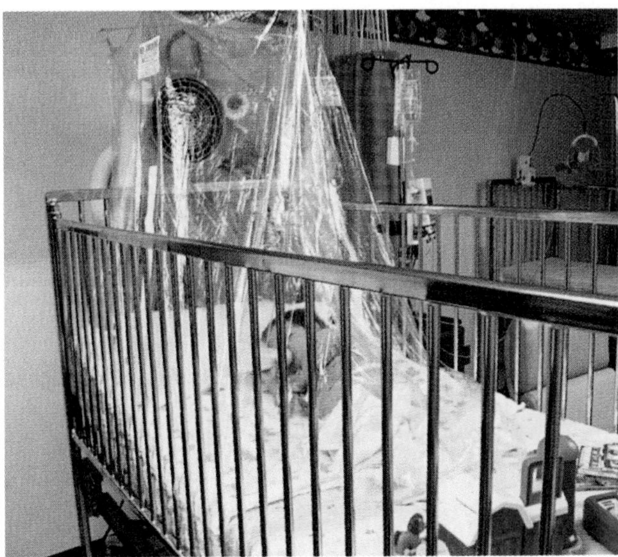

The oxygen tent allows for delivery of between 30% and 50% humidified oxygen.

10. Leave crib sides up for safety.
11. Select toys that are washable, do not produce static electricity, and are appropriate to the child's age.

> **■ CLINICAL ALERT**
>
> Avoid use of friction-type toys or battery-operated devices when oxygen is in use.

12. Place child on cardiac or apnea monitor if ordered by physician.
13. Check dampness of clothes to prevent chilling.
14. Change bed linen and child's clothing as necessary.

USING AN OXYGEN HOOD

Equipment

Oxygen hood
Oxygen source
Oxygen analyzer
Flexible oxygen tubing

Procedure

1. Place hood around child's head and attach tubing to oxygen supply. (Hood may be used alone or with isolette.)
2. Close ports and lid, but do not obstruct neck opening.
3. Infants are cared for through portholes or lid.

Rationale: This avoids decreasing oxygen level.

4. Maintain oxygen levels at 40–50%, and check the amount of moisture that accumulates inside hood.
5. Measure oxygen concentration as you would in isolette.
6. Observe usual oxygen administration precautions.

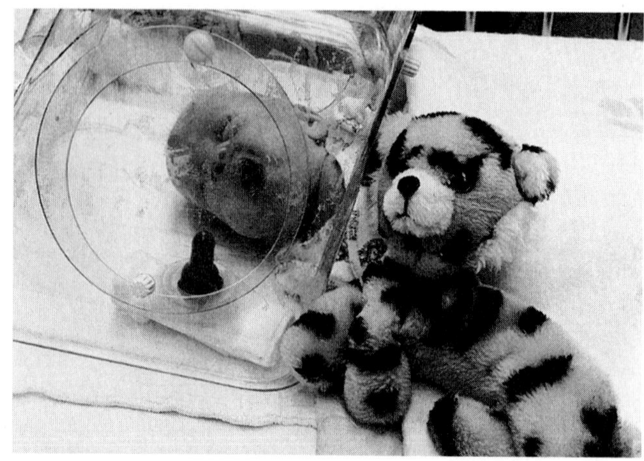

The oxygen hood can be opened to provide care without disturbing oxygen concentration.

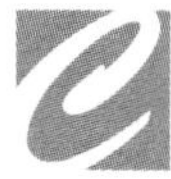

CHARTING for Oxygen Therapy

- Arterial Po_2 or pulse oximetry results
- Vital signs
- Type of equipment used for oxygen administration percentage of FIO_2 and liter flow
- Data from oxygen analyzer
- Client's status regularly

CRITICAL THINKING APPLICATION

CLINICAL PROBLEMS	CRITICAL THINKING OPTIONS
■ Client has difficulty breathing.	• If conscious, the client can usually tell you what he or she is experiencing and cough up mucus. Encourage coughing; suction if necessary. Place in Fowler's or semi-Fowler's position. • If client is unconscious, be alert for wet, gurgling respirations, which indicate need for suctioning. Suction frequently. • Place in side-lying position so that secretions can run out of client's mouth.
■ Client shows these abnormal signs and symptoms: changes in blood pressure, tachycardia, increased respirations, and abnormal color, restlessness, confusion, or altered sensorium.	• Determine if acute acidosis or carbon dioxide narcosis is present, and report. These conditions can occur if hypoxic drive is removed by the administration of high oxygen concentration. a. Check oxygen equipment, and use oxygen analyzer to measure oxygen concentration. b. Reduce oxygen concentration as ordered.

CLINICAL PROBLEMS	CRITICAL THINKING OPTIONS
	• Carbon dioxide retainers may require controlled low oxygen concentration method. Change oxygen therapy from cannula–catheter to Venturi mask as ordered.
■ Client has atelectasis.	• Encourage deep breathing, coughing, frequent position changes, and ambulation if possible. Avoid constrictive dressings, and use sedatives carefully. • Postural drainage and suctioning may be ordered. • Check breath sounds. (They are decreased with this condition, and crackles are frequently heard at the end of inspiration.)
■ Client demonstrates tachypnea.	• Report symptoms, and check oxygen concentration immediately, since inadequate flow rates may be causing the problem. • Increase flow rate as ordered, and monitor with oxygen analyzer. • Monitor vital signs and correlate with client findings as pulmonary embolus may be the cause. • Check client's breathing pattern and breath sounds as mucus plug may be the cause.
■ Client shows retinopathy of prematurity (retrolental fibroplasia).	• Make sure the premature infant receives no more than 40% oxygen unless infant suffers from sustained tachypnea or respiratory distress syndrome.
■ Oxygen toxicity occurs.	• Toxicity occurs 24 hours after initiation of oxygen therapy. • Monitor closely for signs of nausea, restlessness, pallor. • Do not exceed 40% oxygen concentration unless frequent arterial blood gas monitoring occurs.
■ Oxygen saturation findings are inaccurate.	• Check that sensor probes are aligned to prevent photodetector picking up light from sources other than LEDs. • Check that appropriate sensor site was selected for specific probes, e.g., finger site for finger sensor. • Move sensor site away from light source, if possible.
■ Artifact/alarm sounds.	• Encourage client to keep probe site still. Movement scrambles signals from photodetector interfering with readings. • Place sensor on different site.
■ Pulsations are inadequate.	• Check for pressure source interfering with blood flow. • Change sensor sites or change blood pressure cuff site. • Evaluate need for different type of sensor if client is vasoconstricted or edematous. This causes impaired circulation.

unit 4

SUCTIONING

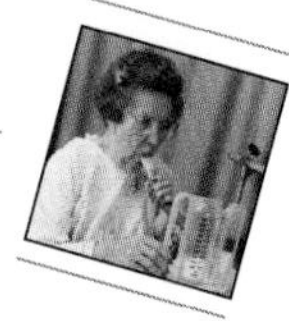

NURSING PROCESS DATA

ASSESSMENT Data Base

Assess client's need for suctioning.

Observe vital signs for increases in pulse and respiration.

Auscultate breath sounds for presence of adventitious sounds.

Observe respiratory status for tachypnea, shortness of breath, and restlessness.

Observe level of consciousness to assess hypoxia.

PLANNING Objectives

To provide patent airway

To remove secretions

To improve ventilation

To decrease breathing rate

To increase tissue oxygenation

IMPLEMENTATION Procedures

Suctioning Using Separate Catheter and Gloves

Suctioning Using Catheter and Sleeve

Suctioning with In-Line Catheter

Suctioning Infants with Bulb Syringe

EVALUATION Expected Outcomes

Secretions removed without complications

Increased respiratory ventilation with increased tissue oxygenation

Breath sounds clear; no adventitious sounds auscultated

SUCTIONING USING SEPARATE CATHETER AND GLOVES

Equipment

Portable suction machine or wall suction unit with Y-connector or release port

Disposable suction catheter (size 6 for infants, size 14 for children, and to size 18 for adults)

Suction Catheters

Adults:	12–18 French
Children:	14 French
Infants:	6–10 French

Suction Machines

Wall Unit Vacuum Setting

Adults:	120–150 mm Hg
Children:	80–120 mm Hg
Infants:	60–100 mm Hg

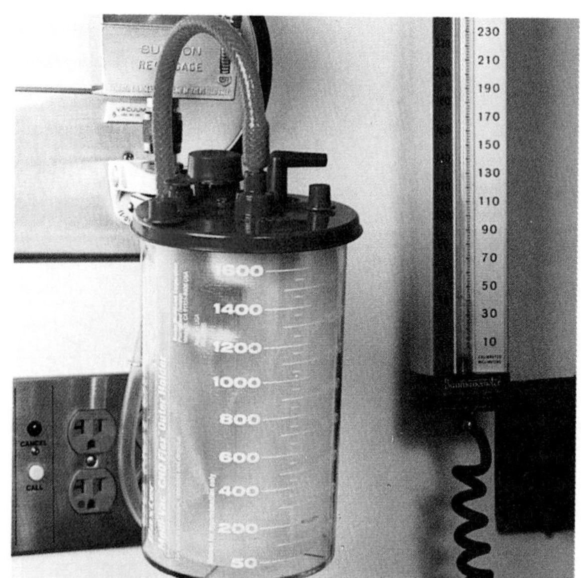

Wall mounted suction machine.

Portable Unit

Adults	7–15 mm Hg
Children:	5–10 mm Hg

Sterile gloves

Container for sterile saline

Sterile saline, labeled with date and time opened (opened bottles should be discarded after 24 hours)

Receptacle for used equipment

Stethoscope

Oxygen source and equipment

Preparation

1. Check physician's orders and client care plan.
2. Gather equipment.
3. Select a catheter that is no larger than one half the diameter of the client's airway. **Rationale:** Larger catheter can occlude trachea and cause hypoxemia.
4. Wash your hands.
5. Assess lung sounds.
6. Open catheter package, and leaving protective covering over catheter, attach distal end to suction tubing.
7. Set regulator to control vacuum level of suctioning. Both portable suction machine and central wall suction are usually marked in millimeters of mercury.
8. Establish normal range for suction: 80–120 mm Hg.
   a. Use lowest pressure level of suction that will clear secretions.
   b. Setting the regulator protects sensitive airway tissue.

INDICATIONS FOR SUCTIONING

- Decreased or ineffective cough
- Semicomatose or comatose client
- Thick, tenacious mucus
- Impaired pulmonary function

Note: Suction catheter is likely to advance into right bronchus due to greater anatomic angulation of left bronchus. Turning and deep breathing help mobilize secretions from left airways to facilitate their removal.

Procedure

1. Explain procedure and rationale to client regardless of level of consciousness.

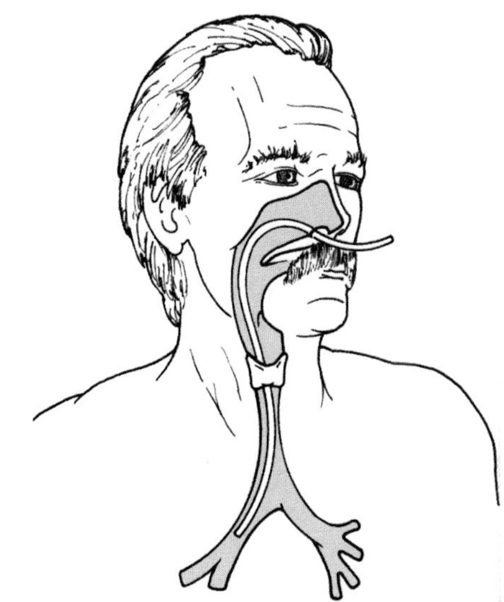

Insert catheter into nares and continue to advance into right bronchus.

2. Place client in semi-Fowler's position. (Or use dorsal recumbent position with client's head tilted backward to open airway.)
3. Use protective gown and goggles if splash anticipated.
4. Turn on suction machine, and set pressure of wall suction.
5. Pour sterile saline into container, and lubricate catheter with sterile normal saline. **Rationale:** This prevents injury to delicate tissue as you are inserting catheter.

■ CLINICAL ALERT

When performing naso-oral suctioning the same procedure is followed, but clean rather than sterile technique is used. The catheter is inserted into the nares or within the oral cavity. The catheter does not extend down to the lower airway.

6. Administer 100% oxygen for 1–2 minutes before suctioning if client is unable to breathe deeply. **Rationale:** During suctioning, lung residual air is removed; this prevents hypoxia.
7. Don sterile gloves.
8. Dip sterile catheter into saline solution to lubricate.
9. Insert catheter through nares. *Do not apply*

suction. **Rationale:** Suctioning during insertion deprives client of oxygen and inhibits catheter advancement.

10. Continue to advance catheter, even if client coughs or "bucks." **Rationale:** Cough is stimulated at the carina (where the bronchi divide).
11. Withdraw catheter slightly when unable to advance further.
12. Begin intermittent suctioning by using a rotating motion as the catheter is withdrawn.
    a. Provide suction (place your thumb over valve or Y-connector on catheter).
    b. Intermittently release pressure (remove your thumb from valve or Y-connector).

Note: Research data indicate that instructing the client to turn his or her head left or right to enter opposite bronchus is not effective. It is simply a matter of chance which bronchus is entered.

13. Limit suction to no more than 10 seconds. **Rationale:** This prevents removal of excessive oxygen.
14. Allow client to breathe deeply between periods of suctioning, and administer 100% oxygen.
15. Rinse catheter in sterile saline. Wrap around gloved hand. Remove glove over catheter and discard.
16. Note character of suctioned secretions.
17. Repeat procedure as necessary using new catheter set-up. Allow 3 minutes between suctioning. **Rationale:** To prevent hypoxemia and cardiac complications.
18. When procedure is completed, turn off suction machine.

Note: Studies show that instillation of saline into airways for suctioning purposes leads to greater hypoxemia than suctioning without saline instillation. In addition, bacteria are dispersed through airways with saline instillation.

19. Cover end of connector tubing with sterile gauze. **Rationale:** This prevents contaminating end that connects to catheter.
20. Offer oral hygiene.
21. Place client in comfortable position.
22. Assess lung sounds for changes.
23. Wash your hands.
24. Empty suction bottle prn or at the end of every shift.

SUCTIONING USING CATHETER AND SLEEVE

Equipment

Portable suction machine or wall suction with Y-connector or release valve

Disposable suction catheter (size 6 for infants, size 14 for children, and to size 18 for adults)

Container for sterile saline

Bottle of sterile saline, labeled with date and time opened (opened bottles should be discarded after 24 hours)

Clean gloves

Receptacle for used equipment

Stethoscope

Oxygen source and equipment

Preparation

1. Check physician's orders and client care plan.
2. Gather equipment.
3. Select a catheter that is one-half the diameter of the client's airway.
4. Wash your hands before starting procedure.
5. Open catheter package, leaving protective covering over catheter.
6. Attach catheter to tubing on suction machine.
7. Explain procedure and rationale to client.
8. Place client in semi-Fowler's position. (Or place in dorsal recumbent position. Tilt head backward to open airway.)
9. Auscultate lung sounds.

Procedure

1. Turn on suction machine. Set pressure of wall unit according to chart.
2. Don gloves.
3. Take container for normal saline out of package and pour 30–50 mL sterile saline into receptacle.
4. Preoxygenate client by asking him or her to deep breathe or breathe normally with 100% oxygen administration for 3 minutes.
5. Lubricate catheter tip with saline.
6. Slide protective covering back over catheter as you

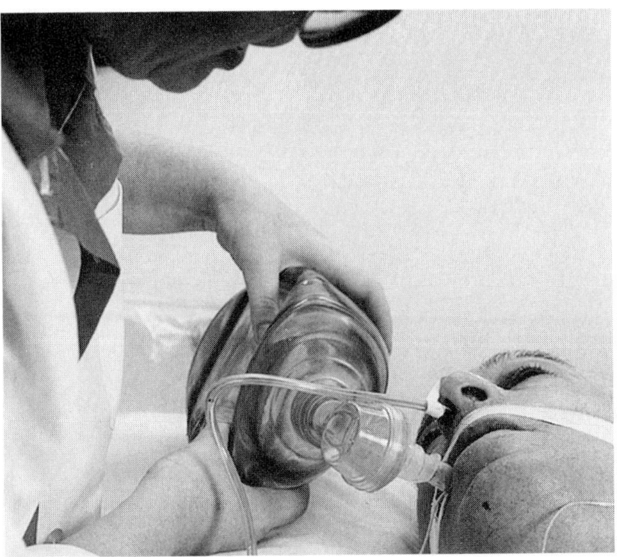

Hyperoxygenate client with a manual resuscitator bag before and after suctioning.

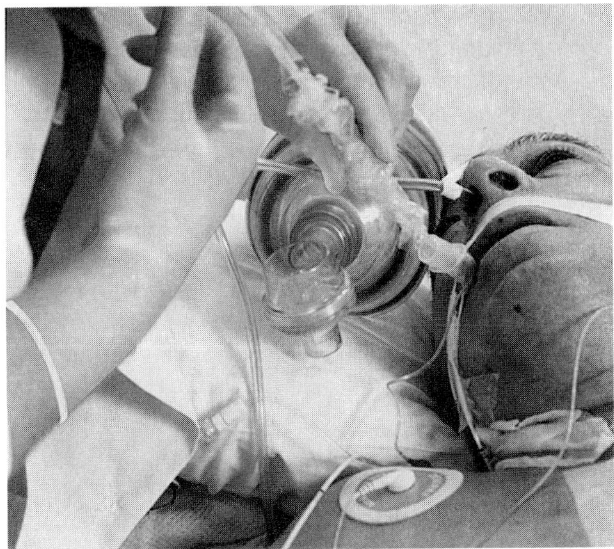

Slide plastic protector back over catheter as it is inserted through endotracheal tube.

insert catheter into client's nose or mouth.

7. Advance catheter as far as possible without applying suction.
8. Withdraw catheter slightly and begin suctioning, using a rotating motion as the catheter is withdrawn back into protective sleeve.
   a. To provide suction, place your thumb over valve or Y-connector on catheter.
   b. To intermittently release pressure, remove your thumb from valve or Y-connector.
9. Limit suctioning to 10 seconds at one time. **Rationale:** To prevent hypoxemia and cardiac complications.
10. To postoxygenate, allow client to deep breathe or breathe normally between periods of suctioning while administering 100% oxygen.
11. Repeat procedure as necessary. If large amounts of secretions are present, allow 3 minutes between suctionings. **Rationale:** This prevents oxygen depletion.
12. Flush suction tubing with sterile saline solution.
13. When procedure is completed, turn off suction machine.
14. Dispose of catheter after each use; dispose of gloves.
15. Offer oral hygiene.
16. Place client in comfortable position.
17. Assess lung sounds for changes.
18. Wash your hands.
19. Empty suction bottle at the end of every shift or more frequently as needed.

SUCTIONING WITH IN-LINE CATHETER

Equipment

Closed system or (ET connected) in-line suction unit with catheter enclosed by plastic sleeve

10 mL normal saline in syringe

Wall suction unit

Connecting tubing

Clean gloves (optional)

Note: In-line suctioning allows rapid suctioning for intubated clients and does not interrupt ventilation or oxygenation in critically ill clients. The nurse does not have to wear gloves because she or he is protected from the client's secretions by the plastic sleeve covering the catheter.

Procedure

1. Wash hands. Donning clean gloves is optional.
2. Check that in-line suction catheter is attached to connecting tubing, attached to suction machine.
3. Turn suction on and set regulator according to

established parameters for client and manufacturer's guide for closed system suction. **Rationale:** In-line systems may require slightly higher regulator setting to maintain adequate pressure.

4. Hyperoxygenate client using ambu-bag or mechanical ventilator.
5. Open port and attach saline syringe or vial, if required.
6. Advance catheter within plastic sleeve with dominant hand and, if required, push syringe with other hand to release 5–10 mL normal saline during inspiration. **Rationale:** As client takes breath or ventilator delivers a breath, saline is dispersed and cough is stimulated.
7. Insert catheter on next breath by pulling plastic sleeve back and pushing catheter forward until resistance is felt. **Rationale:** Sterility is maintained because catheter is enclosed by plastic cover and slides within it.
8. Withdraw catheter completely into plastic sheath. **Rationale:** If not totally out of the airway, the catheter blocks flow of air. Limit suction time to 10 second.
9. Repeat steps 4–8 one or two times to clear secretions; allow 1 minute between suctioning for oxygenation. **Rationale:** Too frequent or long suctioning interferes with ventilation and causes complications such as hypoxia.

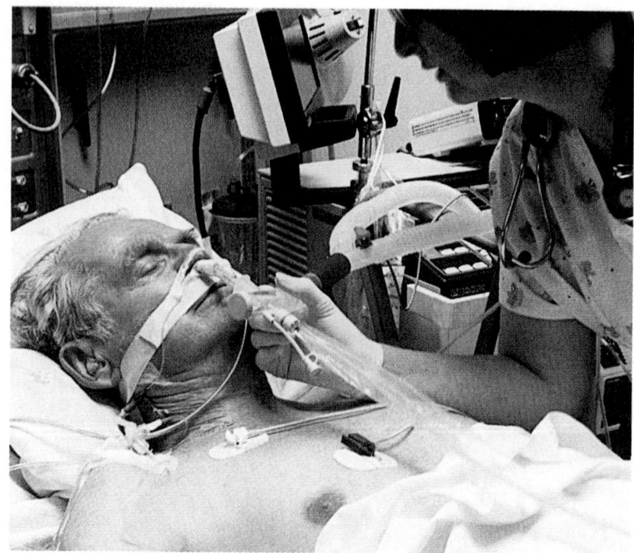

Example of intubated client with in-line suction catheter.

10. Push syringe of normal saline (5–10 mL) to rinse catheter following suctioning. **Rationale:** Rinsing prevents contamination of catheter by bacteria from secretions.
11. Remove syringe and turn off suction. Lock mechanism if appropriate.
12. Remove gloves (if used) and wash hands.

SUCTIONING INFANTS WITH BULB SYRINGE

Equipment

Bulb syringe for infant
Water-soluble lubricant

Procedure

1. Identify infant by checking arm band.
2. Place infant in supine position holding infant's hands together, or use football hold.
3. Squeeze air from bulb of syringe.
4. Insert tip of syringe snugly into infant's nose and slowly release finger pressure from bulb. **Rationale:** It is important to suction nose first, as most infants are nose breathers.

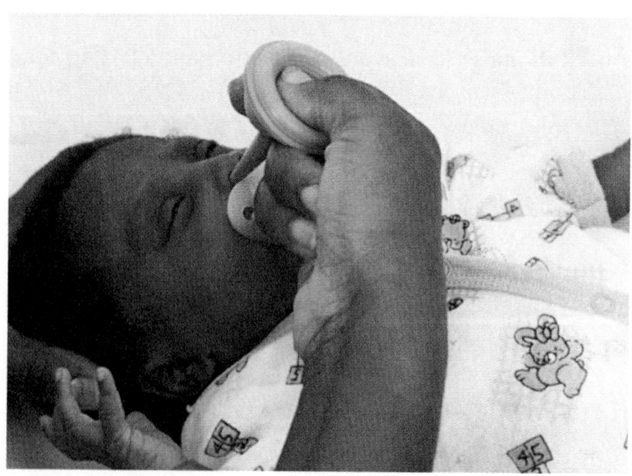

A bulb syringe is used to remove secretions from an infant's nose or mouth.

■ CLINICAL ALERT

With a newborn, it is important to suction mouth first, because delicate receptors in nose may be stimulated and cause infant to inhale mucus from the mouth.

5. Empty bulb contents.
6. Insert into other naris and repeat procedure.
7. Release bulb and squeeze to expel secretions into basin or gauze.
8. Compress bulb, insert into mouth between gum and cheek, suction secretions and expel.
9. Rinse the syringe by immersing tip in water, expanding bulb, and squeezing bulb to expel water.
10. Reposition infant on side or on abdomen with head turned to one side. **Rationale:** This promotes drainage of secretions.

CHARTING for Suctioning

- Amount, color, and consistency of secretions
- Changes in breath sounds
- Breathing rate
- Unanticipated problems and client's response
- Client's tolerance to procedure
- Number of times client was suctioned
- Pre- and post-hyperinflation of oxygen with ambu or Laerdahl suctioning bag
- O_2 flow rate, if used

CRITICAL THINKING APPLICATION

CLINICAL PROBLEMS	CRITICAL THINKING OPTIONS
■ Nares are obstructed.	• Remove catheter from the naris, and insert into the other naris. (Deviated septum is more frequently found on left side of nose.) • If ordered, a nasal airway can be inserted to suction through. • If both nares are obstructed, suction through mouth. (Have client stick tongue out to facilitate.)
■ Frequent nasopharyngeal suctioning may irritate nares and airway.	• Report to physician, obtain order, and insert decongestive nose drops to decrease irritation. • Provide frequent care of nares.
■ Hypoxemia may result if incorrect techniques are used for suctioning. Lethal arrhythmias may occur.	• Observe for signs of increased restlessness while suctioning. • Limit suctioning time to no more than 10 seconds. • Ensure that catheter is no larger than half the diameter of the airway. • Have client deep breathe to preoxygenate and suction once, then reapply oxygen for a couple of minutes before continuing suctioning.

CLINICAL PROBLEMS	CRITICAL THINKING OPTIONS
	• Hyperinflate lungs with oxygen, using ambu or Laerdahl bag and 100% oxygen. • Administer oxygen as ordered.
■ Excessive secretions that require frequent suctioning are present.	• After suctioning, attach new suction catheter to tubing on suction machine so that you have a catheter available in case of an emergency. • Suction more frequently but use ambu or Laerdahl bag to administer 100% oxygen before and after suctioning.
■ Wheezing sounds occur following suctioning due to laryngospasm.	• Do not repeat suctioning. • Administer oxygen with mist if ordered. • Place client in semi-Fowler's position to assist in lung expansion. • Encourage client to take slow, deep breaths.
■ Suctioning equipment is non-functioning.	• Examine suction equipment to determine if it is securely attached to wall outlet or plugged into electric outlet. • Check that suction equipment is turned ON. • If "hissing" sound is present, check that seal is around the top of the bottle. • Observe that connections between catheter and suction equipment are secure and tight without evidence of catheter or tube kinking.

unit 5

INTERMITTENT POSITIVE PRESSURE BREATHING (IPPB)

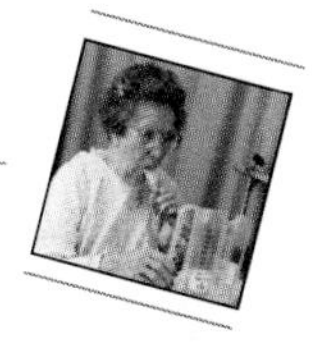

NURSING PROCESS DATA

ASSESSMENT Data Base

Evaluate client's need for IPPB.

Evaluate arterial blood gases, sputum cultures, and chest x-rays.

Review the physician's IPPB order for settings, length of treatment, and medications to be used.

Assess client's lung sounds before and after each treatment.

Observe consistency, amount, and color of expectorated sputum.

Assess need for additional physiotherapy to improve respiratory function.

Assess pulse and respiratory rate to establish baseline data.

PLANNING Objectives

To deliver aerosol medications

To decrease the work of breathing

To promote a better ventilation–perfusion ratio by increasing bronchodilatation and alveolar ventilation

To loosen secretions

To decrease pulmonary edema

IMPLEMENTATION Procedures

Setting up the Puritan–Bennett PR 2

Administering a Nebulized Treatment

Administering Medication by Nebulization

EVALUATION Expected Outcomes

Increased expectoration of secretions occurs.

Client experiences less labored breathing.

Improved blood gas values are documented.

Lung sounds are improved.

Aerosol medications administered into deep air passages and ventilation improves.

SETTING UP THE PURITAN–BENNETT PR 2

Equipment

IPPB machine (Bennett) or pressure-preset ventilator

Ventilator tubing

Nebulizer and manifold

Mouthpiece

Nose piece or clip (optional)

Power source (oxygen, compressed air, or electricity, depending on the machine)

Tidal volume spirometer

Note: IPPB treatments are not as commonly used today due to potential complications. However, these treatments are still given in some parts of the country and, while normally managed by respiratory departments, the nurse is still responsible for monitoring the client.

Preparation

1. Check physician's orders and client care plan.
2. Notify respiratory therapy department regarding the order for IPPB therapy.
3. Gather equipment if nursing performs this activity in

your facility. The PR 2 can be used as an IPPB machine or a pressure-preset ventilator.
4. Identify client via identaband.
5. Explain procedure to client.
6. Wash your hands.

Procedure

1. Connect pressure hose to wall oxygen outlet or compressed air.
2. Attach tubing to the machine.
3. Unscrew the nebulizer cup.
4. Place medication or distilled water in the cup and replace it.
5. Adjust the air mix knob: pull it out to give 100% oxygen, and push it in to administer an air mix.
6. Set the pressure: turn the pressure control knob (in the middle front of the machine) clockwise until the right-hand pressure control gauge reads the ordered pressure.
7. Check that the peak flow knob is completely open (at the maximal counterclockwise position). Do not adjust peak flow without checking with a therapist or physician.
8. Turn the ventilation rate off. **Rationale:** This dial is turned on only for use of the PR 2 in controlled ventilation.
9. Remove the nebulizer from the manifold. Remove the dust cap and lift the drum pin.

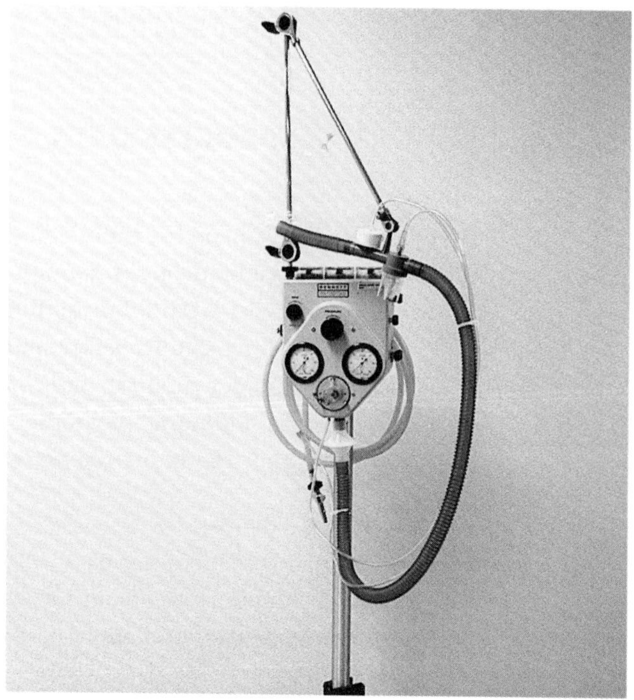

Bennett respirator.

10. Adjust the inspiration nebulization knob until a fine mist appears.
11. Lower the drum pin and replace the dust cap.
12. Replace the nebulizer in the manifold.
13. Set the sensitivity control to off by turning the knob clockwise.

ADMINISTERING A NEBULIZED TREATMENT

Equipment

Puritan–Bennett nebulizer with all appropriate equipment or Bird Mark 7 with all appropriate equipment
Medication or distilled water

Preparation

1. Gather equipment.
2. Identify client.
3. Explain the rationale for the treatment in understandable terms.
4. Assess best position for treatment.
5. Place client on side of bed in sitting position with feet on floor, or have client sit in chair.
6. Instruct client on the following:
    a. Keep lips closed tightly around the mouthpiece.
    b. Breathe only through mouth.
    c. Breathe slowly.
    d. To trigger the machine, breathe in slightly. Then relax and let the machine complete the breath while client expands lower chest and abdomen.
    e. Hold breath briefly at the end of each inspiration.
    f. Exhale normally, around the mouthpiece.
7. Wash your hands.

Procedure

1. Complete client teaching.
2. Administer pain medication about 30 minutes

before treatment if client has postsurgical chest or abdominal pain. **Rationale:** If client is in pain, he or she will be reluctant to use this treatment to facilitate breathing.

3. Post a "No Smoking" sign and alert visitors and other clients in the room not to smoke.
4. Check client's pulse and respiratory rate before, during, and after treatment.
5. Have client inhale through the machine.
6. Provide instruction until client has mastered the correct technique.
7. Gradually increase pressure until client is receiving the ordered pressure.
   a. On the Puritan–Bennett PR 2, turn the pressure control knob until the left-hand delivered pressure gauge reads the ordered pressure.
   b. On the Puritan–Bennett AP 5, turn the pressure control knob until the pressure gauge shows the ordered pressure at the end of inspiration.
8. Observe the chest for full expansion.
9. Encourage periodic coughing to remove secretions.
10. Tap the nebulizer cup periodically. **Rationale:** This action moves moisture to the bottom.

■ **CLINICAL ALERT**

The higher pressure automatically increases sensitivity, so you may need to lower sensitivity by pulling the control level toward the front of the unit (higher number equals less sensitivity). You must also increase flow rate whenever you increase pressure; turn the flow rate dial to a higher number (higher number equals shorter inspiration and increased flow).

11. Continue treatment until the nebulizer is empty, usually about 20 minutes. If the nebulizer becomes empty before the end of the prescribed treatment period, add distilled water.
12. Check pulse, blood pressure, and respiratory rate at the end of treatment.
13. Assist client to a comfortable position. Remind client of the value of the treatment and give positive reinforcement for cooperation.
14. Wash your hands.

ADMINISTERING MEDICATION BY NEBULIZATION

Equipment

Nebulizer medication chamber (nonpressurized aerosol)
T-piece
Mouthpiece or mask
Corrugated tubing
Air flow tubing
Prescribed medication (e.g., bronchodilator)
Prescribed diluent (normal saline)
Wall source (or other source) for compressed air or oxygen (with flowmeter)

Preparation

1. Dilute medication as ordered and place in nebulizer chamber.
2. Attach one end of tubing to compressed air source.
3. Attach other end of tubing to nozzle at side or bottom of nebulizer.

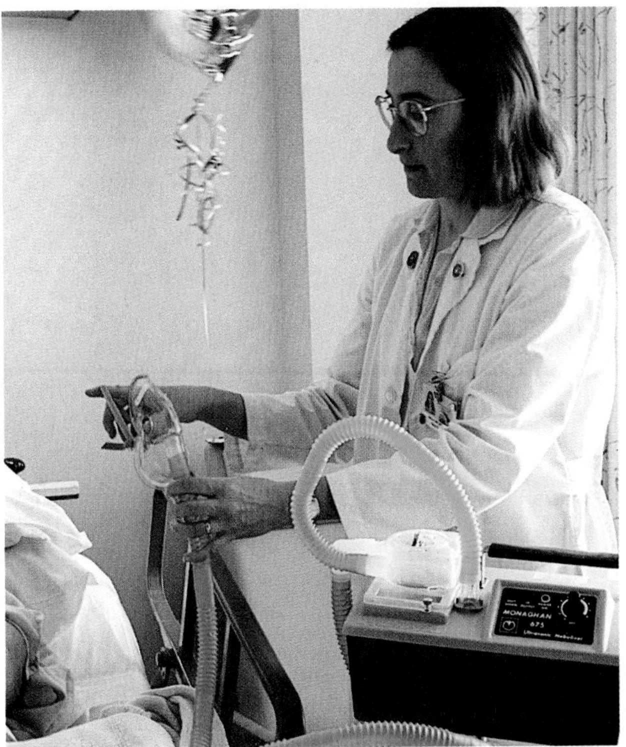

Administering medication with ultrasonic nebulizer.

4. Connect top of nebulizer chamber to mask or T-piece sidearm.
5. Attach mouth piece to one end of T-piece.
6. Attach corrugated tubing to other end of T-piece.

Procedure

1. Place medication in nebulizer chamber.
2. Turn on air or oxygen (8 L/min) source, and observe for mist flow.
3. Instruct client to breathe in and out of mouthpiece or mask normally.
4. Have client take a deep breath and hold for several seconds, then exhale slowly every three to five breaths. (Treatment is complete when all medication is used and no mist is seen.)
5. Turn power (air or O_2 flow) off, and unplug compressor (if used).
6. Clean mouthpiece, and place equipment in plastic bag at bedside. (Dispose of and replace components every 4 days.)

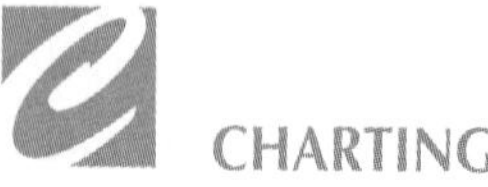

CHARTING

- Medication and dosage
- Settings used on IPPB machine
- Duration of treatment
- Amount, consistency, and color of secretions obtained
- Client's tolerance for treatment
- Vital signs before and after treatment

CRITICAL THINKING APPLICATION

CLINICAL PROBLEMS	CRITICAL THINKING OPTIONS
There is no increase in the expectoration of secretions.	• Check that the nebulizer is expelling a fine mist. • Notify physician for medication order change to a drug that lowers surface tension of sputum, thereby facilitating expectoration. • Encourage deep breathing and coughing between IPPB treatments. • Obtain order for PVD.
Breathing continues to be labored.	• Ensure that client is positioned in Fowler's or at least semi-Fowler's position to facilitate breathing. • Have client expectorate mucus. If unable to cough productively, suction client. • Evaluate need for additional treatments or potential need for assisted mechanical ventilation. • Use relaxation techniques if client is anxious.
Lung sounds do not improve.	• Monitor lung sounds before and after each treatment. • Identify area of lung that contains adventitious sounds, and administer PVD to the specific area. • Obtain order to change medications or increase number of treatments.
Inability to trigger the machine at the usual sensitivity setting.	• On the PR 2, increase sensitivity by turning the sensitivity knob to the left.
Pressure setting reached too quickly.	• Check tubing for kinks. • Encourage client to cough. • Suction client if she or he is unable to expectorate secretions. • Instruct client not to resist the airflow or blow back into the machine. • Decrease the flow rate (and the pressure) in the PR2.

unit 6

TRACHEOSTOMY CARE

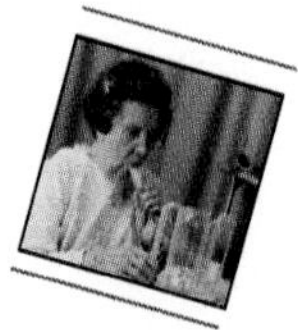

NURSING PROCESS DATA

ASSESSMENT Data Base

Note if there are dried or moist secretions surrounding cannula or on tracheal dressing.

Note excessive expectoration of secretions.

Assess if routine tracheal care is adequate for this client.

Assess respiratory status: breath sounds, respiratory rate, use of accessory muscles for breathing while tracheal tube is plugged.

Observe for labored breathing, flaring of nares, retractions, and color of nail beds.

Observe vital signs for increases in pulse or respirations.

Auscultate for adventitious sounds to evaluate lung field.

Listen for audible hissing sounds indicating an air leak.

Check if pilot balloon is deflated or inflated.

PLANNING Objectives

To prevent airway obstruction

To prevent infections of tracheal site

To improve respiratory function so client can breathe normally, without artificial support

To suction secretions more easily

To deflate tracheostomy cuff to facilitate suctioning

To prevent aspiration while feeding

To prevent tracheal damage

IMPLEMENTATION Procedures

Cleaning the Inner Cannula

Changing Trach Ties

Performing Tracheostomy Suctioning

Using a Manual Resuscitator

Plugging a Tracheostomy

Deflating a Tracheal Cuff

Inflating a Tracheal Cuff

EVALUATION Expected Outcomes

Client adequately ventilated with absence of respiratory distress.

Secretions easily suctioned.

Tracheostomy site remains free of infection.

Client able to eat without aspirating food.

Tracheal necrosis is prevented.

CLEANING THE INNER CANNULA

Equipment

NOTE: Many hospitals use disposable inner cannulas that eliminate the need for cleaning.

Tracheal cleaning tray (includes two sterile basins, pipe cleaners, brush, 4 × 4 gauze pad)
Sterile gloves
Suction equipment
Complete tracheal tube set for emergency use
Interchangeable inner cannula of same size if available or tracheostomy tube and obturator
Sterile normal saline
Sterile nonraveling precut dressings
Clean tracheal ties

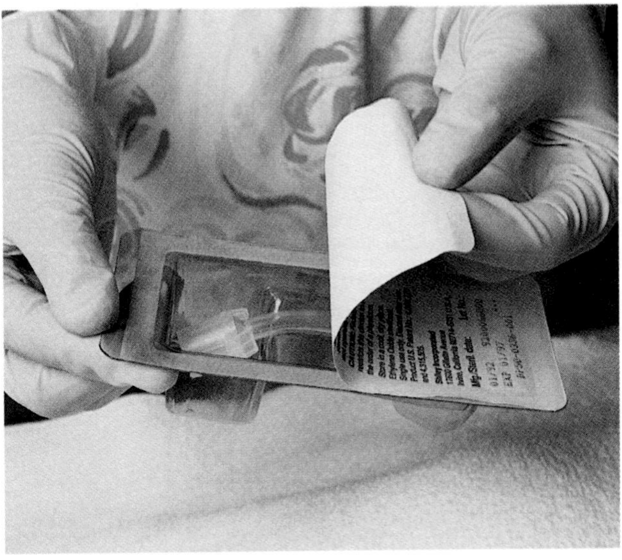

Disposable inner cannula.

Preparation

1. Check physician's orders and client care plan.
2. Assemble equipment.
3. Make sure suction equipment and additional tracheal tubes are available. Suction before cleaning.
4. Wash your hands.

Procedure

1. Explain procedure and rationale to client.
2. Open trach tray, and put on one glove.
3. With gloved hand, separate basins; with ungloved hand, pour each liquid into a basin.
4. Don second glove. Unlock inner cannula by turning left about 90°. Secure outer cannula neck plate with index finger and thumb.
5. Gently pull the inner cannula slightly upward and out toward you.
6. Soak the cannula in a sterile bowl filled with hydrogen peroxide to remove dried secretions.

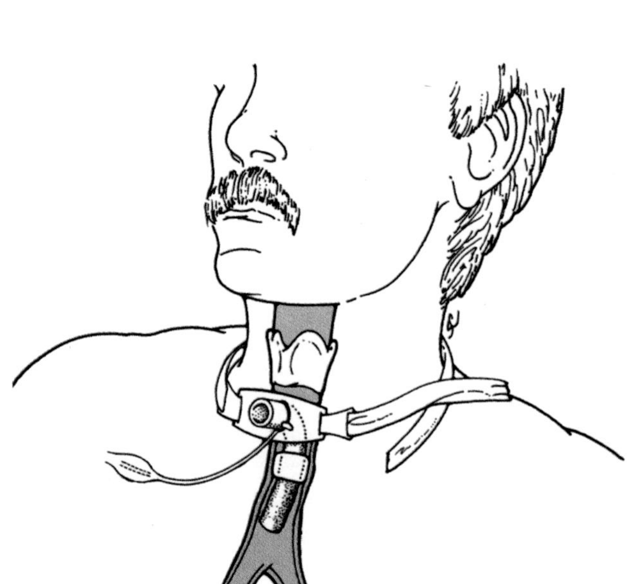

Anatomic placement of a tracheostomy tube.

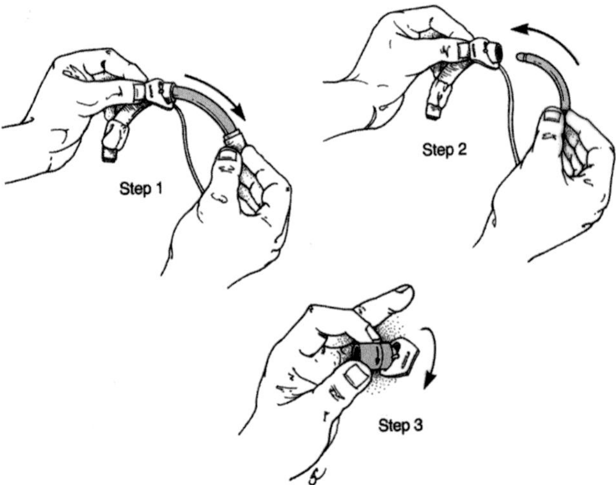

Inner cannula is removed for cleaning. Outer cannula is not.

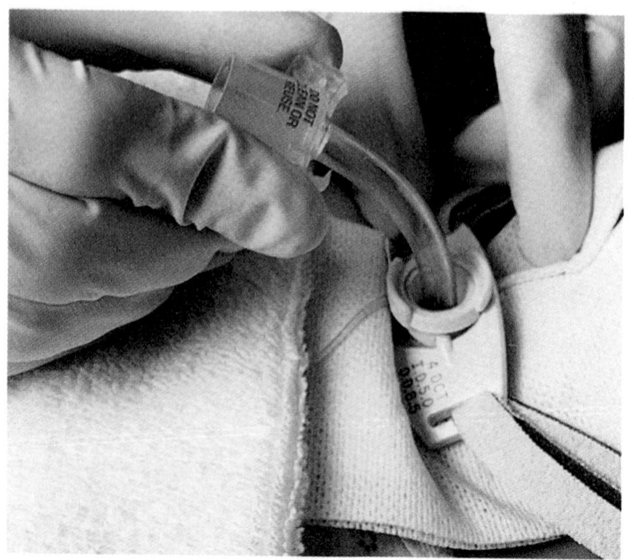

Gently pull inner cannula upward and outward to remove.

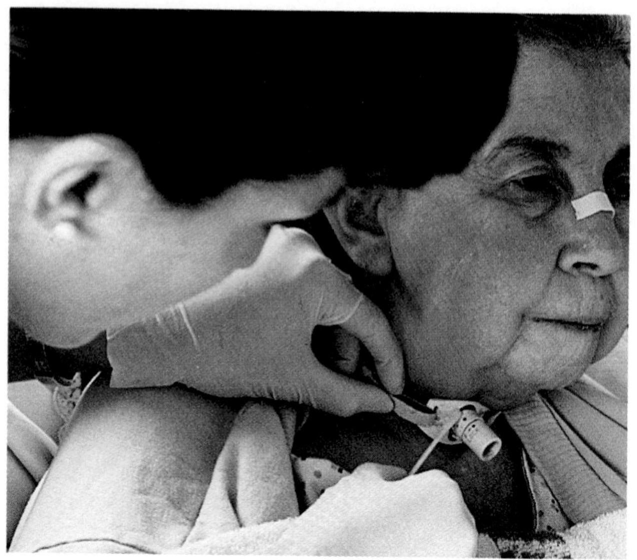

Gently clean around trach opening.

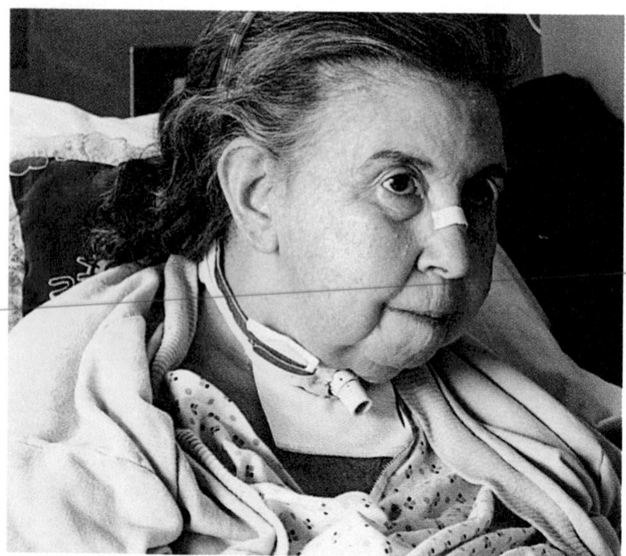

Apply precut nonraveling dressing around trach.

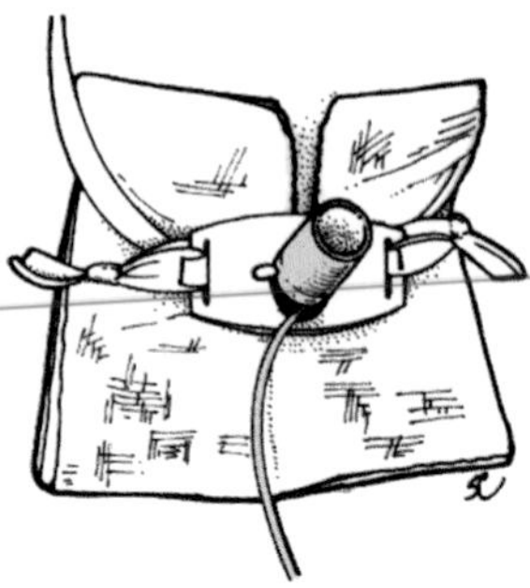

A precut nonraveling material is used for the trach dressing to prevent lint from entering trach tube.

7. Cleanse the lumen and outer surface of the cannula with pipe cleaners or brush moistened with hydrogen peroxide. (Some hospitals use sterile normal saline.) **Rationale:** To remove dried-on secretions.
8. Rinse cannula thoroughly with sterile water or saline.
9. Place clean tube on sterile 4 × 4 gauze pad and dry tube thoroughly.
10. Replace the inner cannula carefully by grasping the outer flange of the cannula with your other hand as you insert the cannula.
11. Lock the inner cannula by turning the lock to the right so that it is in an upright position.
12. Cleanse around the incision site with applicator sticks soaked in normal saline.

■ **CLINICAL ALERT**

A packaged sterile trach tube is kept at the bedside for emergency use. If the trach tube becomes dislodged, the new tube can be immediately inserted.

13. Apply precut, nonraveling trach dressing around insertion site, and change tracheal ties if needed. **Rationale:** Nonraveling dressing prevents lint from entering trach tube.
14. If tracheal ties are to be changed, ask another person to hold the tracheal tube in place while you change the ties. **Rationale:** This procedure prevents accidental extubation if patient coughs.
15. Make client comfortable.
16. Discard soiled dressings, tapes, cleaning equipment, and gloves.
17. Wash your hands.

CHANGING TRACH TIES

Equipment

Scissor
Forceps
Twill tape, foam, or commercial trach ties
Packaged sterile trach tube set-up

Preparation

1. Seek assistance from another person. **Rationale:** It is safer to have someone hold the trach tube in place when changing ties. The client isn't as likely to cough the tube out.
2. Explain procedure to client.
3. Wash your hands.
4. Gather equipment.
5. Place client in semi- to high-Fowler's position as condition warrants.

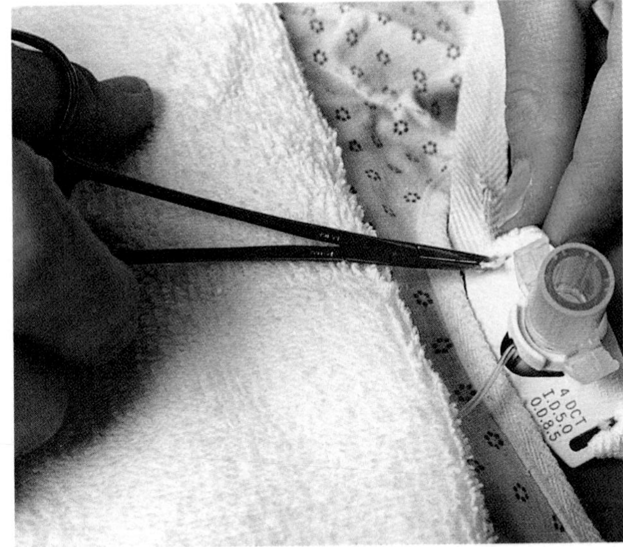

Use forceps to thread tape through trach neck plate.

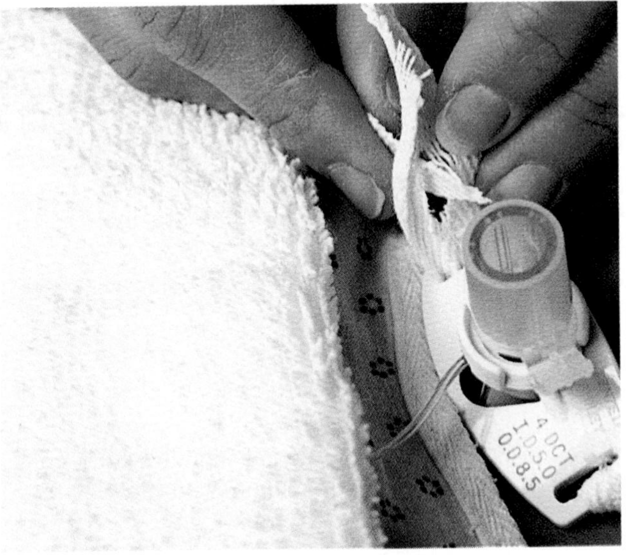

Thread end of tie through slit and pull in place.

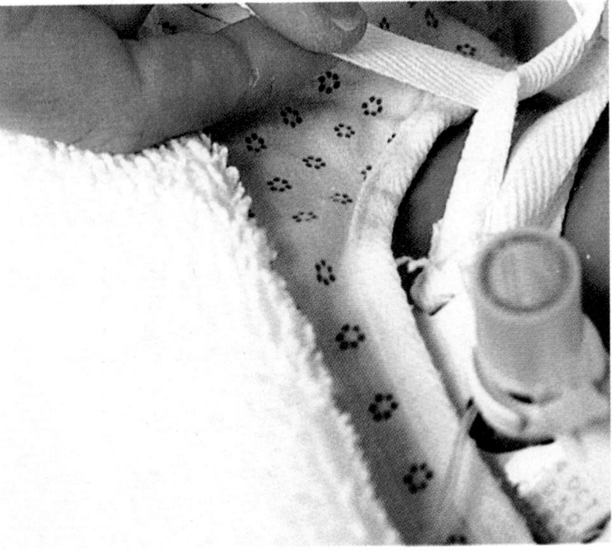
Bring ties around neck and tie in square knot.

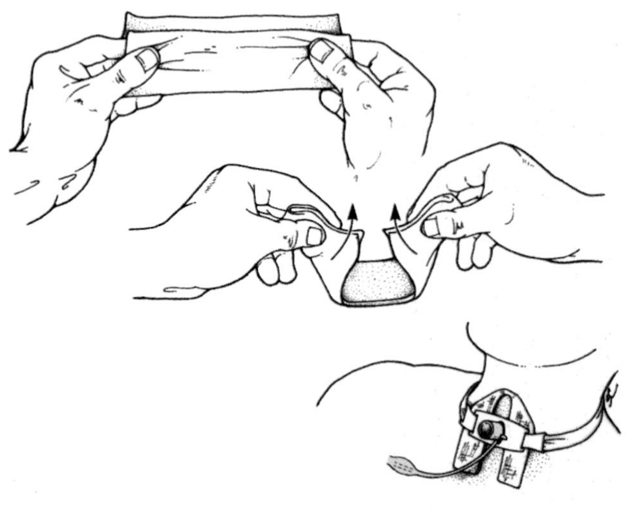

Folded 4 × 4 trach dressing for use if presplit dressing is not available.

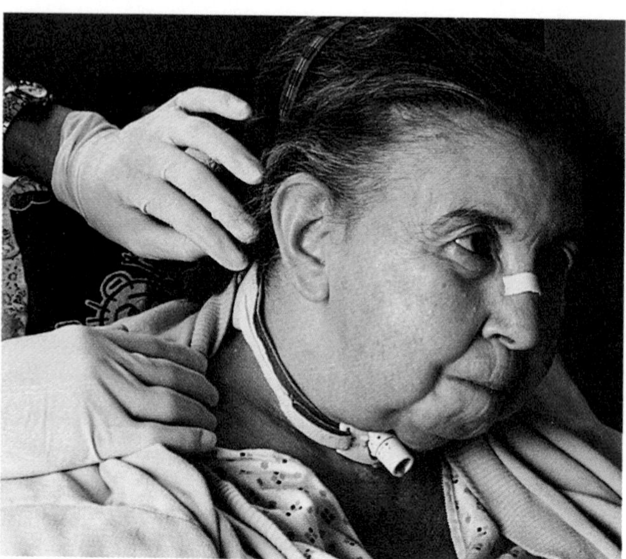

Knot foam trach ties at side of neck allowing one finger-breadth slack.

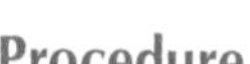

Procedure

For Twill Tape Ties

1. Cut trach ties length you desire, if not precut.
2. Fold ends of the trach ties over $1\frac{1}{2}$ inches, and cut a slit in the piece starting at the folded edge.
3. If assistance is available, have the person hold the trach tube in place. Cut the old trach ties, and remove and discard.
4. Pass the slit end of the ties through the flange loop of the trach tube about 2–3 inches (you may use Kelly forceps to grab tie). **Rationale:** Leave the old trach tie in place if you are changing the ties without assistance. This prevents accidental dislodging of the trach tube.
5. Thread the other end of the tie all the way through the slit. Pull it firmly in place. **Rationale:** This action anchors the tie around the flange loop.
6. Repeat steps 4 and 5 on other flange loop.
7. Bring ties around client's neck and tie in a square knot to one side of neck, leaving one fingerbreadth under tie. **Rationale:** This is more comfortable for the client and prevents pressure on the neck and jugular vein.
8. Cut off soiled trach ties if not already done, and discard.
9. Position client for comfort.
10. Wash your hands.

For Foam Ties

1. Thread "hook" tape through one slot on tracheostomy tube, and attach "hook" fastener to fuzzy side of neck pad or strap.
2. Bring foam neck collar behind client's neck.
3. Thread "hook" tape through other slot in tracheostomy tube.
4. Secure "hook" fastener to fuzzy side of neck strap or neck collar. Neck straps may be knotted to shorten.

PERFORMING TRACHEOSTOMY SUCTIONING

Equipment

Trach suctioning kit or

Disposable saline ampule

2 suction catheters

Sterile gloves

Clean gloves

Goggles, gown, mask as appropriate for client's condition

Portable suction machine or wall suction with Y-connector or release valve—maximum safe suction pressure is −120 mm Hg.

Receptacle for used equipment

Container for sterile saline

Sterile saline
Ambu or Laerdahl bag with trach adaptor
Oxygen source

Preparation

1. Check physician's orders and client care plan.
2. Gather equipment.
3. Explain procedure to client.
4. Wash your hands.
5. Assess lung sounds.
6. Turn suction on to between −80 and −120 mm Hg pressure. **Rationale:** Higher suction pressure increases risk of mucosal damage.
7. Attach resuscitator bag to oxygen tubing.
8. Turn on oxygen supply. The supply must deliver 100% oxygen.
9. Don clean gloves, goggles, mask, and gown as needed. **Rationale:** Type of equipment needed during suction procedure depends on client's condition.
10. Complete nasopharyngeal or oropharyngeal suctioning using clean technique. **Rationale:** This procedure is completed first to obtain the secretions accumulated in the nose, mouth, and above tracheostomy cuff if inflated. **Rationale:** This prevents secretions from moving into bronchus.
11. Change to sterile catheter and glove or obtain new catheter and sleeve package following nasopharyngeal or oropharyngeal suctioning. **Rationale:** Tracheostomy suctioning is a sterile procedure that requires a sterile catheter to prevent contamination of the bronchus. Nasopharyngeal or oropharyngeal suctioning may be completed using the same catheter *after* tracheostomy suctioning. This suction procedure is a clean technique. To prevent contamination, suction from a sterile to a clean environment, not clean to sterile.
12. Remove gloves and discard in appropriate receptacle.

NOTE: This skill is more safely performed with two nurses—one nurse to manage resuscitator bag, the second nurse to perform suctioning procedure.

Procedure

1. Open new suction catheter package. Ensure that catheter size is no greater than half the diameter of the trach tube. **Rationale:** This prevents hypoxia and atelectasis by allowing atmospheric air to be drawn in around catheter.
2. Don sterile gloves. Keep dominant hand sterile and other hand clean.
3. Open sterile container for flushing catheter, and pour in normal saline.
4. Connect suction tubing to catheter, maintaining sterility. **Rationale:** Maintaining sterility prevents

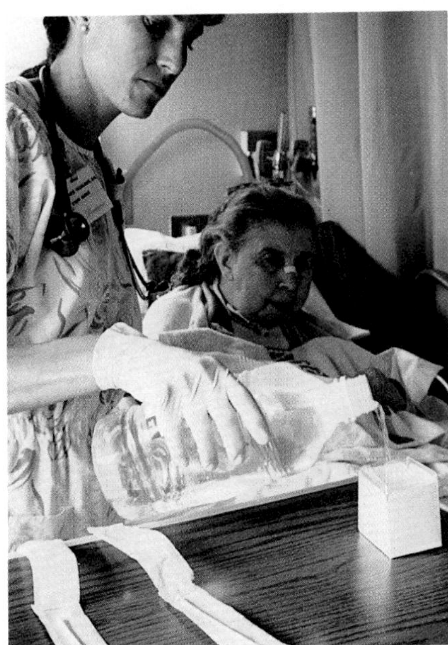

Pour normal saline in sterile container.

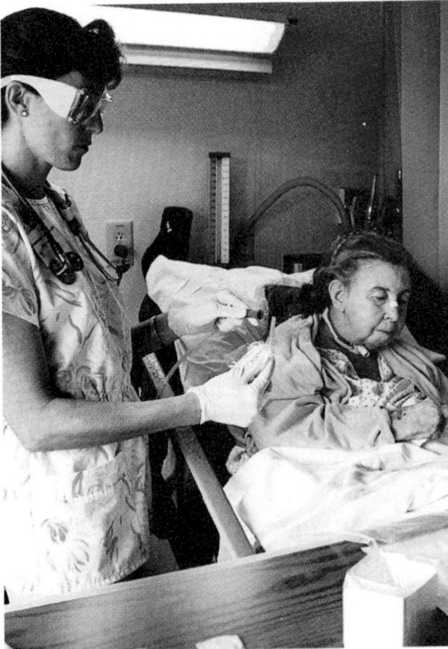

Connect suction tubing to catheter.

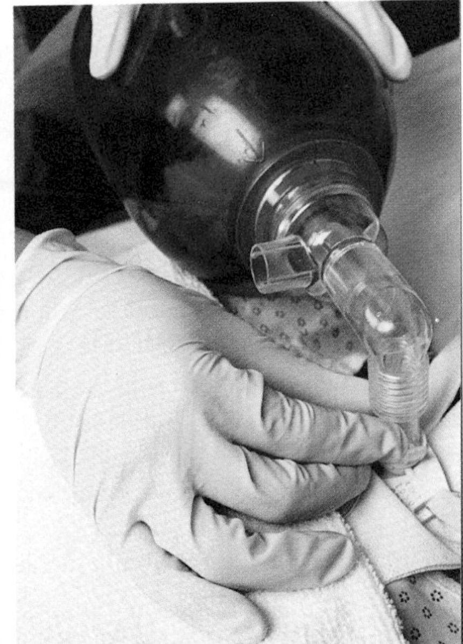

Connect resusitator bag to trach.

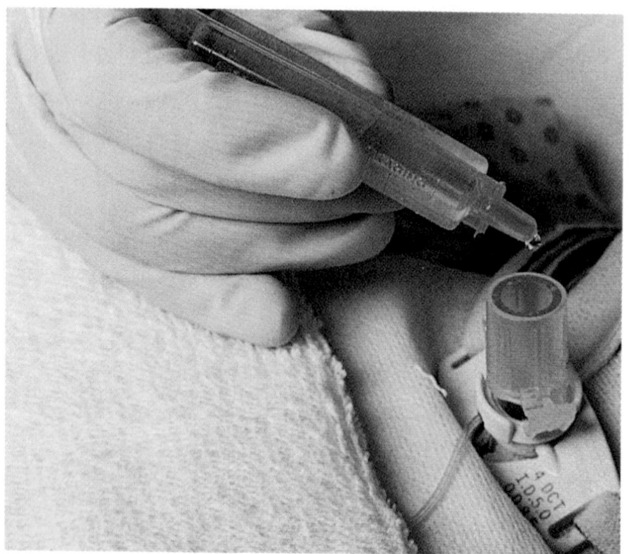

Instill normal saline into trach according to hospital policy.

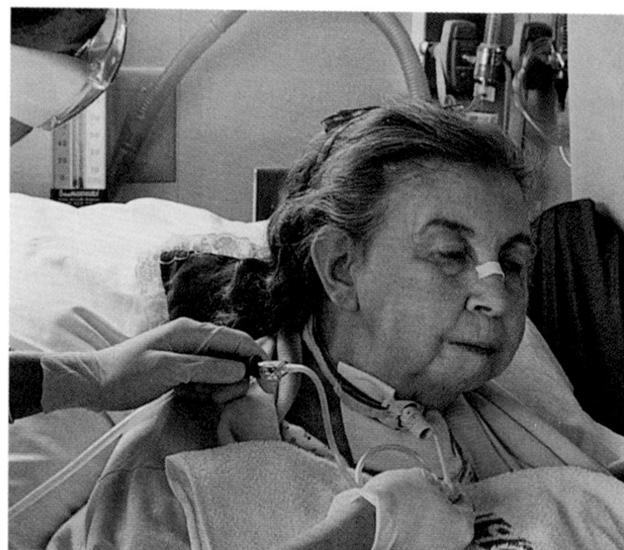

Guide catheter into trach tube using sterile hand.

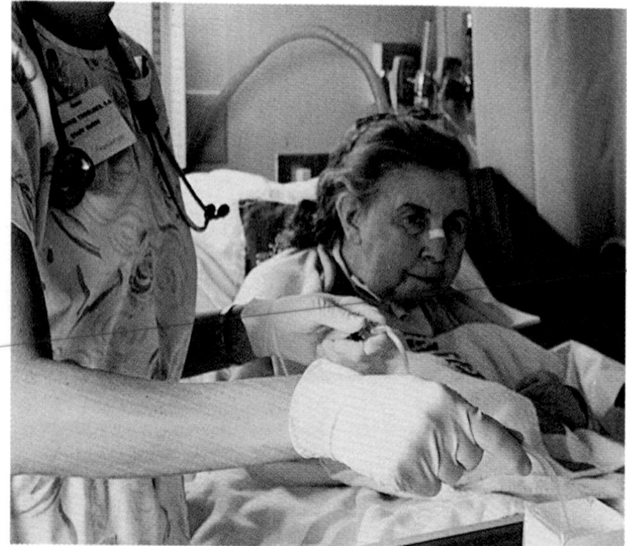

Rinse catheter and connecting tubing with NS to clear.

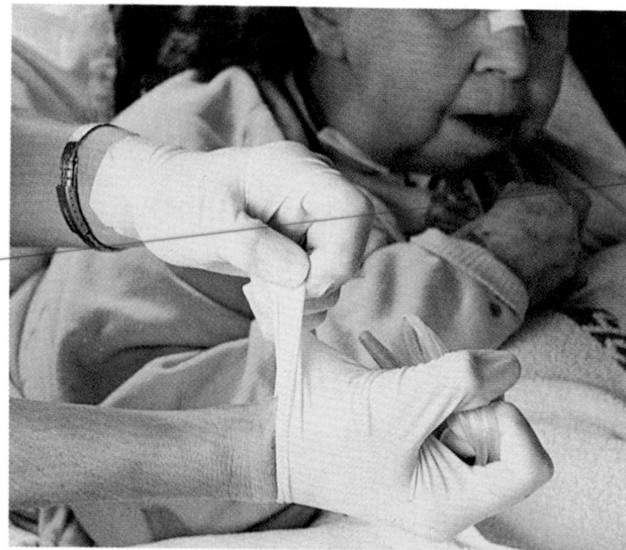

Coil catheter around fingers and pull glove over it.

pathogens from entering bronchus.

5. Disconnect oxygen source from the tracheostomy tube with your clean hand.
6. Pick up manual resuscitator bag with same clean hand. Connect trach adaptor to tracheostomy tube.
7. Hyperoxygenate lungs with five breaths using 100% oxygen, or have client take several deep breaths before disconnecting O_2 source from trach tube. **Rationale:** Suctioning depletes oxygen and causes PO_2 to fall.
8. Disconnect resuscitator bag using clean hand, and place nearby for use after suctioning procedure.
9. Open single-dose ampule of saline. (Hospital protocol dictates if saline is to be used.) Instill 3–10 mL normal saline into tracheostomy tube using clean hand, according to policy.
10. Grasp vented end of suction catheter with clean hand, and guide catheter into tracheostomy tube using sterile hand.
11. Insert catheter, without applying suction, quickly and gently into tracheostomy until you feel resistance. **Rationale:** Suction pressure during insertion may damage tissue.
12. Apply intermittent suction to the catheter as you

rotate and withdraw catheter from tracheostomy. **Rationale:** Intermittent suction and catheter rotation prevents damage to mucosal lining during suctioning.

13. Suction for no more than 10 seconds. **Rationale:** This prevents hypoxia due to oxygen loss through suctioning.
14. Rinse catheter and connecting tubing with normal saline until clear. **Rationale:** This clears tubing of secretions and minimizes spread of microorganisms.
15. Hyperinflate lungs with ambu or Laerdahl bag using 100% oxygen, or have client take several deep breaths.
16. Attach oxygen source to tracheostomy tube.
17. Dispose of catheter by disconnecting it from suction tubing, coiling around fingers, and removing glove back over catheter. Discard the "gloved catheter" into the appropriate receptacle.
18. Discard remaining glove into receptacle.
19. Turn off suction motor, and place tubing in a convenient place for next procedure, or connect new sterile, protected catheter to tubing, according to hospital policy.
20. Position client for comfort.
21. Auscultate lungs and compare presuctioning data.
22. Wash your hands.
23. Empty suction bottle PRN or at end of each shift.

USING A MANUAL RESUSCITATOR

Equipment

Laerdahl or ambu bag
Oxygen source and tubing
Trach adapter or face mask

Preparation

1. Check physician's orders and client care plan.
2. Gather equipment.
3. Connect mask or trach adapter, oxygen tubing, and oxygen flowmeter (reservoir) to bag.
4. Wash your hands.

Procedure

1. Turn on oxygen flowmeter to 15 L/minute as ordered.
2. When using a mask, hyperextend client's neck, and place the apex of the mask over the nose. Place the base of the mask between the lower lip and chin. You may have to open client's mouth by pressing down on the chin. **Rationale:** This ensures a tight seal.
3. When using a trach adapter, attach the universal adapter to the bag. Attach the adapter to the client's endotracheal or tracheostomy tube.
4. Compress the ambu or Laerdahl bag every 5 seconds for an apneic adult and every 3 seconds for an apneic infant.

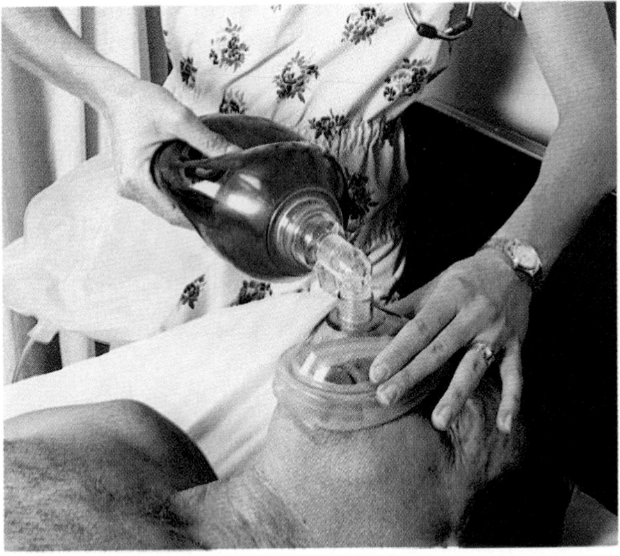

Hyperextend client's neck and place mask apex over nose and base over mouth.

5. If client is able to breathe spontaneously, give the breaths in synchrony with his or her breaths.
6. When using the bag to hyperinflate the lungs following suctioning, compress the bag three to five times each time you suction.
7. To keep the airway open when using a mask, seal mask tightly by pressing down on the mask with

thumb and index finger of one hand and lifting up client's mandible with your remaining fingers.

8. Observe the client's chest rise and fall with each compression. **Rationale:** This ensures adequate ventilation.
9. Observe for possible gastric distention with continued use of the bag.
10. If gastric distention persists, notify physician for nasogastric tube insertion orders.

PLUGGING A TRACHEOSTOMY

Equipment

Trach plug
Suction machine
2 Sterile suction catheters
Clean gloves
Sterile gloves
10-mL syringe

Preparation

1. Check physician's orders and client care plan to determine length of time it should remain plugged.
2. Wash hands.
3. Gather equipment.
4. Explain procedure to client and reassure her that she won't suffocate.
5. Place client in semi- to high-Fowler's position. **Rationale:** This assists with lung expansion and decreases fear of not being able to breathe.
6. Don clean gloves.

Procedure

1. Suction nasopharynx, using clean technique.
2. Change suction catheter, discard clean gloves, and don sterile gloves.
3. Using sterile technique, suction trachea. **Rationale:** If any secretions are above cuff, they would go down trachea if cuff is deflated first.
4. DEFLATE TRACHEAL CUFF; suction again if necessary.

> **■ CLINICAL ALERT**
>
> If tracheostomy is plugged and cuff is not deflated, the client has no airway. Some clinicians recommend cutting the cuff inflation port off completely once trach plugging is begun to prevent client asphyxiation.

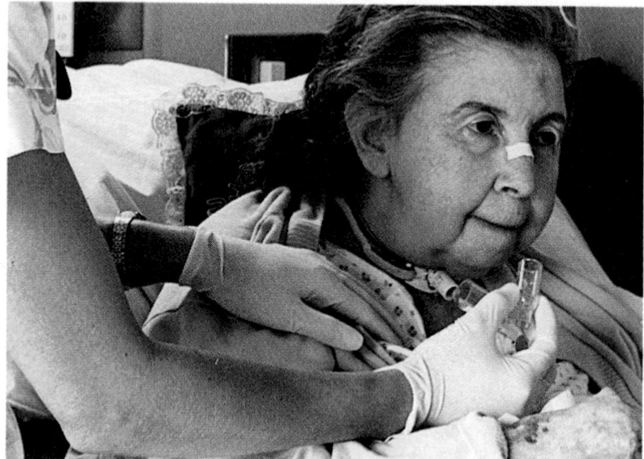

T-piece is inserted to enable client to speak.

5. Place tracheal plug in either the inner cannula or outer cannula with inner cannula removed.
6. Observe client for respiratory distress. **Rationale:** With cuff deflation, the tube's presence increases resistance to airflow dramatically, thus increasing the work of breathing.
7. Stay with client until she is comfortable and exhibits no difficulty breathing.
8. Remove plug when time has elapsed. Cleanse plug and return to clean area for reuse, or discard according to hospital policy.
9. Suction client and replace inner cannula if removed.
10. Reinflate tracheal cuff if ordered.

> **■ CLINICAL ALERT**
>
> Tracheal tube cuff inflation is essential for mechanically ventilated clients. Without cuff inflation, delivered air diverts out through the nose and mouth, and lung is not ventilated.

11. Position client for comfort.
12. Dispose of used equipment and gloves.
13. Wash your hands.

DEFLATING A TRACHEAL CUFF

Equipment

10-mL syringe
Suction equipment

Preparation

1. Check physician's orders and client care plan.
2. Gather equipment.
3. Wash your hands.
4. Prepare client by explaining procedure.
5. Provide client privacy.

Procedure

1. Suction nose or mouth (or both) and tracheostomy before deflating cuff as previously outlined.
2. Attach 10-mL syringe to distal end of inflatable cuff.
3. Slowly withdraw 5 mL of air. **Rationale:** Amount of air withdrawn is determined by type of cuff used and whether minimal air leak is used.
4. Keep syringe attached to end of cuff. **Rationale:** This is present for reinflation.
5. Suction if cough reflex is stimulated.
6. Assess breathing and if labored, reinflate cuff immediately.
7. If high-volume/low-pressure cuff is used, cuff is not routinely deflated. (In fact, deflating cuff does not help tracheal lining. The pooled secretions above the tracheal cuff are the problem.)

INFLATING A TRACHEAL CUFF

Equipment

10-mL syringe
Suction equipment

Procedure

1. If syringe is not already attached, attach 10-mL syringe to distal end of inflatable cuff, making sure seal is tight.
2. Inflate cuff for a minimal occluding volume. Auscultate over suprasternal notch (cuff location in trachea) for *minimal* hissing air flow. **Rationale:** This provides an adequate seal without risking tracheal pressure necrosis.
3. Ask client to speak—if voice is heard, air leak is too great.
4. Remove syringe and apply a one-way valve that prevents air leaks. (Forceps are not recommended, as they can damage the cuff tubing.)
5. Connect ventilator or T-piece as ordered.
6. Assess breath sounds every 2 hours. **Rationale:** Presence of bilateral breath sounds indicates proper tube placement.

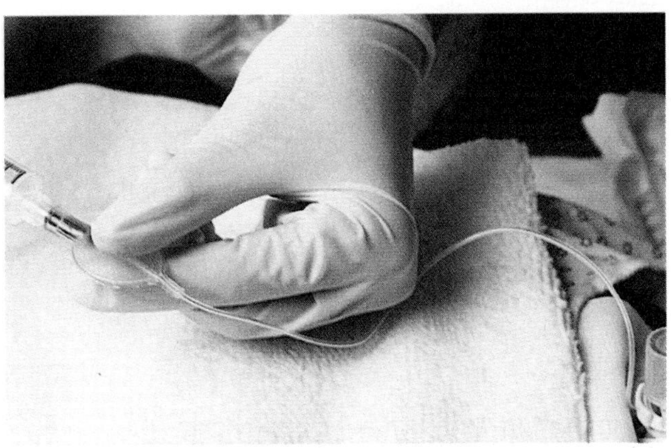

Inflate tracheal cuff by attaching 10 mL syringe.

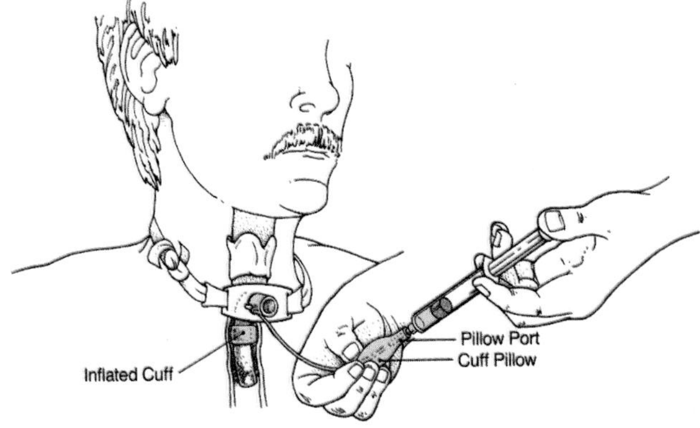

Check pillow port (pilot balloon) for pressure level and tautness to determine if balloon is inflated.

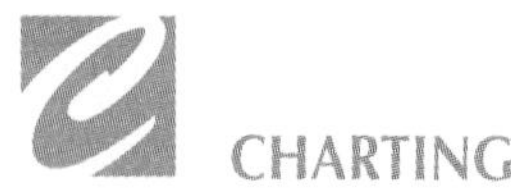

CHARTING

for Tracheostomy Tube Plugging

- Location of plug: outer or inner cannula
- Baseline vital signs before procedure
- Respiratory status during procedure
- Vital signs, any indications of respiratory distress

for Tracheostomy Care

- Trach care completed
- Appearance of site
- Characteristics of secretions
- Trach ties changed
- Client's tolerance of procedure

for Tracheostomy Tube Suctioning

- Amount, color, and consistency of secretions
- Changes in breath sounds
- Respiratory and cardiac rate changes
- Client's tolerance to procedure
- Unanticipated problems and client's response
- Frequency of client suctioning
- Use of ambu or Laerdahl bag for hyperinflation of lungs before and after suctioning

for Tracheal Tube Cuff Deflation

- Tracheal cuff deflation
- Amount of air used for cuff inflation or auscultation for minimal leak
- Changes in respiratory status during deflation–inflation
- Character of secretions

CRITICAL THINKING APPLICATION

CLINICAL PROBLEMS	CRITICAL THINKING OPTIONS
for Tracheostomy Tube Cleaning	
■ Accidental extubation occurs.	• Have second tracheal set available. • Keep airway open by inserting obturator or sterile forceps through trach opening. • Insert new trach tube, or notify physician as hospital policy dictates.
■ Secretions and coughing are excessive while inner cannula is cleansed.	• Perform oral suctioning before removing inner cannula. • Suction lumen, if necessary, while soaking inner cannula. • Place another interchangeable cannula in trach tube, and continue to soak cannula.
■ Inner cannula is dislodged.	• Insert extra cannula from emergency set if cannulas are interchangeable. If not, insert new tracheal set. • If cannula is metal, send it to CSR for autoclaving. If cannula is disposable, discard in trash. If plastic, soak in hydrogen peroxide for 1 hour, then rinse in sterile saline.
■ Client unable to be off ventilator long enough for cleansing of inner cannula.	• Insert new inner cannula (interchangeable), and place client back on ventilator. • Proceed to clean inner cannula and keep it clean for next change.

CLINICAL PROBLEMS	CRITICAL THINKING OPTIONS
for Tracheostomy Tube Suctioning ■ Hypoxia may occur if incorrect techniques are used for suctioning.	• Observe for signs of increased restlessness, tachycardia, bradycardia, or other arrhythmias. • Limit suctioning time to no more than 10 seconds. • Ensure that suction catheter is no larger than half the diameter of the tube. • Hyperinflate lungs with 100% oxygen using ambu or Laerdahl bag before and after suctioning.
■ Excessive secretions are produced that require frequent suctioning.	• Replace suction catheter with new one immediately after suctioning in order to have it ready for next time. • With frequent suctioning, hyperinflate lungs with 100% oxygen using an ambu or Laerdahl bag.
■ After suctioning, intubated client still sounds congested.	• Allow rest period before suctioning again (3 minutes). • Hyperinflate lungs with 100% oxygen using an ambu or Laerdahl bag if ordered. • Encourage deep breathing and coughing exercises. • Notify physician for bronchodilator drugs.
for Tracheostomy Tube Cuff Care ■ Balloon ruptures or herniates over the end of the tube.	• Replace tube immediately and report to physician. • Assess client for respiratory dysfunction. A portion of the cuff may have been aspirated.
■ Client is unable to tolerate cuff deflating for prescribed 5 minutes.	• Release cuff for as long a time as client can tolerate. • May hyperinflate lungs with manual resuscitator while cuff deflated. • Assess need for pressure support.
■ Accidental extubation occurs when the tube is deflated.	• Place client supine with open airway positioning. • Insert oropharyngeal airway • Support tracheostomy stoma open with forceps until reintubation.

unit 7

WATER-SEAL DRAINAGE SYSTEMS

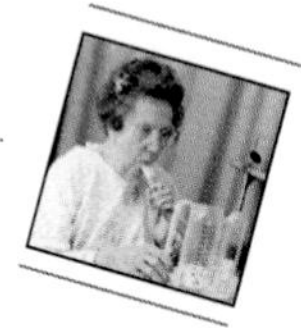

NURSING PROCESS DATA

ASSESSMENT Data Base

Assess client's respiratory status while tubes are inserted.

Check to see that all connections between the water-seal system and the client are securely taped.

Check patency of chest tubes.

Assess if mediastinal shift is present.

Auscultate breath sounds.

Observe for bilateral chest expansion.

Note chest drainage.

PLANNING Objectives

To evacuate air or a combination of air and serosanguineous fluid from the intrapleural space to allow compressed lung to reexpand

To reestablish negative intrapleural pressure after an intrathoracic procedure

To reinfuse autologous blood after surgery

To facilitate drainage of accumulated fluid within the mediastinum after open heart surgery to prevent cardiac tamponade

IMPLEMENTATION Procedures

Maintaining a Three-Bottle System

Setting up and Maintaining a Disposable Water-Seal System

Assisting with Removal of Chest Tubes

Obtaining Chest Drainage Specimen

Administering Blood through Autotransfusion Using the Pleur-evac ATS

EVALUATION Expected Outcomes

Closed water-seal drainage system maintained until client's lung is reexpanded, and air or fluid is removed from pleural space.

Normal respiratory function restored.

Chest tubes remain patent.

Water-seal system remains intact.

MAINTAINING A THREE-BOTTLE SYSTEM

USING BOTTLE SYSTEMS

One Bottle: One bottle functions as a collection bottle as well as water seal. Used mainly to reestablish negative intrapleural pressure to reinflate lung from pneumothorax.

Two Bottles: Water seal bottle and collection bottle are separate. System not usually connected to suction source. Used following thoracic or cardiac surgery.

Three Bottles: Third bottle is connected to an external suction source. The other two bottles are the same as for two-bottle system. Used following thoracic or cardiac surgery.

Procedure

1. Examine the suction regulator bottle (bottle #3) to check if 10–20-cm negative water pressure is maintained, determined by how deep the longest tube is submerged in the water.

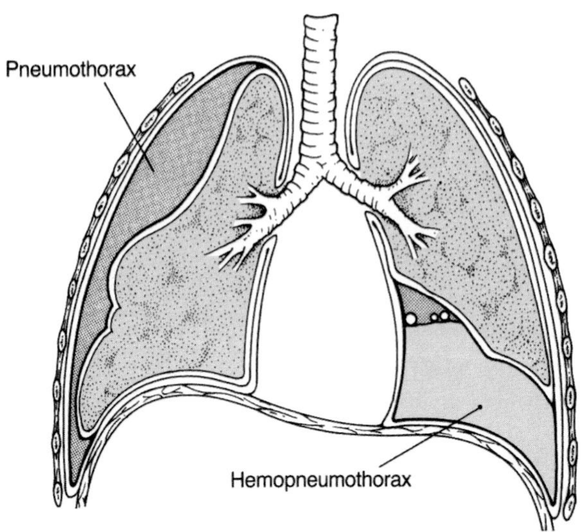

Pneumothorax refers to air in the pleural space and *hemothorax* to blood in the pleural space of the lung; both conditions lead to build-up of positive pressure and collapse of the lung.

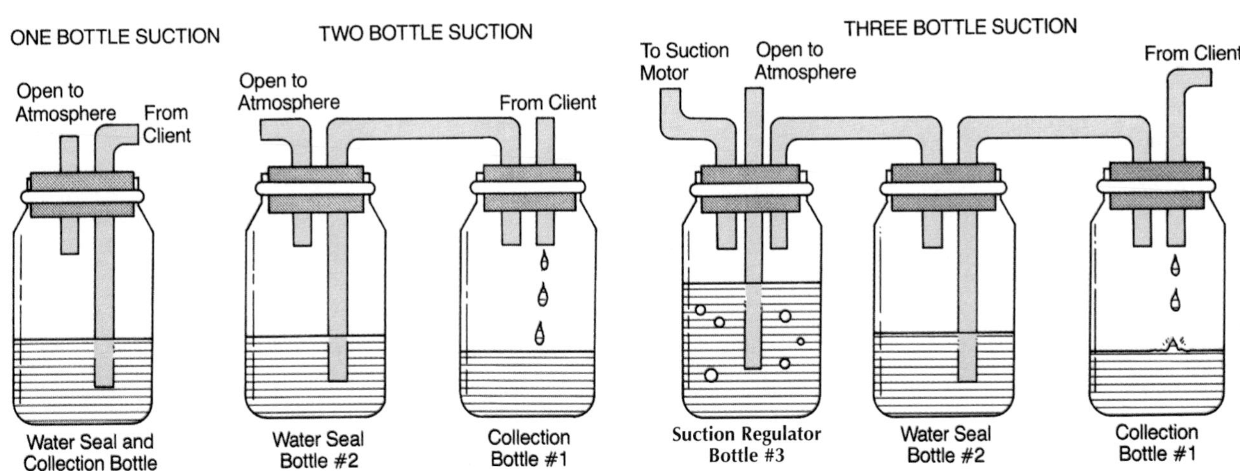

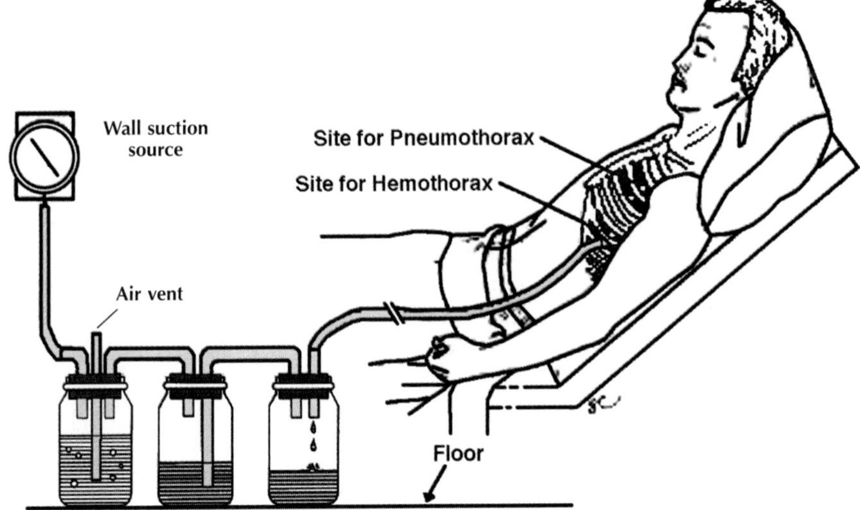

Keep collection system below level of chest tube insertion site.

2. Regulate the wall suction to level where water just bubbles. **Rationale:** Constant bubbling in the control bottle indicates the desired pressure level has been reached.
   a. To increase negative pressure, increase the depth to which the longest tube in the suction control bottle is submerged.
   b. To decrease negative pressure, decrease the depth to which the longest tube is submerged.
3. Examine the water-seal bottle (bottle #2).
   a. Make sure the longer tube is covered with water to maintain the water-seal. **Rationale:** This prevents air from getting into tubing and pleural space, which prevents pneumothorax.
   b. Check water level ($1\frac{1}{2}$ inches) in this bottle to maintain water seal. Ensure that tube is submerged.
   c. Tape all connections between water seal and client to prevent air leaks. You may also band taped connections with wire or plastic cable as an extra precaution against air leaks.
4. Monitor the water-seal bottle for air leaks in system. **Rationale:** These leaks can be identified by constant bubbling in the water-seal bottle.
5. If air leaks occur, clamp tubing close to client's chest (if you have standing orders to do so) and notify the physician immediately.
6. Examine the collection bottle (bottle #1) to determine the amount of drainage per hour. If there is more than 100 mL per hour, notify physician.

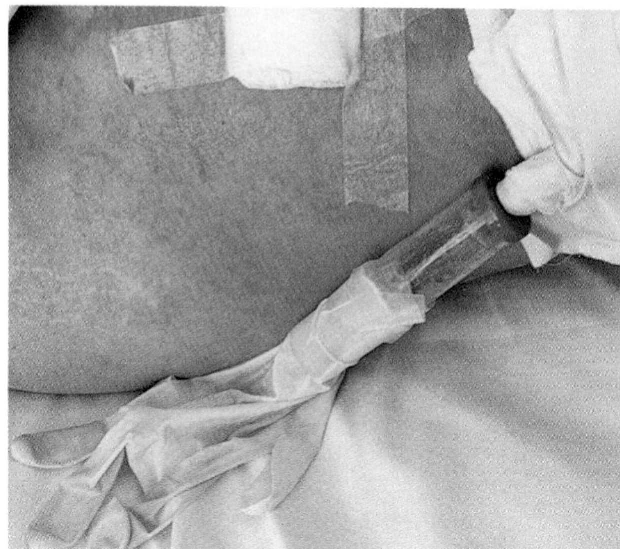

Heimlich valve functions similar to one-bottle suction.

7. Observe and record the drainage level on the collection bottle as ordered:
   a. Every hour immediately after surgery, or if there is a large amount of drainage.
   b. At least every 8 hours while chest tube is inserted; mark the time on the drainage bottle every shift.
8. Whenever the wall suction motor is off, keep the drainage system open to the atmosphere by detaching the tubing from the motor to provide a vent.

SETTING UP AND MAINTAINING A DISPOSABLE WATER-SEAL SYSTEM

Equipment

Disposable water-seal suction, e.g., Pleur-evac, Argyle, Aqua-Seal, Thora-Drain, Thora-Klex
Stand
60-mL Asepto sterile syringe
Sterile water in pouring bottle
Tape or wire
Suction source

Procedure

1. Gather equipment.
2. Unwrap the water-seal system.
3. Place the system on stand at bedside.

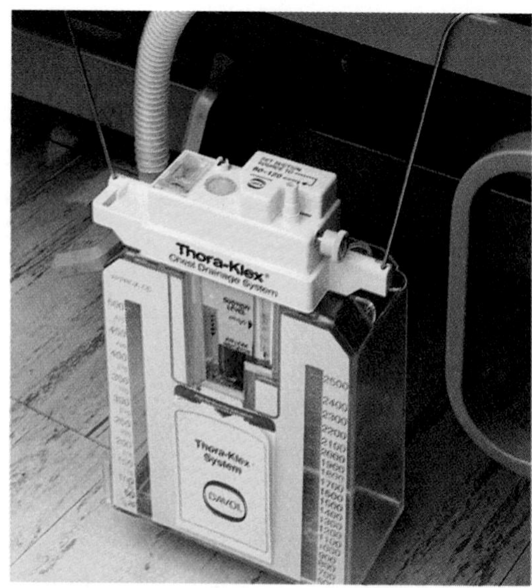

Thora-klex water-seal system.

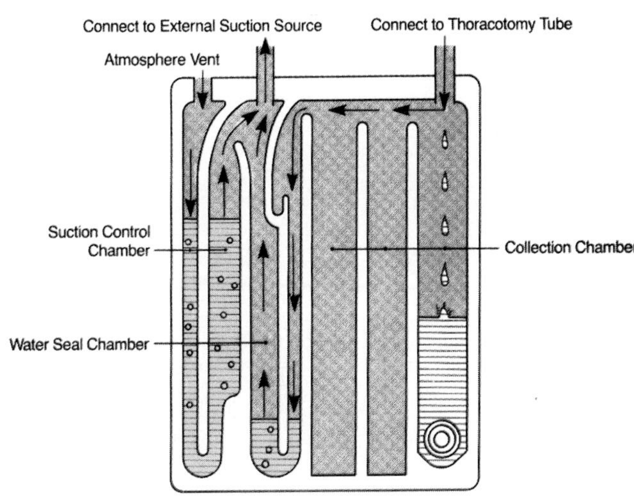

Disposable water-seal system.

4. Remove the plastic connector on the short tube that is attached to the water-seal chamber.
5. Remove the plunger from the large 50–60-mL Asepto syringe. Attach the barrel of the syringe onto short rubber tube to occlude.
6. Pour specified amount of sterile water (according to package directions) into the barrel of the syringe, if not using a pouring bottle of sterile water.
7. Fill the water-seal chamber to the 2-cm level. **Rationale:** This level provides sufficient fluid to create a one-way valve to prevent room air from entering intrapleural space.
8. Remove the plastic plug from the vent to the suction control chamber.
9. Attach the syringe barrel to the vent. Pour sterile water into the chamber. (The tip of the syringe fits into the top of the chamber vent. There is no rubber tubing attached.)
10. Fill the suction control chamber to the 20-cm level.
11. Insert the plastic plug to close the vent.
12. After the physician has inserted chest tubes, remove the long tube adapter from the collection chamber and attach it to the chest tubes.
13. Tape the connector sites.
14. Provide a straight line of tubing from bed to collection system. **Rationale:** Straight-line tubing prevents pooling of fluid.
15. Make sure that tubing is free and not kinked. Do not use pins or restrain tubing. **Rationale:** Pins could puncture tubing causing an air leak.
16. Attach short rubber tube on the water-seal suction to the suction machine (wall or portable), using an adapter connection piece.
17. Turn wall suction device on slowly until bubbling occurs in the suction control chamber.
18. Monitor water levels daily in both the water-seal chamber and the suction control chamber. Refill (20 cm or as ordered) to level with sterile water as needed.
19. Keep rubber-tipped hemostat at the client's bedside. **Rationale:** In emergency, tube can be clamped off nearest to chest insertion site.
20. Maintain pressure.
    a. Keep suction bottles or disposable system below level of bed.
    b. Maintain suction control negative pressure to create gentle bubbling. (Make sure bubbling is not excessive in the control bottle.)
    c. Maintain water-seal level (2 cm). **Rationale:** Water seal prevents room air from entering pleural space.
    d. Maintain suction control chamber water level at 20 cm or as ordered.

CHECK POINTS FOR CHEST TUBE AIR LEAKS

Check Insertion Site: Pinch or briefly clamp with padded hemostat tube at chest insertion site. Bubbling stops in the water-seal chamber if there is an air leak at insertion site.

Check Tubing: Pinch between chest tube and rubber connecting tubing. Bubbling stops if there is a leak at connector site.

Check Water-Seal Drainage System: Pinch between chest tube and rubber connecting tubing. Bubbling continues if there is a leak in water-seal drainage system.

Observe water-seal chamber. There should not be excessive continuous bubbling. A small amount of bubbling is seen in the water seal

- When suction is first initiated.
- As air is displaced by drainage in the collection chambers.
- As client exhales and coughs and air is forced out of pleural space.

When lung has reexpanded, the bubbles cease.

21. Maintain chest tube patency. Only if physician orders, milk chest tubes to maintain drainage and tube patency.
    a. Milk tube away from client toward the drainage receptacle (disposable system or bottles).

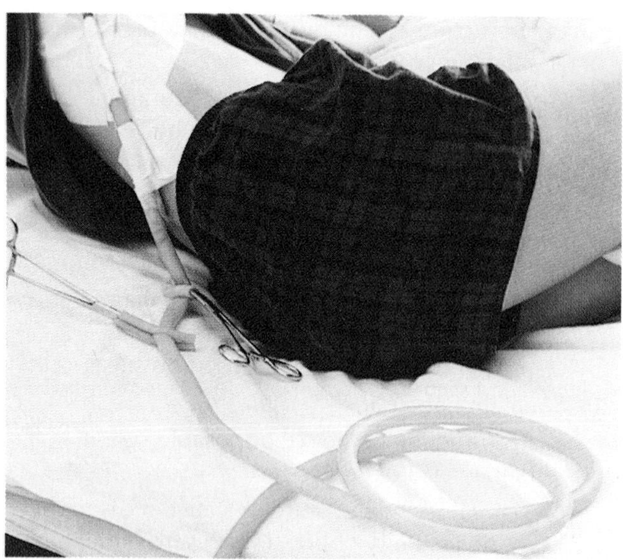

Padded hemostat is used for clamping chest tubes.

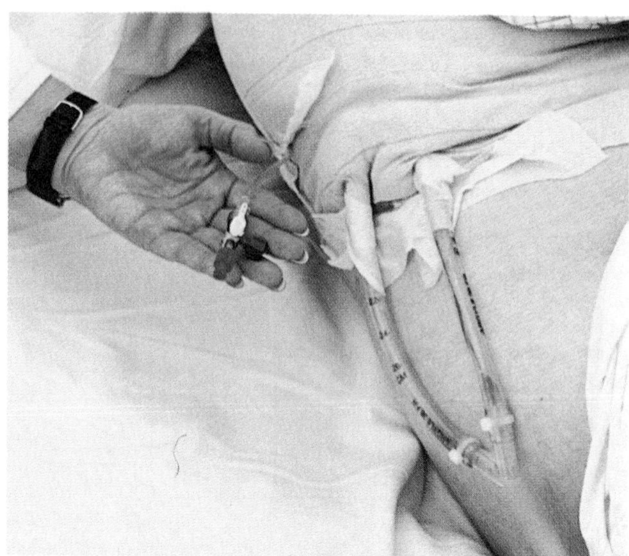

Intrapleural catheter used for pain medication.

b. Milk tube by alternately folding or squeezing and then releasing drainage tubing. **Rationale:** This provides gentle, intermittent suction to the chest tube.

22. Strip chest tubes only if physician orders, following same time frame as milking chest tubes.

> ■ **CLINICAL ALERT**
>
> Strip and milk chest tubes *only* with physician's orders. Excessive negative pressure created by stripping and milking can damage lung tissue.

a. To strip chest tube, pinch tubing close to chest with one hand and, using a lubricated thumb and forefinger, compress and slide fingers down tube toward receptacle. (Lubricant material is usually petrolatum or alcohol swab.)

b. Release pressure on tube and repeat stripping action until reaching receptacle.

23. Keep collection system below level of chest-tube insertion site. **Rationale:** This enables fluid to flow by gravity.
24. Make sure that tubing is free and not kinked. Do not use pins or restrain tubing. **Rationale:** Pins can puncture tubing causing an air leak.
25. Record intake and output. Mark drainage on disposable system collection chamber every shift. Drainage should be measured at eye level. Report drainage exceeding 100 mL/hour.
26. Assess client's status.
    a. Instruct client to deep breathe and cough at frequent intervals. **Rationale:** Frequent deep breathing helps to expand lungs.
    b. Encourage client to change positions frequently. Chest tube drainage does not limit client activity.
    c. Observe and report any unusual respiratory signs or symptoms.
    d. Assess level of pain if present. Note photo with catheter inserted into pleural space for direct administration of pain medication.

ASSISTING WITH REMOVAL OF CHEST TUBES

Equipment

Chest tube removal tray
Suture set
Rubber–tipped clamp
Sterile scissors
Sterile 4 × 4 gauze dressings with petrolatum
Sterile abdominal (ABD) pad
Acclusive dressing
Tape

Procedure

1. Gather equipment and inform client of the steps of the procedure.
2. Assist client to edge of bed.
3. Don sterile gloves.
4. Assist physician to
   a. Remove dressing.
   b. Clip suture of chest tube.
   c. Place clamp on chest tube.
   d. Instruct client to take a deep breath and hold it.
   e. Hold sterile dressing with ABD pad in place

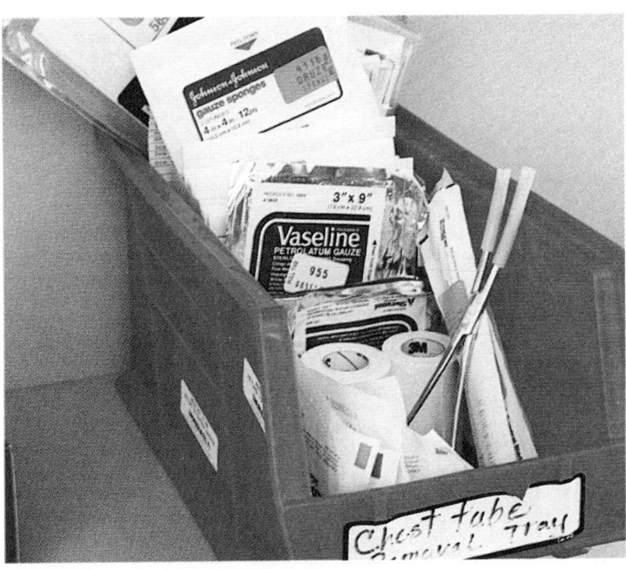

Equipment tray for removal of chest tubes.

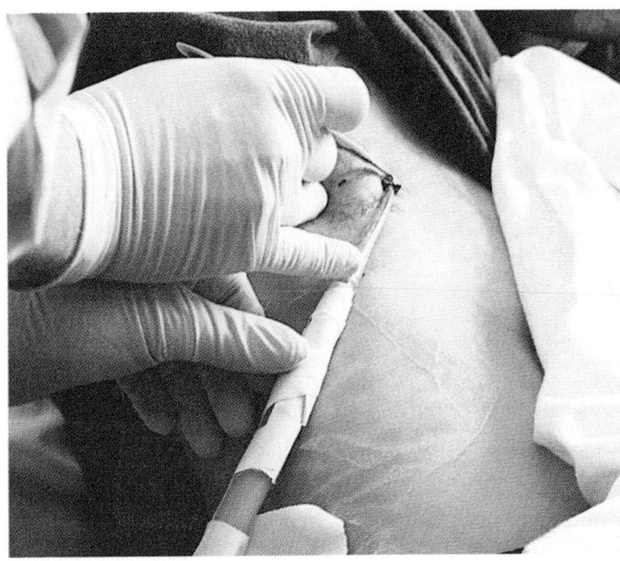

Sutures anchoring chest tube are cut.

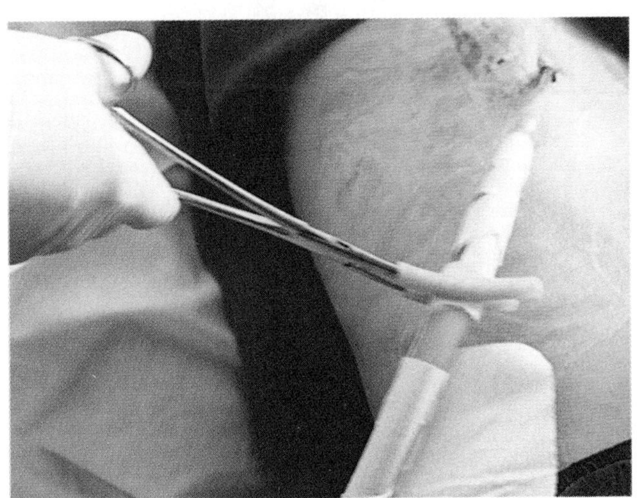

Chest tube is clamped in preparation.

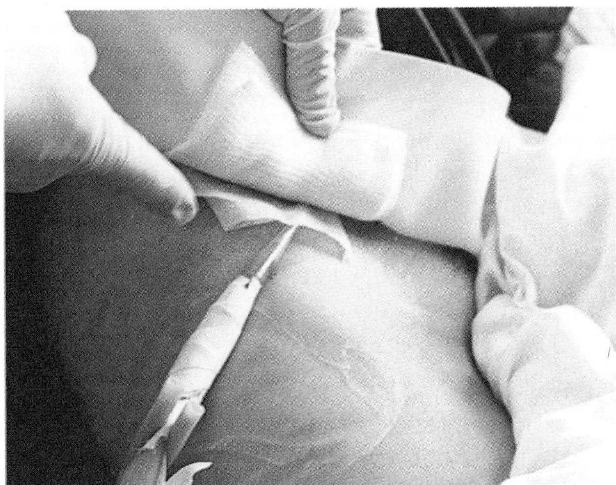

Pressure dressing is applied immediately after tube removal.

while quickly pulling out chest tube.

f. Apply dressing over wound and tape securely.

5. Remove equipment to appropriate area.
6. Remove gloves and discard. Wash hands.
7. Reevaluate client's status for the next 6 hours. **Rationale:** Client should be assessed for unstable vital signs or respiratory distress (pneumothorax) after removal of chest tubes.

OBTAINING CHEST DRAINAGE SPECIMEN

Equipment

10-mL syringe
18–20-gauge needle
Requisition form
Povidone-iodine swab

Procedure

1. Obtain 18- or 20-gauge needle with 10-mL syringe.
2. Swab self-sealing diaphragm on back of the collection chamber with povidone-iodine swab.
3. Insert needle into diaphragm.
4. Withdraw specified amount of drainage.
5. Place needle protector on needle, label specimen with name, hospital number, and source from where specimen was collected.
6. Fill out requisition form, and send to the laboratory with the specimen.

ADMINISTERING BLOOD THROUGH AUTOTRANSFUSION USING PLEUR-EVAC ATS

Equipment

Pleur-evac ATS including blood collection bag
Heparin or citrate phosphate dextrose anticoagulant
18-gauge needle
Replacement bag
Microaggregate filter
Clean gloves

Procedure

1. Wash hands and don gloves.
2. Connect client's chest tube by following steps 1 through 4 printed on Pleur-evac unit. **Rationale:** Tight connection establishes water-seal drainage system.
3. Check that all clamps are open on blood collection bag and tubing and that connections are airtight.
4. Check that chest cavity blood begins collecting in bag.
5. Inject anticoagulant through rubber diaphragm on collection bag's cap, if ordered.
6. Open replacement bag when first bag is nearly full, and close clamps on top of the bag.

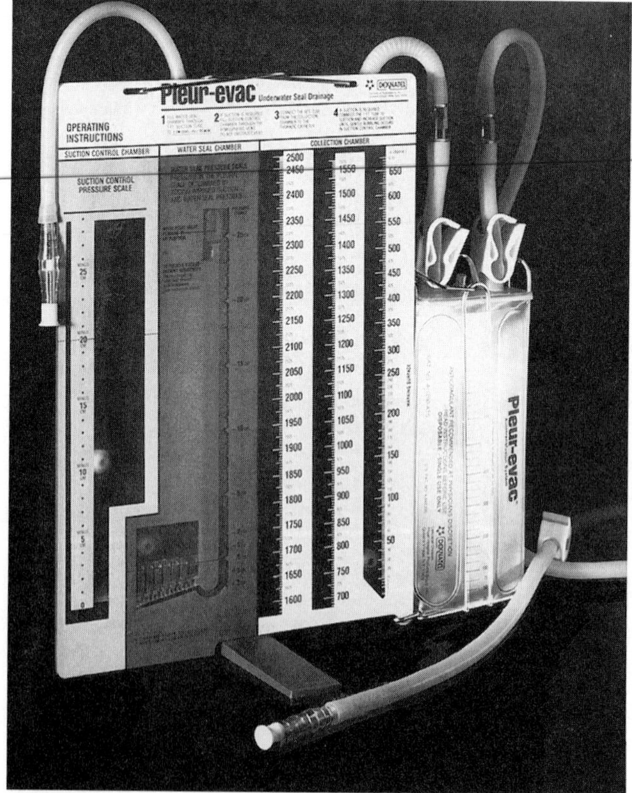

Pleur-evac ATS auto transfusion unit.

7. Depress button on high-negativity relief valve, and release it when negativity drops to desired level. **Rationale:** This reduces excess negativity before removing first collection bag.
8. Close white clamp on client tubing, two white clamps on top of collection bag, and disconnect all connectors on first bag.
9. Remove protective cap from collection tubing on replacement bag. Maintain aseptic technique when changing tubing.
10. Use red connectors to connect collection tubing to client's chest drainage tube.
11. Remove protective cap from replacement bag's suction tube.
12. Use blue connectors to attach replacement bag's suction tube to Pleur-evac unit.
13. Open all clamps, and check that system is airtight.
14. Attach red (female) and blue (male) connector sections on top of autotransfusion bag.
15. Move out and disconnect metal support arms, and disconnect foot hook. **Rationale:** Releasing these connections allows you to remove bag from drainage unit.
16. Attach replacement bag by using foot hook and support arm.
17. Slide bag off support frame and invert bag with spike port pointing up. **Rationale:** This position allows blood to be reinfused from original collection bag.
18. Remove protective cap from spike port, and insert a microaggregate filter. Twist filter into position.
19. Prime filter by gently squeezing inverted bag until drip chamber is half-full.
20. Close clamp on reinfusion line, and remove residual air from bag.
21. Invert bag on IV pole.
22. Flush IV tubing to remove air, and infuse blood according to hospital policy. Blood should be reinfused within 4 hours from start of collection.
23. Remove gloves and wash hands.
24. Assess neurologic signs and pulmonary status every 4 hours. **Rationale:** Microemboli can occur as a result of autotransfusion.
25. Assess pulse rate, temperature every 4 hours. **Rationale:** Sepsis is an infrequent complication.

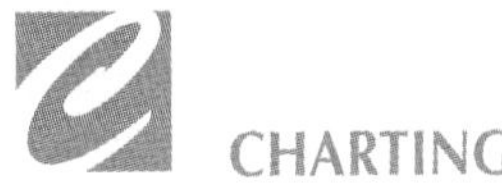

CHARTING

for Chest Tubes

- Size of chest tubes inserted and pressure levels
- Character of drainage
- Client's tolerance of procedure
- Vital signs
- Breath sounds and chest expansion

for Water-Seal Chest Drainage

- Drainage—amount, color, presence of clots
- Any abnormalities in the system and treatment of abnormalities
- Respiratory status, including rate, rhythm, and breath sounds
- Frequency of chest-tube milking

for Autotransfusion

- Amount of blood reinfused
- Signs and symptoms of potential complications, e.g., microemboli, sepsis
- Changes in coagulation times or hemoglobin, hematocrit
- Client's responses to treatment

CRITICAL THINKING APPLICATION

CLINICAL PROBLEMS	CRITICAL THINKING OPTIONS
■ Air leak is present, indicated by bubbling in water-seal bottle or water-seal chamber.	• Check for specific leak area by clamping chest tube (if physician's orders allow) between water-seal bottle or disposable system and client. a. If water-seal bottle continues to bubble, the leak is in the tubing. b. If water-seal bottle stops bubbling, the leak is in the client's chest tube at the site of the insertion. • Secure all connections with tape or wire. • Change tubing if necessary (after obtaining physician's order). • Apply sterile petrolatum gauze and pressure dressing around chest-tube insertion site if air leak is at insertion site.
■ Control bottle is not bubbling.	• Wall suction pressure is too low. Check gauge to wall suction for proper amount.
■ Chest tube becomes dislodged.	• Apply pressure over insertion site with the palm of your hand or any available material, e.g., sheet. Notify physician. • When sterile pressure dressing is obtained, instruct the client to exhale. Then compress the opening, and provide tight seal with dressing. • Observe for signs of respiratory distress: symmetry of chest, respiratory rate, changes in color, or level of consciousness. • Observe for mediastinal shift to unaffected side from tension buildup. (Trachea shifts to unaffected side, and paradoxical pulse develops.)
■ Chest tube becomes disconnected from water-seal drainage system at any one of the connection sites.	• Clamp chest tube near catheter insertion site while replacing extension tubes to prevent pneumothorax from atmospheric air entering intrapleural space during inspiration. • Replace the extension tubing leading from the chest tube with sterile tubing. • Unclamp chest tube as soon as extension tubing is replaced to prevent tension pneumothorax. • Tape or wire new extension connection sites to prevent disconnection. • Observe for signs of respiratory distress due to potential pneumothorax and report.
■ Chest tubes become obstructed by a clot, kink in the chest tube, or pressure on the chest tube.	• Observe for respiratory distress especially if suction is being used to reexpand the lungs, and report immediately. • Observe entire system for kinks in tubing. Loop the tubing on bed. Do not secure with tape. Loop rubber band around the chest tube and put safety pin through rubber band and then pin to linen. Allow sufficient slack. • Observe tubing for signs of clot, decreased flow of fluid through tube, visualization of clotted material in tube. • Obtain order to milk chest tubes.

unit 8 INTUBATION

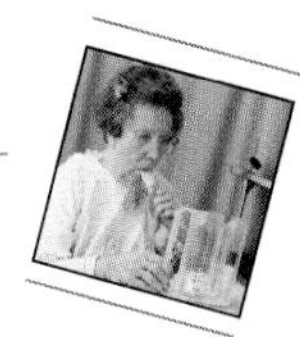

NURSING PROCESS DATA

ASSESSMENT Data Base

Assess client's level of consciousness.

Observe for shortness of breath, labored breathing, tachypnea, or tachycardia.

Note character of secretions.

Check if all lung areas are ventilated adequately.

Note presence of adventitious sounds.

Determine if gag and swallowing reflex are present.

Assess client's ability to understand and cooperate with procedure.

PLANNING Objectives

Oropharyngeal or Nasopharyngeal Intubation

To provide patent airway in an emergency situation

Endotracheal Intubation

To provide patent airway

To provide route for short-term mechanical ventilation

To facilitate removal of pulmonary secretions

To relieve carbon dioxide retention in clients with chronic pulmonary disease

To treat acute respiratory failure

IMPLEMENTATION Procedures

Inserting an Oropharyngeal Airway

Inserting a Nasopharyngeal Airway

Assisting with Endotracheal Intubation

Measuring Cuff Pressure

Providing Care for Client with an Endotracheal Tube

EVALUATION Expected Outcomes

Patent airway maintained in emergency situation.

Route established for mechanical ventilation in either short-term or long-term therapy.

Secretions easily suctioned so that pulmonary complications can be treated or prevented.

Lungs aerated more easily.

Artificial airway provided when upper airway is obstructed.

INSERTING AN OROPHARYNGEAL AIRWAY

Equipment

Oropharyngeal tube

Tongue depressor

Clean gloves

Procedure

1. Select appropriate size airway—length should be from teeth to end of jaw line.
2. Wash your hands; don gloves.
3. Open client's mouth with tongue depressor. You may need to hyperextend client's neck to insert tube.

4. Turn airway upside down (curved upward) and, as airway passes uvula, rotate the airway 180°. **Rationale:** This position facilitates insertion and guides direction of the airway.
5. Check that curve fits over tongue. It should extend from the lips to the pharynx, displacing the tongue anteriorly. **Rationale:** Proper positioning helps prevent injury to lips, teeth, tongue, and posterior pharynx.
6. Tape airway in position. **Rationale:** Stabilization of the tube prevents injuries.
7. Position client on side to facilitate drainage.
8. Remove gloves and discard.
9. Observe position of airway within first hour.

INSERTING A NASOPHARYNGEAL AIRWAY

Equipment

Nasopharyngeal tube
Water-soluble lubricant
Clean gloves

Procedure

1. Select appropriate size tube—should be slightly narrower than client's nares.
2. Wash your hands; don gloves.
3. Lubricate entire length of tube.
4. Insert tube gently through one naris. Follow anatomic line of nasal passage. If obstructed, try other naris.
5. Tape tube in position if necessary.

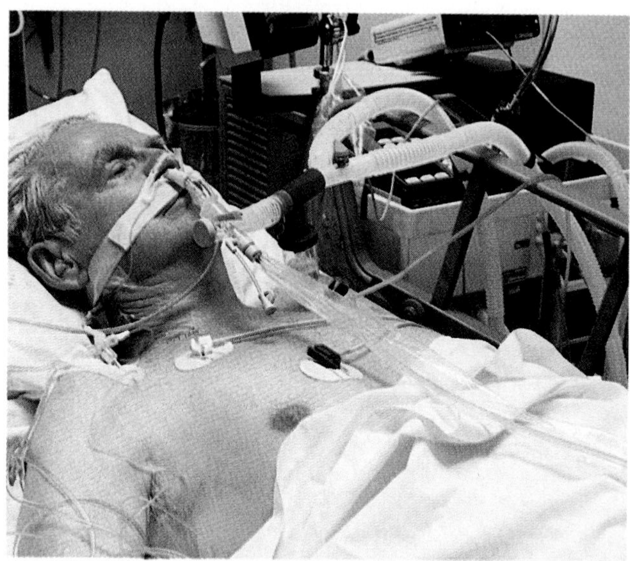

Nasopharyngeal airway in place connected to nebulizer and suction.

ASSISTING WITH ENDOTRACHEAL INTUBATION*

*Only nurses with special preparation or those who are ACLS certified should actually perform endotracheal intubation.

Equipment

Topical and local anesthetic agents: usually 4% lidocaine spray for tongue, gums, and pharynx; 10% cocaine hydrochloride for nares
Laryngoscope with several blade sizes
Water-soluble lubricant
McGill forceps
2.5-cm micropore tape
Disposable plastic syringes (5–10 mL) for cuff inflation
Stylet to guide endotracheal tube, if needed
Clean gloves

Note: New noninvasive positive pressure ventilation methods using nasal pillows, nasal mask, oral mask, or mouthpiece with special headgear provide an appropriate alternative to intubation for many clients with ventilatory insufficiency.

Preparation

1. Explain procedure and rationale to client or to family.
2. Assemble all equipment.
3. Wash your hands; don gloves.
4. Remove client's dentures or bridgework.
5. Check laryngoscope light. (Extra batteries and bulbs should be available.)
6. Inspect tracheal cuff for intactness by inflating cuff.
7. Lubricate tube.
8. Check that all necessary devices for ventilation, oxygenation, and suctioning are functioning.

Procedure

1. Place client in supine position with head and neck hyperextended and a pillow under shoulders. **Rationale:** Proper positioning facilitates intubation and prevents complications, such as erosion and necrosis of nasal septum and turbinates.
2. Restrain client's hands if necessary. Verbally explain why you are using restraints. **Rationale:** Interference during insertion could damage airway.
3. Hyperoxygenate before and after suctioning using an ambu bag with 100% O_2 before intubation.
4. Explain procedure as you proceed. **Rationale:** A clear, step-by-step explanation reduces client's anxiety.
5. Mark tube at level of client's mouth, and tape securely with micropore tape. (Benzoin may be applied before taping to secure tube.) **Rationale:** Secure taping prevents tube displacement.
6. Insert oral airway or bite block when tube is positioned orally.
7. Inflate cuff with 5–10 mL of air after intubation is completed.
8. Auscultate at cuff tracheal site (suprasternal notch) for a slight hissing sound at peak of inspiration. **Rationale:** This ensures adequate cuff inflation.
9. Place client on ventilator or administer humidity or oxygen with T-piece.
10. Auscultate lung fields for ventilation and aeration. **Rationale:** Bilateral breath sounds indicate correct placement.
11. Prepare client for chest x-ray if ordered. **Rationale:** X-ray is used to determine exact placement of tube.
12. Place client in semi-Fowler's or Fowler's position. **Rationale:** This position increases ventilation.
13. Place call bell and writing material within client's reach.
14. Discard disposable equipment and gloves.
15. Clean and return nondisposable equipment to designated place.

MEASURING CUFF PRESSURE

Equipment

Manometer

Procedure

1. Measure cuff pressure every shift. **Rationale:** Regulation prevents overdistention and excess pressure on tracheal wall.
2. Attach pilot balloon tubing to a syringe and mercury manometer by a four-way stopcock.
3. Turn off stopcock to client.
4. Compress syringe until manometer reads 20 mm Hg. **Rationale:** This adds air pressure to system.
5. Turn on stopcock to client, and adjust pressure by syringe. **Rationale:** Manipulation of syringe can set pressure at 20 mm Hg or less, which is preferable setting for client. As pressure exceeds 20 mm Hg, arterial circulation to trachea is severely diminished.
6. Close stopcock to pilot balloon and manometer.
7. Record pressure on ventilator flowsheet.

PROVIDING CARE FOR CLIENT WITH ENDOTRACHEAL TUBE

Procedure

1. Monitor breath sounds every 4 hours. Breath sounds should be heard equally throughout lung fields bilaterally.
2. Check marked points on tube at insertion point. **Rationale:** This determines if tube has moved.
3. Inspect positioning and stabilization of tube. **Rationale:** A change of position can obstruct airway or cause erosion and necrosis of tissues.
4. Inspect and clean mouth and nose. Observe for evidence of pressure areas or ulceration.
5. Provide mouth care every 2 hours. **Rationale:** Because client breathes through mouth, mucous membranes become dry.
6. Support client's head and tube when turning. **Rationale:** This prevents tube from becoming dislodged or airway from becoming obstructed.
7. Place call bell within reach and provide alternative means of communication when cuffed tube is in place. **Rationale:** No air passes over larynx, so client is not able to talk.
8. Support client during this time by spending extra time, using touch, and anticipating client's needs.

CHARTING for Intubation

- Clinical manifestations indicating need for intubation
- Specific reason for intubation
- Size and type of inserted endotracheal, nasopharyngeal, or oropharyngeal tube
- Preoxygenation and postoxygenation with suctioning
- Type and quantity of secretions
- Client's tolerance of procedure
- Type and settings of ventilator connected to tube

CRITICAL THINKING APPLICATION

CLINICAL PROBLEMS	CRITICAL THINKING OPTIONS
■ Pharyngeal airway cannot be inserted.	• Change size of tube. • Relubricate nasopharyngeal airway and attempt to reinsert. • Hyperextend client's neck. • Insert tube at different angle. • Insert oropharyngeal rather than nasopharyngeal airway.
■ Laryngospasm occurs when endotracheal tube is inserted.	• If not severe, remove tube and wait a few minutes. • If severe, give client a muscle relaxant such as succinylcholine chloride. Physician's orders are required for this action. • If severe and causing respiratory distress, you may need to prepare for a tracheostomy.
■ Endotracheal tube is inaccurately placed into right main bronchus.	• Obtain order for chest x-ray to ascertain exact placement of tube. • Pull back slightly on tube, and auscultate for ventilation of lung fields bilaterally.
■ Prolonged endotracheal intubation causes laryngeal damage.	• A cool aerosol mist is helpful in reducing swelling after intubation.
■ Accidental extubation occurs.	• Call physician immediately. Obtain laryngoscope, blades, and extra endotracheal tubes. • Observe the marking on the tube every 2–4 hours to ensure tube placement and to prevent accidental extubation.
■ Client is unable to eat with tube inserted.	• Reassess dietary measures for administering calories. • Weigh daily. • Consider instituting enteral nutrition.

unit 9

TRACHEOSTOMY INTUBATION

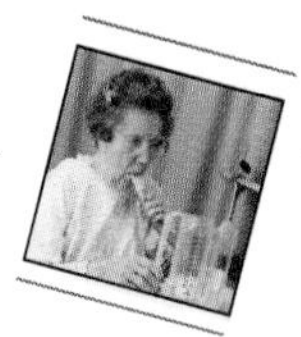

NURSING PROCESS DATA

ASSESSMENT Data Base

Assess severity of respiratory distress.

Determine need for tracheostomy compared with less intrusive methods of providing patent airway.

Assess client's level of consciousness to determine client's ability to understand explanation and instructions.

Observe client's respiratory status: labored breathing, tachypnea, or tachycardia.

Note presence of adventitious breath sounds.

PLANNING Objectives

To provide patent airway

To provide route for long-term mechanical ventilation

To facilitate removal of pulmonary secretions

To increase ventilatory capacity (gas exchange)

IMPLEMENTATION Procedure

Assisting with Tracheostomy Intubation

EVALUATION Expected Outcomes

Artificial airway provided when upper airway is obstructed.

Anatomic dead space decreased.

Route established for long-term ventilatory assistance.

Secretions easily suctioned.

Pulmonary toilet accomplished.

ASSISTING WITH TRACHEOSTOMY INTUBATION

Equipment

Sterile tracheostomy tray
Povidone-iodine solution for cleansing skin
Lidocaine for local anesthesia
Sterile tracheal tube with obturator
Sterile gloves
Clean gloves
Suction equipment
Manual resuscitator bag
Mechanical ventilator
T-piece, mask, oxygen equipment if needed
Humidifier
Applicator sticks
Hydrogen peroxide
Sterile dressing

Preparation

1. Explain procedure and rationale to client or relatives (or both).
2. If not an emergency situation, obtain permission from client or other legally responsible individual prior to tracheostomy.
3. Wash your hands.
4. Assemble all necessary equipment.
5. Set up tracheostomy tray where sterile field may be maintained; open tray when physician is ready.
6. Obtain order for muscle-relaxant premedication if client's condition allows. **Rationale:** A muscle relaxant prevents choking during intubation.

Procedure

1. Explain procedure as it is being done if client is alert.
2. Restrain client, if necessary, with soft hand restraints. **Rationale:** Interference during insertion can contaminate equipment and increase the time required for insertion.
3. Open sterile gloves for physician. Don clean gloves.
4. Assist physician by pouring povidone-iodine solution into sterile containers on tray. To maintain sterile technique, lidocaine is usually held by the nurse while the physician draws it out of vial.
5. Have suction equipment ready when tracheal tube is inserted. Use suction catheter half the diameter of the tracheostomy. **Rationale:** Secretions have accumulated, and client may panic if he feels he is choking.
6. Suction when tube is inserted. If necessary, suction when tube is in place. Preoxygenate before suctioning.
7. Secure tracheal ties using two people. **Rationale:** To prevent dislodging tube, one person is required to hold tracheostomy tube and the other secures ties.
   a. Turn end of twill tape back on itself 1 inch.
   b. Make $\frac{1}{2}$ inch cut horizontally in tape.
   c. Thread one end of tape through flange of tracheal tube.
   d. Pull other end of tape over flange and through slot in the tape.
   e. Repeat steps (a) through (d) for other side of flange.
   f. Tie the ends of tape at the side of client's neck to secure tracheal tube in place. **Rationale:** Ties at back of neck are uncomfortable for client in supine position.
   g. For children, pull tape through each side, doubling it, and tie all pieces at the back of the neck. **Rationale:** This position prevents children from loosening ties.
   h. Insert one finger between neck and tape before securing and knotting ties. **Rationale:** This ensures that ties are not too tight.
8. Attach tracheal tube with an adapter to mechanical ventilator.
9. Cleanse tracheal opening with applicator sticks and hydrogen peroxide or normal saline to remove blood from site. **Rationale:** This measure assists in preventing infection. (This is a clean procedure; gloves may or may not be worn, depending on hospital policy.)
10. Apply sterile tracheal dressing around tracheal opening under tube.
11. Keep a sterile tracheostomy tube of the same size at the bedside. **Rationale:** If tube is dislodged, replacement tube can be immediately inserted.
12. Reposition client for comfort. If not contraindicated, place in semi-Fowler's position. **Rationale:** This position makes breathing easier for client.
13. Place call bell where client can reach it, and provide means of communication.
14. Clean nondisposable equipment, and return to cleaning area.
15. Remove gloves and discard.

PREVENTING INFECTION

- Maintain sterile technique during intubation and suctioning.
- Maintain good handwashing technique.
- Administer good oral care every 4 hours.
- If client is on ventilator, dispose of condensed water from tubing.
- Change ventilatory equipment every 24–48 hours.

CHARTING for Tracheostomy Intubation

- Clinical manifestations and need for intubation
- Size and type of tracheal tube inserted
- Name of physician performing procedure
- Client's tolerance of procedure
- Amount and character of secretions
- Respiratory status before and after procedure
- Any equipment attached to tracheal tube, type of ventilator, and percent oxygen delivered.

CRITICAL THINKING APPLICATION

CLINICAL PROBLEMS	CRITICAL THINKING OPTIONS
■ Artificial airway cannot be inserted due to upper airway obstruction.	• Obtain smaller size tracheostomy tube or change type of tubes. • Hyperextend neck more. • Have CPR cart available for immediate use. • Auscultate all lung fields to assess degree of ventilation.
■ Secretions cannot be easily suctioned.	• Provide postural drainage, percussion, and vibration to help mobilize retained secretions. • Change suction catheter size. • Provide warm, humidified air through ventilator, tracheostomy mask, or T-piece. • Before suctioning, instill 5–10 mL sterile, normal saline into tracheal tube to stimulate cough so as to mobilize secretions.
■ Client becomes dyspneic while tracheal tube is inserted.	• Suction through tracheal opening or through nose. • Remove tube as it may be inaccurately placed in prebronchial tissue. • Until client relaxes, manually ventilate client with resuscitation bag after insertion of tube is complete.
■ Placement of tube is inaccurate.	• Auscultate all lung fields at least every 4 hours to ensure ventilation. • Observe for signs of surgical emphysema or cardiopulmonary collapse. • Obtain physician's order for x-ray to verify tube placement in trachea. • Replace tube with different size.
■ Accidental extubation occurs. (Usually occurs within first 5 days or during suctioning when cuff is deflated.)	• Have emergency equipment at bedside. Sterile tracheal set of same size and style Ties and syringes for inflating cuff Tracheal dilator, scissors, and hemostats Sterile gloves and dressings • Ensure patent airway by one of the following methods: Immediately insert tracheal dilator into stoma to preserve airway. Insert old tube if new one not available to preserve patent airway. Suction stoma, if there is time. Then reinsert new tracheal tube, secure with tapes, and establish ventilation. Oxygenate with ambu bag if signs of respiratory distress are present.

CLINICAL PROBLEMS	CRITICAL THINKING OPTIONS
Hemorrhage from tracheostomy site is noted.	• Apply pressure if hemorrhage site is accessible. • Have physician cauterize bleeding vessels. • Take client to operating room for exploration of site and ligation of bleeding vessel if physician orders surgery.
Tracheostomy is obstructed.	• If no physician available, follow these procedures: Deflate cuff. Cut tracheostomy ties. Remove tube. Insert tracheal dilator (if at bedside). Establish airway. Insert new tube, and reestablish ventilation.

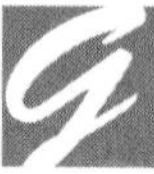

GERIATRIC CONSIDERATIONS

The physiologic age changes that occur in the elderly affect the respiratory system.

- The respiratory muscles lose their strength and the rib cage becomes more rigid.
- Lungs lose their elasticity, breathing capacity decreases, and depth of respirations decrease.
- The alveoli increase in size and decrease in number as well as becoming less elastic and more dilated.
- Gas exchange is reduced; the PaO_2 decreases 1 mm/year after age 60, so a reading of 75 mm Hg is expected in an elderly client.
- Skeletal alterations affect posture and restrict lung expansion.

Pulmonary disorders occur more frequently in the elderly and are the fourth leading cause of death.

- Functional respiratory reserve is reduced with aging; the elderly are at greater risk for respiratory failure.
- Pneumonia may occur spontaneously or as a complication of other conditions. Because it is frequently a cause of death in the elderly, this condition should be assessed for and monitored aggressively.
- COPD, a broad classification of pulmonary disorders, is a major cause of death and disability, especially among the elderly.
- Asthma, included in the COPD group classification, may occur as a problem in the elderly who have never had the disease.
- Cancer of the lung is not uncommon in the elderly.

It is important to implement nursing actions that support the respiratory system in the elderly because of their compromised capability.

- Respiratory activity and exercises are necessary to promote gas exchange: deep breathing, forced expiration, coughing, and moderate exercise.
- Monitor hydration status to liquefy secretions and prevent dehydration.
- Monitor oxygen therapy closely with the elderly—low levels of oxygen with COPD; check for carbon dioxide narcosis.
- The elderly are at especially high risk for hypoxemia with bed rest (PO_2 may drop to 40 mm Hg even with a night's sleep). Position change (supine to sitting) and regular turning must be encouraged in the bedfast.

26

Circulatory Maintenance

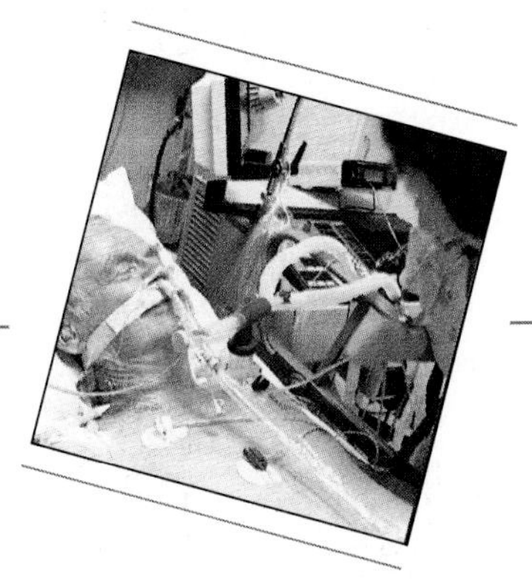

LEARNING OBJECTIVES

- Identify three properties of the cardiac muscle and define cardiac output.
- Define the words "inotropic" and "chronotropic."
- State the reason it is important to minimize the client's stress when hemorrhage occurs.
- Outline the assessment actions for a client who is hemorrhaging.
- Identify two interventions for treating pump failure.
- Define the term "ischemia."
- List the nine pressure points in the body that can be used to control bleeding if hemorrhage occurs.
- Identify two potential problems that could occur in clients who are bleeding, and state one suggested solution for each problem.
- Describe how to measure appropriately for elastic hosiery.
- List at least four potential problems for clients requiring CPR and two suggested solutions for each problem.
- Outline the steps in administering CPR with one rescuer and with two rescuers.
- Compare and contrast the differences in administering CPR to an infant or small child.
- Demonstrate the steps in performing the Heimlich maneuver.
- State two nursing diagnoses relevant to clients with circulatory dysfunction.
- Differentiate between a normal and abnormal ECG pattern.

TERMINOLOGY

Antiembolic: a preventive measure used to help prevent the formation of an embolism, such as elastic hosiery.

Atherosclerosis: a form of arteriosclerosis in which accumulations of lipid-containing material are localized within the surfaces of the blood vessels.

Cardio: pertaining to the heart.

Cardiovascular: pertaining to the heart and blood vessels.

Chronotropic: modification of a repetitive event such as the heartbeat through external causes.

Conductivity: the specific electric conducting capability of a substance.

Congestion: the presence of an excessive amount of blood or fluid in an organ or tissue.

Contractility: having the ability to contract or shorten.

Cyanosis: slightly bluish, grayish, slatelike, or dark purple discoloration of the skin resulting form reduced hemoglobin or oxygen in the blood.

Dilatation: expansion of an organ or vessel.

Dorsiflexion: movement of a part at a joint so as to bend the part toward the dorsum, or posterior, aspect of the body.

Ecchymosis: a form of macula appearing in large, irregularly formed hemorrhagic areas of the skin; color is blue-black, changing to greenish brown or yellow.

Edema: a condition in which the body tissues contain an excessive amount of fluid.

Embolism: obstruction of a blood vessel by foreign substances or a blood clot.

Endocardial: within the heart or arising form the endocardium.

Endocardium: serous lining membrane of the inner surface and cavities of the heart.

Endotracheal: within the trachea.

Epistaxis: hemorrhage from the nose.

Hematemesis: vomiting of blood.

Hematoma: a swelling or mass of blood, usually clotted, confined to a specific space and caused by a break in a blood vessel.

Heme: a prefix meaning blood.

Hemodynamic: the study of the circulation of the blood.

Hemoptysis: expectoration of blood arising from hemorrhage of the larynx, trachea, bronchi, or lungs.

Hemorrhage: abnormal internal or external discharge of blood.

Homan's sign: pain in the calf when the toe is dorsiflexed. An early sign of deep vein thrombosis in the calf.

Hydrostatic: pertaining to the pressure of liquids in equilibrium and that exerted on liquids.

Hypotension: low blood pressure; a deficiency of tone.

Immobilize: the making of a part or limb immovable.

Inotropic: influencing the contractibility of muscle tissue.

Ischemia: local and temporary anemia due to the obstruction of the circulation to a part.

Perfusion: passing of fluid through spaces.

Petechiae: small, purplish, hemorrhagic spots on the skin, which appear in certain severe fevers.

Phlebitis: inflammation of a vein.

Precordial: pertaining to the precordium or epigastrium.

Purpura: hemorrhage into the skin, mucuous membranes, internal organs, and other tissues.

Resuscitation: act of bringing one back to full consciousness.

Sclerosis: hardening or induration of an organ or tissue due to excessive growth of fibrous tissue.

Shock: term used to designate a clinical syndrome with varying degrees of disturbances of oxygen supply to the tissues and return to the heart.

Stasis: standing still; stagnation of normal flow of fluids.

Syncope: fainting, transient loss of consciousness due to inadequate blood flow to the brain.

Thoracentesis: surgical entry into the thoracic cavity in order to remove fluid.

Thrombosis: formation of a blood clot.

Tinnitus: subjective ringing in the ear.

Vertigo: sensation of moving or having objects around you move when they are actually still, due to a disturbance of balance.

THE CIRCULATORY SYSTEM

The heart is a three-layered, four-chambered organ, approximately the size of an adult fist. It weighs close to 600 grams in the normal adult. A thick, fibrous sheath, called the pericardium, surrounds about two-thirds of the heart's surface. Most of the mass lies in the heart's middle layer—the myocardium, or cardiac muscle. The endocardium, a thin, inner layer, lines the four chambers.

In considering the heart's chambers, imagine two major pump systems. The right and left atria contract in one phase, and the right and left ventricles contract in the successive phase. The tricuspid, pulmonary, mitral, and aortic valves are the four flow regulators for the chambers.

Three properties of cardiac muscle best illustrate the heart's specialization. Automaticity physiologically differentiates heart muscle from all other muscle tissue. The other two properties—conductivity and contractility—characterize all muscle; however, a cardiac contraction is normally all or none, as opposed to partial contractions in other muscles.

The heart serves as a pump to maintain blood flow and blood pressure. Adequate blood flow perfuses the lungs for oxygenation. Blood pressure is a driving force for that flow and is normally highest during ventricular contractions. The heart pumps 4–7 L of blood per minute. This constitutes a normal cardiac output, formulated by multiplying contraction volume times ventricular rate.

When the heart maintains a safe blood pressure and blood flow, it is in a state of compensation, regardless of cardiac output. If the heart cannot maintain a safe blood pressure and blood flow, it is in a state of decompensation. Three cardiac reserves allow for compensation: inotropic reserve, increased venous filling pressure, and chronotropic reserve.

Inotropic reserve is under the control of sympathetic nerve stimulation. Adrenergic drugs, as well as some others, exert an inotropic effect by increasing the force of the cardiac contraction and therefore stroke volume. Cardiac output also increases with additional filling pressure in the atria. Starling's law of the heart summarizes the relationship by stating that an increased filling pressure causes an increased force of contraction within the elastic limits of the heart. Finally, chronotropic reserve refers to increased cardiac output. Atropine-like drugs exert a chronotropic effect by increasing the heart rate.

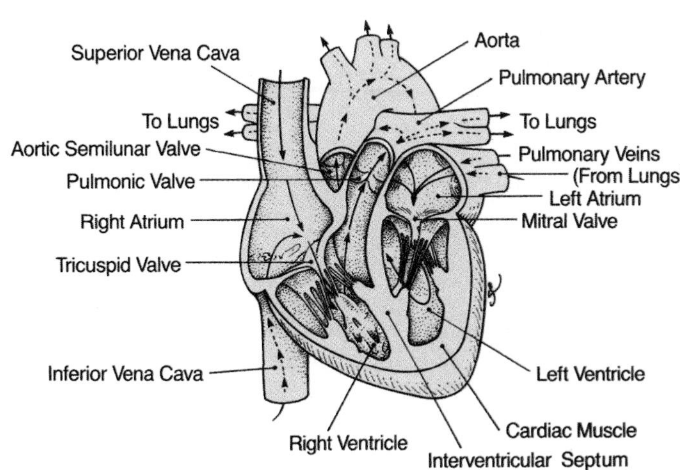

Blood flow pattern through the right and left side of the heart.

Blood vessels, together with the heart, form a closed circulatory system unless there is damage or abnormalities that result in leakage. When the ventricles contract, blood leaves the right ventricle through the pulmonic valve into the pulmonary artery. Blood is now in the pulmonary circulation for oxygenation of the red blood cells, or erythrocytes. After gas exchange occurs at the cellular level, the blood is returned to the left atrium through four pulmonary veins. This is normally the most oxygenated blood in the human body.

On the left side of the heart during a ventricular contraction, blood travels through the aortic valve out of the left ventricle into the ascending aorta. Five percent, or 200–350 mL, of this blood enters coronary circulation for oxygenation and waste removal from the cardiac tissue. Fifteen percent, or 600–1050 mL, travels to the brain and 25%, or 1000–1750 mL, goes to the kidneys, and the same amount to other viscera. The extremities and skin normally receive 30% of the circulating volume.

Arteries carry blood from the heart throughout the body unless obstructed or severed. The largest vessel is the aorta, and the smallest is the arteriole. Similar to the heart, arteries have three layers: endothelium, involuntary muscle, and connective tissue. Capillaries join the arterial system to the venous system and are a single cell layer in thickness. The single layer allows gas, nutrients, and waste exchanges to occur throughout the body. Blood enters the venous system from the capillary beds for eventual return to the right side of the heart via the superior and inferior vena cava.

ELECTRICAL CONDUCTION

Cardiac muscle cells have an inherent rhythmicity that allows for their spontaneous, repetitive self-stimulation. The rate and rhythm of cardiac contractions are primarily determined by this self-generated impulse. The autonomic nervous system affects the heart rate. Sympathetic stimulation increases heart rate and conduction rate through the atrioventricular (AV) node. Parasympathetic stimulation slows the heart rate by decreasing the firing rate of the sinoatrial (SA) note and the speed of conduction through the AV node.

The electrical impulse starts at the SA node located at the junction of the superior vena cava and the right atrium. It functions as the pacemaker for the heart. The SA node initiates approximately 60–100 impulses each minute. The impulse travels to the AV node, located in the right atrial wall near the tricuspid valve. If there is a problem with the impulse being generated in the SA node, the AV node can actually take over as the pacemaker. Over the long term, this may present a problem because the intrinsic rate of the AV node is only 40–60 impulses per minute. The AV node coordinates the incoming electrical impulse from the atria and relays an impulse to the ventricles. The impulse travels in the septum through the bundle of His specialized muscle fibers, which divide into the right and left bundle branches. The impulse continues to the Purkinje fibers, where it terminates. The right bundle reaches out into the right ventricular muscle. The left bundle divides into the left anterior and left posterior bundle branches. These branches reach out into the left ventricular muscle. Further depolarization of the myocardium takes place by conduction through the muscle fibers themselves. If both the SA and AV node are dysfunctional, the myocardium continues to beat, but at a rate of less than 40 BPM. This rate is the intrinsic pacemaker rate of ventricular myocardial cells.

The electrocardiogram (ECG) is used to detect abnormalities associated with the conduction system. The waveforms, which indicate the electrical activity of the myocardium, are analyzed using the ECG printout. The P wave represents atrial muscle depolarization. The QRS complex represents ventricular muscle depolarization. The T wave represents ventricular muscle repolarization. Each segment of the waveform is analyzed for time and configuration of the waveform. Abnormalities in time or configuration indicate a problem is occurring in that specific area of the heart.

Each segment of the heart depicts a different type of waveform termed a dysrhythmia, when abnormalities occur with the myocardial activity in that segment. An atrial dysrhythmia results from a problem with the SA node or atria indicated by an abnormality in the P wave configuration. A ventricular dysrhythmia results from a problem with the ventricle and is indicated by an abnormality in the configuration of the QRS complex. A junctional dysrhythmia occurs when there is a problem associated with the AV node as indicated by a change in the PR interval. A ventricular dysrhythmia is the most life-threatening because it compromises cardiac output.

ALTERATIONS IN CIRCULATION

There are many ways to categorize disorders of the heart, arteries, and veins. Endocarditis, myocarditis, and pericarditis classify cardiac problems according to inflammation of a particular heart layer. Another classification is congenital heart disease, such as tetralogy of Fallot and transposition of the great vessels. For the purpose of this chapter alterations of circulation are divided into hemorrhage, shock, pump failure, ischemia, thrombosis, and embolism.

Hemorrhage

Hemorrhage results when trauma or disease causes leakage in the closed circulatory system. Damage to the heart or arteries usually constitutes the greatest danger because of the high pressure and large volumes. Normally, when a blood vessel ruptures or is severed, compensatory mechanisms protect the body from significant blood loss. The wall of the injured vessel contracts immediately. A platelet plug forms at the site, and blood clotting occurs. New connective tissue penetrates the clot for permanent closure. Interventions for clients who are hemorrhaging are based on one of these compensatory mechanisms.

To prevent, correct, or compensate for hemorrhage, the nurse must assess the client. She identifies the nature of the bleeding as external or internal (or both) and establishes baseline data, which includes blood pressure and vital signs. An assessment is made of the body's response, adaptive, excessive, or deficient, and the nurse assists in formulating and planning appropriate interventions. The first concern is to minimize the client's stress, since sympathetic stimulation of the heart increases heart rate (chronotropic effect) and force of contraction (inotropic effect). Interventions for hemorrhage involve restricting activity, elevating involved body areas above the heart if possible, applying direct pressure, and replacing lost fluid volume. A tourniquet is generally used as a last resort. It is placed proximal to the site of the hemorrhage with the knowledge that the extremity may be sacrificed.

Shock

Unchecked hemorrhage eventually leads to hypovolemic or hemorrhagic shock, a serious state with a poor prognosis. Peripheral resistance is of great significance. In hemorrhagic shock, high peripheral resistance is secondary to pronounced peripheral vasoconstriction in the initial stage. Due to the loss of blood volume it becomes very difficult to start an intravenous line in a superficial vein. Vasoconstrictors, such as Levophed, are undesirable since they cause a further decline in tissue perfusion. Successful recognition and early treatment of hemorrhagic shock depends heavily on sophisticated monitoring devices, the nature of the fluid used for volume replacement, and the use of blood components instead of whole blood. Intervention centers on establishing one or more IV lines for fluid replacement, drug administration, and blood component therapy. Careful monitoring of peripheral pulses, blood pressure, central venous pressure, and even more sophisticated hemodynamic parameters, such as pulmonary arterial wedge pressures, is desirable.

Pump Failure

Heart failure results from any condition that reduces the ability of the heart to pump blood. The heart is no longer in a state of compensation, and cardiac output falls. Cardiac arrhythmias and congestion are the most common types of pump failure.

Effective cardiac contraction depends on correctly timed depolarization of cardiac cells, which is achieved in normal sinus rhythm. When a dysrhythmia (abnormal rhythm) occurs, the ideal timing of depolarization is disrupted, and pump failure can occur, particularly when the dysrhythmia interferes with proper filling and emptying of the ventricles. This problem occurs when the client experiences ventricular fibrillation or tachycardia.

Heart failure has three successive phases of variable duration. The first phase is pathologic cardiac overloading due to excessive pressures, too much fluid, and/or myocardial tissue loss. The second phase of failure is cardiovascular compensatory response, such as dilatation and reflex responses. Finally, the heart fails to compensate, producing a wide variety of signs (objective data base) and symptoms (subjective data base).

Heart failure should not be confused with circulatory overload, a condition in which cardiac output is adequate but blood volume and/or venous return is excessive. Excessive infusion of IV fluids in too short a period of time results in circulatory overload.

Pulmonary edema, the most common result of pump failure, is a life-threatening condition. Pulmonary edema is a disorder in which alveoli fill with fluid. It produces severe abnormalities in gas exchange and can lead to death if not treated immediately. Several disorders can cause pulmonary edema, all of which produce a high hydrostatic pressure in the pulmonary capillaries. Right ventricular output into the pulmonary capillaries depends in part on the volume of venous return to the heart.

Drug therapy for treating and preventing pump failure as a result of fluid overload is long-term therapy. Drugs most often used are digitalis IV, (Lasix) IV or (Edecrin). Two newer drugs, amrinone lactate (Inocor) and milrinone (Primacor), are positive inatropic agents that relax vascular smooth muscle. This action increases cardiac output. These vasodilators act more quickly than digitalis.

Rotating tourniquets had been considered a mainstay of therapy for clients in pulmonary edema. However, with the demonstrated efficacy of IV drug therapy (e.g., Edecrin, Lasix), this treatment has been discontinued in most situations.

Ischemia

Ischemia is a circulatory condition in which blood supply to a body part or region is reduced to a critical level. Relative ischemia occurs with hypotension or the inability to meet increased metabolic demands. Absolute ischemia is usually a sudden, complete occlusion of a blood vessel, resulting in tissue necrosis. Leaving a tourniquet on an extremity for more than 15 minutes may cause tissue necrosis. Other causes of ischemia include Raynaud's disease, Buerger's disease, thromboembolism, mechanical obstruction, arteriosclerosis, and atherosclerosis. Atherosclerosis is always being studied in relation to hypertension, cigarette smoking, genetic factors, obesity, physical activity, hypercholesterolemia, and emotional stress. The actual cause of coronary atherosclerotic disease (CAD) remains a mystery, and the incidence in the United States continues to increase.

Thrombosis and Embolism

Blood clot formation within the circulatory system causes thrombi. Endothelial injury, decreased blood flow, and changes in blood constituency lead to blood clot formation and therefore thrombosis. If veins are inflamed, the condition is termed thrombophlebitis. This phlebitis is usually of bacterial origin, with the thrombi firmly attached in the lower extremities. Thrombophlebitis should be differentiated from phlebothrombosis or thrombus in a vein.

A dislodged, or migrating, thrombus becomes an embolus. Embolism is the process of impaction somewhere within the circulatory system and may be solid, liquid, or air. Liquid emboli are usually injected intravenously by accident such as during a hyperalimentation procedure (TPN). Similarly, air emboli occur when air is not removed from intravenous or arterial lines before infusion of solutions.

Elastic hosiery (TED, Jobst, and others) and sequential stockings are used to prevent venous stasis and avoid thrombus formation and subsequent emboli. They produce compression of peripheral leg veins. This pressure forces the venous blood into deeper, larger leg veins for a more rapid return to the heart.

TABLE 26–1. Assessment Guide for Hemorrhaging

1. Observable bleeding from skin, mucous membranes. Check under the person, clothing, dressing, casts.
2. Observable bleeding into the skin, mucous membranes. Check for petechiae, ecchymosis, hematomas, purpura.
3. Observable bleeding from body orifice. Check for epistaxis, hematemesis, hemoptysis.
4. Observable bleeding from tubes. Check T-tubes, endotracheal tubes, suction drainage, urinary catheters.
5. Generalized signs and symptoms of bleeding.
   a. Low blood pressure (systolic below 90 mm Hg and diastolic below 50 mm Hg).
   b. Progressive drop in blood pressure.
   c. Rapid, weak pulses or absence of pulses.
   d. Clammy skin and central cyanosis.
   e. Deep, rapid respirations (above 24/minute).
   f. Low body temperature (one or more degrees below 98.6°F, or 37°C, for oral temperature).
   g. Reduced urine output (less than 30 mL/hour).
   h. Behavioral changes.
   i. Syncope and visual disturbance.
   j. Loss of consciousness.
6. Localized signs and symptoms of bleeding.
   a. Painful, swollen, tender, or hot joints.
   b. Soft, spongy uterus high in abdominal cavity during postpartum period.
   c. Pupillary and visual changes, behavioral shifts, tinnitus, vertigo, breathing pattern shifts, loss of consciousness following head injury.

ALTERED CIRCULATION

Assessment

Alterations in circulation are indicated by a variety of signs and symptoms. The nurse should not overlook the behavioral manifestations or the more physical signs and symptoms. Systematic client evaluation considers whether or not there is a significant blood loss. If bleeding exists, external and/or internal sites must be identified. Special attention is given to the family history for disease conditions of the heart, vessels, liver, spleen, kidneys, brain, lungs, and coagulation mechanisms. Baseline data is gathered for vital signs and arterial blood pressures. The color, temperature, and condition of the skin are closely noted. Cyanosis is differentiated as peripheral versus central. Weakness and fatigue is significant, as well as physical discomforts, such as pain, pressure, or numbness. Abnormalities of superficial veins often indicate obstruction or pooling. Impaired renal function, especially related to output, is closely considered. Edema is differentiated as dependent versus generalized. Special observations include such findings as clubbing of the fingers, petechiae, and calf tenderness with dorsiflexion of the foot (positive Homan's sign). Information obtained from the client's drug history and present medications may affect the diagnosis and therefore the nursing intervention. Trauma victims require especially close inspection since more overt signs and symptoms may not appear until days later.

Table 26–1 illustrates an assessment of a hemorrhaging client.

Planning and Intervention

Once an initial assessment of a client for alterations in circulation has been made, the nurse develops a prioritized problem list for planning and intervention. Nurses monitor circulatory status with a variety of sophisticated tools. Again, however, the most valuable approach is direct observation of the client. Blood pressure measurements are usually noninvasive, taken with a blood pressure cuff, stethoscope, and sphygmomanometer. The central venous line and the Swan–Ganz catheter for pulmonary arterial pressures (PAP and PAWP) are invasive methods used under certain conditions and by specially trained personnel.

Interventions for circulatory problems cover numerous therapeutic modalities but usually fall into three broad categories: inputs, outputs, and pressure supports. Inputs include arterial lines, venous lines, drug regimens, transfusions, blood component therapies. Outputs include suctioning with specialized equipment like hemovacs and procedures like thoracentesis. Pressure supports include dressings, bandages, digital compression, tourniquets, and cardiopulmonary resuscitation. This chapter outlines some of the most common skills the nurse is required to perform in the management of circulatory problems.

In coping with alterations in circulation, care should be directed toward promoting, maintaining, or regaining the best possible cardiopulmonary function. The design for nursing action is to assess the situation and client for stressors. The client should be interviewed if possible, observed, and examined to identify actual and/or potential circulatory problems. The client's responses are appropriate, deficient, or excessive, and interventions should be planned accordingly. The nurse attempts to reduce client stress, supports adaptive behaviors, replaces deficiencies, modifies or removes excessive responses, and prevents injury and complications. The nurse should always assist in the evaluation of planned actions, report client responses, and assist in modifying the interventions as indicated.

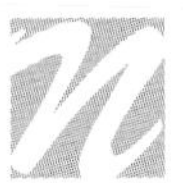

NURSING DIAGNOSES

The following nursing diagnoses are appropriate to use a client care plan when the components are related to circulation.

NURSING DIAGNOSIS	RELATED FACTORS
Decreased Cardiac Output	Cardiac disease states, altered electrical conduction, drug side effects, hypovolemia
Fluid Volume Deficit	Blood loss from lacerations
Altered Tissue Perfusion: cardiopulmonary	Altered blood supply, arterial or venous, hypovolemia, shock

unit 1

CONTROL OF BLEEDING

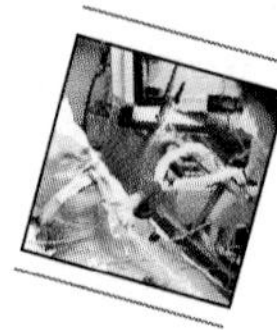

NURSING PROCESS DATA

ASSESSMENT Data Base

Observe the amount of bleeding.
Check for the source of bleeding.
Observe the extent of the wound.
Identify familial history of bleeding disorders.
Assess baseline vital signs and arterial blood pressure readings.
Observe color, temperature, and condition of the skin.
Ask about medications taken routinely by client.

PLANNING Objectives

To detect source of bleeding
To stop or control bleeding or hemorrhage before large blood loss occurs
To provide pressure as an assist (adjunct) to stop bleeding
To minimize capillary seepage, hematoma, and serum accumulation

IMPLEMENTATION Procedures

Using Digital Pressure
Using Pressure Dressing

EVALUATION Expected Outcomes

Early detection of bleeding occurs, and loss of blood is minimized.
Pressure dressing is applied, and bleeding is controlled.
Collateral circulation is minimally inhibited.

USING DIGITAL PRESSURE

Equipment

Towels or gauze dressing if available
Gloves

Procedure

1. Don gloves, sterile preferred.
2. Identify the closest artery proximal to the bleeding site. **Rationale:** The rapid loss of more than 25–30% of the total blood volume leads to death.
3. Apply direct pressure to artery, using your gloved finger.
4. If towels or 4 × 4 gauze pads are available, apply direct pressure to site if wound does not contain glass particles. **Rationale:** If pressure is placed on wound when glass is present, additional tissue damage can occur.

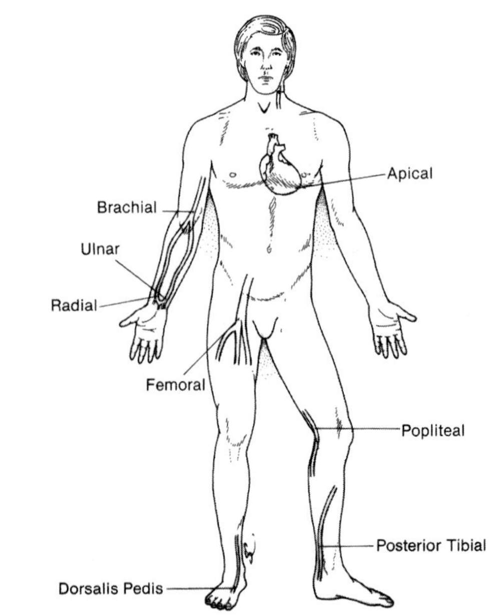

Pulse sites that may be used to control bleeding.

5. Raise the affected limb above the level of the heart about 30°. **Rationale:** This decreases arterial blood flow to area and promotes venous return.
6. Maintain direct pressure for at least 5 minutes.
7. Do not remove pressure before 5 minutes. **Rationale:** Clot formation has not had an opportunity to stabilize.
8. When bleeding has subsided, proceed to clean and dress the wound.
9. To control nose bleeds, place client in sitting position, with head tilted forward. Pinch nose for 5 minutes. If ordered, apply ice pack to assist in vasoconstriction.
10. Remove glove when bleeding subsides.
11. Wash hands immediately. **Rationale:** To protect yourself from possible contamination should the glove have a hole.

USING PRESSURE DRESSING

Equipment

4 × 4 gauze pad
Sterile dressings—number and size depends on wound
Sterile gloves
Cleansing solution
Tape

Preparation

1. Check physician's orders.
2. Assemble necessary supplies according to extent of wound.
3. If time permits, explain procedure to client and provide light and privacy.
4. Wash your hands thoroughly if time permits.
5. Set up sterile field and prepare cleansing solution if time permits.

Procedure

1. Put on sterile gloves.
2. Cleanse wound and apply dressing. Use several layers of 4 × 4 gauze pads.
3. To provide an occlusive dressing, place tape tightly over entire dressing. Do not completely circle an extremity or the body. **Rationale:** To ensure that collateral blood flow is maintained.
4. Place all soiled materials in biohazard bag.
5. Remove gloves and wash your hands thoroughly.
6. Monitor vital signs, and observe for signs of shock.
7. Position client for comfort.
8. Elevate extremity to prevent bleeding.
9. Monitor frequently for signs of bleeding and hematoma. Hematomas feel spongy even under bandages.

CHARTING for Control of Bleeding

- Size, location, condition of wound
- Color, odor, amount of drainage
- Type and number of dressings used
- Approximate amount of blood loss
- Condition of dressing when changed (e.g., soaked with drainage).

CRITICAL THINKING APPLICATION

CLINICAL PROBLEMS	CRITICAL THINKING OPTIONS
■ Even with direct pressure and application of pressure dressing, bleeding continues.	• Reinforce pressure dressing. • Monitor IV flow closely. • Notify physician, and be prepared to send client to surgery for wound closure. • Monitor closely for signs of shock. • Aid with placing tourniquets proximal to the site of the hemorrhage to control bleeding if all other actions are unsuccessful.
■ Wound edges do not approximate.	• Notify physician. • Be prepared to assist with wound closure or to send client to surgery.
■ Glass particles are evident in wound.	• Irrigate wound profusely with sterile saline solution as ordered. • If large amount of glass or if glass is difficult to extract, notify physician, and be prepared to send client to surgery for wound cleansing and debridement. • Do not apply direct pressure or pressure dressing to wound containing glass. • Apply pressure to vessel above wound or, as a last resort, apply a tourniquet.

unit 2

CIRCULATORY MAINTENANCE

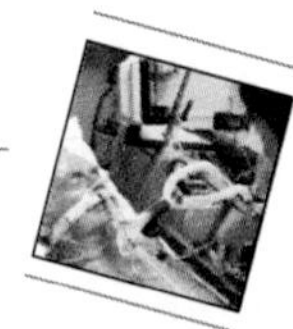

NURSING PROCESS DATA

ASSESSMENT Data Base

Evaluate client's overall physical condition, particularly client's cardiovascular status.

Observe baseline vital signs before procedures are initiated.

Determine if client is at risk for pooling of blood in extremities. Conditions that require use of elastic stockings are leg varicosities, thrombophlebitis, lymphedema, orthostatic hypotension, immediate postcast removal, postoperative venous ligation or stripping, and venous insufficiencies due to muscular inactivity.

Assess for peripheral edema by palpating pulses and observing color and temperature as well as fluid accumulation.

PLANNING Objectives

To prevent venous stasis

To prevent thrombus formation and subsequent emboli

To use elastic hose or sequential stockings to prevent venous stasis

IMPLEMENTATION Procedures

Applying Elastic Hosiery

Applying Sequential Compression Devices

EVALUATION Expected Outcomes

Elastic stockings remain wrinkle-free, and pressure is evenly distributed.

Peripheral pulses are present throughout use of sequential stockings and elastic hosiery.

APPLYING ELASTIC HOSIERY

Equipment

Tape measure

Specific type of hosiery (e.g., below-the-knee or above-the-knee)

Talcum powder

Preparation

1. Check orders for specific reason client needs elastic stockings.
2. Check physician's orders for type and specifications.
3. Gather supplies, identify client, and explain procedure.
4. Wash your hands, and provide for client's privacy and comfort.
5. Apply drape as top linens are removed. Bathe, dry, and powder client's legs.
6. Assess lower extremities for edema, dry skin, and palpable pulses.

Procedure

1. Position client in dorsal recumbent position, and elevate bed to working height.

> **■ CLINICAL ALERT**
>
> It is preferable to place elastic hose on clients before they get out of bed in morning to lessen chance of edema.

2. Measure client for size.
   a. For below-the-knee stockings, measure from the Achilles tendon to the popliteal fold, and measure the midcalf circumference (Table 26–2).
   b. For high stockings, measure midcalf and

TABLE 26–2. Measuring for Elastic Hosiery

Thigh-Hi Measuring		Knee-Hi Measuring	
Circumference	**Length**	**Circumference**	**Length**
Measure calf at largest circumference 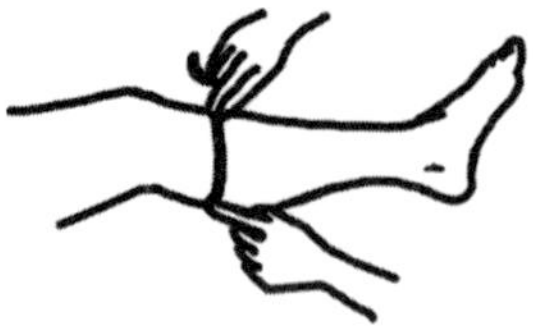	Measure leg from bottom of heel to fold of buttocks 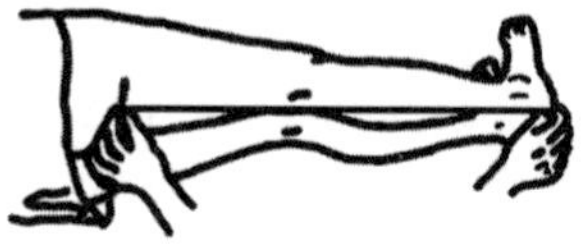	Measure calf at largest circumference 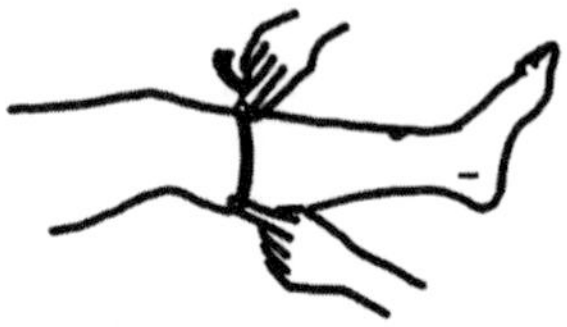	Measure leg form Achilles tendon to popliteal fold 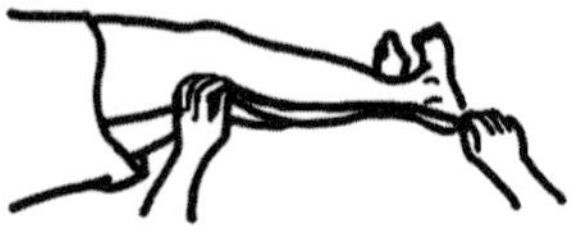

midthigh circumference to determine size. Length is determined by measuring the distance from gluteal furrow to bottom of the heel.

3. Compare your measurements to manufacturer's chart to obtain correct hose size.
4. Powder client's heel and foot.
5. Invert foot of stocking back to heel area.
6. Holding both sides of hose at inverted foot area, pull hose over toes and ease gently toward top of foot.
7. Gather top of hose down to heel area, and with curving motion, cover heel and then pull hose up the leg.
8. Reposition client, and wash your hands.
9. Observe extremities for edema above level of hose.

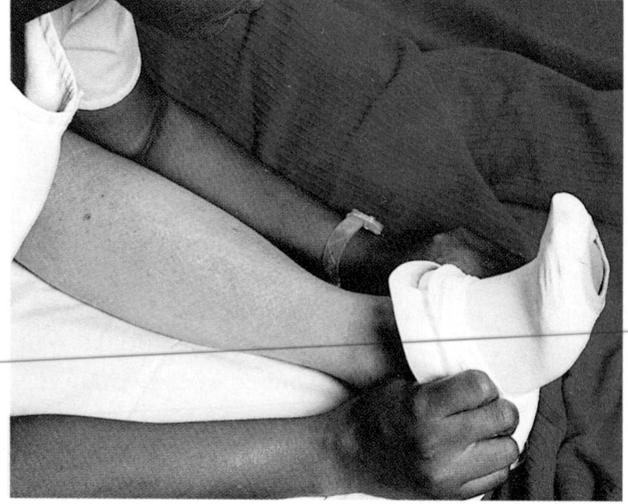

Gather elastic hose and pull hose over toes and then to top of foot.

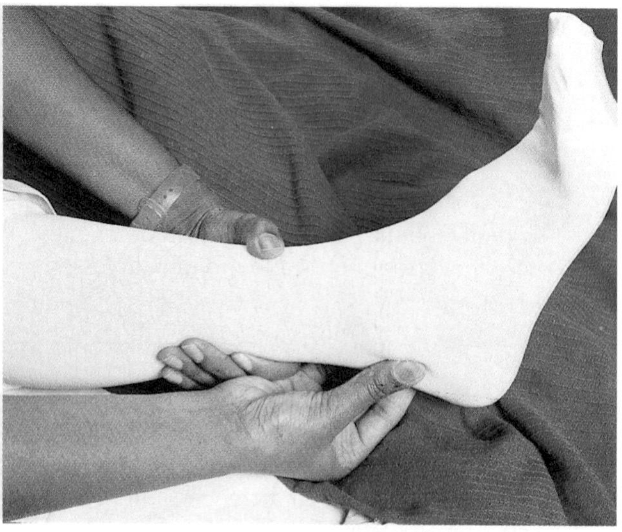

Ensure hose fits properly without wrinkles over toe or heel.

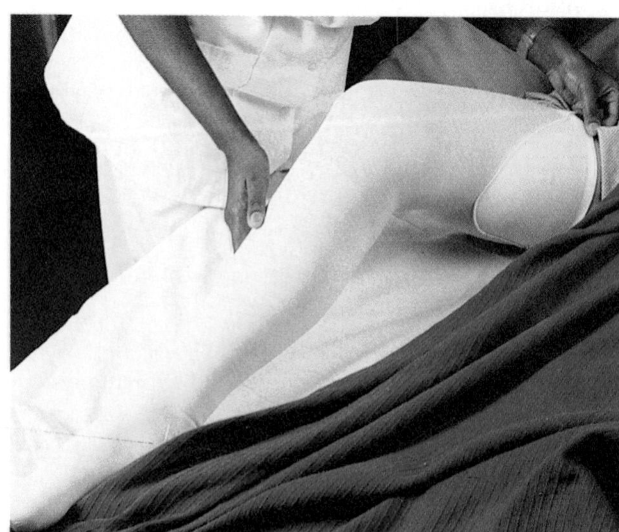

Pull hose to upper thigh and check that support section is on upper thigh.

10. Remove hose two to three times daily for 30 minutes.
11. Wash in mild detergent and warm water as needed.

APPLYING SEQUENTIAL COMPRESSION DEVICES

Equipment

Disposable leg sleeve(s)
 Knee length or thigh length
Tubing Assembly
Controller (motor)

Preparation

1. Review physician's orders for type of disposable leg sleeve needed. **Rationale:** Both knee- and thigh-length sleeves are available.
2. Identify client and explain that this device decreases the risk of developing deep-vein thrombosis for clients following surgery or those on long-term bed rest.
3. Assess client for potential problems, contraindications for use of these devices. **Rationale:** Clients with severe arteriosclerosis, pulmonary edema, or preexisting deep-vein thrombosis are not candidates for these devices, as they could exacerbate the client's condition.
4. Complete a neurovascular assessment. Include an evaluation of skin color, temperature, sensation, capillary refill, and presence and quality of pedal pulses. Document findings. **Rationale:** This assessment provides baseline data for evaluating neurovascular changes while devices are used.
5. Assemble equipment. Read manufacturer's directions for connecting and operating controller and sleeve.
6. Read directions for setting sleeve pressure (between 35 and 55 mm Hg).
7. Locate and identify the indicator lights on the controller for the ankle, calf, and thigh pressure in addition to the cooling light. **Rationale:** Light is on when the pressure is applied to the three leg sleeves and during the cooling time. Pressure is exerted for a total of 11 seconds. The cooling period lasts 60 seconds, during which time there is no compression by the sleeve.

Procedure

1. Remove sleeve from plastic bag.
2. Unfold sleeve and follow directions to fit sleeve to client's leg. Leg is placed on white side of sleeve.

Wrap sleeve securely around client's leg and check for adequate circulation.

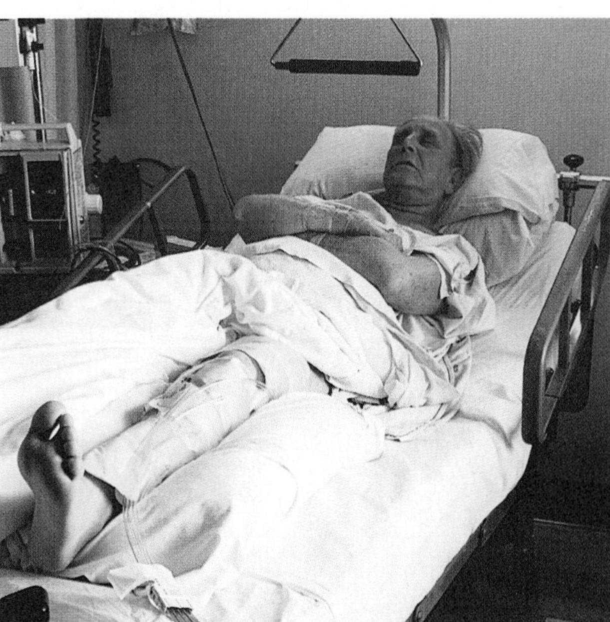

Assess neurovascular status and correct function of equipment every 2 hours.

3. Wrap sleeve securely around client's leg.
4. Attach hook edge securely to the sleeve.
5. Fit two fingers between client's leg and sleeve to prevent tight fit. **Rationale:** To ensure sleeve does not constrict circulation.
6. Remove tubing assembly from package and connect to plugs on leg sleeve. Arrows on both plug and connector must line up to ensure a proper fit.
7. Connect tubing assembly plug to controller at the tubing assembly connector site.
8. Ensure tubing is free of kinks or twists. **Rationale:** Kinks and twists can restrict air flow through system.
9. Plug controller power cable into grounded electric outlet.
10. Turn controller power switch to ON.
11. Check that pressure indicator lights and cooling light are functioning properly. When pressure is applied to each segment of leg, specific light is on. When cooling light is on, the compression lights should be OFF, as this is when no compression is applied to leg.
12. Monitor that compression and cooling cycles are correct. Ankle pressure is applied first, followed by calf pressure and then thigh pressure.
13. Monitor neurovascular checks every 2 hours. Turn machine off immediately if the client complains of numbness.
14. Turn off machine at prescribed time intervals to assess skin and to provide skin care.
15. To remove sleeve, turn power switch OFF, disconnect tubing assembly from sleeve at connection site. Unwrap sleeve from leg.

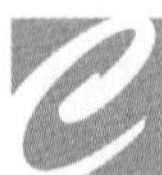

CHARTING for Elastic Hose

- Size and type of elastic hose applied
- Condition of skin
- Presence of pulses
- Edema formation below or above hose
- Time and length of time hose removed

for Compression Devices

- Neurovascular assessment baseline data
- Neurovascular assessment during application
- Condition of skin
- Sleeve pressure
- Time compression devices applied and removed

CRITICAL THINKING APPLICATION

CLINICAL PROBLEMS	CRITICAL THINKING OPTIONS
for Elastic Hosiery	
■ Elastic hosiery are not available.	• If ordered, use elastic (Ace) bandages. Anchor bandages on top of the foot and in front of the leg, using metal clips or tape. Overlap should be one-third of bandage width; for a 4-inch width each turn overlaps by $1\frac{1}{2}$ inches. • Assess that elastic bandages are tight enough for support but do not obstruct arterial flow. • While making each turn, place a finger between the bandage and skin to prevent bandage from becoming too tight.
■ Elastic hosiery are loose and don't provide support.	• Remeasure legs and compare to chart to determine correct size. • Hosiery may be old with no elasticity and should be discarded.
for Sequential Compression Devices	
■ Client complains of numbness or tingling in leg.	• Remove devices immediately. • Complete neurovascular assessment. • Notify physician of assessment findings.
■ Buildup of excess sleeve pressure (above 80 mm Hg).	• Check tubing for kinks or twists. • Turn power switch to OFF position and then ON to restart system.

unit 3

ELECTROCARDIOGRAM (ECG) MONITORING

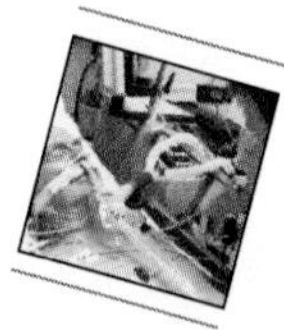

NURSING PROCESS DATA

ASSESSMENT Data Base

Determine if there is preexisting cardiac disease or chest pain.

Assess client's level of understanding and cooperation with procedure.

Determine client's level of fear or anxiety regarding diagnosis, procedure, or outcome.

Identify pharmacologic agents currently prescribed.

Determine other pathologic conditions that may precipitate conditions, such as fever, anxiety, alcohol, tobacco, or caffeine ingestion.

Determine subjective complaints of diaphoresis, palpitations, dizziness, or fainting.

Identify electrolyte abnormalities affecting the electrocardiogram, particularly potassium and calcium deficiencies or excesses.

PLANNING Objectives

To clearly display ECG on oscilloscope

To determine ECG changes

To identify ECG abnormalities reflecting electrolyte abnormalities

To determine cardiac irregularities

To identify and treat potentially dangerous rhythms accordingly

To determine if a relationship exists between chest pain and ECG changes

IMPLEMENTATION Procedures

Monitoring the ECG

Interpreting an ECG Strip

EVALUATION Expected Outcomes

ECG leads applied appropriately and without difficulty.

Abnormal ECG findings interpreted accurately.

Heart rate calculated correctly.

MONITORING THE ECG

Equipment

Electrode discs

Lead wires

Cardiac monitor and cable

Alcohol swab

Wash cloth or 4 × 4s, soap, and towel

Preparation

1. Gather equipment.
2. Wash your hands.
3. Explain procedure to client.
4. Wipe skin areas on client with alcohol where electrodes are to be attached. Allow to dry or wipe with a 4 × 4 pad. **Rationale:** This removes oily substances for better adherence of electrodes.
5. Check that ECG monitor is plugged in and turned ON.
6. Attach cable to monitor.

Procedure

1. Apply electrodes.
   a. Peel off paper backing on electrode disc. Check that sponge pad in center of electrode is moist with conductive jelly. Place electrode on skin with adhesive side down.
   b. Apply electrodes in areas where there will not be excessive movement.
   c. Place near but not directly on bone surfaces; however, if patient is overly obese, electrodes may have to be placed on the bones, since a large amount of adipose tissue results in a poor image on the oscilloscope.
2. Determine the lead placement that gives the best ECG pattern.

   LEAD II:
   Positive (+) *lead*—left side of chest, fourth intercostal space at midclavicular line
   Negative (−) *lead*—right shoulder region, below clavicular hollow
   Ground (G) lead—fourth intercostal space, right sternal border, opposite positive lead

   LEAD MCL_1 (Modified Chest Lead):
   Positive (+) *lead*—right sternal border, fourth intercostal space
   Negative (−) *lead*—left shoulder, below clavicular hollow
   Ground (G) lead—right shoulder, below clavicular hollow, opposite negative lead

   Other leads, such as Lead I and MCL_6, can also be useful in specific situations.
3. Attach the chest electrodes to the lead wires by placing wire level on disc using the appropriate colored lead wires. **Rationale:** The client end of the cable is coded to facilitate connection with the electrodes.

> Common codes are − (neg), + (pos) and G (ground), or RA, LA and LL, or color codes. Be sure that the positive lead wire is connected to the electrode in the positive position, the negative lead wire to the electrode in the negative position, and the ground lead wire to the electrode in the ground position.

4. If lead wires are snapped onto electrodes, you may want to attach lead wires to electrodes before placing disc on client. **Rationale:** To prevent pushing on client's chest when attaching lead wire to disc. This can cause discomfort to client.
5. Set High and Low alarm limits on the monitor.
6. Turn alarm buttons to ON.
7. Observe pattern to determine clarity of image on oscilloscope.
8. Run ECG strip, and place in nurses' notes. **Rationale:** This provides a baseline record of the ECG pattern at the beginning of monitoring. To run the strip, turn the switch on the monitor to RUN. A strip of ECG paper appears with the wave form printed out.
9. Assess skin surrounding electrode disc for signs of irritation every 4 hours.

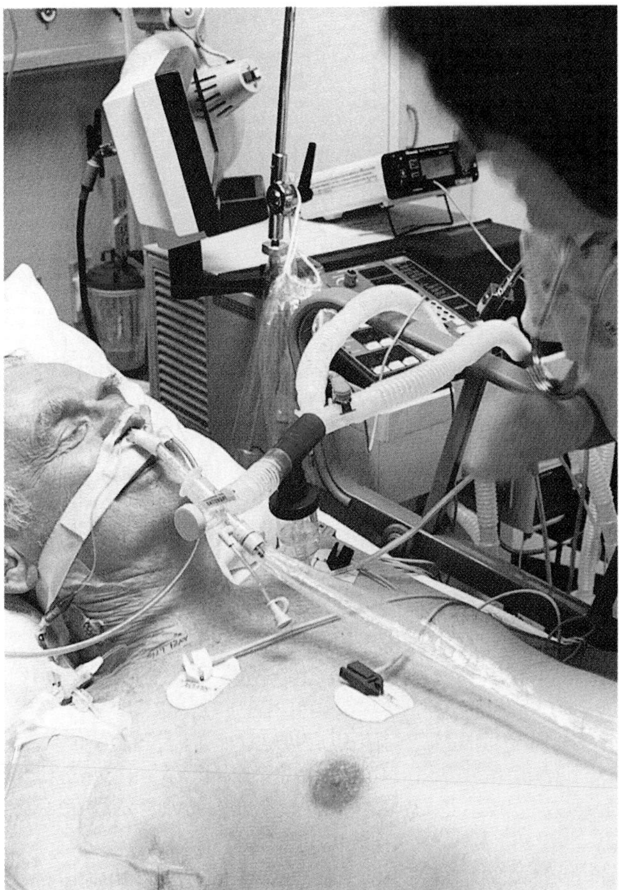

ECG electrode discs are placed on chest according to type of lead placement desired.

INTERPRETING AN ECG STRIP

Equipment

Calipers

Procedure

1. Determine heart rate by calculating atrial rate (PP interval) and ventrical rate (RR interval). Normal pulse is 60–100.
   Heart rate is calculated by:
   a. Counting the number of cardiac cycles (QRS complexes) in a 6-second strip and multiplying that number by 10 to obtain the pulse.
   b. Counting the number of small boxes between R waves, and dividing that number into 1500. The quotient is the ventricular rate.
   c. Counting the number of small boxes between P waves and dividing that number into 1500. The quotient is the atrial rate.
2. Determine regularity of rhythm (atrial and ventricular). Check if complexes look alike and are equally spaced. Use calipers to check this.
3. Measure PR interval to determine conduction time in atria and AV junction (0.12–0.20 seconds).
4. Measure QRS duration to determine ventricular conduction (0.04–0.12 seconds). There are six complexes.
5. Measure QT interval (rate of 70 in 1 minute occurring 0.33–0.44 seconds apart).
6. Check configuration and placement of P waves, QRS complex, ST segment, and T wave.
7. Summarize findings to obtain interpretation.
8. Determine if arrhythmias are potentially life threatening. Immediate intervention must be provided to prevent complications.
9. Document interpretation of findings, and place ECG strip in client's chart.

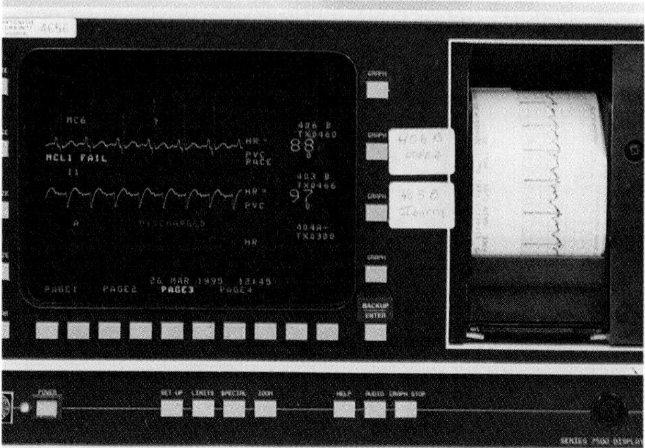

ECG pattern and lead placement are depicted on oscilloscope.

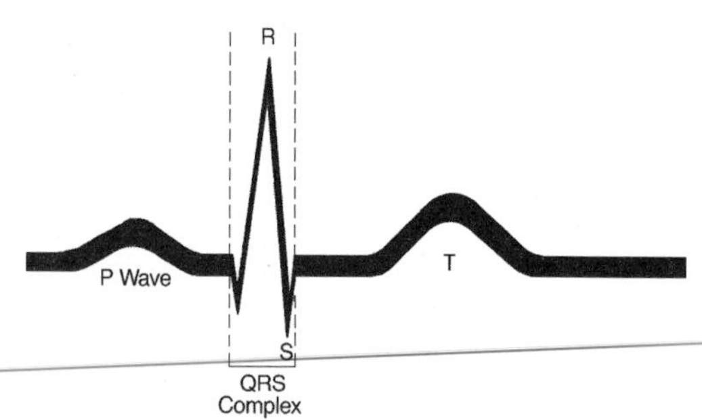

It is important to determine the configuration and location of the wave pattern to interpret an ECG accurately.

TABLE 26–3. Normal Sinus Rhythm

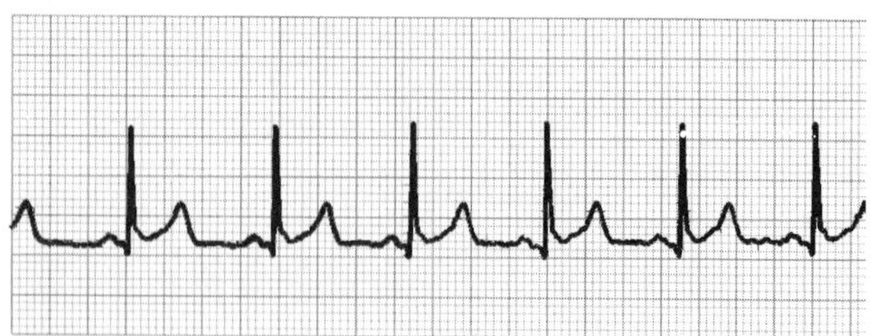

Regular configuration, uniform P wave precedes each QRS
Atrial rate 60–100
PR interval 0.12–0.2 seconds
QRS width 0.08–0.12 seconds
Ventricular rate 60–100

TABLE 26–4. Lead Placements

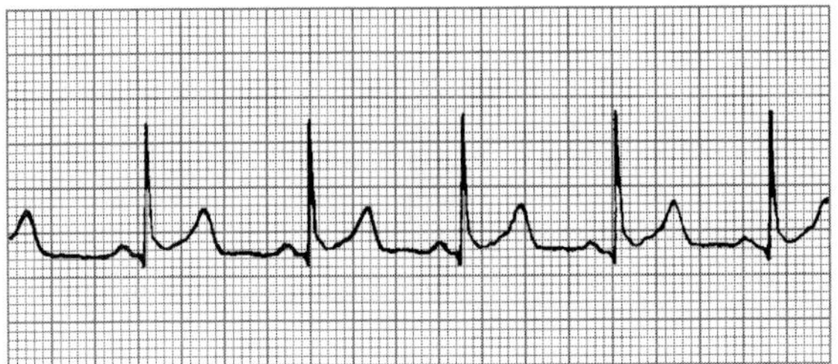

ECG pattern from Lead II placement

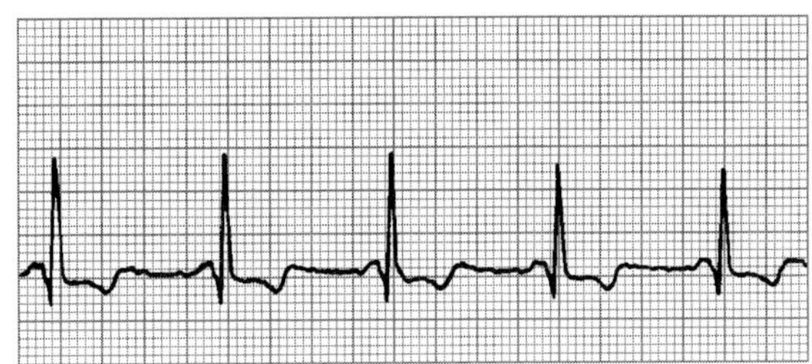

ECG pattern from lead I placement.

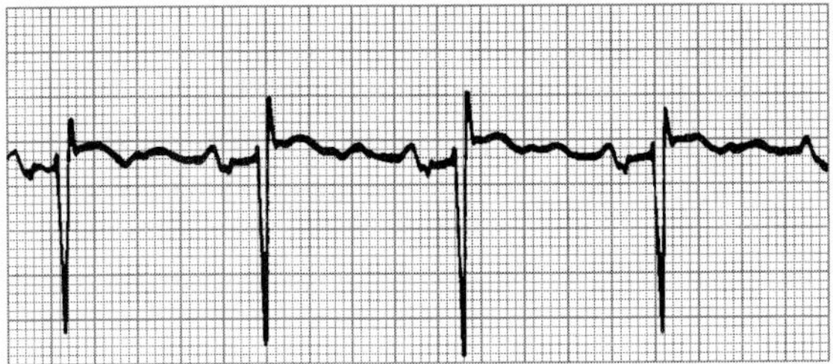

ECG pattern from MCL_1 placement

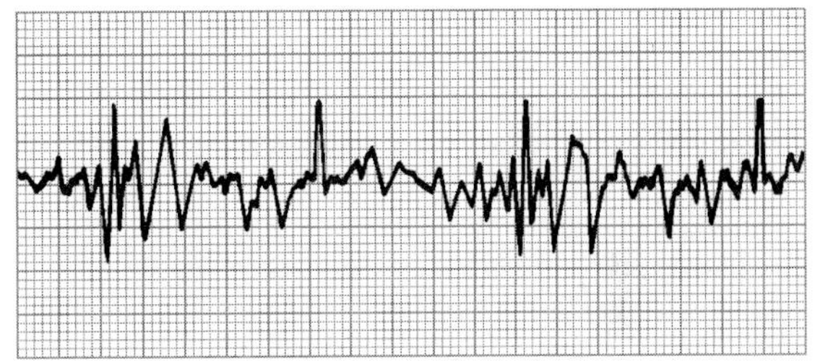

ECG pattern showing artifact.

TABLE 26–5. Potentially Life-Threatening Arrhythmias

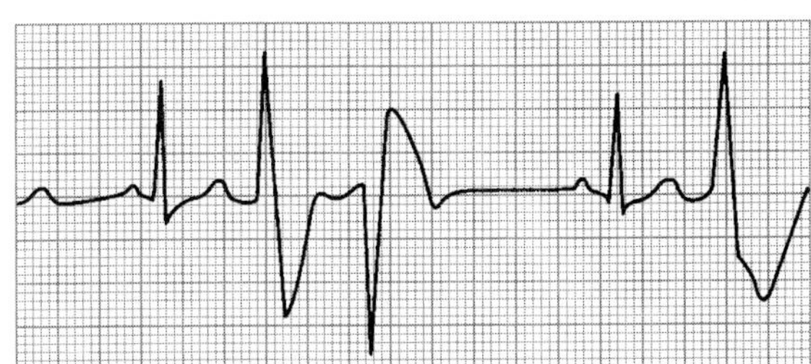

Multifocal Premature Ventricular Contraction (PVCs)
Irregular rhythm
P waves—none with premature beat, impulse originates in ventricle
Atrial rate—undetermined
PR interval—none with premature beat
QRS width—greater than 0.12 seconds for premature beat
Ventricular rate—varies
Note: Each PVC has different configuration as foci are from different areas of heart.
PVCs are result of increased automaticity of ventricular muscle cells.

Etiology
- Digitalis toxicity
- Hypoxia, hypokalemia
- Acidosis

Initial treatment
- Oxygen
- Potassium
- Lidocaine bolus—1–1.5 mg/kg; may repeat doses of 0.5–0.75 mg/kg every 5–10 minutes up to 3 mg/kg
- Continuous IV drip may be started

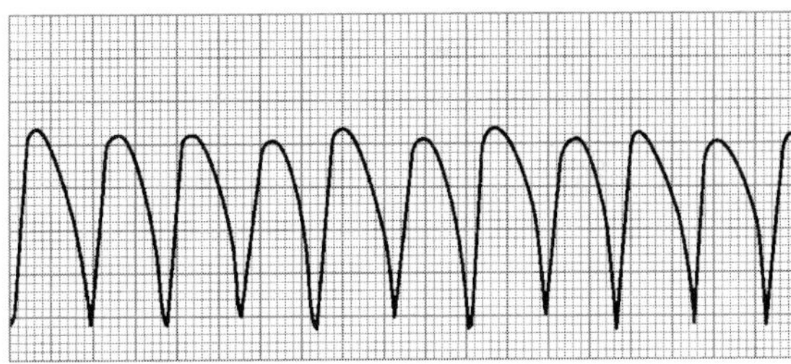

Ventricular Tachycardia
Regular rhythm
Atrial rate—cannot differentiate
PR interval—none
QRS width—greater than 0.12 seconds
Ventricular rate—100–300
Note: Ventricular tachycardia is a result of myocardial irritability.

Etiology
- Coronary artery disease

Initial treatment
- Lidocaine 1.5 mg/kg bolus; may repeat in 3–5 minutes to maximum dose of 3 mg/kg
- Cardioversion of cardiac output is compromised
- Pulseless ventricular tachycardia—follow treatment for ventricular fibrillation

TABLE 26–5. Potentially Life-Threatening Arrhythmias Continued

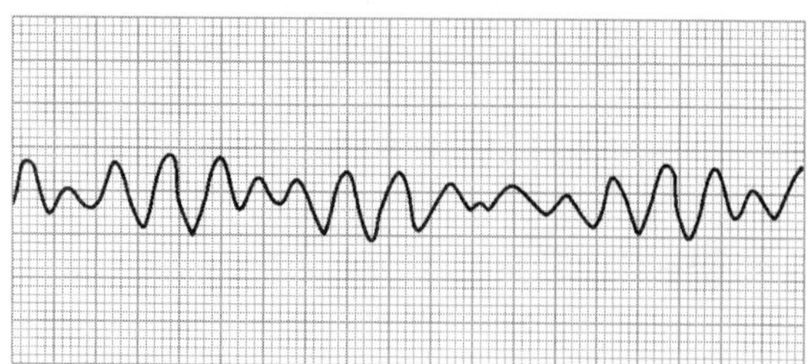

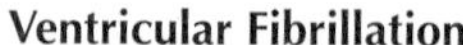

Ventricular Fibrillation
Irregular rhythm
Atrial rate—cannot differentiate
PR interval—none
QRS width—fibrillating waves only
Ventricular rate—cannot differentiate
Note: Ineffective quivering of ventricles with no audible heartbeat, pulse, or respirations

Etiology
- Myocardial ischemia
- Coronary artery disease
- Cardiomyopathy

Initial treatment
- CPR
- Defibrillate; starting at 200 J, defibrillate up to three times, 200–300 J, 360 J
- Ventricular fibrillation continues—epinephrine 1 mg IV push, repeat 3–5 minutes
- Defibrillate—360 J within 30–60 seconds of drug
- Second-line drugs may be used, such as bretylium and procainamide

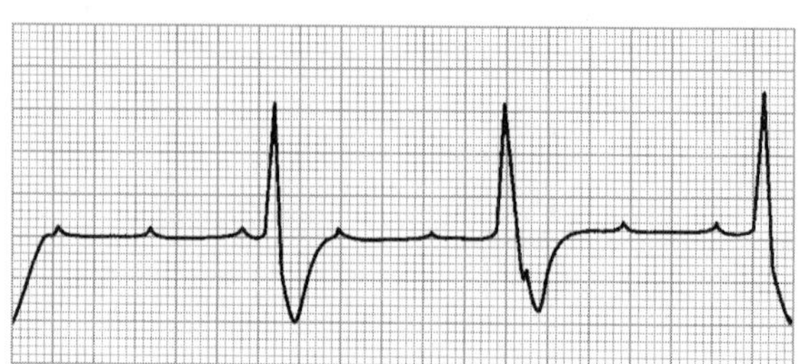

Third-degree Heart Block
Regular atrial and ventricular rhythm
Atrial rate—greater than ventricular rate
PR interval—varies QRS width—less than 0.12 second if pacemaker cell in junction; greater than 0.12 second if cell in ventricle
Ventricular rate—40–60 if escape pacemaker is from junction; 20–40 if escape is from ventricle
Note: Electrical impulse originates in SA node but is blocked to the Purkinje fibers leading to decreased perfusion of vital organs.

Etiology
- Digitalis toxicity
- Myocardial infarction
- Organic heart disease

Initial treatment
- Temporary pacemaker insertion

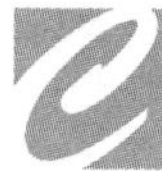

CHARTING for ECG Monitoring

- Findings based on the interpretation of the ECG strip
- Nursing interventions carried out, based on the ECG findings
- Lead placement used in ECG monitoring
- When electrodes were replaced
- Client attitude toward procedure
- Health teaching completed
- When physician was notified of abnormal findings

CRITICAL THINKING APPLICATION

CLINICAL PROBLEMS	CRITICAL THINKING OPTIONS
■ ECG is not clearly displayed on the oscilloscope.	• Ensure that electrodes are applied in correct position and are securely attached. • Observe for electrical interference resulting in a 60-cycle interference on oscilloscope. • Observe for excessive client activity resulting in artifact display on oscilloscope.
■ Electrodes do not adhere to skin, and interference appears on oscilloscope.	• Change placement of electrodes to another area of the body. • Put tincture of benzoin on the skin before placing electrodes. • Recleanse skin thoroughly with alcohol swab.
■ Alarms ring without change in pattern.	• Check HIGH and LOW parameters. They may need to be changed. • Check GAIN. It may be too low to be sensing pattern.
■ ECG pattern is abnormal.	• Recheck each configuration. • Check if pattern is a life-threatening arrhythmia (PVCs, ventricular tachycardia, ventricular fibrillation); if so, notify physician immediately.
■ Electrical interference continues after lead wires and cable connections are secured.	• Check all other electric equipment in the immediate environment. • Check for proper grounding of monitor. • Change electrodes and cable; sometimes poor conduction results in 60-cycle interference. • Check that monitor is calibrated.
■ Skin irritation occurs with use of electrodes.	• Remove electrodes, cleanse site, and reapply electrodes on new site.
■ Chaotic rhythm appears on oscilloscope.	• Check client's other assessment parameters to determine if clinical changes have occurred. • Check electrode contact on skin, and ensure that wires are in contact with cable. • Determine activity level of client.
■ High or low alarms on monitor continue to sound.	• Check for loose electrodes. • Observe activity level of client. • Check that alarm parameters on monitor are not set too close to client's pulse. • Check client's position. • Reposition electrodes, avoiding large muscle masses or bone.
■ Electrodes conduct poorly on diaphoretic client.	• Clean skin sites as usual, apply benzoin to the skin, and let dry and apply electrodes. • Clean skin sites as usual, apply spray deodorant to the skin, allow skin to dry, and apply electrodes.
■ Asystole occurs.	• Before beginning CPR, check client's LOC and electrodes, wires, and cables. • If the client has an arterial line, check for an arterial waveform in the absence of an ECG waveform.

unit 4 EMERGENCY LIFE SUPPORT MEASURES

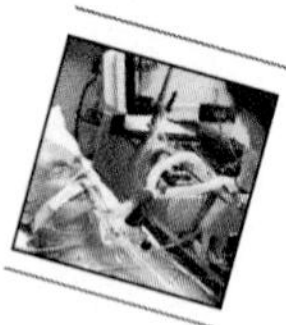

NURSING PROCESS DATA

ASSESSMENT Data Base

Assess client for signs of cardiac or respiratory arrest.

Know your own responsibilities for an arrest situation.

Identify location of resuscitation equipment.

Identify the location of the emergency cart, nearest defibrillator or monitor (if none on cart), and 12-lead ECG machine.

Identify procedure for activation of cardiac arrest team.

PLANNING Objectives

To provide adequate oxygenation of lungs through mechanical support

To provide oxygenated blood to vital organs

To support the client via mechanical intervention or mouth-to-mouth ventilation until other equipment is available

IMPLEMENTATION Procedures

Administering Basic Life Support to Adults

Administering CPR to a Child

Administering the Heimlich Maneuver for Conscious Client

Administering the Heimlich Maneuver for Unconscious Client

Providing Care Following Code

EVALUATION Expected Outcomes

Basic life support measures established within 3 minutes after arrest.

Emergency measures performed according to established protocol.

Client is adequately oxygenated by use of mechanical adjuncts.

No permanent neurologic damage is sustained.

Foreign body is dislodged.

ADMINISTERING BASIC LIFE SUPPORT TO AN ADULT

Equipment

Cardiac board

Procedure

for Unresponsiveness

1. Assess client as the first step in CPR phase. **Rationale:** Assessment ensures expedient rescue.
2. Institute CPR within 3 minutes. **Rationale:** Cardiopulmonary resuscitation is usually not effective in preventing brain damage unless initiated within 4 minutes of an arrest.
3. Quickly approach client.
4. Check responsiveness. Shake shoulders. Shout, "Are you OK?" **Rationale:** To ensure that client has not fainted.
5. Call out for help.
6. Move into proper position. Place victim flat on firm surface, and position yourself next to victim at approximately the same level. **Rationale:** CPR is ineffective if the head is above the level of the heart.

for Airway

1. Take the following measures if you suspect airway obstruction from food or other foreign body.

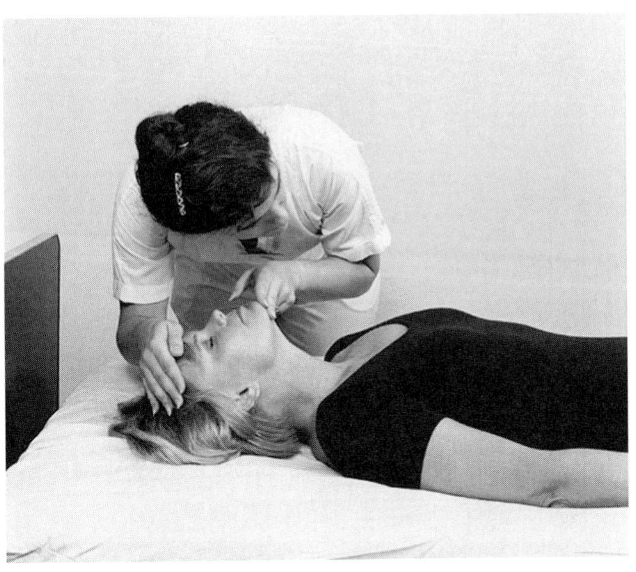

Begin CPR by looking, feeling, and listening for exhalation of breath.

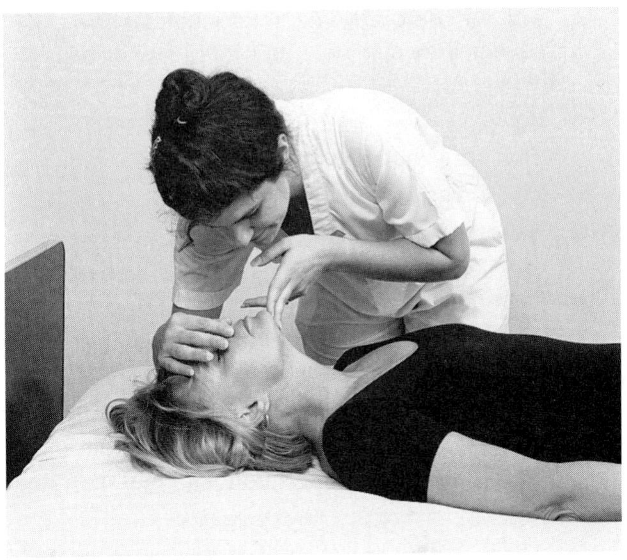

Pinch nose, lift chin, and press backward on forehead.

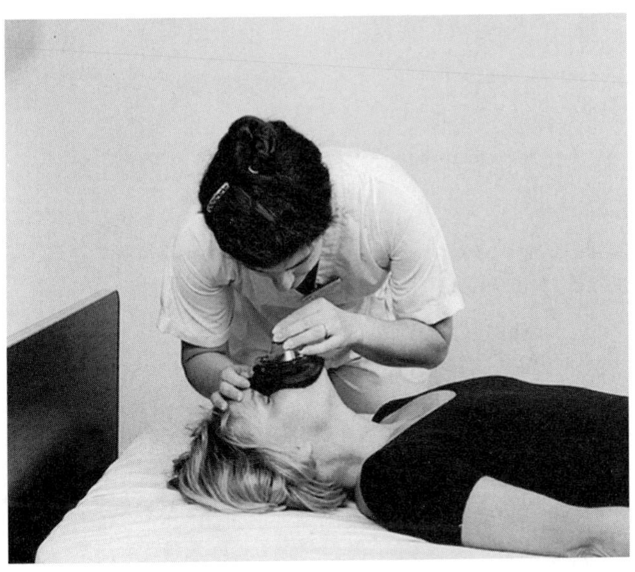

Place mask over mouth and nose and then administer ventilation.

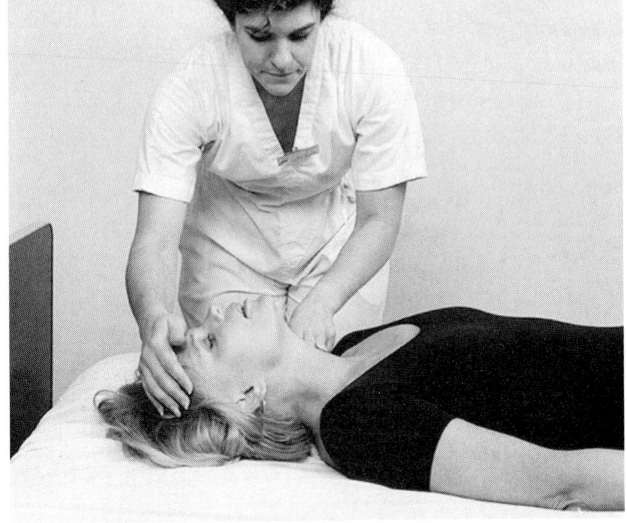

Check carotid pulse 5-10 seconds after administering ventilations.

2. Tilt head by placing palm of hand on victim's forehead.
3. Press backward on forehead. **Rationale:** This causes head to tilt back and open airway.
4. Lift chin by placing fingers of other hand under bony part of jaw on side nearest you.
   a. Place index finger near the chin and next two fingers behind it along the side of the jaw.
   b. Lift chin up and forward until teeth are nearly closed.
5. Assess breathing:
   a. Lean over victim's head, and look at chest to determine if chest rises and falls.
   b. Place ear and cheek near victim's mouth and nose to listen and feel for air movement. **Rationale:** Reliable indicator of adequate patent airway is feeling and hearing air movement. Chest may actually move but breathing could be obstructed.

for Rescue Breathing

1. Evaluate respiratory function:
   a. Put your ear down near client's mouth.

b. Look for chest movement. **Rationale:** If chest movement occurs but you cannot feel or hear air, the airway is obstructed.
c. Feel for air flow against your cheek.
d. Listen for exhalation of breath.

2. Prepare to ventilate if no respirations are present.
   a. Leave dentures in place. **Rationale:** Facilitates airtight seal.
   b. Pinch off nostrils.
   c. Fully cover victim's mouth to form mouth-to-mouth seal.
3. Administer mouth-mouth breathing.
   a. Give a long ventilation ($1\frac{1}{2}$–2 seconds). **Rationale:** Longer ventilation allows time for chest to expand.
   b. Release seal, and turn your head.
   c. Take fresh breath.
   d. Watch for fall of chest.
   e. Give second breath. Provide 800 mL minimum tidal volume per breath.

■ CLINICAL ALERT

CPR Protocol

1. Shake and shout.
2. Open airway.
3. Look, listen, and feel for breathing.
4. Call code.
5. Ventilate client with two slow breaths.
6. Check carotid pulse for 5–10 seconds.
7. Initiate CPR at 15 cardiac compressions to two ventilations at rate of 80–100 compressions/minute.
8. Check for carotid pulse after 1 minute. If absent, continue CPR.

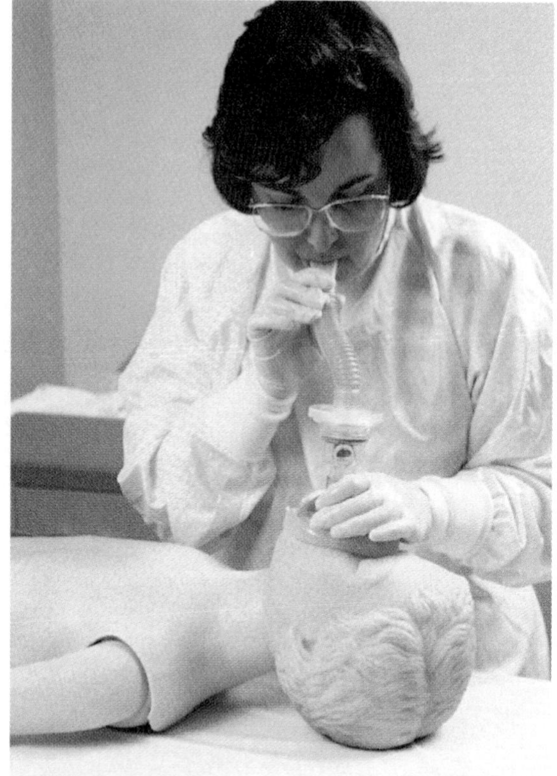

One-way valve mask should be used when performing CPR.

   f. Check carotid pulse for 5–10 seconds.
   g. Call for assistance if pulse is absent.
   h. Continue rescue breaths if pulse is present. Give breaths every 5–6 seconds (10–12 breaths/min).

4. Alternate method: Perform rescue breathing using one-way valve mask. **Rationale:** This method provides an infection-control barrier.
   a. Place mask over mouth and nose to create a tight seal.

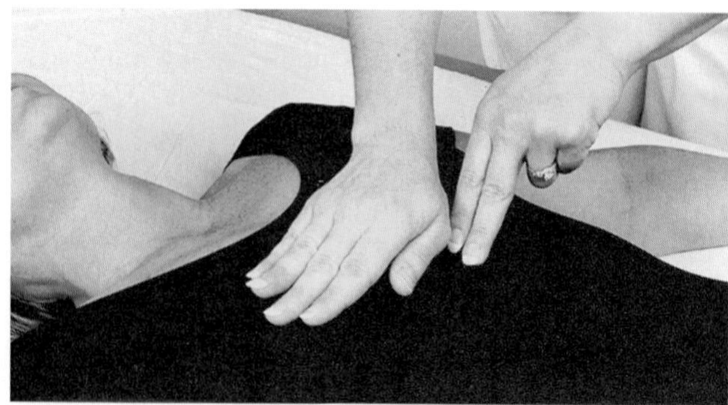

Position hands midline, lower half of sternum, two fingers above xiphoid.

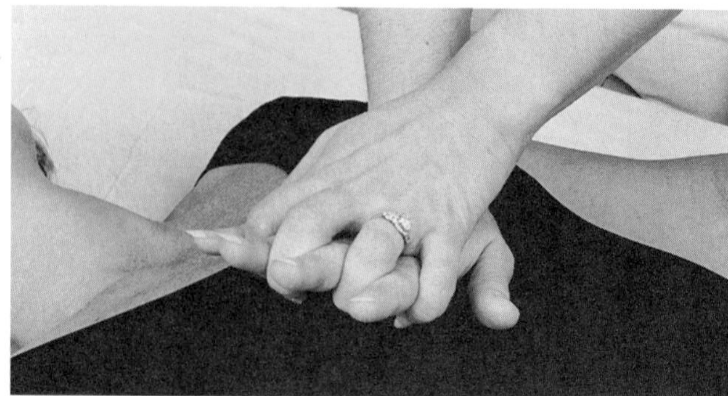

Place heel of one hand on sternum and superimpose second hand on top of first hand.

b. Rescuer takes a deep breath, then gives two slow breaths, $1\frac{1}{2}$–2 seconds to client.

c. Take fresh breath and continue.

for Circulation

Single Rescuer

1. Feel for carotid or femoral pulse, and palpate one side with two fingers for 5–10 seconds.
2. If pulse is absent, begin CPR.
   a. Run finger up rib cage until middle finger reaches xiphoid notch. (Where ribs and sternum meet.)
   b. Position hands midline, lower half of sternum, two fingers above xiphoid. **Rationale:** This location prevents damage to liver.
   c. Place heel of one hand on sternum and other hand superimposed on top of first hand.
   d. Interlace fingers and extend fingers off rib cage.
   e. Administer compressions at a rate of 80–100/minute. Compress chest 1–$1\frac{1}{2}$ inches. **Rationale:** The rate of 80–100 is used because studies show that higher compression rates increase coronary blood flow.
   f. Count compressions: one-and-two-and.
   g. Release pressure between compressions for cardiac refilling but do not take heel of hand off chest. **Rationale:** Leaving the hand on the chest prevents malposition of hands between compressions which could result in injury to the client.
3. Continue CPR at the rate of 15 compressions and two ventilations for single rescuer sequence.
4. Check carotid pulse for 5 seconds after four cycles of compression and ventilation.

Two professionals arrive together to do CPR.

1. a. Rescuer "A" assumes position at head of victim to perform ventilation.
   b. Perform head-tilt/chin-lift maneuver for airway opening.
   c. Assess breathing.
   d. Ventilate with two long slow breaths ($1\frac{1}{2}$–2 seconds). Observe for chest rise and fall. **Rationale:** Longer ventilations allow time for chest to expand and reduce potential for abdominal distention.
   e. Rescuer "A" checks for carotid pulse for 5–10 seconds.
   f. Rescuer "B" assumes position of compressor at level of chest and locates site for chest compression.
   g. If no pulse, rescuer "A" states "no pulse" and "B" begins compressions.
   h. Rescuer "B" completes five compressions ($1\frac{1}{2}$–2 inches) at a rate of 80–100/minute and then pauses after fifth compression.
   i. Rescuer "A" gives one slow breath.
   j. Rescuer "B" counts one-and-two-and. **Rationale:** To maintain smooth rhythm for CPR.
   k. Rescuer "B" begins compressions again at ratio of 5 compressions to 1 ventilation.
   l. Rescuer "A" checks carotid pulse after 1 minute and then after every few minutes.
2. When "Rescuer B" becomes tired, a signal to switch is made. (Complete at least 10 cycles before switching.)
   a. "Rescuer B" (compressor) says "switch" and completes the fifth compression. Each rescuer simultaneously switches.
   b. New "Rescuer A," at head, checks carotid pulse for 5–10 seconds. If no pulse, states, "no pulse" and gives one ventilation.
   c. New "Rescuer B" begins cycle of compressions.

for Continuing CPR

1. Check carotid or femoral pulse every few minutes of CPR.
2. Check pupils every 4–5 minutes (optional if a third trained person is present)—not always a conclusive indicator.
3. Observe for abdominal distention (all age groups). **Rationale:** Longer ventilations reduce chance of abdominal distention.
   a. If evident, reposition airway, and reduce force of ventilation.
   b. Maintain a volume sufficient to elevate ribs.
4. Ventilator: check carotid pulse frequently between breaths to evaluate perfusion.
5. Ventilator: observe each breath for effectiveness.
6. If respiratory arrest only, check major pulse after each minute (12 breaths) to ensure continuation of cardiac function.
7. Terminate CPR under the following conditions:
   a. The resuscitation is successful.
   b. Spontaneous return of vital functions.
   c. Assisted life-support measures are initiated.
   d. Client is transferred to emergency vehicle or code team arrives.
   e. Client is pronounced dead by physician.
   f. Rescuer is exhausted and cannot continue.

ADMINISTERING CPR TO A CHILD

Procedure

1. If you suspect cardiac or respiratory arrest, follow these steps:
   a. Call for help.
   b. Check responsiveness by shaking child, slapping bottom of feet, or rubbing chest to elicit a cry.
   c. Place child on your lap, over your arm, or on a firm surface.
2. If foreign body aspiration is suspected, follow steps for obstructed airway.
3. Clear airway by lowering child's head, turning to side, and sweeping mouth with your little finger.
4. If unable to clear airway with sweeping motion, place child in airway position (chin forward with neck slightly extended). This position usually pulls the tongue from the back of the throat and opens the airway.
5. Place rolled towel under shoulders to maintain chin in a jutting-out position, without causing hyperextension of the neck.
6. Evaluate respiratory function by following these steps:
   a. Place cheek next to child's mouth and nose.
   b. Face infant's chest and observe for chest movement.
   c. Feel for air flow against cheek.
   d. Listen for exhalation.
7. For absent respirations, begin artificial ventilation.
   a. Maintain open airway. Tip head back. **Rationale:** Trachea can collapse if neck is hyperextended.
   b. Form tight seal by encircling nose and mouth of child. **Rationale:** Infant face is too small for nose-pinch/mouth-seal maneuver.
   c. Maintain tight seal.
8. Administer two breaths.
   a. Give breaths slowly.
   b. Fill cheeks with air and use short puffing breaths. Do not use full breaths for children. **Rationale:** Small breaths prevent overinflation of the lungs and abdominal distention.
   c. Between breaths, release seal for exhalation, and turn your head to side.
   d. Take fresh breath; do not allow complete deflation of lungs (stairstep volume).
   e. Maintain position.
9. Do not release the child when giving ventilations; just turn your head to side.
10. Administer ventilations at 20/minute (1 every 3 seconds) for children under 1 year of age, and at 15/minute for children over 1 year of age.
11. Continue ventilations until child is intubated or ambu bag is available.
12. For cardiopulmonary arrest, follow these steps:
    a. Follow procedure for initiating artificial ventilation.
    b. After administering two slow breaths, check carotid for presence of pulse. Palpate for 5–10 seconds. (Infant—check brachial pulse.)
    c. Begin cardiac compression. Maintain patent airway with your hand on infant's forehead.
13. For infants to 1 year of age:
    a. Place tips of index and middle finger at lower sternum. One finger breadth below nipple line.
    b. Alternative method: grasp both hands behind the infant's back for support and overlap your thumbs at midsternum.
14. For children 1–4 years of age, use the heel of one hand at the lower half of the sternum.
15. For children over 4 years of age, use two hands over the lower half of the sternum.
16. Remember that compression depth for children is $1–1\frac{1}{2}$ inches and for infants $\frac{1}{2}–1$ inch.
17. Do not take fingers or heel off skin between compressions.
18. Perform cardiac compression and ventilate at the rate of one breath to five compressions.
    a. For infants under 12 months, administer compression 100 times per minute to depth of $\frac{1}{2}–1$ inch.
    b. For infants over 12 months and up to 8 years, administer compression 100 times per minute to depth of $1–1\frac{1}{2}$ inches.
19. Follow usual steps in CPR for single rescuer until help arrives.
20. Recheck carotid or brachial pulse every 10 cycles.
21. Continue CPR until code team arrives or you are instructed to stop by a physician.

ADMINISTERING THE HEIMLICH MANEUVER FOR CONSCIOUS CLIENT

Procedure

1. Assess choking client for pale color progressing to cyanosis.
2. Be familiar with choking signs.
   a. Ask client if he or she can speak.
   b. Ask client to hold hand on neck if choking.
3. If unable to talk or coughing becomes ineffective, begin abdominal thrusts.
4. Stand behind client. Place your arms around the client's waist.
5. Make a fist with one hand. Place other hand over the fist.
6. Position hands halfway between xiphoid process and umbilicus. (Client will probably fall over your arms.)
7. Press your fist into client's abdomen.
8. Using a rotating motion of the hands, forcefully thrust your hands in an upward direction to assist in expelling the foreign body.
9. Repeat measures until foreign body is expelled.

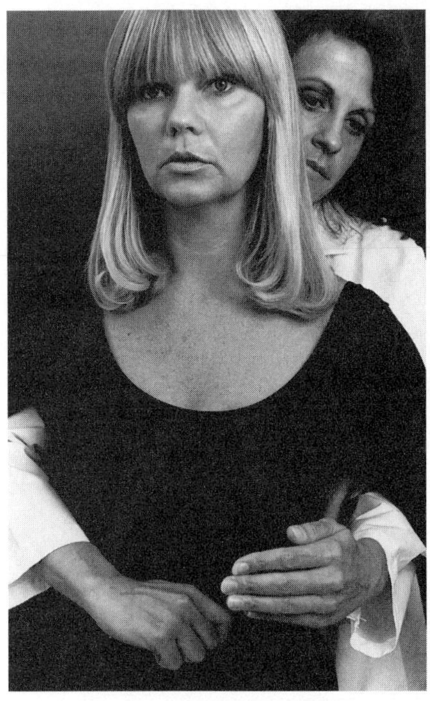

Make a fist and place it between the xiphoid and umbilicus of the client.

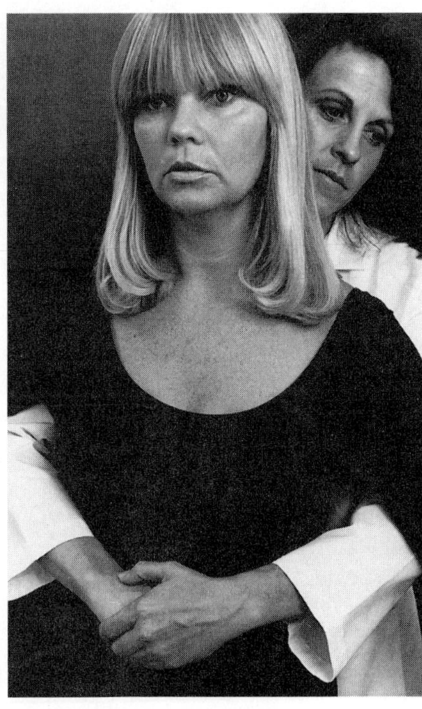

Position second hand over the fist for leverage and a more secure grasp.

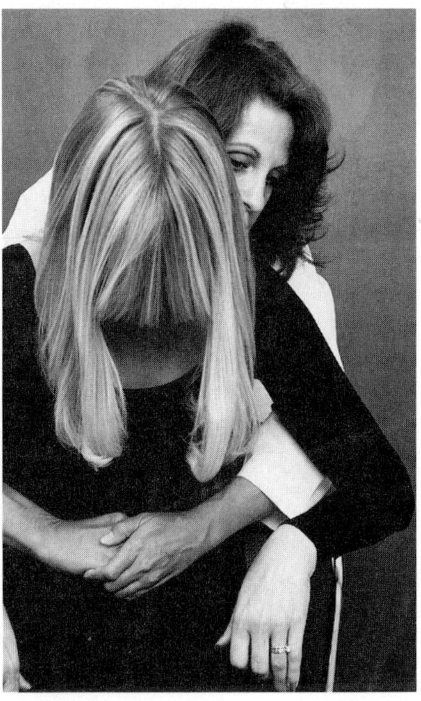

Quickly thrust your hands backwards and up toward you to expel the foreign object.

ADMINISTERING THE HEIMLICH MANEUVER FOR UNCONSCIOUS CLIENT

Procedure

1. Slide client to floor, and place on side if client unconscious.
2. Lift jaw to open mouth. Hold victim's tongue down against lower jaw with your thumb.
3. Finger sweep mouth. Run index finger down inside of cheek toward base of tongue. Scrape across back of throat, and clear debris out other side of mouth with sweeping motion of finger.
4. Roll client onto back.
5. Open the airway and attempt to ventilate.
6. If unable to ventilate, perform Heimlich maneuver.
   a. Kneel and straddle victim's thighs.

b. Find umbilicus and xiphoid process.
c. Place one hand directly over the other slightly above umbilicus.
d. Press heel of hand toward head with 5 quick subdiaphragmatic abdominal thrusts or until foreign object dislodges.
e. Use tongue–jaw lift to open mouth and sweep deeply to remove foreign body.
f. Attempt to ventilate—if not successful, complete steps 5 and 6 again.

7. Repeat steps 5 and 6 until foreign object dislodged.
8. If pulse absent but airway patent, begin CPR.

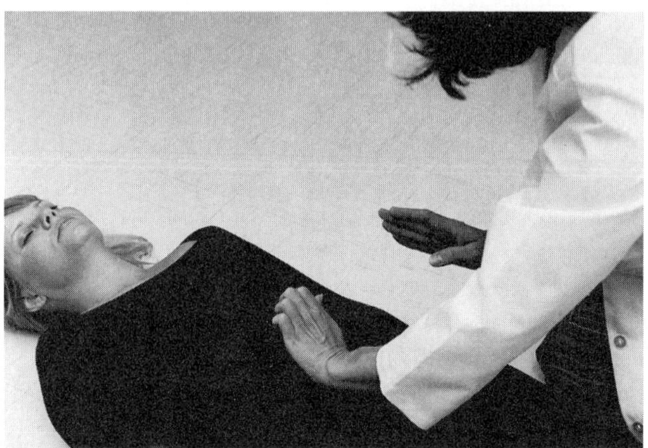

When client is unconscious, kneel and straddle thighs, then place one hand directly over the other above umbilicus.

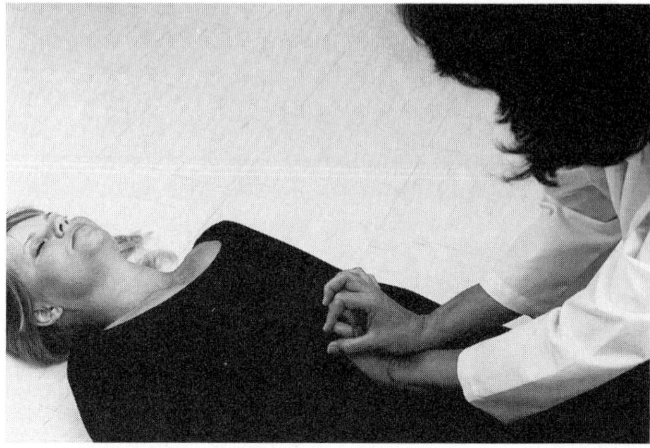

Press heel of hand toward head, and deliver 5 quick thrusts to dislodge foreign object.

PROVIDING CARE FOLLOWING CODE

Procedure

1. Remind physician he or she needs to talk with family.
2. Wash client's face and hands, and provide clean top sheet.
3. Escort family in to see client.
4. Assist in transferring client to ICU (or morgue, if necessary).
5. Provide one-to-one nursing care for client until ICU transfer is accomplished.
6. Update charting.
7. If assigned, restock emergency cart or obtain replacement cart.
8. Return all equipment to original location. Remember to recharge defibrillator.
9. Clean room.
10. Allow other clients to return to room.
11. Participate in staff critique of resuscitation management.

CHARTING for CPR

- Time of arrest
- Type of arrest
- Initial resuscitation efforts before arrival of team
- Resuscitation efforts after arrival of team
- Time of cessation of resuscitation efforts
- Outcome of resuscitation efforts
- Outcome of Heimlich maneuver

CRITICAL THINKING APPLICATION

CLINICAL PROBLEMS	CRITICAL THINKING OPTIONS
Choking client is found on floor. Heimlich maneuver cannot be performed in usual manner.	• Perform procedure for administering the Heimlich maneuver for unconscious client.
Team demonstrates poor coordination efforts.	• Attend practice CPR drills. • Evaluate own performance after every drill.
Client is revived but maintained on life-support system.	• Continually reassess CPR protocol. • Assist in preparing client for serial ECGs if brain hypoxia is suspected. • Reassess for developmental level. • Give custodial care if required.

GERIATRIC CONSIDERATIONS

Stressful physical and emotional conditions may have an especially adverse effect on the elderly client.

- The heart may be unable to respond to these changes with an adequate increase in rate, which could precipitate heart failure.
- Changes in the heart lead to decreased myocardial contractility, increased left ventricular ejection time, and delayed conduction, which plays a role in this phenomenon.

Cardiac output is decreased as a result of tachycardia or atrial fibrillation, which is evidenced on the ECG.

- Tachycardia is caused by a shortened ventricular filling time.
- Atrial fibrillation is caused by the loss of the atrial kick (blood volume delivered to the ventricle as a result of a coordinated atrial contraction).

ECG may be abnormal due to a chronic disease such as congestive heart failure.

- Assess client for behavioral changes, palpitations, dyspnea, fatigue, and falls. These are indicators of a dysrhythmic heart.
- Dysrhythmias, such as PVCs, premature atrial contractions (PACs) may be very common and not cause for alarm unless they change in number or configuration.
- Pacemaker spikes are evident on ECGs for clients with pacemakers.

Client requiring CPR has dentures in place.

- Keep dentures in place to provide for good seal around mouth.
- Rescue breathing is more effective when tight seal around mouth is maintained.

Peripheral vascular assessment is essential when an elderly client is using elastic hosiery or sequential stockings.

- Elderly clients may very well have altered peripheral circulation before this treatment is started.
- Stockings that are too tight can interfere with the already compromised vascular blood flow, leading to ulceration of the lower extremity.
- Check color, warmth, capillary refill, and presence of pedal pulses every 4 hours when client using these devices.

27

Intravenous Therapy

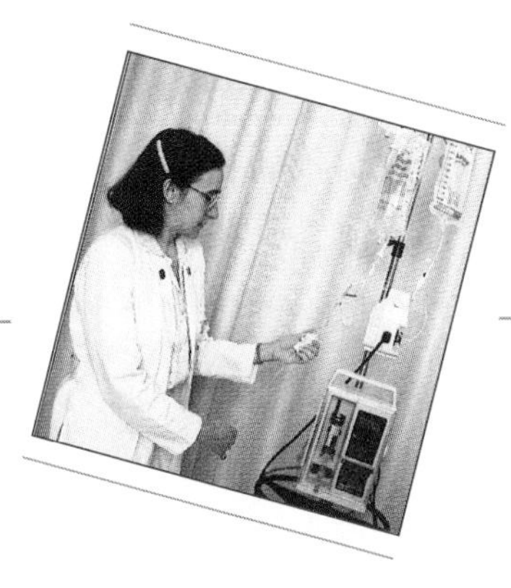

LEARNING OBJECTIVES

- Describe the role the kidneys play in maintaining fluid and electrolyte balance.
- Discuss the two hormonal regulatory systems that influence urinary excretion through the kidneys.
- State the major cations and anions in the body.
- Identify the assessment modalities used to determine a client's fluid balance.
- Compare and contrast the clinical manifestations associated with overhydration and dehydration.
- Describe the steps in the procedure for performing a venipuncture using a wing-tipped needle.
- State at least two potential problems that can occur with IV insertion and one suggested solution for each problem.
- Outline the steps in preparing the IV bag for administration.
- Describe the reason for hanging the partial-fill bag higher than the primary IV bag.
- Calculate an IV flow rate using a standard formula.
- Describe the safety checks utilized to ensure proper blood is administered to the patient.
- Differentiate between the signs and symptoms associated with bacterial, allergic, and hemolytic blood transfusion reactions.

TERMINOLOGY

Anaphylaxis: a hypersensitive state of the body to a foreign protein or drug.

Antiarrhythmic: an agent used to regulate heart rhythm.

Antidiuretic: a drug that decreases urine secretion.

Antimicrobic: preventing the development or pathogenic action of microbes.

Ascites: the excessive accumulation of serous fluid in the peritoneal cavity.

Aspirate: to remove material by suction.

Cardio: pertaining to the heart.

Cardiovascular: pertaining to the heart and blood vessels.

Cyanosis: slightly bluish, grayish, slatelike, or dark purple discoloration.

Diarrhea: frequent passage of watery bowel movements.

Diffusion: spreading or dispersing of molecules in solution, as a gas or liquid.

Diuretic: a chemical agent that increases the secretion of urine.

Dyspnea: air hunger resulting in a subjective feeling of difficulty breathing.

Edema: body tissues containing an excessive amount of fluid.

Electrolyte: a solution that is a conductor of electricity; minerals are common electrolytes.

Evaporation: change from liquid to vapor.

Extracellular: outside the cell.

Girth: the distance around something; circumference, as in measuring abdominal circumference.

Granulocytes: a granular leukocyte (e.g., neutrophil).

Hematoma: a collection of clotted blood confined in a space.

Hematuria: blood in the urine.

Hemo-: prefix meaning blood.

Hemolytic: pertinent to the breaking down of red blood cells.

Homeostatis: state of equilibrium of the internal environment.

Hydration: the chemical combination of a substance with water.

Hydrostatic: pertaining to the pressure of liquids in equilibrium and the pressure exerted on liquids.

Hypersecretion: abnormally large amount of secretion.

Hypovolemia: diminished circulating fluid volume.

Infusion: a liquid substance introduced into the body via a vein for therapeutic purposes.

Intracellular: inside the cell.

Intravascular: within blood vessels.

Metabolism: the sum of all physical and chemical changes that take place within an organism.

Nephro: prefix meaning kidney.

Nephrotoxic: a toxin that destroys renal cells.

Osmosis: the passage of solvent through a partition separating solutions of different concentrations.

Palpate: to examine by touch; to feel.

Pruritis: severe itching.

Purulent: containing pus.

Skin turgor: the tension or fullness of the cells.

Specific gravity: weight of a substance compared with an equal volume of water.

Transfusion: injection of the blood or a blood component of one person into the blood vessels of another.

Urticaria: a vascular reaction of the skin characterized by the eruption of pale raised wheals, which are associated with severe itching.

Valsalva's maneuver: attempt to forcibly exhale with the nose and mouth closed.

Venipuncture: puncture of a vein with a needle.

Viscosity: resistance offered by a fluid; property of a substance that is dependent on the friction of its component molecules as they slide by each other.

FLUID AND ELECTROLYTES

Fluid and electrolytes do not exist independently but rather in a state of dynamic equilibrium that demands a stable composition of the various elements that are essential to life. The primary elements that control this state of equilibrium are fluids, or body water, and electrolytes, most of which are minerals.

Fluids

Body fluid is primarily water. Depending on the amount of body fat, a person's total body weight is usually made up of between 50% and 70% water. Since fat is essentially water-free, an obese adult's body weight is 50% water. In a leaner individual the percentage of body weight due to body water is closer to 70%.

Body water is divided into two main compartments: intracellular and extracellular. The majority of body water, (64%) is located inside the cells. The remaining 36% of body fluid is extracellular. Three-fourths of this extracellular fluid is interstitial (surrounding cells), and the remaining one-fourth is intravascular plasma.

Communication between these fluid compartments varies. Intracellular water does not move out of the cell readily. In contrast, extracellular water (intravascular and interstitial) can diffuse more easily and is similar in electrolyte composition. The flow, or diffusion, of body fluid between the intravascular compartment and the interstitial space is controlled by a variety of factors, such as hydrostatic pressure, osmotic pressure, and the diameter of the vessels.

The overall maintenance of body water is the result of adjustments made between the gains and losses of water that occur on a daily basis. The major sources of water coming into the body are fluids. A small amount of water is also produced as a by-product of cellular metabolism. Most fluid leaves the body through urinary excretion. Water is also lost by fecal elimination, sweating, and diffusion and evaporation through the skin and the lungs (Table 27–1).

The major organ of excretion is the kidney. Because the kidneys handle the end products of cellular metabolism, as well as the elimination of excess fluids, they must excrete a minimum of 500–600 mL of urine every 24 hours. Depending on the amount of fluid intake, the amount of urine usually produced on a daily basis varies from 600–1600 mL.

The regulation of the volume and concentration of body fluids is handled by two mechanisms: thirst and urinary excretion. Thirst is stimulated by receptors in the central nervous system. Under normal circumstances, an individual ingests fluids when these receptors are activated. During an illness or an altered level of consciousness, the thirst response may be depressed, resulting in hypovolemia and increased tonicity or concentration of the extracellular fluids (dehydration).

Urinary excretion through the kidneys is directed or influenced by two hormonal regulatory systems—one of which is the antidiuretic hormone (ADH). An increase or decrease of ADH helps regulate the balance of body water. When extracellular body fluids become concentrated, osmoreceptors located in the hypothalamus stimulate the release of ADH, which acts on the kidney to retain more water. This is a hypotonic gain. As this retained water circulates through the extracellular fluid compartment, the concentration of body fluid is reduced. The osmoreceptors, sensing this change, slow the secretion of ADH, which then causes the kidneys to stop retaining water (negative feedback).

Other conditions that can stimulate the secretion of ADH and lead to increased water retention by the

TABLE 27–1. Fluid Gains and Losses

Intake (mL)	Output (mL)	
Oral intake 1,500–3,000	Urine	600–1,600
Cellular catabolism of proteins, carbohydrates, and fats	Skin	300–600 (insensible loss)
	Lung	350 (insensible loss)
	Feces	200
	Sweat	100–300

kidneys include hemorrhage, decreased cardiac output, trauma, pain, fear, surgery, and dehydration. Drugs, such as morphine, barbiturates, nicotine, and some anesthetics and tranquilizers, also increase the secretion of ADH. The secretion of ADH can be inhibited by alcohol, decreased concentration of body fluids, and hypervolemic states.

The other major regulatory hormone is aldosterone, which is secreted by the adrenal cortex. Aldosterone regulates the levels of sodium in the body. It causes the kidneys to retain sodium and water (an isotonic gain). Under the influence of aldosterone, the kidney reabsorbs sodium in exchange for potassium or hydrogen, therefore, indirectly affecting levels of these electrolytes.

Secretion of aldosterone is increased in response to several stimuli, which include decreased sodium and increased extracellular potassium, hypovolemia, and physical or emotional stress.

When the level of sodium is lowered or when hypovolemia occurs, the receptorlike area in the glomerulus of the nephron releases an enzyme substance called renin. As renin circulates in the body, it converts a plasma protein in the liver into a vasoconstrictor substance called angiotensin I. When this substance enters the lungs, it is converted into angiotensin II. Angiotensin II acts directly on the adrenal cortex and increases the level of aldosterone secretion. Aldosterone then stimulates the kidneys' tubule cells to retain sodium and secrete either hydrogen or potassium. Sodium retention is osmotically accompanied by water retention, thereby creating an isotonic gain. This leads to extracellular volume expansion.

Electrolytes

In partnership with body fluids are substances called electrolytes. These substances, mostly minerals, contribute to body function in many ways and are essential to life (Table 27–2).

Electrolytes are distributed throughout the body, both intracellularly and extracellularly. In the extracellular compartment, the main electrolytes are sodium, chloride, and bicarbonate. Intracellular electrolytes are potassium, magnesium, phosphate, and sulfate.

Electrolytes possess an electric charge when placed in water. Electrolytes with a positive charge are called cations. Negatively charged electrolytes are called anions. Positive cations and negative anions are attracted to each other because of their opposite electric charges. When they combine with each other, they form neutral compounds that either remain in body fluids or dissociate and regain their electric charges.

TABLE 27–2. Major Electrolytes

Cations		Anions	
Na^+	Sodium	Cl^-	Chloride
K^+	Potassium	HCO_3^-	Bicarbonate
Ca^{2+}	Calcium	HPO_4^{2-}	Phosphate
Mg^{2+}	Magnesium		

When they dissociate, or ionize, they are referred to as ions.

Alterations

Alterations in fluid and electrolytes may occur as a primary event or as a secondary response to a preexisting disease state or to a sudden, unexpected traumatic episode. When alterations of fluid and electrolytes exceed the narrow limits consistent with health, the body needs to adjust quickly.

Changes in the composition of body fluid and electrolytes may be relative or absolute. Relative losses or gains can occur when fluids or electrolytes shift from one body space to another. Absolute losses or gains can occur when fluids and electrolytes are lost outside the body or added to the overall body stores by IV fluid.

The kidney has an obligatory urine output, and the body has an insensible water loss. A minimum fluid intake of 1500 mL is essential to balance these losses. If the loss of body water is greater than fluid intake, weight loss results. If the gain of body water is greater than output, weight gain results. One kilogram of body weight gain or loss is equal to 1000 mL (1 L) of fluid.

In addition to methods of assessing fluid balance, this chapter discusses interventions for providing fluid and electrolytes to clients who have experienced alterations in their homeostasis. The rationale for interventions associated with alterations in either fluids or electrolytes is to maintain homeostasis and to regulate and maintain essential fluids and nutrients.

Clients undergoing major surgery or trauma may be subjected to blood loss necessitating replacement therapy. Clients requiring prolonged intravenous therapy may have associated nutritional losses. Support for these clients must be considered.

This chapter presents methods of supplying fluids and electrolytes, blood and blood components, as well as pharmacologic therapy through the IV route. Methods for assessing baseline data and evaluating fluid and electrolyte gains or losses are included in this chapter.

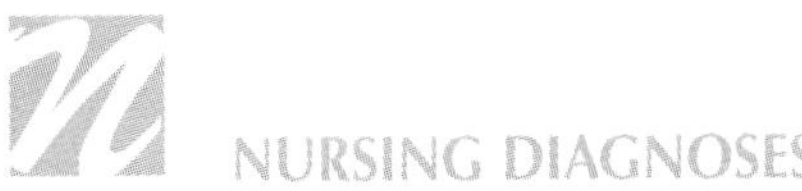

NURSING DIAGNOSES

The following nursing diagnoses may be appropriate to include in a client care plan when the components are related to intravenous therapy.

NURSING DIAGNOSIS	RELATED FACTORS
Fluid Volume Deficit	Excess fluid loss secondary to vomiting, blood loss, surgical drains and tubes, diarrhea, and diuretics
Fluid Volume Excess	Excessive fluid intake secondary to excess sodium intake, medications, renal and cardiac dysfunction; inaccurate IV infusion rate
Risk for Infection	Chronic diseases, invasive lines, immunodeficiency
Noncompliance	Inaccurate I&O records, denial, lack of instruction regarding I&O
Impaired Skin Integrity	Alterations in skin turgor, tissue damage, IV infiltration, infection, immobilization

unit 1

INTRAVENOUS THERAPY

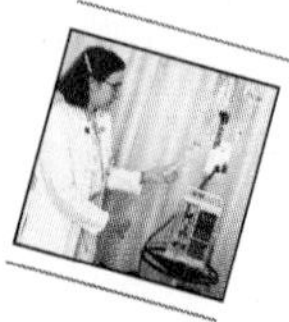

NURSING PROCESS DATA

ASSESSMENT Data Base

Determine physician's order for IV therapy.

Determine client's need for psychologic support.

Assess need for client explanation about IV therapy.

Identify appropriate site for venipuncture. Vein should be distal, superficial, large enough for the needle to be inserted smoothly, rapidly palpated, and easily followed.

Evaluate client for proper placement of needle. Placement is based on client convenience and functional use (left versus right hand).

Assess type and size of needle necessary.

PLANNING Objectives

To maintain fluid and electrolyte balance

To identify the appropriate method for IV infusion

To administer medications through the most therapeutic IV route

To provide a ready access for emergency medications, particularly in critically ill clients

To provide the appropriate means for administering blood and blood products

IMPLEMENTATION Procedures

Preparing IV System

Preparing IV Site

Inserting a Winged-Tip Needle

Inserting an Over-the-Needle Catheter

EVALUATION Expected Outcomes

Appropriate IV equipment is identified.

IV site is prepared appropriately.

IV therapy is initiated without difficulty.

PREPARING IV SYSTEM

Equipment

IV solution in bag as ordered by the physician

Administration set: drip system, which includes drip chamber and IV tubing with clamp or adjuster

Extension tubing to lengthen the original tubing or to provide extra ports for the administration of additional medication

IV pole: free-standing, bed-attached, or ceiling-affixed

IV line filter, if one is not built into the equipment

IV FILTERS

Studies using IV filters have shown that they reduce bacteremia significantly and that the incidence of infusion phlebitis can be reduced as much as 40%. Although the latter condition is usually not life-threatening, it does affect client comfort and attitude toward IV therapy. For these reasons it is important to consider using an in-line IV filter with all IV administration. Many IV catheters now contain an in-line filter, so catheter is sized to maintain adequate flow rate. Size is regulated by use and depends on the substance being infused.

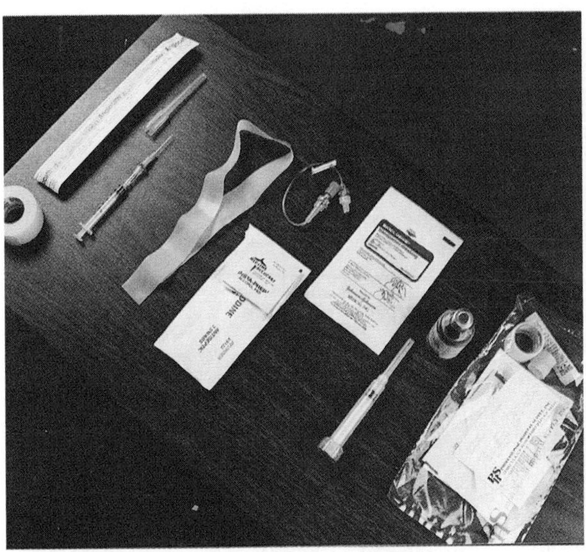
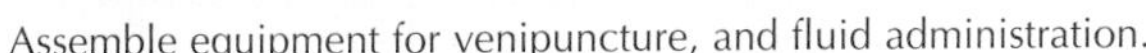

Assemble equipment for venipuncture, and fluid administration.

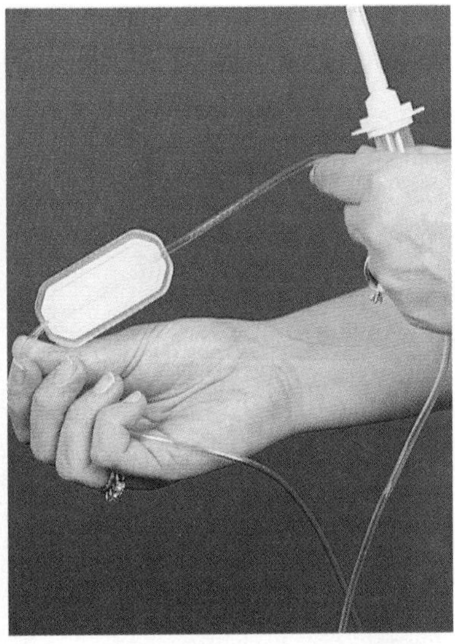

Inline IV filter reduces infection.

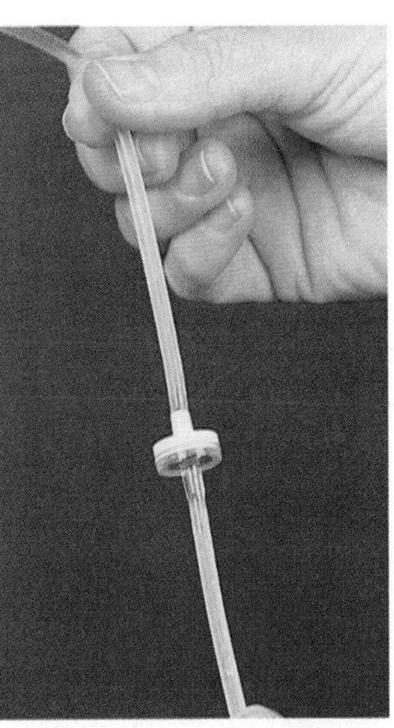

Another type of in-line IV filter.

IV filters come in several sizes or in the catheter; the finer the filter, the more completely it filters the liquid. Sizes range from 5 μm, which filters out most particular matter, to 0.22 μm, which removes most fungi and bacteria. The finer filter does reduce flow rate.

Note: *Some hospitals do not use IV filters due to cost. They are always used for mannitol or if the solution indicates use (blood, hyperalimentation). IV filters are not used for lipids.*

Preparation

1. Wash your hands before preparing IV equipment.
2. Compare the type and amount of solution with physician's orders and client care plan.
3. Check IV solution container for expiration date and for signs of contamination or deterioration.
4. Select IV tubing according to hospital policy.
5. Label IV solution with client's name, date, time, and additives.

Procedure

1. Prepare the IV solution for infusion.
2. Remove outer wrap around the IV container. Bag may be wet due to condensation.
3. Inspect bag carefully for tears or leaks by noting

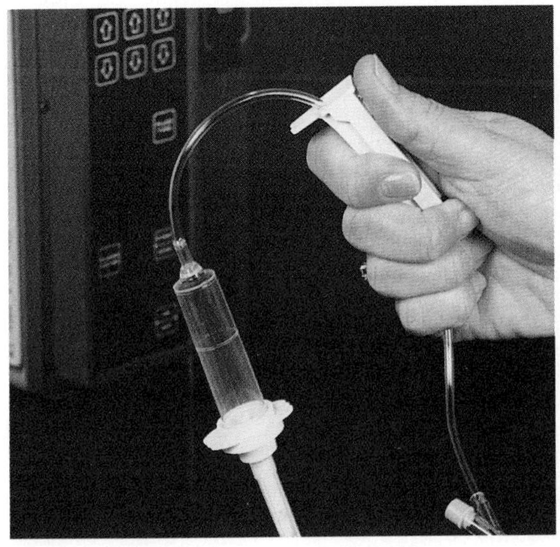

Clamp tubing before spiking IV fluid bag.

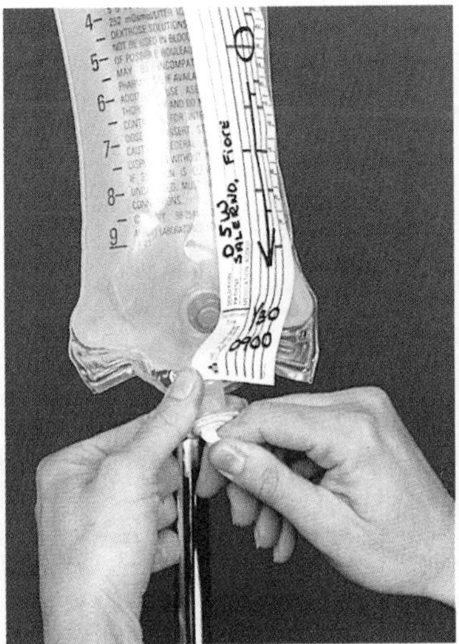

Pull to remove tab on IV bag.

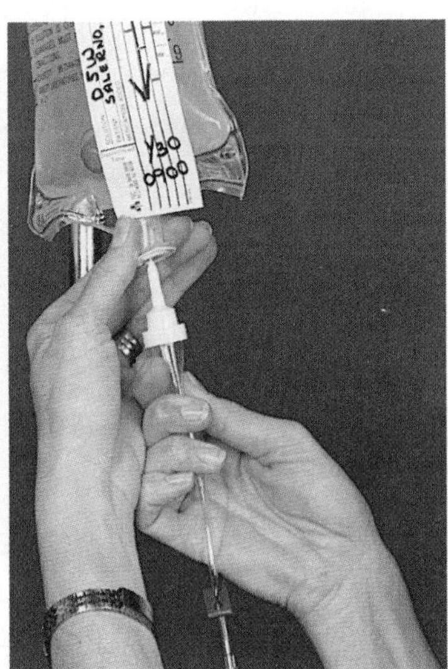

Spike bag port maintaining sterility.

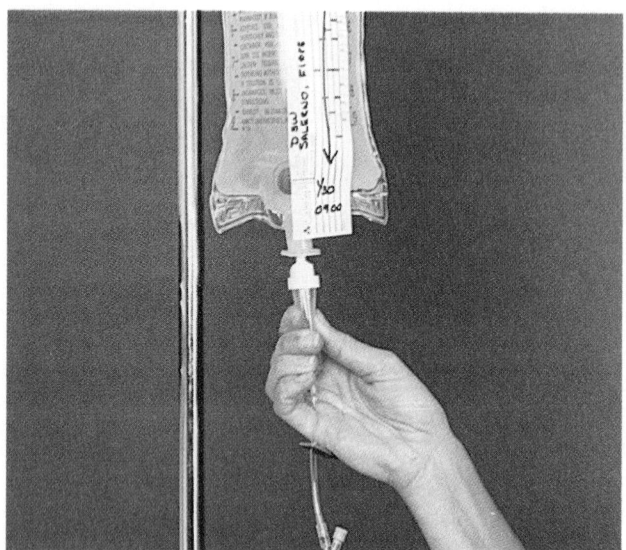

Squeeze and release pressure on drip chamber.

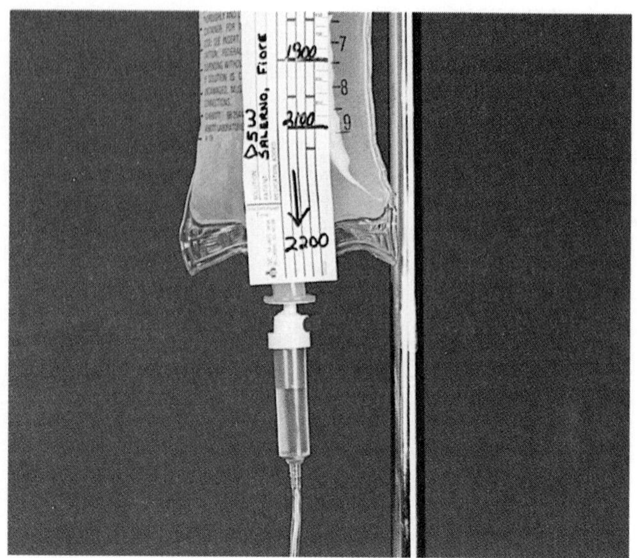

Fill chamber with fluid, one-half to one-third full.

any moisture on protective covering, and by applying gentle pressure to bag. Hold bag up against both a dark and light background to examine for discoloration, cloudiness, or particulate matter. **Rationale:** Any evidence of change may indicate contamination, and bag should be discarded.

4. Hang the IV container on the IV pole.
5. Close tubing roller clamp.
6. Remove plastic protector from the IV container. **Rationale:** Since there is no vacuum in the plastic container, you should not hear any escaping air.
7. Insert tubing spike into the container port, holding the neck of the port securely to prevent possible contamination.
8. Squeeze, then release pressure on the drip chamber until chamber is one-third to one-half full.
9. Remove caps from filter.
10. Fit tubing's male adapter into filter's female connector, and turn to ensure tight connection.
11. Hold filter so connector joint is pointed down.
12. Open clamps on line to prime tubing and filter. Hold tubing tip higher than tubing-dependent loop. **Rationale:** Air rises and passes out as fluid fills tubing.
13. Tap filter as the solution runs through. **Rationale:** This eliminates any air bubbles trapped in the membrane.
14. Close control clamp on IV tubing administration set.
15. Replace the tubing cap or place needleless injec-

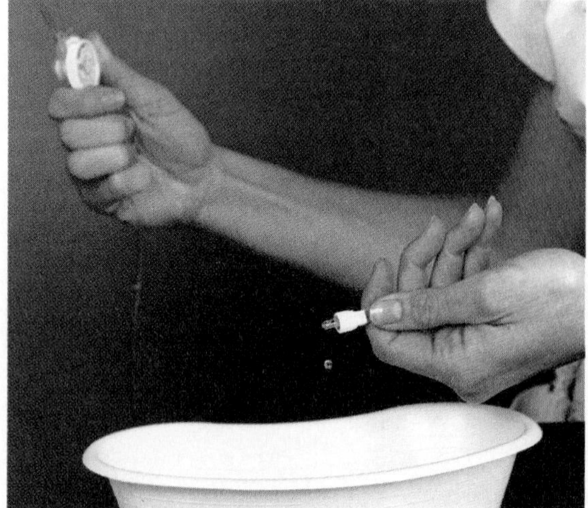
Open clamp on line to clear tubing of air.

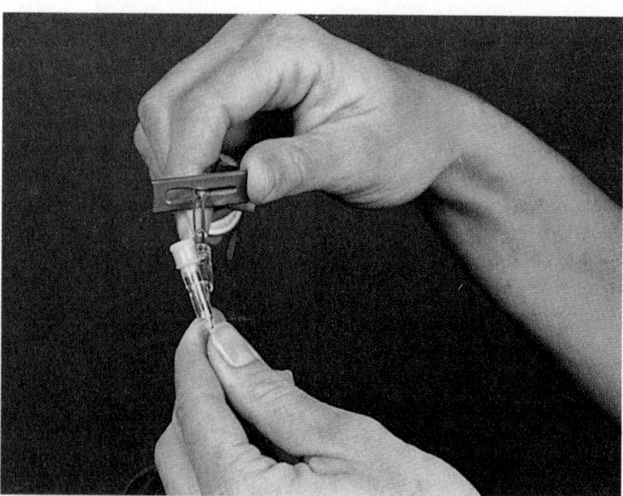
Close clamp on IV tubing.

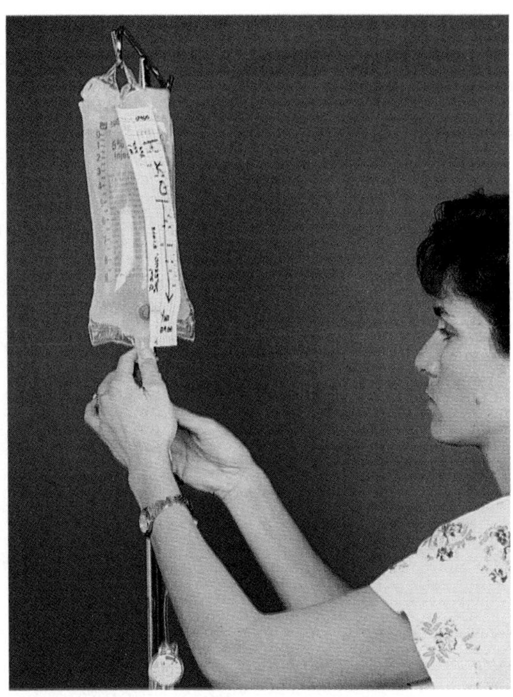

Label bag with client's name, date, time, and additives.

tion cannula over tubing insertion site. **Rationale:** This maintains sterility before infusion is established.

16. Check that IV system is prepared and ready to be used.

Using Glass Bottles

Hospitals still infuse some solutions in glass bottles. Following is the step-by-step skill of using a glass bottle.

- Wash your hands before preparing IV equipment.
- Compare the type and amount of solution with physician's orders and client care plan.
- Check IV solution container for expiration date and for signs of contamination or deterioration.
- Hold against both a dark and bright light background to examine for discoloration, cloudiness, or particulate matter, which indicates contamination.
- Examine bottle for cracks or leaks. **Rationale:** Crack or leak indicates contamination. Return bottle to central supply or pharmacy for manufacturer notification.
- Remove metal cap, metal disc, and rubber diaphragm from IV bottle. If pharmacy has added medications, remove protective additive cap.
- Listen for the escape of air when rubber diaphragm is removed.
- Close control clamp on IV tubing administration set. If indicated, attach IV in-line filter according to manufacturer's directions or procedure included in *Preparing IV System.*
- Place container on a firm surface, and insert spike through appropriate area on bottle cap.
- Invert IV bottle, and place it on IV pole.
- Squeeze drip chamber, then release until it is one-half full of fluid and filter is covered.
- Open tubing control clamp and clear tubing of air over a receptacle, such as an emesis basin or a sink. (It may be necessary to remove adaptor cap at end of tubing so that fluid can flow through tubing.) Reclamp tubing.
- Invert and tap Y injection sites to expel all air as IV tubing is already primed with fluid. **Rationale:** If air remains in the Y, it will be forced into vein.
- Replace adaptor cap, or place covered needleless locking cannula over tubing insertion site. **Rationale:** To maintain sterility before infusion is established.
- Before taking IV equipment to client's room, tell client what you will be doing and what type of equipment you will be using.

PREPARING IV SITE

Equipment

Prepared IV system

Tourniquet or blood pressure cuff

Antimicrobial wipe (povidone-iodine or iodophors are preferred by Centers for Disease Control (CDC); alcohol is acceptable if client is allergic to iodine)

Sterile needle or catheter for venipuncture

Adults use 16- to 19-gauge for viscous solutions and 20- to 25-gauge for less viscous solutions

Neonates use a 25- to 27-gauge needle

Older children use a 21- to 25-gauge needle

Tape (check client for adhesive allergy)

CLINICAL ALERT

Do not shave the venipuncture site. Shaving can facilitate the development of infection through the multiplication of organisms in resulting microabrasions. Hairy sites can be clipped with scissors.

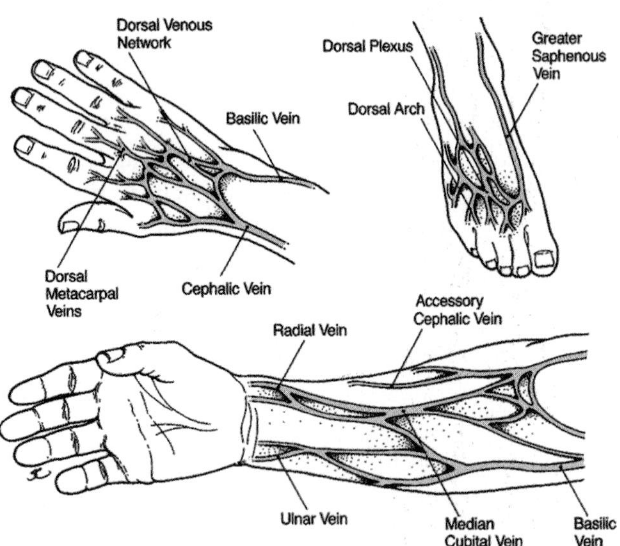

Anatomical sites frequently used for venipunctures.

Sterile 2×2-inch gauze squares or transparent semipermeable adhesive dressing

Antimicrobial or polyantibiotic ointment (according to policy)

Procedure

1. Assemble equipment, and take to bedside.
2. Check client's identaband.
3. Hang bag, and place covered end of administration set within easy reach.
4. Position client, and adjust lighting as necessary.
5. Cut pieces of tape. Open 2×2 gauze pad, and squeeze a dollop of antimicrobial ointment on surface, if indicated.
6. Wash your hands. **Rationale:** Handwashing decreases the numbers of both endogenous and exogenous microorganisms, reducing the risk of cross-contamination of the catheter.
7. Select a vein. Inspect both of the client's arms, palpating and visualizing the exact course of the veins. If the client's skin is thick or darkly colored, you may not be able to visualize the veins easily. Instead, palpate them until you find a vein that feels full and superficial.
   a. Veins should be superficial, easily palpated and followed, and large enough for a needle to be smoothly inserted.
   b. Veins should be free of sclerosis, hematomas, and pain.
   c. Veins should be selected according to the IV solution that is to be infused. Larger veins are preferable for caustic solutions, blood, and viscous fluids.
   d. Distal end of vein should usually be punctured first, reserving more proximal sites for further IV therapy. Client status may dictate choice of a larger, more proximal vein, however.
   e. Catheter placement should be away from mobile joints, such as wrist or elbow. Avoid using veins in affected arm following an axillary dissection (e.g., mastectomy). Select nondominant arm.
   f. If catheter is inserted in leg vein, prompt relocation to upper extremity is advised.
8. Select catheter. Catheter gauge should be smallest size that allows greatest flow, without occluding vessel lumen.
9. Prepare site with povidone-iodine or a 70% ethyl alcohol solution if client is allergic to iodine. **Rationale:** Vigorous skin preparation decreases endogenous and exogenous organisms at the venipuncture site.
10. Let iodine or alcohol solution dry on client's skin before continuing with intervention. Do not use your hand to fan dry skin. **Rationale:** This increases the chance of contamination.

> **CLINICAL ALERT**
>
> For antiseptic effectiveness, allow iodophor to dry on skin at least 30 seconds before using alcohol if better visualization is required.

11. Apply tourniquet or blood pressure cuff to distend client's vein. If using cuff, inflate to a pressure just below diastolic reading. If veins are not palpable, encourage engorgement by using one of these methods:
    a. Ask client to open and close fist several times. You may also tap the vein lightly or stroke vein distal to proximal. Be sure to reprepare site with preparation solution after touching site with your fingers.
    b. Place client in a low- or semi-Fowler's position with arm over edge of mattress for 1–2 minutes.
    c. If the vein is difficult to palpate, release tourniquet and apply warm, moist compresses to arm for 10–20 minutes before reapplying tourniquet.

INSERTING A WINGED-TIP NEEDLE

Equipment

Prepared IV system
Tourniquet or blood pressure cuff
Antimicrobial wipe (povidone-iodine or iodophors are preferred; alcohol is acceptable if client is allergic to iodine)
Sterile winged-tip needle:
- Adults use size 16- to 29-gauge for viscous solutions and 20- to 25-gauge for less viscous solutions
- Neonates use a 25- to 27-gauge needle
- Older children use a 21- to 25-gauge needle

Tape
Transparent dressing or protective wrap (coban)
Antimicrobial ointment (optional)
Clean gloves

Procedure

1. Select a winged-tip needle. (A 20- to 22-gauge needle is adequate for an adult.) **Rationale:** Winged-tip needles are used in short-term therapy with adults and in normal therapy with children, infants, and elderly clients who have small or fragile veins.
2. Carefully affix end of IV administration tubing to end of winged-tip needle. Remove sterile cover from needle. Run fluid through needle.
3. Don gloves.
4. Hold needle by its wings and anchor vein by placing your thumb below the client's vein and gently stretching the skin by pulling down distally.
5. With bevel of needle up, enter client's skin at an angle. You may use either of these methods:
   a. Enter skin at an angle either next to or alongside the vein. Flatten angle once needle is under skin and enter vein from the side.
   b. Enter skin and vein in one smooth motion from above. You feel a gentle "pop" or release as the needle enters the vein. Observe for flashback of blood in needle tubing. **Rationale:** This method requires experience and judgment, since it is easy to put the needle through the vein.
6. Advance needle carefully up the course of the vein.

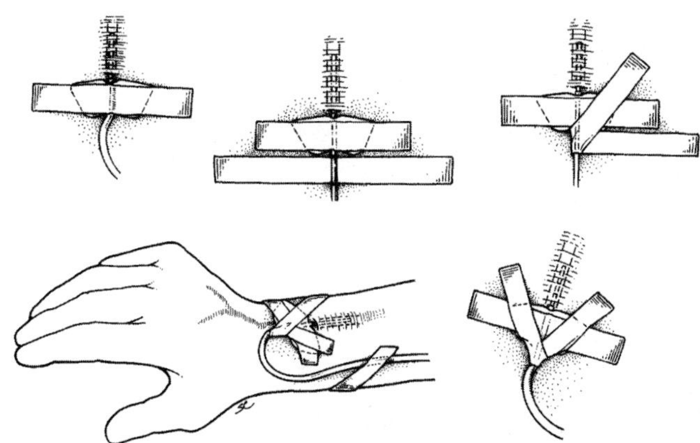

Use chevron method to secure winged-tip needle.

7. Release tourniquet or blood pressure cuff.
8. Open clamp on IV tubing, and observe drip chamber. **Rationale:** Fluid should flow easily, and there should be no sudden swelling around IV site.
9. Reduce flow rate to keep open until you have taped the needle and tubing in place.
10. Apply antimicrobial ointment to needle site (according to agency policy).
11. Tape winged-tip needle and tubing to client's skin.

Each Time the Closed Body System is Entered the Potential for Contamination Exists.

- Strict attention should be directed to maintaining the infusion system aseptically.
- Once the needle has been inserted, it should be anchored with tape to prevent a rocking motion, which may irritate the vein or push bacteria into the bloodstream from the skin.
- The sterile dressing should be applied in such a way that daily dressing changes and venipuncture site inspection can occur without undue problems.
- The IV administration set should be changed every 48–72 hours to decrease risk of infection.
- Infusion solutions should not hang longer than 24 hours.

12. Cover with transparent dressing and tape tubing.
13. Using a watch, set drip rate according to physician's orders.
14. Label IV site with pertinent information, according to hospital policy.

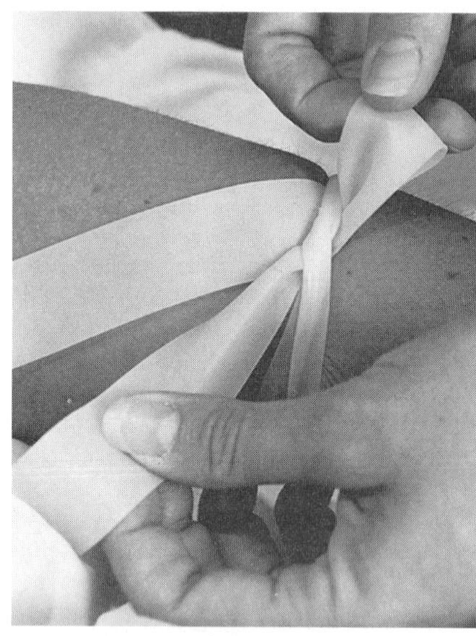
Apply tourniquet proximal to IV puncture site in order to dilate the veins.

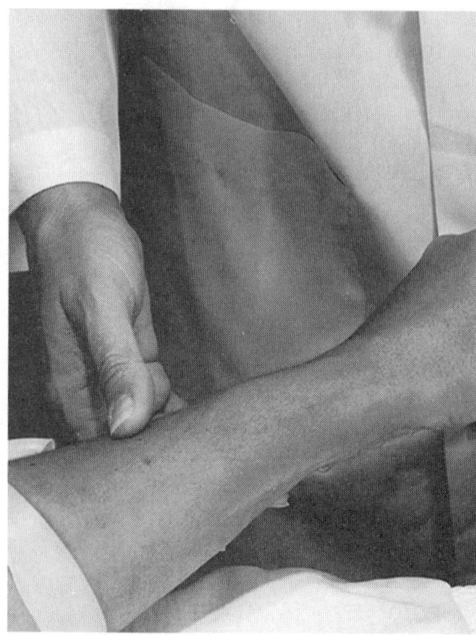
Instruct the client to open and close fist several times to distend the vein.

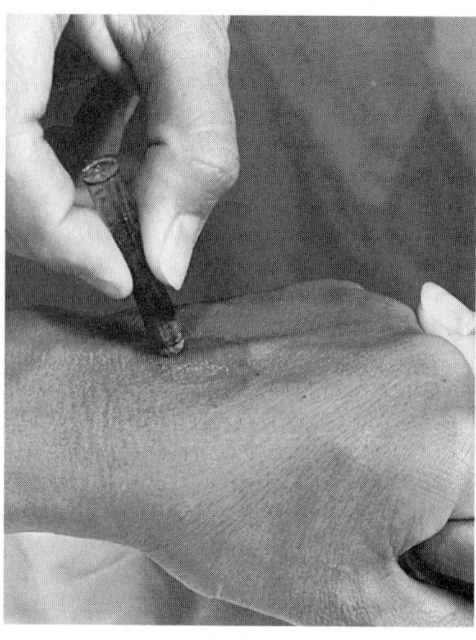
Apply povidone-iodine to puncture site and allow to dry thoroughly.

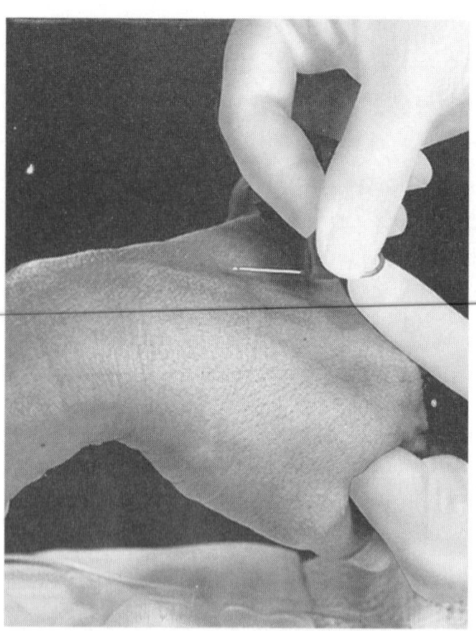
Start venipuncture at distal end of vein to preserve future IV sites.

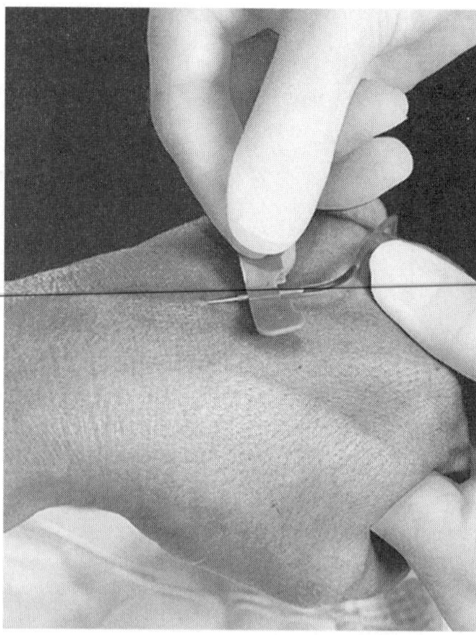
Keep winged-tip needle bevel up and insert needle at 45° angle.

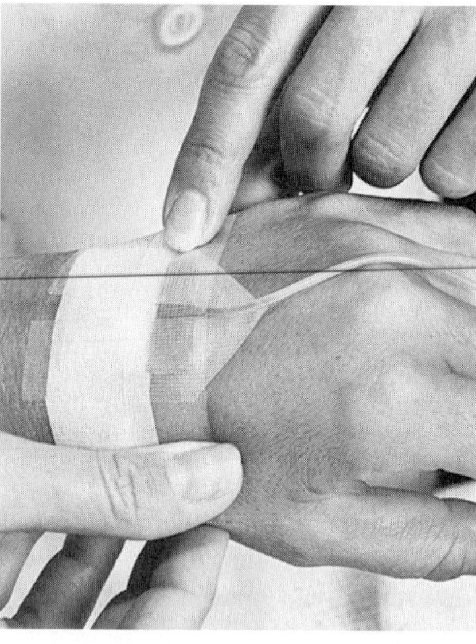
Secure IV site with additional tape, positioning tubing to prevent pulling.

INSERTING AN OVER-THE NEEDLE CATHETER

Equipment

Tourniquet or blood pressure cuff

Antimicrobial wipe (povidone-iodine or iodophors are preferred; alcohol is acceptable if client is allergic to iodine)

Sterile over-the-needle catheter sizes 12- to 22-gauge, $1\frac{1}{4}$–$5\frac{1}{2}$ inch long

Syringe filled with local anesthetic and 25- to 26-gauge needle affixed (check for client sensitivity before using)

IV solution as ordered by physician

Administration set: drip system, which includes drip chamber and IV tubing with needleless cannula

Filter (according to hospital policy)

Extension tubing (if necessary)

Antimicrobial ointment (according to hospital policy)

Sterile 2×2 dressing
Tape (check client for adhesive allergy)
Needleless injection cap
IV controller or pump, if required
Clean gloves

Procedure

1. Prepare IV equipment following steps in preparation. (Whenever possible initiate short-term IV therapy using a safety system with built-in protection against accidental needlesticks.)
2. Select appropriate sized over-the-needle catheter.
3. Prepare IV site following steps 1 through 10 in *Preparing IV Site.*
4. Don gloves.

■ CLINICAL ALERT

Despite excellent aseptic technique and practiced motor skills in establishing an IV line, a nurse may still be at risk from direct contact with client's blood, either via a needle stick or small cuts on nurse's hands; therefore, the nurse should always use gloves when starting an IV line.

5. Inject site intradermally with small wheal of local anesthetic according to client preference and hospital policy. (Allow 90 seconds for anesthetic to take effect.)

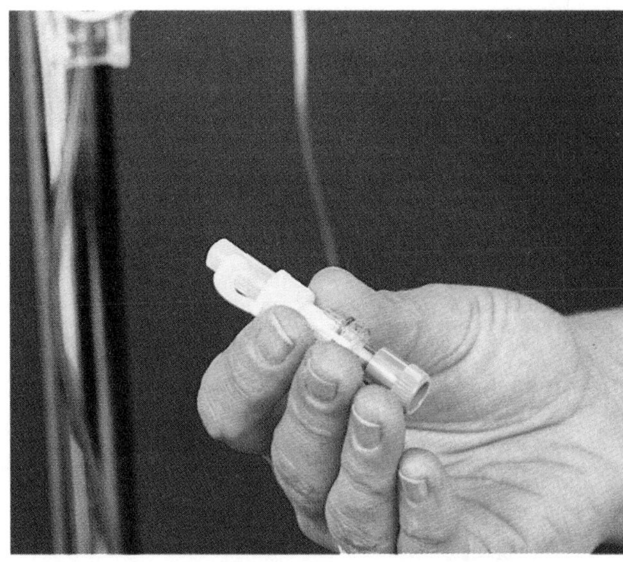

Select appropriate needleless component parts whenever possible.

6. Remove needle cover carefully just prior to insertion. Inspect both needle and catheter. **Rationale:** Barbs or rough edges can occur even with new needle bevels.

■ CLINICAL ALERT

Whenever possible, use needleless access components (caps and cannulas) with all continuous or intermittent IV fluid or drug administration.

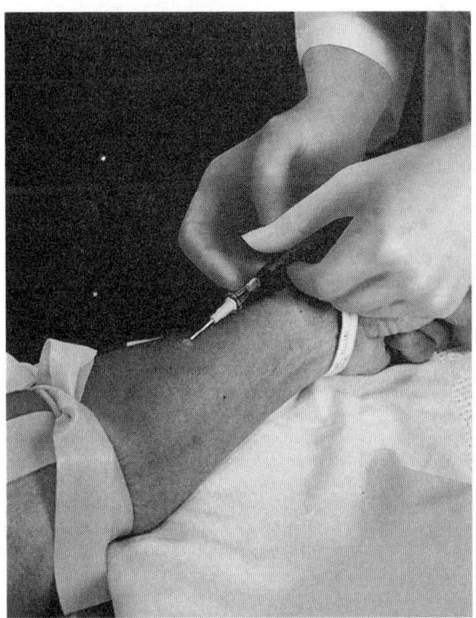

Advance over-the-needle catheter into client's vein.

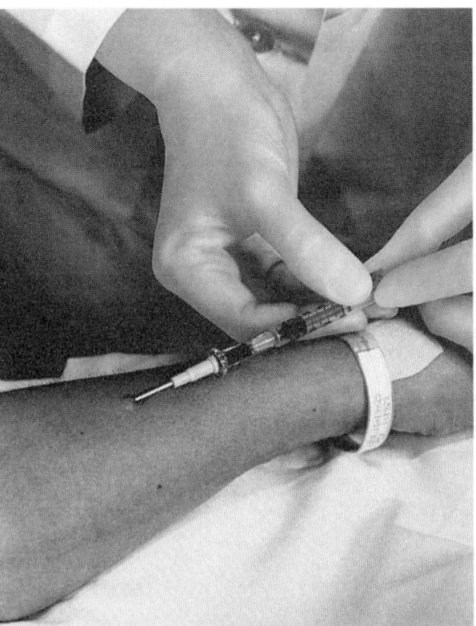

Withdraw needle and observe for blood in hub.

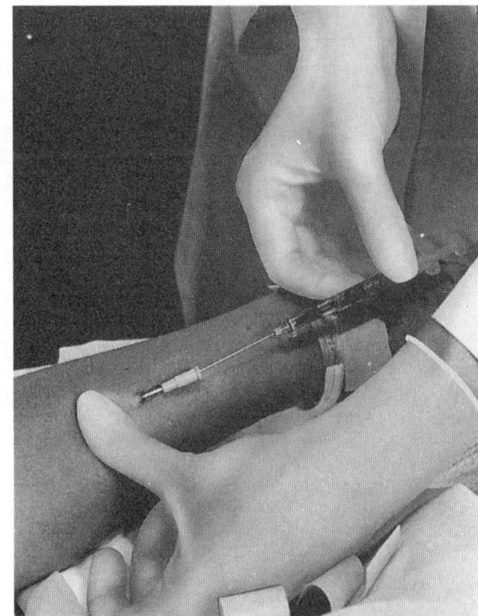

Gently pull needle from inside catheter with one hand.

7. Turn bevel of needle up; insert needle and catheter together as one unit into client's skin—either along side or above vein. **Rationale:** Bevel in the UP position assists with needle insertion.
8. Insert catheter and needle into vein. Advance unit into lumen, making sure that both are inside vein. Observe for backflow of blood in plastic hub of needle. **Rationale:** This indicates you are in the vein.
9. Hold needle hub and gently advance plastic catheter over needle and up vein to desired length. **Rationale:** This method prevents inadvertent puncture of vein. (An alternative method is to advance entire unit up vein to desired length and then remove needle.)
10. DO NOT attempt to replace needle inside catheter if the venipuncture is not successful. This action may sheer off a piece of the catheter.
11. Place small, sterile gauze sponge under hub of over-the-needle unit as an alternative.
12. As soon as catheter is fully in place, release tourniquet.
13. Gently withdraw needle from inside catheter with one hand, placing your fingertip firmly above catheter tip to secure catheter and occlude vein.
14. Affix needleless injection cap.
15. Prep cap with alcohol.
16. Insert IV tubing with needleless cannula.
17. Open clamp on set briefly, and observe drip chamber. Fluid should flow rapidly without obstruction, and there should not be any sudden swelling at IV site.
18. Reduce flow, and proceed with taping, using chevron method.
19. Cover with sterile 2×2 strips, tape, or transparent dressing.
20. Tape tubing to client, using two strips of tape.
21. Using a watch, set drip rate according to physician's orders.
22. Label IV site with pertinent information, according to hospital policy.

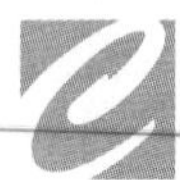

CHARTING for IV Therapy

- Location of insertion site
- Gauge and type of needle or catheter inserted
- Time of insertion
- Type and amount of solution infusing
- Rate of infusion
- Condition of IV site

CRITICAL THINKING APPLICATION

CLINICAL PROBLEMS	CRITICAL THINKING OPTIONS
Venipuncture attempt does not result in insertion into vein.	• Remove needle. Apply Band-Aid. • Move to other side of body for vein assessment. If necessary, move proximally on the same vein. Select new site, and use fresh needle. • After two attempts, ask more experienced personnel to perform venipuncture. • Ensure that the needle enters the skin at 45° angle and to one side of the vein, before proceeding with cannulization.
Veins roll and are difficult to enter.	• Use firmer pressure to anchor skin and vein.
Needle enters vein, but IV flow is not established.	• Check position of needle. • Align needle away from vein wall. • Check the height of the IV bag. May have to *raise* IV pole. • IV tubing may be kinked or roller clamp not open. • Venous flow may be slowed if IV filter is occluded. • Venous spasm may alter flow; allow needle to remain in vein without manipulation to discontinue spasms.
Veins are fragile and appear to "balloon" around the needle once the vein has been entered.	• Loosen tourniquet to reduce pressure in the vein. If possible, use a smaller gauge winged-tip needle.

unit 2

IV MANAGEMENT

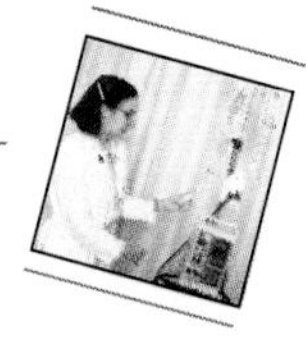

NURSING PROCESS DATA

ASSESSMENT Data Base

Assess flow rate for accuracy.

Determine if pump or controller cassette or administration set needs to be changed.

Assess venipuncture site for edema, erythema, and infiltration.

Assess IV solution for correct solution, amount, and timing.

Assess need to discontinue IV needle or catheter.

Assess need to change client gown while IV infusing.

PLANNING Objectives

To maintain the IV site free from erythema, edema, and purulent drainage

To calculate and monitor the IV infusion rate accurately and to reassess throughout the therapy

To remove IV equipment without complications

To change a gown while maintaining the IV site

IMPLEMENTATION Procedures

Regulating IV Flow Rate

Using an IV Controller

Using an IV Pump

Using a Syringe Pump

Managing IV Site

Changing IV Dressing

Changing Gown for Client with IV

Discontinuing an IV

EVALUATION Expected Outcomes

Fluids, additives, and medications are administered without adverse effects for the client.

IV site remains free from erythema, edema, and purulent drainage.

IV infusion rate is accurately calculated and reassessed throughout the therapy.

Client gown is changed while maintaining IV placement.

IV therapy is discontinued without complications.

REGULATING IV FLOW RATE

Procedure

1. Check manufacturer's drip rate calibration on administration set package. Macrodrip sets vary from 10–20 gtts to equal 1 mL.

IV Calorie Calculation

- 1000 mL D_5W provides 50 g of dextrose
- 50 g of dextrose provides 4 Cal/g (actually 3.4 Cal); therefore, multiply 50 g × 4 Cal.
- 1000 mL D_5W provides 200 Cal.
- Usual IV total/day is 3000 mL (600 Cal/day).

2. Check physician's order for amount of fluids to be delivered per unit of time. Some physicians state 1 L to be given over 8 hours; others specify hourly flow rate, such as 60 mL/hour.
3. Calculate flow rate. Several formulas may be useful. Here is one two-step method.
   a. To find the number of milliliters to be given per hour:

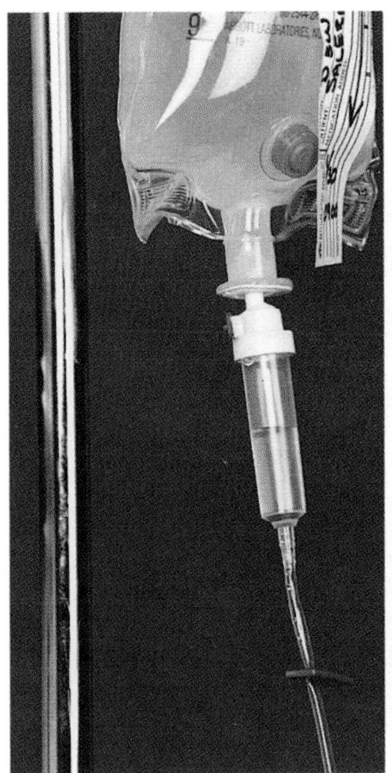
Count drops per minute to check accuracy of drip rate.

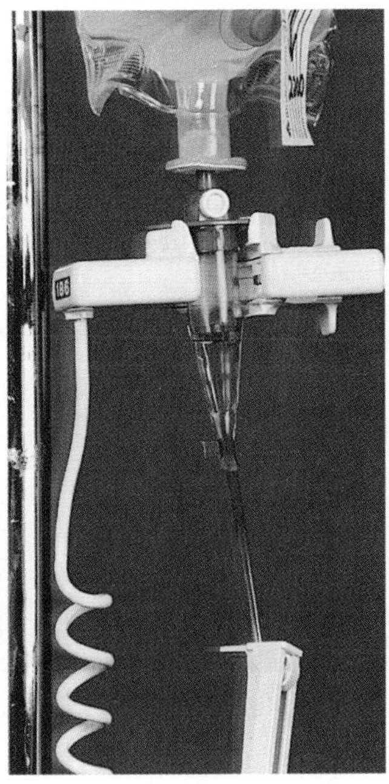
Clamp sensor device over drip chamber for drops per minute.

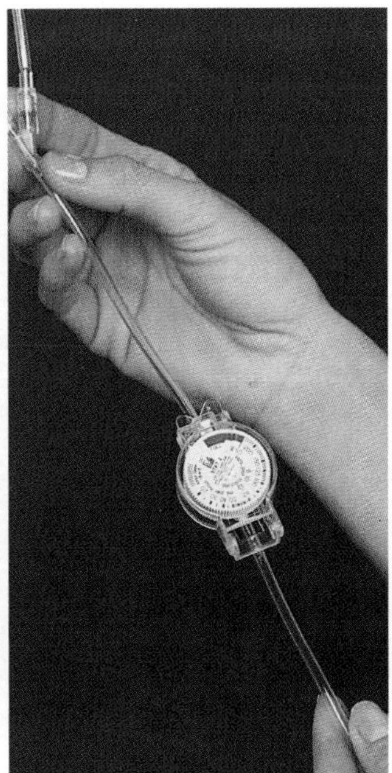
Set dial-a-flow to prescribed drops per minute.

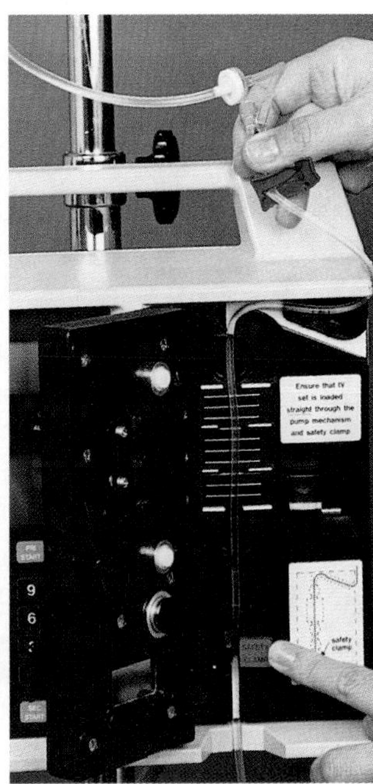
Load delivery system and set drops per minute.

$$\frac{\text{Total solution}}{\text{No. of hours to run}} = \text{mL/hour}$$

b. To find drops per minute:

$$\frac{\text{mL/hr} \times \text{drop factor}}{60 \text{ minutes}} = \text{gtts/minute}$$

4. Stand near the drip chamber and count the drops in 1 minute, using a watch with a sweep hand.
5. Adjust clamp until the chamber drips the desired number of drops.
6. Affix tape to bag and mark the hourly flow rate.

Choice: Controller or Pump

Controller

- Controllers have been described as "electronic flow clamps." They depend on gravity to maintain preselected flow and do not add pressure to system to overcome resistance.
- Resistance develops from:
  a. Use of a large catheter in a small vein.
  b. Administration of viscous fluid.
  c. High venous pressure or a decrease in the height of container from the IV site. Resistance may cause the flow rate to decrease and the controller alarm to sound.
- Older models of controllers, which counted drops/minute, are being replaced by controllers that permit flow rates to be set in milliliters/hour and are called "volumetric" controllers.
- Controllers are the instrument of choice in 80–85% of all drug administration situations requiring close monitoring.

Pump

- Pumps do not depend on gravity for flow; they maintain preselected volume delivery by adding pressure to the system when needed.
- When IV system is working without resistance, pressure used is minimal. When fluid is viscous, or a plug develops in the catheter or tubing, pump adds pressure to maintain its output. Each pump has a maximum pressure limit which, when reached, sounds an alarm.
- Some pumps can deliver up to 14 or 15 psi pressure (723.8–775.5 mm Hg) to the infusion site.
- With pumps there is the danger of developing infiltration or vein irritation caused by a drug or solution administered under high pressure.
- Unless high volumes must be delivered in a short time, pressure pumps are normally not used in place of gravity flow devices.

Note: PCA (patient-controlled analgesia) devices, both electronic and mechanical, are presented in Chapter 17, Pain Management.

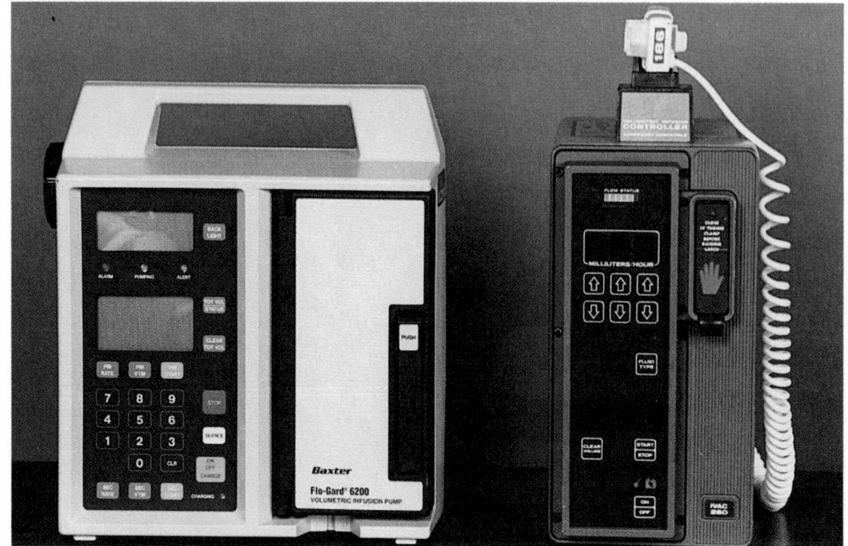

Infusion pump and controller.

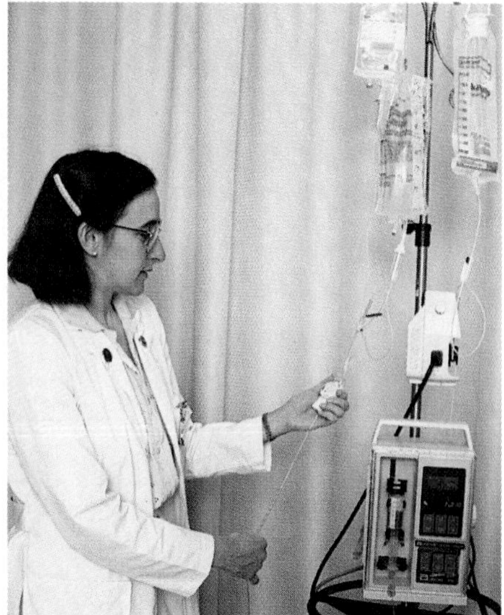

Nurse adjusting IV drip rate.

USING AN IV CONTROLLER

Equipment

Controller
Compatible IV administration tubing

Preparation

1. Identify if type of medication or solution to be infused requires a controller. Infiltration risk needs to be assessed along with condition of the extremity, and age and activity level of client.
2. Bring equipment to the client's room.
3. Explain the use of the machine and alarm system. **Rationale:** This reassures client that machine's alarm may sound occasionally when the sensor senses the rate of flow has decreased.
4. Plug machine into the electric outlet.

Procedure

1. Close tubing regulating clamp.
2. Insert spike of IV administration set into bag.
3. Hang bag on IV pole, and fill drip chamber to no more than one-half full. **Rationale:** This amount allows sufficient air space between the top of the drip chamber and the chamber's fluid level for solution drips to be "sensed."
4. Adjust IV bag height to place the IV drip chamber approximately 36 inches (91 cm) above the infusion site. **Rationale:** This height provides sufficient gravity for flow of solution.
5. Partially open regulating clamp, and slowly prime tubing.
6. Invert, and tap Y injection sites to expel all air. Close clamp.
7. Verify that existing IV is patent. If existing IV is using noncompatible tubing, disconnect and affix appropriate tubing to catheter hub.
8. Partially open clamp to KVO (keep-open) rate.
9. Turn machine ON.
10. Insert tubing into controller mechanism following manufacturer's instructions.
11. Place drip sensor on drip chamber, if required.
12. Open regulating clamp on IV tubing. (After tubing is connected to controller mechanism, with machine not yet functioning, there should be no fluid flow.)
13. Set controller at prescribed rate—either milliliters/hour or drops/minute, and volume to be infused, depending on type of controller.
14. Press START on controller.
15. Observe drip chamber to determine flow has begun.
16. Recheck the infusion site, drip rate, and volume

infused indicator within 15 minutes. **Rationale:** This ensures that controller system is functioning as desired.

17. Observe client regularly to determine that IV system is functioning properly.

USING AN IV PUMP

Equipment

Volumetric pumps

Special IV administration set and tubing, compatible with pump

Procedure

1. Spike IV solution bag.
2. Close regulating clamp on the set tubing before hanging bag.
3. Fill drip chamber to minimum one-third full. **Rationale:** This amount allows sufficient air space in drip chamber.
4. Prime tubing by opening regulating clamp slowly and allow tubing to fill with IV solution. (Follow package instructions to correctly fill the cassette portion of the tubing.)
5. Check that IV is patent and that client's insertion site is free from signs of vein irritation or infiltration.
6. Connect administration set tubing to patent IV.
7. Set rate with regulating clamp to "keep-open" rate.
8. Turn pump ON.
9. Follow manufacturer's instructions, and load administration set into machine, taking care to set tubing or cassette into appropriate mechanism or receptor site.
10. Close pump door, and latch.
11. Open regulating clamp on administration set.
12. Position drip sensor, if one is required.
13. Set pump's parameters for operation, again following manufacturer's instructions or machine's set-up prompts. Parameters may include:
    a. Volume to be infused
    b. Rate (milliliters/hour)
    c. Pressure (unit of measure can vary among manufacturers: mm Hg, cm H_2O, or psi).

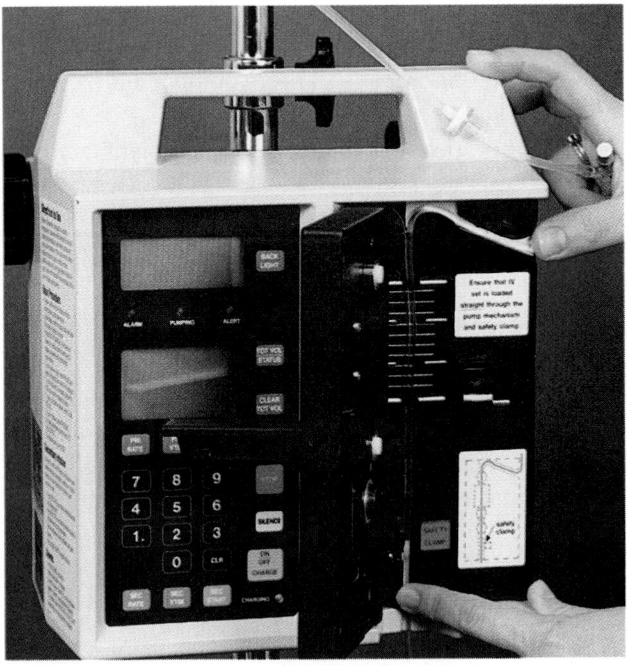

Load administration set into IV pump receptor site.

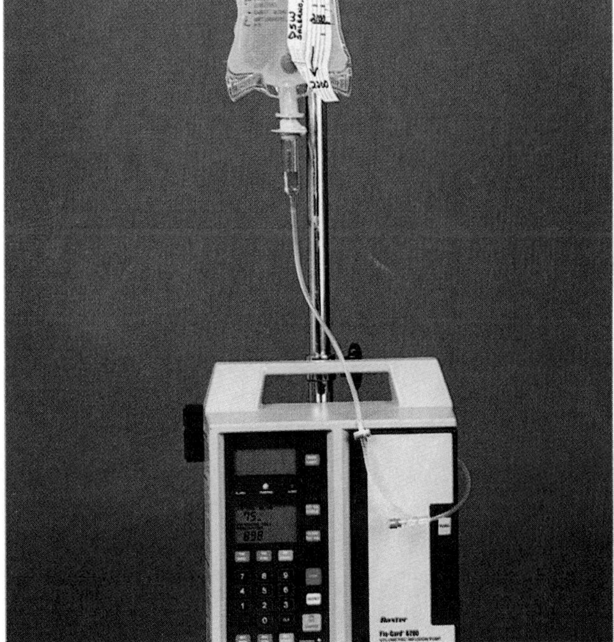

Set pump's parameters for IV operation.

d. Volume limit
14. Start pump when parameters are set.
15. Observe that infusion is running properly.
16. Check client's IV frequently during infusion.

■ CLINICAL ALERT

If using a positive pressure pump, changes in resistance at the insertion site due to infiltration or developing phlebitis are not likely to set off the system's alarm, and site problems could occur.

If Alarm Sounds, Check the Following

Most controllers and pumps have a light or message system that specifies the exact problem. You should be prepared to troubleshoot various components of the system.

- *Infusion Complete:* When the exact volume to be delivered is set and the volume limit has been reached, an alarm sounds and the machine goes to a KVO "keep-open" mode. Establish if the total volume of the container has been delivered; change the solution container if needed, and reset the volume to be infused. With controllers, some machines permit a "volume to be infused" setting and others ask for a "rate" setting when starting the machine. An alarm sounds when the volume to be infused limit is reached.
- *Occlusion:* All controllers sound an alarm when they cannot maintain delivery in the face of increasing resistance. In this instance, check the insertion site for infiltration, look for position problems, pinched tubing, closed clamp, turned stopcock, or clogged filter.
- *Flowrate Variation:* With controllers, the alarms sound when the machine cannot deliver the set flow rate. Start at the catheter insertion site, work backwards to the machine, checking for phlebitis, infiltration, positioning of the arm and catheter, pinched tubing, clogged filter, closed clamp, and height of the bottle (minimum 36 inches). Check position of the drop sensor and the level of fluid in the drip chamber.
- *Other Problems:* Other messages may indicate "air in the line," "low battery," "sensor" (meaning it isn't in correct position), "open door," "cassette" (improperly loaded), "flow rate high."
- *Nursing Action:* Check trouble spot carefully, readjust, and restart the infusion.

USING A SYRINGE PUMP

Equipment

Infusion pump (Harvard is most often used in pediatrics)
Syringes 20 mL, 35 mL, 50 mL (disposable or glass) for use with pump
IV extension tubing with needleless cannula
IV solution
Medication
Diluent for medication (if required)
Syringe 5 mL or 10 mL for drawing up medication

Procedure

1. Check physician's order for drug, dosage, and amount of fluid to be delivered over specified time. Check client's identaband.
2. Identify the amount of medication or fluid to be delivered per minute. (Ensure compatibility of drug and solution.)
3. Select proper syringe, according to manufacturer and equipment directions.
4. Assemble equipment, and plug in machine.
5. Prepare medication in the usual manner, using sterile technique.
6. Draw up prepared medication into syringe filled with appropriate IV fluid for dilution.
7. Attach Leur access pin to end of microbore tubing.
8. Prime tubing and access pin while holding syringe upside-down. (If special sensing devices are part of the tubing, follow manufacturer's instructions to prime tubing.)
9. Insert syringe into cradle of pump, squeeze clamp around designated parts of syringe, and attach to plunger.
10. Swab port closest to client.
11. Insert access pin, twist and lock in place.

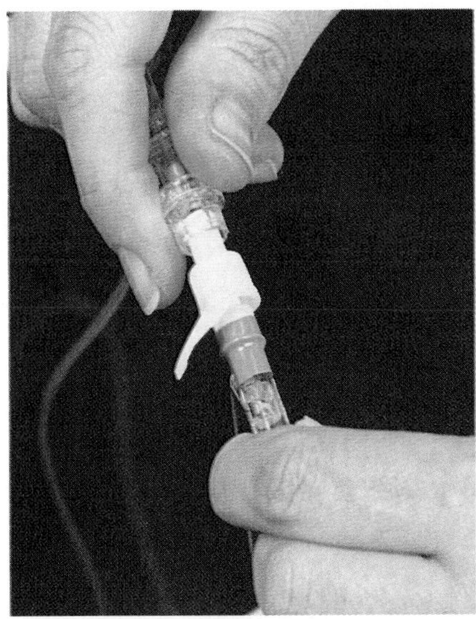
Attach leur access pin to microbore extension tubing.

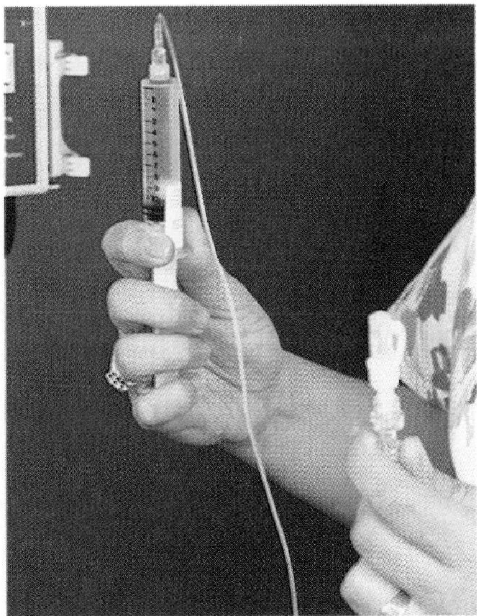
Expell air in syringe before priming tubing and access pin.

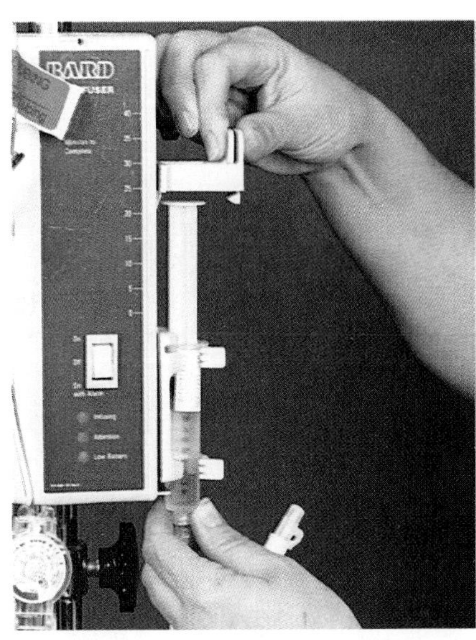

Insert syringe into pump, clamp securely and attach plunger.

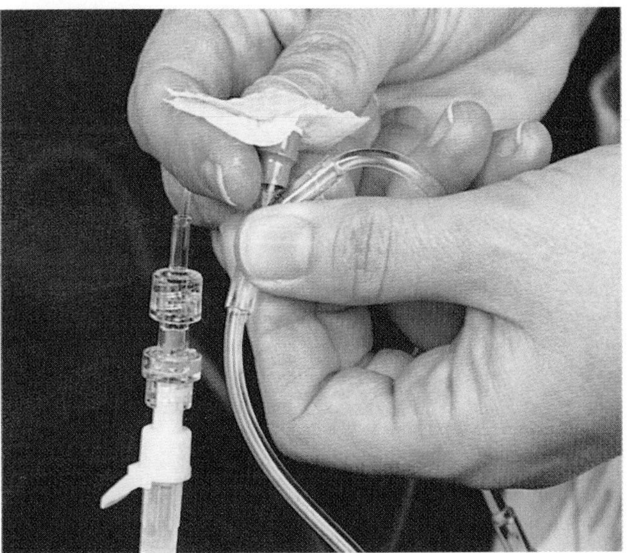
Prep port closest to client before "piggybacking" intermittent syringe pump.

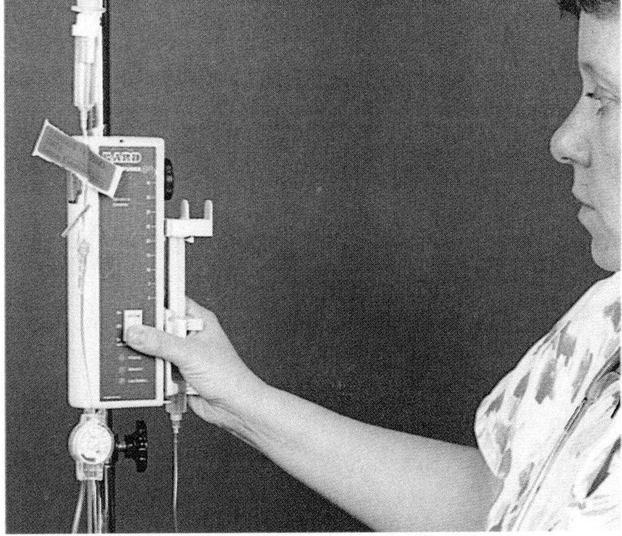

Set amount of volume to be infused—the electronically controlled lever will maintain flow rate.

12. Verify IV site is free from infiltration or vein irritation.
13. Set the amount of volume to be infused (usually in milliliters/hour).
14. Start syringe pump.
15. Check infusion indicator to verify pump is infusing.
16. Monitor site and pump function frequently.

MANAGING IV SITE

■ CLINICAL ALERT

Clients receiving toxic or vesicant drugs, geriatric clients with fragile veins, or pediatric clients who are active are at particular risk for IV site problems.

Procedure

IV Cannula and Dressing

1. Don gloves to evaluate every 8 hours for site related complications (Table 27–3).
2. Include gentle palpation through an intact dressing.
3. Remove dressing and inspect site if client experiences pain or tenderness at insertion site or unexplained fever.
4. Change dressing over the cannula every 24–48 hours, and inspect for any signs of infection.
5. Change dressing immediately if it becomes loose, wet, or soiled.
6. Cleanse skin, apply antimicrobial ointment and sterile dressing (according to agency policy).
7. Remove IV cannula in the periphery, and change to a new site every 48–72 hours.
8. Assess IV site carefully and frequently if client's status prohibits this change.
9. Remove gloves, and wash hands.

IV Administration Sets

1. Change administration sets, including all stopcocks and extension tubings, every 48–72 hours. This can be done routinely at the same time a new container of IV solution is started.
2. Change IV tubing used for hyperalimentation every 24 hours.

"Piggyback" (IVPB) Tubing

1. Change "piggyback" IV tubing every 48–72 hours.
2. Use all "piggyback" sets containing blood, blood products, or lipids only once, then discard.

Converting from Continuous IV to Saline (HEP) Lock Conversion Criteria Procedure:

1. Find patent and functional site.
2. Don clean gloves.
3. Disconnect IV tubing from catheter.

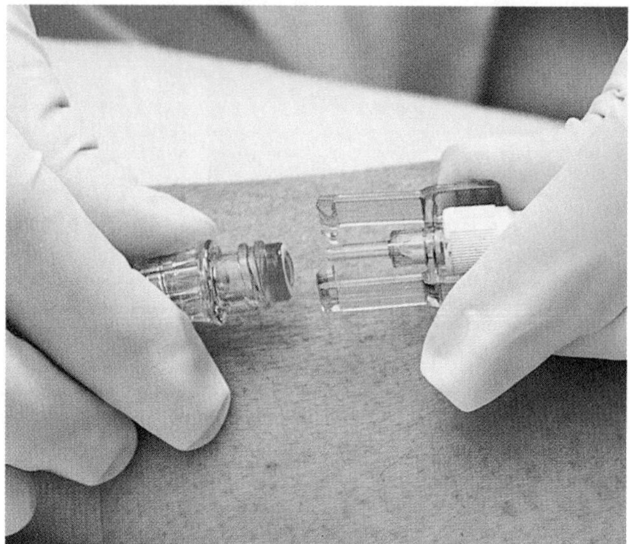

Attach needleless cannula into needleless cap of "HEP lock" for intermittent infusion.

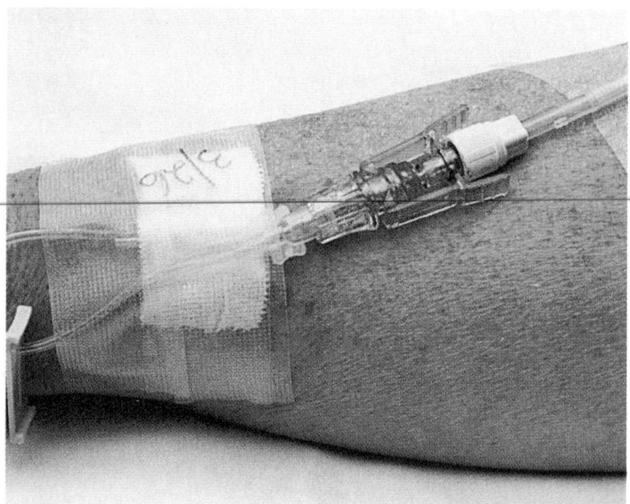

Secure intermittent infusion tubing to arm to prevent strain at "HEP lock" insertion site.

4. Attach needleless injection cap.
5. Inject port with 1 mL sterile normal saline.

Regard IV systems as closed systems and maintain as such. All entries into the tubing, for example, medications, should be made through injection ports that are disinfected just before entry.

CHANGING IV DRESSING

Equipment

Dressing tray

Sterile 2 × 2 gauze dressings, or sterile adhesive dressing

Alternative: sterile transparent semipermeable membrane dressing

Tape (check for client allergy)

70% isopropyl alcohol or povidone-iodine swab

Protective pad

Two pair clean gloves

Procedure

1. Wash your hands.
2. Assemble all equipment, and bring to bedside.
3. Place protective covering under IV site. Don gloves.
4. Remove tape and dressings, keeping pressure over IV site to prevent dislodging needle.
5. Discard dressing and gloves in container.
6. Wash your hands. Don gloves.
7. Inspect IV site for erythema, edema, infiltration.
8. Cleanse IV site with alcohol or povidone-iodine, starting at the puncture site and moving peripherally, using a circular motion.

TABLE 27–3. Complications of IV Therapy

Assessment: Signs and Symptoms	Implementation: Nursing Action
Phlebitis Pain along the vein Erythema—red line above site Edema at insertion site Sluggish flow rate Area is warm to touch	Discontinue infusion, and remove needle Apply warm compresses Notify physician With orders, restart IV at another site Do not irrigate with sluggish flow rate—there may be a clot at the end of the needle and it could be flushed into bloodstream. Document
Infiltration Edema around insertion site—swelling of entire limb Blanching Coolness of skin around site No flashback of blood when tubing is pinched or IV container lowered below IV site Sluggish flow rate	Discontinue infusion and remove needle Apply warm compresses to encourage absorption Lower container below IV site—if blood returns, needle is in vein. Fluid may be leaking into tissue from puncture of vein wall Notify physician With orders, restart IV at another site If IV contains protein hydrolysates, potassium, or sodium lactate, call physician STAT
Infection at Site Erythema Swelling at IV site Client complains of soreness around site Foul-smelling discharge Temperature elevation	Discontinue infusion and remove needle or catheter Aseptically (using sterile scissors) cut needle–catheter tip, place in sterile container, and send to laboratory for culture studies. Culture drainage Clean site, apply prescribed antimicrobial ointment, and cover with sterile gauze Restart IV in another site, as ordered Document
Allergic Reaction Itching Local or generalized rash Dyspnea	Slow infusion to "keep open" rate Notify physician Ask client if he or she has any allergies Follow orders to continue or discontinue infusion

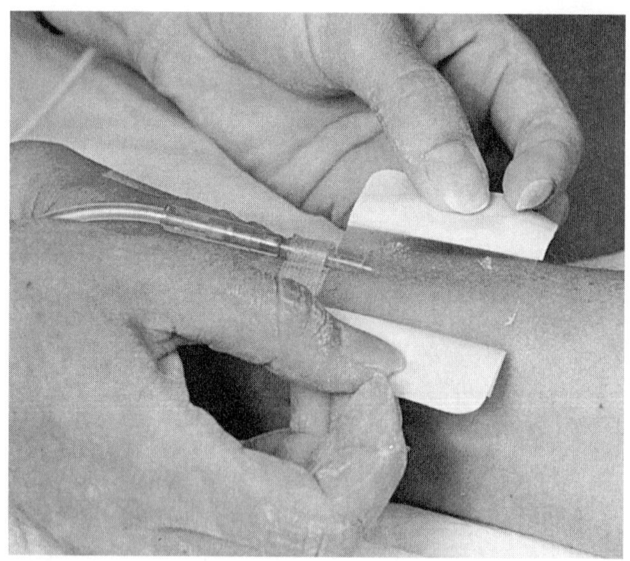

Cover IV insertion site with transparent dressing, according to hospital policy.

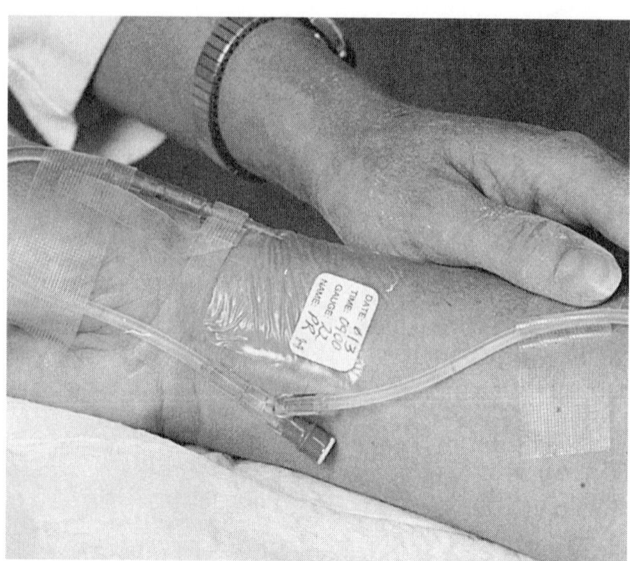

Secure IV tubing to avoid strain at insertion site. Label dressing at site.

9. Apply antimicrobial ointment over IV site, (according to hospital policy).
10. Using transparent dressing, cover IV insertion site with dressing. Use aseptic technique and apply smoothly to avoid wrinkling.
11. Wrap with expanding self-adhering circular wrap according to agency policy.
12. Secure arm to IV arm board if necessary, maintaining good anatomic positioning.

CHANGING GOWN FOR CLIENT WITH IV

Equipment

Clean gown
Bath blanket
Washing equipment, if needed

Procedure

1. Check client care plan for infusion drip rate, type of solution, and any special considerations.
2. Wash your hands.
3. Take equipment to client's room.
4. Explain to client what you are going to do.
5. Raise bed to comfortable working height, and lower side rails.
6. Untie back of gown, and remove gown from unaffected arm. If available, select gown with snap sleeve closure.
7. Support arm with IV and slip gown down arm to IV tubing.
8. Place clean gown over client's chest and abdomen.
9. Remove IV bag from hook and slip sleeve over bag, keeping bag above client's arm. **Rationale:** This prevents backflow of blood into vein. Do not jar or pull tubing. **Rationale:** IV tubing may become dislodged and infiltrate into surrounding tissue.
10. Place your hand up through distal end of clean gown sleeve and grasp IV bag. Pull bag and tubing out through clean gown sleeve.
11. Rehang bag on hook, and check to see that infusion is running according to ordered drip rate.
12. Guide sleeve of gown up client's arm to shoulder.
13. Assist client to put other arm through remaining sleeve.
14. Tie gown at the back.
15. Check IV infusion rate and IV tubing to determine that solution is flowing unimpeded into client's vein. **Rationale:** Kinks in tubing impede solution flow.

16. Return bed to comfortable position for client, and replace side rails.
17. Remove dirty linen from room.
18. Wash your hands.

DISCONTINUING AN IV

Equipment

Band-Aid or two sterile 2 × 2 gauze pads and tape
Clean gloves

Procedure

1. Gather equipment.
2. Wash your hands and don gloves.
3. Explain procedure to client.
4. Stabilize needle or catheter while removing tape. **Rationale:** This action prevents unnecessary movement that could injure the vein.
5. Remove catheter quickly and smoothly. Do not press down on top of needle point while it is in the vein.
6. Quickly press sterile pad over venipuncture site, and hold firmly until bleeding stops.
7. Apply Band-Aid or clean pad and tape in place.
8. Observe venipuncture site for redness, swelling, of formation of hematoma.
9. Check site again in 15–30 minutes.
10. Dispose of equipment and gloves.
11. Wash your hands.

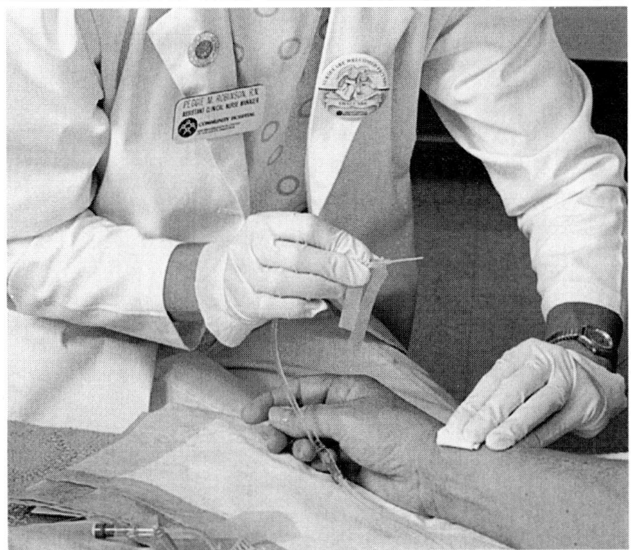

Remove IV needle or catheter and quickly press sterile pad over puncture site.

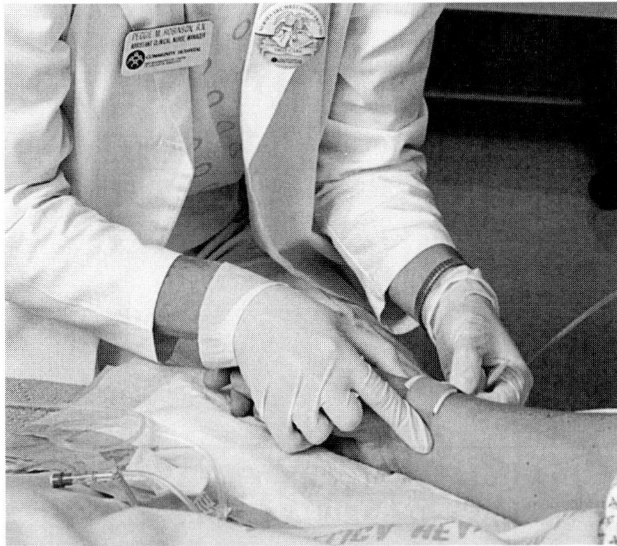

Apply Band-Aid or clean pad and tape in place—observe site in 15 minutes.

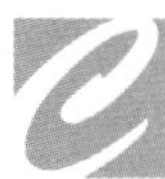

CHARTING for Intravenous Management

- Location of insertion site
- Gauge of needle inserted
- Time of insertion
- Type of controller or pump
- Cassette or module changed
- IV flow rate
- Site care given
- Condition of site
- Time dressing changed
- Any unusual conditions or reactions of skin
- Time IV terminated

CRITICAL THINKING APPLICATION

CLINICAL PROBLEMS	CRITICAL THINKING OPTIONS
Client develops unexplained fever with chills and rising pulse rate.	• Unexplained fever may be associated with catheter-related sepsis. Report to physician. • Check if IV solution has been hanging for more than 24 hours. • Check client's vital signs: temperature usually above 100°F when caused by IV-related sepsis. • Check for other symptoms of pyrogenic reactions (e.g., backache, headache, malaise, nausea, and vomiting). • Stop the infusion. • Obtain blood specimens, if ordered.
IV solution does not flow properly.	• The height of the bag may be too low and therefore the IV fluid does not flow. Raise the bag. • Ensure that the control clamp is open. • Assess that vein is not thrombosed or erythematous. • Check that blood pressure readings are not taken on arm in which IV is running, as flow is impeded and a clot can form on the end of the needle. • Check that correct tubing was used with pump or controller. Most machines require special administration sets. • Check that IV tubing is not compressed in pump or controller.
IV solution appears to be infiltrating into surrounding tissue resulting in pallor and edema.	• Decrease the flow rate, and check for needle placement (follow hospital policy regarding discontinuing the infusion). • Lower bag of IV solution before IV insertion site; if blood returns, needle is in the vein. IV cannula may be in the vein but fluid may be leaking into surrounding tissue via puncture in vein wall.

CLINICAL PROBLEMS	CRITICAL THINKING OPTIONS
Phlebitis is suspected at infusion site (warmth, erythema, and pain).	• Check IV bag for solution and medications being administered. If protein hydrolysates, potassium, or sodium lactate are being infused, call physician immediately. • Discontinue IV according to hospital policy.
Note: Postinfusion phlebitis may also occur after the IV has been discontinued in response to either chemical or mechanical factors of the preexisting IV.	• Check IV solution; hypertonic solution causes irritation necessitating changing IV sites more frequently. • Follow hospital policy for treatment. Hot compresses to the site are generally recommended. • Elevate extremity.

unit 3

INTAKE AND OUTPUT

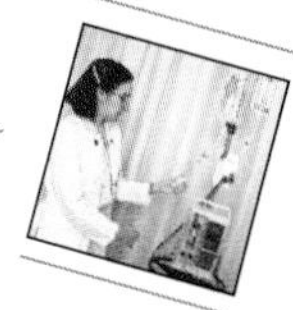

NURSING PROCESS DATA

ASSESSMENT Data Base

Assess client's need for intake and output recording if the client is not taking sufficient fluids, even if there has been no physician's request.

Assess client's ability to keep intake and output fluid records.

Evaluate client for any factors that might affect his or her intake and output (e.g., preexisting disease states, concurrent diagnosed diseases, drug therapies, and current physical status).

Determine all measurable sources of fluid intake: fluids with and between meals, liquid medications, IV fluids, and IV medications as baseline for urinary output.

Determine all measurable sources of fluid output: urine, vomitus, diarrhea, and drainage.

Determine alterations in nonmeasurable sources of fluid intake and loss: food, increased metabolism, rapid respirations, and excessive perspiration.

PLANNING Objectives

To establish a written record of the client's total fluid intake (oral, parenteral, and feeding tubes) and fluid output (urine, stool, GI, and chest drainage, unexpected loss from a wound, diarrhea, vomiting)

To plan fluid replacement or appropriate therapy by assessing deficits and excesses of fluids and electrolytes

To ensure a fluid intake of at least 1500–2000 mL unless contraindicated by diagnosis (e.g., CHF, pulmonary edema)

To monitor the client's hydration state, vital signs, and mental state to determine homeostasis

IMPLEMENTATION Procedures

Monitoring Intake and Output

Monitoring IV Intake

EVALUATION Expected Outcomes

Intake and output, though not exactly equal, are within 200–300 mL of each other.

Fluid intake is at least 2000 mL unless contraindicated by diagnosis.

Client's hydration state, vital signs, and mental status are within normal range.

MONITORING INTAKE AND OUTPUT

Equipment

Graduated container in client's bathroom

Intake and output bedside record and 24-hour record in chart (Table 27–6)

Urinal or bedpan; bedside commode or underseat basin for toilet

Hourly inline urine measurement device for clients requiring frequent monitoring

Posted measurement standards for commonly used drinking and eating utensils (e.g., glasses, mugs, bowls)

Posted signs, dietary slips, and other communication devices to notify hospital personnel about how client's intake and output is to be measured

Procedure

1. Determine if client needs intake and output measurements by checking Kardex or client's chart.
2. Measure intake from all sources.
   a. Oral fluids
   b. IV fluids

TABLE 27–4. Body Sites for Assessment of Hydration

Site	Excess Hydration	Dehydration
Head and Neck		
Face	Eyeballs firm or protruding Edema, especially around eyes	Eyeballs soft or sunken Poor skin turgor over forehead
Mucous Membranes	Excessive salivation Swollen tongue	Dry or sticky mucosa with thick mucous secretions Shrunken tongue with longitudinal fissures Crusted lips
Neck	Jugular vein distention	
Trunk		
Chest	Crackles or rhonchi	Poor skin turgor Dry, flaking skin
Abdomen	Ascites (measure girth at umbilicus)	
Sacrum	Edema	Poor skin turgor
Extremities		
Arms	Edema, particularly of the hands Delayed capillary refill Unequal quality of radial pulses Pulse bounding	Poor skin turgor Delayed capillary refill Dry, flaking skin Pulse weak and thready
Legs	Edema Taut shiny skin Peripheral cyanosis	Poor skin turgor, especially across shins Dry, flaky skin, especially on feet Weak pedal pulse or decreased capillary refill

TABLE 27–5. Objective Data Indicative of the State of Hydration

Data	Excess Hydration	Dehydration
Vital Signs		
Blood Pressure	Increased*	Decreased
Pulse	Increased rate	Increased rate
Temperature	Unchanged	Elevated
Respirations	Increased rate	Unchanged or increased
Laboratory Findings		
Urine Specific Gravity	Decreased, approaching 1.010	Increased, approaching 1.025 or greater
Blood Hematocrit	Less than three times the hemoglobin	Greater than three times the hemoglobin
Serum Sodium (Na)	Less than 135 mEq/L	Greater than 145 mEq/L or normal
Hourly Urine Output	More than 60 mL/hour	Less than 30–60 mL/hour
Weight	A 5% or greater gain	Mild: 2% loss Moderate: 3–5% loss Severe: 6% or greater loss

*If the heart is no longer able to pump the increased blood volume and cardiac decompensation occurs, the blood pressure (reflecting cardiac output) may drop.

   c. Fluids with IV medications
   d. Tube feedings and water used to clear tubing
   e. Correlate with daily weight (a pint gain adds a pound)
3. Measure output from all sources to establish a written record and plan fluid replacement.
   a. Foley and French catheters
   b. Bedpans and urinals
   c. Nasogastric drainage
   d. Drainage tubing (e.g., T tubes)
   e. Diarrheal stools
   f. Draining wounds
   g. Vomitus
4. Record I&O on bedside record each time you take a measurement.
5. Record 24-hour totals of intake and output on bed-

TABLE 27–6. Intake and Output Flow Sheet

Date	Time	IV No.	IV Started	Description	IV Intake	Oral Intake	Urine Output	Other	N/G
1/9/96	9 A			Full liquid breakfast		620			
	9:45 A			Vomitus				400	
	10:30 A	#1	1000						
	12 N						450		
	2:30 P						300		
				7–3 Total	450	620	750	400	100
	6:30 P	#2	1000		550				
	9 P						375		
				3–11 Total	1050	n.p.o.	375		250
1/10/96	2:30 A	#3	1000		450				
	5 A						250		
				11–7 Total	1050	n.p.o.	250		175
				24 hour Total	2550	620	1375	400	525

side record and on graphic sheet in client's chart.

6. Notify physician of any abnormality that could lead to complications. **Rationale:** Hourly urine output less than 25–30 mL/hour or 24-hour urine output less than 500 mL can indicate dehydration, kidney damage, or alterations in hormonal balance.

Fluid Replacement Solutions

Hypertonic Solutions—a solution with higher osmolality than blood serum

- Cell placed in solution shrinks
- Used in severe salt depletion (very rare)
- Used as nutrient source (10% dextrose)
- Examples of solutions: saline solutions greater than 0.9% (e.g., 3% saline or 5% saline), which can be very dangerous; 10% dextrose in normal saline is also hypertronic and irritating to peripheral veins, so central venous administration is preferred.

Hypotonic Solutions—a solution with lower osmolality than blood serum

- Hydrates cells, causes them to expand
- Used in diarrhea, other forms of dehydration
- Examples of solutions: hypotonic saline solutions (e.g., 0.45% NaCl, 0.02% NaCl, or 5% dextrose combined with hypotonic saline); 5% dextrose in water

Isotonic Solutions—a solution with the same osmolality as blood serum.

- Cells remain unchanged
- Used for replacement or maintenance (expands extracellular volume)
- Examples of solutions: Lactated Ringer's, 5% dextrose in normal saline (0.9%); 0.9% saline. *Note:* One liter of normal saline 0.9% NaCl meets the usual daily requirement of these electrolytes in an adult.

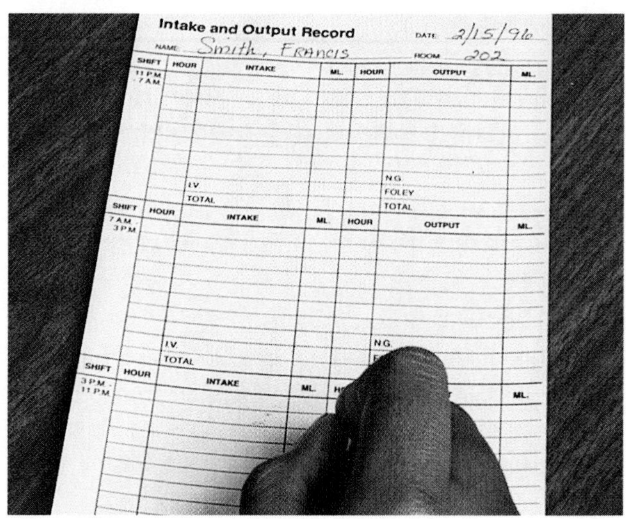

Example of Intake and Output Record.

MONITORING IV INTAKE

Equipment

Volume control set (e.g., Soluset, Metriset, Volu-Trol)
Intake and output record
Graphic sheet
IV container marked with timed intervals

Procedure

1. Place intake and output record at bedside.
2. Determine time interval required for monitoring IV intake.
3. Mark time intervals on IV container according to facility policy (use felt-tip pen, preprinted time strips).
4. Set IV drip rate according to physician's orders.
5. Observe volume control set or IV container and read IV solution level.
6. Record amount of IV solution infused at prescribed time (e.g., every hour, every shift).
7. Record total IV intake on intake and output record at end of each shift.
8. Record 24 hour IV total at midnight. Take into account all sources of IV fluid (all IV sites, IV fluid used for medications).

(For complete I&O Procedure, see Chapter 21.)

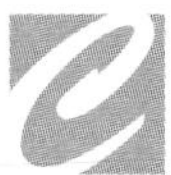

CHARTING for Intake and Output

- Exact measurements of intake and output
- Approximate volume of loss when unable to measure contents (e.g., incontinent of urine in bed)
- Dietary intake (food as well as water)
- Time, amount, and description of all measurable intake and output
- Signs and symptoms of client's state of hydration, including vital signs, urine output, and weight

Note: I&O records are frequently inaccurate due to numerous possibilities for error; it is important to maintain these records accurately.

CRITICAL THINKING APPLICATION

CLINICAL PROBLEMS	CRITICAL THINKING OPTIONS
■ Fluid balance is not correct as stated on intake and output record.	• Report to charge nurse so she can determine if all nurses are keeping accurate records. • Check if client or family can help with keeping the I&O record. • Check the addition on the I&O record to see if an error was made.
■ Client does not maintain an intake of at least 1500 mL.	• Ensure that the diagnosis allows a 1500 mL intake. • Check if the client is able to drink fluids by him or herself, or if he or she needs assistance. • Ensure that adequate fluids are available at the bedside for the client.
■ IV fluids not maintained at appropriate rate to provide adequate intake.	• Monitor IV level hourly. • Observe IV site for infiltration. • Restart IVs immediately when infiltrated to ensure continuous IV fluid intake. • Document IV levels at least every shift.

unit 4 IV MEDICATION ADMINISTRATION

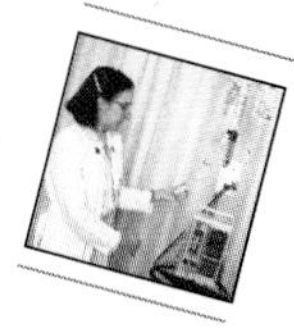

NURSING PROCESS DATA

ASSESSMENT Data Base

Note client's allergies.

Note any drug or solution incompatibilities.

Assess amount and type of diluent needed to mix with medications.

Assess client's general condition to establish a baseline for administering medications.

Assess patency of infusion set and conditions of IV insertion site.

PLANNING Objectives

To maintain a therapeutic level of medication in the client's bloodstream

To administer medication in larger volumes over a longer period of time

To prevent complications associated with bolus administration, such as speed shock and vein irritation

IMPLEMENTATION Procedures

Adding Medication to IV Solution

Using a Secondary, or Partial-Fill, Additive Bag (IV Piggyback)

Using a Volume Control Set

Using a Peripheral Saline Lock

Administering Medications through IV Line Y-site

EVALUATION Expected Outcomes

Solutions from additive bottles or bags infuse without difficulty.

Therapeutic blood level of medication is maintained.

Complications of medication administration are prevented.

Medication is infused over appropriate time span.

ADDING MEDICATION TO IV SOLUTION BAG

Equipment

IV solution bag

Syringe with medications

Alcohol swab

Label with medication, date, time, and initials

Procedure

1. Check physician's orders and Kardex.
2. Wash hands.
3. Gather equipment. Check client identaband.
4. Draw up medication into syringe according to directions on medication label.
5. Check compatibility chart to ensure that prescribed drug is compatible with IV solution.
6. Wipe port on side of IV bag with alcohol swab.
7. Inject medication into bag while maintaining aseptic technique.
8. Mix IV solution and medication by gently squeezing bag.

■ CLINICAL ALERT

Two drugs that must not come in contact with saline solution are diazapam (Valium) and chlordiazepoxide hydrochloride (Librium).

9. Hold bag against a dark and a light background to inspect for any precipitate.
10. Affix medication label to IV bag.
11. Insert IV tubing into bag, and proceed with appropriate method or administration as ordered.

USING A SECONDARY, OR PARTIAL-FILL, ADDITIVE BAG (IV PIGGYBACK)

Equipment

Primary IV set, consisting of IV solution bag and IV administration set with injection port

Medication mixed in syringe, if indicated

Partial-fill additive bag secondary administration set, 20-gauge 1-inch needle or needleless locking cannula, and extension hook or lowering hanger for primary bottle

Label with name of medication, date, time, and nurse's initials

Alcohol swab

Preparation

1. Check physician's orders and Kardex.
2. Wash hands.
3. Gather equipment. Check client identaband.

Procedure

1. Prepare medication following directions on label. Add medication to partial-fill bag using aseptic technique, or use medication bag prepared by pharmacy.

■ CLINICAL ALERT

Do not inject additive medication into *hanging* bag, since medication may not mix, but pool and be delivered to client as a dangerous *bolus*.

2. When hooking on secondary "piggyback" bags, first ensure compatibility with infusing solution.
3. Spike partial-fill bag with administration set. Affix needleless locking cannula to end of tubing. (The CDC strongly recommends using needleless infusion lines to reduce risk of exposure to IV needles.)
4. Cleanse injection port of primary IV with an alcohol swab.
5. Insert needleless locking cannula of partial-fill bag set and secure in place with tape.
6. Hang the partial-fill bag on the IV pole.
7. Use the extension hook to lower primary bag below partial-fill bag.
8. Clear tubing of medication bag by opening clamp, placing bag lower than primary solution bag, and allow primary solution to flow into secondary bag tubing.
9. Backfill until chamber is one-third full. Clamp secondary tubing. **Rationale:** This ensures that no medication is lost in this process.
10. Open clamp on partial-fill (secondary) bag tubing. The solution in partial-fill bag should begin to flow.
11. Program secondary settings into infusion pump if used.
12. Using clamp on primary IV tubing, adjust drip rate to desired rate of administration.
13. Make sure that partial-fill bag is higher than the primary IV bag so the solution drips until partial-fill bag is empty. **Rationale:** The primary solution ceases flow because of an increased hydrostatic pressure in secondary bag.
14. When partial-fill bag and drip chamber are empty, readjust rate of administration in primary solution to desired flow.

■ CLINICAL ALERT

If IV "piggyback" medication is incompatible with primary IV solution, it is necessary to flush IV tubing with sterile NS solution prior to starting IV "piggyback" medication and again after the medication is infused.

15. To hang a new partial-fill bag, prepare the same medication and add it to new bag aseptically. **Rationale:** Medication must be the same as the previously administered drug since some remains in the secondary tubing.

16. Remove old partial-fill bag, and spike new bag. Close clamp on partial-fill bag tubing.
17. Lower partial-fill bag below injection port of primary IV.
18. Open clamp on partial-fill tubing, and allow solution from primary IV set to enter tubing, backfilling the tubing to drip chamber. **Rationale:** This procedure displaces any air left in tubing.
19. Replace new partial-fill bag on IV pole, and proceed with administration.
20. Change partial-fill tubing every 48 hours.

Using a Miniinfuser Pump

A miniinfuser pump is a tandem device that allows a small amount of medication to be given (5–60 mL) as a controlled infusion.

- The prefilled syringe is added to the battery-operated miniinfuser and connected to the main IV line.
- A needleless system is the recommended connection to the primary IV line, although a stopcock or port may be used.
- The infusion pump is hung with the primary IV bag and activated by an ON button.
- Following infusion of medication, the primary infusion automatically begins to flow as the pump stops.
- The primary infusion should be checked and the flow regulated when the miniinfusion pump stops.

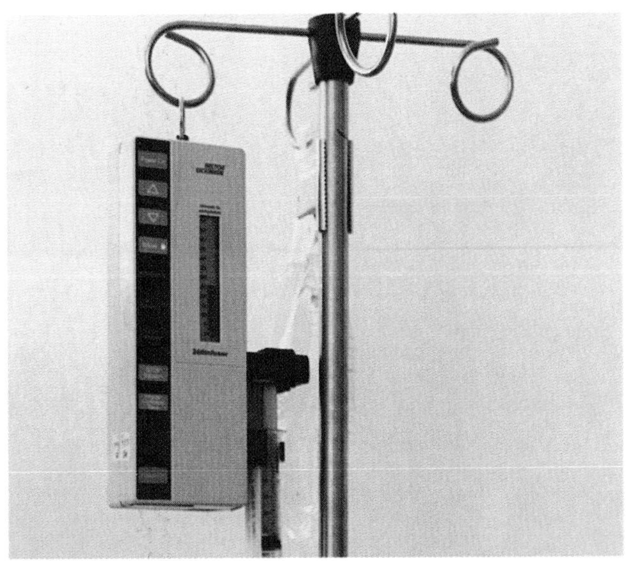

Miniinfuser pump used to "piggyback" secondary infusion—similar to syringe pump.

USING A VOLUME CONTROL SET

Equipment

Primary IV set, consisting of IV solution bag and IV administration set with injection port

Volume control set (Soluset, Metriset, VoluTrol, or Buretrol, depending on need or manufacturer)

Medication mixed in syringe

Alcohol swab

Label with medication, date, time, and nurse's initials

Preparation

1. Check physician's orders. Check client identaband.
2. Wash hands.
3. Obtain volume control set, IV bag, and IV tubing if needed.

Procedure

1. Close clamps on volume control set, both above and below volume chamber.
2. Open air vent by turning clamp located on top of volume chamber.
3. Spike IV bag with volume control set, and then hang bag. Insert IV tubing into volume control set.
4. Open upper clamp (between the bag and volume chamber), and fill chamber with IV solution so that chamber is one-third full.
5. Close upper clamp.
6. Open lower clamp, and squeeze drip chamber (located underneath the volume chamber) until it is one-half full.
7. Allow solution to flow down tubing.
8. Prime tubing and needle affixed to end of tubing. If volume control set has membrane filter instead of floating valve filter, follow manufacturer's instructions for priming so that you do not damage the filter.
9. Close clamp.
10. Swab off injection port (located on top of the volume chamber) with alcohol.

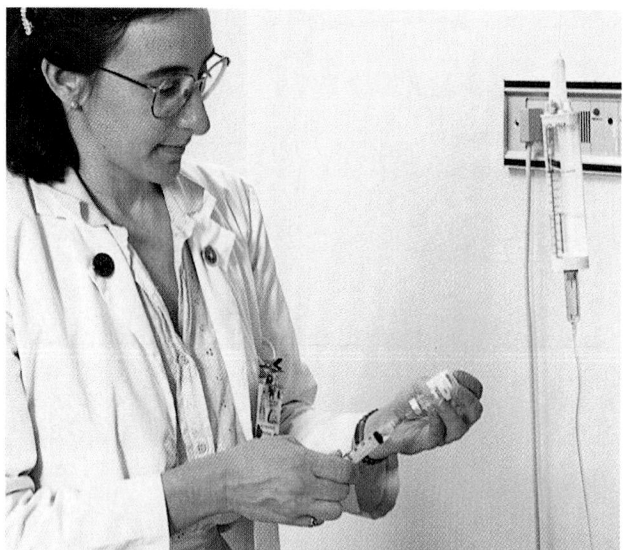
Withdraw prescribed amount of medication to be injected into volume control set.

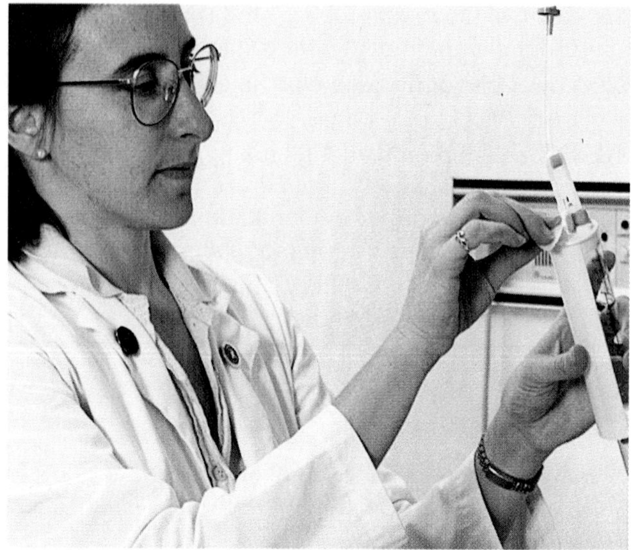
Swab injection port of partially filled volume control set.

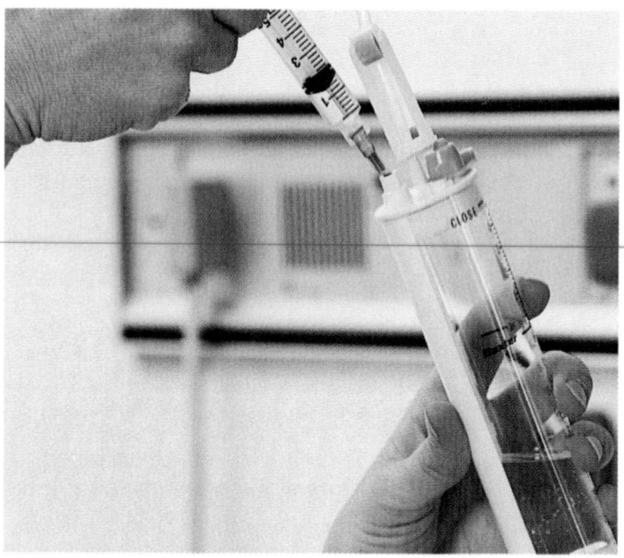
Inject prepared medication into partially filled volume control set.

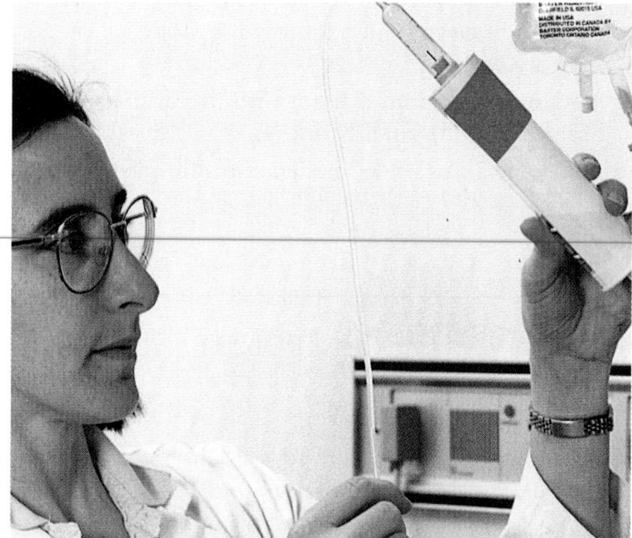
Gently mix medication with solution in volume control chamber.

11. Inject prepared medication into chamber, and agitate gently to mix medication with solution in chamber.
12. Dilute medication, if necessary, by opening upper clamp and adding additional fluid from the IV bag.
13. Open clamp on volume control set and adjust drip rate to desired rate of administration.
14. Place medication label on volume control set. Include patient's name, medication, dose, and time medication infusion began.

USING A PERIPHERAL SALINE LOCK

Equipment

Syringe for medication (if necessary for dilution)
Needleless cannula
Alcohol or iodophor swab
2 normal saline prefilled syringes (2 mL each)
Needleless injection cap (if one not in place)
Clean gloves

Preparation

1. Check physician's orders. Check client identaband.
2. Gather equipment.
3. Wash your hands, and don gloves.
4. Explain procedure to client.
5. If client does not have an intermittent infusion set in place, proceed with venipuncture, selecting veins that are both large enough to receive the bolus of medicine and away from areas of movement (e.g., the elbows and wrists). When taping set in place, secure injection port away from needle insertion site. **Rationale:** This minimizes needle movement when port is being used.

Procedure

1. Prepare medication to be administered, and draw it up into syringe.
2. Fill two syringes with 2 mL of saline each.

> ■ CLINICAL ALERT
>
> Some hospitals still use heparin for flushing; it is usually prepared with 1 mL1:1000 heparin added to 9 mL normal saline to produce 100 U/mL solution.

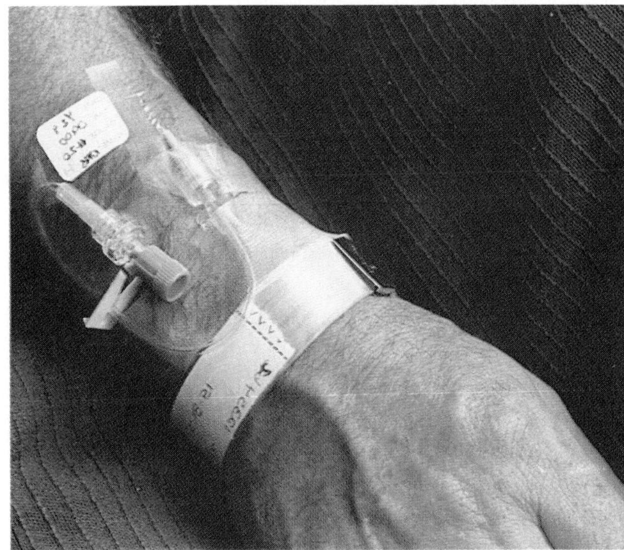

Peripheral saline lock with extension tubing for easy accessibility.

3. Swab needleless injection port with alcohol or idophor swab. Insert saline syringe into port, briefly aspirate to check patency, and flush system. **Rationale:** Presence of blood indicates that needle is probably in vein, not in surrounding tissues.
4. Observe site for swelling and ease of flushing.
5. Insert medication syringe into port, and inject medication into vein, timing flow rate according to physician's orders or drug manufacturer's instructions.
6. Observe client for any adverse reactions.
7. Remove medication syringe.
8. Flush with second saline syringe to clear line, and lock port.
9. Dispose of equipment and gloves.

ADMINISTERING MEDICATIONS THROUGH IV LINE Y-SITE

Equipment

Medication prepared in syringe with needleless cannula
Iodophor swab (preferred by CDC to alcohol)
Clean gloves

Preparation

1. Check physician's orders.
2. Gather equipment.
3. Wash your hands.
4. Prepare medications according to directions on vial or medication insert sheet. **Rationale:** IV bolus is the only way to administer drugs that cannot be diluted: digoxin, diazepam (Valium), furosemide (Lasix). IV

bolus cannot be used to administer medications that must be diluted in a large volume (vitamins or antibiotics) before entering bloodstream.

5. Check medication according to the *Five Rights* (Chapter 16).
6. Take medication to client's bedside.
7. Check that client is not allergic to the IV bolus drug.
8. Don clean gloves.

Procedure

1. Check client's identaband, and ask him or her to state name.
2. Double check drug label. **Rationale:** IV bolus injections can result in complications, so accuracy is imperative.
3. Clean needleless Y-site injection port closest to client with an alcohol swab.
4. Close clamp on IV tubing, or pinch off tubing.
5. Insert cannula into needleless port (Y-site).
6. Pull back on plunger, and observe for blood flash-back. **Rationale:** This ensures the needle or catheter is in vein.
7. Inject medication slowly or according to directions. **Rationale:** Speed shock can occur from administering the drug too rapidly.

> **■ CLINICAL ALERT**
>
> The most common toxic reaction with IV bolus is *speed shock,* caused by administering the drug too rapidly. It is the body's adverse reaction (syncope, shock, or cardiac arrest) to an injection of a foreign substance that raises the drug concentration in the client's blood to a toxic level.

8. Time the length of injection by dividing total amount of medication by prescribed time to inject. Use your watch and administer the medication at the prescribed time. **Rationale:** In addition to avoiding speed shock, this method allows time to observe client for adverse reactions: chills, nausea, localized pain, burning, or itching.
9. Reopen clamp, and readjust flow rate as ordered.
10. Withdraw cannula when medication is infused.
11. Discard cannula in sharps container.
12. Remove gloves, and wash hands.

Note: If medication is to be injected directly into the vein, perform venipuncture, and slowly inject medication into vein. Withdraw needle and apply pressure or a Band-Aid to puncture site.

CHARTING for Medications

- Type and amount of medication administered
- Rate medication administered
- Client's response to medication

CRITICAL THINKING APPLICATION

CLINICAL PROBLEMS	CRITICAL THINKING OPTIONS
■ Partial-fill bag solution does not infuse adequately.	• Check height of IV bag. • Check that primary IV bag is lower than partial-fill bag. • Ensure that cannula is positioned properly in the injection port.
■ Solution in primary IV tubing is incompatible with medication to be administered via secondary additive set.	• Prior to running medication into primary IV tubing, flush tubing with solution that is compatible with medication (e.g., normal saline or 5% dextrose in water). Then proceed with medication administration. • If solution precipitates, discontinue the IV tubing, and place new tubing on additive set. Flush the primary IV tubing with compatible solution, and start the additive set infusing again.
■ Unable to infuse solution through saline lock.	• Gently turn or slightly withdraw lock. • Remove saline lock, and reinsert in another site.

unit 5

BLOOD TRANSFUSIONS

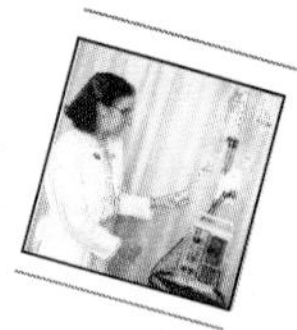

NURSING PROCESS DATA

ASSESSMENT Data Base

Assess if client has an 18- or 19-gauge catheter or needle inserted in the vein.

Assess client's vital signs, especially temperature, for baseline data.

Assess skin for eruptions or rashes to provide baseline data.

Assess for signs and symptoms of blood reactions during the transfusion.

Assess blood type, and label before administration to ensure compatibility.

PLANNING Objectives

To provide blood or blood components, such as red blood cells, platelets, blood protein, and plasma, for clients who have a demonstrated deficiency

To ensure compatibility between client's blood and the whole blood or packed red blood cells that may be transfused

To prevent the infusion of fibrin clots and microaggregates (broken-down blood cells)

To monitor the transfusion of blood or blood components to ensure the blood infuses without complications

To assess that the needle remains patent throughout the transfusion procedure

To monitor for potential complications during and immediately following the blood transfusion

IMPLEMENTATION Procedures

Administering Blood through a Y-Set

Administering Blood through a Straight Line

Monitoring for Potential Complications

Administering Blood Components

EVALUATION Expected Outcomes

Transfusion of blood is performed without complications.

Needle remains patent throughout transfusion procedure.

Equipment is properly used for transfusion.

ADMINISTERING BLOOD THROUGH A Y-Set

Equipment

Blood unit

250-mL bag of normal saline

Y-set IV tubing

Venipuncture supplies if client does not already have an IV in place

18- or 19-gauge needle or 18- to 20-gauge catheter

14-gauge needle, if blood is to be administered rapidly

Needleless injection cap

Alcohol swabs and tape

Infusion pump

Clean gloves

Preparation

1. Check physician's orders for number of units and type of transfusion to be given.
2. Check that type and crossmatch has been completed and that blood is ready in blood bank.
3. Obtain the requisition form for the transfusion.
4. Obtain whole blood unit or packed blood cells unit from blood laboratory or blood bank.
5. Check requisition form with lab technologist and

lab blood record against blood unit for essential data: client's name and identaband number, blood group and type (ABO and Rh), blood unit number, and expiration date of blood unit.

6. Check requisition form with another RN and laboratory blood record with information on client's identaband to make sure that all data match. Essential data include client's name and identaband number, blood group, blood type, blood unit number, and expiration date on blood unit.
7. Sign form with other RN according to hospital policy. Remember that blood must be started within 30 minutes from time it is removed from refrigeration.
8. Check blood bag for bubbles, cloudiness, dark color, or sediment. **Rationale:** These signs indicate bacterial contamination.
9. Prime blood administration set with normal saline.

WARMING BLOOD FOR TRANSFUSION

Routine transfusions should not be warmed. If warming is required, as in massive transfusions, a blood warming coil is inserted into the transfusion line. (Never warm in a microwave.) Immerse coil in a 98.6–100°F water bath. Once blood is warmed, it must be used or disposed of, as it cannot be returned to the blood bank. Hemolysis of the blood occurs at temperatures above 104°F.

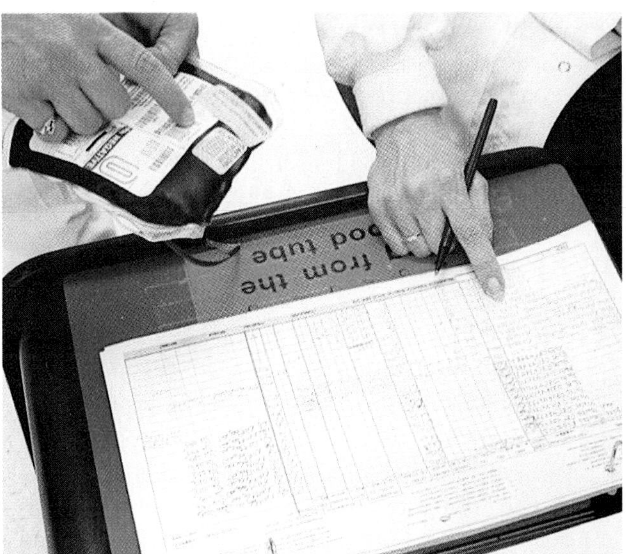

Validate client's name, blood unit number and date on blood tag.

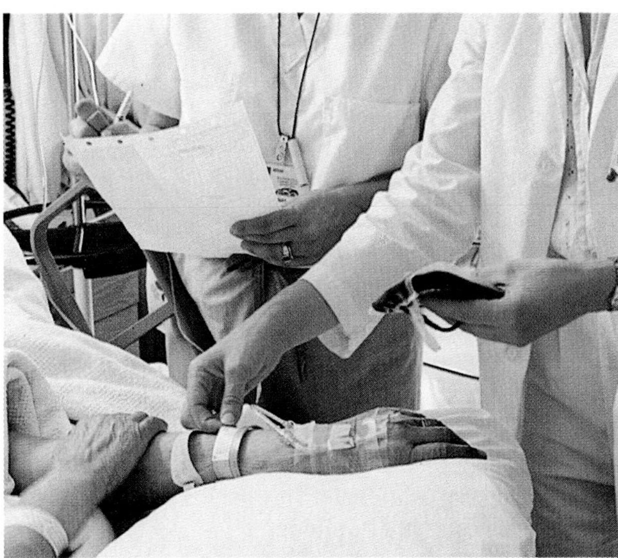

Ascertain that client's name and ID number match number on blood tag.

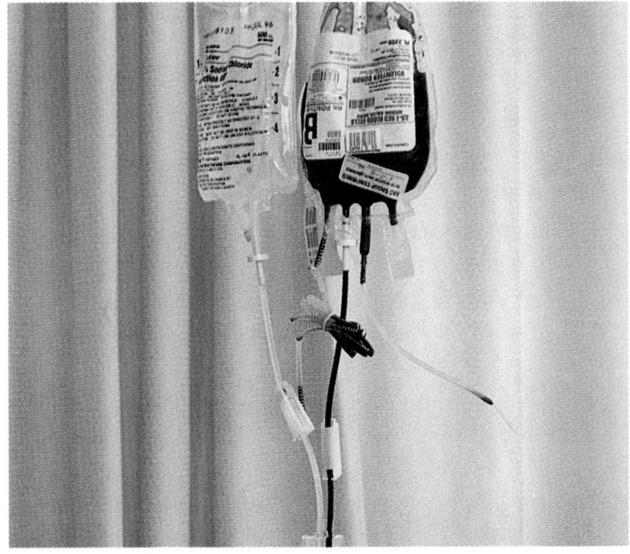

Blood is transfused via Y-set tubing primed with sterile NS.

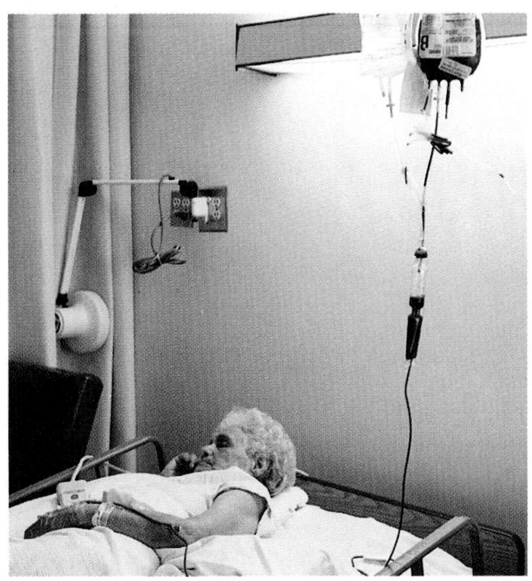

Observe client carefully for first 15 minutes during blood transfusion.

Rationale: This ensures all air bubbles are out of tubing.

10. Check vital signs for baseline data.
11. Don clean gloves.

Procedure

1. Close all clamps on the Y-set.
2. Rotate blood unit bag gently. **Rationale:** Gentle rotation mixes blood cells and plasma.
3. Pull back tabs on blood unit bag, and expose port.
4. Spike port, and carefully hang unit.
5. Spike small saline bag with other spike of the Y-tubing.
6. Hang both saline bag and blood bag, and load infusion pump.
7. Open clamp to saline bag, and squeeze sides of drip chamber until filter is half covered and drip chamber is full.
8. Open main clamp, remove cap that protects end of IV tubing, and prime the rest of the tubing.
9. Replace cap, and close main clamp when tubing is primed.
10. Cleanse injection port on primary IV.
11. Affix a large-gauge needle to end of tubing, and prime needle.
12. Insert needle into injection port, and clamp off primary IV flow.
13. Open clamp to saline bag, and turn clamp on main tubing. **Rationale:** This begins bag flow to clear the primary IV tubing.
14. Clamp off saline bag, and open clamp to blood bag.
15. Squeeze sides of the Y-set drip chamber so that blood covers entire filter.
16. Administer blood slowly for first 15 minutes, approximately 20 gtt minute, which equates to 100 mL/hour. **Rationale:** Slow administration allows time to observe for adverse reactions. Most reactions occur in first 15 minutes.
17. Take vital signs, and observe client closely for reactions. Chilling, backache, headache, nausea or vomiting, tachycardia, tachypnea, skin rash, or hypotension are signs of complications.

■ CLINICAL ALERT

Most clients can tolerate a flow rate of one unit of packed cells in $1^1/_2$–2 hours.

18. Administer blood unit at prescribed rate if no adverse effects occur.
19. Complete the blood transfusion in less than 4 hours. **Rationale:** Blood deteriorates rapidly after a 2-hour exposure to room temperature.
20. Monitor client throughout transfusion. Complete transfusion record.
21. Check that transfusion is completed, then flush line with normal saline.
22. Reattach primary IV solution, and adjust drip to desired rate.
23. Remove blood unit bag and administration set. If you are going to transfuse a second unit of blood, obtain that unit and a new administration set, and repeat the procedure described above.
24. Obtain posttransfusion vital signs.

ADMINISTERING BLOOD THROUGH A STRAIGHT LINE

Equipment

Blood unit
250-mL bag of normal saline
Blood administration straight-line set
Needleless cannula (15 gauge)
Clean gloves

Procedure

1. Obtain and check blood as stated in preparation for *Administering Blood through a Y-Set.*
2. Don gloves.
3. Spike blood bag port carefully, and hang unit. (Be sure clamp on set is closed.)
4. Open clamp, and fill drip chamber by gently squeezing its flexible sides. Make sure filter is submerged in the blood.
5. Open clamp on tubing, carefully run blood through tubing, and place needleless cannula on end of tubing.
6. Check if client has a primary IV in place with an appropriate-sized needle. If not, place an 18-gauge needle (or larger needle) in the end of the blood

TABLE 27–7. Transfusion Reactions

Type	Clinical Manifestations	Nursing Interventions
Bacterial	Sudden increase in temperature Hypotension Dry, flushed skin Abdominal pain Headache Lumbar pain Sudden chill	Stop transfusion immediately. Maintain IV site; change tubing as soon as possible. Observe for shock. Monitor vital signs every 15 minutes until stable. Obtain urine specimen. Insert Foley (retention) catheter if necessary. Notify physician, and obtain order for broad-spectrum antibiotic. Draw blood cultures before antibiotic administration. Send blood tubing and bag to laboratory for culture and sensitivity. Control hyperthermia.
Allergic	Urticaria and hives, pruritus Respiratory wheezing, laryngeal edema Anaphylactic reaction	Stop transfusion immediately if symptoms are severe. Monitor vital signs for possible anaphylactic shock. If symptoms are mild, slow down transfusion and obtain order for antihistamine. Monitor for signs of progressive allergic reaction as transfusion continues.
Hemolytic	Severe pain in kidney region and chest Pain at needle insertion site	Stop transfusion immediately. Change IV tubing as soon as possible, maintaining patent IV. If necessary, disconnect IV tubing from needle, and run normal saline through IV tubing into emesis basin. Reconnect tubing to needle, and obtain new tubing as soon as possible.
	Fever (may reach 105°F), chills Dyspnea and cyanosis	Administer oxygen. Send two blood samples, from different sites, urine sample (catheterize if necessary), blood, and transfusion record to laboratory.
	Headache	Obtain orders for IV volume expansion and diuretic (mannitol) to ensure flushing of kidneys to prevent acute renal tubular necrosis.
	Hypotension Hematuria	Monitor vital signs every 15 minutes for shock. Monitor urine output hourly for possible renal failure. Foley catheter may need to be inserted.

unit tubing port, and perform venipuncture.

7. Check to determine if primary IV solution is compatible with blood to be infused. If not, remove primary IV solution.
8. Spike small bag of normal saline, and run this solution through the tubing. **Rationale:** Normal saline prevents cell hemolysis. (Never use dextrose solutions.)
9. Prime blood unit tubing.
10. Swab needleless injection port of the primary IV administration set with alcohol.
11. Carefully insert blood tubing with needleless cannula into IV tubing and tape it into place.
12. Shut off primary IV, and begin the blood transfusion.
13. Follow procedure as you did for previous bag.
14. When blood bag is empty, clamp off tubing to bag, open clamp to normal saline bag, and flush line.
15. Close all clamps and remove blood tubing cannula from injection port.
16. Open clamp on primary IV, and establish desired rate of administration.
17. Monitor client for signs and symptoms of blood transfusion reactions (Table 27–7) throughout procedure.

MONITORING FOR POTENTIAL COMPLICATIONS

Equipment

Sphygmomanometer
Stethoscope
Thermometer

Procedure

1. Check temperature, blood pressure, pulse, and respiration before transfusion is started.
2. Check vital signs every 5–15 minutes for the first 100 mL after transfusion has started. **Rationale:** Most blood transfusion reactions occur during this time.

Blood Transfusion Protocol

The nurse is responsible for early assessment of possible transfusion reactions by completing the following interventions.

- Identify client and blood bag.
  Identaband number matches transfusion record number.
  Name spelled correctly on transfusion record.
  Blood bag number and pilot tube number are the same.
  Blood type matches on transfusion record and blood bag.
- Check blood with an RN before infusing.
- Ask client about allergy history, and report any previous blood reactions.
- Establish baseline vital sign data.
- Start transfusion slowly to observe for severe reactions.
- Maintain aseptic technique during procedure.
- Observe time rules for administering blood. (Hang no longer than 4 hours.)
- Observe blood bag for bubbles, cloudiness, dark color, or black sediment, which is indicative of bacterial invasion.

3. Maintain vital sign assessment throughout blood infusion according to hospital policy.
4. Monitor client for possible transfusion reactions.
   a. Hemolytic or incompatibility reaction—most severe reaction
   b. Bacterial contamination
   c. Allergic reaction
5. If any severe untoward sign occurs (sudden increase in temperature, severe pain in kidney region), stop transfusion immediately.
6. Remove blood and any blood-filled tubing, and replace with saline bag and new tubing to keep line open. Return blood bag and administration set to blood bank or laboratory.
7. Notify physician immediately after stopping IV for signs of transfusion reaction. Also notify physician if any unusual sign (itching or hives) occurs.

ADMINISTERING BLOOD COMPONENTS

Equipment

Blood component
Appropriate IV administration set
Clean gloves

Procedure

1. Check physician's orders and Kardex.
2. Obtain blood component from laboratory or appropriate source.
3. Obtain appropriate administration set.
4. Wash hands, and don gloves.
5. Read directions for proper administration of the solution.
6. Identify rate at which blood component should infuse.
7. Check Table 27–8 for appropriate rate, risk factors, and possible complications.

TABLE 27–8. Blood Component Therapy

Type	Use	Alerts	Administration Equipment
Fresh Plasma	To replace deficient coagulation factors To increase intravascular compartment	Hepatitis is a risk. Administer as rapidly as possible. Use within 6 hours.	Any straight-line administration set
Platelets	To prevent or treat bleeding problems, especially in surgical clients To replace platelets in clients with acquired or inherited deficiencies (thrombocytope-i nia, aplastic anemia) To replace when platelets drop below 20,000 mL/mm (normal 150,000–350,000 mL/mm)	Administer at rate of 10 minutes a unit (usually come in multiple platelet packs).	Platelet transfusion set with special filter to allow platelets to infuse through filter
Granulocytes	To treat oncology clients with severe bone marrow depression and progressive infections	Administer slowly, over 2–4 hours.	Use Y-type blood filters and prime with physiologic saline. A microaggregate filter is not used as it filters out platelets.
	To treat granulocytopenic clients with infections that are unresponsive to antibiotics	Give one transfusion daily until granulocytes increase or infection clears.	
	To treat clients with gram-negative bacteremia or infections where marrow recovery does not develop	Use within 48 hours after drawn. Observe for shaking, fever, chills Observe for hives and laryngeal edema (treat with antihistamines)	
Serum Albumin	To treat shock	Available as 5% or 25% solution.	Special tubing accompanies albumin solution in individual boxes
	To treat hypoproteinemia	Infuse 25% solution slowly 1 mL/minute to prevent circulatory overload. Administer 100–200 mL (25% solution) for shock clients and 200–300 mL for hypoproteinemia.	
Gamma Globulin	To treat agammaglobulinemia	Pooled plasma contains antibodies to infectious agents.	Given IM
	To act as a prophylaxis for hepatitis exposure	Administer 0.25–0.50 mL of immune serum globulin/kg of body weight every 2–4 weeks.	
Coagulation Factors	To treat clients with von Willebrand's disease	Made from fresh-frozen plasma.	Standard syringe or component drip set only
Factor VIII (cryoprecipitate)	To treat clients with factor VIII, hemophilia A	Administer one unit cryoprecipitate for each 6 kg of body weight initially, followed by 1 U/3 kg of body weight at 6–12-hour intervals until treatment discontinued. Administer 1 unit/5 minutes. Observe for febrile reactions.	
Factor IX	To treat clients with factor IX, hemophilia B	Administer in 12–24-hour cycle. Preparation for administration is 400–500 U/vial. Must reconstitute in 10–20 mL diluent. One unit/pound of body weight increases the circulating factor activity by 5%. Serum hepatitis can be transmitted.	Any straight-line set

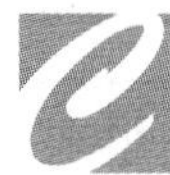

CHARTING for Blood Transfusions

- Type and amount of blood administered
- Amount of normal saline used
- Size of needle inserted for administration
- Time transfusion began and ended
- Vital signs before transfusion begins; 15, 30, and 60 minutes after infusion begins; and then hourly until infusion completed
- Blood bank slip may have space for vital sign information as well
- Client's response to procedure
- Any unusual clinical manifestations; any nursing interventions

CRITICAL THINKING APPLICATION

CLINICAL PROBLEMS	CRITICAL THINKING OPTIONS
■ Transfusion reaction or nursing alert conditions occur.	• Check transfusion chart for appropriate nursing intervention. • Complete all relevant nursing actions.
■ Blood does not flow through tubing.	• Check site where IV needle has been inserted to make sure it is in place. • Gently agitate blood bag to mix blood cells with the plasma. • Raise blood bag to a higher location on IV pole. Squeeze flexible tubing to promote blood flow. • Adjust clamp on tubing. As the blood passes over the filter, more blood microaggregates clog the filter and slow drip rate. • Replace tubing.
■ Blood has been hanging for more than 4 hours.	• Take down blood bag, and send to laboratory. • Maintain IV with normal saline or ordered IV solution. • Monitor vital signs for complications.
■ Pain, redness, discharge.	• Infection. Follow hospital policy. Report to physician.

GERIATRIC CONSIDERATIONS

Elderly clients' veins are fragile, roll easily, and frequently the needle punctures the wall of the vessel.

- Insert IV needle in distal vein first to preserve proximal vessel.
- Maintain close assessment of IV sites to promote long-term use of vessel.

Elderly clients are prone to fluid and electrolyte disorders as a result of the normal aging process.

- Thirst mechanism is decreased.
- Renal threshold is altered.
- Total body fluid is less.
- Fluid replacement therapy requires close monitoring to prevent fluid overload, leading to pulmonary edema.

Chronic conditions of the elderly lead to repetitive use of IV therapy.

- Vessels may be sclerosed from earlier use and not available.

28

Vascular Access Devices

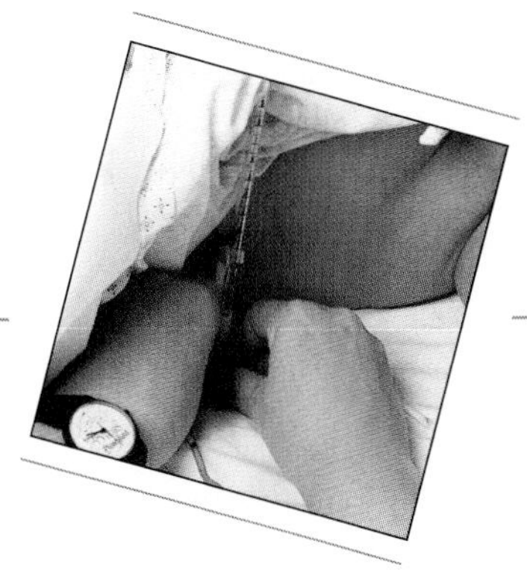

LEARNING OBJECTIVES

- Identify the common types of vascular access devices (VADs).
- Discuss the rationale for using central venous catheters for long-term IV therapy.
- Discuss the special needs of clients with central venous lines (prevention of infection, maintenance, etc.).
- Contrast tunneled and nontunneled central venous catheters.
- Outline the steps for inserting a peripherally inserted central catheter (PICC).
- Describe how an implanted infusion port is used to administer an injection infusion.
- State the steps necessary to care for a VAD.
- Outline the nurse's responsibility for assisting the physician with a central venous port insertion.
- Explain the protocol for maintaining sterility during a central venous port dressing change.

TERMINOLOGY

Antiarrhythmic: an agent used to regulate heart rhythm.

Antimicrobic: preventing the development of pathogenic action of microbes.

Aspirate: to check for blood return with IV needle insertion.

Calorie: the amount of heat necessary to raise the temperature of 1 kilogram of water 1°C. One thousand (1 kcal) of these calories equals 1 dietary calorie (or calorie).

Carbohydrates: a group of chemical substances, including sugars, glycogen, starches, dextrins, and celluloses, that contain only carbon, oxygen and hydrogen.

Cardio: word part that pertains to the heart.

Cardiovascular: term that pertains to the heart and blood vessels, as cardiovascular system.

Central venous catheter: a catheter that accesses a central vein (internal jugular of subclavian vein) that empties into the vena cava.

Central venous pressure (CVP) measurement: monitors circulating blood volume, right ventricular function, and central venous return.

Cyanosis: slightly bluish, grayish, slatelike, or dark purple discoloration.

Digestion: the process by which food is broken down mechanically and chemically in the gastrointestinal tract.

Dyspnea: air hunger resulting in a subjective feeling of difficulty in breathing.

Electrolyte: a solution that is a conductor of electricity; minerals are common electrolytes.

Erythema: redness of the skin produced by capillary congestion as in a sunburn.

Extracellular: fluid outside the cell.

Fat: substance made up of carbon, hydrogen, and oxygen, occurring naturally in most foods but especially in meats and dairy products.

Gastrointestinal: term that pertains to the stomach and intestines.

Hemo-: prefix meaning blood.

Hemodynamic: study of circulation of blood.

Hemolytic: pertinent to the breaking down of red blood cells.

Huber needle: a right-angled (90° or straight, noncoring needle.

Hydrostatic: pertaining to the pressure of liquids in equilibrium and the pressure exerted on liquids.

Hyperalimentation: the process of nourishing the body through parenteral means.

Hyperglycemia: condition characterized by an increase in blood glucose levels.

Hypertonic: solution having a higher osmotic pressure or tonicity than a solution to which it is compared.

Hypovolemia: diminished circulating fluid volume.

Implanted: inserted under the skin.

Implanted infusion port: device placed in subcutaneous tissue with a tunneled catheter that goes into the central venous system.

Infusion: a liquid substance introduced into the body via a vein for therapeutic purposes.

Intracellular: fluid inside the cell.

Intralipids: emulsion containing fats used to correct fatty acid deficiencies via parenteral nutrition.

Intravascular: within blood vessels.

Irrigate: to rinse or wash out with a fluid.

Isotonic: a solution that has the same concentration of salts, or tonicity, as another solution to which it is compared.

Lumen: the inner open space of a tube or blood vessel.

Malnutrition: a condition characterized by a lack of essential food substances or improper absorption and distribution of food substances in the body.

Minerals: inorganic elements or compounds.

Nutrient: nourishing; food item that supplies the body with necessary elements.

Obstruction: blocking of a structure that prevents it from functioning normally; obstacle.

Osmosis: the passage of solvent through a partition separating solutions of different concentrations.

Palpate: to examine by touch; to feel.

Peripherally inserted central catheter (PICC): soft, flexible catheter placed in an arm vein.

Phlebitis: inflammation of a vein.

Polyunsaturates: a long chain of carbon compounds with more than one double bond between the carbons; especially refers to fats.

Port: plastic or metal case that provides access to the venous system through a self-sealing silicone septum.

Proteins: substances that contain amino acids essential for growth and repair of tissues.

Sepsis: pathologic state usually febrile, resulting form the presence of microorganisms or their poisonous products in the bloodstream.

Thrombo: a clot of blood; a thrombus.

Thrombophlebitis: an inflammation of a vein due to the presence of a thrombus.

Transfusion: injection of blood or a blood component of one person into the blood vessels of another.

Tunneled catheter: a thin-walled silicone rubber catheter that is radiopaque and ends with a Luer-Loc mechanism.

Valsalva's maneuver: attempt to forcibly exhale with the glottis closed.

Vascular access device (VAD): An array of infusion ports, catheters, and cannulas that allow long-term intravenous therapy or repeated access to the central venous system.

Venipuncture: puncture of a vein with a needle.

Viscosity: resistance offered by a fluid; property of a substance that is dependent on the friction of its component molecules as they slide by each other.

Vitamins: a group of organic substances essential for life.

VASCULAR ACCESS DEVICES

Long-term intravenous therapy is best accomplished through the use of vascular access devices (VADs), which include infusion ports, catheters, and cannulas. The specific form of venous access devices used depends on the type and length of time of treatment, as well as the diagnosis. Clients requiring chemotherapy, nutritional supplements, blood products, and fluids can benefit from an implantable device. These devices provide for repeated access to the venous system without venipuncture and multiple intravenous lines. VADs protect clients from vein sclerosis, infection, bleeding, and pain.

Central venous catheters, or triple-lumen, nontunneled catheters, such as the Hohn or Deseret catheter, are for short-term fluid or blood administration, obtaining blood specimens, and administering medications. Catheter insertion into the superior vena cava minimizes vessel irritation and sclerosis of the vessel. Tunneled catheters, such as the Hickman, Broviac, and Groshong catheters, are single or double lumens and are used for long-term fluid replacement therapy, medication administration, nutritional supplement, and blood specimen withdrawal. These catheters can remain in place from months to years. A tunnel is made through the subcutaneous tissue, usually between the nipple and clavicle. The catheter tip is inserted through the cephalic internal or external jugular vein and threaded to the right atrium. The tunnel creates a space between the end of the catheter and the actual vein.

Client Selection for VADs

- Long-term intravenous therapy
- Need for frequent venous access
- Impaired peripheral venous flow
- Sclerosed peripheral veins
- Elderly client requiring multiple venipunctures

TOTAL PARENTERAL NUTRITION

Parenteral nutrition is a method whereby nutrients may be introduced into the system via the enteral route. Bypassing the normal gastrointestinal system, this route provides a nitrogen source for those unable to ingest protein, carbohydrates (adequate calories), or fats. A balanced blend of nutrients, including vitamins and minerals, can be administered peripherally, using isotonic concentrations of glucose, crystalline amino acids, and fats; or, because the solution may be irritating to the veins, nutrients can be administered through a central, high-flow vein. Hypertonic glucose, along with crystalline amino acids, fats, electrolytes, vitamins, and trace elements, is given through central vein access. This technique requires special handling and management of the client and is the most expensive method of feeding. It should be used only if the intestines do not work adequately, if the client has an obstruction or has a fistula, if a bowel rest is required, or if the client is so debilitated that the gastrointestinal tract is nonfunctional.

Implantable vascular access devices are placed under the skin in a subcutaneous pocket and a surgically tunneled silicone catheter is placed in the cephalic or external jugular vein and threaded to the superior vena cava. Access to the port is through placement of a Huber needle (a right-angle noncoring needle) through a self-sealing injection port sitting in a plastic or metal case. This needle can remain in place for 5–7 days.

PERIPHERAL INSERTION OF A CENTRAL VENOUS CATHETER (PICC)

Peripheral insertion of a central venous catheter (PICC) in the subclavian vein is becoming more frequent for administering chemotherapy, antibiotics, blood, IV fluids, and controlled narcotics. These access devices may be inserted by specially trained nurses. A chest x-ray is taken to verify placement of the catheter tip. If solutions are irritating or sclerosing, the PICC must be advanced to the superior vena cava.

Nursing responsibilities for clients receiving long-term IV therapy whether for medications or fluids is a major component of nursing care today.

Sterile technique must be maintained throughout all procedures associated with VADs and PICC lines. Infection can occur if contamination results from poor technique in cleaning insertion sites, flushing catheters, or inserting the Huber needle. Transparent dressings are placed over the insertion site for easy assessment and monitoring.

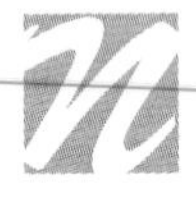

NURSING DIAGNOSES

The following nursing diagnoses may be appropriate to include in a client care plan when the components are related to intravenous therapy.

NURSING DIAGNOSIS	RELATED FACTORS
Activity intolerance	Change in setting—intensive care Compromised cardiac reserve
Altered nutrition: less than body requirements	Chronic fatigue states, fatigue, nausea and vomiting, inadequate absorption, faulty metabolism, eating disorders, side effects of chemotherapy
Anxiety	Lifestyle modification, pain, chronic conditions Uncertainty related to illness and diagnosis
Fluid volume excess	Excess fluid replacement, medications, renal and cardiac dysfunction
Decreased cardiac output	Impaired myocardial function due to disease states, altered electrical conduction, hypovolemia
Risk for infection	Invasive procedures, inadequate site care, tissue trauma, use of high glucose IV solutions, catheter-related infections
Altered tissue perfusion	Altered blood supply, arterial or venous, impaired myocardial contractility, hypovolemia, shock

unit 1

NONTUNNELED CENTRAL VENOUS CATHETERS

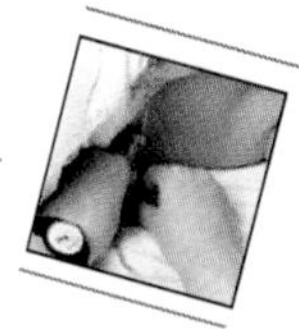

NURSING PROCESS DATA

ASSESSMENT Data Base

Determine client's level of consciousness so full explanation of procedure can be done to allay anxiety.

Assess level of anxiety to determine need for possible premedication.

Assess skin and surrounding tissue for erythema, edema, and warmth.

PLANNING Objectives

To assist the physician with central venous catheter insertion

To maintain patency of central venous line

To change central venous catheter dressing without complications

To maintain the insertion site free of infection and the catheter free of clots

IMPLEMENTATION Procedures

Assisting with Central Venous Catheterization

Changing a Central Venous Catheter Dressing

Measuring and Monitoring CVP

EVALUATION Expected Outcomes

Central venous line is properly placed.

Central venous line remains open.

Central venous catheter dressing is changed without complications.

ASSISTING WITH CENTRAL VENOUS CATHETERIZATION

Equipment

Routine IV setup

Tape

Through-the-needle radiopaque central catheter

Local anesthetic, sterile syringes, and needles

Sterile gloves, sterile gown, masks, drapes, and sutures

Central catheter dressing kit

Procedure

1. Explain procedure to client.
2. Place client in Trendelenburg's position (approximately 15–30° angle). **Rationale:** This position prevents air embolism and helps fill subclavian vein.
3. Extend client's neck and upper chest by placing a rolled pillow or blanket under shoulders. Make sure that side of client's neck or chest where the central venous line is to be inserted is closest to physician. **Rationale:** Usual insertion sites are subclavian or jugular veins.
4. Place mask on client, and turn client's head away from site of venipuncture. **Rationale:** This facilitates filling the vessel with blood and prevents contamination.
5. Maintain sterility when you open glove packet and sterile drape pack. (Physician must wear sterile gloves, gown, and mask for this procedure.)
6. Open povidone-iodine (Betadine) prep pads.
7. Assist with central catheter insertion.
   a. Physician dons mask, gown, and sterile gloves for this procedure.
   b. Physician prepares the client's skin, drapes area, and, using a sterile syringe and needle, draws up anesthetic to infiltrate the site.
   c. As physician inserts catheter, have client per-

form Valsalva's maneuver to prevent air embolism.
(1) Instruct client to exhale against a closed glottis.
(2) If client is unable to do this, compress client's abdomen. **Rationale:** Both these procedures help to decrease chances of air embolism.
8. When physician has completed catheterization, primed IV tubing is attached (use needleless components) and infusion drip set to desired rate of administration. Physician sutures catheter into place.
9. Tape all connections on tubing.
10. Cover insertion site and sutures with povidone-iodine ointment, sterile 2 × 2 gauze pads, and tape occlusively. (*Optional:* sterile transparent dressing according to hospital policy.)
11. Secure dressing and tubing with tape.
12. Label insertion site dressing with date, nurse's initials, and time of insertion.

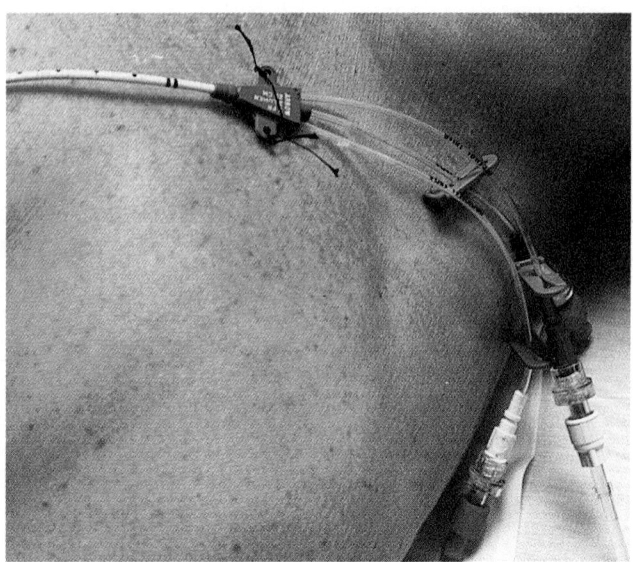

Multilumen central venous catheter depicting insertion location (yellow portion would be inserted internally).

13. Client usually sent to x-ray for catheter position validation.

CHANGING A CENTRAL VENOUS CATHETER DRESSING

Equipment

Tape
Central catheter dressing kit
or sterile gloves, mask(s), 70% alcohol
or povidone-iodine (Betadine) swabs, povidone-iodine ointment, sterile 2 × 2 gauze pads with precut slits and tape, or transparent dressing (according to hospital policy)
Receptacle for soiled dressing
Clean gloves

Preparation

1. Check client care plan and Kardex for last dressing change.
2. Gather equipment.
3. Check the location of the central vein catheter.
4. If located in client's neck or subclavian area, position client flat on back. **Rationale:** This eliminates the risk of air embolism.
5. Turn the client's head away from the insertion site, and mask the client's nose and mouth if necessary.
6. Wash your hands thoroughly.
7. Explain procedure to client.
8. Make sure that all personnel don masks.

Procedure

1. Don clean gloves.
2. Carefully remove old dressing and tape without pulling on catheter.
3. Discard old dressing and gloves in proper receptacle.
4. Put on sterile gloves.
5. Inspect site for loose sutures and signs of infection, inflammation, or infiltration.
6. If skin, insertion site, and catheter look normal, cleanse insertion site, sutures, and catheter with alcohol or iodine swabs, working from insertion site outward in a circular motion. **Rationale:** Working from cleanest area to least clean prevents contamination.
7. Cleanse site with circular motion three times with three different swabs.
8. Apply povidone-iodine ointment directly on insertion site (according to hospital policy).
9. Place preslit sterile 2 × 2 gauze pads around insertion site. The catheter should protrude through center of pads. *Alternative:* One gauze pad may be

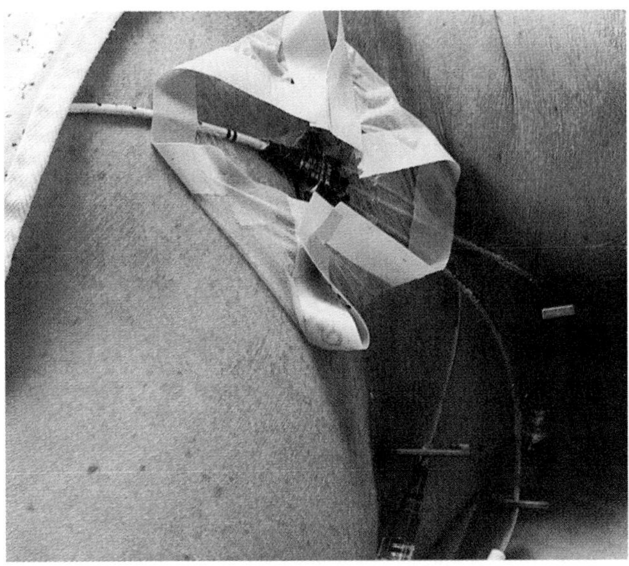

Carefully remove old dressing and tape.

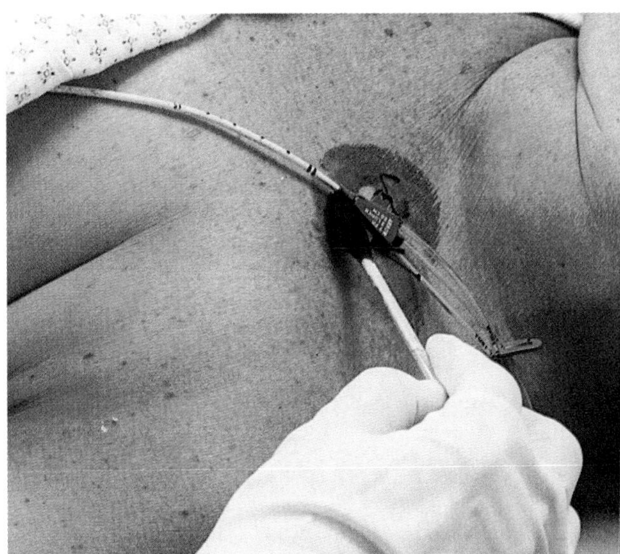

Swab insertion site with iodine swabs.

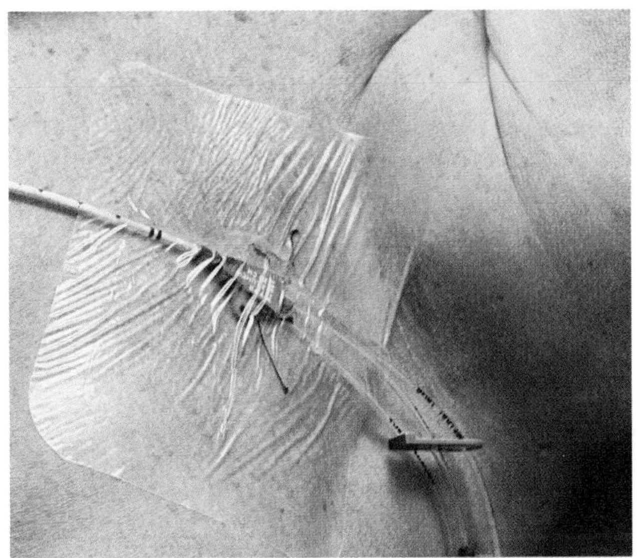

Apply transparent dressing.

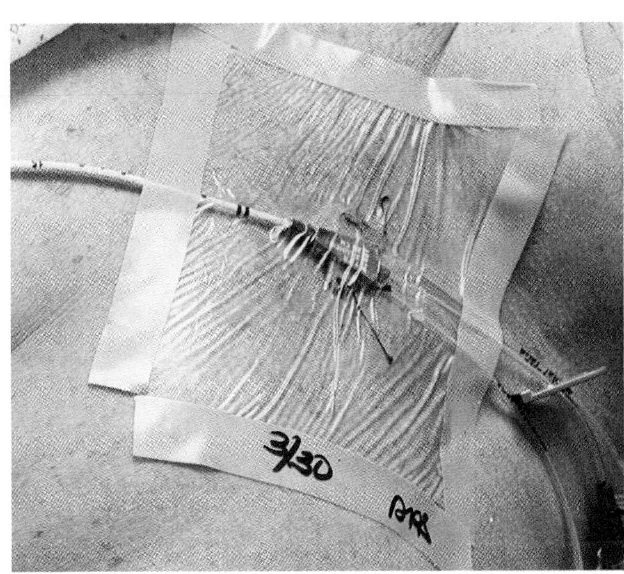

Label dressing with date and initials.

placed between catheter and skin, then covered with a sterile transparent dressing over insertion site, or transparent dressing may be used alone.

10. Tape dressing. Window pane dressing with tape to secure edge of dressing.
11. Change IV tubing, if hospital policy requires dressing and tubing to be changed at same time.
    a. Clamp central catheter using on-line slide or squeeze clamp.
    b. Change needleless access cap.
    c. Prepare site with Betadine.
    d. Insert new tubing with needleless connector.
12. Label dressing with date and your initials.
13. Change dressing if it becomes loose, wet, or soiled. **Rationale:** if it is wet, soiled, or loose, it is contaminated. Follow hospital policy regarding the length of time a transparent dressing may remain in place.
14. Discard equipment and gloves, and wash hands.

MEASURING AND MONITORING CVP

Equipment

Stopcock
Manometer
IV solution bag
Administration set (with extension tubing)
IV pole with C arm
Carpenter's level

> ■ CLINICAL ALERT
>
> Central venous pressure (CVP) is a measure of the pressure of blood in the right atrium or vena cava. It is measured in centimeters of water pressure, which vary within the normal range of values cited.

Procedure

1. Determine desired CVP parameters. Check client care plan, physician's orders, and Kardex. **Rationale:** When changes occur beyond the values established for client, check CVP system and client's vital signs. If CVP system is functioning correctly, report changes in values to physician.
2. Establish baseline by taking client's vital signs and by checking client's hydration status.
3. Spike IV solution bag with IV administration set using sterile technique.
4. Prime tubing with solution, making certain that no air bubbles are present in tubing.
5. Close clamp on tubing.
6. If you are using a one-piece disposable manometer and stopcock, affix unit to an IV pole with a C-shaped clamp. Attach IV pole to client's bed or a

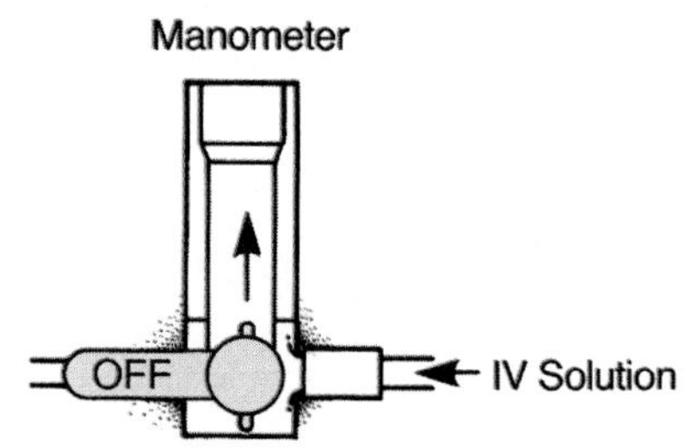

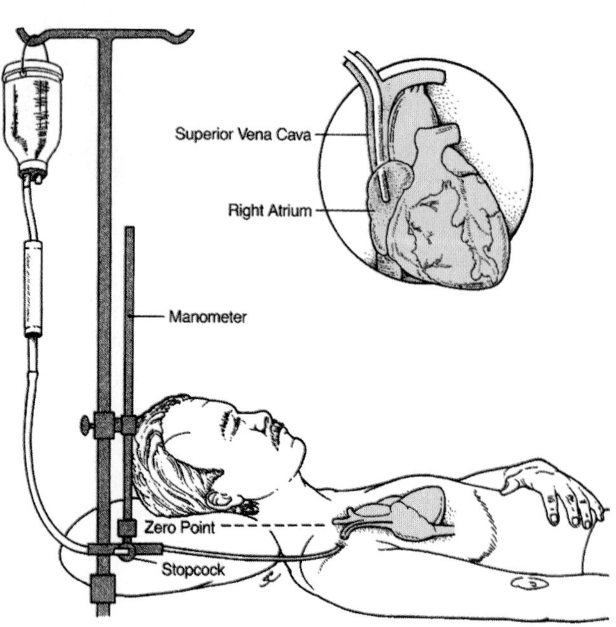

When a CVP reading is taken, the zero of the manometer is level with the client's right atrium.

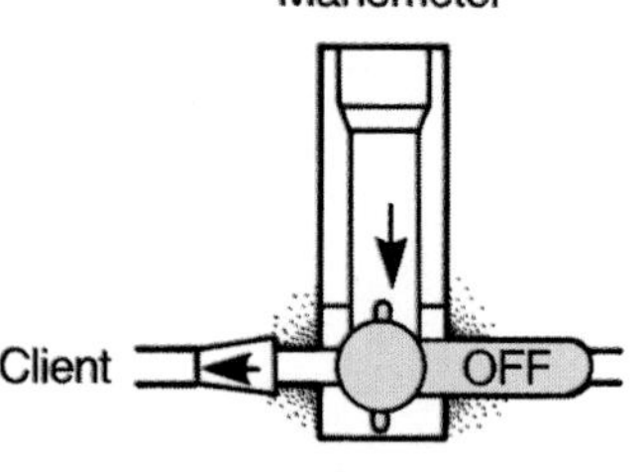

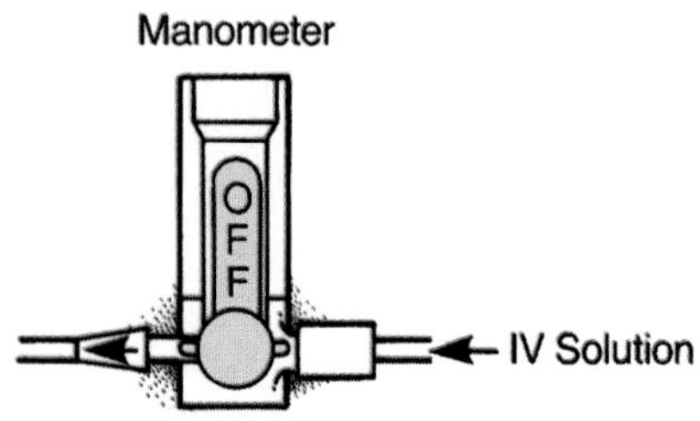

Top stopcock: Fill the manometer by turning stopcock OFF to the patient. This allows solution to flow from the bottle to the manometer. Middle stopcock: Measue CVP by turning stopcock OFF to IV solution allowing fluid to flow from manometer to patient. Bottom stopcock: Reinstitute flow from IV bottle to patient by turning stopcock OFF to the manometer.

pole that fits under mattress. **Rationale:** A floor stand IV pole is unstable and can affect CVP readings.

7. Push male end of IV administration set into female end of stopcock, connecting the IV set to stopcock.
8. Turning stopcock so that manometer and IV solution are open to each other, open clamp on IV tubing and fill manometer with IV solution to between 18 and 20 cm. **Rationale:** Overfilling the manometer may expose the client to contamination resulting from overflow.
9. Close clamp, and rotate stopcock so that IV solution is open to client.
10. With IV solution, prime the rest of IV tubing that extends from stopcock, and connect tubing to CVP catheter.
11. Place client flat in bed, without a pillow, if client can tolerate this position. If not, place client in position of comfort (e.g., head of bed at 15–30°). Record position so that same position can be used each time a CVP reading is made. **Rationale:** This allows accurate summary of CVP findings.
12. Locate client's right atrium (midaxillary at fourth intercostal space). Mark this location on client's skin.
13. Adjust level of manometer (using carpenter's level) so that zero on manometer scale is at the same level as client's right atrium, 5 cm on manometer level to sternal notch. **Rationale:** Using level of right atrium reflects blood volume and cardiac function of client.
14. Turn stopcock to open position for manometer IV solution, filling manometer with additional solution if needed.
15. Turn the stopcock to the manometer–client position, and watch the level of the solution in the manometer fall to the pressure level existing in the right atrium. **Rationale:** Normally this pressure should be between 5 and 10 cm. Remember, however, there are no absolute values and trends—the rise and fall of CVP readings are more important than one pressure level reading. For example, if CVP goes from 5 to 10 cm in 30 minutes, something is wrong—even though 10 cm is a normal reading.
16. Observe meniscus at eye level, and watch rise and fall of fluid column in response to client's breathing. **Rationale:** Fluctuations reflect changes in intrathoracic pressures during respiratory cycle and indicate that manometer is functioning properly.

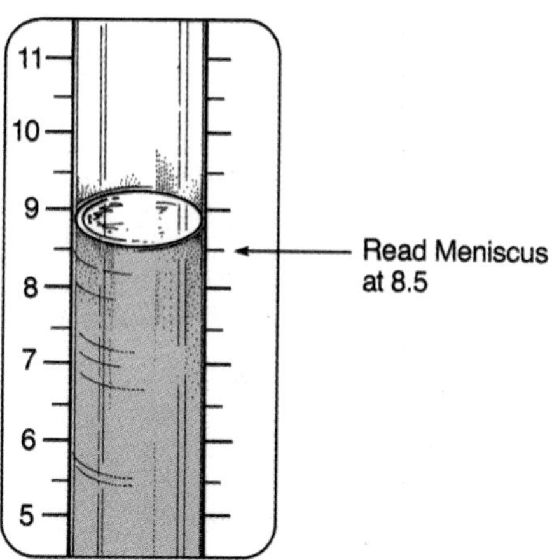

Take CVP reading at highest level of meniscus and at end of expiration.

17. Take reading at end of respiratory cycle—expiration.
18. Turn off stopcock to manometer, and adjust rate of infusion with clamp.
19. Return client to desired position, and record CVP readings.

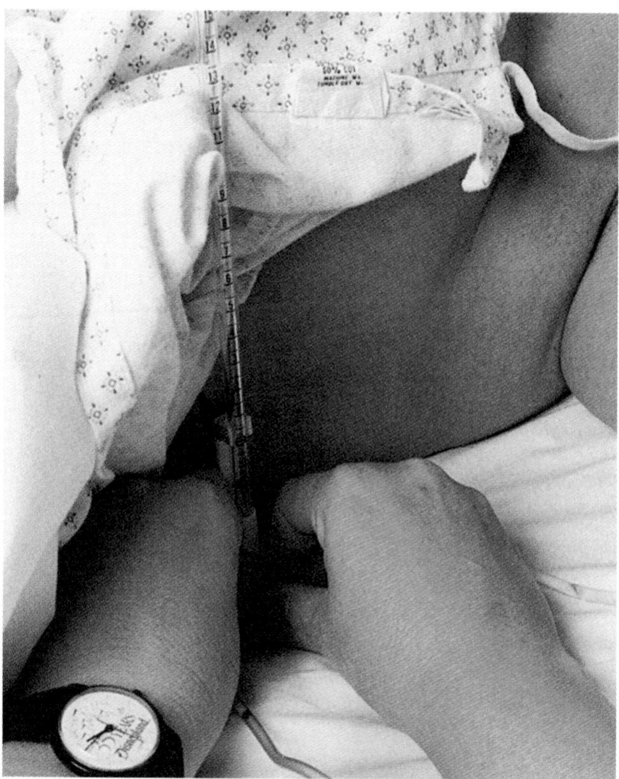

CVP reading is taken midaxillary at the fourth intercostal space.

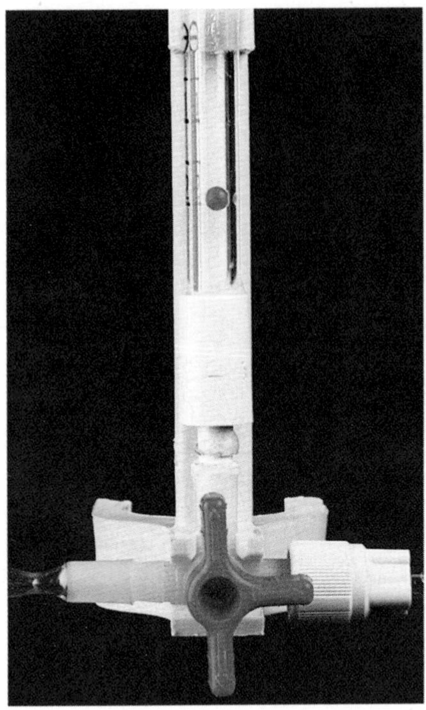

Solution to manometer.

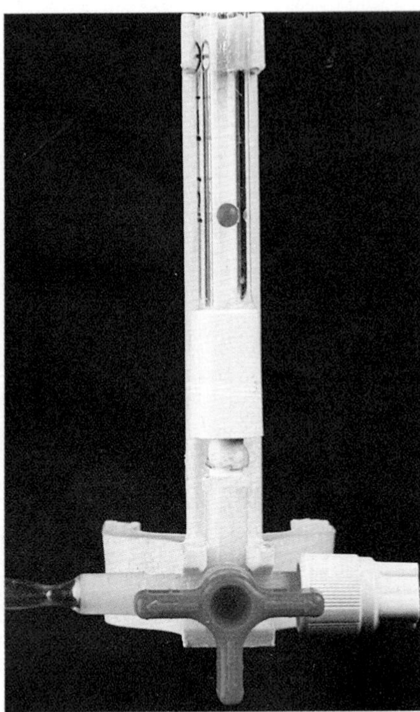

Solution to client.

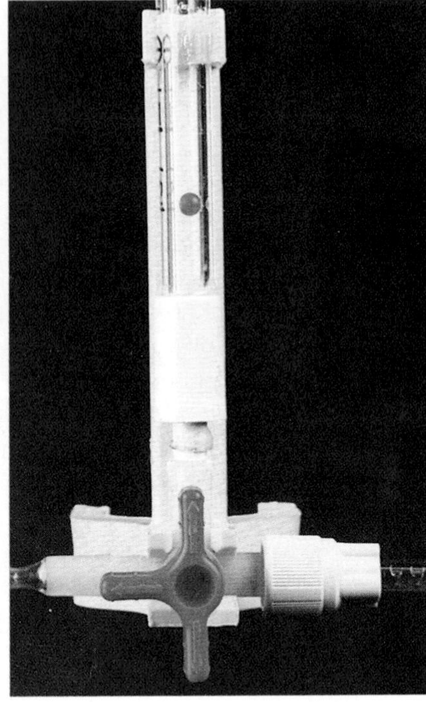

Manometer to client.

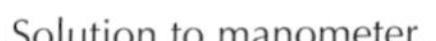

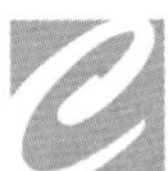

CHARTING for CVP Catheterization

- Location of insertion site
- Type and size of needle or cannula used for insertion
- Time of insertion
- Appearance of needle insertion site
- Name of physician performing catheterization
- Types of solutions used, including all additives listed in sequence used
- Amount of solution infused
- Time x-ray was performed to check position of radiopaque catheter
- Time and date dressing or tubing changed
- Initials of person changing the dressing
- Condition of catheter insertion site when dressing changed
- Date and time of CVP reading (record subsequent CVP readings on appropriate forms)
- Client's response to treatment
- Any unusual conditions or reactions

CRITICAL THINKING APPLICATION

CLINICAL PROBLEMS	CRITICAL THINKING OPTIONS
■ Air enters central vein, producing air embolism, from a break in the catheter.	• Inform physician immediately; clamp catheter as ordered. • Place client in a head-down position with the right atrium uppermost. Monitor until physician arrives. • Administer high flow O_2 as necessary.
■ CVP system does not drip.	• Check the entire line for kinks in the tubing. Change client's position. Check to make sure the manometer stopcock is in the IV–client position. • Notify physician, and gather equipment for catheter aspiration or irrigation. • Obtain order for placing heparin in IV bottle to prevent clotting at tip of catheter. • Prepare for possible reinsertion.
■ CVP readings appear to be inaccurate.	• Assess patency of setup. • Assess client's level of pain; pain increases the CVP reading. • Assess if position of client has been changed; raising the head of the bed alters the reading. • Check that the marked area at midaxillary level is at the level of the client's right atrium. • If client has COPD, CHF (especially right-sided), or hypovolemia, expect readings to differ from normal range. However, once baseline is established for individual client, changes and trends should be watched and judged against the baseline.
■ Sepsis.	• Prepare for catheter removal and possible reinsertion. • If catheter is removed, send tip to laboratory for culture. • Administer antibiotics, as ordered.
■ Dysrhythmia detected.	• Change client's position. • Notify physician. • Verify catheter position on chest x-ray. • Prepare for catheter repositioning or removal of catheter by physician.
■ CVP dressing is wet following dressing change.	• If leakage around the catheter has wet the dressing and skin, check all connections. • Lower the solution and check for backflow of blood in the tubing. • Tape the dressing securely to ensure connections do not become loosened.

unit 2

TOTAL PARENTERAL NUTRITION

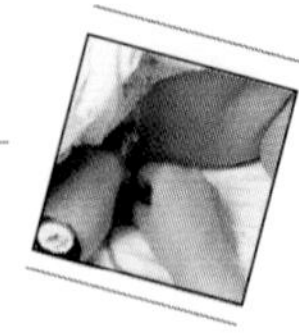

NURSING PROCESS DATA

ASSESSMENT Data Base

Complete a physical assessment and client history.

Assess weight and take a weight history.

Identify any condition that would affect TPN (renal or cardiac disease).

Assess nutritional needs of clients who are unable to ingest nutrients normally.

Identify the caloric intake necessary to promote positive nitrogen balance, tissue repair, and growth.

Observe for correct additives in each hyperalimentation bottle.

Check label of solution with physician's orders.

Check rate of infusion on physician's orders.

Assess ability of client to understand instructions during procedure.

Ensure patency of central venous line following insertion.

Observe catheter insertion site for signs of infection, thrombophlebitis, or possible infiltration.

Inspect dressing over central line to ensure a dry, noncontaminated dressing.

PLANNING Objectives

To provide a nitrogen source for clients unable to ingest protein normally

To provide adequate calories for clients unable to tolerate oral feedings

To provide nutrients for clients requiring bypass of the gastrointestinal tract

To provide increased calories where regular IV solutions are insufficient

To prevent or correct a deficiency of essential fatty acids

To provide a contamination-free mode of delivering the hyperalimentation solution

IMPLEMENTATION Procedures

Assisting with Catheter Insertion

Maintaining Central Vein Infusions

Changing Parenteral Hyperalimentation Dressing and Tubing

Maintaining Hyperalimentation for Children

EVALUATION Expected Outcomes

Catheter is placed correctly with no infiltration.

Solution is infused at prescribed flow rate and tolerated by patient.

Dressing remains dry and intact during interval between changes.

Insertion site remains free of infection and inflammation sepsis does not occur.

Client receives nutrients necessary for tissue repair and sustenance.

ASSISTING WITH CATHETER INSERTION

Equipment

Intracath (20 cm, 16-gauge, radiopaque, polyvinyl chloride) or peripheral line catheter
Povidone-iodine (Betadine) solution
Betadine ointment and swabs
Alcohol sponges
Acetone solution (optional)
Sterile 4×4 gauze pads
Sterile gloves
Sterile towels or drapes
Sterile gown
Masks (2)
3-mL syringe with 25-gauge needle
Lidocaine (Xylocaine) or local anesthetic agent
Sterile 00 or 000 black silk suture with needle
IV filter and tubing
Plastic tape and micropore tape or occlusive dressing material
IV extension tubing
500 mL normal saline IV bag or D_5W
Hyperalimentation solution from pharmacy
IV infusion pump and cassette (for some equipment)
Bath blanket to provide roll under shoulders

Composition of Hyperalimentation Solutions

- Amino acid (Freamine or Aminosol: 10% amino acid solution)
- Carbohydrates—monohydrous glucose
- Vitamins
- Minerals and trace elements
- Hypertonic glucose/dextrose (20–50%): calories (1000–2000 Cal/L)
- Electrolytes
- Water
- Hyperalimentation solution is prepared in the pharmacy under a laminar flow hood

Preparation

1. Explain procedure to client to allay anxiety.
2. Obtain consent from client or family.
3. Teach Valsalva's maneuver for use during catheter insertion procedure, if client does not have a cardiac disorder. **Rationale:** This maneuver prevents air from entering the catheter during catheter insertion or tubing changes.
   a. Ask client to take a deep breath and bear down without exhaling.

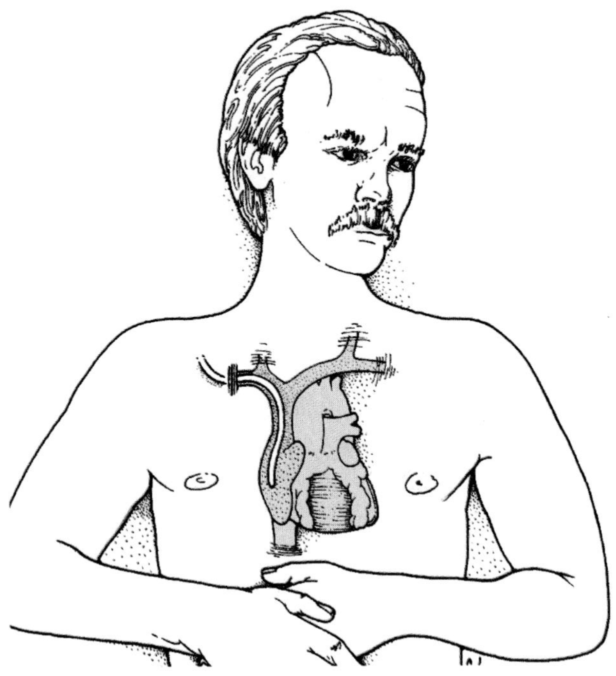

Central venous catheter inserted via right subclavian vein.

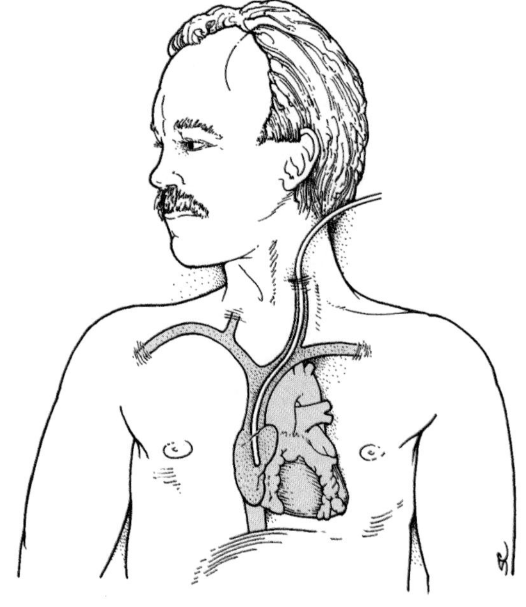

Central venous catheter inserted via left jugular vein.

TABLE 28–1. Complications with Total Parenteral Nutrition

Complication	Symptoms	Implementation	
		Prevention	**Nursing Action**
Air embolus Air enters catheter during catheter insertion or tubing changes, or from undetected hairline cracks in tubing	Potentially fatal Respiratory distress, apprehension Chest pain, dyspnea Blood pressure drop Pulse weak and rapid CVP rises—cardiac arrest	Instruct client in Valsalva's maneuver Check all catheter connections Place client in position of head down with head turned opposite direction of insertion site (increases intrathoracic venous pressure)	Clamp catheter Place client in left Trendelenburg's position (to allow air to pass from pulmonary artery) Notify physician Administer oxygen as ordered
Catheter-related infection (sepsis) Because the TPN solution is high-concentrate glucose, it is a medium for bacterial growth and CV line provides systemic access	Fever (early sign), chills Insertion site—evidence of infection with erythema or drainage Elevated white blood cell count Septic shock	Use strict aseptic technique Change solution every 12 hours Change tubing as ordered (every 24 hours using aseptic technique) Change dressing every 48 hours	Remove tip of catheter, and send to laboratory for culture Administer antibiotics as ordered
Hyperglycemia Increased sugar level after day one (positive urine acetone and urine 3+ or 4+) from infusion solution	Elevated glucose levels (more than 200 mg/dL) Excessive thirst, fatigue, restlessness, confusion, weakness, diuresis When severe—coma	Check history for glucose intolerance; frequent glucose monitoring—check rate of infusion Begin infusion at slow rate (usually 40 mL/hour) to reduce risk of hyperglycemia Do not "catch-up" if infusion rate falls behind	Start insulin therapy as ordered Request physician slow infusion rate Monitor blood glucose levels every 4–6 hours
Hypoglycemia TPN is discontinued abruptly or client is receiving too much insulin	Client is shaky, weak, anxious, and irritable May be hungry Decreased blood glucose (less than 80 mg/dL)	Continue blood glucose monitoring to check insulin levels Gradually decrease infusion—avoid discontinuing TPH abruptly	Infuse dextrose 10% in water (restart IV if necessary) Assess blood glucose level 1 hour after discontinuing TPN

b. Note how long client can hold breath. **Rationale:** Nurse can judge the time available for insertion.

c. Apply gentle pressure to the abdomen.

4. Review physician's order for correct hyperalimentation solution additives. Check solution content with orders. **Rationale:** Incompatible additives can cause a severe reaction or complication.
   a. TPN bottles come directly from the pharmacy and are numbered sequentially.
   b. Each TPN bottle label includes client's name, room number, additives, IV number, start time, date, and stop time.
5. Inspect TPN bottle for cracks, turbidity, or precipitates. ("Cracking" may occur in solution when there are layers—return to pharmacy. TPN formula may have to be adjusted to remove additive-causing cracking.)
6. Assemble IV insertion tray or kit, normal saline solution bottle or D_5W, IV tubing, extension tubing, and filter. **Rationale:** Filter removes crystals/microorganisms from solution. Do not use filter to administer intralipids.
7. Wash hands.
8. Flush IV tubing with IV solution.
9. Place IV tubing through infusion pump. (IV tubing may be placed through an infusion cassette with some equipment.)
10. Place catheter insertion equipment on bedside stand.

Procedure

1. Position client in head-down position with head turned to opposite direction of catheter insertion site. Place a small roll between client's shoulders

to expose insertion site. **Rationale:** This position increases intrathoracic venous pressure and reduces risk of air embolism.

2. Cleanse insertion area with Betadine solution. (If allergic to Betadine, use 70% isopropyl alcohol.)
   a. Cleanse a large area around insertion site.
   b. Use a circular motion to cleanse from insertion site to periphery.
3. Assist physician to gown, put on mask and gloves prior to beginning procedure.
4. Don mask and sterile gloves.
5. Assist physician as needed during catheter insertion.
6. Instruct client in Valsalva's maneuver when stylet is removed from catheter and when IV tubing is connected to catheter.
   a. Instruct client to exhale against a closed glottis.
   b. If client is unable to do this, compress client's abdomen. **Rationale:** Both these procedures help decrease possibility of air embolism.
7. After tubing is connected, instruct client to breathe normally.
8. Tape area between tubing and catheter hub. **Rationale:** Secure taping holds connection together and lessens chance of contamination.
9. Turn on IV infusion pump, using normal saline solution, at slow rate, 10 gtt/minute, until x-ray ensures accurate catheter placement.
10. Place Betadine over catheter insertion site. Apply transparent dressing.
11. Order portable chest x-ray to verify correct catheter placement.
12. Following confirmation of catheter placement, change IV solution to hyperalimentation solution and adjust flow rate as ordered.
13. Time tape the bottle after adjusting flow rate. Be prepared to document on IV hourly infusion record.
14. Observe for signs of complications (Table 28–1).
15. Take vital signs every 4 hours. **Rationale:** If signs change or temperature rises significantly, the client may be developing complications.

Monitoring Guidelines for TPN

- Monitor for signs of infection or sepsis at the insertion site—the most common complication of TPN.
- Weigh client daily (1–3 lbs/week)—observe for fluid gain or loss. Weight gain may indicate fluid overload rather than increased nutritional gain.
- Monitor electrolyte and protein levels daily in the beginning of treatment. Magnesium and calcium imbalances may occur.
- Monitor serum glucose levels observing for hyperglycemia (thirst, polyuria).
- Assess blood urea nitrogen and creatinine levels—increases may indicate excess amino acid intake.
- Check liver function test results—abnormal values may indicate an excess of lipids or problems in protein or glucose metabolism.

MAINTAINING CENTRAL VEIN INFUSIONS

Equipment

Hyperalimentation solution (refrigerated)
IV tubing, filter, and infusion pump
Extension tubing
Sugar and acetone testing equipment
Specific gravity urometer
I&O record
TPN record sheet

Procedure

1. Store hyperalimentation solution in refrigerator until 30 minutes before use. (Some pharmacies deliver the solution before each infusion.) **Rationale:** Solution is refrigerated to prevent growth of organisms, but should be left at room temperature one hour prior to use.
2. Change IV tubing, filter, and infusion pump cassette (if used) every 24 hours. **Rationale:** This is recommended for TPN infusions to prevent infection.
3. Maintain IV flow rate at prescribed rate.
   a. If rate is too rapid, hyperosmolar diuresis occurs (excess sugar is excreted); if severe enough, intractable seizures, coma, and death can occur.
   b. If rate is too slow, little benefit is derived from the calories and nitrogen.
4. Monitor IV flow rate every 30–60 minutes even though you are using an IV pump.

CLINICAL ALERT

Do not correct an overload or deficit in flow, as doing so could result in complications for the client. Notify physician if this occurs.

5. Change solution every 12–24 hours according to hospital policy if dextrose is used. **Rationale:** Changing the solution prevents growth of bacterial organisms that proliferate in a sugar solution.
6. Check urine specific gravity, sugar, and acetone every 4 hours. **Rationale:** Solution is composed of glucose as well as protein, vitamins, and minerals.
7. If necessary, administer insulin according to prescribed "rainbow" coverage.
8. Notify physician of urine sugars of 3+ or 4+ and positive urine acetone. **Rationale:** Most clients show a sugar level as high as 2+ during the first few days of treatment.
9. Maintain accurate I&O. Record on special total parenteral nutrition (TPN) sheet at least every 4 hours.
10. Weigh client daily, and record on graphic sheet and TPN sheet.
11. Observe for complications, such as air embolus, hyperglycemia, osmotic diuresis, infiltration, or sepsis. (See Table 28–1.)

CHANGING PARENTERAL HYPERALIMENTATION DRESSING AND TUBING

Equipment

Hyperalimentation dressing tray
Sterile towels or drapes
Clean and sterile gloves
Mask
IV tubing and filter
TPN solution
2×2 sterile gauze pads
Povidone-iodine swabs and ointment
Micropore tape
Sterile transparent tape
Paper bag

Preparation

1. Gather equipment, and wash hands thoroughly.
2. Add IV tubing and filter to parenteral hyperalimentation solution bottle.
3. Flush tubing to force out air.
4. Place IV tubing through IV pump or insert pump cassette into infusion pump, and then prime cassette if used.
5. Prepare dressing material or open dressing kit containing povidone-iodine swabs, sterile 2 × 2 gauze pads, and sterile transparent dressing.
6. Place the client with head flat and turned in the opposite direction of the insertion site. Instruct the client not to talk or cough. (Place mask on client if client cannot cooperate.) **Rationale:** These instructions reduce risk of contamination.

Procedure

1. Place mask on (according to institutional policy), and don clean gloves.

CLINICAL ALERT

When central-line dressings are loose, wet, or soiled, they are considered contaminated and must be changed.

2. Take off old dressing and dispose of it in paper bag. (Do not touch the insertion site.) Remove gloves.
3. Drape area with sterile towels (according to institutional policy).
4. Put on sterile gloves.
5. Observe insertion site for signs of erythema, drainage, or possible swelling.
6. Cleanse around the insertion site with povidone-iodine swabs, using a circular movement from inside out. **Rationale:** This action cleanses the site of dried blood or serum.
7. Apply povidone-iodine swabs in same circular motion, working outward from catheter site. Allow at least 2 minutes for drying.
8. Place precut 2×2 sterile gauze pads under catheter hub and around the insertion site, with the catheter protruding through the center of the pad according to hospital policy. More commonly,

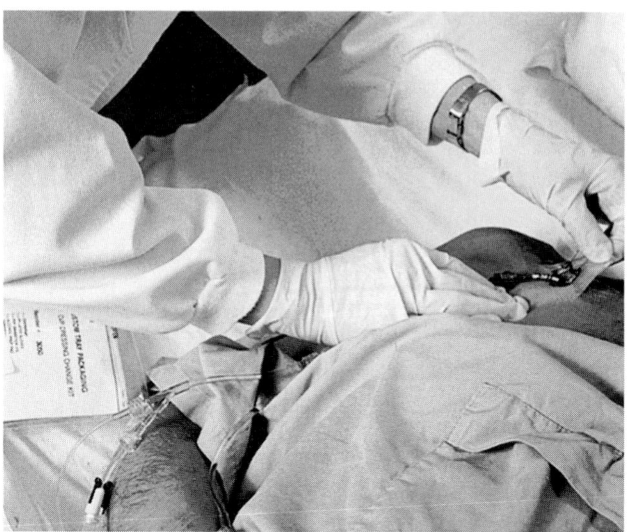
Remove old dressing, discard and remove clean gloves.

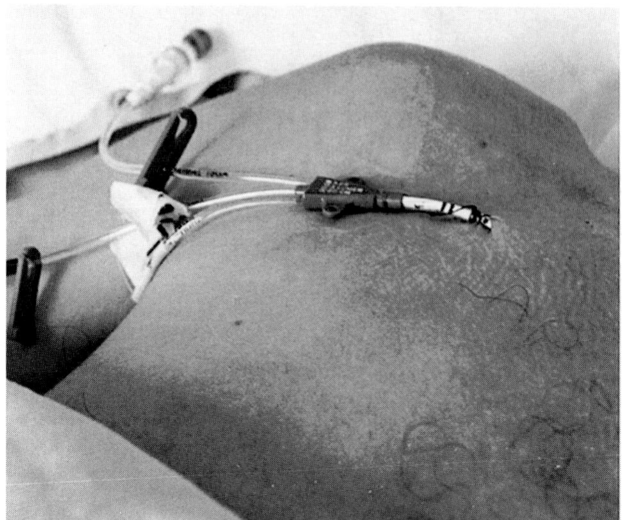
Assess triple lumen caatheter, hub, and insertion site.

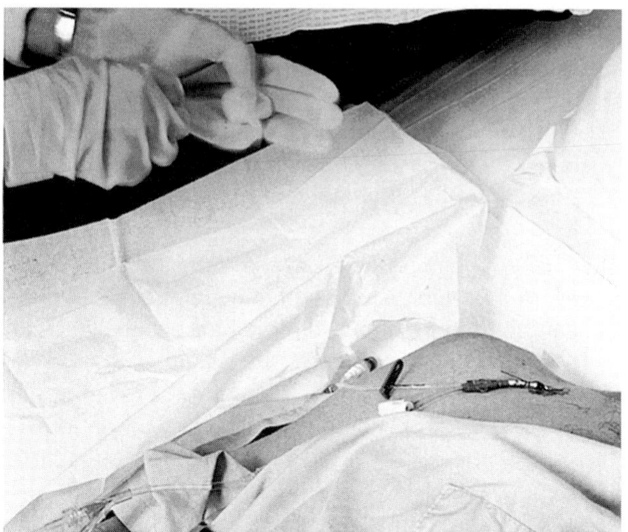
Prepare sterile field on the bed and don sterile gloves.

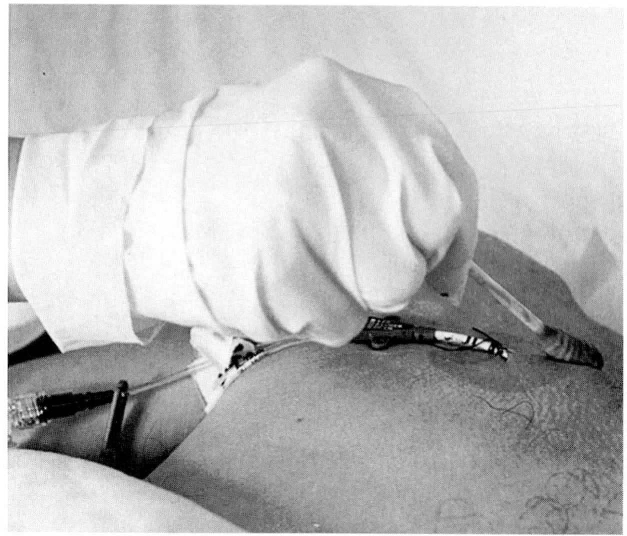
Clean site with alcohol, followed by Povidone-iodine swabs.

a sterile transparent dressing is applied.

9. Change the tubing if hospital policy dictates that tubing is changed at the same time as the dressing.
   a. Slide clamp catheter.
   b. Loosen the tubing in the catheter hub. Policy may dictate that the hub be wiped with Betadine.
   c. Insert primed tubing.
   d. Tape the connection between the tubing and catheter hub.
   e. Discard equipment in biohazard container or bag.
10. Remove gloves.
11. Tape down the dressing around the catheter site or place tape around edges of transparent dressing. Tape the connection (tubing–catheter hub) to the skin. If a filter is part of the central line tubing, as with a hyperalimentation catheter, secure the filter onto the dressing with tape.
12. Label the dressing with the date and your initials.
13. Answer any questions the client may have about the procedure, and make client comfortable before leaving the room.
14. Wash hands.

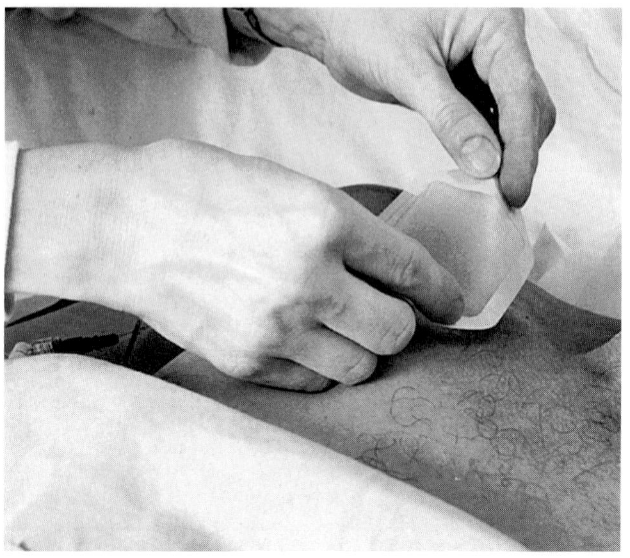

Center transparent dressing over catheter insertion site.

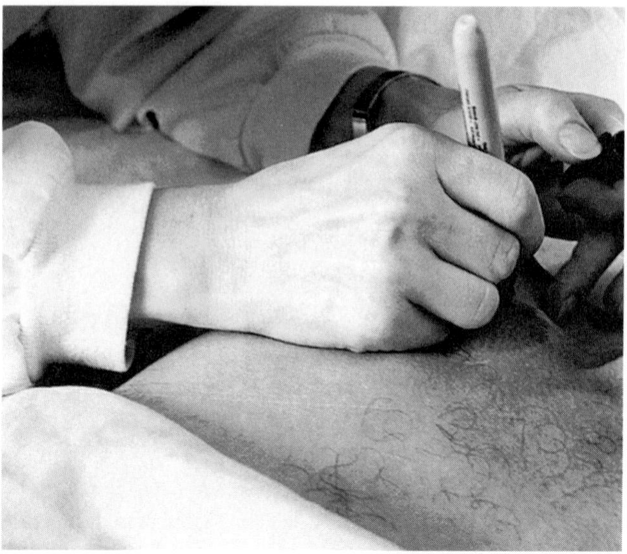

Label dressing with date, time and initials of nurse.

MAINTAINING HYPERALIMENTATION FOR CHILDREN

Equipment

Same as for adult hyperalimentation with these additions:

Intracath, 22-gauge needle

Microdrip IV tubing administration set

Restraints, if necessary

Procedure

1. Examine solution. Generally, there is a higher concentration of calcium, phosphorus, magnesium, and vitamins. Usually, a 10% solution of dextrose is started. It can be increased to 25% if tolerated.
2. Monitor patency of catheter (usually placed through internal or external jugular or scalp veins). Stopcocks are never used. Monitor constant infusion pump and filter.
3. Obtain urine sugar and acetone samples. **Rationale:** Sugar level rises, but usually exogenous insulin is not required as the pancreas adapts to high-glucose loads.
4. Change the dressing every 48 hours and the tubing every 24 hours using aseptic technique. Stockinette can be used to keep scalp dressing secure. Tight-fitting T-shirt can keep chest site secure.
5. Monitor for accurate rate of infusion. Do not "catch up" if infusion is behind. Positive pressure pumps can be used to maintain infusion rates, particularly when small amounts of solution are being infused.
6. Observe the child when ambulating for accidents, such as twisting or kinking the tubing, getting the tubing caught in the crib, or stepping on it.
7. Instruct parents on rationale for treatment and methods to prevent accidental dislodging of the tubing.
8. Provide play therapy and sources of stimulation to distract the child from thinking about the catheter.

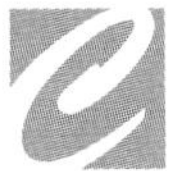

CHARTING for Hyperalimentation

- Special TPN sheet may be used. If so, charting is done directly on the sheet
- Catheter insertion site, size, physician's name, and any difficulty in insertion
- X-ray, following insertion
- Type of hyperalimentation solution and flow rate
- Specific gravity
- Results of urine sugar and acetone
- If insulin administered, type, amount, and site
- Time of dressing or tubing change date, and condition of catheter insertion site, along with name or initials of person who did the change
- Condition of insertion site
- Client's tolerance of procedure
- Signs of hypoglycemia or hyperglycemia
- Daily weights
- Vital signs every 4 hours

CRITICAL THINKING APPLICATION

CLINICAL PROBLEMS	CRITICAL THINKING OPTIONS
■ Hyperalimentation solution is not infused at the prescribed rate.	• Observe filter to ensure patency. A plugged filter is the most common cause of infusion failure. Replace the plugged filter. • Ensure that the next hyperalimentation bottle is ready to be superimposed. If bottle is not ready, add a bottle of $D_{10}W$ until the hyperalimentation solution can be superimposed. • Observe for signs of hypoglycemia caused by sudden change in dextrose concentration—weakness, trembling, sweating, hunger. • Adjust flow rate to that which was ordered. Do not attempt to "catch up" the amount not infused as this action could lead to osmotic diuresis from hyperglycemia.
■ Catheter insertion site does not remain free of infection, inflammation, or infiltration.	• Notify physician immediately so catheter can be discontinued. • Cut tip of catheter off with sterile scissors and place in sterile container. Send to laboratory for culture and sensitivity for specific causative organism. • Cleanse site of catheter insertion with povidone-iodine, and place sterile dressing over site. • Obtain order for and administer antibiotics as needed.
■ The dressing does not remain dry and intact during the interval between changes.	• Change the dressing as soon as moisture is observed, following aseptic technique. • If the dressing is exposed to moisture or secretions, a plastic, adhesive-like Steridrape or plastic wrap can be applied over sterile dressing.

unit 3

INTRALIPID THERAPY

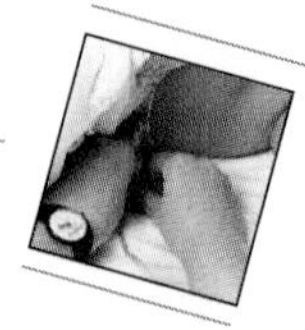

NURSING PROCESS DATA

ASSESSMENT Data Base

Observe for signs of essential fatty acid deficits; rash; eczema; dry, scaly skin; poor wound healing; sparse hair.

Assess pancreatic function.

Assess client for predisposing factors that could promote fat emboli, such as anemia, coagulation disorders, abnormal liver, or pulmonary function.

Check IV site for patency erythema, and edema before infusing solution.

Assess vital signs to establish baseline.

PLANNING Objectives

To spare protein in critically ill client

To provide a source of energy for clients with deficient protein intake

To provide essential fatty acids

IMPLEMENTATION Procedure

Infusing IV Lipids

EVALUATION Expected Outcomes

Adequate calories and essential fatty acids are provided to clients unable to ingest them by usual means.

No untoward effects or complications are experienced as a result of procedure.

Parenteral nutrients are provided without complications.

INFUSING IV LIPIDS

Equipment

IV fat solution (Intralipid 10%: soybean oil; Liposyn 10%: safflower oil)

Nonphthalate IV tubing infusion set (to prevent pooling of fat on IV tubing)

Iodophor sponges

Alcohol swabs

Volume control device

20-gauge needle

Small-gauge needle if piggybacking into dual injection site

Micropore tape

Preparation

1. Explain procedure to client.
2. Review physician's orders.
3. Obtain Intralipid (refrigerated) from the pharmacy and warm the solution to room temperature, or obtain Liposyn (nonrefrigerated) from the pharmacy.
4. Examine bottle for separation of emulsion into layers or fat globules or for accumulation of froth. Do not use if any of these appear.
5. Label bottle with correct client name, room number, date, time, flow rate, bottle number, and start and stop times.

Guidelines for IV Fat Infusion

- IV fat solutions are isotonic and provide 1.1 Cal/mL of solution. 1 mL of Intralipid equals 0.1 g.
- Putting additives into IV bottle is contraindicated as additives might be incompatible.
- Use of an IV filter is contraindicated as the particles are large and the infusion cannot pass through the filter, thereby clogging it.

Procedure

1. Take vital signs for baseline assessment. **Rationale:** Baseline information is needed because an immediate reaction can occur.
2. Wash hands, and then swab stopper on IV bottle with iodophor sponge and allow to dry.
3. Attach special IV tubing to bottle, twisting the spike to prevent particles from the stopper falling into the emulsion.
4. Hang IV bottle at least 30 inches above IV site. **Rationale:** Due to the solution viscosity, fat emulsion needs to be at this height to prevent backing up into infusion tubing.
5. Fill drip chamber two-thirds full, slightly open clamp on the tubing, and prime the tubing slowly. **Rationale:** Priming more slowly reduces chance of air bubbles with this solution.
6. Attach the tubing to the IV site, and tape connectors to prevent dislodging of the tubing.
7. Infuse fat solutions initially at 1.0 mL/min for adults and 0.1 mL/min for children. Time period for initial infusions varies from 15–30 minutes for Intralipid to 30 minutes for Liposyn.
8. Monitor vital signs every 10 minutes, and observe for side effects during first 30 minutes of the infusion. If side effects occur, stop the infusion and notify the physician.

■ CLINICAL ALERT

Observe for IV lipid side effects after starting lipid infusion:

- chills
- fever
- flushing
- diaphoresis
- dyspnea
- cyanosis
- allergic reactions
- chest and back pain
- nausea and vomiting
- headache
- pressure over the eyes
- vertigo
- sleepiness
- thrombophlebitis

9. Adjust flow to prescribed IV rate if no adverse reactions occur.
10. Monitor and maintain the infusion at the following rates:

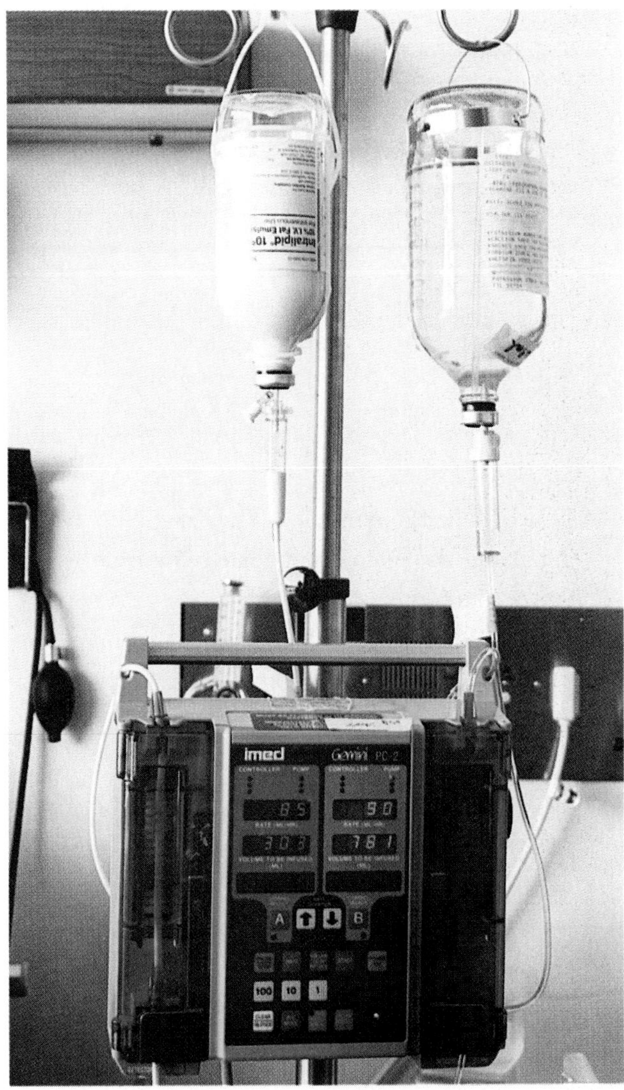

Intralipids (left) infusing with hyperalimentation fluids (right).

for Adults

Intralipid 10%: Up to 500 mL 4–6 hours on first day to maximum of 2.5 g/kg body weight per day. Do not exceed 60% of client's total caloric intake per day.

Liposyn 10%: No more than 500 mL/day in 4–6 hours.

for Children

Intralipid 10%: Up to 1 g/Kg in 4 hours. Do not exceed 60% of total caloric intake.

11. Monitor serum lipids 4 hours after discontinuing infusion. **Rationale:** If you draw blood too soon after infusion is completed, incorrect blood values result.

12. Monitor liver function tests for evidence of impaired liver function. **Rationale:** These tests indicate the liver's ability to metabolize the lipids.
13. Discard partially used bottles. **Rationale:** This action prevents contamination.
14. Continue to monitor vital signs, and observe client for adverse reactions during the entire process of infusion.
15. Flush tubing with normal saline when infusion is completed.
16. Answer any questions the client may have about the procedure, and make client comfortable before leaving room.

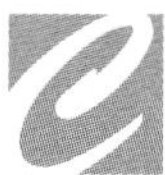

CHARTING for Fat Emulsion Therapy

- Type of solution infused
- Initial rate and maintenance rate of infusion
- Site of infusion
- Adverse clinical manifestations and appropriate nursing intervention

CRITICAL THINKING APPLICATION

CLINICAL PROBLEMS	CRITICAL THINKING OPTIONS
Client experiences difficulty and cannot continue with lipid infusion.	• Reassess client's ability to tolerate fat solution. • Notify physician for order to discontinue fat solution, and administer hyperalimentation solution. • Observe liver function tests.
Client develops dyspnea, cyanosis, or allergic reaction, such as nausea, vomiting, increased temperature, or headache.	• Stop infusion immediately, and notify physician.
Client's serum triglyceride and liver function tests remain elevated.	• Attach the IV tubing to the Luer adapter. • Hang the solution bottle on an IV standard as you would an IV bottle. • Begin the feeding with a weaker concentration of formula, and increase the concentration slowly as ordered.
Client develops hyperlipemia or hypercoagulability.	• Monitor laboratory results, particularly liver function tests, and notify physician when any abnormality occurs.

unit 4

TUNNELED VENOUS ACCESS DEVICES (VADS)

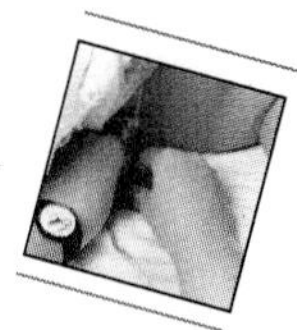

NURSING PROCESS DATA

ASSESSMENT Data Base

Assess patency of catheter.

Assess insertion site for signs of infection.

Assess the tubing for accidental breaks.

Assess injection cap at the end of catheter to ensure tightness.

PLANNING Objectives

To provide a patent catheter

To clear a nonpatent catheter

To provide an access for blood drawing

To provide an access for chemotherapeutic infusions

To provide total parenteral nutrition

IMPLEMENTATION Procedures

Maintaining the Hickman or Broviac CV Catheter

Changing the Hickman or Broviac CV Catheter Dressing

Drawing Blood from a Hickman or Broviac Catheter

Maintaining the Groshong CV Catheter

Changing the Groshong CV Catheter Dressing

Drawing Blood from the Groshong CV Catheter

EVALUATION Expected Outcomes

The catheter remains patent.

The catheter site is infection-free.

Blood samples are obtained without difficulty.

Infusions of medications or fluids are accomplished without difficulty.

MAINTAINING THE HICKMAN OR BROVIAC CV CATHETER

Equipment

Syringe with needleless cannula with 3-mL heparin 100 U/mL solution

Povidone-iodine swab

Clean gloves

Three tuberculin syringes

10-mL syringe

Preparation

1. Check client care plan.
2. Prepare syringe with dilute heparin.
3. Explain procedure to client.
4. Provide privacy for client.

Procedure

for Flushing Intermittently Used Line

1. Wipe catheter cap with povidone-iodine.
2. Insert syringe cannula into needleless access cap and unsnap catheter squeeze clamp.
3. Inject heparin solution slowly through catheter until almost empty.
4. Clamp catheter squeeze clamp as plunger is moving forward. **Rationale:** This promotes positive pressure

VENOUS ACCESS DEVICES (VADS)

- Venous access devices (VADs) provide long-term access to a central vein for the purpose of drawing blood, administering drugs (chemotherapy, antibiotics), administering total parenteral nutrition (TPN), or administering blood and blood products.
- Long-term catheters have one, two, or three lumens.
- They are inserted into the subclavian or external jugular vein.
- Three common tunneled central VADs are the Hickman, Broviac, and Groshong.
- Clients with tunneled VADs are advised to display medical-alert information.

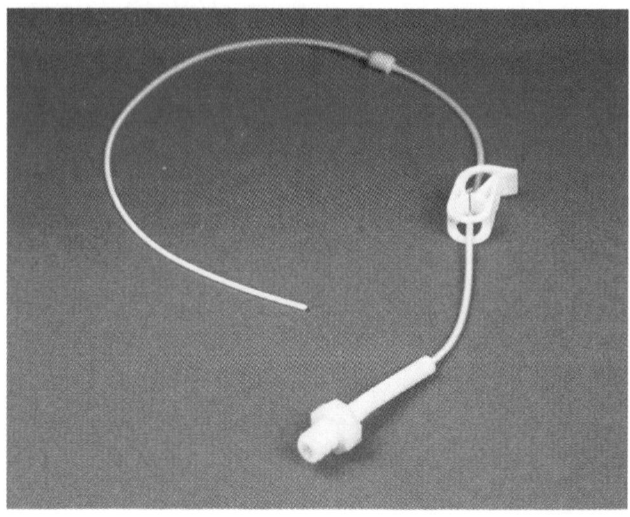

The Broviac catheter, single, double or triple lumen, is the most common catheter used for children.

in catheter and prevents clotting by preventing backflow of blood into catheter.

5. Withdraw syringe.
6. Flush nonused capped lines daily.

for Irrigating a Nonpatent Catheter

1. Prepare three tuberculin syringes with heparin. **Rationale:** The size of this syringe increases pressure exerted in the system.
2. Swab catheter cap with povidone-iodine.
3. Insert syringe with needleless cannula, and unclamp catheter.
4. Inject heparin from syringes, to a total of 3 mL.
5. Leave heparin in catheter tubing for 1 hour.
6. Check that hour is completed, then use a 10-mL syringe to aspirate solution from catheter by gently pulling back on plunger.
7. Follow with an irrigation of 5–10 mL of heparinized solution if aspiration is successful. Use same dilution factor (100 u/mL) for irrigation solution as with maintenance solution.
8. Repeat procedure once. If unsuccessful, notify physician.

CHANGING THE HICKMAN OR BROVIAC CV CATHETER DRESSING

Equipment

Povidone-iodine (Betadine) ointment or antimicrobial ointment
Alcohol swab
Cleansing solution (e.g., Betadine solution)
2×2 sterile dressings, or transparent, semipermeable dressing
Nonallergic tape
Sterile cotton-tipped swabs
Clean gloves
Sterile gloves

Procedure

1. Wash hands, and don gloves.
2. Remove old dressing.

CLINICAL ALERT

Never use scissors near central venous catheters.

3. Observe for signs and symptoms of infection and crepitus at insertion site. **Rationale:** Signs most frequently observed are erythema, edema, and drainage for infection; crackling under the skin denotes crepitus.
4. Discard dressing and gloves.

5. Set up supplies on a sterile field.
6. Don sterile gloves.
7. Clean exit site using povidone-iodine swabs (may use alcohol initially to remove exudate). Start from inner aspect, move out toward periphery approximately 1–2 inches from exit site. Do not go over same area twice. **Rationale:** This prevents contamination at the insertion site.
8. Clean catheter tubing starting from exit site down toward the cap.
9. Apply antibacterial or Betadine ointment around exit site.
10. Place sterile 2×2 gauze under catheter and over site, and tape occlusively. *Alternative:* Apply sterile transparent dressing.
11. Remove gloves, and discard.
12. Secure catheter to prevent dislodging; tape to chest. *Note: Nonhospitalized clients may protect exit site with a Band-Aid or leave the site undressed. To prevent accidental dislodgement, the catheter should be taped to the chest.*

CLINICAL ALERT

The dressing should be changed daily when the client is immunosuppressed. Strict aseptic technique must be used.

DRAWING BLOOD FROM A CV CATHETER

Equipment

10-mL syringe filled with sterile normal saline
3-mL syringe with 3 mL of heparinized saline (100 u/mL heparin)
Two 10-mL syringes (or larger size if needed) with needleless cannula
Povidone-iodine swabs
Blood tubes appropriate for tests ordered
Clean gloves

Procedure

1. Wash hands, and don gloves.
2. Swab cap or hub with povidone-iodine and allow to dry.
3. Remove cap from catheter end, insert 10-mL syringe, and unclamp catheter. *Alternative:* Use syringe with needleless cannula.
4. Slowly withdraw 6 mL of blood from catheter, and clamp catheter.
5. Discard syringe in appropriate place. **Rationale:** This prevents contamination of blood sample with heparin.
6. Attach 10-mL syringe to catheter, and withdraw required amount of blood for laboratory tests. **Rationale:** Each laboratory test requires a specific number of milliliters of blood for test. Check laboratory manual for exact amount needed for each test.

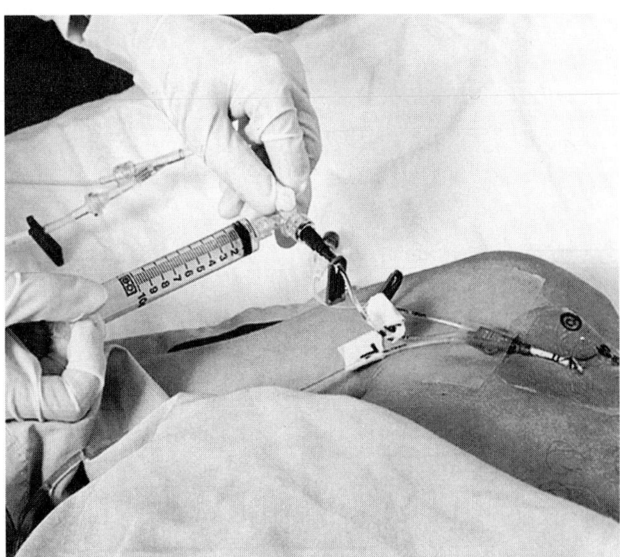

Stopcock may be used when withdrawing blood.

7. Clamp catheter, and withdraw syringe. Inject blood into laboratory blood tubes by taking cap off tubes and gently filling the tubes with blood. **Rationale:** Blood cells are easily damaged if put through needles into laboratory tubes, which causes hemolysis and abnormal laboratory results.
8. Attach saline syringe, unclamp catheter.

9. Flush the line with 10 mL of saline, clamp catheter, and remove syringe.
10. Attach 3-mL syringe filled with heparin solution into catheter.
11. Unclamp catheter, and gently infuse solution.
12. Clamp catheter according to procedure, and withdraw syringe.
13. Replace cap at end of catheter.
14. Secure catheter.
15. Remove gloves, and wash hands.

CLINICAL ALERT

Heparin, used as a flushing solution for IV lines, central venous catheters, and subcutaneous ports, may cause serious side effects: thrombocytopenia, abnormal clotting, and severe bleeding. Any client at risk for bleeding who is receiving frequent heparin flushes should have PTT times checked frequently and consistently. The *Groshong CV* catheter is irrigated with saline, thus preventing bleeding complications.

Heparinizing Central Venous Catheters (CVCs)

Amount of Heparin used for flushing

Equal to two times the filling volume of catheter—usually 3 mL (each lumen of triple-lumen catheter); implanted ports—5 mL.

Concentration 10 U/mL to 100 U/mL (high enough to prevent blood clotting in lumen without increasing client's PT).

Frequency of irrigating

Triple-lumen short-term—every 12 hours to once a day.

Long-term CVCs—daily to once a week (more recent practice).

Implanted ports—once every 4 weeks.

Flushing after infusions

Flush and heparinize all CVCs.

Exception—Groshong catheter does not require heparinization.

Changing injection cap

Change once or twice a week.

Cleanse catheter hub and cap with povidone-iodine, allow to dry, then wipe with alcohol.

Clamp catheter and change cap.

MAINTAINING THE GROSHONG CV CATHETER

Equipment

Normal saline
Alcohol or povidone-iodine swab
Needleless cannula
Appropriate syringe: 5 mL, 10 mL, or 20 mL
Clean gloves
Sterile gloves

Recommendations for Irrigating the Groshong CV Catheter

Using 5 mL of Saline

- Irrigate catheter every 7 days when not in use.
- Irrigate catheter after every use.

Using 10 mL of Saline

- Irrigate catheter after any aspiration, infusion, or transfusion of blood or when blood is seen in the catheter.

Using 20 mL of Saline

- Irrigate catheter after the infusion of TPN or hyperalimentation solutions and just prior to taking blood sample.

Note: Regardless of the volume of saline used, ALWAYS irrigate in a VIGOROUS manner.

Preparation

1. Check physician's orders and client care plan.
2. Gather equipment.
3. Wash hands, and don gloves.

Procedure

for 5-mL Irrigation

1. Wipe top of Luer-Lok injection cap with alcohol or povidone-iodine swab. DO NOT LET GO of cap. **Rationale:** This helps to maintain asepsis of injection cap.
2. Insert needleless cannula of syringe into cap.
3. Inject 5 mL of normal saline rapidly into lumen.
4. Maintain positive pressure on syringe plunger as syringe is withdrawn following injection. **Rationale:** Keeping pressure on the plunger does not permit irrigation solution to push back into syringe.
5. Check to see if injection cap needs to be changed. Recommended times for change: every 7 days; when cap has been removed (irrigation and blood sampling procedures); p.r.n.
6. Remove cap by holding catheter connector between thumb and forefinger of one hand and grasping barrel of cap with other hand.
7. Twist and pull counterclockwise to separate cap from connector.
8. Continue to hold connector with one hand. **Rationale:** Holding connector avoids inadvertent contamination by placing connector on dirty surface.
9. Discard old cap.
10. Clean liberally around connector using alcohol or povidone-iodine wipe.

TABLE 28–2. Flushing Intervals for Vascular Access Devices

Device	Flushing Solution/Amount	Flushing Schedule
Hickman or Broviac	3 mL heparinized saline	After each use or daily
Groshong	5 mL normal saline	After each use or weekly
Implanted Port	5 mL heparinized saline	After each use or every 4 weeks
PICC	2 mL or 3 mL heparinized saline	After each use or daily
	10 mL normal saline	After blood sampling

11. Twist and insert into connector clockwise while holding new injection cap by the barrel.

for 10- or 20-mL Irrigation

1. Remove needle from syringe.
2. Remove injection cap carefully from connector and discard.
3. Clean connector with alcohol or povidone-iodine wipe. DO NOT allow alcohol to enter connector, and DO NOT let go of connector. **Rationale:** Holding connector prevents inadvertent contamination.
4. Insert syringe barrel directly into catheter connector, twisting slightly to ensure good connection.
5. Irrigate lumen vigorously (Table 28–2).
6. Maintain positive pressure on syringe barrel as syringe is removed from connector. DO NOT clamp the catheter following irrigation. **Rationale:** The Groshong CV catheter does not require clamping to keep blood from entering the lumen. Clamping the catheter damages it.
7. Change injection cap as discussed under the 5-mL irrigation procedure.

CHANGING THE GROSHONG CV CATHETER DRESSING

Equipment

Povidone-iodine (Betadine) ointment or other antibiotic ointment
Alcohol wipe
Cleansing solution (e.g., Betadine)
Sterile transparent semi-permeable dressing
Nonallergic tape
Sterile cotton-tipped swabs
Clean gloves

Procedure

1. Don gloves, and remove old dressing.
2. Follow routine dressing change procedure. See *Changing the Hickman or Broviac CV Catheter Dressing*.

> **■ CLINICAL ALERT**
>
> Nursing attention to catheter during dressing change is important to ensure catheter is not pinched, kinked, occluded, cut, or dislodged. It is recommended that the external end of catheter be curved and then taped to avoid a straight pull on catheter.

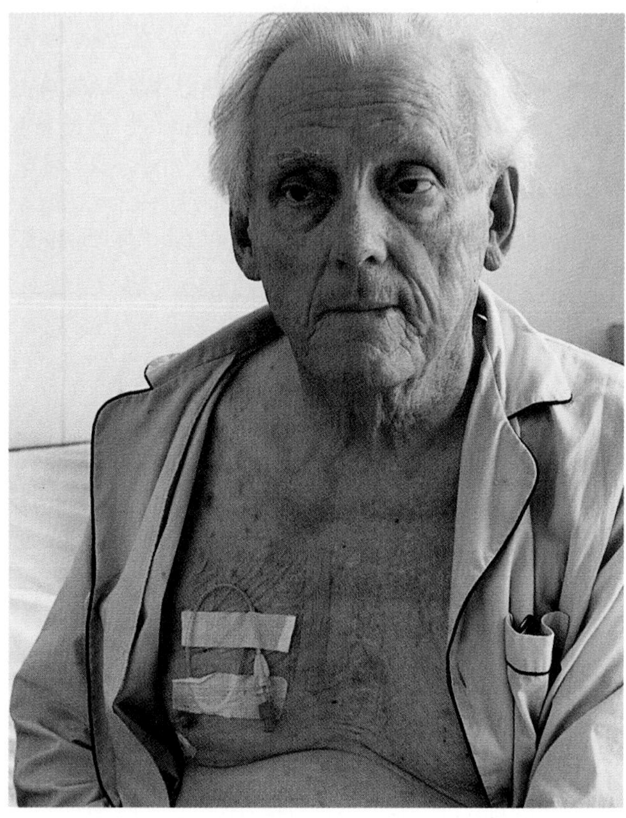

The Groshong is a tunneled CV catheter for long-term therapy.

DRAWING BLOOD FROM THE GROSHONG CV CATHETER

Equipment

Sterile heparin lock
Two 10-mL syringes for drawing blood
One 20-mL syringe, filled with normal saline
Blood tubes appropriate for tests ordered. *Note:* Vacuum tubes should not be used with the Groshong CV catheter
Alcohol or povidone-iodine
Clean gloves

Procedure

1. Don gloves, then remove and discard injection cap.
2. Clean outside of connector using alcohol wipe.
3. Continue to hold connector so that it does not make contact with any surface. DO NOT clamp connector. **Rationale:** Clamping might damage

catheter and is not necessary with the Groshong CV catheter.

4. Insert first 10-mL syringe directly into catheter, twisting slightly to ensure connection.
5. Pull back plunger 0.5 mL, pause 2 seconds, and then continue aspirating until 3–5 mL of blood and saline is in syringe.
6. Remove syringe, set aside; continue to hold connector.
7. Connect second 10-mL syringe directly to catheter connector, twisting slightly to ensure connection.
8. Proceed to aspirate blood volume needed for sample following same aspiration procedure of pulling 0.5 mL and waiting for 2 seconds.
9. Remove syringe, and continue to hold connector.
10. Proceed with irrigation procedure and attach new injection cap.
11. Place blood sample into appropriate tube(s), and label.
12. Discard first syringe containing blood and saline into specified container according to hospital policy.

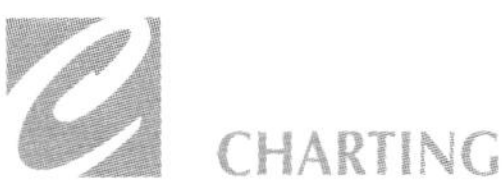

CHARTING

for Hickman Catheter

- Irrigation performed with heparinized solution
- Dressings changed with type of ointment applied
- Patency of catheter
- Amount of blood withdrawn for testing
- Color of blood withdrawn
- Exit site condition
- Any medications or solutions administered through the catheter

for Groshong CV Catheter

- Irrigation performed—include specific number of milliliters and if injection cap is changed
- Dressing changed—type of ointment applied
- Condition and patency of catheter
- Amount of blood withdrawn and label
- Exit site condition
- Any medications or solutions administered

CRITICAL THINKING APPLICATION

CLINICAL PROBLEMS	CRITICAL THINKING OPTIONS
CV Catheter:	
Unable to aspirate blood even though solution flows through the catheter.	• Use less pressure on barrel of syringe when aspirating blood. Tip of catheter is probably lodged against wall of right atrium. • Have client raise arms above head. This can alter position of catheter. • Have client perform Valsalva's maneuver. • Change client's position.
Clotting of catheter occurs.	• Use irrigating procedure for catheter clotted only a brief time. Instill 1 mL of 1:1000 mL heparin solution followed by 1 mL normal saline. Allow 15 minutes of clamping to see if declotting occurs. You may need to repeat this procedure several times.
Hickman Catheter:	
Catheter breaks or is pierced by clamp.	• Clamp catheter proximal to break site, if necessary. • Obtain repair kit for catheter. • If kit not available, place 14-gauge blunt-ended needle or intracath into broken catheter. Tape securely.
Air enters catheter when cap is removed, or catheter becomes disconnected.	• Turn client on left side with head lower than rest of body. • Call physician immediately. • Instruct staff in proper methods of connecting or capping catheter.
Infection develops at the exit site.	• Catheter may have to be removed. (Always use sterile supplies and technique.)
Catheter is dislodged.	• Take x-ray to determine position of catheter.

CLINICAL PROBLEMS	CRITICAL THINKING OPTIONS
Groshong Catheter:	
Catheter or connector is damaged or connector appears worn.	• Obtain connector package with sleeve and stylet, package of sterile gloves and sterile scissors. Using sterile technique, cut catheter just below old connector. Place sleeve over catheter, insert connector firmly into lumen of catheter and then slide sleeve back towards connector hub, seating sleeve firmly against connector hub. • Remove stylet from connector, and discard. Irrigate catheter, and replace injection cap.

unit 5

IMPLANTED SUBCUTANEOUS INFUSION PORT

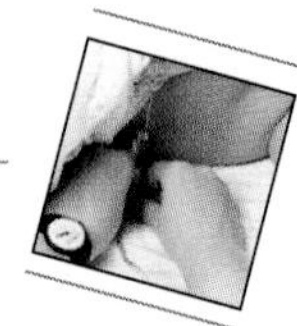

NURSING PROCESS DATA

ASSESSMENT Data Base

Assess site.

Assess patency of port.

PLANNING Objectives

To provide an access for blood drawing

To provide an access for blood or blood products administration

To provide an access for chemotherapy

To provide an access for IV drugs and solutions

IMPLEMENTATION Procedures

Accessing and Flushing an Implanted Infusion Port Using a Huber Needle

Administering IV Drugs via an Implanted Infusion Port

Administering Solutions or Drugs via Continuous Infusion

Drawing Blood from an Implanted Port

EVALUATION Expected Outcomes

Implantation site remains free from bruising, swelling, redness, or tenderness.

Port is easily accessible.

Infusions of drugs and fluids are accomplished without difficulty.

Blood samples are obtained without difficulty.

ACCESSING AND FLUSHING AN IMPLANTED INFUSION PORT USING A HUBER NEEDLE

Implanted venous access ports, such as Port-a-Cath or Medi-Port, are usually placed in the chest wall, require minimal maintenance, and may be used for months to years.

Equipment

Huber Needle

- This specially designed needle (usually bent at 90° angle) has a sharp-angled bevel and attached extension tubing with clamp and needleless cap.
- Prevents coring of the port.
- Produces straight-line tear that seals itself when needle is removed.
- Inserted through skin and rubber septum into reservoir.

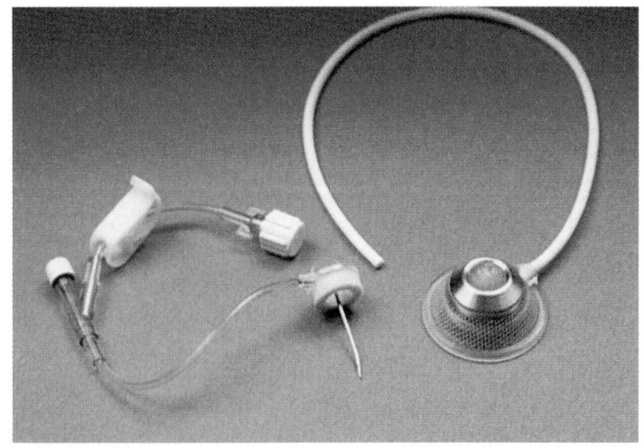

Example of Huber needle and stainless steel port which is surgically implanted under the skin.

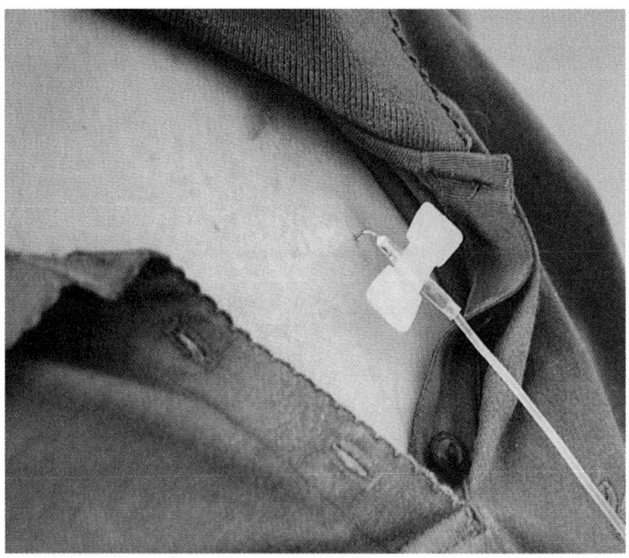

A non-coring, 90° angle Huber needle is used to access the implanted port.

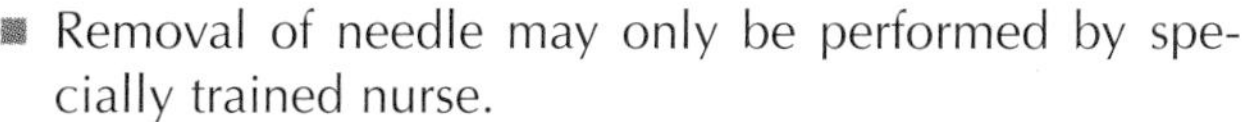

- Removal of needle may only be performed by specially trained nurse.

Huber needle with attached extension tubing or Luer-Lok extension tubing
Intermittent infusion (INT) cap
5-mL syringe with needleless cannula
10-mL syringe with needleless cannula
Povidone-iodine swabs
Sterile gloves
Mask
Normal saline
Heparin (100 U/mL, or 10 U/mL, varies with hospital policy)
Dry sterile swab

Preparation

1. Check physician's orders and client care plan.
2. Gather equipment.
3. Wash hands, using germicide solution.
4. Draw up 10 mL normal saline into 10-mL syringe.
5. Draw up 5 mL dilute heparin (100 U/mL) into 5-mL syringe.
6. Explain procedure to client.
7. Provide privacy.
8. Raise bed to working position.

Procedure

1. Don mask.
2. Palpate skin over subcutaneous infusion port.

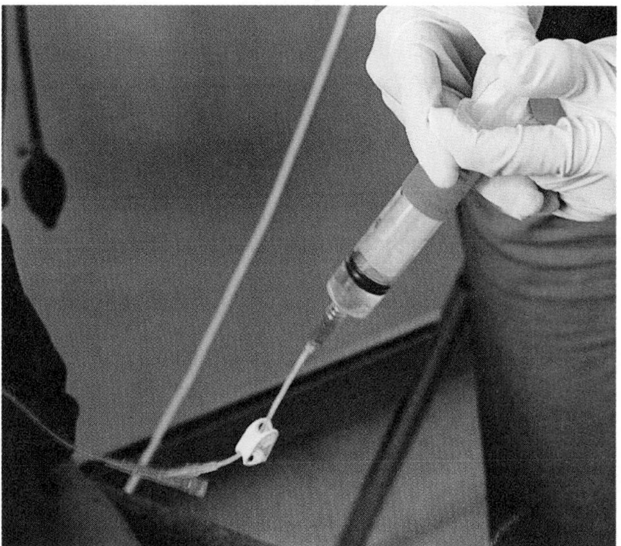

Hold syringe like a dart and, after aspirating, inject saline.

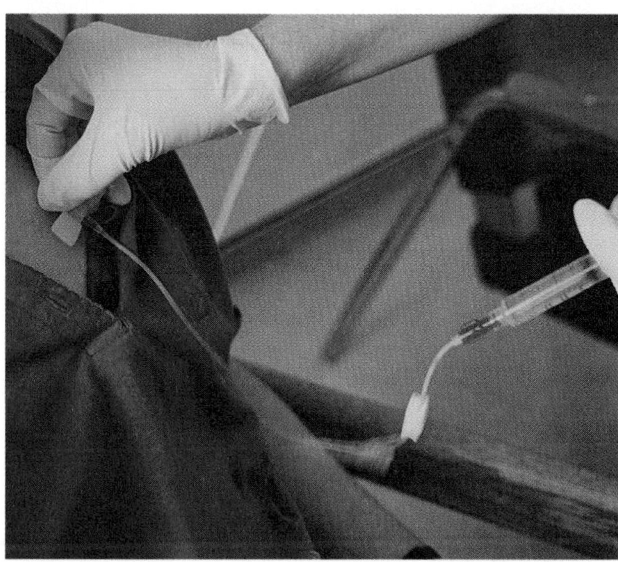

Inject last of herapin flush while maintaining pressure on port.

Rationale: This identifies location and contours of the device.

3. Place thumb and forefinger of left hand on port (right hand if left-handed) and feel for septum with right hand. **Rationale:** This position stabilizes the port.
4. Clean skin with povidone-iodine swab starting from center of septum, working outwards to a diameter of 3 inches. Use brisk circular movement.
5. Repeat twice or scrub for 3 minutes. Allow site to air dry. **Rationale:** Drying permits solution to work best against bacteria, fungi, and spores.
6. Don sterile gloves.

7. Affix Huber needle with extension tubing and syringe with 10 mL normal saline to the other end and prime tubing.
8. Stabilize port with free hand.
9. Hold syringe like a dart and insert needle down into port at a 90° angle.
10. Push needle into port until it hits bottom of port chamber.
11. Check for correct placement by aspirating for blood return. If placement is correct, inject priming solution of saline. **Rationale:** There should be no sign of infiltration into the tissue if placement is correct.
12. Close clamp of small extension tubing.
13. Exchange syringe of normal saline for syringe filled with heparin flush, then open clamp.
14. Instill entire volume of heparin flush except for 0.5 mL.
15. Inject remaining volume of flush (0.5 mL) simultaneously while removing needle from port and maintaining pressure on the port with free hand. **Rationale:** This prevents reflux and possible clotting in the catheter.
16. Remove Huber needle if ordered after flushing with 20 mL normal saline. While removing needle, apply pressure using 3-mL saline-filled syringe, and withdraw needle quickly. (Skill only to be done by specially trained nurse.)

> **CLINICAL ALERT**
>
> Flush system after every treatment. If the port is not used regularly, flush with 5 mL of heparinized saline (100 U/mL) once every 4 weeks if placed in a vein; flush once a week if placed in an artery.

17. Wipe skin gently with dry swab to remove any solution.
18. Dispose of equipment; remove gloves.
19. Wash hands.

ADMINISTERING IV DRUGS VIA AN IMPLANTED INFUSION PORT

Equipment

Syringe filled with medication
Equipment as listed in previous skill
10-mL syringe filled with saline
5-mL syringe with heparin flush solution, according to hospital policy

Procedure

1. Follow procedure listed in previous skill. (Using sterile gloves, access port verifying correct placement, i.e., blood return on aspiration, ability to infuse normal saline flush, and no infiltration.)
2. Clamp short IV extension tubing.
3. Exchange saline syringe for syringe filled with ordered medication.
4. Unclamp tubing.
5. Administer medication at prescribed rate.
6. Flush port between drugs with 5 mL of saline if giving more than one drug. **Rationale:** This prevents the possibility of drug-to-drug interactions.
7. Flush system with heparin flush after administration of drug(s).
8. Inject remaining 0.5 mL of heparin flush while simultaneously withdrawing needle and pressing down on port.
9. Wipe skin gently with dry swab to remove any solution.

ADMINISTERING SOLUTIONS OR DRUGS VIA CONTINUOUS INFUSION

Equipment

Right-angled Huber needle with short IV extension tubing with clamp
Locking cap for needleless access
Sterile towel
Sterile gloves
2×2 sterile gauze pad
Povidone-iodine swabs
Steri-strips

Semipermeable transparent dressing
10-mL syringe (needleless cannula) with NS
Syringe with heparin flush
Alcohol wipe
Ordered solutions, drugs, or blood products

Preparation

1. Check physician's orders and client care plan.
2. Gather equipment.
3. Wash hands.
4. Explain procedure to client.
5. Provide privacy.
6. Raise bed to good working position.

Procedure

1. Spread sterile towel, and place all equipment on field using sterile technique.
2. Cleanse skin with povidone-iodine. (Use cleansing method described previously.)
3. Don sterile gloves.
4. Attach saline-filled syringe to short extension tubing.
5. Flush tubing with saline to expel all air.
6. Clamp tubing.
7. Stabilize port with nondominant hand.
8. Insert right-angled Huber needle into skin and port septum using other hand.
9. Stabilize needle by exerting pressure against the angle. **Rationale:** Needle can rotate at the hub, which could traumatize either skin or port septum.
10. Assess needle placement.
11. Use normal saline flush.
12. Clamp extension tube, and secure Huber needle.
13. Secure needle hub by using Steri-strips. If right angle of needle does not lie just above skin's surface but protrudes 0.5 cm or greater above skin, secure the needle's position by placing folded sterile 2×2 under hub.
14. Apply antimicrobial ointment at insertion site (per agency policy).
15. Continue to secure rest of proximal portion of IV extension tubing.
16. Place transparent dressing over needle and proximal IV tubing.
17. Proceed with administration of ordered solution(s), drug(s), blood, or blood products.
18. Flush system with normal saline followed by dilute heparin after administration is complete.

If client is to receive a series of intermittent IV drugs or solutions, the Huber needle, if properly secured and dressed, may remain in place for 7–10 days. Convert end of IV extension tubing to "heparin lock" by inserting a male injection port into distal end. As discussed, the system should be flushed and heparinized at the end of each drug administration. Replace Huber needle weekly.

19. Check that system is secure.
20. Dispose of needles according to hospital policy.
21. Dispose of gloves and equipment.
22. Evaluate client following completion of procedure.

DRAWING BLOOD FROM AN IMPLANTED INFUSION PORT

Equipment

Huber 19-gauge needle with short extension tubing
Luer-Lok adapter with needleless injection cap
Vacutainer holder with needleless cannula
Vacutainer collection tubes (red and other colored tops as ordered)
Heparin and saline flush solutions
Povidone-iodine swabs
2×2 gauze pads and tape
Alcohol wipes
Sterile gloves

Procedure

1. Gather equipment.
2. Check physician's orders for type of blood test ordered.
3. Explain procedure to client.
4. Wash hands, and don sterile gloves.
5. Access implanted port using Huber needle with capped extension tubing as discussed previously.
   a. Clean tubing cap with alcohol wipes using circular motion from inside outward.
   b. Repeat cleaning with povidone-iodine.
   c. Wipe off excess with 2×2 gauze pad.
6. Insert vacutainer holder into tubing injection cap.
7. Unclamp tubing.

8. Fill red-topped or extra collection tube and discard. **Rationale:** This discards the filling volume of the catheter—studies show that about 5 mL of blood is enough to discard.
9. Fill remaining tubes according to blood tests ordered.
10. Remove vacutainer holder.
11. Clean the cap.
12. Flush catheter with normal saline after obtaining the necessary blood. If lumen is not to be used for an infusion, heparinize the catheter as discussed previously.
13. Discard equipment.
14. Remove gloves and wash hands.

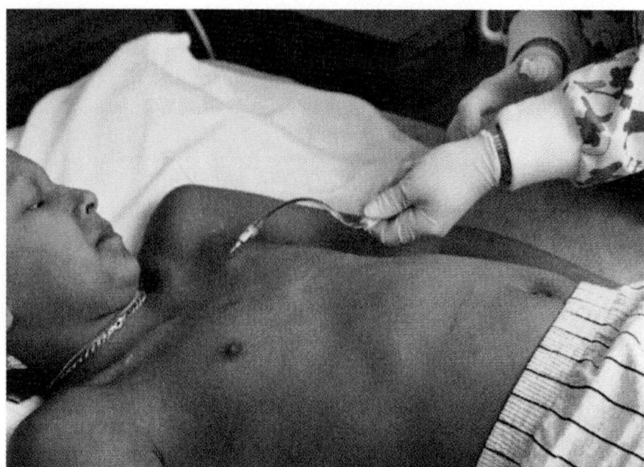

Blood is drawn from an implanted port by piercing the skin directly over the port.

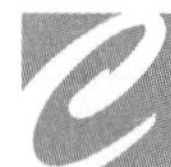

CHARTING for Subcutaneous Infusion Port

- Condition of implantation site
- Correct placement of port verified
- Port flushed with heparinized solution
- Amount and name of drugs or solutions administered via port or continuous infusion
- Presence of Huber needle, if left in place
- Dressing type
- Amount of blood withdrawn

CRITICAL THINKING APPLICATION

CLINICAL PROBLEMS	CRITICAL THINKING OPTIONS
■ Needle entry is painful.	• Use topical anesthetic or apply ice before accessing. • Use local anesthetic injected subcutaneously before inserting needle.
■ Occluded catheter due to: Packed red blood cell infusion.	• Transfuse packed red blood cells along with continuous infusion of normal saline; consider using an infusion pump; flush catheter well with NS between units.
Plugged needle.	• Change needle. If no improvement, suspect occluded catheter.
Occluded catheter.	• Use a large (35- to 50-mL) syringe half-filled with heparinized saline; gently aspirate, alternating with irrigation. If unsuccessful, fibrinolytic agents, such as streptokinase or urokinase, can be instilled into the catheter via a tuberculin syringe. Leave in place 10 minutes, then retry aspirating the clot. If still unsuccessful, retry procedure every 5 minutes, until clot is aspirated.
■ Inability to aspirate blood.	• Tip of catheter may be against vessel wall. Try changing client's position from sitting up to lying down or ask client to raise one or both arms. If appropriate, have client bear down or cough in Valsalva's maneuver while irrigating with normal saline. • Heparinize the catheter, and return in 40 minutes to aspirate. • Formation of a fibrin sleeve at the tip of catheter is another reason for inability to aspirate blood. If demonstrated during fluoroscopy, fibrin sleeve prohibits any further blood drawing and can't be dissolved. Do blood sampling in the conventional manner. • Needle may not be in port reservoir.
■ Pain, swelling at site.	• Suspect catheter rupture. Report to physician. Port misplaced due to client's habitual manipulation—"twiddler's syndrome." Report to physician.

unit 6

PERIPHERALLY INSERTED CENTRAL CATHETER (PICC)

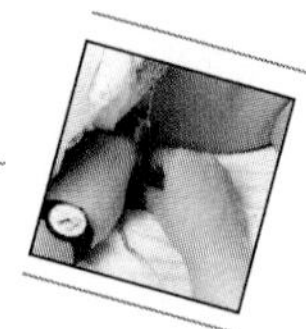

NURSING PROCESS DATA

ASSESSMENT Data Base

Assess length of exposed catheter.

Assess that catheter is secure.

Assess insertion site.

Assess catheter patency.

PLANNING Objectives

To provide access for infusion, hyperalimentation, or irritating drugs

To provide access for blood sampling

To provide catheter patency

IMPLEMENTATION Procedures

Maintaining the PICC

Changing the PICC Dressing

Drawing Blood form the PICC

EVALUATION Expected Outcomes

PICC remains patent.

Arm vein site remains free of infection.

Sterile technique is maintained when dressing change is completed.

Peripherally Inserted Central Catheter

PICCs are soft, flexible catheters placed in an arm vein by way of the antecubital space and advanced to a central vein—length of catheter is documented. (Central venous pressure measurement is possible with a PICC.) Placement is less invasive and costs less than other VADs. These catheters may be used for several months. Either saline *or* dilute heparin is used for maintenance.

MAINTAINING THE PICC

Equipment

Syringe with 10 mL normal saline *or*

Syringe with 2 mL dilute heparin (100 U/mL) solution (per hospital policy)

Clean gloves

Povidone-iodine swabs

Preparation

1. Check client care plan.
2. Explain procedure to client.
3. Provide privacy for client.

Procedure

1. Don gloves.
2. Withdraw irrigating solution into syringe.
3. Swab catheter port with povidone-iodine swab. Allow to dry.
4. Insert flush solution (heparin or saline) slowly through catheter until almost empty.
5. Use positive pressure on syringe plunger while removing from catheter port.
6. For intermittent use (e.g., intravenous piggyback [IVPB]).
   a. Flush catheter with 10 mL normal saline.

b. Administer infusion or medication.
c. Flush catheter with 10 mL normal saline.
d. Flush with 2 mL dilute heparin (per hospital policy).

7. Flush nonused catheter daily.
8. Place discarded equipment in appropriate receptacle. Place needle and syringe in sharps container.
9. Remove gloves and wash hands.

■ CLINICAL ALERT

Chemotherapeutic agents should be administered only by registered nurses who have been *educated specifically* to perform the procedure; nurses must also be IV certified.

CHANGING THE PICC DRESSING

Equipment

Sterile dressing kit that includes

Povidone-iodine (Betadine) ointment or antimicrobial ointment

Povidone-iodine swabs

2 × 2 sterile dressings or transparent semipermeable dressing

Tape or SteriStrips skin closure tape

Sterile gloves

Clean gloves

■ CLINICAL ALERT

Avoid blood pressure measurement in the arm with a PICC. Catheter damage may occur.

Procedure

1. Wash hands, and don clean gloves.
2. Very carefully remove old dressing. *Note*: The catheter is secured by tape only and is *not sutured*. Approximately 1 inch of catheter extends from the insertion site.
3. Note site for bleeding, signs of phlebitis, or pain. **Rationale:** Bleeding may occur with arm use. Phlebitis is the most common complication.
4. Discard old dressing and gloves.
5. Set up sterile equipment.
6. Don sterile gloves.
7. Clean exit site and catheter with povidone-iodone swabs or alcohol using circular movement from inner to outer edge three times with three swabs. Carefully stabilize catheter with nondominant gloved hand, if necessary. (Some facilities use

Carefully remove soiled dressing with clean gloves.

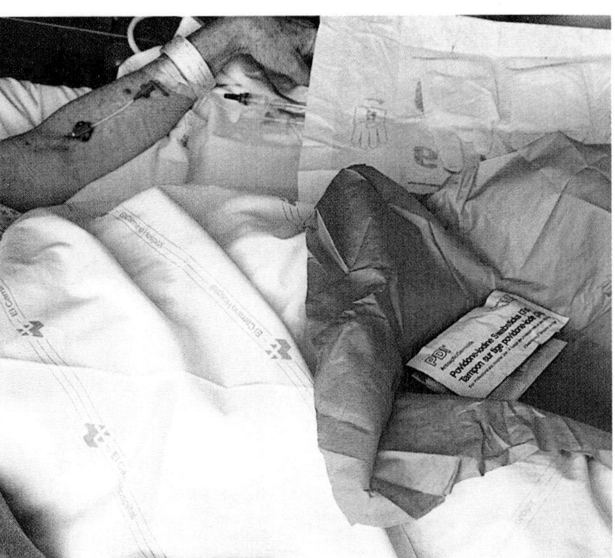

Set up sterile dressing pack and sterile gloves.

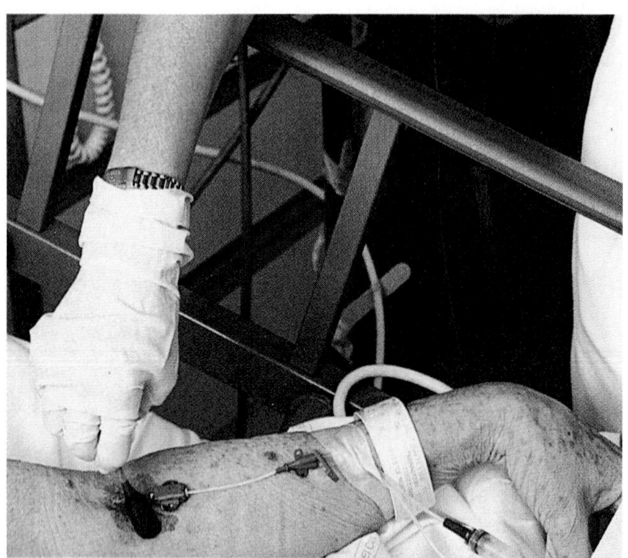

Cleanse exit site with povidone-iodine swabs three times.

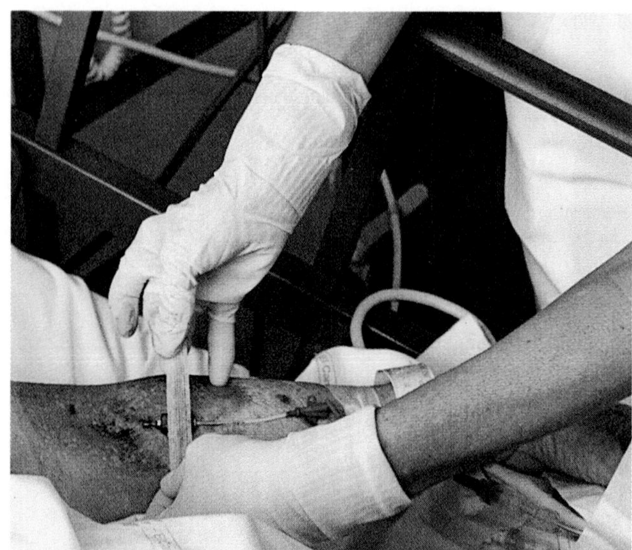

Apply tape on SteriStrips to catheter hub to stabilize.

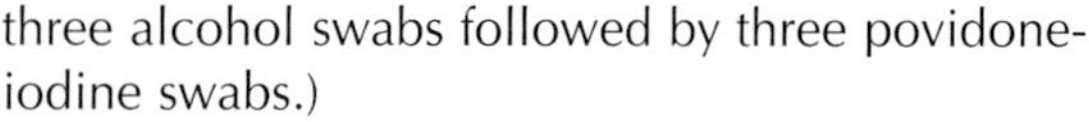

three alcohol swabs followed by three povidone-iodine swabs.)

8. Allow time for povidone-iodine to dry. Do not blow on arm or wave hand to hasten drying. **Rationale:** Waving hand or blowing may contaminate site—antibacterial action does not take effect until it is dry.
9. Apply antimicrobial ointment (only per hospital policy).
10. Apply SteriStrip to catheter hub to stabilize. **Rationale:** Catheter is not sutured so tape prevents dislodgement.
11. Cover exit site with transparent semipermeable dressing (e.g., OpSite 3000.). Alternatively, place sterile 2 × 2 dressing over exit site, and tape occlusively and securely.
12. Remove gloves, and discard.
13. Secure extension catheter to prevent dislodgement.
14. Change transparent dressing every 3 days or whenever soiled or loose, and change dry gauze dressing every other day.
15. Document dressing change and date.
16. Discard equipment, and wash hands.

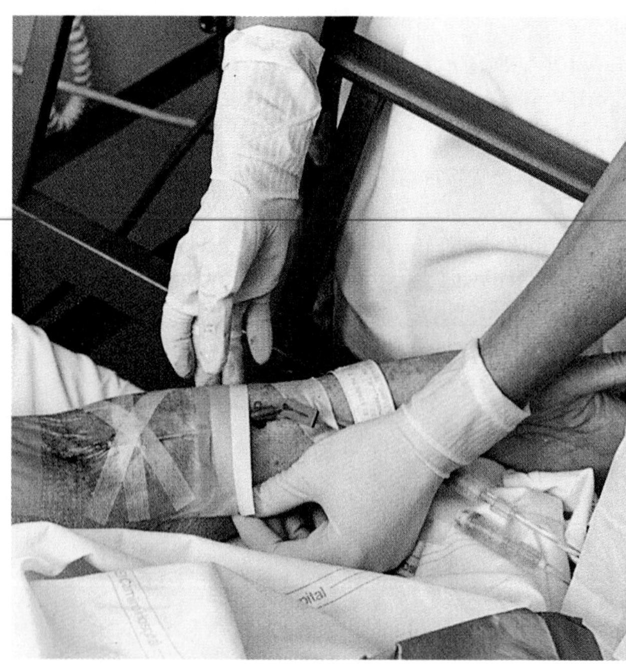

Cover exit site with transparent semipermeable dressing.

DRAWING BLOOD FROM THE PICC

Equipment

Povidone-iodine swabs

5-mL syringe with needleless cannula

10-mL syringe with needleless cannula for specimen

10-mL syringe with needleless cannula filled with saline

Syringe with 2 mL dilute heparin (per hospital policy) and needleless cannula

Clean gloves

Procedure

1. Wash hands, and don gloves.
2. Swab catheter cap with povidone-iodine, and allow to dry.
3. Using 5-mL syringe, withdraw 5 mL of blood and discard appropriately.
4. Using 10-mL syringe with needleless cannula, withdraw required amount of blood for laboratory tests.
5. Flush with 10 mL saline solution to clear catheter.
6. Complete procedure with 2 mL dilute heparin (per hospital policy).
7. Discard equipment and gloves; wash hands.

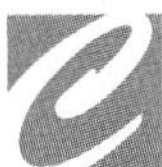

CHARTING for the PICC

- Flush performed (saline or heparin)
- Dressing applied
- Site assessment
- Length of exposed catheter
- Amount of blood withdrawn
- Solutions or drugs administered

CRITICAL THINKING APPLICATION

CLINICAL PROBLEMS	CRITICAL THINKING OPTIONS
Mechanical phlebitis—trauma to the endothelial lining of the vein. (Occurs 15% of the time within 1 week of insertion.)	• Apply warm, moist compresses for 20 minutes every hour throughout the day. • Elevate the arm. • If not resolved within 72 hours, catheter should be removed.
Bleeding occurs at insertion site.	• Apply direct pressure on insertion site, or apply a pressure dressing. • Check prothrombin time of client to check for coagulation problems.
Fluid does not infuse.	• Flush catheter if possible. • If unable to flush, attach a 3-mL saline-filled syringe, and gently pull back on syringe hub. • Request physician to declot catheter with urokinase.
Pain occurs during infusion.	• Pull catheter back 1–3 cm to move catheter from the vein wall or valve. • Slow rate of infusion. • Apply warm compresses to dilate lumen of vein.
Sepsis occurs.	• Monitor insertion site for drainage, fever, tenderness. • Obtain blood samples for culture. • PICC may be removed—send tip to laboratory for culture.

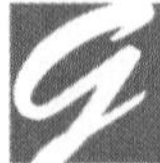

GERIATRIC CONSIDERATIONS

Elderly clients requiring chemotherapy or parenteral nutrition are good candidates for implanted vascular access devices.

- Decreased amounts of fluids can be administered to prevent fluid overload.
- Risk of infection is decreased, and in the elderly infection is a concern. Frequency and severity of infection tends to increase with age due to a decline in the immune response. T-cell (immune) function decreases with age and increases a person's likelihood of infection.
- Repeated IV punctures are not necessary so veins are preserved and discomfort minimized.
- Greater client mobility is achieved.

With aging epidermal turnover decreases and skin fragility increases. Even minimal trauma may result in serious erosion.

Health care providers or family members can be instructed to provide medication administration, fluid therapy, or parenteral nutrition at home.

Elderly clients, especially on anticoagulant therapy, should have a Groshong catheter inserted. It is the central venous catheter of choice because it does not require heparin for maintenance.

29

Orthopedic Measures

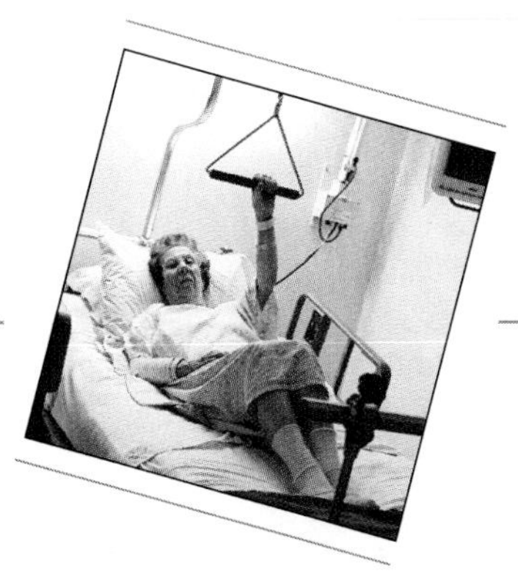

LEARNING OBJECTIVES

- Define the mnemonic ICE.
- Differentiate between four types of fractures.
- Compare and contrast skeletal and skin traction.
- Write three nursing diagnoses that would be appropriate for clients requiring special orthopedic procedures.
- Demonstrate the application of a circular and figure-eight bandage.
- Demonstrate the procedure of applying an air splint.
- Compare and contrast plaster and synthetic casts.
- Describe the steps in assessing a casted extremity.
- Complete a client teaching guide for clients requiring a synthetic cast.
- Outline the procedure for monitoring a client in traction.
- Discuss the nursing care necessary for clients in a halo traction.
- List the relevant charting data for halo traction.
- Explain the rationale for applying a shrink bandage to an amputated limb.
- Demonstrate the various bed positions for the Nelson bed.
- Demonstrate a client turn on a CircOlectric bed.
- State one potential problem of turning a client on a Stryker frame, and describe at least two suggested solutions.
- Discuss the nursing care for clients on special beds.

TERMINOLOGY

Abduction: movement of a bone away from the midline of the body or body part, as in raising the arm or spreading the fingers.

Adduction: movement of a bone toward the midline of the body or part.

Alignment: arranged in a straight line.

Ambulate: walking; able to walk.

Amputation: surgical removal of a diseased limb, part, or organ.

Bryant's traction: a type of skin traction used to treat small children with fractures of the femur.

Buck's traction: a type of skin traction used occasionally in the elderly client with a hip fracture prior to surgery.

Callus: localized hyperplasia of the horny layer of the epidermis usually due to pressure or friction.

Cardiovascular: pertaining to heart and blood vessels.

Circulation: movement in a circular course, as the movement of blood.

Comminuted: broken in pieces.

Contusion: soft tissue injury as a result of a blow.

Diaphysis: the part of the long bone between the ends, also known as the shaft.

Edema: a condition in which body tissues contain an excessive amount of fluid.

Embolus: a mass of undissolved matter present in a blood or lymphatic vessel brought there by the blood or lymph current.

Epiphysis: the end of a long bone.

Evisceration: protrusion of the viscera; removal of the viscera.

Extension: a movement that increases the angle between two bones, straightening a joint.

Fibroblasts: an immature fiber-producing cell of connective tissue.

Flexion: a movement that decreases the angle between two bones; the act of bending a joint.

Hyperextension: continuation of extension beyond the anatomic position, as in bending the head backward.

Metaphysis: wide part of bone at end of shaft adjacent to the epiphyseal disk.

Mobility: state or quality of being mobile; facility of movement.

Musculo: pertaining to muscles.

Musculoskeletal: pertaining to the muscles and bones.

Osteoblasts: immature cell, which on maturation plays a role in bone production.

Orthostatic: concerning an erect or standing position.

Orthostatic hypotension: low blood pressure in a standing or upright position.

Paralysis: temporary or permanent loss of function, especially loss of sensation or voluntary motion.

Paresthesis: pertains to an abnormal sensation.

Pearson attachment: an attachment to skeletal traction that allows continuous traction in line of the femur by the use of cords and weights.

Prosthesis: replacement of a missing part by an artificial substitute.

Restorative: promoting a return to health.

Russell's traction: type of skeletal traction to treat fractures of the shaft of the femur.

Sprain: injury caused by wrenching or twisting of a joint that results in tearing or stretching of the associated ligaments.

Strain: injury caused by excessive force or stretching of muscles or tendons around the joint.

Stryker frame: a special bed used to treat clients with spinal cord injuries.

Syncope: a transient loss of consciousness due to inadequate blood flow to the brain.

Thomas splint: skeletal traction used for long-term immobilization of fractures.

Torque: a rotary force.

Traction: process of drawing or pulling, often by weights, to keep the body or parts in proper alignment.

RESTORING FUNCTION

Orthopedic nursing involves the prevention and correction of alterations in the musculoskeletal system. To help clients achieve and maintain optimal mobility, nurses use preventative, restorative, and rehabilitative methods. Preventative and restorative measures include the use of bandages, splints, traction, and casts. Rehabilitative treatments include the use of special beds and halo traction.

The usual cause of injury to the musculoskeletal system is trauma from accidents. These accidents result in soft tissue injuries, fractures, and dislocations. Injuries occurring from falls in the home account for many admissions to health care facilities.

Sprains and strains are the two most common causes of musculoskeletal injuries. The usual treatment is application of a pressure bandage, elevation, and ice.

Bandages are used for applying pressure over an area; immobilizing a body part; preventing or reducing edema; correcting a deformity; and securing splints in place. Several types of material are used as bandages. Woven cotton, elastic webbing, and gauze are the most common materials.

When sprains, strains, contusions, or dislocations occur, remember the mnemonic ICE. "I" refers to immobilization, usually with a bandage or by splinting. "C" stands for application of cold treatments, such as ice packs. Cold is applied for 24–48 hours. "E" refers to elevation of the affected extremity. These initial interventions prevent edema formation and other complications.

Fractures

The long bone, the most common type involved in fractures, is composed of the shaft, or diaphysis, and the flared end of the bone, termed the metaphysis. In children the metaphysis is in two important segments: the physis, which is the growth region, and the epiphysis, which is directly adjacent to joints. The epiphysis fuses to the metaphysis at the end of the growth period. Injuries to long bones in childhood can result in growth retardation or arrest in the longitudinal growth of the limb.

When a bone is fractured, a specific repair process takes place, beginning with the formation of a blood clot at the site of the fracture. Once this clot is formed, osteoblasts and fibroblasts converge on the site and start laying down the organic matrix. Together, the fibrin net, the osteoblasts, and the organic matrix form a callus into which calcium salts are deposited. This callus evolves into regular bone tissue, which connects the pieces of original bone. In the final stage of the repair process, osteoblasts and osteoclasts remodel the callus area into a permanent and strong bone.

Fractures are classified in a variety of ways. One classification is by the type of injury to the bone or surrounding tissue. Examples of these fractures include a transverse fracture, which proceeds directly across the bone; an oblique fracture, which proceeds at an angle across the bone; and, a comminuted fracture, which results in more than two fragments of bone being displaced.

Fractures can also be classified as open or closed. An open fracture is one in which the skin has been broken due to penetration of a bone fragment or external trauma. An open fracture requires additional treatment to prevent infection as a result of the skin puncture. Surgical debridement and irrigation must be completed within hours of the fracture. A closed fracture indicates that the fracture is contained under the skin surface.

Soft tissue injury is also a probability with fractures. Immediate splinting and elevation of the extremity can prevent complications.

TYPES OF FRACTURE

Greenstick	A crack; the bending of a bone with incomplete fracture. Only affects one side of the periosteum. Common in skull fractures or in young children when bones are pliable.
Comminuted	Bone completely broken in a transverse, spiral, or oblique direction (indicates the direction of the fracture in relation to the long axis of the fracture bone). Bone broken into several fragments.
Open, or compound	Bone is exposed to the air through a break in the skin. Can be associated with soft tissue injury as well. Infection is common complication due to exposure to bacterial invasion.
Closed, or simple	Skin remains intact. Chances are greatly decreased for infection.
Compression	Frequently seen with vertebral fractures. Fractured bone has been compressed by other bones.
Complete	Bone is broken with a disruption of both sides of the periosteum.
Impacted	One part of fractured bone is driven into another.
Depressed fracture	Usually seen in skull or facial fractures. Bone or fragments of bone are driven inward.
Pathologic	Break caused by disease process.

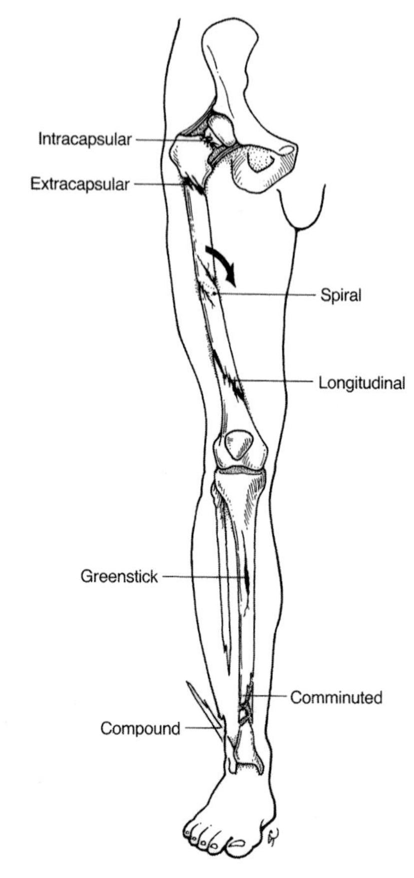

Types of fractures.

Fractures can be treated by manipulation or closed reduction. This results in manipulating broken bones to return to their normal anatomic position. Closed fractures are treated in this manner. Casts are generally applied to maintain the reduced fracture in proper alignment. Casts are made from plaster of Paris or synthetic materials, such as polyester, polyurethane, fiberglass, or plastic. The synthetic casts dry faster, weigh less, and can get wet without fear of cracking or disintegration. One major disadvantage of synthetic casts is their cost. Another disadvantage is their inability to mold easily, which prevents their use for immobilizing severely displaced bones or unstable fractures. Casted extremities need to be observed frequently during the drying process. When assessing the client in a cast, remember to check for *p*ulse distal to the cast, *p*ain, *p*allor, and *p*aresthesia (the four Ps).

Open reductions, the correction of bone alignment through a surgical incision, includes internal fixation of the fracture with rods, wires, screws, pins, or nails. External fixator apparatus is used to compress fracture fragments and immobilize reduced fractures. These are usually used when casts or traction are not appropriate. The fixator is attached to the bone by the use of percutaneous pins.

Traction

Traction is another method of treating fractures. It is most effective and useful when reduction of the bone fracture is required. Two types of traction are used: skin traction and skeletal traction. Skeletal traction is usually more reliable and effective because it maintains the reduction of the fractured limb. To provide the traction, a steel pin or wire is inserted through the distal fragment and attached to the traction apparatus. The affected limb is maintained in an elevated position, which decreases edema and promotes healing. The most common type of skeletal traction is the Thomas splint with Pearson attachment. Other types are Dunlop's traction, side-arm traction, and tongs, such as Crutchfield and Vinke.

Many types of skin traction are seen in hospital settings. The oldest and simplest type is Buck's traction. This type of traction is usually applied for short periods, 48–72 hours. Elderly clients may require Buck's traction prior to surgical repair for a fracture hip. Buck's traction is a boot with Velcro straps. Superficial peroneal nerve compression can result if the straps are too tight. Frequent release of the straps prevents this complication.

Bryant's traction, another type of skin traction, is used primarily for children under 3 years of age who have sustained a fractured femur. Neck halters and pelvic traction are also forms of skin traction. Neurovascular and skin complications can occur with each of these modalities of treatment; therefore, frequent observations by the nurse are required.

Clients who require the more sophisticated orthopedic procedures may be immobilized by the use of several pieces of equipment. The halo traction, the Jewett–Taylor brace, and the Stryker frame or kinetic therapy Rotorest bed are used to immobilize clients with spinal cord injury.

Clients with spinal cord injury are immobilized to prevent further complications and to promote healing. Cervical traction can be maintained most easily with the Stryker frame or Rotorest bed. Skeletal traction may be necessary and is applied by placing tongs through burr holes in the outer layer of the skull. Weights are applied to ropes connected to the tongs to provide constant hyperextension of the head.

Following surgical immobilization of the spinal cord with Harrington rods, clients are usually placed on the Stryker frame or Rotorest bed. Some clients may be placed in a regular hospital bed. When placed in the hospital bed, clients are turned in log-roll fashion to prevent torsion of the spine. Generally, a Jewett–Taylor brace is applied before getting the client out of bed. The brace maintains spinal cord alignment.

Halo traction is popular because this form of immobilization allows early mobility of clients. When the client is able to be up in the wheelchair, physical complications, such as pneumonia and circulatory impairment can be avoided. Some spinal cord fractures can be immobilized with the halo, but others require surgical intervention. Application of the halo follows surgery and functions as a stabilizing modality.

Special Beds

The Nelson bed is used when movement of a body part could result in a complication. Following total hip replacement surgery, clients are often placed in this bed to prevent hip flexion when getting out of bed.

The CircOlectric bed can be helpful in the treatment of immobility when the client requires turning and positioning. To facilitate positioning and dressing changes, burn clients are sometimes placed on these beds. This bed also provides optimal care for immobilized clients.

Clients on long-term bed rest are prone to the following complications: respiratory problems, especially pneumonia; thrombophlebitis or embolus due to stasis in circulation; muscle atrophy and contractures; skin breakdown; urinary retention and calculi; constipation; and altered body image. Nursing measures to prevent complications are a major factor in providing care for orthopedic clients.

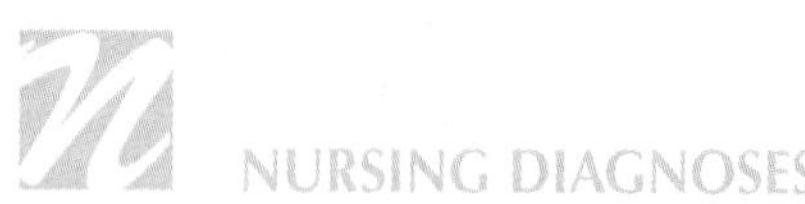

NURSING DIAGNOSES

The following nursing diagnoses may be appropriate to include in a client care plan when the components relate to a client who requires special orthopedic procedures.

NURSING DIAGNOSIS	RELATED FACTORS
Body Image Disturbance	Surgery, chronic illness, chronic pain.
Ineffective individual coping	Restriction in activity, ability to perform ADLs independently
Pain	Improper position or application of equipment (cast, sling, Stryker frame), surgical procedure, improper alignment, neurologic injury
Impaired Physical Mobility	Decreased motor function or interruption of central nervous system, physical injury, disease process (spinal cord injury or surgical intervention), joint contractures, inappropriate or inadequately performed range-of-motion exercises
Bathing/Hygiene Self-Care Deficit	Physical limitations, immobilized body or limb, pain, decreased strength and endurance
Impaired Skin Integrity	Pressure points, improper application of cast, sling, or traction, immobility, altered circulation
Social Isolation	Decreased opportunity for communication or interaction with peers, long-term confinement, limited physical ability, life style changes

unit 1

BANDAGE APPLICATION

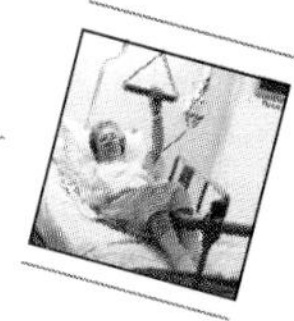

NURSING PROCESS DATA

ASSESSMENT Data Base

Assess need for bandages.

Identify appropriate type of bandage required.

Assess surrounding area of bandage to ensure it is not restrictive.

Evaluate bandage for tightness and evenness of pressure.

Evaluate the affected extremity for circulation, sensation, and movement.

Assess skin under bandage for abrasions, erythema, or discoloration.

PLANNING Objectives

To immobilize a joint or extremity

To provide support to an injured extremity or surgical site

To prevent edema to injured extremity

To secure a dressing in place

IMPLEMENTATION Procedures

Applying a Sling

Applying a Circular Bandage

Applying a Spiral Bandage

Applying a Figure-Eight Bandage

EVALUATION Expected Outcomes

Affected joint or extremity is immobilized.

Edema is decreased in affected extremity.

Dressings are held securely in place.

Skin remains free of complications.

APPLYING A SLING

Equipment

Sling or

Triangular bandage

Safety pin

Procedure

1. Check physician's orders for sling.
2. If commercial slings are not available, obtain a triangular cloth or bandage.
3. Explain use of sling to client.
4. Place one end of triangular cloth over the shoulder on the unaffected arm.

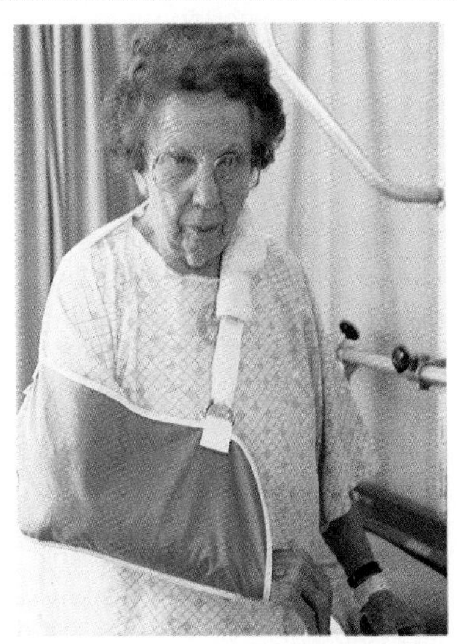

This commercial sling supports the arm and hand and immobilizes the shoulder.

5. Place cloth against the body and under the affected arm.
6. Place the apex, or point, of the triangle toward the elbow.
7. Bring the opposite end of the triangle around the affected arm and over the affected shoulder.
8. Tie the sling at the side of the neck.
9. Fold the apex of the triangle over the elbow in the front, and secure with a safety pin.
10. Assess client for comfort and for support of the affected arm.
11. Monitor for adequate circulation every 2 hours.

Note: If using commercial sling, check directions on package for proper application.

APPLYING A CIRCULAR BANDAGE

Equipment

Roller bandages
Metal clip or safety pin

Procedure

1. Gather necessary roller bandages. The number and size of the bandages depends on the extent and area of the extremity to be bandaged.
2. Explain the use of the bandage to the client.
3. Elevate the extremity. **Rationale:** This position prevents the bandage from becoming too tight after wrapping.
4. Begin to wrap the extremity at the distal end. Anchor the bandage with at least two circular turns. A moderate amount of tension should be maintained on the bandage during the application.
5. Continue to unroll the bandage and overlap the previous circle until the designated area is covered.
6. Secure the bandage with tape, safety pin, or metal clip.
7. Observe for even, tight fit of the bandage, and ensure the bandage is not occluding circulation. **Rationale:** Uneven wrapping can result in circulatory impairment and skin disruption.
8. Assess extremity every 2 hours for circulation, and ensure that the bandage is wrinkle-free.
9. Rewrap bandage at least every 8 hours.

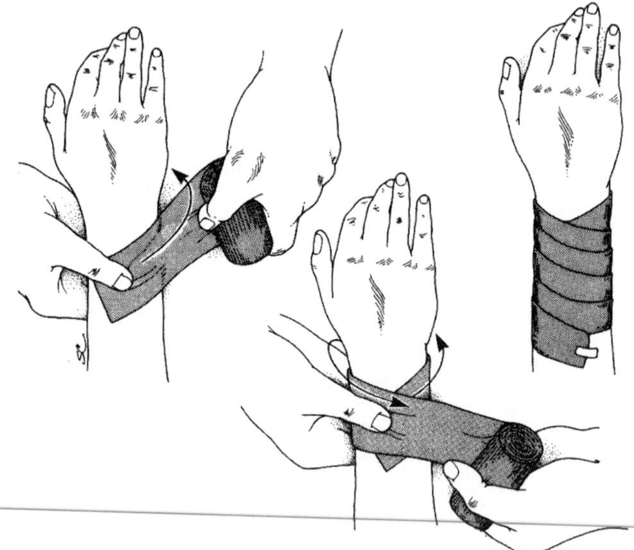

A circular turn is used for anchoring and securing a bandage.

APPLYING A SPIRAL BANDAGE

Equipment

Roller bandages
Metal clip or safety pin

Procedure

1. Gather necessary roller bandages.
2. Explain necessity for bandage to client.
3. Elevate the extremity to be bandaged.
4. Anchor the bandage with two circular turns at the distal end of the extremity.
5. After anchoring the bandage, begin the spiral turns by moving up the extremity on the first turn, then straight around the extremity toward the back and then down the extremity. Complete the turn by encircling extremity.

6. With each turn of the bandage, overlap the preceding turn by at least one-half the bandage width.
7. After wrapping the extremity, assess for adequate circulation, evenness of pressure, and comfort of client. **Rationale:** Uneven or too much pressure can impede circulation; therefore, pulses should be monitored.
8. Secure bandage with tape, safety pin, or metal clip.
9. Assess client for circulation, fit of bandage, and comfort every 2–4 hours.
10. Rewrap bandage every 8 hours.

APPLYING A FIGURE-EIGHT BANDAGE

Equipment

Roller bandage
Metal clip or safety pin

Procedure

1. Gather necessary bandages.
2. Explain necessity for bandage to client.
3. Anchor bandage around the distal end of the extremity using circular turns.

> ■ **CLINICAL ALERT**
>
> For all bandages assess extremity for circulation after the first 20 minutes and then every 2 hours. Ensure that the bandage is wrinkle-free. **Rationale:** Partial occlusion of the vessels can occur within 20 minutes of application.

4. Make a circular turn around the foot and ankle.
5. Make a spiral turn down over the ankle and around the foot.
6. Continue to make alternate turns around the ankle and foot. Overlap the preceding bandage by at least one-half or two-thirds of the bandage.
7. Wrap the entire area below and above the involved point. **Rationale:** This immobilizes the affected area.

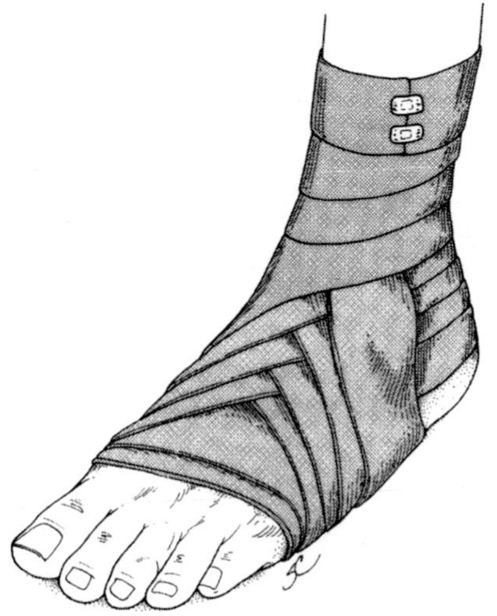

A figure-eight turn is used to support and limit joint movement.

8. Assess extremity for circulation and evenness of pressure as well as comfort of client.
9. Assess extremity at least every 4 hours, and rewrap every 8 hours.

Note: Edema can result if the heel is not enclosed within bandage. An alternative wrap is to enclose the heel as the bandage is being applied.

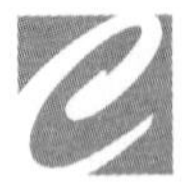

CHARTING for Bandage Application

- Type of bandage applied
- Condition of extremity following application, skin color, and temperature
- Note drainage, if any, from wound
- Effectiveness of bandage
- Client's tolerance of bandage

CRITICAL THINKING APPLICATION

CLINICAL PROBLEMS	CRITICAL THINKING OPTIONS
Affected joint or extremity is not immobilized with bandage.	• Assess if type of bandage is effective or if an alternative type of bandage would provide more support. • Assess the need for a possible cast or immobilizer in place of the bandage. • Evaluate if the bandage is applied tightly enough to immobilize the extremity.
Edema is noted in the area surrounding the bandage.	• Take bandage off, and check circulation and skin condition. • Keep extremity elevated. • Rewrap bandage after edema has subsided. • If edema persists, notify physician for orders.
Distal pulses are diminished or absent.	• Take off bandages immediately and reassess pulses. If pulses are present, rewrap bandage, keeping pressure even and bandage loose. • If pulses remain diminished or absent, notify physician immediately.

unit 2

SPLINTING A FRACTURE

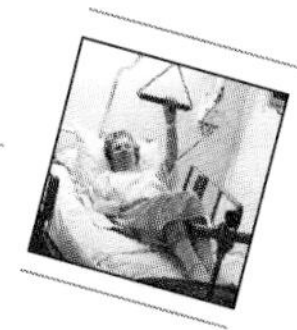

NURSING PROCESS DATA

ASSESSMENT Data Base

Note location of fracture.

Determine whether the fracture is open or closed.

Note presence and amount of hemorrhage.

Assess for deformities of fractured extremity.

Assess for signs of fat emboli.

- Classic sign: petechiae deposits across chest, shoulders, and axilla
- Pulmonary signs: dyspnea, pallor, cyanosis
- Cardiac signs: tachycardia, shock
- Neurologic signs: restlessness, change in level of consciousness, confusion

PLANNING Objectives

To immobilize a fractured limb and maintain good alignment
To minimize pain and injury to soft tissue
To prevent complications associated with a fracture (e.g., hemorrhage, edema, shock, emboli)
To monitor circulation and neurologic status of the affected extremity

IMPLEMENTATION Procedures

Applying a Splint
Applying an Air Splint

EVALUATION Expected Outcomes

Client experiences minimal pain and injury to soft tissues.

Complications associated with a fractured limb are minimized.

Circulation and neurologic status are maintained.

APPLYING A SPLINT

Equipment

Splint materials: pieces of wood or pillows, magazines, blankets

Padding materials: pieces of cloth or towels, blankets

Strapping materials: strips of cloth, rope, tape

Procedure

1. If the client's life is in danger, move the client to a safe place.
2. Control hemorrhage by applying direct pressure and by using pressure dressings.
3. Explain the rationale for the intervention to client.
4. Move the affected extremity as little as possible.
   a. Splint legs in an extended position.
   b. Splint arms in a flexed or extended position.
5. Pad joints, bony prominences, and skin areas as much as possible. **Rationale:** This prevents skin damage. Also make sure that the padding does not affect the client's circulation (e.g., don't put padding in the axilla).
6. If splint material is not available, use the client's body for support.
   a. Splint the legs together.
   b. Splint an arm to the torso.
   c. Splint toes or fingers together.
7. Reinforce soft splint materials (pillows, blankets)

■ CLINICAL ALERT

Splinting, using these materials, is usually done in a prehospital setting.

with something to make them firmer, such as magazines.

8. Strap the splint and extremity together tightly so that the extremity is immobile. Try to include the proximal and distal joints in the splint.
9. Check the client's circulation by assessing pulse, capillary refill, color, and temperature.
10. Arrange to transport client to medical facility as soon as possible.

APPLYING AN AIR SPLINT

Equipment

Appropriate size air splint
Dressings for wound if necessary

Procedure

1. Cover compound fracture with absorbent dressings.
2. Place air splint over fractured extremity. **Rationale:** This splint is used most often to splint the forearm or lower leg.
3. Inflate splint by blowing into mouth piece. Pressure should be about 30 mm Hg in the splint.
4. Check the tension in the splint. Press a finger into the splint; it should dimple to the depth of $\frac{1}{2}$ inch.

■ CLINICAL ALERT

Once inflated, do not deflate splint. Only physicians may deflate air splints.

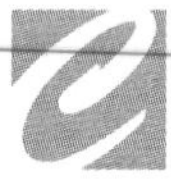

CHARTING for Splinting

- Location of the fracture
- Time splint applied
- Materials used in splinting
- Circulatory and neurologic status of the extremity
- Any change in client's condition
- Client's comfort and reactions to the fracture
- Presence and treatment of open wound

CRITICAL THINKING APPLICATION

CLINICAL PROBLEMS	CRITICAL THINKING OPTIONS
■ Client complains of pain or numbness in splinted extremity.	• Elevate extremity above level of heart to decrease edema. • Check for padding, straps, or splint material that is impinging on a major nerve or blood vessel. Correct the problem.
■ Extremity still moves in the splint.	• Apply more padding if possible. • Tighten straps slightly. Observe condition of client's extremity: color, temperature, and sensation.

unit 3

CAST CARE

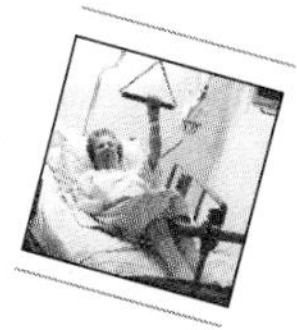

NURSING PROCESS DATA

ASSESSMENT Data Base

Identify type of cast applied.

Note condition for which the cast was applied.

Observe condition of the cast.

Assess for neurovascular complications.

PLANNING Objectives

To increase the client's level of activity after injury or disease

To maintain normal sensation, movement, and circulation in a casted extremity

To improve muscle tone and joint flexibility

To strengthen muscles weakened by immobility, trauma, or surgery

To increase client's psychologic sense of freedom

IMPLEMENTATION Procedures

Caring for a Wet Cast

Assessing a Casted Extremity

Instructing in Care of a Synthetic Cast

EVALUATION Expected Outcomes

Complications are prevented during the casting procedure.

Cast dries without cracking or indentation areas on the cast.

The client experiences minimal discomfort from pain or swelling.

TABLE 29–1. Comparison of Casts

	Plaster	Synthetic
Material	Plaster of Paris, comprised of powdered calcium sulfate crystals impregnated into the bandages	Polyester and cotton, fiberglass or plastic. Polyester and cotton is impregnated with water-activated polyurethane resin.
Drying time	24–48 hours No weight bearing until dried	7–15 minutes for setting 15–30 minutes for weight bearing
Advantages	Less costly More effective for immobilizing severely displaced bones Smooth surface Doesn't require expensive equipment for application	Less likely to indent into skin Lighter in weight Less restrictive Doesn't crumble Nonabsorbent; can be immersed in water

CARING FOR A WET CAST

Equipment

Bedboard
Pillows covered with plastic

Procedure

1. Explain to the client that the cast feels warm as the plaster dries.
2. Use ONLY the palms of your hands on the cast when turning and positioning for the first 24 hours. **Rationale:** Fingers can cause dents in the cast, which may create pressure areas on the inside of the cast.
3. Support the cast with pillows as necessary.
    a. Keep the casted extremity above the level of the heart. **Rationale:** This position decreases venous pooling and edema.
    b. Maintain the angles that were built into the cast.
    c. Prevent cracking from undue pressure.
    d. Prevent flat spots in the cast caused by pressure on the bed. For example, when the client has a long leg cast, place pillows under knees to maintain the angle of the cast and under lower leg to prevent pressure and flattening of heel area.

■ **CLINICAL ALERT**

If client is wearing a spica or body cast, place a bedboard under the mattress to provide firm support.

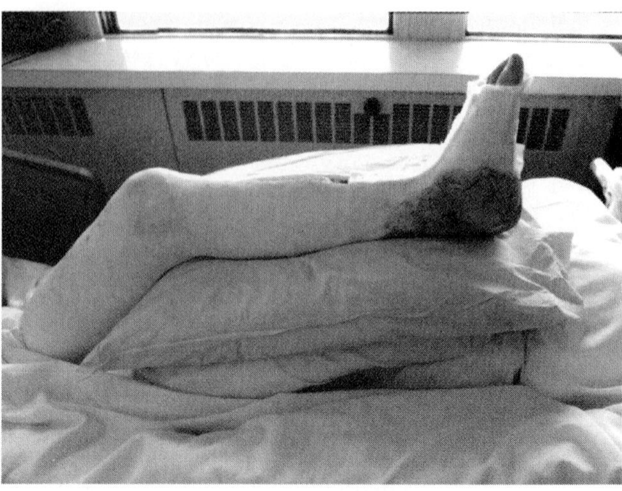

Position casted extremity above level of heart to prevent edema.

4. Keep the cast uncovered. **Rationale:** This allows heat and moisture to dissipate and air to circulate.
5. If the cast is near the client's groin, protect this area with plastic to avoid soiling the edges of the cast.
6. If edges of cast are rough or crumbling, pull stockinette over edge of cast and tape down.
7. Turn client according to facility policy. **Rationale:** Turning promotes even drying of cast.

■ **CLINICAL ALERT**

Cast is dry when dampness is gone and cast is white and shiny. When tapped, a resonant sound is heard.

ASSESSING A CASTED EXTREMITY

Equipment

Pen to mark drainage on cast

Procedure

1. Explain the rationale for the procedure to the client.
2. Encourage the client to notify you of any unusual sensations or changes in sensations in the casted extremity.
3. Check the client's fingers or toes to make sure they are pink in color.
4. Feel the client's fingers or toes to make sure they are warm.
5. Ask what the client feels when you touch his or her toes. The client should have normal sensation and be able to identify which digit you are touching. He or she should not have a "pins-and-needles" sensation. **Rationale:** Changes in color, temperature, and sensation indicate inadequate blood supply or nerve damage.
6. Assess for capillary refill by applying pressure to

one of the client's toenails or fingernails. After you stop the pressure, observe the nail to see how rapidly the color returns. **Rationale:** Comparing one of your nails to the client's nail is a check on how quickly color should return.

7. Ask the client to move the fingers or toes that are affected by the cast. The client should be able to move them without difficulty.
8. Ask the client to identify the exact location of any pain. Assess for adequate blood supply or nerve paralysis.

> **■ CLINICAL ALERT**
>
> Casted extremity should be assessed every $\frac{1}{2}$ hour for 2 hours, then every hour for 24 hours, then every 4 hours for 48 hours.

9. Check for any drainage from a wound under the cast. Note the color and amount of drainage.
10. Report any unusual odor or increase in drainage.

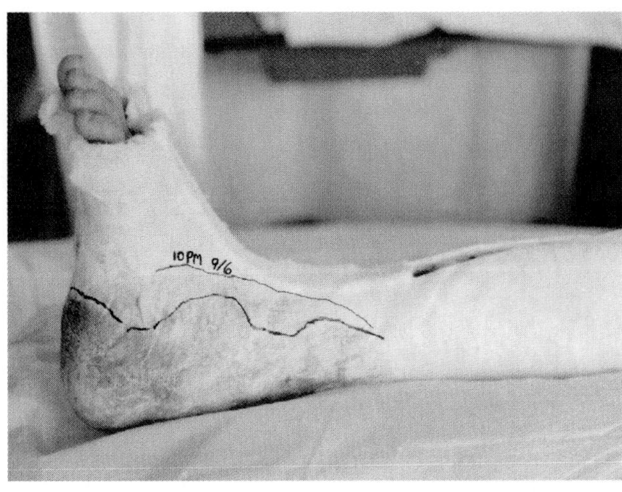

Observe casted extremity frequently for signs of drainage.

INSTRUCTING IN CARE OF A SYNTHETIC CAST

Equipment

Pamphlet on cast care

Procedure

1. Explain necessity for neurovascular check.
   a. Check temperature, color, and blanching of extremity.
   b. Observe for edema, numbness, or tingling sensations.
2. Check cast daily for
   a. Odor or drainage
   b. Cracks or position change
3. Instruct client to avoid overly rigorous activities. **Rationale:** This prevents dislodging or malaligning of the fracture.
4. Instruct in bathing procedures when cast can be wet.
   a. Use only mild soap and water when bathing.
   b. Avoid getting soap on cast.
   c. Flush cast with water following bathing. **Rationale:** This prevents skin irritation and maceration from soap.
   d. Place nonslip mat on floor to prevent slipping when getting out of shower or tub.
5. Instruct on drying cast.
   a. Remove excess water by blotting with towel.
   b. Set blow dryer on cool setting and dry cast by moving dryer along all aspects of cast. **Rationale:** If cast remains wet the client will feel a cold, clammy sensation.
6. Explain necessity for keeping particles and dirt out of cast. Cast can be flushed with water to remove debris. Dry cast thoroughly.

CHARTING for Cast Care

- Type of cast applied
- Positioning of cast
- Client's complaints and nursing responses
- Color, warmth, movement, and sensation in casted extremity
- Presence, location, and amount of drainage from wound
- Client's acceptance of the cast

CRITICAL THINKING APPLICATION

CLINICAL PROBLEMS	CRITICAL THINKING OPTIONS
Client complains of numbness, discomfort, or pain.	• Notify physician immediately. • Reevaluate condition of casted extremity every 15 minutes. • Reassess circulation, movement, and sensation (CMS).
Cast cracks from improper drying procedure or stress.	• Notify physician immediately. • Reassure client. • Do not reposition client until physician assesses.
Synthetic cast has rough edges.	• Smooth edges by filing with nail file. • Make sure furniture and clothing are protected from scratches and snags by covering cast with a cloth.
Cast edges begin to crumble.	• "Petal" edges of cast with 1- to 2-inch strips of adhesive tape. • Place half of tape inside cast, pull tape over cast, and anchor on outside of cast. • Continue to petal cast until all edges are covered.

unit 4

TRACTION

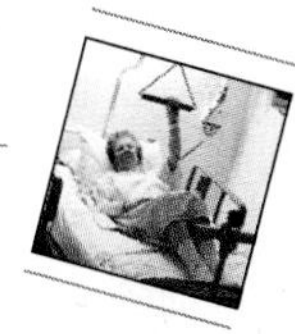

NURSING PROCESS DATA

ASSESSMENT Data Base

Determine type of traction used.

Note the amount of weight ordered.

Note any conditions requiring special treatment.

Assess for circulation, movement, and sensation of affected extremity.

PLANNING Objectives

To maintain correct alignment of bone ends

To prevent unnecessary injury to soft tissue

To prevent ischemia and necrosis, which can be caused by continued pressure on the soft tissues

IMPLEMENTATION Procedures

Monitoring Skin Traction

Monitoring Skeletal Traction

EVALUATION Expected Outcomes

Extremity is maintained in correct alignment.

Bone ends are approximated and do not override.

Skin of affected extremity remains intact.

Client maintains correct position while in bed.

MONITORING SKIN TRACTION

Procedure

1. Examine the material (tape, foam rubber, or plastic) that attaches the weights to the extremity.
   a. Material should be held firmly in place, not slipping.
   b. Material should fit comfortably, neither too loose nor too tight.
2. Examine all bony prominences of the involved extremity for abrasions or pressure areas.
   a. Traction should be removed at least every 8 hours.
   b. Wash, dry thoroughly, and powder skin before reapplying traction. Check hospital policy or physician orders regarding which skin traction can be removed by the nursing staff.
   c. Remove straps on Buck's traction every 4 hours to prevent compression of superficial peroneal nerve.

CLINICAL ALERT

It is best to have another nurse assist with traction removal. The second nurse maintains traction pull on the limb as the traction is slowly removed. This prevents muscle spasms. Reapply traction slowly. This consideration is for clients in pelvic, head halter, or Dunlop's traction.

3. Examine the extremity distal to the traction.
   a. Note any presence of edema.
   b. Take and record peripheral pulses.
   c. Check temperature and color to see if both are normal.
4. Observe for possible neurologic impediment from traction slings encroaching on popliteal space or axilla. **Rationale:** Numbness or tingling, if present, indicates neurologic problems have occurred.

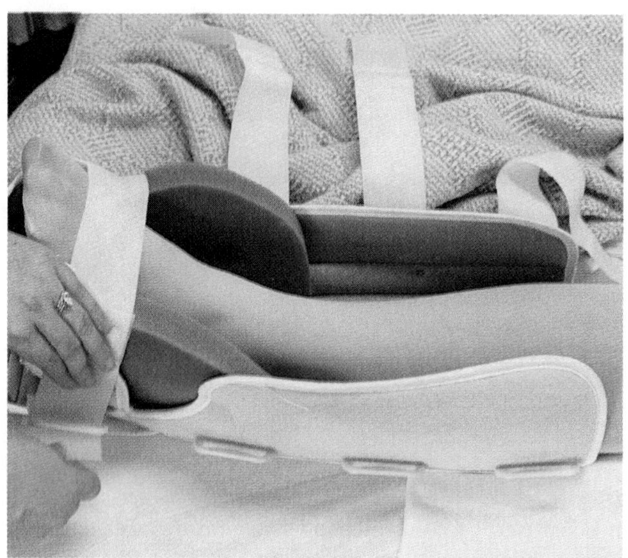

Remove straps on Buck's traction every four hours to prevent nerve compression.

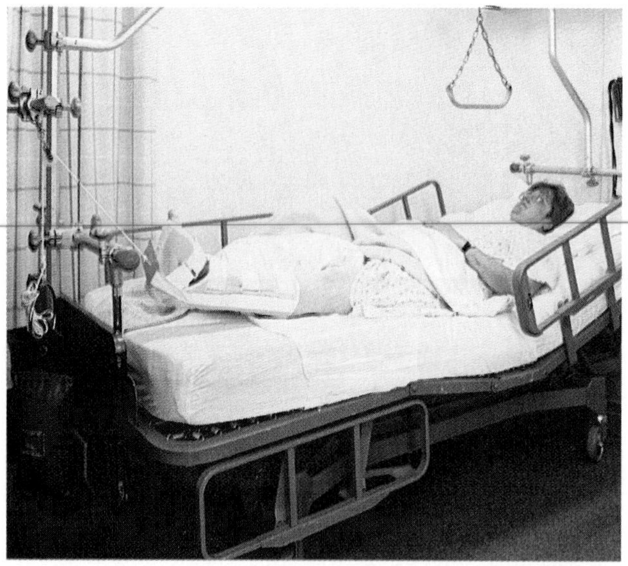

Ensure client is positioned correctly in bed to prevent complications.

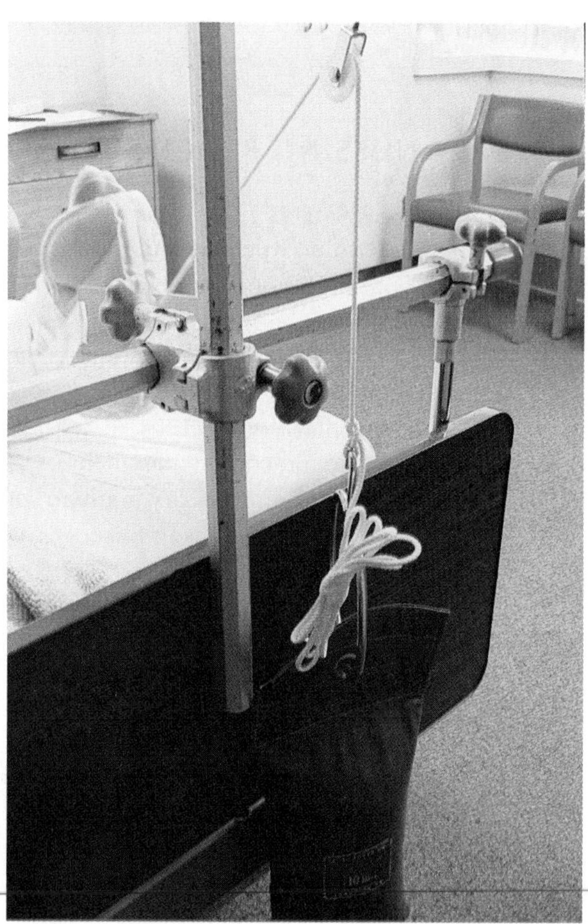

Maintain traction pull by ensuring weights hang freely.

5. Ask the client to move the extremity that is distal to the traction.
   a. Note if full range of motion is present.
   b. Ask the client if he or she has any decreased or unusual sensations.
6. Examine the rope and weights to see that the pull goes directly through the long axis of the fractured bone.
7. Check the traction mechanism.
   a. Weights should hang freely, off the floor and bed.

PRINCIPLES OF TRACTION MAINTENANCE

- Maintain traction pull by ensuring weights are hanging freely.
- Maintain ropes in pulley system and ensure rope moves freely through system and knots do not interfere with movement.
- Maintain countetraction, keep client aligned in center of bed.
- Maintain traction either continuous or intermittent, according to physician's orders.

   b. Weights are 5–10 pounds for adult clients.
   c. Knots should be secure in all ropes.
   d. Ropes should move freely through pulleys.
   e. Pulleys should not be constrained by knots.

TABLE 29–2. Skin Traction

Type	Purpose	Bed Position
Buck's extension	Preop for fractured hip; to prevent muscle spasms and dislocation	Flat in bed; head elevated 10–20° for ADLs
Cervical	Degenerative or arthritic conditions of cervical vertebrae, neck strain	Flat in bed or head can be elevated 15–20°
Dunlop's	Fractured humerus	Flat in bed
Pelvic girdle	Low back pain, muscle spasm, ruptured or herniated disc	Head of bed and knee gatch raised so hips flexed at 45° angle (William's position)
Russell's	Preop for fractured shaft of femur in adolescents, and some knee injuries	Head of bed elevated 30–45°
Bryant's	Preop for fractured femur, children weighing less than 40 lbs.	Flat in bed with hips flexed at 90° angle to body and buttocks raised 1 inch from mattress.

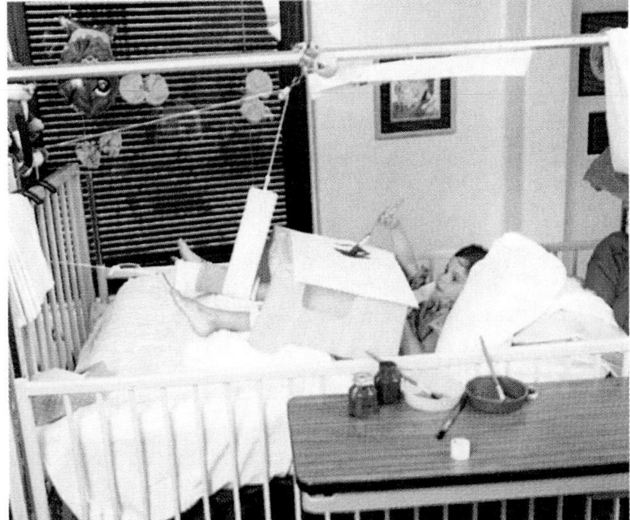

Russell traction is used for fractures of the femur and lower leg before surgery.

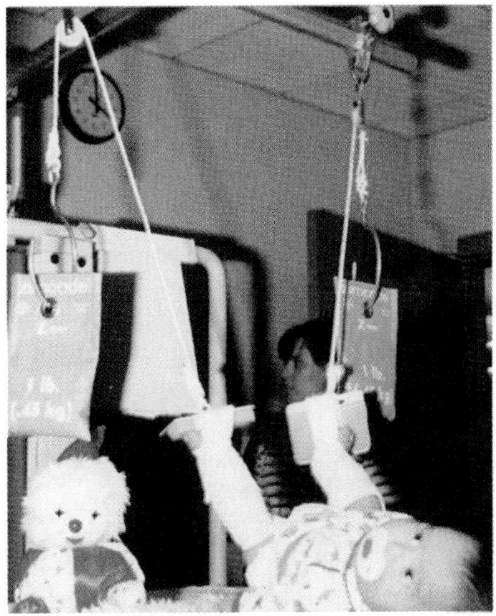

Bryant traction is used for children under 2 years and weighing less than 14 kg.

8. Position correctly in bed: the client should be positioned in the center of the bed. Affected leg or arm should be aligned with trunk of body. **Rationale:** Misalignment is the leading cause of pain for traction clients. The client should not be pulled down to the end of the bed because this negates the traction.
9. Place sheepskin or an alternative material under the affected extremity if appropriate. **Rationale:** This helps prevent pressure areas.
10. Provide foot plates for the affected side to prevent footdrop. Remove foot plate every 2 hours and have client perform foot exercises, flexion and extension, and circular rotation of ankle.

MONITORING SKELETAL TRACTION

Equipment

Sterile cotton-tipped applicators
Normal saline *or*
Hydrogen peroxide
Antibacterial ointment (optional)
Gauze dressing (optional)
Sterile gloves

Procedure

1. Check the pin and the pin site surrounding the pin.
   a. Pin should be immobile.
   b. Pin site should be clean and dry.
2. Assess for infection at the pin site. Note any local pain, redness, heat, or drainage.
3. Provide pin site care if ordered.
   a. Open applicator sticks.
   b. Open solution container.
   c. Don sterile gloves.
   d. Clean area with normal saline or hydrogen peroxide-soaked cotton-tipped applicators. Dip stick into solution bottle, or pour solution over sticks.
   e. Use new applicator stick for each pin site. **Rationale:** This prevents cross-contamination of sites.

TABLE 29–3. Skeletal Traction

Type	Purpose	Position and Activity
Balanced suspension with Thomas splint and Pearson attachment	Align bone and promote effective line of pull	Bed rest in supine position; may turn side to side for care; knee is flexed
External fixation devices Hoffman Synthes	Manage open fractures with soft tissue damage; provide stability for severe comminuted fractures	Early mobility and active exercise of uninvolved joints
Skeletal tongs Crutchfield Vinke Gardner–Well	Traction is used to immobilize and reduce cervical roll fractures Tongs maintain alignment of cervical spine	Bed rest, supine position; may turn on special frames or log-roll
Halo	Device provides immobilization of cervical spine	Early ambulation

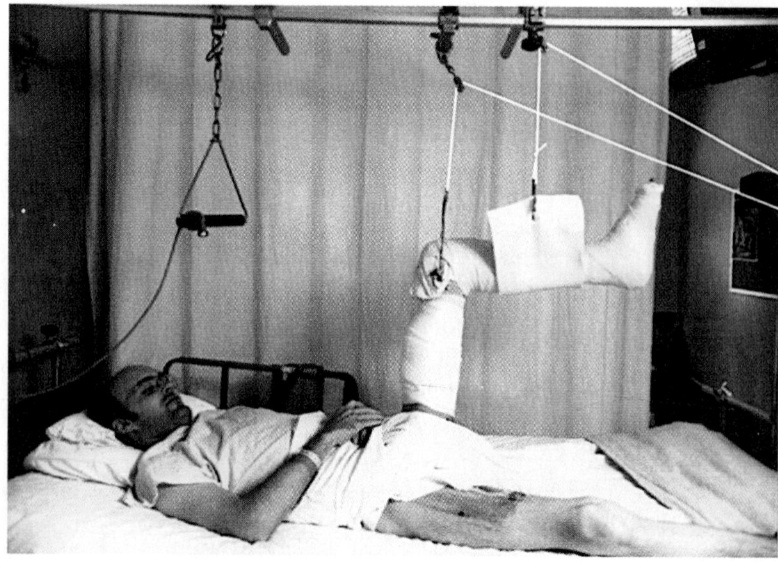

Russell skeletal traction.

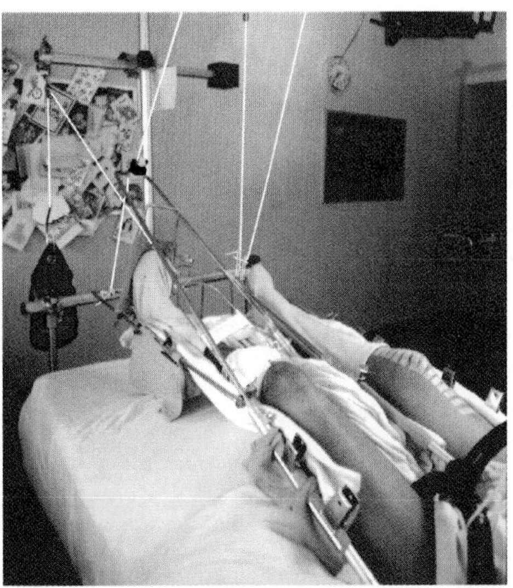
Thomas leg splint with Pearson attachment.

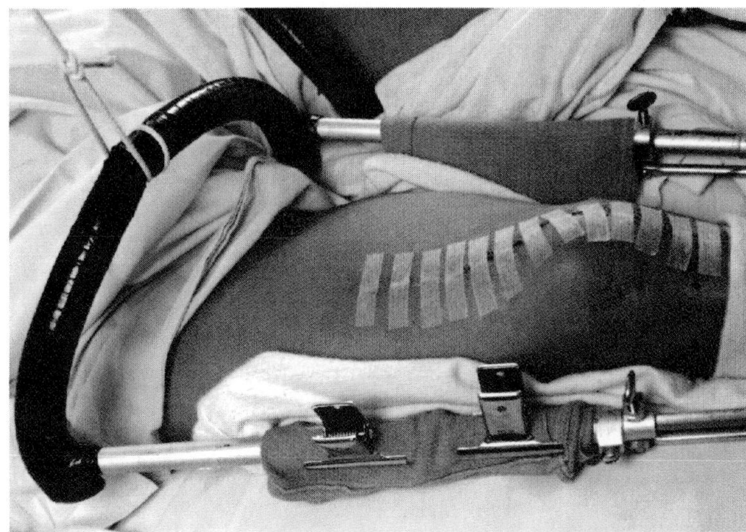
Thomas leg splint.

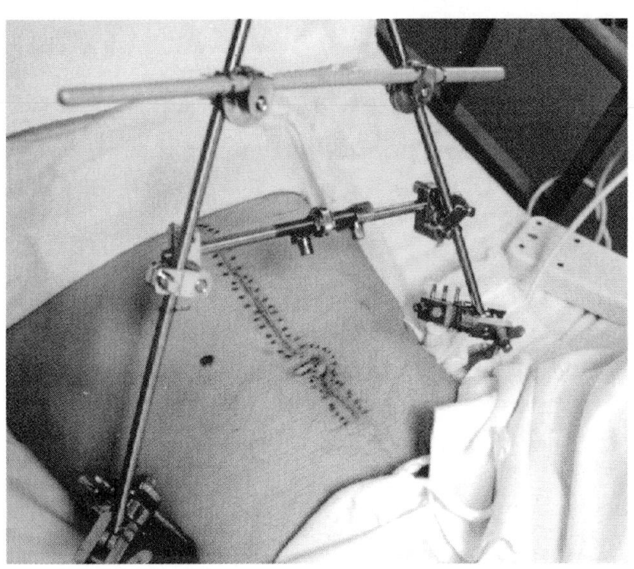
Hoffman Colles frame.

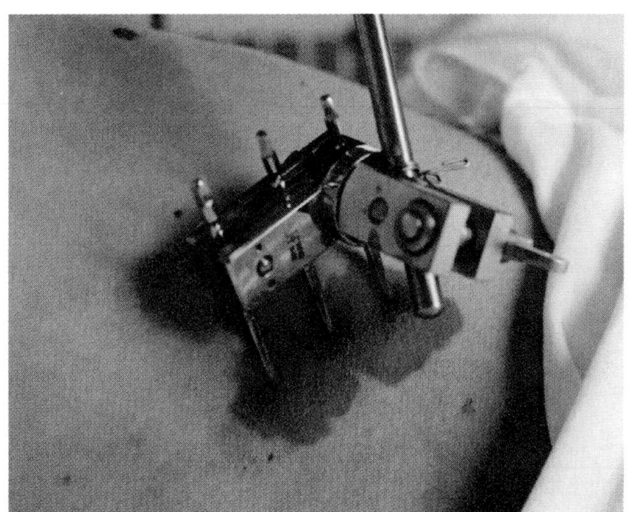
Pin sites for Hoffman Colles frame.

   f. Rinse pin site with sterile water or normal saline.
   g. Apply antibacterial ointment to site as ordered.
   h. Apply sterile, gauze dressing, according to hospital policy.
   i. Remove gloves, and discard sticks.
4. Examine all bony prominences for pressure areas or abrasions.
5. Assess distal extremity for pulses, temperature, color, and edema.
6. Check for normal range of motion and sensation in the affected extremity.
7. Check the ropes and weights to make sure the pull goes directly through the long axis of the fractured bone. **Rationale:** This pull maintains the fracture in alignment.
8. Check the traction mechanism.
   a. Weights should hang freely, off the floor and bed.
   b. Knots should be secure in all ropes.
   c. Rope should move freely through pulleys.
   d. Pulleys should not be constrained by knots.
9. Instruct client to use trapeze to assist in moving in bed, during linen change and back care.
10. Make sure the client is positioned correctly in bed.

Rationale: If the client is pulled down to the foot of the bed, the traction is negated.

11. Check placement of the foot rest. The client's foot should be correctly positioned to prevent footdrop.
12. Check groin area for skin irritation when Thomas splint is used.

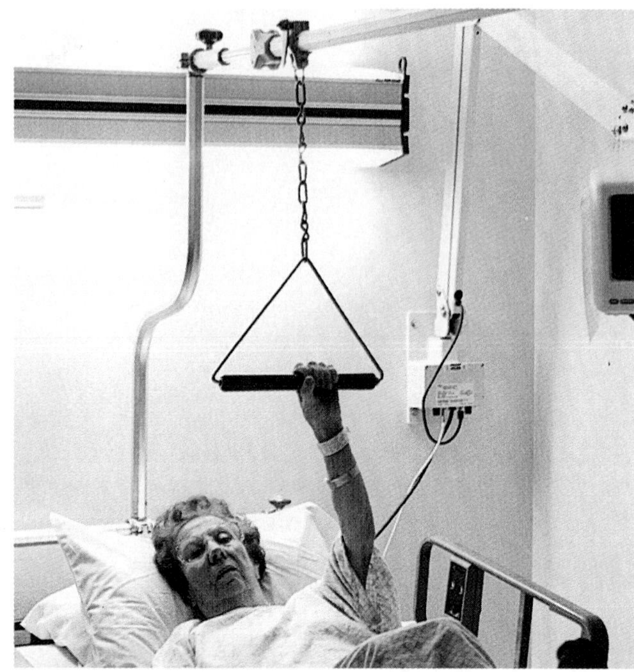

Trapeze is used to assist client to move in bed.

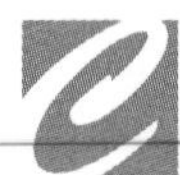

CHARTING for Traction

- Type of traction
- Alignment of traction
- Integrity of the skin
- Temperature, color, pulse, and range of motion in extremity
- Specific complaints by client and nursing actions taken to solve problems
- Client's comfort and overall feelings

CRITICAL THINKING APPLICATION

CLINICAL PROBLEMS	CRITICAL THINKING OPTIONS
■ There is a change in the temperature, color, or pulses of the extremity.	• Notify physician at once. • If the client has a fractured femur, measure the size of the thigh with a tape measure every 15–30 minutes. Look for areas of ecchymosis. (It is possible for several units of blood to be sequestered in the thigh if a vessel has been torn.) • Assess for circulatory shock.
■ Countertraction is not maintained for clients in Buck's traction.	• Check alignment to ensure client is placed in center of bed and not touching head- or footboard. • Instruct client to stay flat on back; turning from waist down or sitting up interferes with countertraction.

unit 5

HALO TRACTION AND BACK BRACE

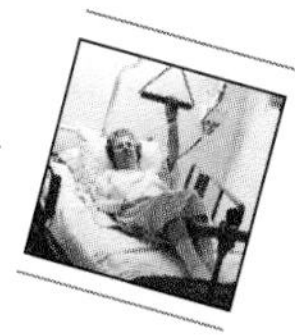

NURSING PROCESS DATA

ASSESSMENT Data Base

Assess for respiratory impairment: absence of breath sounds or adventitious sounds.
Assess for orthostatic hypotension while placing client in sitting position.
Assess pin sites for infection.
Assess skin under vest for erythema or skin breakdown.
Assess alignment of vest and position of traction.

PLANNING Objectives

To promote adequate respiratory function
To prevent orthostatic hypotension
To maintain pin site free of infection
To maintain skin integrity

IMPLEMENTATION Procedures

Placing a Jewett–Taylor Back Brace
Monitoring Halo Traction

EVALUATION Expected Outcomes

Complications are prevented or identified early.
Immobilization and proper alignment are maintained.

PLACING A JEWETT–TAYLOR BACK BRACE

Equipment

Front and back brace with Velcro straps
T-shirt
ABD dressings

Procedure

1. Wash your hands.
2. Explain procedure to client.
3. Provide privacy.
4. Put T-shirt on client. **Rationale:** This protects the skin from the brace rubbing on bare skin. This brace is used frequently with clients with spinal cord injuries who already have potential skin problems.
5. Place the bed in a flat position. Keep side rail in UP position on side of bed opposite from you.
6. Log-roll or ask client to turn to side farthest away from you. **Rationale:** This position prevents torque on the spinal cord.

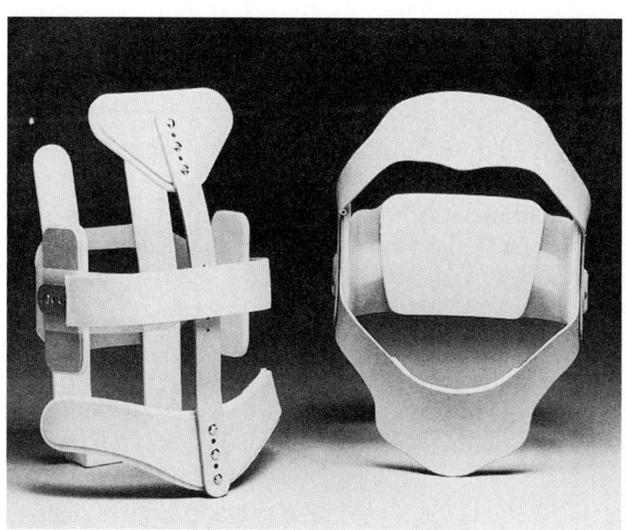

Jewett–Taylor braces are used to provide back support without exerting pressure following spinal cord surgery.

7. Position brace on back so that struts fit on either side of the spinal cord and it fits the natural lumbar curve of the back. **Rationale:** The struts provide an open space along the spinal cord so pressure is not exerted on a surgical site or on the vertebrae.
8. Log-roll the client to a supine position.
9. Place the front section of the brace by positioning the iliac wings (made of plastic material) over the iliac crest. Adjust the triangular sternum piece, the metal struts will fall into place.
10. Secure the brace with the Velcro straps.
11. Observe under the brace for pressure areas. If pressure areas are present, pad the area under the brace with ABD pads until the brace can be readjusted. **Rationale:** The physician should be notified immediately so the brace can be adjusted before complications occur.

MONITORING HALO TRACTION

Equipment

Allen wrench
Tracheostomy tray
Hydrogen peroxide
Antibacterial ointment (e.g., Neosporin, bacitracin)
Normal saline
Sterile cotton-tipped applicators
Antiembolic stockings, if needed
Abdominal binder, if needed
Wheelchair, if needed

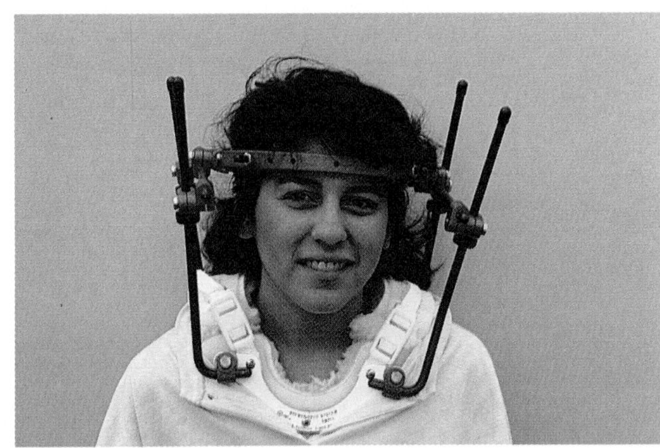

Halo traction provides support to neck following cervical spine injury.

Procedure

1. Evaluate client's psychologic status and knowledge base. Explain procedure at client's level of understanding.
2. Evaluate respiratory status.
   a. Check respiratory rate and rhythm at least every 2–4 hours.
   b. Observe respiratory excursion.
   c. Monitor breath sounds every shift for presence of adventitious sounds or absence of breath sounds. **Rationale:** Pulmonary embolus is a common complication associated with spinal cord injury. Due to sensory loss, the client is unable to feel the pain associated with an embolus.
   d. Keep Allen wrench and tracheostomy tray at bedside. **Rationale:** The Allen wrench is used to remove screws from the vest in order to perform CPR in the advent of respiratory or cardiac arrest. Endotracheal intubation is contraindicated in these clients, so a tracheostomy would be required.
3. Monitor alignment of cast and vest. If traction is intact the neck should not be flexed or extended. **Rationale:** Traction is maintained by anterior metal bars. Do not pull on anterior bars; use posterior bars for positioning clients.
4. Prevent orthostatic hypotension when placing client in sitting position.
   a. Apply antiembolic stockings. **Rationale:** Stockings promote venous return to heart.
   b. Apply abdominal binder. **Rationale:** Binders increase venous return to the heart.
   c. Raise client to 90° sitting position over period of 20–30 minutes. Take vital signs with each increment.
   d. Administer medications such as ephedrine 30 minutes before client is scheduled to move to a wheelchair. **Rationale:** Medication prevents hypotension.
   e. If hypotension persists, keep client in bed for 1 hour and attempt procedure again.
5. Prevent skin breakdown under vest.
   a. Open vest at both sides during bath.
   b. Wash skin and dry thoroughly.

c. Check skin for reddened area of skin breakdown. Treat skin problems immediately. **Rationale:** With poor vasomotor action, skin breakdown is difficult to treat.
d. Remove sheepskin lining once a week for cleaning.

6. Prevent pin site infection.
   a. Observe pin sites for drainage, edema, or erythema. If present, take specimen and send to lab for culture. **Rationale:** Clinical signs of infection should be treated immediately, as brain abscess can occur from pin site infections.
   b. Cleanse pin sites with sterile cotton-tipped applicators and hydrogen peroxide or normal saline. **Rationale:** Hydrogen peroxide has a tendency to remove tissue and loosen pins; therefore, check with hospital procedure for cleaning policy.
   c. Rinse sites with sterile saline if hydrogen peroxide is used.
   d. Apply light covering of antibacterial ointment to site. **Rationale:** Povidone-iodine (Betadine) tends to corrode the pins so it should not be used.
   e. Hair should be shaved around the pin sites to allow easy observation and cleaning.

■ CLINICAL ALERT

If pins are loose, notify physician immediately; keep client immobilized until physician arrives.

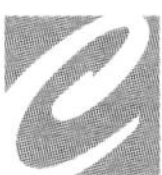

CHARTING for Halo Traction

- Pin site assessment
- Pin site care
- Skin condition under vest
- Stability of traction
- Presence of signs or symptoms of orthostatic hypotension
- Nursing measures used to prevent orthostatic hypotension
- Respiratory status

CRITICAL THINKING APPLICATION

CLINICAL PROBLEMS	CRITICAL THINKING OPTIONS
■ Infection at pin site.	• Monitor neurologic signs closely, as brain abscess is a major complication. • Obtain culture of drainage. • Call physician for systemic antibiotic order. • Cleanse sites more frequently. • Apply dressing over pin site to absorb drainage.
■ Pins are loose.	• Immobilize client immediately. • Contact physician. • Have Allen wrench available for physician.

unit 6

CLIENTS WITH AMPUTATED LIMBS

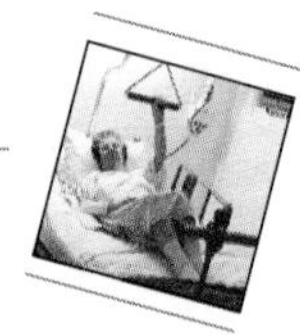

NURSING PROCESS DATA

ASSESSMENT Data Base

Assess incision for intactness.

Assess range of motion and muscle strength.

Note condition of client's skin (e.g., pressure areas, edema).

Assess for phantom limb pain.

Assess for signs of hemorrhage or infection.

PLANNING Objectives

To provide the stump with full range of motion

To ensure adequate muscle strength in both extremities for optimal use of the prosthesis

To promote a smooth conical stump that fits into a prosthesis comfortably

To assist the client in accepting the disability

To decrease the incidence of phantom limb pain

To prevent edema and pressure areas

IMPLEMENTATION Procedures

Positioning and Exercising

Applying a Shrink Bandage

EVALUATION Expected Outcomes

Stump exhibits full range of motion and adequate muscle strength.

Smooth conical stump that fits into prosthesis comfortably.

Stump incision is kept clean, dry, and free of infection.

POSITIONING AND EXERCISING

Equipment

Bedboard

Procedure

1. Explain the rationale for the intervention to client.
2. Place a bedboard under mattress, preferably at the time of surgery. **Rationale:** The client cannot sag into the mattress and develop contractures.
3. For the first 24 hours, elevate foot of bed. **Rationale:** Do not place pillow under stump as this leads to hip contracture.
4. Place client in prone position every shift for at least 1 hour.
5. Explain the importance of the exercises to the client. Tell client that because the flexor muscles are stronger than the extensors, the stump will be permanently flexed and abducted unless the client practices the range-of-motion exercises. **Rationale:** Range-of-motion exercises increase muscle strength and improve mobility of amputated extremity.
6. If ordered, assist the client with quadriceps-setting exercises with a below-the-knee amputation.
   a. Extend leg and try to push the popliteal area of the knee into the bed; try to move the patella proximally.
   b. Contract quadriceps and hold the contraction for 10 seconds.
   c. Repeat this procedure four or five times.
   d. Repeat the exercise at least four times a day.
7. Teach stump extension exercises.
   a. Lie in a prone position with foot hanging over the end of the bed.

b. Keep stump next to intact leg to extend stump and to contract gluteal muscles.
c. Hold the contraction for 10 seconds.
d. Repeat this exercise at least four times a day.
8. Teach adduction exercise.
a. Place a pillow between the client's thighs.
b. Squeeze the pillow for 10 seconds and then relax for 10 seconds.
c. Repeat this exercise at least four times a day.
9. Have the client keep track of time spent with the stump flexed and then spend an equal amount of time with the stump extended.

APPLYING A SHRINK BANDAGE

Equipment

Elastic bandages: two or three 4- to 6-inch bandages, sewn together if possible for lower extremity

Elastic bandages: one or two 3- to 4-inch bandages for upper extremity

> Commercial stump shrink bandages are sometimes used to apply pressure, reduce edema formation, and help shape stump for prosthesis fitting.

Procedure

1. Explain the rationale for the intervention to client.
2. For amputations above the knee, apply 3- to 4-inch shrink bandages as illustrated.
   a. Ask the client to hold the loops of bandage at the top of the thigh.
   b. Apply pressure evenly. **Rationale:** This allows tissues to be shaped properly.
   c. Apply the bandage smoothly, making sure there are no wrinkles to cause pressure areas.
   d. Extend the bandage as high as possible into the groin. **Rationale:** This prevents formation of an abrasion or loose roll of tissue which can hamper the fit and use of a prosthesis.
   e. If you use spica turns, make sure that the stump is not pulled into a flexed position by the bandages.
3. For amputations below the knee, apply a shrink bandage using same principles, anchoring bandage on thigh.
4. Carefully observe the bandages you have applied to ensure proper tension and molding of the stump.
5. Rewrap bandages three to four times a day.
6. Wash skin, dry thoroughly, and after assessing skin, rewrap stump.

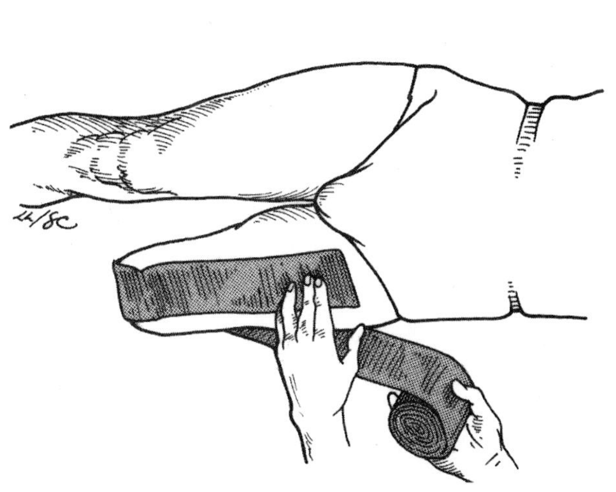

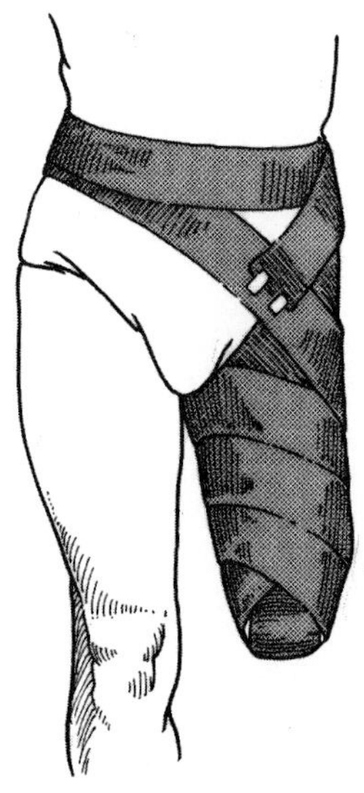

Shrink bandage is used following amputation to mold stump in preparation for prothesis.

CHARTING for Shrink Bandaging

- When bandage was changed
- Condition of client's skin and incision
- Extent of range of motion
- Any changes in how the bandage has been applied
- Client's response to seeing the stump and assisting with the care

CRITICAL THINKING APPLICATION

CLINICAL PROBLEMS	CRITICAL THINKING OPTIONS
Stump edema occurs even with application of shrink bandage.	• When on bed rest, elevate foot of bed to increase venous blood flow and decrease edema. • Assess for possible complications of infection or obstruction in blood flow. • Evaluate wrapping procedure. Ensure bandages are properly applied.
Shrinkage of stump is delayed or doesn't occur as expected.	• Continue treatment as ordered. • Observe carefully for signs of infection or edema.
Stump is unable to be put through full range of motion.	• Observe the client to see which positions he or she uses most often. Assess stump for continued flexion or abduction. • Explain why the client should practice full range-of-motion exercises and demonstrate exercises again if necessary. • Show the client how to position the stump to attain optimal stump movement. Help the client assume these positions several times a day. • Notify the physician.

unit 7

NELSON BED

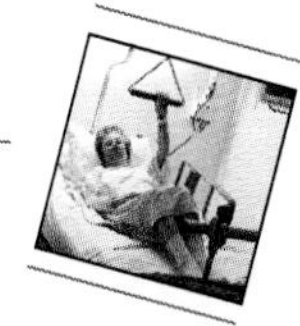

NURSING PROCESS DATA

ASSESSMENT Data Base

Assess client's vital signs, including peripheral pulses and circulation.

Determine if symptoms of orthostatic hypotension are present.

Determine client's ability to maintain balance.

Assess client's knowledge of the bed and its function.

Ascertain client's previous experience with the bed.

PLANNING Objectives

To maintain optimal functioning of body systems by putting client's body in positions of normal activity

To assist the client with total hip replacement in ambulation without flexion of the affected hip

To allow clients with spinal surgery to ambulate without torsion of the spine

To provide a vertical position at intervals to maintain stress on bone. This prevents loss of calcium

To change a client on bed rest from a horizontal to a vertical position without symptoms of orthostatic hypotension

To maintain or attain normal movement of ankles, knees, and hips while clients are on bed rest

IMPLEMENTATION Procedures

Using a Nelson Bed

Moving to Chair Position

Moving to Contour Position

Tilting Bed to Vertical Position

Tilting Bed to Trendelenburg's Position

EVALUATION Expected Outcomes

Clients with total hip replacement are able to get out of bed and ambulate without flexion of the affected hip.

Spinal surgery clients are able to get out of bed and ambulate without torsion of the spine.

Clients are able to change from horizontal to vertical position without symptoms of orthostatic hypotension.

Client maintains normal movement of ankles, knees, and hips.

USING A NELSON BED

Equipment

Nelson bed

Safety restraining straps

Procedure

1. Explain the function of bed to client.
2. Adjust seat section of the bed to the height of the individual client. This is most easily done before the client is put into bed, but it may be done afterward.
   a. Unscrew knobs at each side of the bed at the area marked "To adjust for client height."
   b. Slide head section until knob position corresponds to the height of the client as printed on the side of the bed.
   c. Tighten knobs securely.
3. Place client on the bed.

4. Familiarize client with the bed controls for section changes.
   a. Tilt: whole bed goes up at head end.
   b. Head.
   c. Knee.
   d. Foot: whole bed goes up at foot end.
5. Instruct client how to change height position of bed.
6. Instruct client how to control UP and DOWN for each section and height of bed.
7. Place safety straps across client when tilting bed.

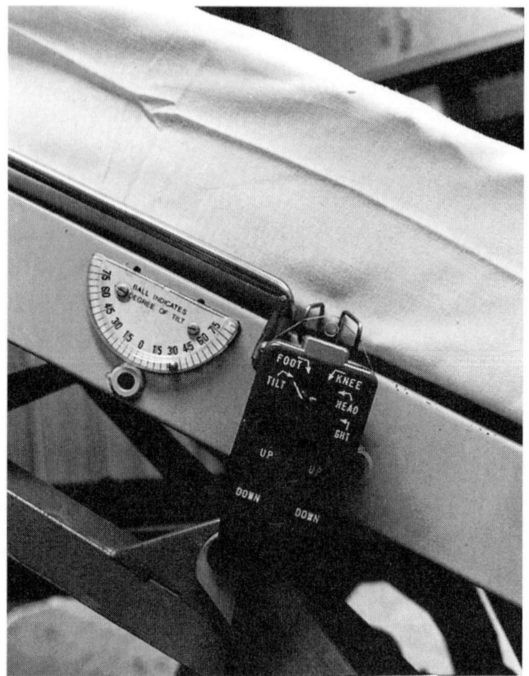

The Nelson bed provides position variation. Control knobs allow clients to maintain mobility.

MOVING TO CHAIR POSITION

Equipment

Nelson bed
Safety restraining straps

Procedure

1. Explain the procedure to client.
2. Put the side rails in UP position.
3. Adjust the footboard to client's need.
   a. To move toward client, push the footboard forward by holding the middle of the supporting legs.
   b. To move away from client, tilt the footboard slightly forward and then pull downward to the desired position. **Rationale:** The client's weight locks the footboard in position.
4. Adjust the casters at the foot of the bed so they are parallel to the bed and locked in place.
5. Put safety straps around client if necessary.
6. Put head section up to vertical position.
7. Put knee section down until the foot of the bed is vertical.

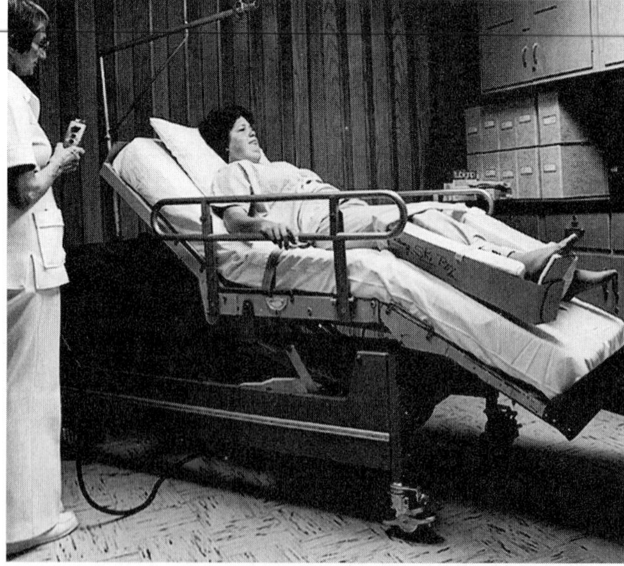
Facilitate self-care by positioning Nelson bed in a sitting position.

8. Lower the bed by choosing HEIGHT and DOWN until the footboard is on the floor.
9. To return the bed to a horizontal position, reverse the procedure.

MOVING TO CONTOUR POSITION

Procedure

1. Explain the procedure to client.
2. Put the side rails up.
3. Put the head of bed up to a comfortable position.
4. Put knee section down as desired.
5. Use the FOOT control to tilt the whole bed back (head end down).
6. Adjust all parts as necessary for comfort.
7. To return to a flat position, reverse the procedure.

TILTING BED TO VERTICAL POSITION

Procedure

1. Explain the procedure to client.
2. Align and lock the foot casters parallel to the bed frame.
3. Place the bed in the flat position.
4. Put height up to highest position.
5. Put the footboard down to farthest position.
6. Slide client down until feet are on the footboard.
7. Apply safety restraining straps around the client as needed.

Step *one* in assisting a client out of bed is to pull client down toward footboard.

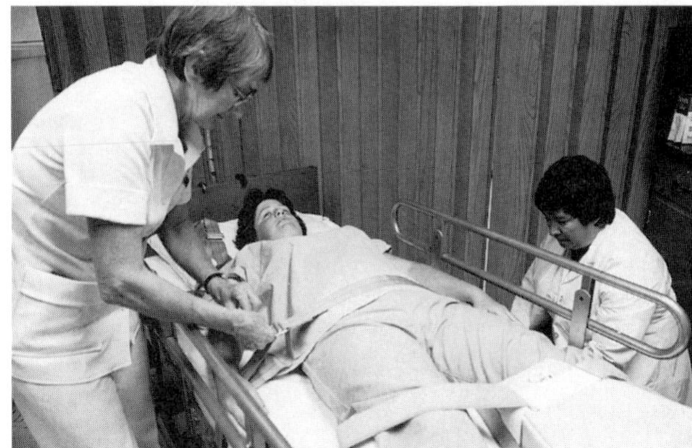

Step *two* is to place straps across abdomen and legs to prevent sliding down.

Step *three* is to place bed in vertical position.

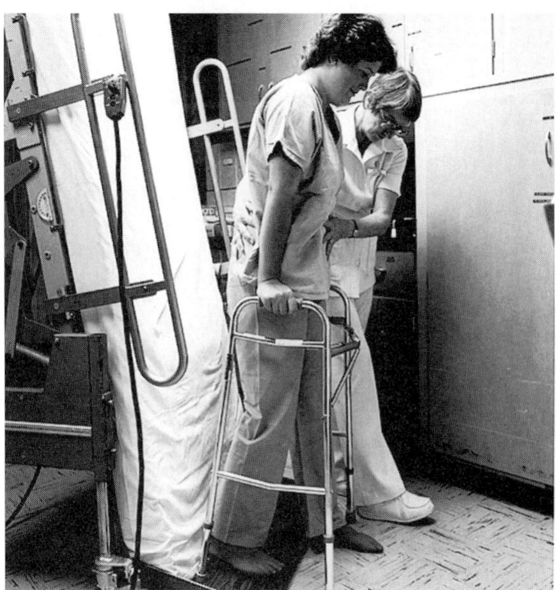

Step *four* is to assist client to walk.

8. Put the side rails up.
9. Select TILT, and put the bed up to full tilt (82°) or to a level the client can tolerate.
10. When bed is in vertical position, support client with your knee to prevent fall.
11. Assist client to step from bed with support of walker.
12. To place the client back to a horizontal position, reverse the procedure.

TILTING BED TO TRENDELENBURG'S POSITION

Procedure

1. Explain the procedure to the client.
2. Place the mattress flat.
3. Set the controls to FOOT, and press UP button.
4. To place client back to a flat position, set controls to FOOT and press DOWN button.

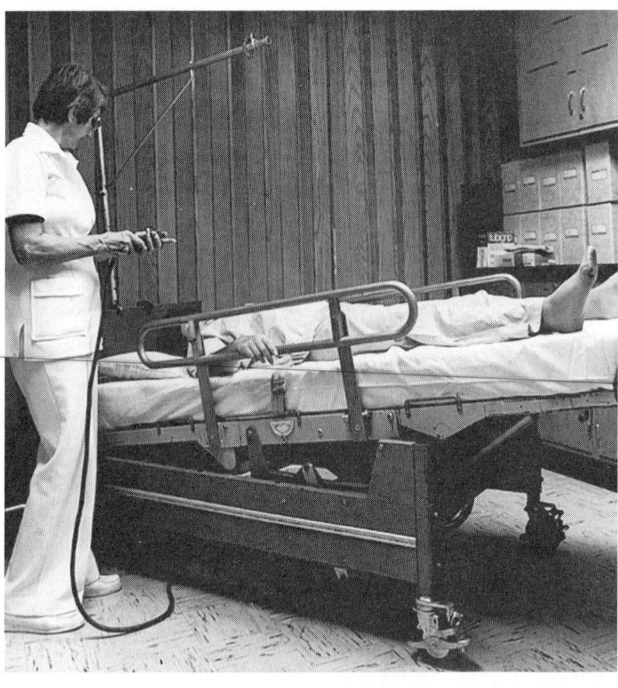

Nelson bed can be placed in Trendelenburg's position with control.

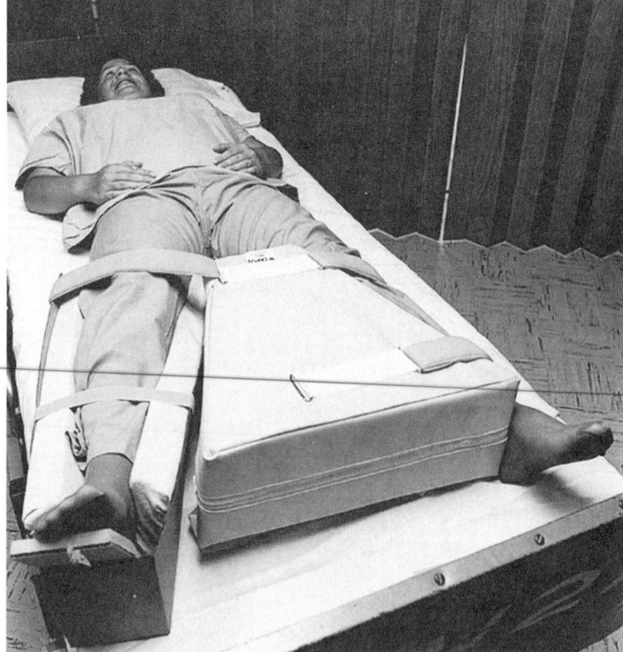

Charnley pillow maintains abduction and external rotation of the hips.

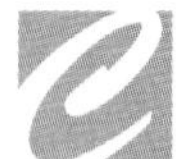

CHARTING for Nelson Bed

- Bed position used
- Degree of tilt
- Time client was in a specific position
- Vital signs
- Client's emotional reaction
- Signs and symptoms of untoward reactions
- Straps used, if any

CRITICAL THINKING APPLICATION

CLINICAL PROBLEMS	CRITICAL THINKING OPTIONS
The client experiences syncope when the body's position is made more vertical.	• Lower the head of the bed at once. • Check blood pressure and pulse every 5–10 minutes until stable. • When raising bed next time, raise client to a lower degree of tilt and keep client in that position for a longer time before continuing to raise bed. • Increase degree of tilt in small increments, checking blood pressure and pulse with each increment.
The client is not strapped in and falls from the bed.	• Have client checked by physician. • Obtain x-rays if ordered. • Complete unusual occurrence report. • Assess client's ability to maintain balance while tilting the bed. • Use safety straps until sure of client's ability to maintain balance. • Strap client's legs if they are weak before changing bed's position.
The client is fearful of the movement of the bed.	• Fully explain the reasons for using the bed. • Answer all the client's questions. • Let the client control movement of the bed. • Stay while the client moves the bed. • Strap client in place while moving the bed. • Change bed positions slowly.

unit 8 STRYKER FRAME

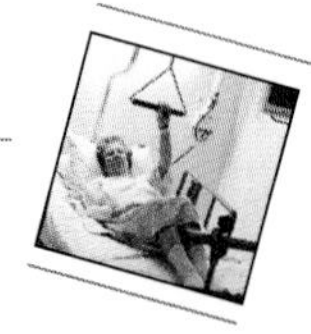

NURSING PROCESS DATA

ASSESSMENT Data Base

Determine client's level of movement and sensation.

Evaluate client's ability to understand explanation of turning procedure.

Assess condition of traction apparatus.

Evaluate client's ability to assist with turning.

PLANNING Objectives

To assist the client in turning horizontally from supine to prone to supine without torsion or abnormal flexion/extension of the spinal column

To provide optimal skin care for clients who require immobility

To prevent pressure areas and decubitus ulcers

To provide optimal nursing care to clients with skin grafts or other conditions that require minimum client movement

IMPLEMENTATION Procedures

Using a Stryker Wedge Turning Frame

Turning from Supine to Prone

Using a Stryker Parallel Frame

Assisting Client with Bedpan

Attaching Fixed Traction

Attaching Skeletal Traction

EVALUATION Expected Outcomes

Client turns horizontally without torsion or abnormal flexion/extension of the spinal column.

Client receives optimal skin care without developing decubiti.

Client receives optimal nursing care for skin grafts or similar conditions.

USING A STRYKER WEDGE TURNING FRAME

Equipment

Stryker wedge turning frame

Arm rests and footboard

Software: mattress, canvases, linen, straps

Safety straps

Pillows and sheepskins

Procedure

1. Explain procedure to client.
2. Show client the Stryker frame before placing on the frame.
3. Position the posterior frame at the bottom of the turning circle.
4. Place client supine on the posterior frame using the three-man carry transfer method.
5. If client is on a backboard, place client and board on the posterior frame.
6. Attach the anterior frame.
7. Turn client and remove the back board.
8. Reverse the procedure, and turn client to his or her back.

TURNING FROM SUPINE TO PRONE

Procedure

1. Explain procedure to client. This procedure requires only one person; however, it is advisable to have two people when possible.
2. Position sheepskin, pillows, or comfort aids on top of client.
3. With client on the posterior frame, open the turning circle and put the head end of the anterior frame on the securing bolt and fasten it with the nut.
4. Fasten the foot end of the anterior frame with the nut, making sure that client's legs and feet are correctly positioned.
5. Have client clasp hands around the anterior frame. If client is unable to do this, put a safety strap around the whole frame at elbow level to keep arms contained.
6. Close the turning circle until it locks.
7. Move the arm rests down out of the way of the turn.
8. Pull out the bed-turning lock.
9. Turn the frame toward the client's right until it locks automatically. The narrow side of the wedge (at the client's right) always turns down. The frame automatically locks when the bottom frame is horizontal.
10. Open the turning circle, unscrew the nuts, and

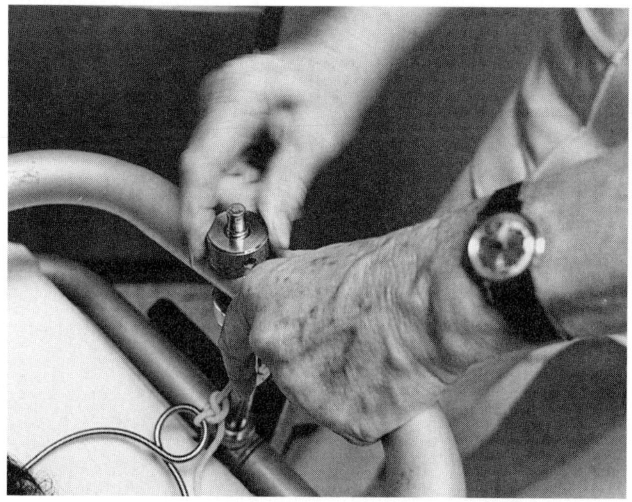

Before turning, fasten nut securely at head and foot of frame.

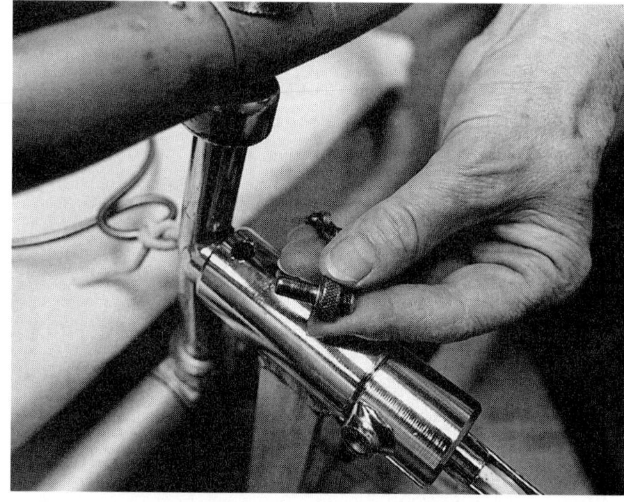

Pull out the turning lock before beginning the turning process.

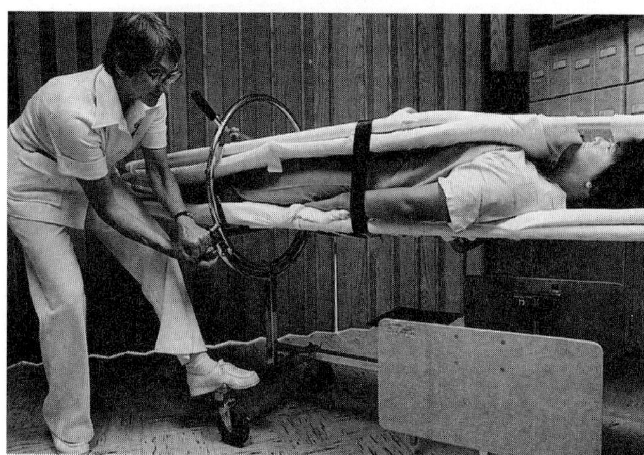

Fasten straps securely around Stryker frame before turning.

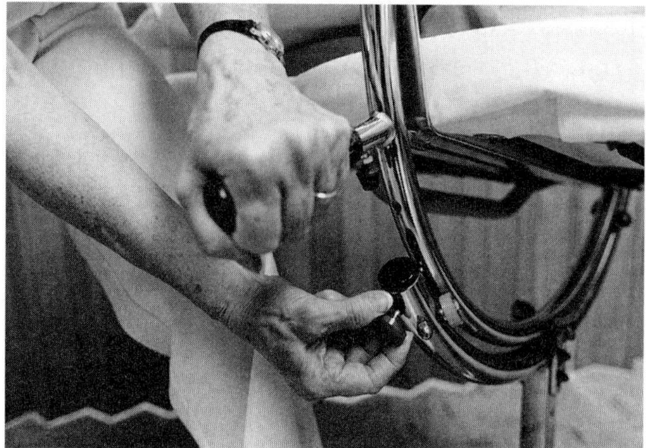

Hold handle while pulling knob and begin turn.

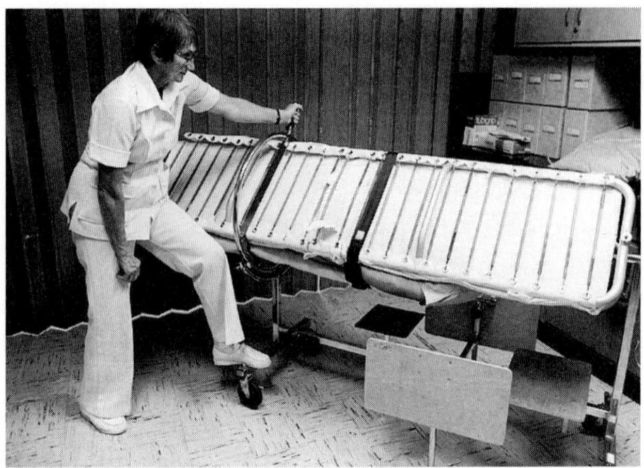

Clients can be turned safely by one person.

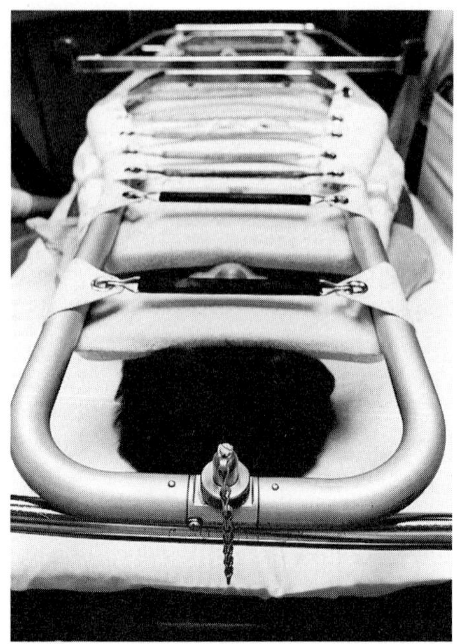

Unscrew nut and lift frame to remove.

remove the upper posterior frame. Relock the turning circle for safety.

11. To turn the client on the Stryker wedge from prone to supine, reverse procedure for turning from supine to prone. Remember that the narrow side of the wedge (on client's right) always turns down so client cannot slip out.

USING A STRYKER PARALLEL FRAME

Equipment

Stryker parallel frame
Arm rests and footboard
Software: mattress, canvases, linen, straps
Safety straps
Pillows and sheepskins

Procedure

1. Place a pillow lengthwise over the client's legs to prevent moving during turning.
2. Attach the anterior frame to the main frame using the two nuts on the turning circle. Make sure the client is held firmly between the frames.
3. Put three safety straps around the frame at level of knees, waist, and elbows. Tighten securely.
4. With a person at each end of the frame, pull out the locking pins at the center of each end, turn the frame slightly to hold the lock open, and then quickly finish turning the client. The bed automatically locks when the bottom frame is horizontal.
5. Remove the top frame, and reposition the client for comfort.

ASSISTING CLIENT WITH BEDPAN

Equipment

Special bedpan
Plastic drape
Towels
Clean gloves

Procedure

1. Explain procedure to client.
2. Place client in a supine position.
3. Don clean gloves.
4. Drop the center section of the posterior frame by releasing the hooks or rubber bands from the sides of the frame.

5. Protect the linen by putting plastic or towels around the edges.
6. Insert the bedpan into the opening and hold securely with hands or with the arm supports.
7. Remove the bedpan, clean the client, and reattach the center section of the frame.
8. Clean bedpan, and replace in storage area.
9. Remove gloves, and discard.
10. Wash your hands.

ATTACHING FIXED TRACTION

Equipment

Traction halter
Weights
Pulleys
Rope

Procedure

1. Explain procedure to client.
2. Attach the rope to the frame of the Stryker through the hole in the center pin of the disc.
3. Apply a traction halter or belt to the client. (Client's body forms counterweight.)
4. Attach the rope from the frame to the halter or belt.
5. Determine the number of centimeters the end of the frame must be elevated to provide for sufficient traction. Determine the client's weight, and use the table provided in the operating instructions to obtain the number of centimeters.
6. Lift up the head or foot of the Stryker frame, depending on the type of traction. Put the stop pins into the holes corresponding to the elevation needed.
7. Check that the client's body is positioned so the feet or head is free to maintain traction.

ATTACHING SKELETAL TRACTION

Equipment

Weights
Rope
Pulley

Procedure

1. Explain procedure to client.
2. Attach the rope to weights by placing it through the hole in the center of the disc and laying it over the pulley.
3. Attach the rope to the skeletal traction and tape all knots. Traction is applied to head or lower extremities.
4. Assess that weights are clear of frame and remain above the floor.

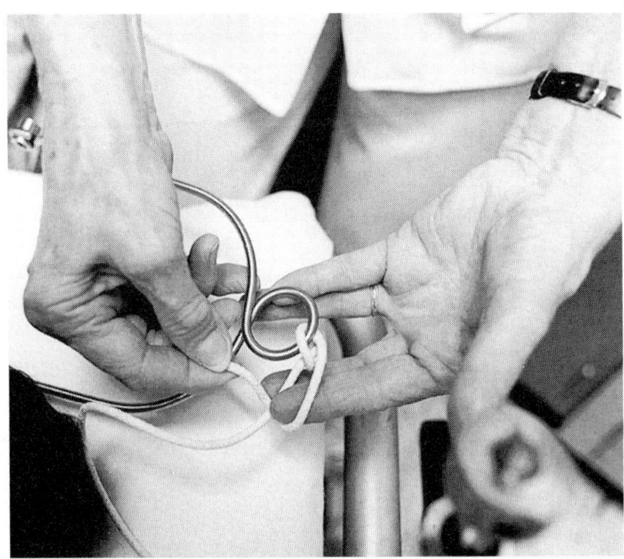

Tie knot through the loop in tongs to prevent rope from slipping.

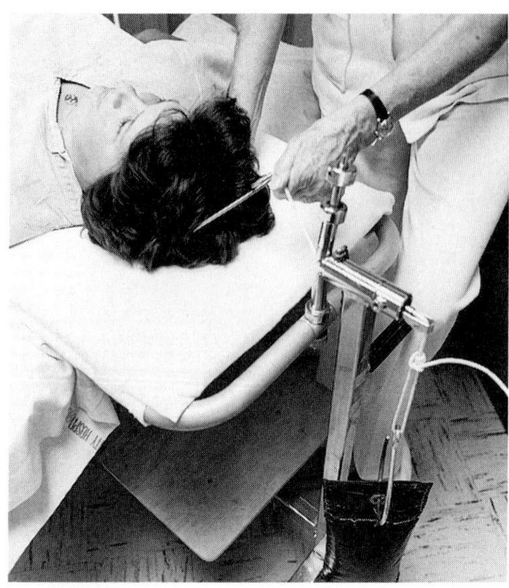
Ensure that weights hang freely and do not touch bed or floor.

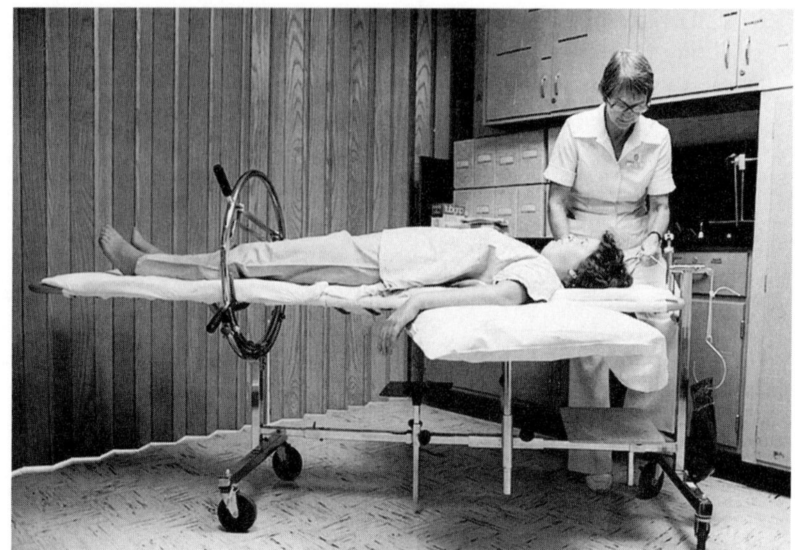
Cervical spine immobilization is accomplished through use of tongs.

CHARTING for Stryker Frame

- Length of time spent on each side
- How client tolerates turning procedure
- Complaints of physical discomfort despite frequent position changes
- Status of the traction apparatus
- Vital signs

CRITICAL THINKING APPLICATION

CLINICAL PROBLEMS	CRITICAL THINKING OPTIONS
The client expresses fear of being turned.	• Encourage client to lie on the frame and be turned before being placed on it after surgery. • Carefully explain each step of the turning process and the use of each piece of equipment. • Allow the client to express fears and concerns. • Carefully answer all questions in a way that the client can understand.
The client experiences unusual pain or discomfort when turned.	• Have the client describe details of pain. • Assess the client's neurologic status, and compare it with the client's status before turning. • Ensure that the traction apparatus is intact. • Assess for psychologic component of pain. • Notify physician if pain persists or if there is a change in neurologic status.

unit 9

CIRCOLECTRIC BED

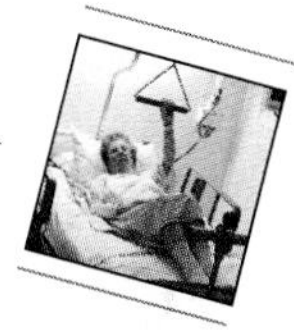

NURSING PROCESS DATA

ASSESSMENT Data Base

Determine client's level of movement and sensation.

Evaluate client's ability to understand the procedure.

Assess the client's ability to control his or her own turning.

PLANNING Objectives

To turn from supine to prone to supine without excess client movement

To provide optimal skin care for immobilized clients

To maintain good skin condition for clients on long-term bed rest

IMPLEMENTATION Procedures

Preparing to Operate Bed

Placing Ambulatory Client on Bed

Placing Nonambulatory Client on Bed

Turning from Supine to Prone

Assisting Client with Bedpan

EVALUATION Expected Outcomes

Client turns from supine to prone to supine without excess movement.

Client receives optimal skin care.

PREPARING TO OPERATE BED

Equipment

CircOlectric bed

Hand control unit

Procedure

1. Learn the mechanical aspects of operating the CircOlectric bed.
2. Hand control unit has two parts: a toggle switch designated FACE or BACK and a push-button switch for actual movement.
3. Bed is operated by selecting FACE or BACK position and pressing button until bed is in desired position.
4. A crank is stored in a tray at the head of the bed to adjust the bed if the electricity is off.
5. Two wheel locks are located on opposite corners of the bed.
6. Two automatic stops are on the bottom rail of the bed. They should be set whenever the anterior frame is not in use.
   a. The sitting stop, on the client's right side, prevents rotation beyond an upright sitting position.
   b. The standing stop, the client's left side, prevents rotation beyond a semierect position.
7. The gatch lever, at the client's right hip, changes the posterior frame from a flat to a semisitting position.

PLACING AMBULATORY CLIENT ON BED

Equipment

CircOlectric bed
Hand control unit

Procedure

1. Explain procedure to client.
2. Demonstrate bed movement by using the controls.
3. Place bed in a vertical position.
4. Have client step backward onto the footboard with his or her back toward the posterior frame.
5. Rotate the bed backward to the desired position.
6. Adjust client's position so that hips are at level of gatch.

PLACING NONAMBULATORY CLIENT ON BED

Equipment

CircOlectric bed

Procedure

1. Explain transfer to client.
2. Demonstrate bed movement to client if he or she is alert.
3. Position bed or gurney parallel to CircOlectric bed.
4. Alert client when you are ready to move him or her to the CircOlectric bed.
5. Transfer client using a standard sheet or the three-man carry method.

TURNING FROM SUPINE TO PRONE

Equipment

CircOlectric bed
Bed linen

Procedure

1. Explain procedure to client.
2. Move the footboard from the client's feet to the foot of the bed.

The CircOlectric bed provides position change for clients with restricted mobility.

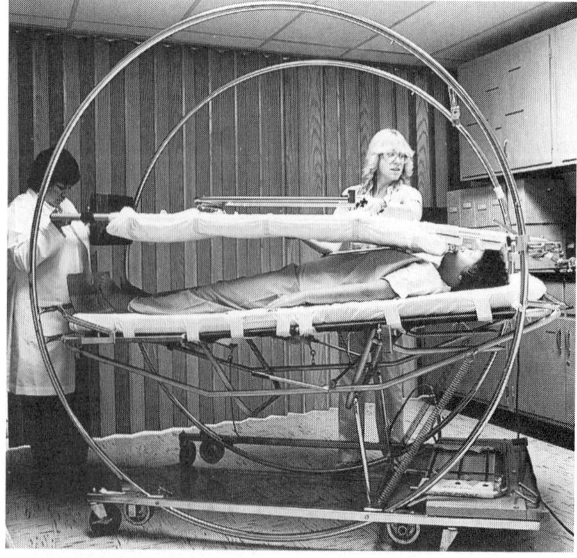

Place frame on bed and secure bolt at head of bed first, before attaching footboard.

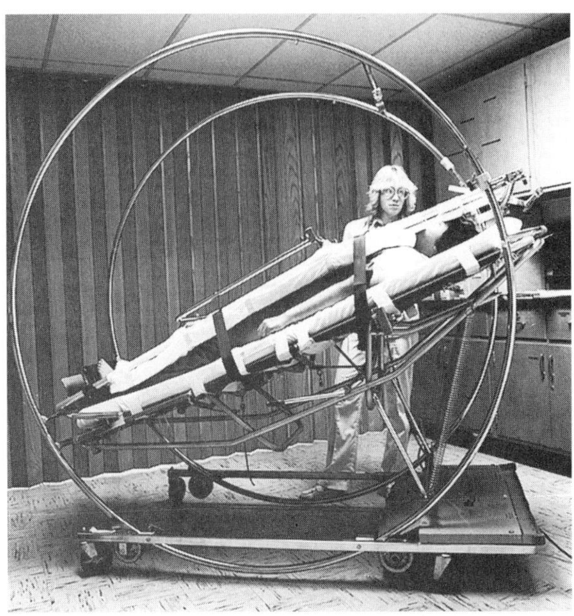

Complete securing anterior frame before turning.

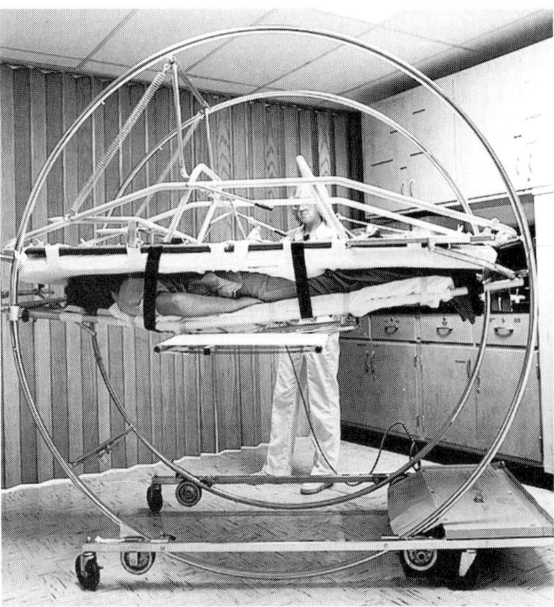

Stop turn with client in prone position with head slightly down.

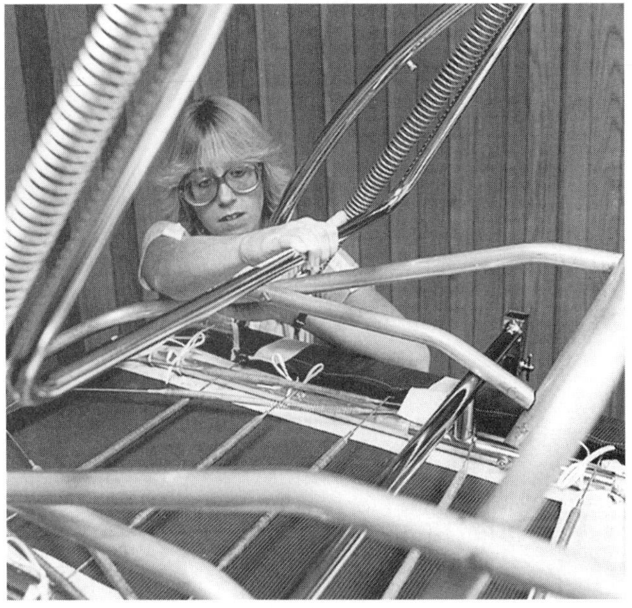

Pull support bar outward to raise frame off client.

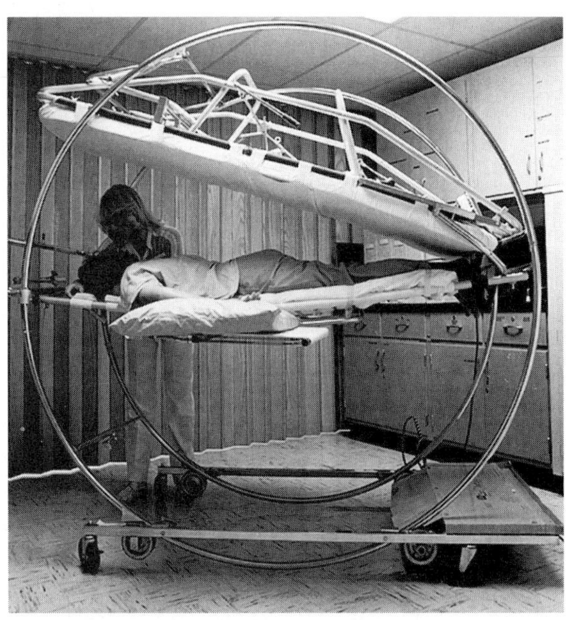

Lock frame with support bar to complete turn.

3. Place the anterior frame through the large rings one end at a time.
4. Attach the anterior frame on bolt at the head of the client, and secure it with a nut.
5. Adjust the footboard of the anterior frame to the client.
6. Attach the anterior frame to the foot of the bed with a bolt and nut as at the head of the bed.
7. Adjust the support bar (at the head of the anterior frame) at the level of the chest to hold client firmly but comfortably.
8. Adjust the security collar knobs against the support bar.
9. Adjust the headbands to client's forehead and chin.
10. Put client's arms into the slings attached to the anterior frame.
11. Double-check all attachments, and release all stops.

12. Turn client to slightly head-down position.
13. Raise the posterior frame by removing the nut, pulling the support bar in the frame outward, and lifting the frame until it locks with the support bar.
14. Gatch the posterior frame to remove pressure from the client's feet.
15. Rotate bed backward to a prone or a slightly upright position.
16. To turn the client from a prone to a supine position, reverse the procedure.

ASSISTING WITH BEDPAN

Equipment

CircOlectric bed
Absorbent pads
Stryker bedpan
Clean gloves

Procedure

1. Explain procedure to client.
2. Provide privacy.
3. Don clean gloves.
4. Place client on the posterior frame in a flat or semisitting position.
5. Pull apart the elastic cords under the posterior frame, and remove the round mattress insert.
6. Insert the bedpan into the opening, and hold it there with the elastic cord.
7. Place absorbent pads at the edges of the opening to prevent soiling linen (optional).
8. Remove the bedpan when the client is finished, and replace the mattress insert.
9. Clean bedpan, and replace to storage area.
10. Remove gloves, and discard.
11. Wash hands.

CHARTING for CircOlectric Bed

- Length of time client spends on each side
- How client tolerates the turning procedure
- If applicable, how client tolerates being in a relatively vertical position
- Complaints of physical discomfort despite frequent position changes
- Status of condition for which client is on the CircOlectric bed
- Vital signs

CRITICAL THINKING APPLICATION

CLINICAL PROBLEMS	CRITICAL THINKING OPTIONS
■ The client expresses a fear of turning.	• If possible, ensure that client has preoperative teaching. Encourage the client to lie on the bed and be turned. • Carefully explain each step of the turning process and the use of each piece of equipment. • Allow client to express fears and concerns. • Carefully answer all the client's questions in a way that the client can understand. • Change positions slowly to allow the client to adjust to the turning position.
■ The client experiences unusual pain or discomfort when turned.	• Have client describe details of the pain. • Assess the client's neurologic status and compare it with the status before turning. • Assess for psychologic component of pain. Notify the physician if pain persists or if there is a change in neurologic status.

GERIATRIC CONSIDERATIONS

Normal aging processes affect the musculoskeletal system and, when orthopedic measures are implemented, must be considered.

- Decreased height
- More brittle bones
- Muscle atrophy
- Diminished strength
- Joint stiffening
- Weakness and slowed movement

Usual fractures associated with the elderly client with osteoporosis are related to acute trauma (i.e., falls or repetitive stress injuries):

- Hip fractures
- Vertebral fractures
- Forearm fractures

Elderly clients are at high risk for falls and musculoskeletal injury as a result of

- Weakness and being easily fatigued
- Unsteady balance
- Poor eyesight
- Altered mobility resulting from medications
- Increased time on bed rest, leading to muscle weakness

30

Operative Care

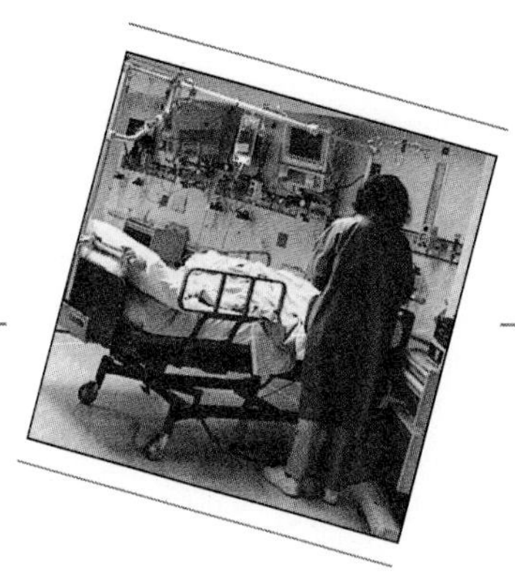

LEARNING OBJECTIVES

- Define the word "perioperative."
- Discuss the nursing care focus in each of the three stages of the perioperative period.
- Identify at least three factors that influence the surgical client's degree of stress.
- Explain why postoperative complications are reduced by decreasing the stress level.
- Describe at least one potential problem and the suggested solution for clients demonstrating high stress levels in the preoperative period.
- State the primary purpose of providing preoperative care for clients.
- Discuss how preoperative teaching can reduce the surgical client's stress.
- Describe the information contained in the surgical permit.
- Outline the essential steps in physically preparing a client for surgery.
- Explain the purpose for administering the three classifications of drugs used for preoperative medications.
- Outline the essential postoperative nursing interventions completed in the surgical unit.
- Summarize the major categories of postoperative pain medications, and describe the general side effects of each category.
- Discuss at least three major postoperative complications and the nursing interventions to prevent and treat the complications.

TERMINOLOGY

Adaptation: ability of an organism to adjust to a change in environment.

Analgesia: absence of the normal sense of pain.

Analgesic: a drug that relieves pain without altering the conscious state.

Anesthesia: partial or complete loss of sensation by administration of a drug or gas.

Anxiety: a troubled feeling; experiencing a sense of dread or fear without a stimulus. A condition associated with physiologic changes.

Arthritis: inflammation of a joint, usually accompanied by pain and sometimes by change in structure.

Asepsis: sterile, a condition free from germs.

Atelectasis: a collapsed or airless condition of the lungs.

Bronchitis: inflammation of the bronchial mucous membrane.

Bronchoscopy: examination of the bronchi with a scope.

Contamination: the introduction of disease, germs, or infectious materials into or on normally sterile objects.

Dehydration: to deprive the body or tissues of water.

Diplopia: double vision.

Egophony: a nasal sound heard while auscultating the lungs of a person as he speaks; a sound heard in pleural effusion.

Emesis: vomiting.

Emphysema: a condition in which the alveoli of the lungs become distended or ruptured.

Enema: injection of water or fluid into rectum and colon to empty the lower intestine or to introduce medicine or food for therapeutic purposes.

Euphoria: an exaggerated feeling of well-being.

Exudate: accumulation of fluid in a cavity.

Hernia: the protrusion or projection of an organ or part of an organ through the wall of the cavity that normally contains it.

Hypertension: higher blood pressure than normal; usually above 140 mm Hg/90 mm Hg.

Hypnotic: drugs that cause insensibility to pain or partial to complete unconsciousness; includes sedatives, analgesics, anesthetics, and intoxicants.

Hypothermia: the state of low body temperature.

Hypovolemia: diminished blood supply.

Immunosuppressive: acting to suppress the body's natural immune response to an antigen.

Induction: the process of causing or producing; in anesthesia, the period from the initial inhalation or injection until optimum level of anesthesia is reached.

Intervention: the act of coming in or between so as to modify.

Lethargy: a condition of sluggishness; stupor.

Maladaptive: poorly adjusted; inability to adapt.

Mesentery: a peritoneal fold connecting the intestine with the postabdominal wall.

Narcotic: producing stupor or sleep; a drug that depresses the central nervous system.

Neurohormonal: concerning the interaction between nerves and hormones.

Orthopedic: concerning the prevention or correction of deformities of the musculoskeletal system.

Palpitation: rapid, violent, or throbbing pulsation, as an abnormally rapid, throbbing, or fluttering heart.

Peritonitis: inflammation of the peritoneum.

Pneumonia: inflammation of the lungs caused primarily by bacteria, viruses, and chemical agents; can be characterized by chills, high fever, pain in the chest, cough, and purulent and often bloody sputum.

Stress: a mentally or emotionally disruptive or disquieting influence; distress.

Therapeutic: having medicinal or healing properties.

Thrombophlebitis: inflammation of a vein associated with thrombus.

Topical: pertinent to a particular area; local.

Trauma: a physical injury or wound caused by external force or violence; an emotional or psychologic shock that may produce disordered feelings to behavior.

Vaso: a word part meaning vessel, as a blood vessel.

Vasoconstriction: constriction of a blood vessel.

NURSE'S ROLE

Nurses take an active role in the psychologic and physiologic preparation of the surgical client. Nurses instruct the preoperative client in stress-reduction techniques, expectations for the postoperative period, and use of special postoperative equipment. In fact, many hospitals provide time for the operating room nurse to make postoperative visits to clients to assess the client's evaluation of the surgical intervention.

PERIOPERATIVE STAGES

The first stage of the perioperative period is the *preoperative stage.* During this stage a thorough physical assessment of the client is completed. The nurse records all baseline data and reports any alteration from normal to the surgeon and anesthesiologist. Client teaching and interviewing are also completed during this period. The physical preparation of the client includes preoperative skin preparation, identifying the correct client in the operating room, and the preoperative scrub.

The *intraoperative stage* is the period from the surgery until the client is admitted to the recovery room. During the intraoperative stage, nursing interventions focus on the surgical scrub, positioning, and safety measures.

The *postoperative stage* can be divided into three segments. The immediate postoperative period includes the care given to the client in the recovery room and in the first few hours on the surgical floor. The intermediate period usually involves the care given during the course of surgical convalescence to the time of discharge. The third segment in the postoperative stage is discharge planning, teaching, and referral.

Besides nursing care, nursing management during the postoperative period centers on assessing the client's postoperative condition and monitoring for complications. It also includes client teaching, pain control, and psychologic support of both the client and family.

In each phase of the client's perioperative experience—preoperative, intraoperative, and postoperative—physiologic elements are affected by the threat of the surgical trauma, the actual trauma, and the response to the trauma. The predominance of each element varies in each operative phase.

PREOPERATIVE ANXIETY

Admission to the hospital and anticipation of surgery result in some degree of anxiety and stress. Stress is a physiologic and psychologic response to a stressor—a demand to adapt. Anxiety is a stress response to an existing stressor. The degree of anxiety and stress depends on many factors.

- The client's likelihood of reacting to anticipated stressors with high anxiety.
- The number of stress-producing events that have occurred recently in the client's life or within the client's family.
- The client's perceptions of the hospitalization and surgical experience.

TABLE 30–1. Responses to Anxiety States

Low Anxiety	High Anxiety
Less likely to react with high anxiety to stressors	Likely to react with high anxiety to stressors
Few changes in personal situation in recent past	Many changes in personal situation in recent past
Perceives hospital and surgical experience as beneficial	Perceives hospital and surgical experience as threatening
Believes surgery will end chronic problem	Fears that surgery may lead to pain, disability, and possibly death
Regards admission procedures as friendly and supportive	Regards admission procedures as strange and frightening
Finds hospital conditions comfortable and the nursing staff supportive and informative	Finds hospital conditions unbearable and the nursing staff nonsupportive

- The significance of the surgery to the client.
- The number of unknowns that confront the client on admission.
- The client's degree of self-esteem and self-image.
- The client's belief system and religious conviction.

The body responds physiologically to an actual or perceived threat. The hypothalamus controls a neurohormonal response. The heart rate is increased, and the heart contracts more forcefully. Blood volume is redistributed by vasoconstriction of the vessels in the skin, stomach, mesentery, and kidneys. Increased blood volume increases cardiac output. Increased blood flow to the skeletal muscles results in the muscles becoming tensed for action. The bronchi dilate, and the increased respiratory rate increases oxygenation. Mechanisms that provide energy include increased glucose release and decreased insulin production.

Behavioral responses to stress or anxiety can be adaptive or maladaptive (Table 30–1). Adaptive behaviors are purposeful. The client adapts to a stressful situation by preparing to face it or by removing the threat. Maladaptive behaviors result from the inability to adapt to a stressful situation.

One of the objectives of providing preoperative care is to identify the level of stress present in the client. If nursing interventions can be planned that reduce high anxiety levels, the result is a safer intraoperative period. High levels of anxiety can prevent successful preoperative adaptation and can negatively influence postoperative recovery. Mild anxiety, on the other hand, increases alertness, increases the ability to learn, and increases the ability to assess and to adjust to one's environment. Mild anxiety also increases the ability to adjust to several simultaneous stressors. In the preoperative client this level of anxiety is adaptive in nature, while a high level is maladaptive. When levels of anxiety or stress become intolerably high, defense mechanisms are unconsciously implemented to reduce the distress by concealing, falsifying, or distorting reality.

Preoperative anxiety is increased by ambiguity, conflicting perceptions, misconceptions, fears of the unknown, and bombardment by many simultaneous stressors. Ambiguity occurs from uncertainty or vagueness concerning the hospital environment, preoperative procedures, intraoperative procedures, or postoperative events.

Conflicting perceptions occur when preconceived notions about the operative experience are different from those actually encountered. The client who thought that a herniorrhaphy would be a quick, safe cure can become quite anxious after the anesthesiologist informs him or her of potential complications.

Misconceptions arise when inaccurate information is given, when terminology is not understood, and when events are not explained clearly. A client who is scheduled for a bronchoscopy in the morning, and whose nurse silently places an n.p.o. sign over the bed, may believe that he is destined for the same hospital regimen as his roommate, who had a gastrectomy.

The stress responses are additive. An increasing number of stressors can eventually drain adaptive energy. The newly admitted surgical client who has been confronted with many stressors before admission is more likely to respond with a higher level of stress as each new stressor is encountered.

Psychologic preparation includes preoperative teaching of the client and the family as well as the administration of preoperative medications (Table 30–2). Preoperative teaching prepares the client by explaining the events that will occur preoperatively and postoperatively. Preoperative teaching reduces stress by minimizing the client's fears—fears of the unknown, pain, anesthesia, and loss of control. Many hospitals have teaching programs developed for the surgical client. Group teaching sessions are valuable ways of disseminating information.

TABLE 30–2. Managing Surgical Clients

Conscientious preoperative care of clients prevents postoperative complications.
▪ Preparing the client psychologically reduces the client's stress level and helps to prevent postoperative complications.
▪ Teaching coughing and deep breathing exercises, procedures for getting out of bed, and uses of specialized equipment enhance the client's cooperation and prevents postoperative complications.
▪ Completing the surgical scrub reduces microorganisms on the body surface and the possibility of wound infections postoperatively.
Scrupulous asepsis throughout the perioperative period reduces complications.
▪ Maintaining strict asepsis reduces cross-contamination.
▪ Identifying breaks in sterile technique and taking appropriate action decrease the risk of postoperative complications.

Postoperative complications can also be decreased by reducing stress levels. Prolonged high stress levels are associated with deficient immune systems, stress ulcers, hypertension, life-threatening arrhythmias, sodium and water retention, and congestive heart failure.

The need for frequent and high doses of analgesia is reduced when stress levels are low and when clients are assured of pain relief when they need it. Levels of stress closely correlate with levels of perceived pain. Reduction of stress reduces perceived pain. Anxiety levels are increased when the client envisions having to endure pain without relief. Assurance that medication is available and encouragement to use the medication for relief reduces anxiety significantly.

The degree of client participation in recovery affects the complication rate. Effective pulmonary care significantly curtails the most frequent postoperative complications—atelectasis and pneumonia. The client's active and willing participation in deep breathing, coughing, use of incentive spirometers, and early ambulation enhance a rapid recovery and thus shorten hospitalization.

The influence of the family can also affect the client's recovery. In many cases, the client's strongest support system is the family. To be an effective support system, the family must be informed. Also, the anxiety and stress of each family member must be within tolerable limits. Knowledge of the client's problems, type of surgery proposed, and recovery rate allow the family to provide support. The knowledgeable family can reinforce preoperative teaching for each other and the client.

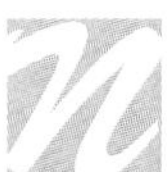

NURSING DIAGNOSES

The following nursing diagnoses are appropriate to use on client care plans when the components are related to perioperative care.

NURSING DIAGNOSIS	RELATED FACTORS
Ineffective Airway Clearance	Pulmonary secretions, allergic response, medications, suppressed cough reflex, decreased oxygen intake, pain, mechanical obstruction
Anxiety	Surgical outcome, helplessness, threat to body image
Ineffective Denial	Impending surgery, diagnosis, and expected outcome
Ineffective Individual Coping	Inadequate support system, change in body integrity, unrealistic expectations regarding surgical outcome, stress from surgery
Knowledge Deficit	Inadequate preoperative teaching, lack of motivation, cognitive limitation
Pain	Surgical incision, trauma, stress, immobility

unit 1

STRESS IN PREOPERATIVE CLIENTS

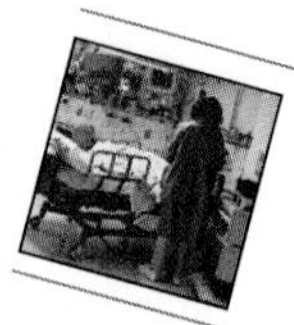

NURSING PROCESS DATA

ASSESSMENT Data Base

Identify if high level of stress exists.

Assess exaggerated anxiety or stress behaviors.

Evaluate defensive behaviors.

Assess client's vulnerability to number and significance of changes in life before admission.

Evaluate client's level of knowledge and perceptions of the impending surgery and perioperative period.

PLANNING Objectives

To identify the level of stress and anxiety present in preoperative clients

To provide interventions that decrease stress levels and promote optimal preoperative behavioral and physiologic responses

To observe for use of defensive behaviors that mask a failure to adapt appropriately in stressful situations

To prepare the client for a smooth preoperative and postoperative period

To prevent postoperative complications

IMPLEMENTATION Procedures

Preventing Anxiety and Stress

Reducing Anxiety and Stress

Assisting the Client Who Uses Denial

EVALUATION Expected Outcomes

Client's level of stress and anxiety is identified.

Nursing interventions are provided that decrease stress levels and promote optimal preoperative responses.

Denial, as a defense mechanism, is identified in the client.

PREVENTING ANXIETY AND STRESS

Procedure

1. Establish a trusting relationship.
2. Encourage verbalization of feelings.
3. Listen attentively.
4. Communicate acceptance of the client as an individual.
5. Identify the client's needs (Table 30–3) and keep the charge nurse informed of them.
6. Give adequate information regarding hospital procedures.
   a. Hospital environment, including sights, sounds, and equipment
   b. Hospital personnel and routine procedures: mealtimes, telephone usage, call light
   c. Ordered preoperative procedures: lab tests, diagnostic procedures (explain the sensory experiences that will be encountered)
   d. Scheduled time of surgery
   e. Hospital regulations: visiting hours, children's age for visiting
   f. Preoperative procedures: skin preparation,

TABLE 30–3. Preoperative Stress Assessment

Physiologic Responses	Emotional and Defensive Responses	Anxiety and Activity Responses
Heart rate: rate increases 10 BPM over baseline during three observations	Withdrawal: daydreaming, increased time in sleep, unwillingness to talk, disinterest	Hyperactivity: pacing, hand-wringing, lip or nail biting, finger-tapping, impatience, irritability, insomnia
Presence of palpitations	Anger: resentment, aggressiveness, noncompliance, swearing, boasting, attempts to gain control and independence	Disorganization of thought: repetitive speech, constant conversation, difficulty concentrating
Blood pressure: increases more than 10 mm Hg over baseline during three observations	Denial: joking, carefree attitude, inappropriate laughter, refusal to discuss impending surgery	Increased sensitivity to environmental noise, light, temperature, activity
Respiratory rate: increases more than five per minute over baseline during three observations.		Increased muscle tensing: furrowed eyebrows, facial tics, clenched jaws, loud or high-pitched voice, stammering, rapid speech, elevated shoulders, clenched fists, urinary frequency, tension or inability to relax
Vasoconstriction of blood vessels near the skin: cool, pale fingers and toes; increased capillary filling time of more than 3 seconds		Increased energy and preparedness: restlessness, easily startled, increased activity level
Vasoconstriction of renal vessels: decreased urine output compared with baseline and fluid intake		
Vasoconstriction of gastric and mesenteric vessels: anorexia, nausea, vomiting, abdominal distention with flatus, decreased bowel sounds, hyperactivity, diarrhea		

n.p.o., medications, side rails, dentures, nail polish

g. Anticipated postoperative events: recovery room, pain and pain medications, coughing and deep breathing exercises, dressings, IVs

REDUCING ANXIETY AND STRESS

Equipment

Cassette tape player

Appropriate relaxation tape

Procedure

1. Establish a trusting relationship.
2. Encourage verbalization of feelings.
3. Use touch to communicate caring and genuine interest.
4. Avoid false reassurance.
5. Use realistic outcomes.
6. Assist client in exploring effective coping methods to reduce anxiety and/or stress.
   a. Ask the client or the family what method the client normally uses to successfully reduce stress.
   b. Provide activity: walking, range of motion.
   c. Provide a back rub to loosen tense muscles. **Rationale:** Physical relaxation will often lead to mental relaxation.
   d. Teach client relaxation techniques. One technique is to ask the client to picture a blue sky that is clear except for one white, fluffy cloud. Tell client to concentrate on this scene for 10 minutes. This technique often relaxes the mind and the body.
   e. An alternative is to ask the client to picture a favorite place (e.g., a warm, sunny beach with sand and gentle surf).
7. As the client begins to relax, reinforce success. Assist client in recognizing his or her strengths and progress.
8. Encourage self-awareness of increasing tension and immediate reversal of escalation.

ASSISTING THE CLIENT WHO USES DENIAL

Procedure

1. Establish a trusting relationship.
2. Encourage verbalization of feelings.
3. Use touch to communicate caring and genuine interest.
4. Do not attempt to enforce reality. The client is denying reality to prevent outright panic. Allow use of this defense.
5. Use techniques to reduce anxiety and stress to manageable proportions.
6. Attempt to determine the cause of the need for denial.
7. Listen for cues that indicate readiness to discuss the stressors causing the need for denial.
8. Notify physician of your findings.

CHARTING for Preoperative Stress

- Observed and subjective indications of anxiety or stress levels
- Nursing interventions used to decrease stress and the results of the intervention
- Changes that occurred as a result of the nursing interventions
- Specific fears verbalized by the client
- Nonverbal indications of stress or anxiety

CRITICAL THINKING APPLICATION

CLINICAL PROBLEMS	CRITICAL THINKING OPTIONS
■ Anxiety level increases rapidly.	• Maintain calm composure, and speak in a soft, caring manner. • Use touch to communicate caring and peacefulness. • Reinforce client self-acceptance as an individual. • If unable to achieve success with stress-reducing techniques, notify physician.
■ Client becomes angry or hostile.	• Maintain calm composure. • Accept anger, but place limits on how it may be expressed (e.g., no destructive behavior). Understand that anger is usually the result of feeling helpless and powerless to change an intolerable situation. • Do not reward this behavior, but explore other means of meeting client's needs. • Do not isolate client, but continue to respond to needs. • Notify physician of client's behaviors and the actions you used to decrease anger or hostility.
■ Client becomes depressed because of overwhelming anxiety and feelings of helplessness or hopelessness.	• Convey respect and belief that the client is worthwhile. Question the client's appraisal of reality, and provide support while the client works through his or her feelings. • Provide positive feedback and recognition of strengths, progress, and improved self-esteem. • Spend additional time with the client to allow time to verbalize fears.

unit 2

PREOPERATIVE TEACHING

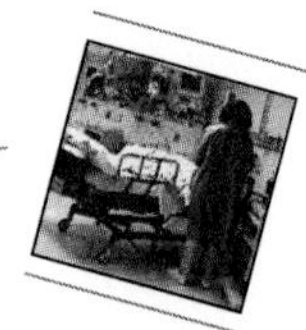

NURSING PROCESS DATA

ASSESSMENT Data Base

Identify type of surgical procedure client will experience.

Determine type of anesthesia client will use.

Assess client's learning needs.

Determine most appropriate method of client teaching.

Assess client's willingness and ability to learn.

Determine availability of prepared audiovisual material or printed information regarding surgical procedure.

PLANNING Objectives

To reinforce physician's explanation of surgical procedure and answer questions regarding treatment

To identify client's readiness to learn about surgical treatment

To select appropriate time and place for client instruction regarding surgery

To provide instruction in measures to prevent postoperative complications

To provide a time for client to ask questions regarding surgical procedure

To instruct client in use of special equipment required during the postoperative period

To provide tour of specialty units, such as critical care unit, lithotripsy, or laser rooms

IMPLEMENTATION Procedures

Providing Surgical Information

for the Preoperative Client

for the Intraoperative Client

for the Postoperative Client

Providing Client Teaching

Providing Family Teaching

Providing Teaching for Laser Therapy

Providing Teaching for Lithotripsy

Instructing in Deep Breathing Exercises

Instructing in Coughing Exercises

Providing Instruction to Turn in Bed

Instructing in Leg Exercises

EVALUATION Expected Outcomes

Client is psychologically and physically prepared for surgery.

Client is able to demonstrate deep breathing, coughing, turning, and leg exercises accurately.

Client is able to verbalize knowledge of operative procedure, potential problems, and expected nursing actions postoperatively.

Client's family is informed about what to expect during perioperative period.

Appropriate audiovisual and written materials are used for client understanding of perioperative experience.

Client's fears are allayed regarding special equipment used during perioperative experience.

Client is aware of safety precautions used with laser and lithotripsy surgery.

PROVIDING SURGICAL INFORMATION

Equipment

Quiet room for client and family where there will be no interruptions during the teaching program

Equipment that may be used postoperatively by the client (e.g., IV bag and tubing, drainage tubes, nasogastric tube, cardiac monitor and electrodes)

Procedure

for the Preoperative Client

1. Blood work, ECG, urinalysis, chest x-ray.
2. Preoperative skin preparation.
3. Placement of nasogastric tube, Foley catheter, as indicated.
4. Enema or special bowel preparation as ordered.
5. Use of medications preoperatively and postoperatively.
6. Deep breathing and coughing exercises (use of spirometer or Triflow if indicated).
7. Leg exercises and antiembolic stockings.
8. Turning and moving in bed.
9. Use of postoperative medications for pain control; PCA.
10. Reason for n.p.o. and when it begins.
11. Alterations in diet preoperatively or postoperatively.
12. Activities and preparation the morning of surgery.
13. Need for quiet environment after medications have been given.
14. Information usually provided by anesthesiologist and surgeon.
15. Tour and explanation of monitoring devices and special equipment in ICU if client is to be transferred there postoperatively.

for the Intraoperative Client

1. Mode of transportation to operating room.
2. Discussion of procedure in preinduction room or operating room suite in relationship to anesthesia.
3. Reinforce physician's explanation of surgery.
4. Description of dressings, tubes, or equipment that will be used postoperatively.
5. Recovery room physical environment and procedures.
6. Administration of oxygen.
7. Administration of medications.

for the Postoperative Client

1. Assessment procedures.
2. Routine procedures of vital signs.
3. Deep breathing, turning, and coughing exercises.
4. IV therapy if indicated.
5. Irrigation of tubes when directed.
6. Catheter care.
7. Dietary alterations.
8. Observation and changes of dressing.
9. Ambulation or restrictions in ambulation.
10. Medications.
11. Anticipated discharge and plans for referral.

PROVIDING CLIENT TEACHING

Equipment

Prepared teaching aids when available: audio-visual, filmstrips, pamphlets, pictures, posters, programmed learning modules, slides, cassette tapes, overhead transparencies

Procedure

1. Assess client's knowledge base and readiness to learn. **Rationale:** This provides framework for client education at the level client can understand.
   a. Determine the information provided to client by physician by reading physician's progress notes and asking client specific questions.
   b. Identify client's psychosocial status and ability to listen to teaching by communicating with client and asking direct questions.
   c. Be alert for cultural or religious beliefs that may influence client's surgical experience.
2. Develop individualized teaching plan based on client's needs.
   a. Choose appropriate equipment for teaching, based on client's level of understanding and knowledge base.

b. Review information previously provided. **Rationale:** To determine retention of information and needless repetition of information already mastered.
c. Choose a quiet environment, and provide for sufficient time to allow client to ask questions. **Rationale:** To ensure client understands impending surgical experience.
d. Be alert for clues indicating client confusion or misunderstanding of information. **Rationale:** Misunderstanding information can be detrimental to the client's sense of well-being.

3. Select appropriate audiovisual materials to assist with teaching.
4. Demonstrate use of special equipment or devices (e.g., incentive spirometer, chest tubes, suction equipment).
5. Evaluate client teaching by assessing client's ability to return demonstration of exercises and verbally answer specific questions. Reinforce information or provide additional data as needed.

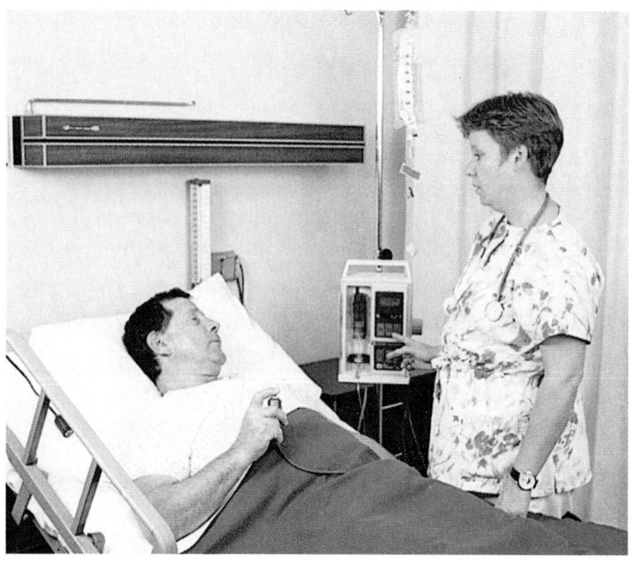

Demonstrate use of special equipment in preoperative teaching plan.

PROVIDING FAMILY TEACHING

Procedure

1. Include family in teaching provided to client.
2. Instructions to family members should include:
   a. Visiting hours
   b. Where to wait during surgery
   c. Where the surgeon will meet with them, and when
   d. Where they can find bathrooms, telephones, and food and beverage service
   e. When they can see the client after surgery.
3. How to contact a spiritual or religious resource person.
4. How they can best get information regarding the client's condition while they are at home or in the hospital.
5. Whether they will be called if there is a change in the client's condition.
6. What to expect: client's behavior, which may be regressive; attitude which may be depressed or angry; physical condition, which may appear worse than it is, and postrecovery period.

PROVIDING TEACHING FOR LASER THERAPY

Procedure

1. Determine type of laser (Table 30–4) to be used for surgery.
2. Identify client and introduce yourself.
3. Determine client's willingness to accept instruction.
4. Determine most appropriate time and place for instruction.
5. Identify client's level of understanding of surgical procedure and what information physician has provided (Table 30–5).
6. Reinforce explanation of surgical procedure by physician as needed.
7. Describe operating room setting or outpatient setting, including the environment.
8. Explain that client and operating room staff will wear goggles. **Rationale:** Goggles protect eyes from the laser beam.

9. Explain the use of wet drapes placed over client's skin if required. **Rationale:** Wet drapes prevent skin from burns when some types of laser therapy are used.
10. Describe that laser machine may be very noisy.
11. Describe physician's actions during laser therapy. Physician will discharge laser by using a foot pedal while at the same time issuing instructions to nurses using terms such as, "fire," "watt seconds," and "standby." **Rationale:** Describing these words to client allays fear of unfamiliar terms or actual fire. It also describes nurses' role of regulating power and duration of laser beam use.
12. Caution client, if under local anesthesia, he or she may feel heat and smell smoke and a burning odor from tissue being lased.
13. Instruct client to tell physician if pain occurs. **Rationale:** Additional anesthetic may need to be administered as patient should not feel pain.
14. Instruct client to maintain n.p.o. status 6–8 hours before surgery.
15. Instruct client in postoperative care specific to procedure performed.

TABLE 30–4. Types of Laser*

Types	Uses
Carbon dioxide	High-precision cutting instrument used in areas where function must be preserved (e.g., vocal cords, brain)
Nd:YAG	Laser made of a neodymium alloy, yttrium, aluminum, and garnet crystals. Beam penetrates deeply; can be passed through flexible fibers for cardiovascular laser therapy and scopes (e.g., cystoscope, bronchoscope, and endoscope to treat bladder and lung tumors and coagulate esophageal varices)
Argon	Used for ophthalmic and dermatologic procedures (e.g., treating glaucoma, cataract, retinal detachment, and removing birthmarks, hemangiomas)
Liquid dye	Used for diagnostic procedures and in conjunction with drugs for photodynamic treatment (e.g., lithotripsy)

* Light amplification by the stimulated emission of radiation. Choice of laser type is determined by procedure required for treatment.

TABLE 30–5. Common Types of Laser Surgical Procedures and Complications

Procedure	Client Teaching	Assessment Findings for Potential Complications
Pulmonary	Gag reflex returns in 2–4 hours Begin taking fluids when gag reflex returns Expect hoarseness, dyspnea, sore throat, difficulty swallowing for 48–72 hours	Bright red blood expectorated related to hemorrhage. Use of accessory muscles for breathing related to tracheal edema Wheezing related to airway obstruction. Pneumonia and respiratory insufficiency related to aspiration of secretions. Altered arterial blood gases and sudden pain causing altered vital signs related to pneumothorax.
Upper GI	May experience burning sensation in esophagus May experience difficulty swallowing Heartburn present for 3 days	Poor skin turgor and decreased urine output related to dysphagia or dehydration. Vomiting bright red blood related to colon perforation Vomiting and abdominal distention related to obstruction of GI tract due to edema.
Urology	May experience traces of blood or sooty material in urine for 24 hours Catheter may be left in place for 24 hours Urinary frequency and urgency may occur for 1 week	Bright red urine related to hemorrhage. Abdominal pain related to perforated bladder.
Cardiovascular	May experience slight burning or chest pain over coronary vessels	Arrhythmias related to hypoxia or laser treatment. Bleeding at site of percutaneous laser angioplasty area related to catheter insertion Intake and output values altered related to osmotic contract media used for laser treatment.

16. Instruct client to notify physician if temperature is above 100°F for more than 24 hours following laser therapy. **Rationale:** Infections are unlikely but can occur, therefore, client needs to monitor for presence of symptoms.

PROVIDING TEACHING FOR LITHOTRIPSY

Preparation

1. Identify type of extracorporeal shock wave lithotripsy (ESWL) used: for gallstones or kidney stones.
2. Identify type of anesthesia that will be used: epidural, spinal, or general. General anesthesia is usually used to prevent pain as stones are crumbled and expelled.

Procedure

1. Identify client, and introduce yourself.
2. Determine client's knowledge base and information provided by physician.
3. Reinforce physician's description of procedure, as needed.
4. Answer client's questions regarding procedure.
5. Explain that lithotriptor discharges a series of shock waves through water or water-filled cushion.
6. Describe to client that he or she may feel fluttering or mild blows where shock waves are beamed. From 500–2400 shocks are required to disintegrate stones.
7. Discuss use of specialized equipment that will be used. Client may sit in tank of water or lie with water-filled cushion pressed against area of abdomen where stones are present.
8. Describe use of monitoring equipment throughout procedure. **Rationale:** The heart rate and rhythm is monitored throughout procedure and shocks synchronized with the rhythm to prevent arrhythmias.
9. Explain that the procedure takes 45 minutes to 2 hours, depending on type of procedure.
10. Describe postlithotripsy care.
    a. Following procedure, client is removed from tub, covered with warm blanket, and taken to recovery room.
    b. Vital signs are monitored as with any surgical client.
    c. Urine output is monitored for hematuria. **Rationale:** To determine kidney damage from procedure.
    d. Liver function studies are performed following lithotripsy for gallstones. **Rationale:** To assess if shock waves have damaged liver.
    e. Pain management is monitored and maintained as gravel is passed following disintegration of stones.
    f. Medication is provided for nausea and vomiting. **Rationale:** Nausea and vomiting often accompany pain.
    g. Intake and output measurements are taken. **Rationale:** Fluids are encouraged to hydrate clients with kidney stones to assist in the excretion of gravel.
    h. Catheter care is provided for kidney clients requiring indwelling catheters. **Rationale:** Indwelling catheters and ureteral stents, if used, are left in place for 24 hours to assist with passage of gravel or if second ESWL treatment is required.
    i. Exercise is encouraged to assist with passing gravel.
    j. Ecchymoses and discomfort may be felt over area of the body that experienced shock waves.
11. Provide tour of lithotriptor room, if possible.

INSTRUCTING IN DEEP BREATHING EXERCISES

Procedure

1. Identify client, and introduce yourself.
2. Explain procedure and purpose of exercises. **Rationale:** Deep breathing and coughing exercises promote lung expansion; lower the risk of pneumonia, atelectasis, and pulmonary emboli.
3. Instruct and have client demonstrate deep breathing exercises. **Rationale:** Encouraging the client to practice and return the demonstration before surgery assists him or her to deep breath more effectively after surgery.

4. Have client sit in upright position.
5. Place client's hands along lower borders of rib cage. **Rationale:** This assists client to feel adequate chest movement.
6. Instruct client to breathe through nose slowly, take a deep breath, hold 1–2 seconds, then exhale through mouth. **Rationale:** This expands alveoli and prevents hyperventilation if client is breathing too quickly.
7. Repeat exercise sequence three to four times, at least every 2 hours when awake.

INSTRUCTING IN COUGHING EXERCISES

Procedure

1. Identify client, and introduce yourself.
2. Explain procedure and purpose of exercises.
3. Instruct and have client demonstrate coughing exercises.
4. Have client sit in upright position.
5. Instruct client to splint incision when deep breathing and coughing.
6. Demonstrate placement of hands on either side of incision. Instruct client to press hands firmly toward incision during exercises. **Rationale:** This prevents tension on the suture line and diminishes pain.
7. Instruct in use of cough pillow. Place folded bath towel in pillowcase. Hold pillow directly over incision and press on pillow when performing exercises. **Rationale:** This prevents pain and discomfort by splinting the incision and reducing stress on suture line.
8. Demonstrate technique for inhaling deeply and holding breath for 1–2 seconds.
9. Instruct client to take two to three breaths slowly and exhale passively; on third breath, hold for 2–3 seconds.
10. Encourage client to cough forcefully two to three times by using abdominal and other respiratory muscles to assist with coughing. **Rationale:** This extra force provides a more effective cough.
11. Have client cough a second time.
12. Instruct client to do coughing exercises following deep breathing exercises at least every 2 hours when awake.

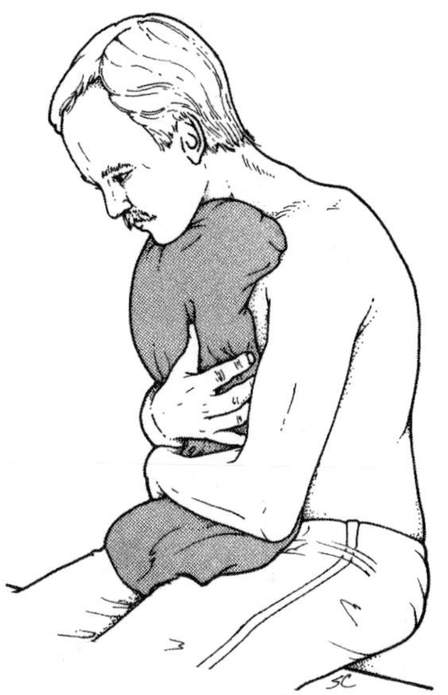

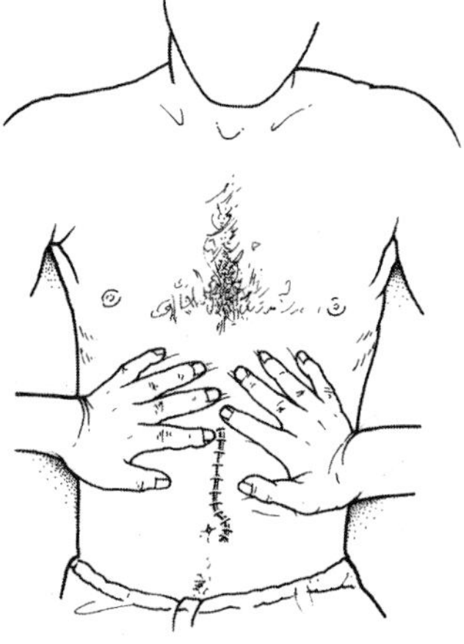

Instruct client in coughing exercises using cough pillow or demonstrate placement of hands on either side of incision for support during coughing.

PROVIDING INSTRUCTION TO TURN IN BED

Procedure

1. Identify client, and introduce yourself.
2. Explain turning procedure and purpose. **Rationale:** Turning assists in the prevention of thrombophlebitis, pressure ulcer formation, and respiratory complications.
3. Instruct and demonstrate turning procedure.
4. Instruct client to splint incision whenever turning.
5. Have client move to far side of bed with side rails up. **Rationale:** This position allows client to turn without rolling to edge of bed.
6. Instruct client to splint incision with hand on side toward which he or she will be turning. **Rationale:** This leaves the uppermost hand available to grasp side rail or trapeze to assist with turning.
7. Instruct client to keep leg straight on side to which he or she will turn.
8. Flex other leg over straight lower leg. **Rationale:** Flexing the leg assists in shifting the weight when turning to opposite side.
9. Instruct client to turn on side and grasp side rail.
10. Instruct client to move pillow into comfortable position under head and place arm into comfortable position.

INSTRUCTING IN LEG EXERCISES

Procedure

1. Identify client, and introduce yourself.
2. Explain exercise and purpose. **Rationale:** These exercises assist in preventing stasis of blood in lower extremities and thus thrombophlebitis.
3. Place client in supine or semi-Fowler's position.
4. Instruct client to bend knee, raise foot in air, and hold this position for 2–3 seconds.
5. Have client extend the leg and lower it to bed.
6. Repeat procedure with other leg.
7. Complete sequence 5–10 times each hour while awake.
8. Have client extend toes (plantar flexion) toward bottom of bed, then flex (dorsiflexion) toward head of bed.
9. Repeat foot extension and flexion with other side.
10. Repeat sequence five times each hour while awake.
11. Instruct client to make circles with the ankle moving first to the left and then to the right.
12. Repeat sequence five times each hour while awake.

CHARTING for Preoperative Teaching

- Type of instruction provided
- Amount of time provided for instruction
- Type of audiovisual materials or written information used
- Client's response to teaching
- Accuracy and participation in return demonstration exercises
- Areas of instruction that need to be reinforced
- Psychologic response to preoperative teaching and impending surgery

CRITICAL THINKING APPLICATION

CLINICAL PROBLEMS	CRITICAL THINKING OPTIONS
Client refuses to participate in preoperative teaching.	• Encourage client to state reasons for refusal. • Encourage client to discuss knowledge of surgery. • Assess if client is experiencing fear or denial regarding impending surgery. • Ask client to provide a time frame more acceptable for teaching. • Notify physician of client's refusal if facility policy.
Client unable to understand directions.	• Identify client's learning capabilities. • Determine if a language barrier exists. If so, find person who speaks client's primary language and ask for assistance with teaching. • Use different words to explain information. • Determine a different teaching strategy that the client can understand. • Evaluate client's stress level to determine if it is interfering with learning. • Establish a new time for teaching when client may be able to concentrate on teaching. • Develop a slower pace for instruction and present less information at one time.
Client not adequately prepared for surgery.	• Ascertain where data are insufficient or unclear and provide additional instruction in that area. • Use a different approach or teaching style to provide information. • Select different teaching materials that may explain information in a more useful way.
Client becomes angry or hostile.	• Maintain calm composure. • Accept anger, but place limits on how it may be expressed (e.g., destructive behavior). Understand that anger is usually the result of feeling helpless and powerless to change an intolerable situation. • Do not reward this behavior but explore other means of meeting client's needs. • Do not isolate client, but continue to respond to needs. • Notify physician of client's behaviors and actions used to decrease anger or hostility.
Client becomes depressed because of overwhelming anxiety and feelings of helplessness or hopelessness.	• Convey respect and belief that client is worthwhile. Question client's appraisal of reality; provide support while client works through feelings. • Provide positive feedback and recognition of strengths, progress, and improved self-esteem. • Spend additional time with the client to allow time to verbalize fears.

unit 3

PREOPERATIVE CARE

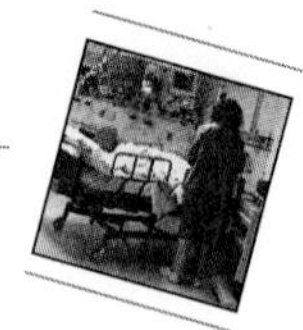

NURSING PROCESS DATA

ASSESSMENT Data Base

Assess type of surgical procedure to be carried out and extent of data base needed.

Evaluate the client's ability to provide accurate information.

Assess level of anxiety present that may interfere in the transmission of information at that moment.

Identify the appropriate physical care needed for the specific surgical intervention.

Assess special needs for the surgical shave.

Check if a special permit is needed for shaving, such as the head for neurosurgic clients, extremities for orthopedic clients, or children.

Check for need for special soap or antiseptic scrub prior to shave.

Check if sterile drape is required following shave.

Check if a policy exists in the hospital for disposing or handling of scalp hair.

Assess surgical site before preparing; observe for unusual cuts, abrasions, or markings, and report findings to charge nurse.

PLANNING Objectives

To assist with monitoring the client's progress through the operative experience

To assist in identifying deviations from the client's baseline data that may occur as a result of anxiety or stress of admission, preoperative events, diagnostic procedures, the surgical trauma, postoperative complications, responses to and side effects of drugs

To provide appropriate preoperative physical care to enable the client to have a safe intraoperative and postoperative period

To report client's statements about allergies or chronic problems that could affect postoperative nursing care

To complete a surgical prep correctly

IMPLEMENTATION Procedures

Obtaining Baseline Data

Preparing the Surgical Site

Preparing the Client for Surgery

Administering Preoperative Medications

EVALUATION Expected Outcomes

The client's physical or emotional deviations from normal are identified preoperatively.

Preoperative baseline data is obtained.

Explicit preoperative care is provided to ensure a safe intraoperative and postoperative course.

Surgical site is prepared correctly.

OBTAINING BASELINE DATA

Equipment

Thermometer
Sphygmomanometer and stethoscope
Chart for documenting findings

Procedure

1. Establish rapport with the client.
2. Ask about allergies to drugs or food.
3. Take and record vital signs and weight of client.
4. Check if client wears dentures, hearing aid, or glasses, or has an artificial eye.
5. Record any unusual stress or anxiety exhibited by the client.
6. Complete a physical assessment and health history. Report unusual findings to physician.
7. Evaluate lab values for abnormalities (ECG, x-rays, blood work, and urinalysis).
8. Identify areas requiring client teaching.

PREPARING THE SURGICAL SITE

Equipment

Wash cloth and towels
Absorbent pad
Bath blanket or drape
Scissors or clippers
Disposable prep kit (for shaving)
If kit not available:
- Disposable razor (number according to area to be shaved)
- 2 sterile bowls
- 4 × 4 gauze pads
- Emesis basin
- Applicator sticks
- Cleansing solution
- Sterile water

Clean gloves
Depilatory
Antiseptic soap
Tongue blade
4 × 4 gauze pad

Procedure

1. Refer to physician's orders for specific operative site or area to be prepared. If orders do not state preference for site, refer to procedure manual for appropriate area to be prepared, based on surgical procedure.
2. Determine type of preparation to be done: clipping of hair, shaving site, or hair removal using depilatory. Gather equipment.
3. Explain procedure to client, and provide privacy.
4. Adjust light to ensure good visualization.
5. Wash your hands.
6. Position client for maximum comfort and site exposure.
7. Drape client for comfort and to prevent undue exposure.
8. Protect bed with absorbent pad.
9. Arrange equipment for your convenience.
10. Put on clean gloves.
11. Prepare site using scissors or clippers.
    a. Use scissors or clippers and cut hair 1 cm above skin site.
    b. Clip small amount of hair each time.
    c. Cut in direction hair grows.
    d. Remove all hair from site, and discard.
12. Prepare site using depilatory.
    a. Clip hair before applying cream.
    b. Apply cream to designated area using tongue blade or gloved hand.
    c. Leave on skin for designated time, according to directions on package, usually 10 minutes.
    d. Remove cream by rubbing off with tongue blade or moistened 4 × 4 gauze pads.
    e. Wash skin with antiseptic soap; dry area thoroughly.
    f. Remove all hair with washing. **Rationale:** This provides a clean, smooth, skin free of abrasions and cuts.

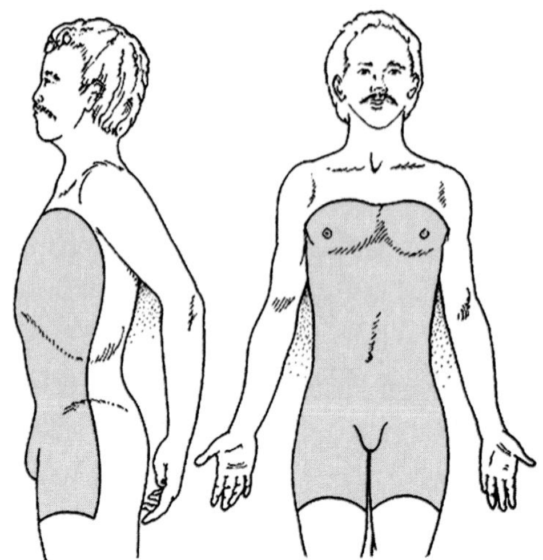

The area shaved for abdominal surgeries.

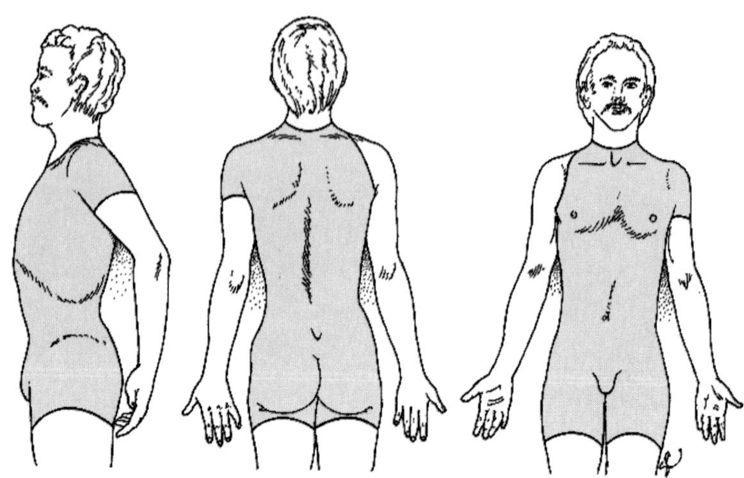

Areas shaved for thoracotomy and upper abdominal surgeries.

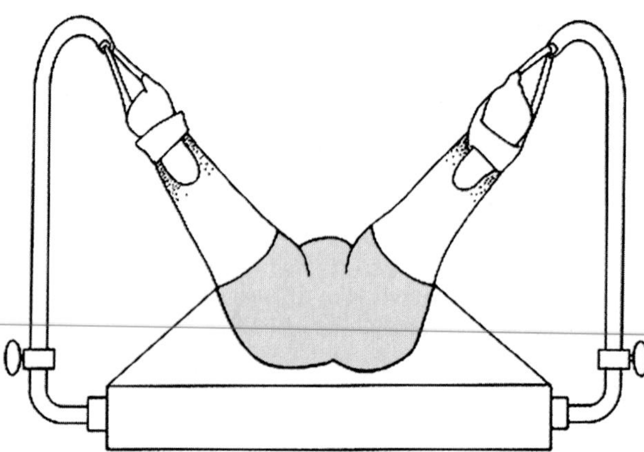

Shaved area for gynecological surgery.

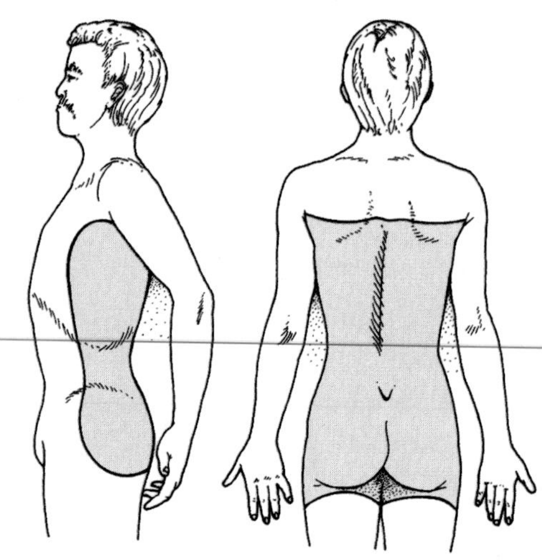

Shaved areas for laminectomy and renal surgery.

13. Prepare site using razor.
    a. Lather skin with antiseptic solution and 4 × 4 gauze pads.
    b. Discard soiled sponges frequently.
    c. Using sharp razor, shave hair moving away from incision site. With free hand, stretch skin taut and shave, following the hair growth pattern and using firm, steady strokes. Shave small area at one time. **Rationale:** Shave is closer and nicks are prevented.
    d. Change razor as often as necessary. Avoid nicking the skin. Report if skin is nicked. **Rationale:** Nicks, if severe, can cause infection by bacteria normally found on the skin.
    e. Wash all hair off site with 4 × 4 gauze pads.
14. After removing hair, apply cleansing solution with 4 × 4 pads.
15. Begin at incision site and, with light friction, make ever-widening circles, moving outward from the center to the most distant line of area. **Rationale:** Working from most clean to least clean area prevents contamination. Scrub area for 2–3 minutes.
16. Rinse area with warm water and blot dry with 4 × 4 gauze pads.
17. Remove gloves, and discard.
18. Assist client to put on clean gown.
19. Remove and dispose of equipment; scissors and razors are disposed of in sharps container.
20. Position the client for comfort.

PREPARING THE CLIENT FOR SURGERY

Equipment

Preoperative check list

Specific equipment needed to provide physical care as ordered, such as enema equipment, nasogastric tube, Foley catheter

Operative permit

Procedure

1. Obtain client's signature on preoperative permit.
2. Administer enema if ordered.
3. Complete skin prep if ordered.

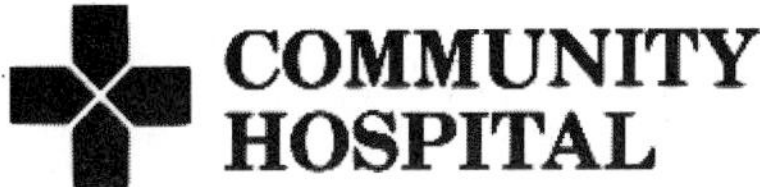

COMMUNITY HOSPITAL

Client Information

AUTHORIZATION FOR AND CONSENT TO SURGERY, ADMINISTRATION OF ANESTHETICS, SPECIAL DIAGNOSTIC OR THERAPEUTIC PROCEDURES

Date ______________ Time ______________

Your admitting physician is ______________________________, M. D.

Your surgeon is ______________________________, M. D.

1. The hospital staff and facilities assist your physicians and surgeons in the performance of various surgical operations and other diagnostic and therapeutic procedures. These surgical operations and special diagnostic or therapeutic procedures all may involve calculated risks of complications, injury or even death, from both known and unknown causes and no warranty or guarantee has been made as to result or cure. Except in a case of emergency or exceptional circumstances, these operations and procedures are not performed upon clients unless and until the client has had an opportunity to discuss them with his/her physician. Each client has the right to consent to or refuse any proposed operation or special procedure (based upon the description or explanation received).
2. Your physicians and surgeons have determined that the operations or special procedures listed below may be beneficial in the diagnosis or treatment of your condition. Upon your authorization and consent, the operations or special procedures will be performed by your physicians and surgeons and their staff. The persons in attendance for the purpose of administering anesthesia or performing other specialized professional services, such as radiology, pathology and the like, are not the agents, servants or employees of the hospital or your physician or surgeon, but are independent contractors performing specialized services on your behalf and, as such, are your agents, servants, or employees. Any tissue or member severed in any operation will be disposed of in the discretion of the pathologist, except ______________________ and those body parts specified as donor organs.
3. Your signature opposite the operations or special procedures listed below constitutes your acknowledgement (a) that you have read and agreed to the foregoing, (b) that the operations or special procedures have been adequately explained to you by your attending physicians or surgeons and that you have all of the information that you desire, and (c) that you authorize and consent to the performance of the operations or special procedures.

Operation or Procedure

____

____

Signature ______________________ Signature ______________________
Client Witness

(If client is a minor or unable to sign, complete the following): Client is a minor, is unable to sign because

____

____
Father Guardian

____
Mother Other person and relationship

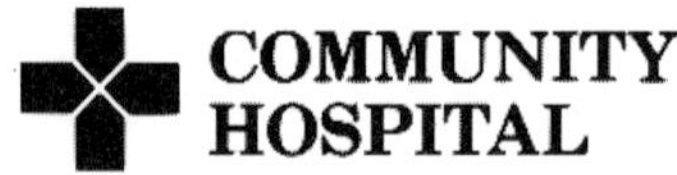

Client Information

SURGICAL CHECK LIST

Unit Check List — PLEASE PRINT

1. Surgical Procedure scheduled: ______ Rt. Lt. (circle)
2. Consent for surgery ______ Yes or No
3. Consent for Sterilization or Special Procedure ______ Yes or No
4. Consultation ______ Yes or No
5. Surgical Prep done by ______ (Signature)
6. History and Physical ______ Yes or No
7. Urinalysis ______ Yes or No CBC ______ Yes or No Type & Xmatch ______ Yes or No
8. Chest X-ray ______ Yes or No EKG ______ Yes or No
9. List allergies (if none, state "none") ______
10. Allergy Band ______ Yes or No
11. TPR ______ BP ______
12. Voided ______ Time ______ Retention Cath. ______ Yes or No
13. Pre-op medication and times ______
14. Condition after pre-op medication: ______ awake asleep drowsy (circle)

15. Prosthesis:	None	Removed	Disposition	Left In
a. Bridge				
b. Partial				
c. Plates				
d. Artificial limbs				
e. Artificial eyes				
f. Contact lenses				
g. Hearing aid				
h. Pacemaker				
i. Hairpieces, Hairpins, Eyelashes				

16. Valuables	Removed Yes or No	Disposition, if yes
a. Rings		
b. Watch		
c. Medal and chain		
d. Glasses		
e. Radio		
f. Wallet		
g. Other		

17. Identification band checked with chart ______ Yes or No

Signature ______ R.N.

Operating Room Check List

Check — Comment

1. ______
2. ______
3. ______
4. ______
5. ______
6. ______
7. ______
8. ______
9. ______
10. ______
11. ______
12. ______
13. ______
14. ______
15. ______
 a. ______
 b. ______
 c. ______
 d. ______
 e. ______
 f. ______
 g. ______
 h. ______
 i. ______
16. ______
17. ______

Signature ______ Circulating Nurse

POSTOPERATIVE

Sponge Count ______

Needle Count ______

Drains Left In ______

Catheter In ______

Scrub Nurse ______

Signature ______ Circulating Nurse

4. Observe for signs of cold or upper respiratory infection.
5. Explain need for client to be n.p.o. for 8–10 hours preoperatively.
6. Remove lipstick and nail polish.
7. Provide preoperative showers with bacteriostatic soap.
8. Insert Foley catheter if ordered.
9. Take and record vital signs.
10. Remove earrings, necklaces, medals, watch, rings (ring may be taped to finger in some facilities).
11. Remove contact lenses, glasses, hair pieces, and dentures.
12. Assist client to void if catheter not inserted, and record time and amount.
13. Place surgical cap on client's head.
14. Administer preoperative medications.
15. Place side rails in UP position following administration of medications.
16. Darken room, and provide quiet environment following administration of medications.
17. Check client 15 minutes after medication administered to observe for side effects.

CONDITIONS THAT PLACE CLIENTS AT RISK FOR POSTOPERATIVE INFECTION

- Uncontrolled diabetes
- Renal failure
- Obesity
- Receiving corticosteroids
- Receiving immunosuppressive agents
- Prolonged antibiotic therapy
- Protein or ascorbic acid deficiencies
- Marked dehydration and hypovolemia
- Decreased cardiac output
- Edema and fluid and electrolyte imbalances
- Anemia
- Preoperative infection

ADMINISTERING PREOPERATIVE MEDICATIONS

Equipment

Preoperative check list
Preoperative medications

Procedure

1. Complete preoperative check list.
2. Check orders for medication, dosage, route, and time.
3. Check history for allergy to ordered medication.
4. Explain the purpose of the medication to the client.
5. Warn the client that the injection may sting or burn.
6. Follow procedure for administration of injections.
7. Administer medication.
8. Raise side rails to UP position.
9. Explain why the client should not get out of bed after the medications have been given. **Rationale:** Medication makes the client drowsy and affects equilibrium.
10. Place the call light within reach, and encourage the client to use it.
11. Ask if there are any questions or assistance you can offer before leaving the room. Darken the room or close curtains.
12. Give the client the estimated time of surgery.

PREOPERATIVE MEDICATIONS: TYPE AND ACTION

Hypnotic or opiate—given night before surgery

- Decreases anxiety
- Promotes good night's sleep

Hypnotic or opiate—preoperative medication

- Decreases anxiety
- Allows smooth anesthetic induction
- Provides amnesia for immediate perioperative period

Anticholinergic—preoperative medication

- Decreases secretions
- Counteracts vagal effects during anesthesia

CHARTING for Preoperative Care

- Safety measures carried out preoperatively.
- Completion of preoperative shave and area involved
- Solution used and length of time of scrub
- Operative checklist completed
- Review physician's explanation of potential surgical complications
- Physical care completed prior to surgery
- Preoperative medications given and effects of medications
- Time and method of transportation to operating room
- Preoperative teaching completed

CRITICAL THINKING APPLICATION

CLINICAL PROBLEMS	CRITICAL THINKING OPTIONS
Factors that can affect the postoperative course are identified during the preoperative care (e.g., arthritic changes in client's back, history of thrombophlebitis).	• Place information on client's care plan, and inform charge nurse about findings. • Write a note on client's chart, and alert the operating room and recovery room staff of the findings so that they can assess for the problems.
Client refuses to go to operating room without dentures.	• Explain to client that dentures are likely to be lost, broken, or inadvertently pushed to back of mouth if not removed. • If client refuses to remove dentures, alert anesthesiologist that dentures are in place.
Client unable to void before surgery.	• Run water so client can hear trickling sound to stimulate voiding. • Run warm water over perineum. • Place ammonia or oil of wintergreen on a cotton ball in urinal or bedpan.
Client appears to be abnormally stressed.	• Explore feelings and reasons for client's or family's stressed behaviors. • Explore more effective methods to reduce stress for client and family. • Provide additional stress reduction exercises. • Clarify misconceptions and inappropriate perceptions. • Introduce client to another client who has had similar surgery. • Have physician speak to client and answer questions.
Client's preoperative laboratory findings are abnormal.	• Check with laboratory to have them reevaluate if lab results are accurate. • Have laboratory rerun tests if extremely abnormal. • Notify physician of abnormal findings.

unit 4 RECOVERY ROOM CARE AND DISCHARGE

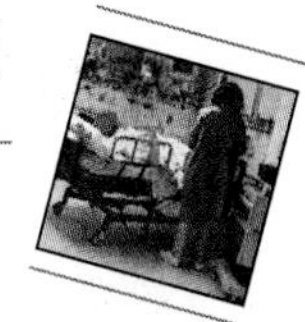

NURSING PROCESS DATA

ASSESSMENT Data Base

Assess for patent airway.

Assess for order and type of oxygen administration set.

Check gag reflex, and remove endotracheal tube as ordered.

Assess vital signs.

Assess body temperature.

Check all IVs for type, amount of fluid, and infusion rate.

Observe all dressings, tubes, and drains.

Monitor urine output, color, consistency, and odor.

Assess color, skin temperature, and condition.

Assess monitor findings if ordered.

Assess neurologic status if necessary.

Assess heart and lung sounds.

Assess bowel sounds.

PLANNING Objectives

To provide safe effective nursing care during the immediate postoperative period for clients in the recovery room

To promote and maintain adequate airway function

To monitor and maintain adequate circulatory status

To identify potential postoperative complications and initiate nursing interventions to prevent complications

To identify client's readiness to return to nursing unit or to be discharged if an outpatient

IMPLEMENTATION Procedures

Providing Recovery Room Care

Discharging Client from Recovery Room

EVALUATION Expected Outcomes

Client experiences no untoward effects during recovery room period.

Potential postoperative complications are identified early, and appropriate nursing actions are taken to prevent occurrence of complications.

Client is discharged from recovery room at appropriate time.

PROVIDING RECOVERY ROOM CARE

Equipment

Blood pressure cuff and stethoscope

Oxygen administration device: nasal cannula or mask

IV pole

Suction catheters

Gloves

Special equipment needed—based on surgical procedure

Procedure

1. Identify client, and determine surgical procedure performed.

2. Obtain report, and review chart with anesthesiologist and operating room nurse.
3. Connect client to monitoring system if needed.
4. Assess for patent airway. Leave airway in place until gag reflex returns and client attempts to remove it. **Rationale:** This promotes adequate airway exchange and prevents tongue from falling back and occluding airway.
5. Administer humidified oxygen by mask or nasal cannula at 6 L/min or as ordered. **Rationale:** Humidified oxygen prevents drying of the tracheobronchial tree and liquefies secretions to facilitate expectoration.
6. Monitor oxygen saturation using finger probe monitor.
7. Encourage client to cough and deep breathe when awake.
8. Suction client as needed.
9. Position client to ensure adequate ventilation. Side-lying position is best if not contraindicated. Turn every hour if not contraindicated. **Rationale:** This prevents pooling of secretions in lungs and assists with ventilation.
10. Monitor vital signs every 5–15 minutes as condition warrants. Vital signs are sometimes difficult to obtain due to hypothermia and movement from operating room to recovery room.
    a. Check pulse rate, quality, and rhythm.
    b. Check blood pressure, pulse pressure, and quality.
    c. Check respiratory rate, rhythm, depth, and pattern.
11. Maintain body temperature by applying warm blankets. **Rationale:** Operating rooms are cold, which promotes vasoconstriction.
12. Observe for adverse signs of general or spinal anesthesia:
    a. Level of consciousness
    b. Movement of extremities
13. Monitor IV fluids.
    a. Check type and amount of solution being administered.
    b. Set appropriate flow rate using IV pump or controller if needed.
    c. Observe IV site for signs of infiltration.
    d. Maintain accurate IV intake record.
14. Monitor blood or blood component infusions.
    a. Identify appropriate replacement fluid.
    b. Check client's name and identification number with fluid.
    c. Check blood type, blood bank number, and expiration date.
    d. Check time infusion initiated.
    e. Observe and record amount of fluid remaining in bag when admitted to recovery room.
    f. Determine time frame for completion of fluid.
15. Monitor and measure urine output hourly if

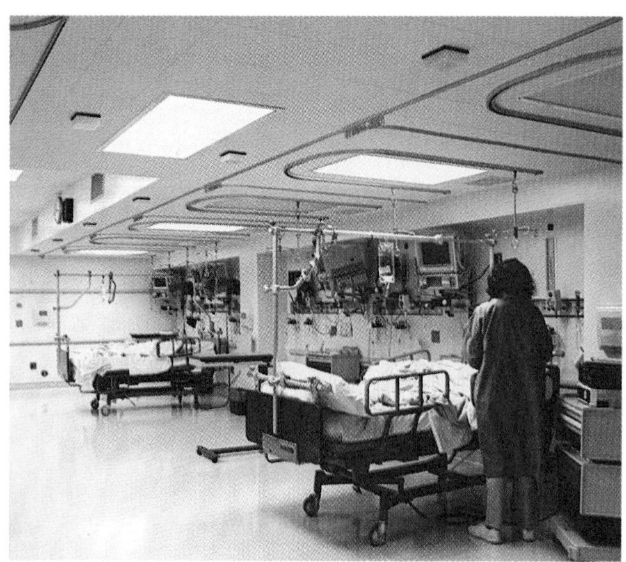

Recovery room is usually an open space for easy receiving of all clients.

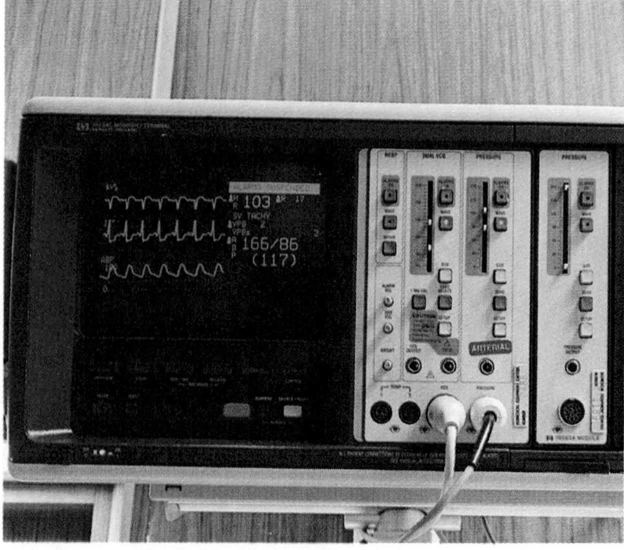

Clients may be connected to monitoring system for cardiac surveilance.

indwelling catheter is in place or before client leaves recovery room.

16. Observe surgical dressings and drains hourly.
    a. Follow hospital policy for marking drainage on dressings.
    b. Note color and amount of drainage on dressings and from drains or tubes.
    c. Check that dressings are secure.
    d. Reinforce dressings as needed.
    e. Report unusual amount or type of drainage to physician before client leaves recovery room.
17. Monitor skin for warmth, color, and moisture.
18. Check nailbeds and mucous membranes for color and blanching. Report unusual findings or signs of cyanosis to physician immediately.
19. Orient client to surroundings and relieve anxiety and fear.
20. Observe for return of reflexes, especially if client received spinal or epidural anesthesia.
21. Monitor for pain and medicate as needed.
22. Administer all STAT drugs.
23. Assess parameters for discharge from recovery room.

DISCHARGING CLIENT FROM RECOVERY ROOM

Procedure

1. Assess that lung sounds are clear to auscultation and airway is maintained without artificial measures (unless client is to remain on mechanical assistance).
2. Assess that vital signs are within normal range for at least 1 hour and appropriate for client's condition.
3. Observe that client is awake, alert, and responds to command and that reflexes are present (if spinal anesthesia used).
4. Ensure IVs are patent, infusing with correct solution and at prescribed rate. Record total amount of IV fluid infused and amount remaining in bags.
5. Check that all dressings are intact, and there is no excessive drainage from drains or tubes. Reinforce dressings if needed before returning to nursing unit.
6. Ensure urinary output is adequate. Record all urine output and empty drainage bag before transporting to nursing unit.
7. Record all medications administered in recovery room.
8. Medicate client $\frac{1}{2}$ hour before transport if vital signs are stable and client requires pain medication. **Rationale:** Transporting clients from recovery room can increase pain due to moving and transfer from gurney to bed.
9. Call anesthesiologist for discharge orders or use Aldrete Postanesthesia Recovery Scoring System if allowed.
10. Call for transport assistance if available. Recovery room nurse accompanies client to nursing unit.

ALDRETE POSTANESTHESIA RECOVERY SCORING SYSTEM

This is one method for determining if recovery room discharge criteria have been met. In addition to stable vital signs, a total score of 10 for the 5 assessed areas must be achieved for nurses to discharge clients without a physician's order. The areas assessed include:

- Ability to move extremities voluntarily or on command
- Ability to cough and deep breathe freely
- Blood pressure maintained within 20 mm Hg of preanesthesia values
- Fully awake
- Normal skin color

11. Call nursing unit, and provide information on equipment needs for client (e.g., oxygen, IVs).
12. Document all findings in computer before discharge.
13. Provide report to unit nurse.
    a. Type of surgical procedure performed
    b. Type of anesthesia and length of procedure
    c. Length of time in recovery room

d. Condition of client at time of discharge from recovery room
e. Report on vital signs, IVs, dressings, drains, tubes, need for special equipment, medications received and time given

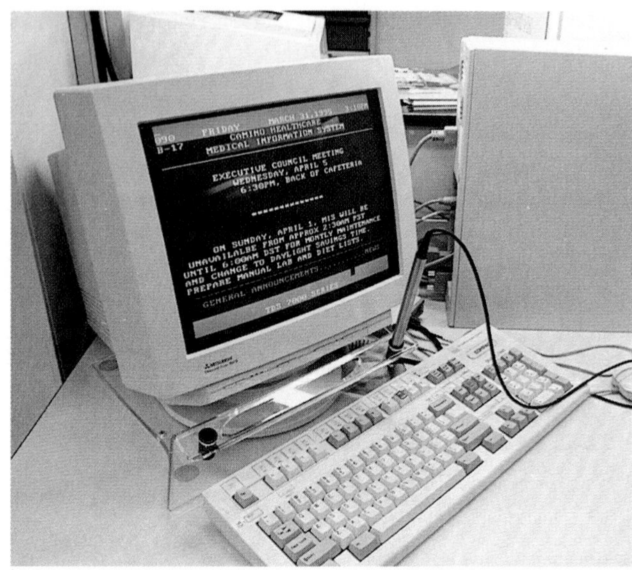

Recovery room documentation is accomplished using computerized system.

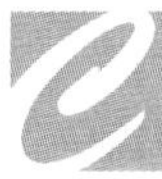

CHARTING for Recovery Room Care

- Assessment findings
- Effects of anesthesia
- Status of airway management
- Need for oxygen administration
- Status of neurologic signs and reflexes
- Fluid replacement—type and amount
- Blood and blood product replacement
- Medications administered
- Condition of dressings, drains, and tubes
- Intake and output from all sources: urine, drains, tubes, IVs
- Vital signs
- Description of pain and interventions for relief of pain
- Response to recovery room activities

CRITICAL THINKING APPLICATION

CLINICAL PROBLEMS	CRITICAL THINKING OPTIONS
Client experiences untoward effects in recovery room.	• Complete physical assessment. • Identify and initiate appropriate nursing interventions within allowed guidelines and parameters of the facility. • Contact physician for additional orders.
Client does not awaken easily.	• Retain client in recovery room. • Continue to provide oxygen. • Arouse every 15 minutes. • Check for pain.

unit 5

POSTOPERATIVE CARE

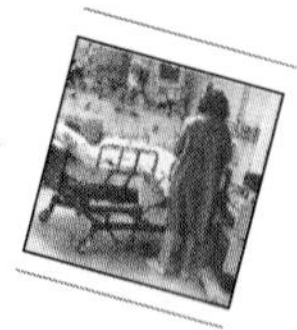

NURSING PROCESS DATA

ASSESSMENT Data Base

Assess for patent airway.

Check if oxygen is ordered.

Check gag reflex.

Observe for adverse signs of general anesthesia or spinal anesthesia.

Take vital signs.

Check client's temperature for heat control.

Observe dressings and surgical drains.

Check IVs for type and amount of fluid to be infused.

Observe color and amount of urine.

Observe client's overall condition.

PLANNING Objectives

To ensure that the client experiences an uneventful postoperative course

To provide safe, effective nursing care in the immediate postoperative period

To ensure that postoperative pain is relieved promptly

To be aware of the common postoperative drugs for pain control

IMPLEMENTATION Procedures

Providing Postoperative Care

Administering Postoperative Medications

EVALUATION Expected Outcomes

Client experiences an uneventful postoperative course.

Postoperative pain is relieved promptly.

Postoperative nursing interventions are carried out effectively and in a timely manner.

Medications control postoperative pain.

PROVIDING POSTOPERATIVE CARE

Equipment

Surgical bed

Absorbent pads

Warm blankets

IV pole

Oxygen source, tubing, and equipment

Emesis basin and tissues

Sphygmomanometer and stethoscope

Thermometer (rectal or oral)

Nurses' notes

Intake and output record

Special equipment depending on type of surgery

Procedure

1. Assess for patent airway and level of consciousness; administer oxygen if ordered.
2. Take vital signs: usual orders are every 15 minutes until stable; then every half hour for 2 hours; every hour for 4 hours; then every 4 hours for 24–48 hours.
3. Check IV site and patency frequently.
4. Observe, and record urine output.

5. Measure intake and output.
6. Observe skin color and moisture.
7. Position client for comfort and maximum airway ventilation according to orders.
8. Turn every 2 hours and p.r.n.
9. Give back care at least every 4 hours.
10. Encourage coughing and deep breathing every 2 hours (may use IPPB or blow bottles if ordered).
11. Keep client comfortable with medications.
12. Check dressings and drainage tubes every 2–4 hours; if abnormal amount of drainage, check more frequently.
13. Give oral hygiene at least every 4 hours; if nasogastric tube, nasal oxygen, or endotracheal tube is inserted, give oral hygiene every 2 hours.
14. Bathe client when temperature can be maintained. **Rationale:** Bathing removes the antiseptic solution and stimulates circulation.
15. Keep client warm and avoid chilling, but do not increase temperature above normal. **Rationale:** Increased temperature increases metabolic rate and need for oxygen. Excessive perspiration causes fluid and electrolyte loss.
16. Irrigate nasogastric tube every 2 hours and p.r.n., as ordered, with normal saline to keep patent and to prevent electrolyte imbalance.
17. Maintain dietary intake: type of diet depends on type and extent of surgical procedure.
    a. Minor surgical conditions: client may drink or eat as soon as he or she is awake, desires food or drink, and has gag reflex present.
    b. Major surgical conditions: n.p.o. until bowel sounds return. Clear liquid advanced to full diet as tolerated.
18. Place client on bedpan 2–4 hours postoperatively if catheter not inserted.
19. Check physician's orders when to begin the client's postoperative activity. Most clients are ambulated within first 24 hours.
20. Observe for signs and symptoms of possible postoperative complications.

ADMINISTERING POSTOPERATIVE MEDICATIONS*

Equipment

Medication as ordered

Appropriate syringe and needle for parenteral medications

Procedure

1. Evaluate client's need for pain relief.
2. Provide nonmedication measures for relief of pain, such as relaxation techniques, back care, positioning.
3. Identify the pharmacologic action of the ordered medication.
4. Review the general side effects of the medication.
    a. Drowsiness
    b. Euphoria
    c. Sleep
    d. Respiratory depression
    e. Nausea and vomiting
5. Administer medications as ordered, usually at 3- to 4-hour intervals for first 24–48 hours for better action and pain relief. Assess for pain relief.
6. Instruct in use of PCA pump, if ordered.
7. Know the action of the following drugs.
    a. Opiates
    b. Synthetic opiate-like drugs
    c. Nonnarcotic pain relievers
    d. Narcotic antagonists
    e. Antiemetics

*See Chapter 17, Pain Management, for PCA and epidural pain control.

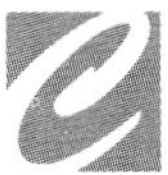

CHARTING for Postoperative Care

- Postoperative nursing interventions
- Fluid replacement—type and amount of solution
- Condition of dressings and drains
- Urine output, intake and output
- Vital signs
- Signs and symptoms of potential complications
- Preventive nursing measures
- Client's activity level
- Clinical manifestations indicating pain
- Type, time, and amount of pain medication administered
- Site of injection
- Any side effects of medications observed
- Effectiveness of pain medication

CRITICAL THINKING APPLICATION

CLINICAL PROBLEMS	CRITICAL THINKING OPTIONS
■ Client develops abnormal breath sounds.	• Increase deep breathing and coughing exercises to every 2 hours. • Medicate for pain before coughing or ambulating to prevent splinting. • Encourage use of incentive spirometer. • Turn every 1–2 hours, and ambulate if allowed. • Place client in Fowler's position to expand lungs. • Increase fluid intake to liquify secretions, if not contraindicated. • Obtain physician's order for nebulizer treatments if indicated.
■ Bowel sounds are absent.	• Do not give ice chips or fluids, keep on n.p.o. status until discussed with physician. • Obtain order for nasogastric tube if abdomen is distended and absent bowel sounds persist. • Encourage frequent turning and ambulation, if allowed.
■ Thrombophlebitis occurs.	• Place on bed rest. • Remove antiembolic stockings on affected leg. • Do not massage legs. • Monitor clotting times and titrate anticoagulants according to physician's orders. • Measure circumference of both legs each shift to determine effectiveness of treatment. • Encourage leg exercises on unaffected leg.
■ Temperature increases after second postoperative day.	• Assess incision for possible infection. • Observe urine for potential infection. • Check breath sounds for adventitious sounds. • Increase fluids, if not contraindicated. • Monitor temperature frequently, until it returns to normal.

CLINICAL PROBLEMS	CRITICAL THINKING OPTIONS
Blood pressure decreases; pulse and respiration increase.	• Assess client for hypovolemia. • Check skin turgor and urine output. • Observe dressings for signs of bleeding. • Check intake and output values to determine hydration status.

GERIATRIC CONSIDERATIONS

Statistics for elderly clients requiring surgery are important to consider when providing care.

- Fifty percent of clients over 60 years of age require surgery before they die.
- Forty percent of elderly clients admitted to hospitals undergo a surgical procedure before discharge.
- The most common surgical procedures for elderly clients involve tissue biopsy and pacemaker insertion. Fractures comprise a large percentage of surgical interventions, particularly hip fractures.

Elderly clients are more prone to fluid and electrolyte imbalance.

- Dehydration is the most common cause of fluid and electrolyte imbalance.
- Check IV fluid type and amount to ensure adequate hydration.
- Elderly clients require 1.5–2.5 L of fluid every 24 hours.
- Monitor intake and output carefully to ensure adequate hydration.
- Monitor neurologic status for possible electrolyte imbalance.
- Fluid loss occurs with nasogastric tube placement and preop bowel preparation; clients requiring either of these interventions should be observed for dehydration.
- Evaluate electrolyte lab values for abnormal levels. (Hyperkalemia is common as a response to age-related alterations in the renin–aldosterone system.)

Elderly clients are at risk for complications associated with immobility following surgical interventions.

- Turn client frequently, at least every 2 hours.
- Ambulate as soon as possible postoperatively.
- Encourage deep breathing and coughing exercises every 1–2 hours. Instruct in use of incentive spirometer if ordered.
- Encourage leg exercises every hour when awake.

Preoperative teaching should be individualized keeping in mind the following:

- Elderly clients may have chronic conditions that make movement more difficult, altering preventative measures such as turning.
- Clients may have visual or auditory alterations requiring a quiet environment for teaching.
- Larger print or brochures with photos and large print should be used when teaching elderly clients.

Chronic conditions may alter normal vital signs, which may be misinterpreted during the perioperative phases.

- Document abnormalities in vital signs on client care plan so that all health care workers are alerted to client's usual values. Blood pressure and pulse alterations can be different for this age group.
- Monitor peripheral pulses to ensure adequate circulation.

Altered physiologic states need to be communicated to all health care workers.

- Document if client has an artificial eye or other prosthesis.
- Document client's visual or auditory alterations. If hearing aide is necessary for client to hear, indicate clearly on care plan.
- Identify if client has any condition that can interfere with postoperative care.

Consent forms must be signed by legally competent client.

- Signing of consent form can only be done if client is considered competent to understand directions given and explanation of procedure.
- Signing of consent form must be voluntary.
- Client must be informed about procedure and must understand what he or she is signing.
- A court-appointed conservator may need to be obtained for clients not considered mentally competent to sign for themselves.
- Family members may not sign for client unless they are legally considered the client's guardian.
- In emergency situations permission may be obtained from family members, but not for routine procedures.

31

Client Education and Discharge Planning

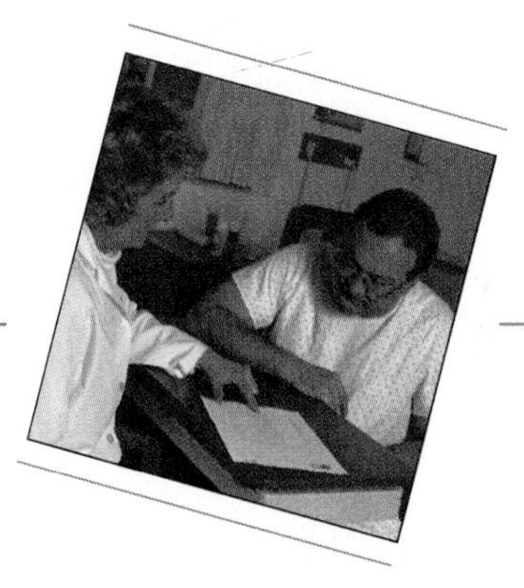

LEARNING OBJECTIVES

- Define the process of client education.
- Describe what is meant by the term "learning theory."
- Outline the process of collecting client data.
- Explain how the nursing process relates to client education.
- List two factors to consider when you are determining the appropriate teaching strategy.
- List and describe two specific teaching strategies.
- Describe how to develop an evaluation tool.
- Discuss what is meant by the term "discharge planning."
- List three risk factors that require discharge planning.
- Identify the steps necessary to complete a discharge summary.

TERMINOLOGY

Acceptance: favorable reception; basic acknowledgment.

Anxiety: a state of uneasiness and distress; diffuse apprehension.

Assessment: critical evaluation of information; the first step in the nursing process.

Assistance: aiding, helping, or giving support.

Attitude: a state of mind or feeling with regard to some matter; disposition.

Behavior: the actions or reactions of persons under specified circumstances.

Client Care Plan: a plan for care of a specific client or one designed especially for one client.

Client education: the process of influencing behavior and teaching the client self-care techniques so that he or she can resume responsibility for certain aspects of health care following discharge from the health facility.

Comprehensive health care: a total system of health care that takes the whole person into account.

Counseling: to give support or to provide guidance.

Diagnosis-related groups (DRGs): categorization of disease diagnoses that standardizes the reimbursement of government funds for number of days in the hospital.

Discharge: to let go, as in discharging a client from the hospital; the flowing away of a secretion or excretion of pus, feces, urine.

Discharge planning: systematic process of planning for client care following discharge; includes client needs, goals of care, and strategies for implementation.

Evaluation tool: a test, questionnaire, or direct observation that evaluates the effectiveness of the teaching.

Health: the state of physical, psychologic, and sociologic well-being.

Helping relationship: an interaction of individuals that sets the climate for movement of the participants toward common goals.

Home care assistance: nursing care given in the client's home.

Maladaptive: inability to, or faulty adjustment or adaptation.

Readiness to learn: a component of the learning process; referring to the psychologic state of being open and accepting of new information and the learning process.

Relationship: an interaction of individuals over time.

Resistance: opposition to or the ability to oppose.

Support: to lend strength or give assistance to.

Termination: the end of something; a limit or boundary; conclusion or cessation.

Therapeutic: having medicinal or healing properties; a healing agent.

Transfer: to convey or shift from one person or place to another.

Transition: the process or an instance of changing from one form, state, activity, or place to another.

Transitional care: the process of facilitating the transition or move between hospital and home to maintain continuity of health care.

Understanding: to perceive and comprehend the nature and significance of; to know.

Validate: to substantiate or verify.

CLIENT EDUCATION

Client teaching became an important component of the health care system during the 1970s. Numerous factors contributed to the advancement of client education: A shift from the treatment focus on acute, infectious, and curable diseases to the treatment of chronic, degenerative, noncurable diseases with multiple causes; increased involvement of consumers in their health care, including issues such as client rights, informed consent, and client access to records; recognition of the cost benefits of client education; emergence of the self-care movement with its emphasis on the individual's responsibility for his or her state of health; and finally, the development of health education and client teaching theories through scientific research.

Escalating health care costs resulted in implementation of diagnosis-related groups (DRGs), requiring subsequent shorter hospital stays as well as affecting client education practices. Although shortened hospital stays may save health care costs, they place a burden on health care professionals to provide adequate teaching before the client is discharged from the hospital. This practice becomes a special problem when the discharged client falls into a high-risk group, such as elderly, illiterate, or highly anxious.

The goal of client education is to influence behavioral changes that promote the person's health status. The dynamics of human behavior and the forces that influence behavioral changes are highly complex, and there is simply no "one right way" to go about the process of educating clients in order to achieve this goal.

Although there are different models of client education, traditional health care professionals tend to adhere to the medical model; that is, diagnosis, prognosis, and therapeutic regimen. Educating the client is oriented toward imparting knowledge in these three areas.

A client education plan is a component of the total plan of care for that client. And, since this plan is based on the nursing process, this model is also appropriate for client education. Client education, when viewed as a process rather than the simple action of imparting information, assists the client to actively participate in his or her health plan for wellness. Individualized to the client and included as part of a total care plan, client education contributes to continuity of care following discharge. Another advantage of using this approach is that all nursing personnel may participate in a coordinated effort to implement teaching and evaluation of care can be accomplished.

Readiness to Learn

Readiness to learn is an essential component of the learning process. One of the principles of client education and adult learning is that the goals are constructed mutually with the nurse, the client, and the family. When goals are negotiated between nurse and client, the readiness to learn is enhanced. Desired outcomes of client education are formulated as goals. Objectives can be stated as specific statements related to a goal. The more clearly stated the goals and objectives, the more directed the planned interventions. Written as behavioral objectives, evaluating the outcome is easier.

Most nurses recognize that the client may resist learning and cannot be forced to learn; the nurse can only assist the client, encourage him or her, and facilitate learning. To master information, the client must have internalized some form of motivation to learn; that is, he or she realizes that to adequately control diabetes (for example) and feel better, the client must understand the relationship of insulin and food to body needs.

Resistance to Change

Many clients appear to resist change, even when changing would result in a positive outcome. When this occurs, the process of learning is blocked. As a nurse educator, you are functioning as an agent of change and dealing with resistance to change is a necessary task. There are several reasons underlying resistance: one of the most common is that change is frightening, even when a person consciously wishes to alter his or her behavior. Also, if a person perceives change as a possible threat, he or she may resist. Another cause of resistance is inaccurately perceiving the reason for or effect of change. Other sources of resistance include psychologic inflexibility, inability to tolerate change, and not believing that change will have a positive effect.

The nurse is both an educator and an agent of change. If the client resists change (the teaching process), attempting to identify the reason for that resistance and altering the teaching approach accordingly may assist the nurse to accomplish the goals of client education.

Barriers to Change	**Nursing Approaches**
Perceived threat or fear of change	Identify specific fears or threats and impart accurate information that may reduce fears. Focus on the positive outcome of change.

Inaccurate perceptions of effect of change	Clarify client perceptions. Impart accurate information, and discuss results of behavior change.
Disagreement that change is positive	Work to agree on mutual goals and demonstrate positive outcomes so client views change as positive rather than negative.
Psychologic resistance or perceived loss of freedoms or behaviors	Focus on discussion of client's perceived loss of freedom and demonstrate willingness to alter plan or adapt to client's needs.
Inability to tolerate change	Recognize that low tolerance is often caused by fear—allaying fear through developing trust, being supportive when client attempts to change, and giving positive feedback decreases fear of change.

Malcolm Knowles, author of *The Modern Practice of Adult Education*, discusses strategies for adult learning. He suggests that adult learning and readiness to learn are influenced by developmental tasks. It may be useful for the nurse to review Erik Erikson's eight stages of human development and the tasks associated with each stage when determining the client's readiness to learn.

Client education is more than imparting information to a client; it is the process of influencing behavior. As such, it needs to be directed toward behavioral change. When goals are mutually agreed on and clearly stated, the learner understands what is expected, the nurse understands his or her role and can evaluate it, and the results can more easily be measured.

Student Nurse's Role in Client Education

As we discussed in the beginning of the chapter, the nurse's role has changed during the last 20 years. Now, a major constituent of the nurse's responsibility is to follow through on client care and implement discharge planning. Client education is an important component of the planning, especially since the majority of clients require assistance to maintain their health status when they leave the hospital. Learning new skills, understanding the disease process, medications, and treatments provide a self-care means to return to a wellness state. Nursing students are learning to be practitioners; their learning takes place in a curriculum that is based on the nursing process. Since client education is considered a part of total client care within this framework, student nurses should understand the principles of client education and learn to include this process as part of the nursing care they administer to their clients.

Tips to Facilitate Client Education

- Assess client's motivation to learn.
- Determine readiness to learn.
- Assess client's developmental level and interact on this level.
- Understand the client's expectations for the learning situation; correct misconceptions.
- Agree on goals; mutual formulation enhances positive outcome.
- Discuss steps to achieve goals so that outcomes are anticipated.
- Direct client education toward behavioral change.
- Formulate outcome criteria for goal evaluation.

DISCHARGE PLANNING

Recent changes in health care delivery and the introduction of diagnosis-related groups (DRGs) as an attempt to contain rapidly rising costs, has altered client care. The number of hospital days for clients in acute care hospitals has decreased; frequently, these clients are discharged still needing care; and this care is frequently delivered in the home setting. Most clients, especially those who are high risk, benefit from the process of discharge planning. *Discharge planning* is defined as the systematic process of planning for client care after discharge from the hospital. The emphasis and goal of discharge planning is to meet client needs through continuity of care—from an acute care setting to a discharge facility.

When the client is admitted and the care plan formulated, discharge planning should be initiated. The process includes an assessment of the client and family needs; the physical, emotional, and psychosocial status; home environment; and family and community resources.

Risk Factors for Discharge Planning

- Elderly age group
- Multisystem disease process
- Major surgical procedure
- Chronic or terminal illness
- Emotional or mental instability
- Inadequate or inappropriate living arrangement

- Lack of transportation
- Financial insecurity
- Unsafe features in the home

Discharge planning involves multidisciplinary action with participation by all members of the health care team, the client and family. Many of the larger hospitals have discharge planners or coordinators. These staff are considered part of the health care team; they orchestrate the discharge planning. This is especially important when the client is considered high risk. More often, however, the staff or head nurse is responsible for discharge planning. With the assistance of social workers or community-based nurses, the staff identifies and anticipates client needs and formulates a plan for meeting these needs after discharge from the hospital.

Successful discharge planning includes

1. A total plan of care from the acute care setting to recovery at home.
2. Appropriate teaching for family and client in self-care.
3. Knowledge of the necessary procedures for self-care, as well as emergency procedures.
4. Appropriate agencies involved in transition to the home care setting.

A new approach to discharge planning is transitional care using transition specialists. This category of practitioner was implemented to facilitate the transition from hospital (where discharge planning is initiated) to recovery (in the home). The transition specialist meets with the family and client in the acute setting, begins discharge planning, and usually makes a home visit before the client is discharged. Following discharge to the home, this specialist is available to the client and family. This type of transitional care and coordination has proven to be cost-effective and has improved the quality of care.

Communication between the client, family, and health care agencies is essential for effective discharge planning. The nurse establishes a dialogue between these various people and coordinates the discharge plan before the client leaves the hospital. When referrals to other agencies are necessary, these are initiated before the client is discharged. The nurse, if there is no discharge planner available, is responsible for coordinating such referrals—including signed physician's orders for specific care, treatments, or medications, so that the client can be reimbursed by third-party payment.

Included in the discharge plan is a discharge summary. This summary includes the client's learning needs, how well they have been met, the client teaching completed, short- and long-term goals of care, referrals made, and coordinated care plan to be implemented after discharge.

From 1988 onward, hospitals have been mandated by federal requirements to provide a discharge planning process for all Medicare clients. These same requirements now apply to all clients within hospitals in the United States.

Federal Requirements for Discharge Planning Process

- Hospitals must identify at an early stage of hospitalization all Medicare clients who are likely to suffer adverse health consequences on discharge if there is no planning.
- The hospital must provide a discharge planning evaluation.
- A registered nurse, social worker, or other qualified person must develop or supervise development of the evaluation.
- Discharge planning must include an evaluation of the likelihood of needing posthospital services and of the availability of the services.
- The evaluation must include the client's capacity for self-care or the possibility of the client being cared for in the environment from which the client entered the hospital.
- The evaluation must be completed on a timely basis so that appropriate arrangements for posthospital care are made before discharge.
- The discharge planning evaluation must be in the client's medical record.

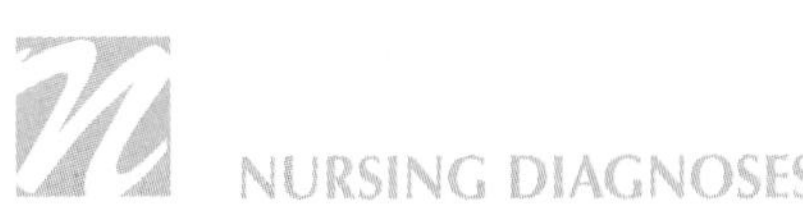

NURSING DIAGNOSES

The following nursing diagnoses may be appropriate to include in a client care plan when the components are related to establishing and maintaining client teaching and discharge planning.

NURSING DIAGNOSIS	RELATED FACTORS
Impaired Verbal Communication	Cognitive impairment, auditory impairment, language barrier
Altered Health Maintenance	Cultural and religious beliefs, information misinterpretation, lack of education, lack of motivation, inadequate health care services
Knowledge Deficit	Inadequate understanding of condition, misinformation, language differences
Noncompliance	Impaired ability to perform tasks, poor self-esteem, lack of motivation
Relocation Stress Syndrome	Changes associated with transfer between facilities or facility and home, effects of losses associated with moving, stress in family members

unit 1

CLIENT EDUCATION

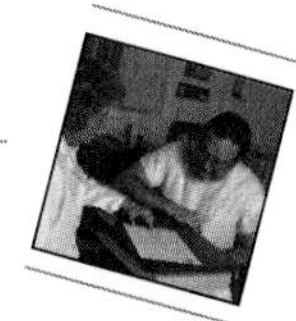

NURSING PROCESS DATA

ASSESSMENT Data Base

Assess high-risk criteria for client education.

Determine the need for client teaching program.

Identify client learning requirements and expectations.

Assess knowledge and skill level of client.

Assess motivation to learn.

Assess readiness and openness to learning.

Identify health beliefs and practices.

Assess developmental and educational level of client.

Determine appropriate methodology for client teaching sessions.

Identify appropriate adjunctive materials, such as audiovisual aids, to enhance learning process.

Assess appropriate setting for the individual client.

PLANNING Objectives

To develop a plan in the nursing process framework

To determine teaching priorities and establish learning objectives

To select appropriate teaching strategies

To increase client's knowledge so as to positively affect health status

To increase client's self-esteem by encouraging participation in goal selection and implementation program

To encourage client to acknowledge individual responsibility for health behaviors and health status

To improve client's ability to make informed decisions affecting health status

To facilitate behavioral changes that are conducive to optimum health status

To provide continuity of care when the client is moving from one health care setting to another

IMPLEMENTATION Procedures

Collecting Data

Determining Readiness to Learn

Identifying Learning Needs

Determining Appropriate Teaching Strategy

Selecting the Educational Setting

Implementing the Teaching Strategy

Developing an Evaluation Tool

EVALUATION Expected Outcomes

Client's knowledge regarding his or her health status has increased.

Client's ability to make informed and effective health-related decisions, based on accurate information and awareness of self, has improved.

Effective use of the health care delivery system has been promoted.

Continuity of care and information exchange has occurred between health agencies or between the hospital and client's home and family.

The nurse has evaluated his or her teaching effectiveness and revised the plan, teaching style, and content as necessary.

COLLECTING DATA

Equipment

Nursing care plan in the nursing process
Room or suitable setting to complete assessment
Adjunct materials, such as audiovisual equipment, charts, and illustrations
Written materials, such as outlines or other handouts
Equipment for demonstration and return demonstration
Documentation forms: Kardex, client's chart

Preparation

1. Develop a nursing care plan in the nursing process format.
2. Use communication and relationship skills. **Rationale:** These skills encourage client's participation in the plan.
3. Avoid a judgmental attitude to prevent client telling the nurse what client thinks the nurse wants to hear. **Rationale:** An open nonjudgmental attitude assists client to be honest with feelings.
   a. Use "how" questions to facilitate communication. **Rationale:** "How" is more effective than "why" in a question, as "why" tends to set up a defensive reaction to the question.
   b. Use verbal and nonverbal behavior and congruence of both to build relationship with the client.
4. Use assessment (observation) skills. **Rationale:** This establishes a data base.
5. Request demonstration of a skill previously learned or currently used (e.g., giving self an insulin injection). **Rationale:** Client's ability to demonstrate skill assists you to evaluate ability to perform, as well as mastery of previous teaching principles.

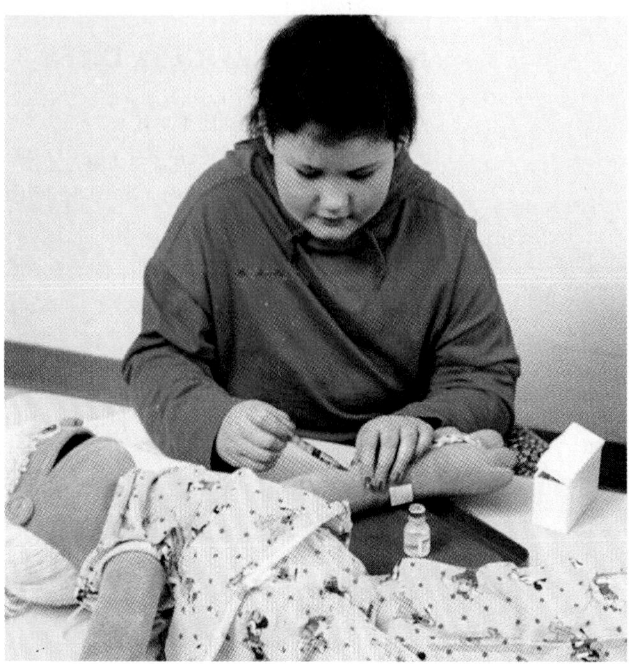

When collecting data to determine learning needs and strategies use age-appropriate materials.

Procedure

1. Identify personal characteristics.
   a. Age and sex
   b. Educational level
   c. Marital status
   d. Family composition and living situation
   e. Ethnic group and cultural practices pertinent to learning
2. Identify support systems available, both personal and community.
3. Identify values and attitudes toward self and others having his or her particular disease or condition.
4. Assess knowledge base—anatomy and physiology (normal and disease-related) and the disease process—by asking specific questions.
5. Evaluate capacity and ability to perform specific skills, including those previously learned.
6. Assess knowledge of rationale behind specific skills.
7. Evaluate patterns of coping.
   a. Past experiences of self and others in relation to the disease
   b. Perception by client of how ill he or she is at this time
   c. Reactions to stress and ways of managing anxiety
   d. Current level of self-management
   e. Willingness of client to change behavior

DETERMINING READINESS TO LEARN

Procedure

1. Determine client's physiologic readiness.
   a. Degree of physical comfort of client (level of pain), level of alertness, ability to concentrate, degree of interest
   b. Acuteness of the illness and its influence on client's ability to learn
   c. Environmental factors that may affect client's degree of readiness
   d. Safety issues and need for supervision
2. Evaluate client's psychologic readiness.
   a. State of client's feelings and their influence on receptivity to learning. **Rationale:** An angry and hostile client is not going to absorb information until his or her anger is acknowledged or worked through.
   b. Psychologic barriers (for example, the presence of denial) and their influence on the learning process.
   c. Client's intellectual capacity and level of comprehension.

IDENTIFYING LEARNING NEEDS

Procedure

1. Use assessment data and assessment instrument to jointly determine client's learning needs: educational, physical, psychosocial, and financial needs.
2. Formulate needs as goals.
3. Prioritize learning needs or goals.
4. Review with client alternative resources available to accomplish goals.
5. Determine ability of the facility, family, staff, or multidisciplinary team to meet goals or learning needs.
6. Obtain verbal or written contract with client for educational program.
7. Refer client to other resources or agencies when appropriate.

DETERMINING APPROPRIATE TEACHING STRATEGY

Procedure

1. Consider the following factors when determining appropriate strategy:
   a. Input from client about how he or she learns best
   b. Specific task or nature of the content to be transmitted and how it is best learned
   c. Client attention span and retention ability
   d. Teaching materials and resources available
   e. Time, availability, skills, and abilities of staff; appropriate use of paraprofessional and professional staff
   f. Participation by members of other health care disciplines as part of a team
   g. Determination of most appropriate time for teaching
2. Determine which type of teaching strategy will be effective in a given situation.
   a. Group process: use of principles from group dynamics, mental health, or other related fields to enhance learning or behavior changes in a small group setting
   b. Lecture–discussion: presentation of content in a didactic fashion with opportunity for questions and interaction during or at the conclusion of the presentation
   c. Demonstration–return demonstration: demonstration (videotape) by the instructor with practice by the learner and return demonstration of mastery of the skill

d. Role playing: assumption of roles by various participants or learners for the purpose of clarifying various aspects of a situation.
e. Games: structured game situation with rules designed for the learner to accomplish specific educational objectives.

3. Select appropriate teaching adjuncts.
   a. Videotape or videocassette programs
   b. Films
   c. Slide and tape presentations
   d. Programmed instruction materials
   e. Books
   f. Pamphlets and other written handouts
   g. Diagrams, charts, and illustrations

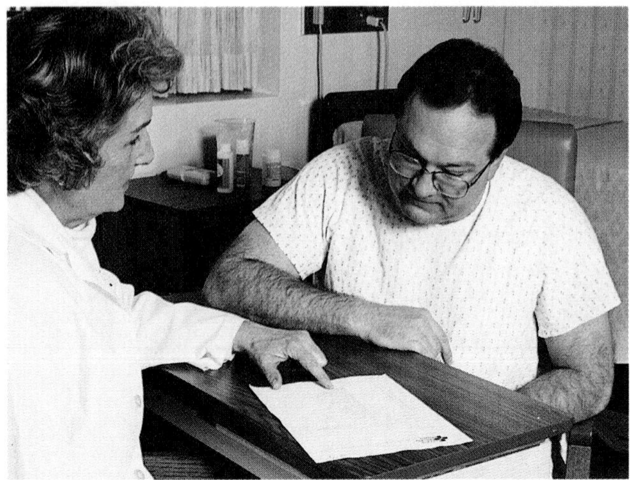

Determine which teaching strategy will be most effective for client.

SELECTING THE EDUCATIONAL SETTING

Procedure

1. Choose an appropriate setting based on selected teaching strategy and available facility space.
2. Evaluate types of setting most appropriate to individual client and client's learning needs.
3. Consider an informal setting.
   a. Spontaneous teaching interactions between nurse and client can occur at any time in any setting.
   b. Usually no formal plan or evaluation tool is used.
4. Consider a formal setting.
   a. Teaching is carried out in a specified area of the facility such as an in-service classroom.
   b. Teaching can occur independently, such as with audiovisual programmed instruction modules or in a group setting.
   c. Formal plan for the teaching program includes written goals, objectives, teaching strategies, content, and evaluation method.

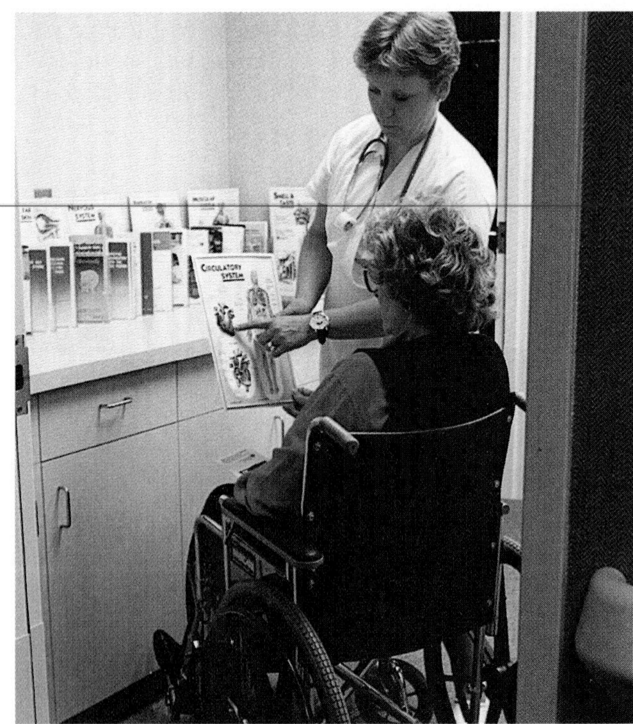

After selecting the appropriate setting, choose the teaching adjuncts.

IMPLEMENTING THE TEACHING STRATEGY

Procedure

1. Gather teaching materials appropriate for client's learning needs and teaching strategy.
2. Sit with client in the designated setting, and establish a warm and accepting relationship. **Rationale:** This is conducive to teaching and assists the client in learning.
3. Specify previously established mutual goals and behavioral objectives of the program. **Rationale:** Mutually agreed on goals promote acceptance of teaching strategy by the client.
4. Clarify or reclarify contract, agreements, or expected outcomes with the individual or group. **Rationale:** Beginning at the level of understanding of the person or group facilitates the process.
5. Assess teaching situation for any modifications needed and adjust plans accordingly.
6. Teach content or components of the plan to client. **Rationale:** Sticking to the plan and not deviating or going off on a tangent reinforces your commitment to help the client master the content.
7. Use appropriate communication skills throughout session. **Rationale:** Therapeutic communication techniques enhance learning environment.
8. Request feedback (evaluation interchange) during teaching process. **Rationale:** Feedback lets you know how client is understanding the content and allows for modification as indicated.
9. Adhere to agreed-on starting and ending times; negotiate any changes. **Rationale:** This encourages client to trust you.
10. Provide closure to teaching situation by summarizing and reiterating agreements made, actions to be taken, or subsequent events to follow.
11. Provide positive reinforcement if not done previously. **Rationale:** This approach increases self-esteem and encourages learning in client.
12. Terminate teaching session by establishing time for next client contact.
13. Do postassessment of your own participation, and plan for corrections and improvements in presentation. **Rationale:** Ongoing evaluation assists in final step of nursing process evaluation.

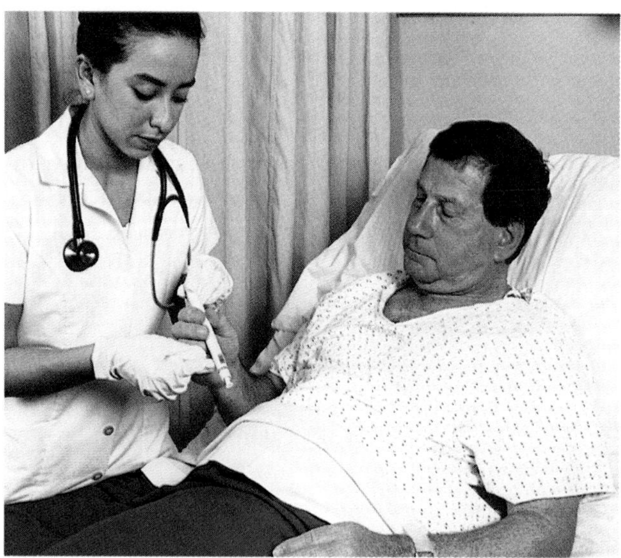

Demonstration is an important component of teaching strategy.

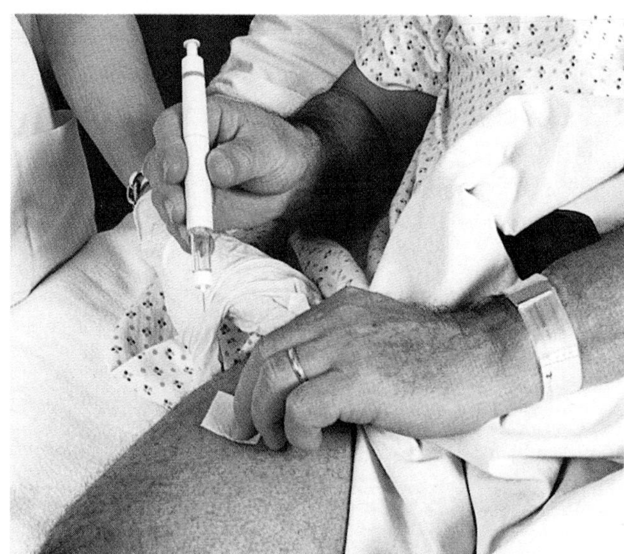

Request client to do return demonstration to evaluate client understanding.

DEVELOPING AN EVALUATION TOOL

Procedure

1. Use an evaluation tool. **Rationale:** Evaluating with a specific tool focuses the evaluation phase better.
2. Evaluate forms, format, and types of tools available for evaluation.
   a. Pretest–posttest: measures changes in (e.g., knowledge level, attitudes, values).
   b. Questionnaire: completed by client to report attitudes, certain behaviors, and, most frequently, level of satisfaction with the teaching program.
   c. Physiologic tracers: determined prior to teaching episode to be the criterion of measurement of success (i.e., changes in blood pressure values after teaching program for hypertensive clients).
   d. Direct observation of behavior changes: report of level of performance during return demonstrations.
3. Choose an evaluative tool based on the goals and objectives of the teaching program. **Rationale:** The purpose is to achieve goals, thus evaluative tool should be based on goals.

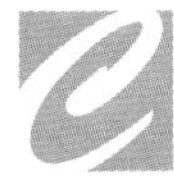

CHARTING for Client Education

- Topics or subjects covered as a part of client education process, such as medications, procedures, dietary plan, activity restrictions, or follow-up care
- Degree of client's participation in the teaching activity
- Progress in meeting the expected outcomes of teaching
- Client's emotional response to the learning process
- Information or equipment sent home with client

CRITICAL THINKING APPLICATION

CLINICAL PROBLEMS	CRITICAL THINKING OPTIONS
Client's health status has not improved as a result of the teaching program.	• Reevaluate nursing care plan in the nursing process. • Reassess client for barriers to learning. • Reevaluate testing tool. • Problem solve with client as to next step to take. • Request assistance from in-service consultant for determining which aspects of the teaching program were not successful and why. • Assist in revising parts of the program and restructure for individual client needs.
Client is hostile to teaching program.	• Attempt to determine underlying reason for hostility. • Terminate this session of teaching program, but tell client you will return tomorrow or at a later time. • Bring another nurse along to assist you in teaching as well as to help you evaluate reason for hostility.
Client's ability to make informed and effective health-related decisions, based on accurate information and awareness of self, has not improved.	• Assist client to take realistic responsibility for ineffective decisions without guilt and shame attached. • Assist client to identify those areas in which he or she is willing to make changes and support development of a plan of action. • Refer to other resources such as mental health therapy as appropriate.

unit 2

DISCHARGE PLANNING

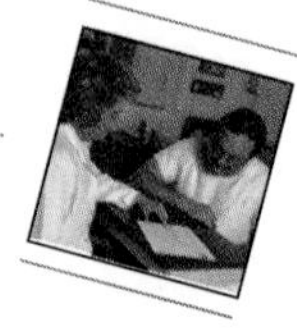

NURSING PROCESS DATA

ASSESSMENT Data Base

Determine if client requires discharge planning.

Determine if client is in a high-risk category.

Assess special needs of client for individualized planning.

Assess need for multidisciplinary health care workers.

Determine information needed for compiling discharge summary.

PLANNING Objectives

To complete a discharge risk factor assessment when admitting a client

To determine health care workers needed for discharge planning

To make appropriate referrals for client discharge

To complete discharge teaching

To develop a discharge plan

To complete a discharge summary

IMPLEMENTATION Procedures

Preparing a Client for Discharge

Completing a Discharge Summary

EVALUATION Expected Outcomes

Discharge teaching is completed.

Discharge planning is effective.

Discharge summary is completed.

PREPARING A CLIENT FOR DISCHARGE

Procedure

1. Obtain admission history, physical, and hospital progress notes.
2. Determine risk factors for discharge planning.
3. Refer high-risk clients to discharge coordinator or social service department, if appropriate.
4. Develop discharge plan (if not already completed) including short- and long-term goals in conjunction with physician and client.
5. Evaluate degree to which client education plan was implemented; reinforce aspects that were incomplete or refer to home agency.
6. Identify need for follow-up care after discharge in conjunction with physician.
7. Make appropriate agency referrals.

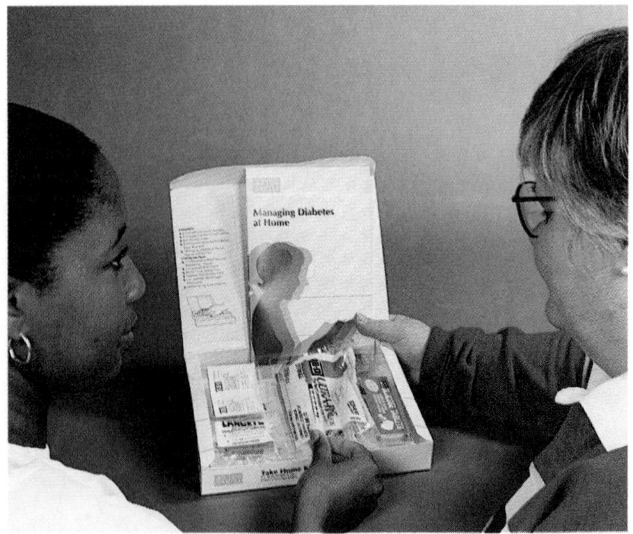

Discharge teaching is an important component of the discharge plan.

8. Complete a discharge referral form, and communicate directly with referral agency about client.

   (Health care agency may prefer their own discharge form to be completed rather than documentation in the nurse's notes.)

9. Update client care plan, and send copy to referral agency.
10. Document discharge summary.

COMPLETING A DISCHARGE SUMMARY

Procedure

1. Document a complete physical, psychosocial assessment at time of discharge.
2. Review vital sign ranges, and state latest vital signs.
3. Identify activity level of client.
4. Describe use of adaptive devices or equipment needs.
5. Review client teaching plan. Provide explanation of areas where teaching was adequate and where additional reinforcement is required.
6. Identify prescribed medications, dosage, and administration times. Provide information on client's knowledge of medication.
7. Describe goal achievement based on client care plan. Describe action taken if goal not achieved.
8. Identify referral agencies contacted.
9. Provide information regarding instructions on physician office visits, appointments to health care agencies, or support services.
10. Describe client's condition at time of discharge.
11. Document discharge instructions provided to client and family.
12. Describe method of discharge (i.e., wheelchair) and person accompanying client at discharge.
13. State means of discharge transportation (e.g., private car, ambulance).
14. Specify discharge facility where client is going.

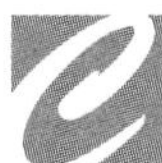

CHARTING for Discharge Planning

- Discharge teaching completed.
- Discharge plan completed.
- Referral agencies contacted.
- Discharge summary form completed.

Discharge Plan (Sample)

Medicare No. ____________________
MediCal No. ____________________

Name ____
Admission Date ____________________ Discharge Date ____________________

1. Living arrangement: Alone ____________________ With ____________________
2. Residence after discharge: ____________________
   Name and address of nearest relative or friend:
   ____
3. Financial situation: Needs assistance __________ Covered ____________________
4. Agency Referrals: Discharge Coordinator ____________________
   Home Health: ____________________

DISCHARGE INSTRUCTIONS

Medications

Name/Dose	Time	Special Instructions

Potential Side Effects ____________________

Nutrition

Special Diet ____________________
Restrictions ____________________

Treatments

Special Equipment Resources and Instructions ____________________
____
____

Discharge Nursing Evaluation

	Independent	**Needs Assistance**	**Dependent**	**Plan**
Personal Needs (ADLs)				
Dressing self				
Bathing				
Skin condition				
Mobility				
Walking				
Bed rest				
Sensory capability				
Glasses				
Hearing aid				
Mental State				
Confused				
Alert				
Oriented				

SUMMARY OF CARE PLAN

Follow-up appointments scheduled

Other relevant information

CRITICAL THINKING APPLICATION

CLINICAL PROBLEMS	CRITICAL THINKING OPTIONS
■ Client is discharged before discharge plan is completed.	• Continue to complete discharge plan, and send to referral agency. • Verbally communicate to referral agency and discuss discharge needs of client.
■ Discharge plan does not contain adequate data.	• Reassess parameters of a discharge plan, and revise accordingly. • Elicit assistance from another nurse or supervisor to revise discharge plan.
■ Goals of discharge plan were not accomplished.	• Attempt to assess reason goals were not met. • Reformulate or revise goals so that they are mutually agreed on and more realistic. • Request assistance from expert health care workers or in-service consultant.
■ Discharge referral plan is not implemented and client receives no referral notice before discharge.	• Attempt to contact other referral agencies to provide continuity of care for client. • Notify physician and discharge coordinator (if available) of necessity of providing follow-through care after discharge.

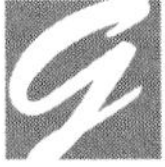

GERIATRIC CONSIDERATIONS

Teaching Strategies

Memory changes occur with the elderly population.

- There is better short-term memory with auditory rather than visual presentation of information.
- Structure should be brief and simple.
- Repetition is important.
- Older clients learn better by doing, using multiple senses, than by reading instructions.
- Memory is better for things considered important.
- Clients remember best what is told *first.*
- Declining mentation is not inevitable with aging, but some memory loss is usual.

Retention facts that underlie teaching strategies. People remember

- 5–10% of what they read
- 10–20% of what they hear
- 30–50% of what they hear and verbalize
- 70% of what they verbalize and write
- 90% of what they say as they perform a task

Interventions for teaching the elderly

- Speak distinctly and sit close to learner.
- Face the learner so that lip reading can supplement hearing.
- Use visual aids and verbal teaching.
- Decrease extraneous noise.
- Use printed materials with large type and high contrast.
- Limit use of blue, green, and violet illustrations. Use red.
- Avoid totally dark room for audiovisual presentations.
- Increase time allowed for psychomotor skills, and allow time for repetition.
- Slow the pace of presentation.
- Give small amounts of information at one time.
- Use analogies and examples to explain information. Mnemonic devices are helpful to compensate for imperfect memory.

- Establish attainable short-term goals.
- Encourage participation in goal setting and planning.
- Integrate new behaviors with previously learned ones.
- Focus on problem solving, not just delivery of facts.
- Apply teaching to present situation.
- Bolster self-esteem and self-confidence in self-care.
- Stress the "why" of what is presented.
- Recognize that the elderly client may prefer to be alone when learning.

Discharge Planning

A discharge plan for the elderly contains some of the same components as a plan for a younger adult; at every step in the plan, however, the coordinator must remember that this is an elderly person and he or she must be evaluated for the ability and resources to manage at home. This is especially so if the elderly person lives alone or with another elderly person. Following are several issues that the discharge planner must consider when formulating the plan:

1. Was the person functioning independently at home before hospitalization, and is it realistic to expect them to do so again?
2. Does this person have capable family or friend resources to assist with functioning in the home (in addition to the necessary professional resources)?
3. What is the baseline health status of the person (assuming they recover from the current hospitalization), and does this status allow for independent functioning following hospitalization?
4. What are the long-term financial resources of the elderly person and do special measures need to be initiated for coverage?
5. If the elderly person cannot return to the facility he or she was in prior to hospitalization, what special arrangements need to be made?
6. Special considerations the discharge planner must take into account when coordinating a plan for an elderly individual:

- Does the person have a hearing or visual impairment that interferes with learning?
- Does the teaching need to be done in written form (not just verbal)?
- Would a return demonstration of care procedures by the home health nurse be beneficial after the client has returned home?
- Will the anxiety level of the client to be discharged interfere with understanding and learning?
- Is the health status of the client a way of gaining attention? If so, this need should be separated from the needs of self-care following discharge. It is important to convey this need to the follow-up caregiver.

32

Care of the Dying Client

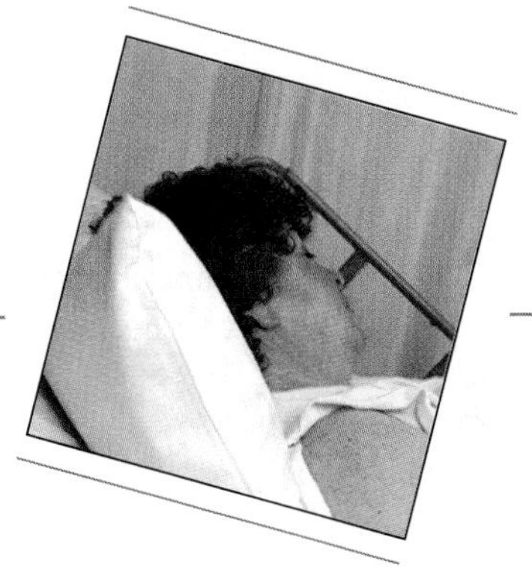

LEARNING OBJECTIVES

- Discuss the stages of the grief process.
- State the main characteristics observed in a person experiencing grief.
- Identify the factors that influence the outcome of the grieving process.
- Explain three assessment parameters for observing psychologic and somatic symptoms that accompany the grief process.
- Discuss at least two nursing interventions for each stage of grief.
- Describe the phases of dying outlined by Elisabeth Kübler-Ross.
- Explain what is meant by providing emotional care for the dying client.
- Discuss at least four nursing interventions that assist the dying client.
- Describe the steps of providing postmortem care.

TERMINOLOGY

Agitation: excessive restlessness; increased mental and physical activity.

Anger: a feeling of extreme displeasure, hostility, indignation, or exasperation toward someone or something.

Anorexia: loss of appetite occurring from a variety of possible reasons.

Anxiety: a troubled or apprehensive feeling; experiencing a sense of dread or fear.

Cope: to contend with, strive, or handle.

Corneal reflex: closure of eyelids resulting from direct corneal irritation or touch.

Counseling: giving assistance to or guidance.

Crisis: a crucial point or situation in the course of anything; turning point.

Denial: refusal to grant the truth of a statement or allegation.

Depression: being dispirited, saddened; low in mood.

Empathy: objective awareness of an insight into the feelings, emotions, and behavior of another person.

Esteem: regard, respect.

Grief: intense mental anguish, deep remorse, sorrow.

Homeostasis: an internal state of equilibrium or balance.

Idealization: to regard as ideal; to make or regard someone or something as perfect.

Insomnia: inability to sleep; difficulty with sleeping.

Pain: suffering, distress, or discomfort.

Psychosomatic: pertaining to phenomena that are both physiologic and psychologic in origin.

Resolution: the state of having made a firm determination; a course decided on.

Restitution: a return to a former status.

Shock: a clinical syndrome with varying degrees of disturbances of oxygen supply to the tissues.

Somatic: referring to the body.

Stress: a mentally or emotionally disruptive or disquieting influence; distress.

Therapeutic: having medicinal or healing properties.

Withdrawal: to pull back or away.

LOSS AND GRIEVING

Grief is an emotion experienced in relation to loss; it can also be viewed as a behavioral response to death and dying. Human beings experience loss as the emotion of grief and must withdraw from the painful stimulus to recuperate. Emotions allow us to experience our environment—they are the means of cognition. When we are grieving, we experience the emotion of grief; this experience is accompanied by a definite syndrome with somatic and psychologic symptoms.

Stages of Grief

George Engle, in a classic article in the American Journal of Nursing, 1964, describes progression of the grief process in stages. These stages may occur in order, or an individual may skip a stage, become locked in a particular stage, or even return to an earlier stage already worked through.

The first stage is *shock and disbelief,* denial and numbness. The first response on learning of a death is shock and a refusal to accept or comprehend the fact. This reaction is followed by a stunned, numb feeling and does not allow the person to acknowledge the reality of death. This initial phase is characterized by attempts to protect oneself against severe stress by blocking recognition of the death.

Developing awareness is the second stage. Within minutes or hours the individual becomes acutely and increasingly aware of the anguish of loss. Anger may be present during this time and may be directed toward persons or circumstances held to be responsible for the death. Behavior that frequently accompanies this stage is crying and a regression to a more helpless and childlike state. The crying and regression appear to acknowledge the loss, indicating that conscious awareness is now present.

The third stage is *restitution,* in which the various rituals of the culture, such as the funeral, attire, wake, particular folkways, and mores, help to initiate the recovery process. These rituals serve the function of emphasizing the reality of death and the very act of experiencing them assists the mourner to face the loss.

As the reality of death becomes accepted, the *resolution* of the loss begins. This stage involves a number of steps. First, the mourner attempts to deal with the painful void created by the loss of a loved one. At this time the thoughts of the mourner are occupied almost exclusively with the deceased. Then the mourner becomes more aware of his or her own body and bodily sensations. Finally, the mourner begins to talk about the dead person, recalling the dead person's attributes and personality and reminiscing about the memories they shared. Resolving the loss is a long and painful phase that continues until the mourner remembers the positive aspects of the dead person.

The next stage that is frequently experienced is that of *idealization.* All hostile and negative feelings toward the dead person are repressed. As the process proceeds, two important changes are taking place: the recurring thoughts about the dead person bring a distinct image of the loss to mind and these memories serve to bring out the more positive aspects of the lost relationship. At the same time the mourner begins to assume certain admired qualities of the dead person through the mechanisms of identification or incorporation. The mourner may begin to dress, speak, or develop mannerisms or beliefs similar to the person who was lost. Often, many months are required for this process to be experienced, and as it dissipates, the mourner's preoccupation with the dead person lessens. It may be at this point that the person begins to reinvest intimate feelings toward other relationships.

The outcome of the mourning process usually takes a year or more. The clearest evidence of healing is the ability to remember the deceased comfortably and realistically, with both the pleasures and disappointments of the relationship. At this stage the obsession with the loss is ended and the person accepts the responsibility of living his or her own life.

Each individual who experiences loss moves through at least some of these stages as he or she attempts to cope with loss. The stages of grief are the means human beings have of moving through the loss to resolution.

STAGES OF DYING

Elisabeth Kübler-Ross has beautifully described the phases of dying, which mirror those of the grieving process. As a person learns of his or her own impending death, he or she experiences grief in relation to his or her own loss.

The first stage, as Dr. Ross views this process, is that of *denial.* The denial may be partial or complete and may occur not only during the first stages of illness or confrontation but later on from time to time. This initial denial is usually a temporary defense and is used as a buffer until such time as the person is able to collect him or herself, mobilize his or her defenses, and face the inevitability of death.

The second stage is often *anger.* The person feels violent anger at having to give up life. This emotion may be directed toward persons in the environment or even projected into the environment at random. Dr. Ross discusses this reaction and the difficulty in handling it for those close to the person by explaining that we should put ourselves in the client's position and consider how we might feel intense anger at having our life interrupted abruptly.

The third stage is *bargaining.* The person attempts to strike a bargain for more time to live or more time to be without pain in return for doing something for God. Often during this stage the person turns or returns to religion.

Depression is the fourth stage. Usually, when people have completed the processes of denial, anger, and bargaining, they move into depression. Dr. Ross writes about two kinds of depression. One is preparatory depression; this is a tool for dealing with the impending loss. The second type is reactive depression. In this form of depression, the person is reacting against the impending loss of life and grieves for him or herself.

The final stage of dying is that of *acceptance.* This occurs when the person has worked through the previous stages and accepts his or her own inevitable death. With full acceptance of impending death comes the preparation for it; however, even with acceptance, hope is still present and needs to be supported realistically.

Many factors influence how individuals accept death. Personal values and beliefs about life; views of personal successes, both financial and emotional; the way they look physically when experiencing the dying process; their family and friends and their families' attitudes and reactions; their past experiences in coping with difficult or traumatic situations; and, finally, the health care staff who are caring for them during this process—all affect an individual's attitude toward dying.

NURSING DIAGNOSES

The following nursing diagnoses may be appropriate to include in a client care plan when a client is in the process of grieving or dying.

NURSING DIAGNOSIS	RELATED FACTORS
Decisional Conflict	Surgery, diagnostic tests, treatments, perceived threat to value system, lack of experience in making critical decisions
Anticipatory Grieving	Loss of significant other, chronic illness, threat of death, perceived loss of biologic integrity
Altered Health Maintenance	Lack of motivation, lack of education, religious and cultural beliefs, cognitive impairment
Ineffective Family Coping, Disabling	Terminal illness, acute disability of family member, changes in body integrity.
Spiritual Distress	Hospital barriers to practicing spiritual rituals, loss of body part or function, terminal illness, debilitating disease, death or illness of significant other, challenge to belief or value systems.

unit 1

THE GRIEF PROCESS

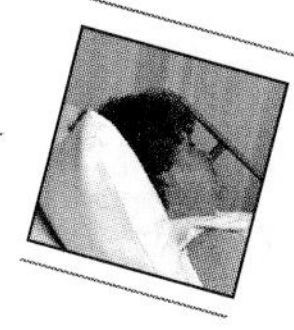

NURSING PROCESS DATA

ASSESSMENT Data Base

Observe for presence of psychologic symptoms:
- Weeping
- Guilt
- Anger and irritability toward others and the deceased
- Depression
- Inability to initiate meaningful activity

Observe for somatic symptoms:
- Physical exhaustion
- Insomnia
- Restlessness and agitation
- Digestive disturbance
- Anorexia

Determine client's complaints:
- Sense of unreality
- Sense of detachment
- Lack of strength

Observe stage of grief response client is experiencing:
- Shock and disbelief
- Developing awareness
- Restitution
- Resolution
- Idealization
- Outcome of grieving process—positive or negative

Observe for morbid reaction to grief:
- Delay of reaction
- Distorted reaction: acquisition of symptoms of the deceased (e.g., psychosomatic illness, or disease)

Atypical grief syndrome manifested by distorted pictures of grief.

PLANNING Objectives

To assist the client who is experiencing the grief process

To intervene therapeutically and provide support

To allow the client to express feelings of loss openly

To understand and tolerate client's behavior that is related to loss

To assist the client to move successfully through stages of the grief process

IMPLEMENTATION Procedures

Understanding Grief

Assisting with Grief

EVALUATION Expected Outcomes

The client's experience of the grieving process is therapeutic.

Client moves through grieving process.

Client accepts loss, and outcome of grieving process is positive.

UNDERSTANDING GRIEF

Procedure

1. Understand the importance of the person lost as a source of support.
2. Observe the degree of dependency of the relationship. **Rationale:** The more dependent, the more difficult is the task of resolution.
3. Identify the degree of ambivalence felt toward the deceased. **Rationale:** When there are persistent hostile feelings, guilt may interfere with the work of mourning.
4. Check on the number and nature of other relationships the mourner has to depend on. **Rationale:** A client with few other meaningful relationships has a more difficult time and is less willing to give up the attachment to the deceased.
5. Check on the number and nature of previous grief experiences. **Rationale:** Losses tend to be cumulative in their effects, and unsuccessfully resolved previous losses only aggravate the current loss.
6. Determine the degree of preparation for the loss. **Rationale:** In terminal illness, grief work may have begun long before the actual death of the person.
7. Determine the capacity to cope with loss. The more inner resources the client has available, the better his or her coping ability. **Rationale:** The physical and psychologic health of the mourner at the time of the loss determines capacity.

ASSISTING WITH GRIEF

Procedure

1. Become familiar with the grief process, the stages of grief, and natural responses to grief so you can provide the client with optimal support.
2. Denial stage
   a. Allow client denial of grief to give him or her time to move through shock and to mobilize defenses.
   b. Encourage client to talk when he or she is ready to do so.
   c. Understand that shock and disbelief may be first response, and anticipate that behavior may be inappropriate or disturbed.
   d. Accept client's inability to face reality, and allow mood swings and expressions of happier times (which may seem inappropriate at this time).
3. Anger stage
   a. Allow "acting-out" of feelings and verbalization of anger.
   b. Anticipate expression of anger toward others, loved ones, and the environment.
   c. Understand that unreasonable, insatiable demands are an expression of this stage of grief, and attempt to meet the demands. Anticipate client's needs before demanded.
   d. Encourage client to take as much control as possible over care and environment. Avoid criticism and negative feedback at this time.
   e. Avoid false reassurance and false cheerfulness, which lead to distrust. Also, avoid diversion by introducing cheerful activities or stories. These actions lead client to believe you do not care about his or her feelings.
   f. Explain and clarify all procedures and treatments to decrease misinterpretation and expansion of fears.
4. Bargaining stage
   a. Allow client to move through bargaining stage; listen to verbal expressions without judgment or pointing out reality.
   b. Encourage client to talk about bargaining with God. This may assist client to cope with guilt and not lose faith.
5. Reactive depression stage
   a. Encourage verbalizations about loss, its meaning in client's life, and feelings about the loss.
   b. Support client's self-esteem and understand that it is affected with awareness of the loss.
   c. Encourage and reassure as appropriate; do not give false reassurance at this stage but assist client to be realistic.
   d. Be aware of your own feelings of sadness and loss so that they do not interfere with therapy.
6. Preparatory depression

a. Allow client to be quiet and silent in order to internalize feelings.
b. Remain with client and share on a nonverbal level.
c. Verbalize feelings to client when they are appropriate; do not deny yourself expressions of sadness or empathy (crying) when appropriate.
d. Limit association with cheerful, insincere staff, friends, or family.

7. Resolution–acceptance stage
   a. Allow client to express whatever feelings are present, knowing that he or she has moved through the above stages and may now be feeling totally empty of emotion.
   b. Spend quiet time with client, interacting on a nonverbal, nondemanding level.
   c. Encourage client to make preparations for impending death by supporting requests to finish tasks and discussing options for plans to complete areas in his or her life.
   d. Honor client's requests to be alone, and do not overload client with external information. Client may need a lot of quiet contemplation to prepare for death.
8. Show respect for cultural, religious, and social customs throughout stages of mourning.
9. Offer support and reassurance to family.

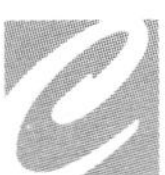

CHARTING for the Grief Process

- Stage of grief the client is experiencing and client's ability to cope
- Behavioral manifestations of grief
- Support systems available to client
- Measures nurse has taken to assist client to cope with grief
- Client's response to psychosocial interventions

CRITICAL THINKING APPLICATION

CLINICAL PROBLEMS	CRITICAL THINKING OPTIONS
The client experiences a morbid reaction to grief.	• Recognize distorted symptoms and be accepting but firm with client. • Request further assistance from the staff.
Family cannot support grief of client or handle their own grief.	• Know the general response to death by recognizing the stages of the grief process. • Understand that the behavior of the mourner may be unstable and disturbed. • Request assistance from nursing staff to cope with the family.

unit 2

THE DYING CLIENT

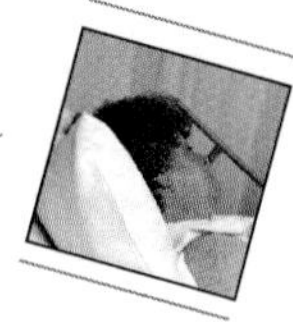

NURSING PROCESS DATA

ASSESSMENT Data Base

Observe the physical symptoms.
- Evidence of circulatory collapse
- Variations in blood pressure and pulse
- Disequilibrium of body mechanisms
- Deterioration of physical and mental capabilities
- Absence of corneal reflex

Observe the client's ability to fulfill basic needs without complete assistance.
Assess the nature and degree of pain the client is experiencing.
Observe for impending crisis or emergency situation.
Observe for psychosocial condition.
- Need to establish a relationship for support
- Grief pattern and stage of grief the client is experiencing
- Need to express feelings and verbalize fears and concerns

Determine anxiety level, which may be expressed in physical or emotional behavior.
- Sleep disturbance
- Palpitations
- Digestive complaints
- Anger or hostility
- Withdrawal

Determine depression level that client may be experiencing.
- High fatigue level or lethargy
- Poor appetite, nausea, or vomiting
- Inability to concentrate
- Expressions of sadness, hopelessness, or uselessness

PLANNING Objectives

To assist the dying client to cope with the dying process
To handle own feelings of loss and sadness that arise when caring for a client who is dying
To provide support for the client and the client's family during the dying process
To complete the actions necessary to care for the client who has died

IMPLEMENTATION Procedure

Assisting the Dying Client

EVALUATION Expected Outcomes

Client finds internal resources to accept death.
Client is able to verbalize feelings and needs.
Physical discomfort is minimized.

ASSISTING THE DYING CLIENT

Procedure

1. Minimize the client's discomfort as much as possible.
   a. Provide warmth.
   b. Provide assistance in moving, and position client frequently.
   c. Provide assistance in bathing and personal hygiene.
   d. Administer the appropriate medications before the pain becomes severe.
2. Recognize the symptoms of urgency or emergency conditions and seek immediate assistance.
3. Notify the charge nurse if there is an impending crisis and perform emergency actions until help arrives.
4. Encourage dying clients to do as much as they can for themselves so that they do not just give up—a state that only reinforces low self-esteem.
5. Provide emotional nursing care for the client.
   a. Form a relationship with the dying client. Be willing to be involved, to care, and to be committed to caring for a dying client.
   b. Allocate time to spend with the client so that not only physical care is administered.
   c. Recognize the grief pattern and support the client as he or she moves through it.
   d. Recognize that your physical presence is comforting by staying physically close to the client if

TO MY FAMILY, MY PHYSICIAN, MY LAWYER, MY CLERGYMAN
TO ANY MEDICAL FACILITY IN WHOSE CARE I HAPPEN TO BE
TO ANY INDIVIDUAL WHO MAY BECOME RESPONSIBLE FOR MY HEALTH, WELFARE OR AFFAIRS

Death is as much a reality as birth, growth, maturity and old age—it is the one certainty of life. If the time comes when I, ______________________ can no longer take part in decisions for my own future, let this statement stand as an expression of my wishes, while I am still of sound mind.

If the situation should arise in which there is no reasonable expectation of my recovery from physical or mental disability, I request that I be allowed to die and not be kept alive by artificial means or "heroic measures". I do not fear death itself as much as the indignities of deterioration, dependence and hopeless pain. I, therefore, ask that medication be mercifully administered to me to alleviate suffering even though this may hasten the moment of death.

This request is made after careful consideration. I hope you who care for me will feel morally bound to follow its mandate. I recognize that this appears to place a heavy responsibility upon you, but it is with the intention of relieving you of such responsibility and of placing it upon myself in accordance with my strong convictions, that this statement is made.

Signed ______________________

Date ______________________

Witness ______________________

Witness ______________________

Copies of this request have been given to ______________________

____

____

____

In case of terminal illness, Euthanasia Council's "Living Will" can clarify client's wishes. (Copies can be obtained by writing the Council at 250 W. 57th St., New York, NY 10019.)

he or she is frightened. Use touch if appropriate and nonverbal communication.

   e. Respect the client's need for privacy, and withdraw if the client has a need to be alone or to disengage from personal relationships.
   f. Be tuned into client's cues that he or she wants to talk and express feelings, cry, or even intellectually discuss the dying process.
   g. Accept the client at the level on which he or she is functioning without making judgments.

6. Provide the level of care that encourages the client to retain confidence in the health care team.
7. Assist the client through the experience of dying in whatever way you are able to do so.
8. Support the family of the dying client.
   a. Understand that the family may be going through anticipatory grief before the actual event of dying.
   b. Understand that different family members react differently to the impending death and support the different reactions.
   c. Be aware that demonstrating your concern and caring assists the family to cope with the grief process.
9. Be aware of your own personal orientation toward the dying process.
   a. Explore your own feelings about death and dying with the understanding that until you have faced the subject of death you will be inadequate to support the client or the family as they experience the dying process.
   b. Share your feelings about dying with the staff and others; actively work through them so that negativity does not get transferred to the client.

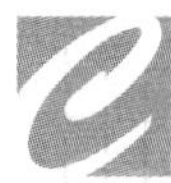

CHARTING for the Dying Client

- Client's physical symptoms
- Stage of dying and acceptance of client
- Support systems available to client
- Nursing care measures that make the client the most comfortable
- Family acceptance and interaction with client

CRITICAL THINKING APPLICATION

CLINICAL PROBLEMS	CRITICAL THINKING OPTIONS
Nurse is unable to care for the dying client due to her or his own emotional reaction.	• Request that other staff members take over, as the objective is to be able to give good nursing care. • Request assistance from skilled professional so you can work through your own feelings about death in order to be able to cope with the next death experience.
Client loses confidence in the health care team.	• Attempt to ascertain exactly what occurred to cause client to lose confidence in the team. • Report to charge nurse so that staff caring for client may be changed. Be sure to choose experienced personnel who are equipped to cope with a dying client.
Client lingers on and does not fulfill expectation that death would occur in the near future.	• Report status to staff so arrangements may be made for respite–supportive care for family who is having a difficult time coping. • Discuss hospice care with the client's family.
Pain cannot be controlled adequately with ordered medication.	• Report to physician so alternative pain relief methods may be used. • Assist the client to cope by spending additional time and meeting physical needs.

unit 3

POSTMORTEM CARE

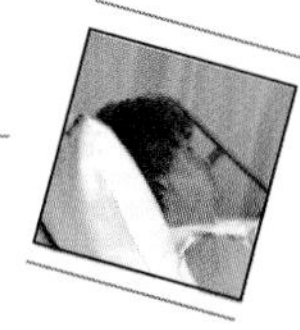

NURSING PROCESS DATA

ASSESSMENT Data Base

Verify that client has been pronounced dead by the physician.

Complete your own observations that client has no observable responses to stimuli.

Identify client by name and client's belongings for labeling.

PLANNING Objectives

To prepare body for removal from clinical unit

To protect the condition of the body for the purpose of respect for the deceased and his or her family during final viewing

To document facts and time relating to death

To identify and label client and client's belongings

IMPLEMENTATION Procedure

Providing Postmortem Care

EVALUATION Expected Outcomes

Postmortem care is completed by assigned staff member.

Client's personal items have been identified and labeled properly.

Family is supported through grief process by staff.

PROVIDING POSTMORTEM CARE

Equipment

Bathing supplies
Shroud or morgue bag
Identification tags
Protective pads, if necessary
Rolls of gauze and abdominal pads, if necessary to secure limbs together
Paper bags or plastic bags for personal belongings
Gurney or specialized morgue cart
Clean gloves

Procedure

1. If there are other clients or visitors in the room, carefully explain the situation and ask them to temporarily leave the room if possible. Provide privacy.
2. Collect necessary equipment.
3. Follow hospital procedure regarding notification of various departments and personnel.

Signed by the donor and the following two witnesses in the presence of each other:

Signature of Donor ______ Date of Birth of Donor ______

Date Signed ______ City & State ______

Witness ______ Witness ______

This is a legal document under the Uniform Anatomical Gift Act or similar laws.

For further information consult your physician or

National Kidney Foundation
116 East 27th Street, New York, N.Y. 10016

To ensure that organs are donated appropriately, instruct client to fill out and keep donor card available at all times.

   a. Determine if client has signed a donor card and/or has made a decision to donate any organs.

b. Check client's Advanced Directives on file at the hospital for donor instructions.
c. Notify appropriate hospital personnel or local procurement organization (OPO) for assistance with organ donation.
d. Follow specific procedures for organ transplant according to hospital policy.

4. Maintain proper alignment of the body. Raise the head of the bed slightly to prevent pooling of fluids in the head or face.
5. Don gloves.
6. If possible, place dentures in mouth to maintain original shape of face and mouth.
7. Remove any external objects causing pressure or injury to the skin (e.g., oxygen mask).
8. Following hospital policy, remove, cut, or secure any tubes, drains, or monitoring lines.
9. Following hospital policy, secure or replace dressings.
10. Cleanse the body as needed. A partial bath may be required to remove secretions, wound drainage, stains.
11. Close the eyes. If necessary, use paper tape or gauze pads. You may do this after the family has visited the deceased.
12. Place protective incontinent pad under buttocks and between legs diaper fashion.
13. If family is to visit the deceased, provide clean linen and gown for client.
14. Remove equipment used for cleansing client.
15. If previously determined or requested by client or family, notify the appropriate clergy or religious support person.
16. After family and clergy have visited, label the body, attaching ID tags to the big toe, wrist, and morgue bag or as determined by standard procedure.
17. Tie limbs loosely together, using padding and gauze roll. Attach wrist and ankles, using proper alignment.

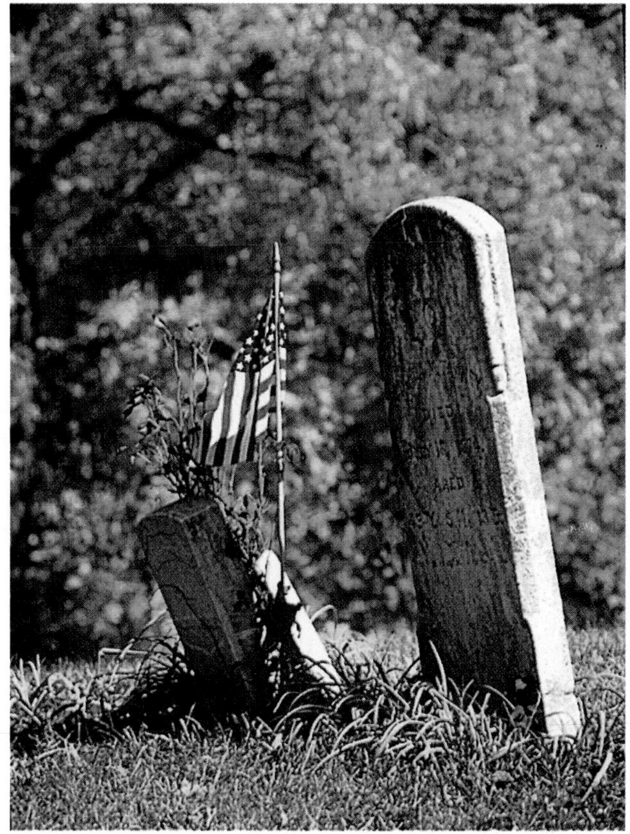

18. Place the body in the shroud or in morgue bag.
19. Label all personal belongings, and place them in a bag.
20. Remove gloves, and wash hands.
21. Close doors to client's room, and clear hallways in preparation to transfer the body to the morgue.
22. Transfer the body to the morgue on a gurney or a special morgue cart.
23. Place client's personal belongings in the appropriate place determined by hospital policy.
24. Support family members as needed.

CHARTING for Postmortem Care

- The events leading to the actual death (i.e., termination of vital signs)
- The exact time the physician was informed and death was pronounced
- When family members or significant others were notified
- Consent forms signed
- Condition of the body and postmortem care delivered
- Time the body and belongings were sent to the morgue

CRITICAL THINKING APPLICATION

CLINICAL PROBLEMS	CRITICAL THINKING OPTIONS
■ Client is not identified properly when sent to the morgue.	• Check identaband and shroud label before releasing client to mortician. • Request another nurse to check labels.
■ Donated organs are needed.	• Provide support to family and give an opportunity for questions. • Obtain signatures for consent form. (Kidneys should be removed within 1 hour after death. Eyes should be removed within 6–24 hours after death.) • Examine reverse side of driver's license, or remind the charge nurse to call mortician if burial plans have been made previously, to check on permission for organ donation through a living will.

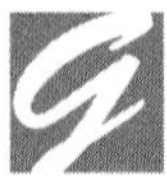

GERIATRIC CONSIDERATIONS

Three out of four elderly people die of heart disease, cancer, or stroke.

- Heart disease is leading cause of death, although it has declined since 1968.
- Death rates from cancer continue to rise, especially lung cancer.
- Death statistics for people in the 65–74 age group: heart disease accounted for 38%; cancer, 30% of deaths.

Death in the life cycle.

- In American culture death is not considered a positive process.
- Elderly may see death as an end to suffering and loneliness.
- Death is usually not feared if the person has lived a long and fulfilled life, having completed all developmental tasks.
- Religious beliefs or philosophy of life are important.

33

Advanced Skills in Nursing Practice

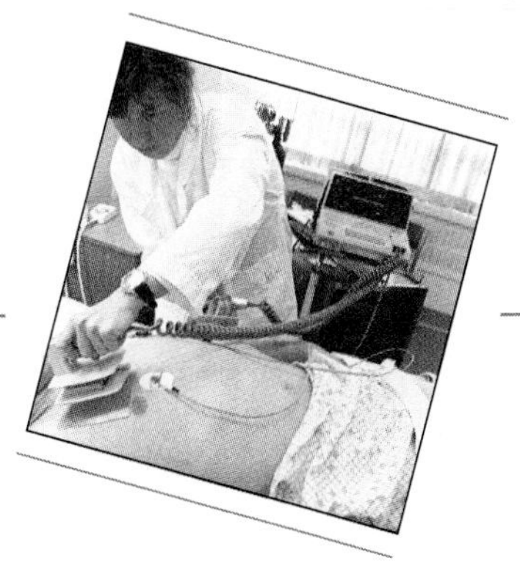

LEARNING OBJECTIVES

- Discuss the nursing actions required for treating clients requiring mechanical ventilation.
- Compare and contrast the changes in the ECG that indicate pacemaker failure to pace, sense, or capture.
- Describe the purpose of arterial line monitoring.
- Outline the steps in performing Allen's test.
- Explain the rationale for expelling all air from the syringe after drawing ABGs.
- Identify a normal arterial waveform.
- Explain what hemodynamic information is obtained when the client has a Swan–Ganz (balloon-tipped flow-directed) catheter.
- Discuss the purpose and method for calibrating and balancing the transducer.
- State three solutions for trouble shooting abnormal pulmonary artery catheter waveforms.

TERMINOLOGY

Adjunctive: accessory to or assisting with.

Allen's test: manual test to determine occlusion of the ulnar or radial artery. Digital pressure is applied directly over the radial and ulnar arteries. When pressure on one vessel is released, blood flow to palm and fingers indicates obstruction is not present in that vessel.

Aspiration: removal of fluid or air by applying suction.

Bipolar leads: electrocardiographic recording in which two poles are used: one positive, one negative. Leads I, II, and III of the 12-lead ECG are bipolar.

Bolus: a concentrated medication given intravenously directly or through an IV injection port.

Calibrate: to check or adjust the transducer to a standard measurement.

Cannulation: insertion of a tube into a vessel for purposes of invasive pressure monitoring. The cannula is attached to a transducer, which in turn displays the pressure on a monitor.

Cardiac index: the cardiac output in relation to body surface area.

Cardiac output: amount of blood ejected by the heart per minute. Determined by multiplying heart rate by stroke volume.

Central venous pressure: reflects diastolic pressure of right ventricle and filling pressure of right heart.

Diastole: Period when ventricles are relaxed; a period of ventricular filling.

Dicrotic notch: represents closure of aortic valve. Visualized on arterial waveform.

Distal: area farthest away from point of reference; fingers are most distal part of upper extremity.

Dysrhythmia: abnormal heart rhythm or rate.

Electrocardiogram: graphic representation of the variations in electrical potential caused by excitation of heart muscles.

Electrical potential: charges on cell membrane are separated into negative and positive charged particles.

Electrode: a medium used between an electric conductor and the object to which the current is applied.

Hemodynamic: movement of blood.

Left ventricular end-diastolic pressure: pressure of blood remaining in the left ventricle at end of diastole; preload.

Inherent: implanted by nature.

Invasive: puncture or incision through skin; insertion of tube or instrument into body.

Low cardiac output: decreased effectiveness or pumping ability of ventricle, leading to diminished amount of blood being ejected into systemic circulation with each heart beat. Can be due to disease states, such as CHF or dehydration.

Lumen: the inside, channel, or opening of the blood vessel.

Mean arterial blood pressure: average pressure within cardiovascular system throughout one cardiac cycle.

Oscilloscope: instrument that displays a visual representation of electrical activity on a screen.

Perfusion: blood flow to the tissues.

Peripheral resistance: constriction of the vessel lumen, decreasing blood flow to an area.

Precipitate: causes a substance in solution to settle in solid particles.

Proximal: refers to an area closest to the point of reference; humerus of upper extremity is more proximal to the body than the finger.

Pulmonary artery pressure: pressure in pulmonary artery

caused by tension in walls of pulmonary vascular bed.

Pulmonary artery wedge pressure: reflects left atrial mean pressure and left ventricular end diastolic pressure.

Repolarization: restoration of the heart to the original resting potential.

Thermodilution: method of calculating cardiac output through injection of solution into the proximal port of a pulmonary artery catheter.

Transducer: device that converts one form of energy into another (i.e., pressure is converted into electrical waveform, which is displayed on the monitor).

Vasculature: vascular system of the body.

Vasodilator: causes dilation of the blood vessels.

Vasopressor: causes contraction of the muscular tissue of the arteries and veins.

Vasospasm: constriction of a vessel due to spasm.

Ventricular systole: ejection of blood from ventricles.

Voltage: electromagnetic force measured in volts.

Waveform: pictorial representation of the arterial or pulmonary artery pressure, or electrical activity of the heart, depicted on an oscilloscope.

ADVANCED SKILLS IN NURSING PRACTICE

This chapter presents a nursing process framework for interventions used in the diagnosis and maintenance of homeostasis during life-threatening conditions. Provision for competent care during critical periods requires a knowledge of monitoring techniques. Working with monitors and providing client care at the same time can be a challenging experience for the nurse.

All of these monitoring techniques are useful adjunctive tools that provide the practitioner with critical information. Interpretation of the clinical information assists in rapid documentation of the pathophysiologic status of the major systems. In particular, data can identify shock states, alterations in cardiac output, fluid deficit or overload, or alterations in blood pressure. Pressure readings and other data serve as guides for identifying appropriate nursing diagnoses, developing a plan of care, and evaluating therapy.

In the clinical setting, nurses are constantly faced with new equipment, new techniques, and better and more sophisticated evaluative methods. To keep pace in the area of technologic advancement can be a monumental task, one that challenges the nurse's energy, patience, and abilities. The nurse's role in assessment, planning, intervention, and evaluation is based in part on the nurse's familiarity with monitoring data.

Hemodynamic monitoring has evolved over the years from continuous ECG monitoring, measuring CVPs (right heart pressures) and indirect measurements of left-side filling pressures through the Swan–Ganz pulmonary artery catheter to sophisticated multilumen flow-directed catheters. The nurse's role in monitoring clients has increased dramatically as the monitoring equipment has expanded and become more intricate.

Nurses are responsible for measuring cardiac output, inserting PICC lines, removing CVP lines, and defibrillating clients with life-threatening arrhythmias. Bedside monitoring has become as commonplace in the nurse's daily routine as starting IVs and reading ECGs. Nurses, particularly in the critical care unit, are responsible for monitoring clients, validating hemodynamic data, and making decisions about titrating medications.

Hemodynamic pressure-monitoring techniques require that the equipment is properly inserted, functions correctly, and that the monitor waveforms are interpreted correctly.

Catheters used to measure pressures are inserted into the right side of the heart and the multilumen, balloon-tipped, flow-directed catheters. The two-lumen (port) catheters are used to measure pulmonary artery or pulmonary artery wedge pressures. Three-lumen catheters also monitor right atrial pressure. Four- and five-lumen catheters measure cardiac output and have one port for infusion of medications or fluids. Unfortunately, as the number of ports increases the transmitted pressure waveforms are less accurate. Waveforms, or pressure signals, are transmitted to monitors via a fluid-filled catheter called a transducer. Digital display on the monitors provides necessary data for nurses to make critical assessments necessary for safe, effective care.

Ability to integrate monitoring data with other physiologic parameters is essential to providing excellent nursing care. Monitoring is a method of providing additional data, which, although important, does not obviate the need for quality care based on the nursing process. In fact, it is important that monitors not become more important than the client. The first objective then is to care for the client, not tend the monitor.

One of the ways to achieve both goals, the mastery over monitoring procedures and the attainment of high-quality client care, is to become familiar with the technical equipment so that it no longer causes anxiety and uncertainty. Once this level of understanding is realized, the focus can be on the client, not the monitoring equipment. The monitoring modalities presented in this section can easily be learned and assimilated into clinical practice.

unit 1 CARDIAC EMERGENCIES

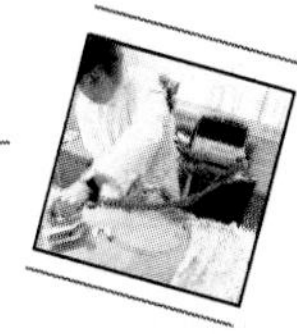

Early identification of the signs of cardiac pump failure will lead to prompt and effective treatment. If left untreatred, ventricular arrhythmias and some atrial arrhythmias may develop into reduced cardiac output and pump failure.

Interventions for treating cardiac failure and pulmonary edema focus on correcting the arrhythmias and removing excess body fluid. One way to restore ideal timing is to terminate the dysrhythmia by delivering an electrical countershock. This countershock causes simultaneous depolarization of the entire myocardium. It thus interrupts the dysrhythmia, allowing the sinoatrial node to resume control of the sequence and coordination of depolarization. Two types of electrical countershock are used—defibrillation and cardioversion.

Defibrillation is an emergency procedure in which the maximum dose of electricity possible is delivered, and the timing of the shock is not synchronized with ventricular depolarization. Cardioversion is an elective procedure. An electrical countershock is synchronized with ventricular depolarization for the purpose of converting a pathological cardiac rhythm to normal sinus rhythm. Cardioversion is contraindicated in rhythms due to digitalis toxicity, because of the danger of inducing lethal ventricular dysrhythmias.

Essential for treating emergency situations in the hospital setting is the crash cart. Being required to know the location of the crash cart, its contents, and knowledge of the available emergency drugs will assist the hospital staff to provide quick, competent care to clients in cardiac arrest. The crash carts should be kept uncluttered, easily accessible and located in an area that is obvious to all of the staff. Nurses must be familiar with the contents of each drawer of the cart to quickly find the emergency equipment.

NURSING PROCESS DATA

ASSESSMENT Data Base

Assess heart rate and rhythm.

Identify ventricular or atrial arrhythmias on ECG recording.

Assess need to use the emergency cart.

Identify appropriate drugs needed for an emergency situation.

Assess need for defibrillation.

Assess that safety factors are maintained during cardioversion and defibrillation.

PLANNING Objectives

To provide low-voltage, direct current treatment to convert ventricular or atrial arrhythmias to normal sinus rhythm

To provide a systematic method of organizing emergency equipment and medications for easy access and use

To identify appropriate drugs used in emergency situations

IMPLEMENTATION Procedures

Using the Emergency Cart

Contents of Typical Emergency Cart

Performing Defibrillation

Assisting with Synchronized Elective Cardioversion

EVALUATION Expected Outcomes

All necessary equipment is easily accessible from the cart in an emergency situation.

Appropriate medications are obtained during an emergency situation.

Heart rhythm and rate return to normal following defibrillation or cardioversion.

Safety factors are maintained during cardioversion and defibrillation.

USING THE EMERGENCY CART

Equipment

Emergency cart with locking drawers
Emergency cart checklist
Airway equipment
Oxygen equipment
Suction equipment
Monitor leads
Defibrillator
Oscilloscope
IV equipment
Emergency drugs

Procedure

1. Identify equipment and medications commonly used in emergency situations.
2. Gather equipment.
3. Place equipment in drawers according to priority use in the most commonly occurring emergency situations.
4. Lock drawers when cart is not in use. **Rationale:** This prevents personnel from using equipment for situations other than emergencies and not replacing it.
5. Place emergency cart checklist on outside of cart in visible area. **Rationale:** Cart contents are checked on a daily basis to ensure medications are not outdated, equipment is in working condition, and cart is locked.
6. Place cart in designated, easily accessible, and visible area of the nursing unit. **Rationale:** Provides for less confusion if the cart is needed.
7. Familiarize all personnel with location and contents of cart, function of equipment, and emergency procedures.
8. Practice retrieving and setting up equipment through mock situations. **Rationale:** This ensures that all personnel are able to use cart during an emergency situation.
9. Check cart daily, and restock immediately after use. **Rationale:** If cart is not completely stocked, delays can occur during an emergency situation jeopardizing client care.

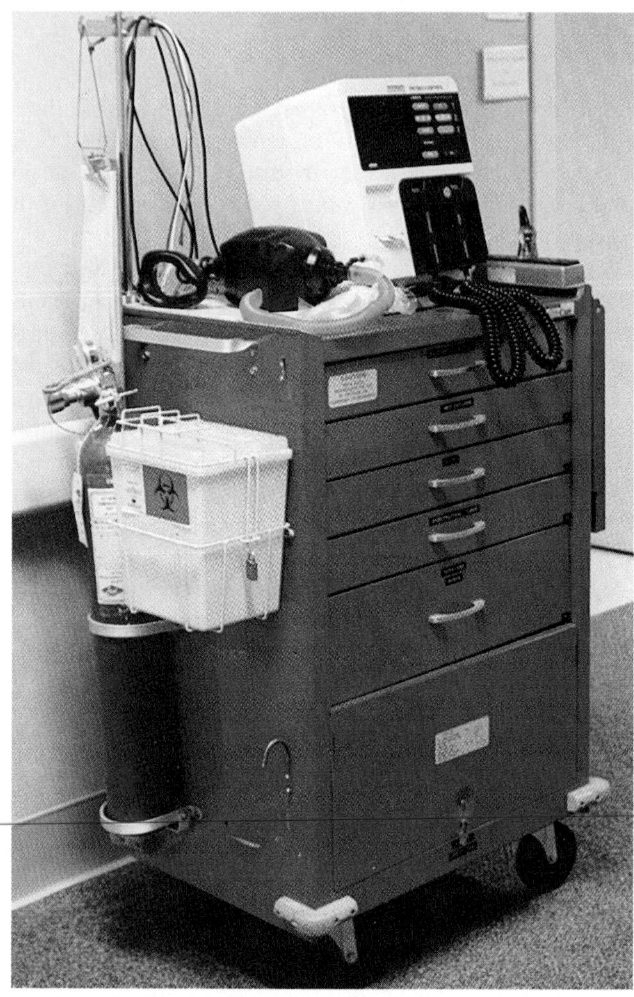

Fully equipped emergency cart is placed in easily accessible and visible area.

CONTENTS OF TYPICAL EMERGENCY CART

Top of Cart
ECG monitor with readout
ECG electrodes and extra roll of recording paper
Defibrillator
Defibrillator paddles and conductive medium
First drawer
Intubation equipment
Second Drawer
Emergency medications

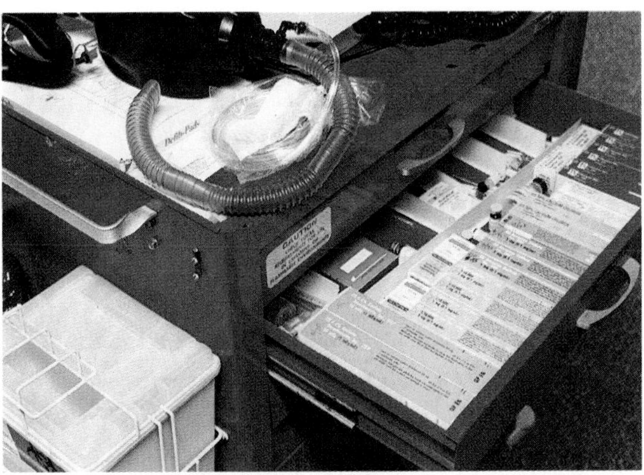

Stock drugs for emergency use are checked daily and restocked immediately after use.

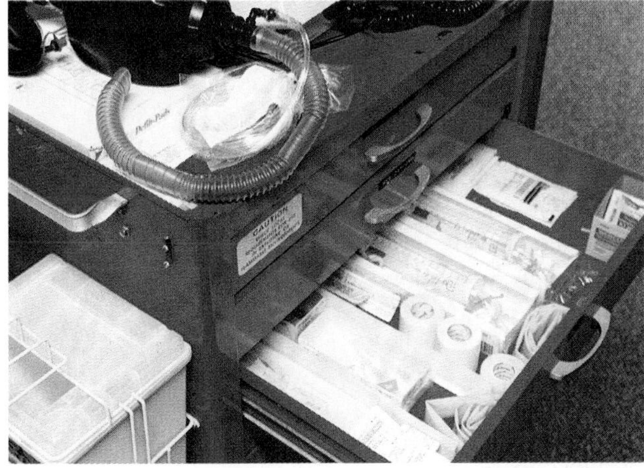

Supplies for initiating IV access are included in the emergency cart.

Third Drawer

Venipuncture supplies: Steel needles, over-the-needle catheters, inside-the-needle catheters, short intracatheters, macrodrop administration sets, microdrop administration sets, extension tubing, stopcocks, syringes, tape, alcohol swabs, tourniquets, tincture of benzoin, gauze pads

Blood sampling supplies: Venous blood tubes, arterial blood gas kits or glass syringes

Spinal needles for intracardiac injections

Scalpels with blades attached

Alligator clips

Fourth Drawer

Oral airways

Endotracheal tubes

Laryngoscope handle, curved blades, straight blades, extra batteries, extra bulbs, stylet

McGill forceps

Tonsil suction

Surgical lubricant

Hand-held self-inflating resuscitation bag

Oxygen masks, connecting tubing, flowmeter

Suction catheters

Nasogastric tubes

Bottom Shelf

Tracheostomy tray

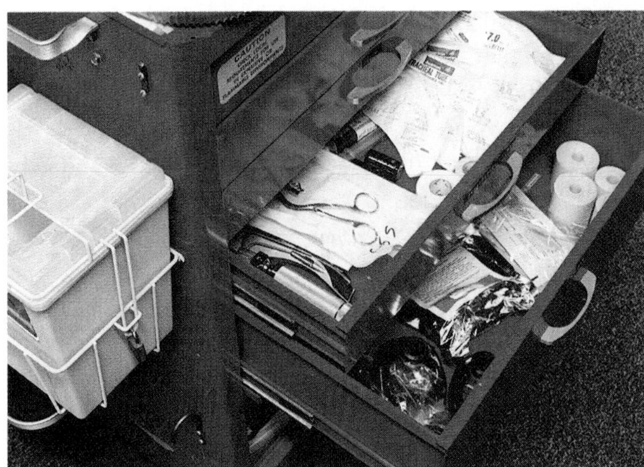

Airways and endotracheal tubes are stored in the fourth drawer.

Cutdown tray and sutures

IV solutions, armboards

Portable suction device

Pacemaker and electrodes

Back of Cart

Cardiac arrest board

Side of Cart

CVP catheters or long intracatheters

Emergency cart checklist

Cardiac resuscitation recording sheet and clipboard

PERFORMING DEFIBRILLATION

Equipment

ECG monitor
Defibrillator with external paddles
Saline pads or conducting gel or paste
Airway
Cardiac board
Resuscitator bag
Emergency cart
Oxygen equipment

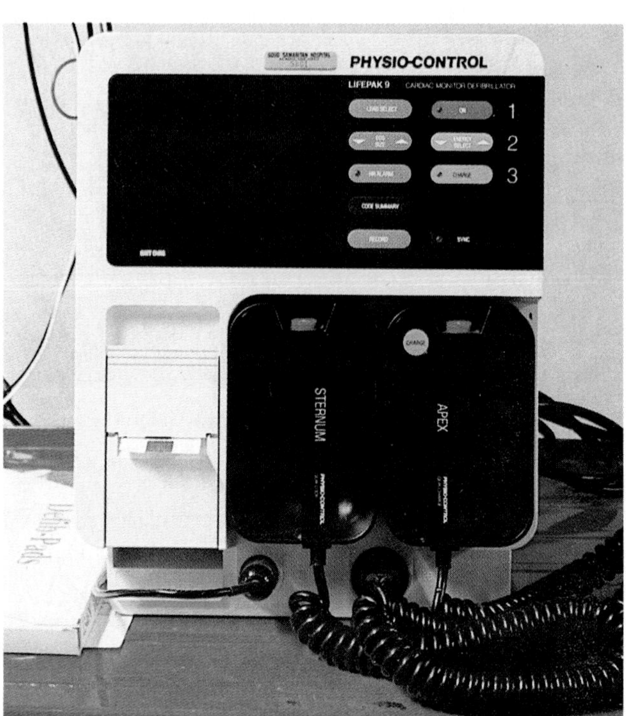

Defibrillator with monitor screen is stored on top of the emergency cart.

Preparation

1. Verify ECG reading of ventricular fibrillation (or ventricular tachycardia in nonresponsive client). **Rationale:** Artifact can mimic ventricular fibrillation.
2. Validate client nonresponsiveness.
3. Gather equipment.
4. Plug defibrillator or emergency cart into electric outlet.
5. Turn defibrillator power ON, and allow to warm up.
6. Place cardiac board under client's torso, if not already present from CPR.
7. Dry client's chest if necessary.
8. Place saline-soaked pads on client's chest, or spread thin coat of conductive paste to surface of paddles. One pad is placed below right clavicle near sternum and second pad is placed to left of cardiac apex (below and to the left of left nipple) in anterior axillary line. **Rationale:** Conductive medium decreases skin resistance and prevents burns.
9. Set defibrillator in nonsynchronized mode. **Rationale:** The machine does not function in synchronized mode as there are no R waves in ventricular fibrillation. The synchronized mode is used for cardioversion.

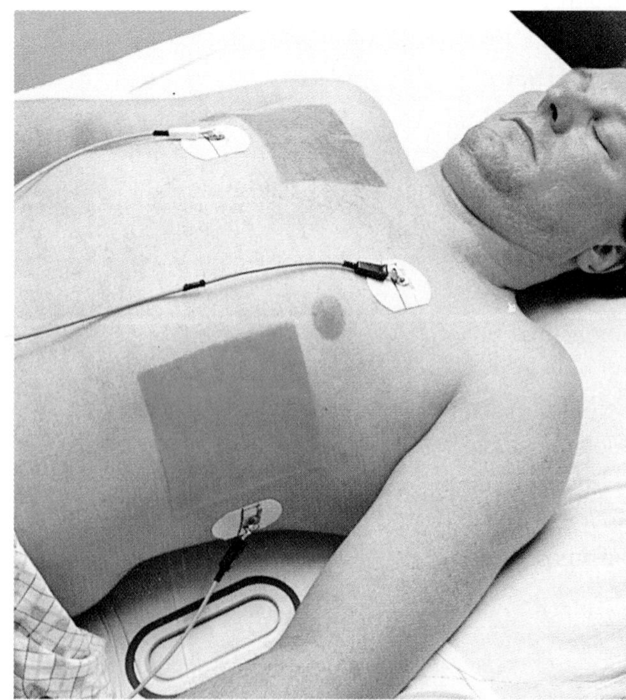

Conducting pads are placed below right clavicle and left of cardiac apex.

■ CLINICAL ALERT

Before beginning defibrillation procedure remove all transdermal medication patches on chest. Defibrillation over nitroglycerin could cause an explosion.

TABLE 33–1. Energy Levels for Cardioversion and Defibrillation

Type of Arrhythmia	Energy Level (J)*
Cardioversion	
Paroxysmal supra ventricular tachycardia	75–100
Atrial flutter	25–50
Atrial fibrillation	100 to 200 to 360J
Unstable ventricular tachycardia	50 to 100 to 200 to 360J
Defibrillation	
Pulseless ventricular tachycardia, ventricular fibrillation	200 to 200–300 to 360J Alternate with advanced cardiac life support (ACLS) drugs

*1 joule = 1 watt second

10. Dial defibrillator to charge at 200 watt seconds. **Rationale:** Electric shock is damaging to myocardium. Start with 200 J, then proceed if necessary to 300 J, then 360 J (Table 33–1).

Procedure

1. After identifying urgent situation, call for defibrillation and begin CPR.
2. Ensure that defibrillator is charged to 200 watt seconds *initially*.
3. Instruct all persons to move away from bed area and any equipment connected to client.
4. Stand away from bed area yourself.
5. Apply paddles with firm pressure (20 lb).
6. Depress discharge buttons on defibrillator simultaneously to ensure appropriate energy discharge.
7. Check ECG pattern to determine effects of defibrillation. Reinstitute CPR and administer appropriate medications if ventricular fibrillation continues.
8. Prepare defibrillator equipment for second attempt.
9. Instruct all persons to move away from bed area.
10. Repeat defibrillation procedure.
11. Monitor client every 15 minutes after defibrillation until stable:
    a. Monitored heart rhythm
    b. Level of consciousness
    c. Vital signs
    d. Presence of peripheral pulses
    e. Heart and lung sounds
12. Continue oxygen administration.
13. Continue IV medication administration (e.g., sympathomimetics antiarrhythmics).

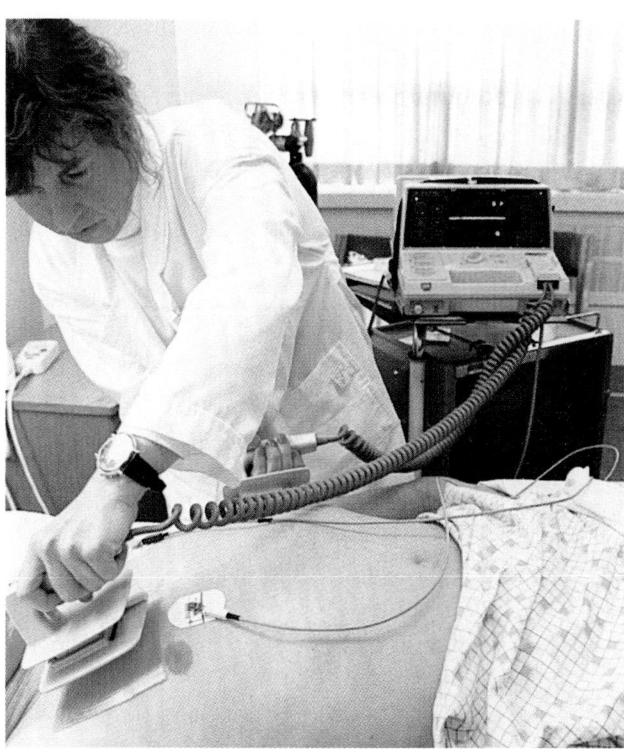

Apply paddles with firm pressure over conducting pads.

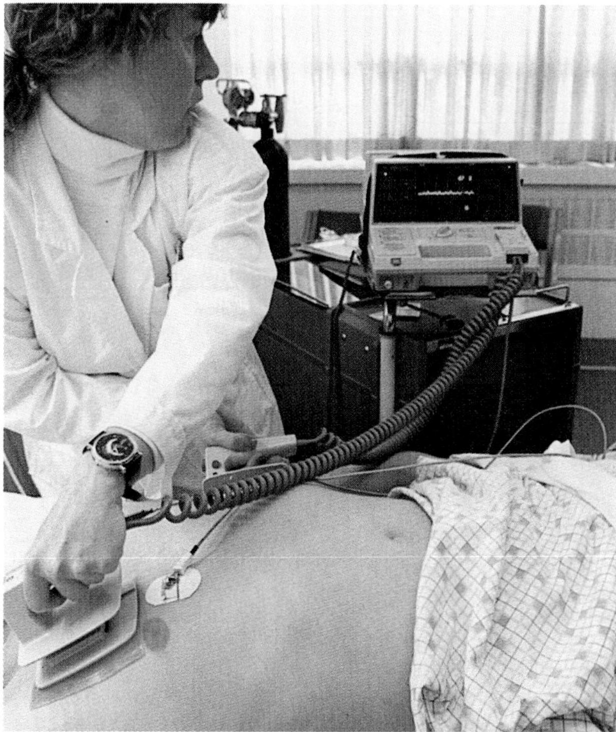

After discharge, check ECG monitor to evaluate client's response.

ASSISTING WITH SYNCHRONIZED ELECTIVE CARDIOVERSION

Equipment

Cardioverter (defibrillator unit set in synchronization mode)
Paddles—anteroposterior or anterolateral
ECG monitor and recorder
12-lead ECG machine
Conductive paste or saline gauze pads
Emergency cart, drugs, and equipment
IV solution of D_5W, administration set, and medium-gauge IV needle or catheter
IV sedative medication as ordered

Synchronized cardioversion is also used for emergency management of supraventricular and ventricular tachycardia.

Preparation

1. Review cardioversion orders, and check that equipment is functioning properly.
2. Review ordered laboratory values or drug levels, particularly potassium level. **Rationale:** Hypokalemia or drug toxicity may increase risk of dysrhythmias after cardioversion.
3. Check that digitalis was discontinued 24 hours or more before cardioversion, or as ordered by physician.
4. Withhold food and fluids for 6–12 hours before elective cardioversion.
5. Determine client's understanding of procedure, and clarify information as needed.
6. Validate signed consent form.
7. Remove dentures.
8. Have client void before procedure.
9. Administer prophylactic atropine or quinidine if ordered.
10. Obtain baseline 12-lead ECG, and label it "precardioversion."
11. Place emergency cart in room or immediately outside.
12. Verify that emergency drugs are prepared and available on a "standby" basis. Emergency drugs are atropine and lidocaine.
13. Obtain baseline assessment values for vital signs and ECG rhythms.
14. Notify anesthesia department of readiness.

Procedure

1. Place client in supine position.
2. Establish IV line, and administer fluids at "keep open" rate.
3. Administer oxygen per nasal cannula precardioversion.
4. Connect client to ECG monitor (lead I or lead II for good R waves).
5. Check monitor pattern for size and clarity of pattern.
6. Plug cardioverter in, and turn power switch ON.
7. Turn **synchronizer** switch ON.
8. Test synchronization by pushing manual synchronization button.
9. Charge machine to level specified by physician, usually 25–50 J to start (1 joule = 1 watt second). Note that designated charge is reached.
10. Disconnect all electric equipment from client except ECG monitor and cardioverter.
11. Administer sedative as ordered by physician (anesthesiologist may do this).
12. Administer oxygen as ordered, then D.C. and remove oxygen from client area.
13. Apply conductive paste to surface of paddles, or use saline pads on chest.
14. Make sure chest is dry, and place paddles on chest.
    a. Anterolateral paddles are placed as in defibrillation, one over second intercostal space to right of sternum and other over fifth intercostal space in left midclavicular line.
    b. Anteroposterior paddles are placed with flat paddle posteriorly between scapulae and anterior handheld paddle over fifth intercostal space in left midclavicular line.
15. Observe ECG rhythm on monitor.
16. Start ECG recorder.
17. Note whether synchronization indicator is superimposed on R wave of ECG.
18. Give command to "stand clear," and stand clear yourself.

19. The **physician** depresses discharge buttons on paddles and keeps them depressed until countershock is delivered. The shock may not occur instantly, since machine waits until the next R wave in the ECG to discharge.
20. Observe postcardioversion rhythm.
21. Provide postcardioversion care.
    a. Evaluate vital signs, ECG, level of consciousness, peripheral pulses, neurologic status, and vital signs every 15 minutes until stable, then routinely. **Rationale:** Thromboemboli to the lungs or systemic circulation may occur, especially if client has been in long-standing atrial fibrillation.
    b. Support airway and ventilation, and oxygenate as needed.
    c. Monitor heart rhythm continuously.
    d. Obtain 12-lead ECG, and label it "postcardioversion."
    e. Keep client under observation for 12–24 hours. **Rationale:** Transient hypotension and minor dysrhythmias are common.

CHARTING

for Defibrillation

- Time of arrest or discovery
- Client symptoms
- Predefibrillation rhythm
- Number of defibrillation attempts and watt seconds used
- Postdefibrillation rhythm
- Other resuscitative measures
- Time resuscitation discontinued
- Outcome of resuscitation
- Drugs administered

for Cardioversion

- Precardioversion rhythm
- Precardioversion client preparation completed
- Number of cardioversion attempts
- Watt seconds for each attempt
- Postcardioversion rhythm
- Postcardioversion problems, if any
- Drugs administered

CRITICAL THINKING APPLICATION

CLINICAL PROBLEMS	CRITICAL THINKING OPTIONS
for Emergency Cart	
■ Equipment is missing from cart.	• Immediately notify charge nurse or pharmacist, and obtain replacement from pharmacy, floor stock, or nearby unit. • If any delay in obtaining item, tape warning notice to chart that item is missing.
■ Additional useful equipment is not included on cart.	• When emergency is over ask to obtain approval to add item to cart on a trial basis.
■ Equipment cannot be located promptly on cart.	• During resuscitation, ask assistance in locating items.

	CLINICAL PROBLEMS	CRITICAL THINKING OPTIONS
		• After resuscitation, suggest more logical placement of item (e.g., alphabetize or with similar equipment). • After resuscitation, practice mock codes to retrieve items.
■	Equipment is inaccessible or malfunctions.	• Replace malfunctioning equipment immediately. • Obtain care from the nearest unit.
	for Defibrillation	
■	Carotid pulse is present and client is conscious, although monitor shows pattern of ventricular fibrillation.	• Check client monitor electrodes and wires for contact with client, cable, or telemetry connections and adjust or replace as needed.
■	Defibrillator fails to discharge.	• Check that defibrillator is plugged in. • Check that unit is turned ON. • Make sure synchronizer switch is OFF.
■	There is an electric arc across chest when paddle buttons are depressed.	• Avoid excessive gel on paddles. • Wipe off any conductive paste or perspiration between the paddle sites, and defibrillate again. • Remove all transdermal medication patches. Defibrillation over nitroglycerin can cause explosion.
■	After defibrillation, rhythm changes to standstill or rhythm appears on monitor, but carotid pulse is absent (pulseless electrical activity).	• Institute CPR. • Administer calcium as ordered by physician to improve excitation–contraction coupling.
	for Cardioversion	
■	On precardioversion laboratory assessment there is elevation of serum digitalis level.	• Notify physician of findings. • Reassure client that there is not a life-threatening problem.
■	Ventricular fibrillation occurs.	• Anticipate that physician will immediately turn off synchronizer switch. Increase energy setting to 200 J, and defibrillate.
■	Asystole occurs.	• Immediately institute CPR. • Assist physician in advanced cardiac life-support measures.

unit 2 PACEMAKER MANAGEMENT

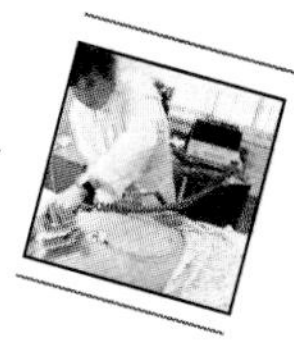

PACEMAKER

A pacemaker is a device that provides electrical stimulation to the heart muscle to maintain effective cardiac output. Pacemakers are used when normal initiation or conduction of electrical impulses fails. Pacemakers have two primary parts: the pulse generator and the electrodes. When temporary pacing is desired, the pulse generator is external. When permanent pacing is needed, the pulse generator is placed internally. Advanced degrees of heart block usually require permanent pacemaker placement. We focus primarily on the use of pacemakers for temporary cardiac rhythm support.

The temporary pacemaker is inserted for temporary conditions, such as severe bradycardias, drug toxicity, myocardial infarction, and in cardiac surgery. The temporary pacemaker is a device that provides a low-voltage electrical stimulus to the endocardial surface of the right atrium or ventricle (transvenous method) or to the epicardium (transthoracic, or epicardial, method). Either chamber can be paced alone, or both chambers paced sequentially. In addition, the pacemaker can be used to suppress or overdrive tachyarrhythmias.

All methods of temporary pacing use a pulse generator with rechargeable or replaceable batteries and some type of electrode or impulse conductor. These electrodes may be either unipolar or bipolar and differ in sensitivity. Unipolor (single-pole) catheter electrodes have a single cathode tip and are more sensitive to the client's generated impulses. The catheter electrode wire fits into the negative output terminal on the generator. Bipolar (double-pole) catheter electrodes have both an anode and cathode at the tip and fit into both positive and negative output terminals on the generator. The pace rate determines the number of beats per minute (BPM) provided by the generator.

Demand (synchronous) pacing is the most frequently used. The electrode is triggered to stimulate the heart only when the heart's intrinsic or natural atrial or ventricular stimulation fails to occur by a predetermined time. The atrial synchronous electrode's discharge is *inhibited* if natural atrial depolarization occurs, or is *triggered* to stimulate atrial depolarization if this does not occur naturally within a specified period. The ventricular inhibited pacemaker senses when the ventricle naturally depolarizes, and is inhibited or is triggered to discharge to activate the ventricle if the client's ventricular rate falls below the preset rate.

Initiation of temporary pacing by attaching electrode wires to an external generator source may be accomplished by the following routes:

Transvenous

Pacemaker wires are threaded percutaneously through the subclavian or femoral vein or through a cutdown in the brachial or external jugular vein. With either method, the electrode is advanced through the vena cava, to the right atrium, or advanced through the tricuspid valve and positioned at the apex of the right ventricle on the endocardial surface. The electrode is then attached to the generator.

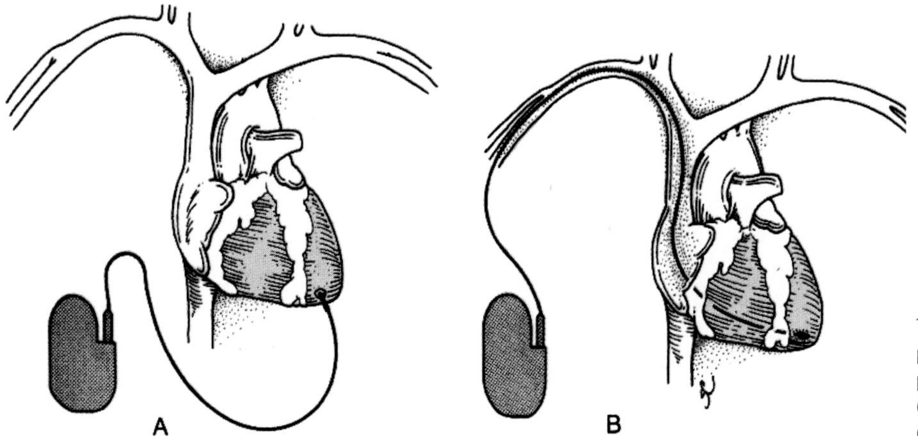

Temporary pacemakers have two parts, the pulse generator and the electrode. The pulse generator is external to the body. **(A)** Transthoracic pericardial pacemaker **(B)** Transvenous pacemaker.

Transthoracic

Electrodes are attached to the pericardial surface of the right atrium and right ventricle and threaded externally via a needle through the chest wall. Pacemaker wires are frequently inserted in this manner during cardiac surgery. Instead of being connected to the generator, the wires are covered, and are then available for use. If pacing is necessary, the atrial or ventricular electrode is connected to the respective output terminal on the generator, or both are connected for dual-chamber pacing, which best mimics normal cardiac electrophysiology.

NURSING PROCESS DATA

ASSESSMENT Data Base

Assess preexisting cardiovascular status.

Identify client's or family's knowledge of and cooperation with procedure.

Assess cardiac monitor rhythm and rate.

Assess heart sounds.

Observe client's general appearance for pallor, dyspnea, or edema.

Assess for hemodynamic abnormalities related to low cardiac output, including dizziness, weakness, altered level of consciousness, low blood pressure, and decreased urinary output.

Ensure placement of intravenous route for administration of fluids and drugs during an emergency.

PLANNING Objectives

To provide temporary cardiac electrical stimulation for conditions resulting in alterations of heart rate

To prevent bradycardia

To improve cardiac function, thereby improving cardiac output

To provide a treatment modality for those cardiac dysfunctions impervious to drug therapy

IMPLEMENTATION Procedures

Assisting with Pacemaker Insertion

Maintaining Pacemaker Function

Providing Client Teaching

EVALUATION Expected Outcomes

Client's cardiac rate is maintained through use of a pacemaker.

Client is prepared psychologically and physically for insertion of the pacemaker.

Pacemaker is inserted without complications.

Heart rate and cardiac output improve.

ASSISTING WITH PACEMAKER INSERTION

Equipment

Emergency cart with defibrillator
External pacemaker pulse generator
Pacing catheter electrodes
ECG monitor
Client cable
Rubber glove
Skin antiseptic solution (povidone-iodine)
Sterile gloves, gown, and mask
Sterile towels
Lidocaine, 1–2%
Alcohol wipes
Syringe
Needles
Suture with attached needle
Sterile 4 × 4 gauze pads

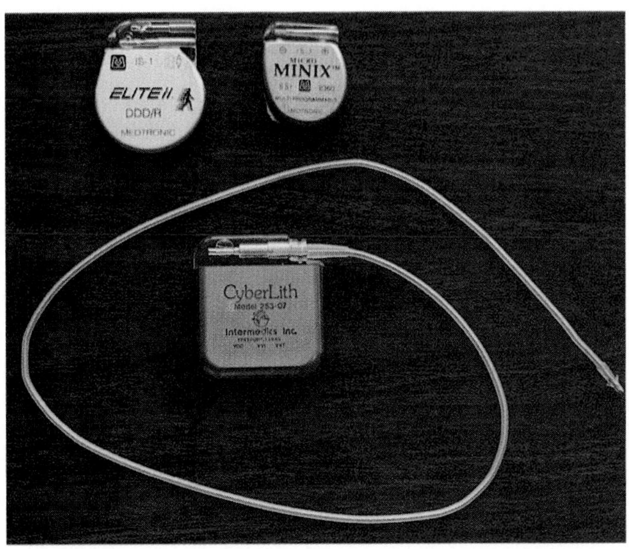

Permanent pacemaker and electrode for internal implant.

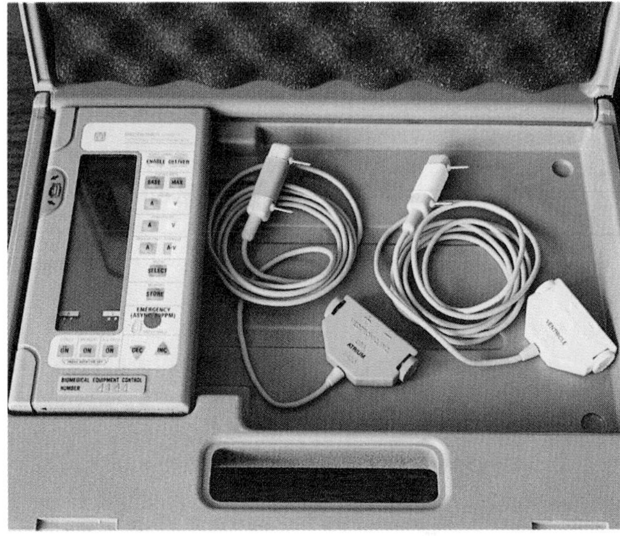
Type of external pacemaker in case.

Tape
Cutdown tray
Gloves

Preparation

1. Wash hands.
2. Provide sedation as necessary. Diazepam (Valium) is frequently used.
3. Connect client to a continuous ECG monitor.
4. Place the client in a supine position with head flat, or slightly lower than body.
5. If either the subclavian or external jugular vein is to be used, place a towel roll under the client's shoulders to provide better exposure of the insertion site.

Electrical Safety Alert

- Use only grounded equipment; use common ground.
- Remove and tag any defective equipment.
- Maintain environmental humidity at 50–60%
- Ground all metal beds.
- Validate electrical safety of beds.
- Avoid placing wet articles on electrical equipment.
- Insulate exposed pacing electrodes at all times.
- Wear rubber gloves when handling pacing electrodes or terminals.
- Do not touch any electric equipment while handling wire or terminals.

Procedure

1. Assist physician as needed.
   a. Physician dons mask, sterile gown, and gloves.
   b. Insertion site is cleansed with sterile antiseptic solution.
   c. Area is draped with sterile towels.

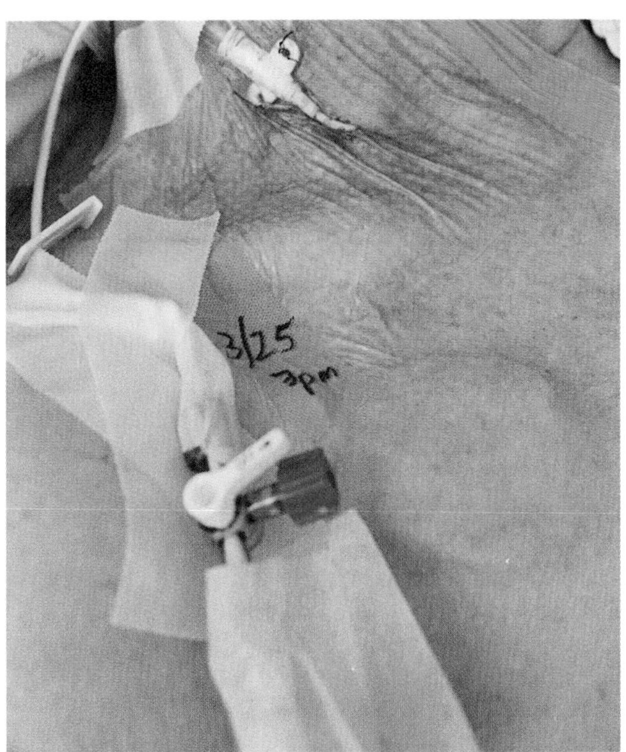

Implanted pacemaker outline is visible under the skin.

d. Top of lidocaine is cleansed with alcohol wipe.
e. Physician withdraws lidocaine, and skin is injected with 25-gauge needle.
f. Insertion is accomplished (transvenous method via cutdown or percutaneously). Catheter electrode wires are positioned, and skin sutures are applied.

2. Continuously monitor the ECG and client status during the insertion.
3. Don gloves to prevent microshock to client.
4. Connect the pacing electrode to the appropriate outlet terminal (unipolar to negative and bipolar to both the positive and negative terminals).
5. Turn on power switch on external pacemaker.
6. Set rate according to physician's orders.
7. Set milliamperes (ma) by determining threshold. To do this, observe the ECG while slowly increasing the number of milliamperes from its lowest setting to a point where a QRS complex is detected following each stimulus.
8. Multiply the threshold level according to hospital policy (usually two to four times) to adjust the milliampere setting.
9. Set sensitivity mode according to physician's order. (Usually 1.5 mV.)
10. Secure all connections. Put plastic cover back over pacemaker controls if required.
11. Place external pacemaker and exposed wires in a rubber glove to ensure insulation against electric shock to client.
12. Apply sterile dressings to insertion site, and tape securely.
13. Obtain chest x-ray following insertion to validate lead placement.
14. Obtain 12-lead ECG.

MAINTAINING TEMPORARY PACEMAKER FUNCTION

Equipment

9V batteries
Rubber gloves

Procedure

1. Observe for failure to sense.
   a. Observe the oscilloscope for presence of pacemaker artifact (spikes). Artifact before QRS complex in ventricular paced or preceding the P waves and QRS waves in AV sequential pacing.
   b. Check connections for secure, tight fit.
   c. Observe that pace–sense needle deflects to right, indicating pacing is occurring.
   d. Check sensitivity dial to determine if sensitivity threshold is set correctly.
2. Observe for failure to pace.
   a. Check that external generator is ON.
   b. Check battery to ensure it is functioning.
   c. Check lead connector sites.
   d. Check pace–sense indicator. (Absence of or slight deflection of the pace–sense indicator reveals battery failure.)
3. Observe for failure to capture.
   a. Observe for pacing artifact not followed by QRS complex. **Rationale:** This indicates a failure of the stimulus to trigger a ventricular response.
   b. Check the setting of the ma, or output dial, to determine if setting should be increased. **Rationale:** The myocardial threshold may be altered as a result of disease or drugs.
   c. Check all connector sites for secure, tight fit.

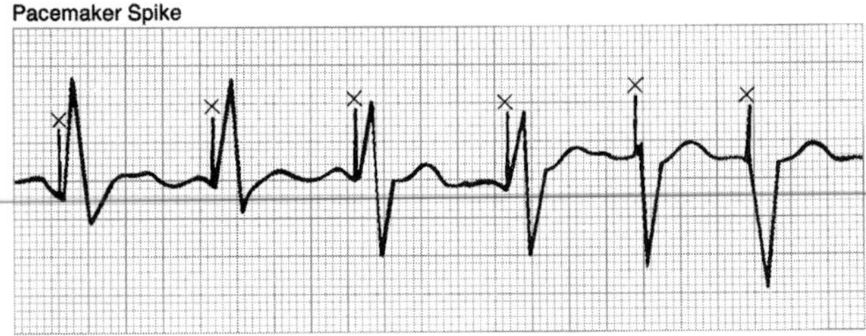

ECG tracing showing pacemaker spike triggering ventricular depolarization (QRS).

■ CLINICAL ALERT

Observe for pacemaker failure:
- Decreased urine output
- ECG pattern change
- Decreased blood pressure
- Bradycardia
- Shortness of breath

4. Observe that sutures are intact.
5. Obtain CXR at every observation stage.
6. Monitor client's response to therapy.
   a. Assess urine output. **Rationale:** Decreased urine output indicates poor cardiac output.
   b. Observe for dyspnea, crackles, bradycardia, hypotension.
   c. Monitor temperature.
   d. Observe client for signs of anxiety or fear. Complete pacemaker teaching as necessary.

PROVIDING CLIENT TEACHING

Equipment

Audiovisual aids
Written material

Procedure

1. Ascertain what client already knows and understands.
2. Determine client's ability and level of interest in learning about pacemaker.
3. Recognize client's fears, and provide opportunity to talk about them.
4. Review facts: heart anatomy and physiology and pacemaker information. Use illustrations and audiovisual aids.
5. Clarify misconceptions and allay fears.
6. Describe insertion procedure.
7. Provide rationale for any mobility restrictions.
8. Answer questions, and provide additional opportunities to discuss impending procedure.

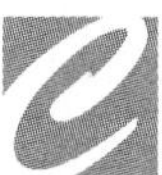

CHARTING for Client with a Temporary Pacemaker

- Date and time of insertion
- Model and type of pacemaker used
- Type of catheter electrode wires
- Method of insertion
- Mode of pacing
- Pacemaker settings (rate, outputs, sensitivity, AV interval)
- Client's response to treatment
- Vital signs
- Rhythm strips of pacing obtained during insertion

CRITICAL THINKING APPLICATION

CLINICAL PROBLEMS	CRITICAL THINKING OPTIONS
■ Client's cardiac rate is not stabilized.	• Check sensitivity setting. (If too high, P or T wave may be sensed; if too low, fixed-rate pacing occurs.) • Check ma setting (may be too high). • Check pace indicator for movement. • Check rate setting. • Check all connections. • Check catheter insertion site.

CLINICAL PROBLEMS	CRITICAL THINKING OPTIONS
	• Check for battery depletion, and change if necessary (9-V batteries). • Check for electromagnetic interference. • Insulate generator in rubber glove. • Obtain 12-lead ECG and chest x-ray. • Anticipate repositioning of pacing lead.
■ Client is unprepared for pacemaker insertion.	• If client is frightened, reassure him or her that a pacemaker is not dangerous. • If client does not understand explanation of how the pacemaker or the heart functions, reexplain the procedure, using illustrated learning aids. • Demonstrate the pacemaker and electrode, and allow time for questions and further explanations. • Describe insertion procedure, allowing time for questions. • Orient your teaching to the client's intellectual and interest level.
■ Electromagnetic interference occurs.	• Check all electric equipment for proper grounding. Use common ground. • Remove unnecessary electric equipment from vicinity of client. • Insulate generator, terminals, and exposed electrodes in a rubber glove.
■ Inflammation occurs at insertion site.	• Provide daily site care using strict aseptic technique. • Keep dressings dry at all times. • Monitor vital signs. • Instruct client to limit extremity movement.
■ Diaphragmatic pacing occurs.	• Observe for hiccoughs or muscle twitching. • Change client's position. • Decrease the amperage (ma). • Notify physician that endocardial perforation may have occurred.
■ Failure to capture is suspected.	• Check client's heart rate. If heart rate less than the rate set on generator, and if pace indicator shows firing, suspect failure to capture. • Check all connections. • Anticipate that pacer wires are dislodged. • Check battery. • Change position of extremity. • Turn client on left side; catheter may float back to epicardial wall. • Increase amperage (ma) after checking threshold.

CLINICAL PROBLEMS	CRITICAL THINKING OPTIONS
	• Obtain chest x-ray and 12-lead ECG. • Anticipate change of batteries, electrode terminals, or generator.
■ Battery depletion occurs.	• Have atropine and isoproterenol on stand-by. • Anticipate possible CPR. • Turn on power switch, and observe pace indicator. If there is little or no movement, replace battery immediately. • Record clock hours of battery usage. (Record should be taped to back of generator.) • Determine rate fluctuations. • Label each pacemaker with the date battery is inserted. • Store extra batteries in refrigerator, and put new battery in pacemaker before use. • Disconnect catheter from pacemaker before replacing battery. Contact with battery terminal may be dangerous to the client.

unit 3 ARTERIAL LINES

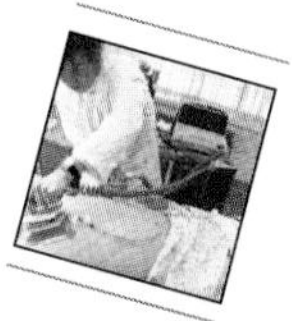

ARTERIAL LINE MONITORING

An intraarterial line is an invasive catheter used to provide a continuous measurement of a client's systolic, diastolic, and mean arterial blood pressure. This is a direct measure of blood pressure (as opposed to the indirect measure using a sphygmomanometer and stethoscope). Indirect measurements are most useful when cardiac output and peripheral resistance are normal. During critical situations when peripheral vasoconstriction occurs (e.g., shock, hypovolemia, decreased cardiac output), indirect cuff sounds are faint and measurements are inaccurately low. In these situations, direct blood pressure (arterial) measurement is more indicative of perfusion pressures.

Invasive arterial pressure measurement provides for early detection of altered hemodynamic status in clients with low cardiac output, excessive vasoconstriction, or unstable condition. Invasive monitoring is appropriate for surgical clients, clients on mechanical ventilators, or those requiring vasodilator or vasopressor drugs, or frequent arterial blood gas studies.

The radial artery is the site of choice for cannulation and direct monitoring. Other sites less commonly used for arterial catheter insertion include the brachial or femoral arteries.

Catheter placement in the more distal sites yields higher systolic pressures than catheters placed in the aorta. Although normal arterial blood pressure varies among clients, significant variations should be checked by recalibrating the monitor, balancing the transducer, and checking cuff pressures. To preserve the patency of the intraarterial catheter, a continuous flush mechanism identical to that for the pulmonary artery catheter is used.

Continuous direct monitoring of intraarterial blood pressure is possible with the arterial catheter attached via a pressure transducer to an arterial monitor.

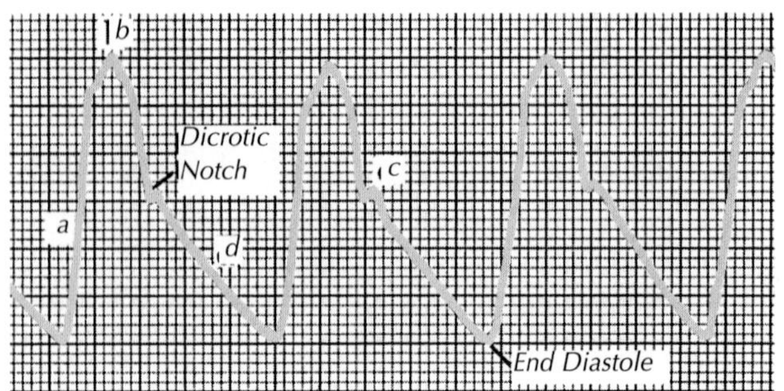

Arterial line—normal waveform. The dicrotic notch indicates aortic valve closure.

Waveform representation of cardiac function is represented by the symbols shown in the figure.

- *a* represents a sharp ascent correlating with left ventricular systole and the QRS complex found on the electrocardiogram.
- *b* represents peak systole; its numerical value is the systolic pressure recorded.
- *c* represents the notch on the downstroke of the waveform. This notch is called the *dicrotic notch* and represents closure of the aortic valve.
- *d* is diastole and is represented by a continuous decline in pressure. The numerical value at the lowest point is the diastolic pressure.

TABLE 33–2. Causes of Imbalance

Acidosis	Alkalosis
Hypoventilation	Hyperventilation
COPD	Hypokalemia
Cardiac arrest	Pulmonary embolus
Narcotic or barbiturate overdose	Mechanical ventilatory assistance
Diabetic ketoacidosis	Diuretics/dehydration
Severe diarrhea	Prolonged vomiting
Renal failure	Prolonged NG suction

TABLE 33–3. Laboratory Values in Acid–Base Imbalances

Respiratory Acidosis		Compensation
pH: decreased	<7.35	7.35
Pco_2: increased	>45 mm Hg	
HCO_3^-: normal	24	>26 mEq
Respiratory Alkalosis		**Compensation**
pH: increased	>7.45	7.45
Pco_2: decreased	<35 mm Hg	
HCO_3^-: normal	24	<22 mEq
Metabolic Acidosis		**Compensation**
pH: decreased	<7.35	7.35
HCO_3^-: decreased	<22 mEq	
Pco_2: normal	40	<35 mm Hg
Metabolic Alkalosis		**Compensation**
pH: increased	>7.45	7.45
HCO_3^-: increased	>26 mEq	
Pco_2: normal	40	>45 mm Hg
Normal ABG Values		
pH	7.35–7.45	
Pco_2	35–45 mm Hg	
HCO_3	22–26 mEq	

Continuous arterial waveforms are observed on the oscilloscope, and numerical pressures are observed on a digital readout. Blood pressure deviations can immediately be detected and appropriate therapy instituted without delay.

Blood Gas Analysis

Arterial blood gas analysis provides important clinical data. The blood gas studies assist in determining the respiratory and metabolic acid–base status (Tables 33–2 and 33–3) of the client and reveal the lung capacity to provide oxygen. The measurements serve as a guide for evaluating treatment.

NURSING PROCESS DATA

ASSESSMENT Data Base

Determine preexisting cardiovascular disease.

Assess client's level of understanding and ability to cooperate with staff.

Determine client's level of fear or anxiety about the procedure.

Assess distal peripheral perfusion using Allen's test.

Observe the mean arterial pressure on the monitor.

Measure the systolic and diastolic pressure reading on the monitor.
Observe for trends in arterial pressure readings.
Evaluate the patency of the arterial catheter.
Assess catheter insertion site for signs of infection or bleeding.
Determine pressure in flush bag. (Pressure should be 300 mm Hg.)
Assess for presence of peripheral pulses distal to catheter insertion site.

PLANNING Objectives

To directly collect data related to systolic, diastolic, and mean arterial pressures
To provide essential information regarding impending shock states, low cardiac output, vasoconstriction, oxygen concentration
To provide immediate access for arterial blood gas samples
To assess adequacy of oxygenation
To assess adequacy of alveolar ventilation
To evaluate acid–base balance
To evaluate effectiveness of ventilatory treatment modalities
To maintain a patent arterial catheter
To allay the client's fear and anxiety, and provide comfort measures

IMPLEMENTATION Procedures

Performing Allen's Test
Assisting with Arterial Line Insertion
Maintaining Arterial Line Function
Withdrawing Arterial Blood Samples
Removing Arterial Line

EVALUATION Expected Outcomes

Blood supply to hand is assessed before arterial line insertion.
Clear arterial pressure waveforms are observable on monitor.
Arterial catheter remains patent.
Puncture site remains free of complications.
Distal peripheral perfusion remains intact.
Arterial blood samples are obtained.
Pressure readings are accurately obtained and recorded.

PERFORMING ALLEN'S TEST

Procedure

1. Perform Allen's test to determine distal peripheral perfusion. **Rationale:** This procedure assesses blood supply to client's hand to determine how well the radial and ulnar arteries are functioning before an arterial line is inserted.
2. Compress both arteries at client's wrist for about 1 minute.
3. Instruct client to clench and unclench fists several times. **Rationale:** This causes blanching in the hand and palm.
4. With client's hand in open, relaxed position, release pressure on ulnar artery. **Rationale:** If ulnar artery cannot support distal peripheral perfusion,

another site must be chosen for arterial line insertion.

5. Observe how quickly the palm returns to normal color. **Rationale:** If normal color does not return within 5 seconds, there may be occlusion or poor capillary refill.
6. Repeat procedure with the radial artery.
7. Report to physician if both arteries are not functioning well.

ASSISTING WITH ARTERIAL LINE INSERTION

Equipment

Arterial catheter with introducer
Intravenous solution (usually 500 mL D_5W or normal saline)
Heparin (1–2 U/mL of IV solution)
One 5-mL syringe
Pressure infusion bag
IV tubing with microdrip
Three-way stopcocks
Pressure transducer, dome, and amplifier
Flush valve
Pressure monitor
IV pole
Clean gloves
Sterile gloves
Sterile towels and drape
Skin antiseptic solution (povidone-iodine)
Sterile 4×4 gauze pads
Sterile 2×2 gauze pads
Lidocaine 1–2%
Syringe with 18- and 25-gauge needle for *topical* anesthetic
Alcohol wipes
000 silk suture
Antiseptic ointment
Tape
Cutdown tray
Sphygmomanometer with proper sized cuff
Carpenter's level

Preparation

1. Explain rationale for procedure to client.
2. Verbally reassure client.
3. Gather equipment.
4. Wash your hands.
5. Add heparin to D_5W solution, and label bag with medication and date (commonly 1–2 U heparin/1 mL fluid).
6. Connect IV tubing to solution bag.
7. Insert IV bag into pressure infusion bag, and hang bag on IV pole.
8. Prepare and assemble pressurized monitoring system (transducer, flush system device, and stopcocks) following manufacturer's instructions.
9. Level, calibrate, and balance transducer at the level of client's right atrium (fourth intercostal space, midaxillary line).
10. Shave or prepare site as needed.
11. Inflate pressure infusion bag to 300 mm Hg, using hand pump on bag.

Procedure

1. Don gloves, and prepare to assist the physician as needed.
   a. Skin is prepped with povidone-iodine solution.
   b. Lidocaine vial is cleansed with alcohol wipe.
   c. Physician dons sterile gloves.
   d. Sterile drape is placed over arterial insertion site.
   e. Physician aspirates lidocaine with 18-gauge needle, changes needle, and injects client's skin with 25-gauge needle.
   f. Percutaneous insertion is made at arterial insertion site, and arterial catheter is inserted.
   g. Physician advances catheter in artery.
   h. Arterial catheter is sutured in place with 000 silk suture.
2. Observe for pulsating bright-red blood spurting retrograde in catheter. **Rationale:** This evidence ensures accurate catheter position.
3. Attach catheter to pressure-monitoring system tubing.
4. Press on flush valve for 3 seconds to clear system.

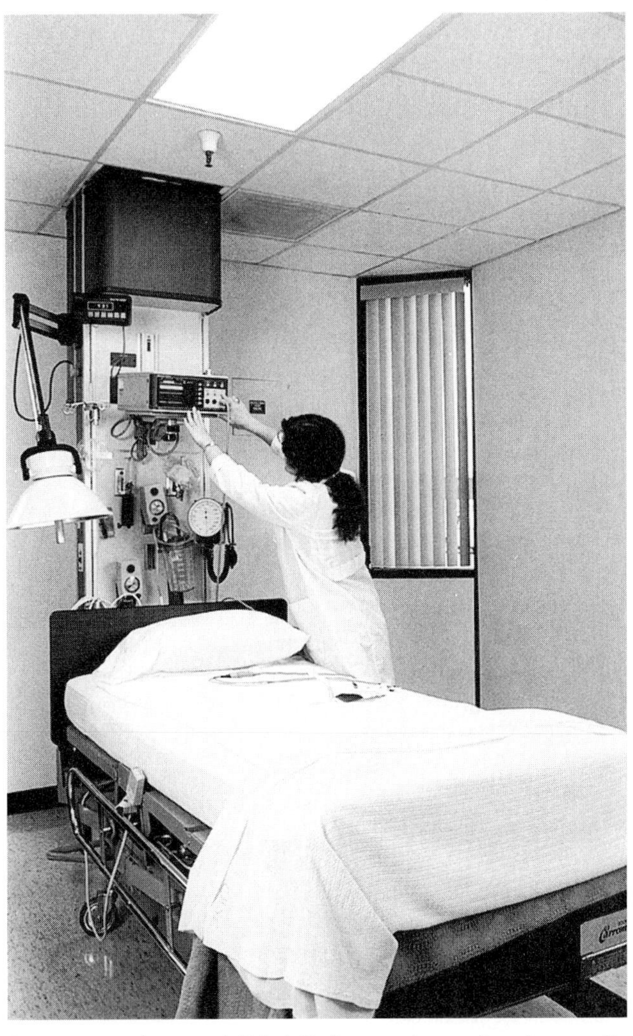

Pressure wave forms and digital displays can be monitored on a calibrated oscilloscope.

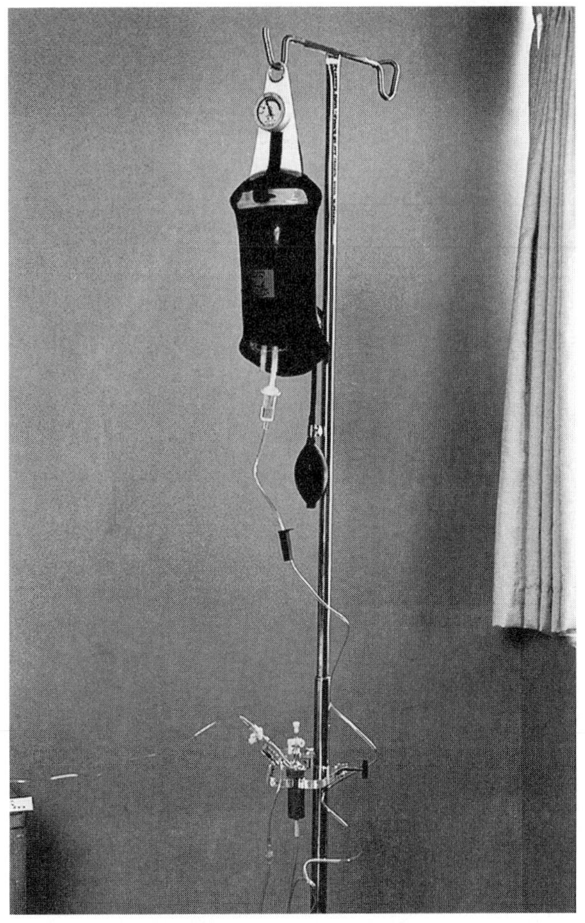

Heparin is added to solution and labeled with medication and date.

5. Observe oscilloscope for arterial waveform tracing.
6. Apply sterile antiseptic ointment, sterile dressings, and tape.
7. Reassure client during arterial catheter insertion.
8. Set monitor alarms for both HIGH and LOW parameters.

MAINTAINING ARTERIAL LINE FUNCTION

Equipment

Pressure transducer, dome, and amplifier
Flush valve with flush valve device
Pressure monitor
Sphygmomanometer with proper sized cuff
2×2 gauze pads
Tape
Gloves
Carpenter's level

Procedure

1. Determine pressure reading.
    a. Calibrate and balance transducer at appropriate intervals to maintain continuity. Transducer to be calibrated at level of right atrium. (Calibrate according to manufacturer's direction.)

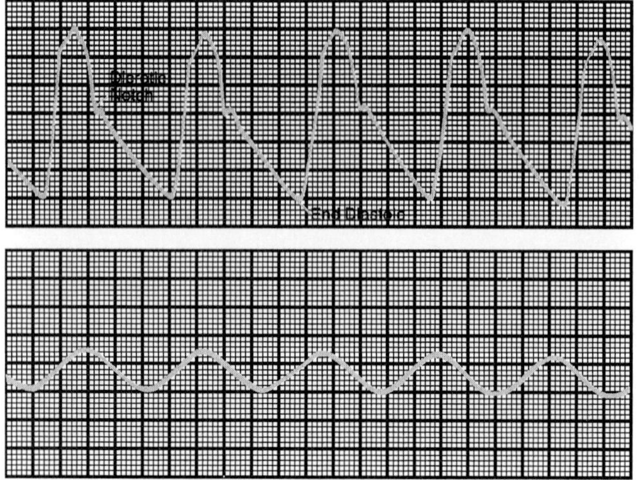

(**A**) Arterial line–normal waveform. (**B**) Arterial line–flattened waveform. Flattened arterial waveform indicates damping. Damping results from obstruction in arterial line or imbalance of transducer.

b. Determine systolic, diastolic, or mean arterial pressures by selecting the appropriate position on pressure monitor.

c. Flush line by pressing on flush valve for 3 seconds.

d. Record readings as indicated.

2. Calibrate and balance transducer at least every 8 hours. **Rationale:** Unbalanced transducers or monitors can lead to erroneous results.
3. Compare direct and indirect blood pressure measurements at least every 4 hours. **Rationale:** Dysrhythmias, vasospasm, or peripheral vasoconstriction can lead to discrepancies between direct and indirect methods.
4. Observe waveform at eye level for the sharp upward stroke, peak, dicrotic notch, and end diastole.
5. Flush line with valve device as necessary to promote patent system.
6. Ensure pressure infusion bag is maintained at 300 mm Hg.
7. Keep limb with arterial catheter uncovered at all times. **Rationale:** This allows for observation of dislodging or disruption of catheter.
8. Change dressing every 24–48 hours or if it becomes wet. **Rationale:** Wet dressings increase risk of infection at site.
   a. Put on gloves.
   b. Remove dressing, and discard in appropriate container.
   c. Apply antiseptic ointment directly over cannula site.
   d. Cover with 2×2 sterile gauze pad.
   e. Tape securely.

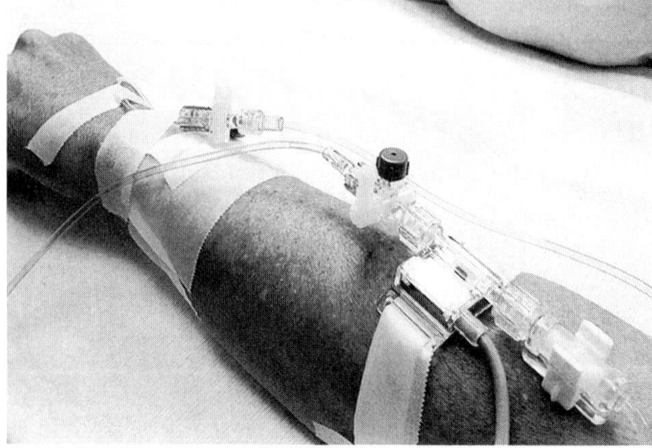

Arterial line transducer with flush device in client's radial artery.

WITHDRAWING ARTERIAL BLOOD SAMPLES

Equipment

2 5-mL syringes
21-gauge needle
Heparin 1:1000
Alcohol wipe
Container with ice (plastic bag, emesis basin)
Label
Laboratory slip

Preparation

1. Gather equipment.
2. Explain procedure to client.

3. Wash hands.
4. Cleanse heparin vial with alcohol wipe. Insert needle into vial.
5. Withdraw 1 mL heparin into specimen syringe with 21-gauge needle, and then withdraw needle from vial.
6. Withdraw plunger to coat barrel of syringe.
7. Expel air and all but 0.1 mL heparin from syringe.
8. Attach label to specimen syringe with client's name, hospital number, room number, time, and date.
9. Fill plastic bag or emesis basin with ice.

Procedure

1. Remove protective cap from open port on three-way stopcock closest to insertion site.
2. Attach nonheparinized 5-mL sterile syringe without needle to open port of three-way stopcock.
3. Turn stopcock off to transducer.
4. Aspirate 5 mL blood.
5. Turn stopcock midway between open port and IV tubing. **Rationale:** This prevents escape of blood or introduction of IV solution into line.
6. Discard blood-filled syringe.
7. Remove 21-gauge needle from specimen syringe.
8. Attach specimen syringe to stopcock.
9. Turn stopcock to open port to syringe.
10. Withdraw 5 mL for arterial blood gas specimen.
11. Turn stopcock off to open port. **Rationale:** This reestablishes flow between IV solution and client.
12. Remove syringe and expel all air and gas bubbles. **Rationale:** Air and gas bubbles interfere with accuracy of specimen analysis.

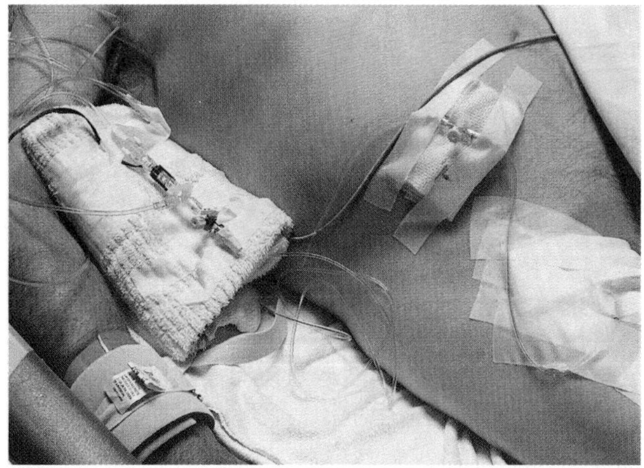

Client with femoral arterial access for immediate arterial blood gas samples.

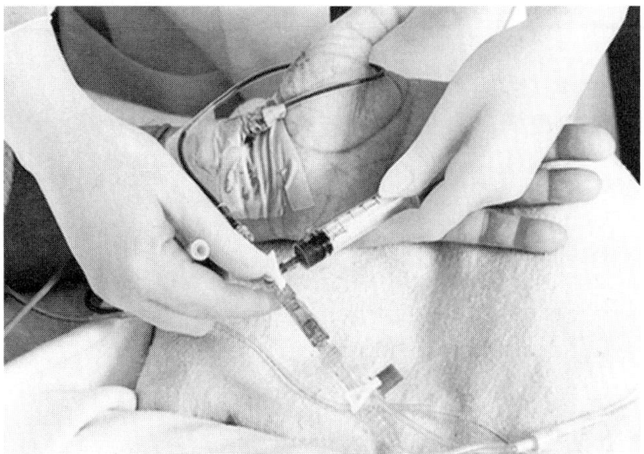

Discard first blood-filled syringe when collecting arterial blood gas sample.

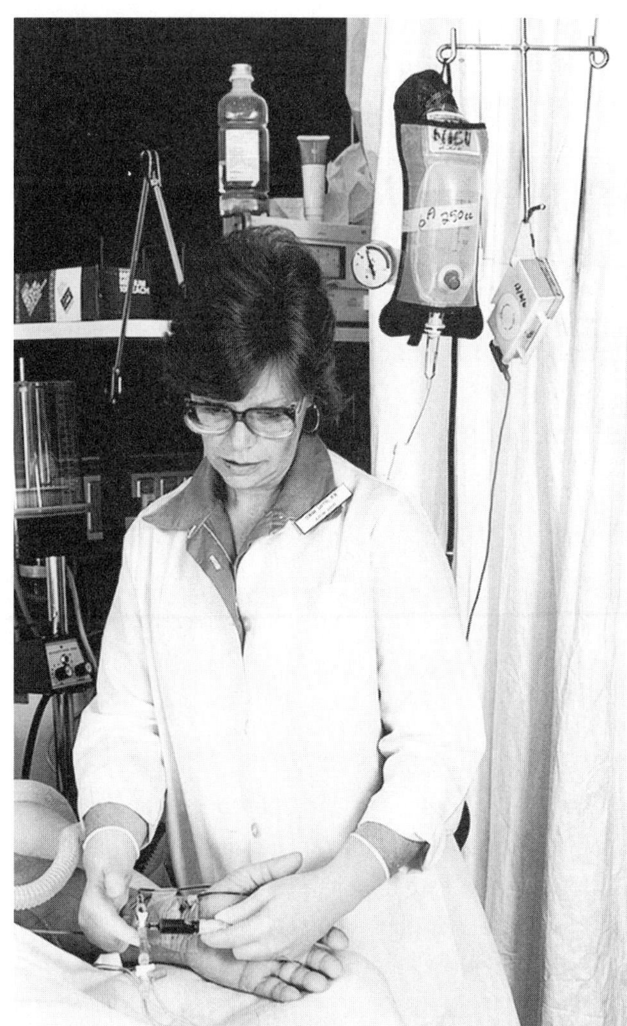

After attaching specimen syringe, withdraw 5 mL for arterial blood gas specimen.

13. Place arterial blood gas specimen in container filled with ice.
14. Irrigate line with valve flush device.
15. Reattach protective cap on open port.
16. Ensure good arterial waveform on monitor.
17. Write client's current temperature and fractional inspired oxygen (FIO_2) on laboratory slip.
18. Send to laboratory immediately.

REMOVING ARTERIAL LINE

Equipment

Gloves
4×4 gauze pad
Tape
Alcohol wipe
Specimen tube
Laboratory slip

Preparation

1. Check physician's orders.
2. Gather equipment.
3. Wash hands.
4. Explain procedure to client.

Procedure

1. Remove tape from site. **Rationale:** Tape is difficult to remove with gloves on; however, if dressing is soiled, don gloves before removing tape to protect from accidental blood exposure.
2. Don gloves.
3. Remove dressing, and place in appropriate container.
4. Place alcohol wipe over cannula site with nondominant hand, and apply gentle pressure.
5. Pull cannula straight out of artery with quick, even pressure.
6. Apply firm pressure over cannula site for at least 5 minutes. **Rationale:** This action prevents formation of a hematoma at puncture site.

> **■ CLINICAL ALERT**
>
> Pressure needs to be applied for at least 10 minutes if client is on anticoagulation therapy.

7. Place folded 4×4 gauze pad over puncture site, and tape tightly. **Rationale:** This provides additional pressure to site to prevent bleeding.
8. Complete laboratory slip, and send cannula to laboratory for culture and sensitivity if infection present and physician orders.
9. Check cannula site in 15 minutes. **Rationale:** To observe for bleeding at site.

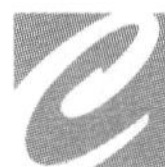

CHARTING for Arterial Lines

- Size of arterial catheter inserted
- Technique used to insert catheter
- Pressure readings
- Unexpected outcomes and appropriate interventions
- Client response and tolerance of procedure
- Condition of extremity in which catheter is inserted
- Presence of peripheral pulses
- Appearance of catheter insertion site

for Arterial Blood Gas Studies

- Time specimen obtained
- Client's temperature and FIO_2 at the time blood was drawn

for Dressing Change

- Condition of insertion site
- Dressing applied

for Removing Arterial Line

- Condition of insertion site
- Cannula disposal (i.e., to laboratory)
- Condition of peripheral pulses
- Color and warmth of extremity

CRITICAL THINKING APPLICATION

CLINICAL PROBLEMS	CRITICAL THINKING OPTIONS
▪ Absence of collateral or distal peripheral pulse when performing Allen's test (negative Allen's test).	• Choose brachial artery. • Choose femoral artery. • Notify physician.
▪ Damped pressures observed on oscilloscope.	• Check for beginning thrombus formation by aspirating blood through stopcock and then flushing system. • Check for presence of air in system. • Check that there is 300 mm Hg pressure in pressure bag. • Ensure secure fit of all stopcocks and connections. • Change position of extremity in which catheter is placed. • Be sure to flush arterial line thoroughly after arterial blood samples are obtained.
▪ Hematoma or hemorrhage at insertion site.	• Apply direct pressure over artery while you check for leaks in the system. Check all stopcocks, and see if catheter is inserted in artery as far as it should be. • Remove catheter if oozing or hemorrhage continues.
▪ Infection or inflammation at insertion site.	• Cleanse site, and change dressing every 24 hours using strict aseptic technique to prevent infection. • Change tubing every 24–48 hours using sterile technique. • Flush open port after aspirating blood to prevent build-up of old blood. • Cover open port on stopcock to maintain asepsis. • Prepare for catheter removal if infection occurs. • Notify physician for antibiotic order.
▪ Diminished or absent distal peripheral perfusion.	• Check periphery for changes in color, warmth, movement, and pain resulting from thrombus occlusion. • Prepare for removal of catheter.
▪ Arterial catheter not patent.	• Assess insertion site for signs of hemorrhage or infection. • Attempt to aspirate blood from the arterial line using a syringe. If blood can be aspirated, then flush the arterial line using valve flush device. • If unable to flush arterial catheter, remove catheter, and apply direct pressure over artery for 5–10 minutes. Apply pressure dressing over artery.

CLINICAL PROBLEMS	CRITICAL THINKING OPTIONS
■ Arterial blood samples unable to be withdrawn.	• Release pressure on syringe, allow spasm of artery to stop, and then attempt to aspirate blood with gentle pressure. • Check that catheter is in artery (observe waveform on oscilloscope). If catheter is malfunctioning, attempt to aspirate blood from the catheter. If blood is aspirated, flush the catheter using valve flush device. Then, try to obtain the sample again. • Reposition catheter and arm, gently pulling back on plunger. • If necessary, remove dressing, and check if any pressure was applied at the site. • Notify physician, who may need to remove sutures and reposition catheter.
■ Oscilloscope readings are abnormally high or low.	• Recheck transducer and client position to ensure accurate data. • Calibrate transducer. • Flush system with IV solution.

unit 4

HEMO-DYNAMIC MONITORING USING A PULMONARY ARTERY CATHETER

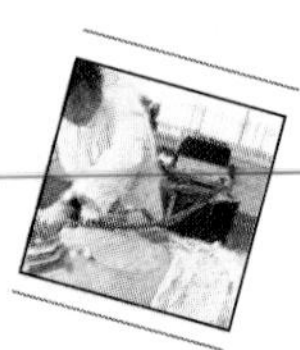

Systemic perfusion depends on adequate blood volume and left ventricular performance. Shock, cardiac failure, or other conditions alter the left ventricle's ability to pump, resulting in a change in the intracardiac pressures. Since direct measurement of left atrial or ventricular pressure is not usually done in the clinical setting, an indication of these measures must be obtained by indirect means via the right side of the heart.

A balloon-tipped, flow-directed catheter inserted transvenously into the pulmonary artery permits a continuous, *indirect* diagnostic measurement of left ventricular function for detecting and managing cardiopulmonary changes. Clients that require monitoring include those receiving fluid replacement therapy and those with altered cardiac or pulmonary function. Reduction of cardiac function is manifested primarily by two hemodynamic abnormalities: decreased cardiac output and increased left ventricular end-diastolic pressure (LVEDP). The pulmonary artery catheter indirectly measures the LVEDP by directly measuring pulmonary artery and pulmonary artery wedge pressures.

At the end of diastole (filling), the mitral valve is open, and the left atrium, left ventricle, and pulmonary vasculature momentarily act as a single chamber in which the pressure is equal throughout. Since the normal pressures of these chambers and vessels are known, pressure changes in the pulmonary artery can be used to reflect changes in the LVEDP. Abnormal pressures can indicate changes in a client's fluid balance, vascular tone, or heart pumping action. The catheter measures central venous pressure (CVP), or right atrial pressure (RAP), pulmonary artery pressure (PAP), and pulmonary artery wedge pressure (PAWP). Cardiac output and other hemodynamic parameters are also calculated using this catheter (Table 33–4).

The catheter is inserted percutaneously or through a cutdown and threaded transvenously through the right atrium, the tricuspid valve, the right ventricle, and the pulmonary valve to the pulmonary artery. When the balloon at the tip of the catheter is inflated, the catheter is carried by blood flow through the pulmonary circulation until it wedges in a pulmonary capillary. During this brief wedge time, pressure reflected back on the tip of the catheter allows indirect measurement of LVEDP.

The pulmonary artery catheter typically has four or five lumens. Two lumens are used for pressure measurements. A proximal lumen is available to measure central venous pressure (right atrial pressure), assist in measuring cardiac output, and inject selected solutions. The distal lumen is used to measure pulmonary artery pressure and pulmonary artery wedge pressure. A third lumen is used for balloon inflation. A fourth lumen is attached to a thermister tip that assists in the measurement of cardiac output.

The advantage of pulmonary artery catheter readings over CVP readings is that CVPs do not provide information about left ventricular function or pulmonary vascular pressure changes until they are significant enough to be reflected back to the right atrium.

TABLE 33–4. Normal Pressures

Right atrial (RAP): 2–5 mm Hg

Right ventricle (RV): $\frac{25}{5}$ mm Hg

Pulmonary artery pressure (PAP): $\frac{25}{10}$ mm Hg

PA mean ($\overline{PA}$): <15 mm Hg

PAWP: 10

Left atrial (LA): 5–10 mm Hg

Left ventricle (LV): $\frac{130}{5\text{–}10}$ mm Hg

Aorta: $\frac{130}{80}$

Mean arterial pressure (MAP): 70–90 (Diastolic × 2) + (Systolic × 1)÷3

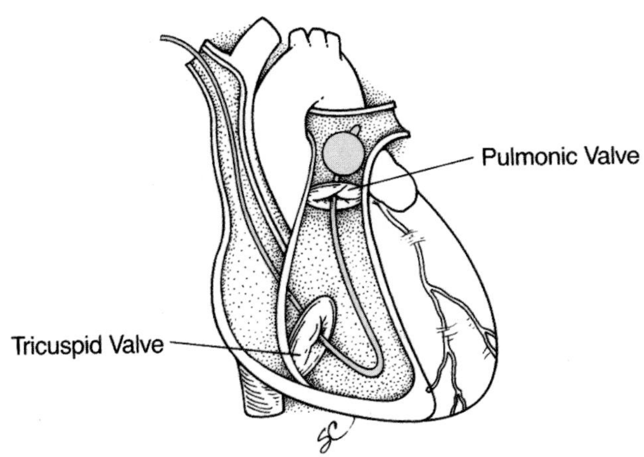

Balloon-tipped, flow-directed catheter with balloon inflated for pulmonary wedge pressure determination.

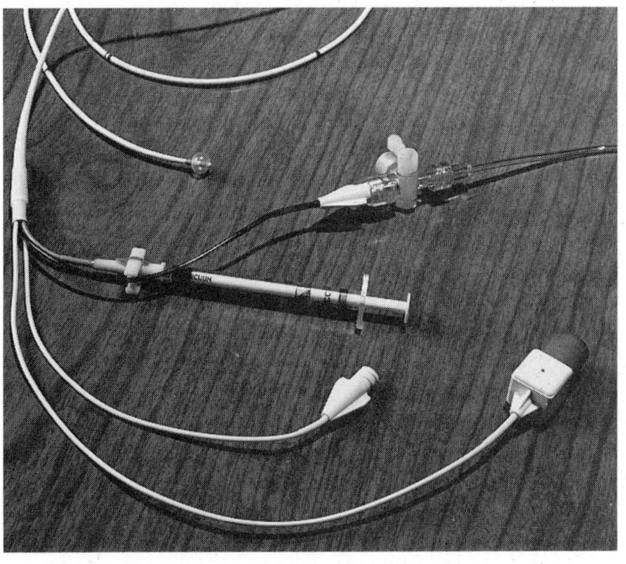

Swan-Ganz catheter or pulmonary artery catheter. Syringe is attached to the port used for balloon inflation. The proximal lumen is attached to the pressure line which measures right atrial pressure.

NURSING PROCESS DATA

ASSESSMENT Data Base

Evaluate client's understanding and cooperation with the procedure.

Assess for preexisting cardiovascular disease.

Determine client's level of fear or anxiety regarding the procedure.

Determine baseline vital signs.

Obtain a 12-lead electrocardiogram.

Assess systolic PA, diastolic PA, mean PA, PCWP, and RA pressures.

Assess cardiac output using thermodilution technique.

Assess insertion site for inflammation or infection.

Assess patency of all lines.

Determine pressure in flush bag.

Determine calibration and balancing of transducer and monitor.

PLANNING Objectives

To indirectly assess left ventricular end-diastolic pressure (LVEDP)

To provide essential information regarding shock syndromes and intravascular fluid volumes

To obtain samples of mixed venous blood (mixed due to blood from systemic and coronary veins)

To administer intravenous solutions and determine response to fluid therapy

To measure cardiac output

To assess data related to central venous pressure

To determine need for drug therapy

To maintain a patent pulmonary artery catheter

IMPLEMENTATION Procedure

Assisting Physician with Insertion

Obtaining Pressure Readings

Obtaining Cardiac Output Measurements

Balancing the Transducer

Calibrating the Monitor and Transducer

Balancing and Calibrating the Oscilloscope

EVALUATION Expected Outcomes

Clear pulmonary artery waveforms depicted on the oscilloscope.

Pulmonary artery catheter remains patent.

Systolic, diastolic, mean pulmonary artery, and pulmonary artery wedge pressure measurements recorded accurately.

Cardiac output measurements recorded accurately.

Pulmonary artery waveforms and pressures maintained within normal limits.

Pressure in flush bag remains at 300 mm Hg.

Altered cardiovascular status is detected early.

ASSISTING PHYSICIAN WITH INSERTION

Equipment

Pulmonary artery catheter (size 5–7.5)

Catheter introducer (size depending on catheter size)

Intravenous solution (usually 500 mL D_5W or sterile normal saline solution)

Heparin (1–2 U/mL of IV solution)

Tuberculin syringe

Pressure infusion bag

IV tubing

Pressure monitor

Transducer

Valve device for system flush

High-pressure tubing

Three-way stopcocks

IV pole

CVP solution if required

12- to 16-gauge intracatheter

Sterile gloves

Clean gloves
Sterile towels
Skin antiseptic solution (povidone-iodine)
Razor
Sterile 4×4 pads
Sterile basin and sterile irrigating solution
Lidocaine 1–2%
Syringe with 18- and 25-gauge needle for topical anesthetic
Alcohol wipes
Sterile antiseptic ointment (see agency policy)
Occlusive dressing or tape
Suture with attached needle
Sterile needle holder or clamp
Cutdown tray, sterile gown, mask, and cap
Defibrillator
Emergency cart
Lidocaine bolus for arrhythmias (50–100 mg)
10-mL sterile syringes filled with 5 mL or 10 mL D_5W (cardiac output)

Preparation

1. Bring emergency cart and defibrillator to area near client's room.
2. Explain rationale for procedure to client.
3. Verbally reassure client.
4. Wash hands.
5. Inject heparin into IV solution bag (usually 1 mL heparin/1 mL solution). Remove all air from bag by withdrawing the air with a 10–20-mL syringe. **Rationale:** Air in the line gives inaccurate readings.
6. Label IV bag with client's name, date, time, amount of heparin added, and your initials.
7. Connect rigid IV tubing to flush fluid bag.
8. Place prepared IV solution in pressure bag, and inflate to 300 mm Hg pressure. **Rationale:** This facilitates solution flowing through the system against an arterial pressure.
9. Prepare and assemble pressurized monitoring system (transducer, system flush device, and stopcocks) following manufacturer's instructions. Attach stopcocks to proximal and distal ports. Fill all lumens with flush solution.
10. Attach distal port stopcock to connecting tubing and heparinized flush solution, then attach to pressure monitoring unit.
11. Place client in a supine position. **Rationale:** This position provides for consistency in readings.
12. Calibrate and balance transducer according to manufacturer's instructions. The transducer must be at the level of client's right atrium or phlebostatic axis (fourth intercostal space at the midaxillary line).
13. Shave and scrub skin with antiseptic solution.
14. Open sterile gloves for physician.
15. Open drape for physician.

Right Atrial (RA) Pressure

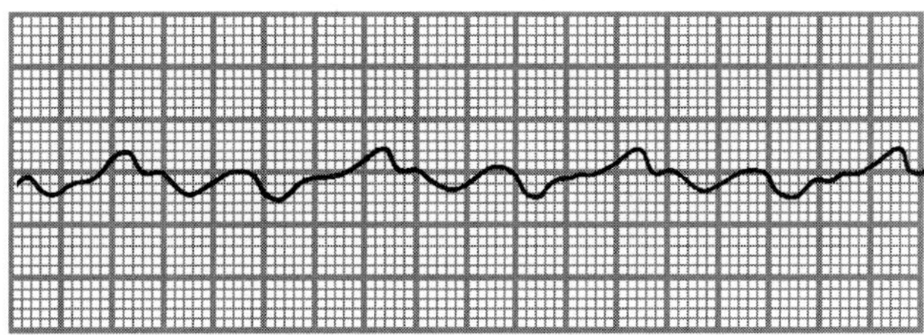

Right Ventricular (RV) Pressure

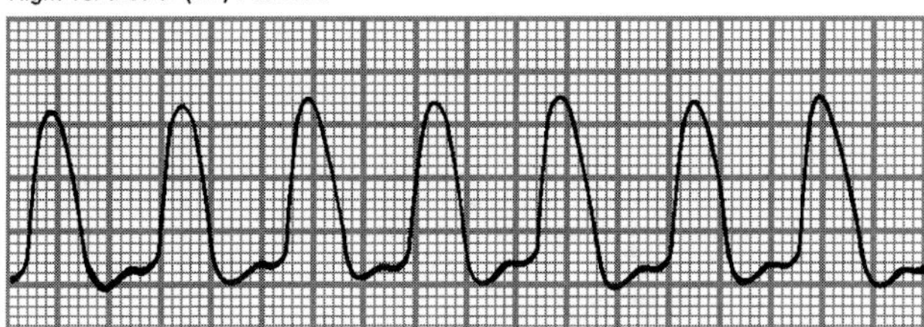

Pulmonary Artery Pressure (PAP)

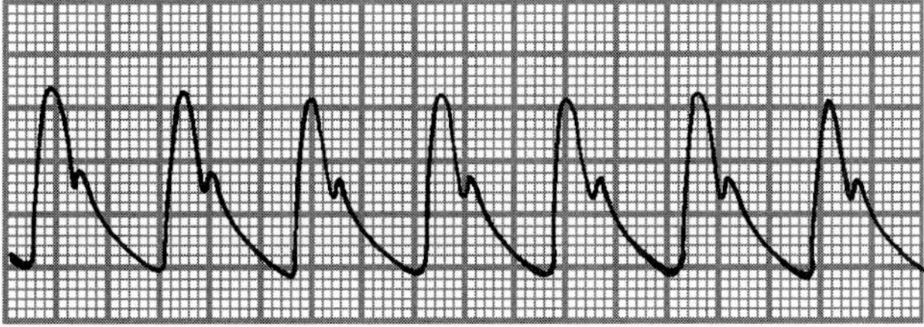

Pulmonary Artery Wedge Pressure (PAWP)

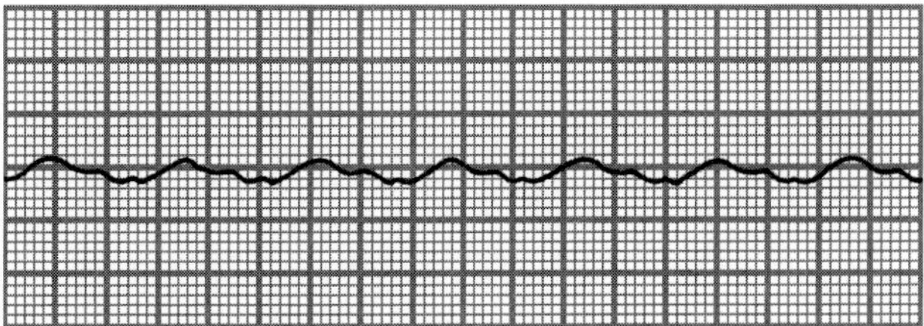

Waveform changes depicted on monitor as Swan-Ganz catheter traverses heart.

16. Cleanse lidocaine vial with alcohol wipe.
17. Continuously monitor client's ECG throughout insertion of catheter.

Procedure

1. Don gloves, and be prepared to assist physician as necessary.
   a. Physician dons sterile mask, cap, gown, and gloves. Catheter is tested for air leaks by inflating balloon with 0.5–1.5 mL (amount determined by catheter size) of air, not fluid, while balloon is submerged in sterile basin filled with sterile irrigating solution. **Rationale:** Fluid is difficult to retrieve and, because it cannot be compressed, may cause pressure on walls of pulmonary vessels.
   b. Physician aspirates lidocaine with 18-gauge needle, changes to 25-gauge needle, and injects lidocaine under skin.
   c. Physician flushes catheter with sterile normal saline before insertion. **Rationale:** This clears air from catheter, preventing air embolus.
   d. Physician performs cutdown or percutaneous insertion. Subclavian vein usually used; however, jugular vein may be selected.
   e. Catheter is attached to pressure monitoring system.
   f. Catheter is flushed using flush valve device. **Rationale:** This prevents air embolism from occurring.
   g. Catheter is advanced with balloon deflated or partially inflated until correct right atrial waveform and pressure appear on monitor.
   h. Record right atrial pressure.
   i. Physician fully inflates balloon to assist in catheter's flow through tricuspid valve into right ventricle.
2. Observe for higher and more pronounced pressure waveform, indicating catheter's presence in right ventricle.
3. Record right ventricular pressure (systolic and diastolic reading), and observe for dysrhythmias: premature ventricular contractions (PVCs) or ventricular tachycardia.
4. Inflate balloon with minimal amount of air to assist with catheter's passage into pulmonary artery.
5. Observe monitor for higher diastolic pressure waveform and pulmonary arterial waveform.
6. Record pulmonary artery systolic (PAS), diastolic (PAD), and mean pressures. *Note: Measure pulmonary artery pressures at end of expiration.*
7. Inflate balloon fully (1.5 mL maximum) or until a change is seen in waveform or pulmonary artery capillary wedge pressure. **Rationale:** Inflated balloon assists passage of catheter into a distal pulmonary capillary.

> **■ CLINICAL ALERT**
>
> Do not exceed manufacturer's recommended amount of air when inflating balloon.

8. Record PCW mean pressure.
9. Deflate balloon by removing syringe and allowing air to escape. **Rationale:** Aspiration of air from balloon with a syringe can lead to rupture of balloon.
10. Determine balloon deflation by observing pulmonary artery waveform tracing.
11. Repeat steps to ensure that catheter is wedging and deflating properly.
12. Replace empty syringe in place on balloon port.
13. Use locking device on balloon lumen port if present. **Rationale:** This prevents accidental inflation of balloon.
14. Clear catheter using flush device.
15. Apply sterile antiseptic ointment, and secure occlusive dressing to site after physician secures catheter with sutures.
16. Reassure client, and position as needed.
17. Ensure placement by chest x-ray as ordered.

OBTAINING PRESSURE READINGS

Preparation

1. Calibrate and balance transducer, and monitor every 4 hours. **Rationale:** This ensures accurate and consistent readings.
2. Check catheter, tubing, and connection points to ensure patency.
3. Verbally reassure client.
4. Wash hands.
5. Place client in horizontal position.

Procedure

1. Check that pressure transducer is at level of client's right atrium. **Rationale:** This ensures accurate pressure reading.
2. Expose distal port to the transducer. **Rationale:** All pulmonary artery pressure readings are taken from distal lumen of catheter, and right atrial pressures are taken from proximal lumen.
3. Change monitor switch to determine pulmonary artery systolic, diastolic, and mean pressure. Use "mean" designation when determining pulmonary artery wedge pressure. (Newer equipment calculates and displays MAP.)
4. Open balloon inflation port-locking device.
5. Remove syringe from balloon port. **Rationale:** This ensures there is no air in balloon.
6. Reattach syringe filled with proper amount of air, and align valve to open position.
7. Slowly inject 0.8 or 1.5 mL air into balloon, depending on size of catheter—inflate sufficient volume to support float and change in waveform. Discontinue attempt to inflate if resistance is met, and notify physician.
8. Observe waveform change from pulmonary artery to pulmonary artery wedge pressure on the monitor. Pulmonary wedge tracing depicts an "a" wave (left atrial contraction and left ventricular relaxation) and a "v" wave (left atrial relaxation and left ventricular contraction).
9. Balloon should not be inflated longer than 5–10 seconds. **Rationale:** This can cause overwedging (falsely high pressure readings) and damage to pulmonary artery.

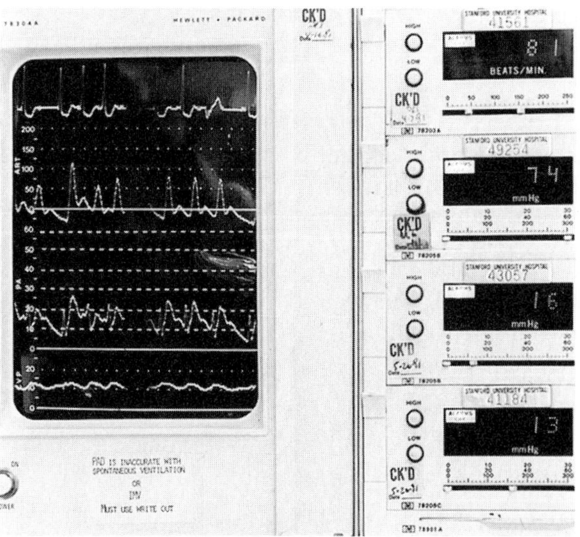

Monitor display of ECG and pressure waveforms for continuous client assessment.

> **■ CLINICAL ALERT**
>
> To prevent air from entering the system, CO_2 is used at some institutions to inflate the balloon. *Note: Suspect balloon rupture if no resistance is encountered on inflation or blood returns from balloon lumen. Do not inflate.*

10. Allow balloon to deflate passively, and close valve once pulmonary artery wedge pressure reading is obtained. **Rationale:** Aspirating air with syringe damages the balloon wall.
11. Ensure readings are always taken at end of expiration whether or not client is on ventilator (document if client is on ventilator). **Rationale:** Slightly higher readings are obtained if client is on a ventilator.
12. Replace empty syringe on balloon port.
13. Check that locking device is in place. **Rationale:** This device prevents accidental inflation of balloon.
14. Flush line with flush device system.
15. Record readings as ordered, and report unusual findings to physician.
16. Place client in comfortable position.
17. Change dressings daily, and observe for infection at site of catheter insertion.

OBTAINING CARDIAC OUTPUT MEASUREMENTS

Equipment

Four to six 10-mL "control syringes" filled with D_5W (Store filled syringes in refrigerator or on tray if room temperature injectate is used.)

Four to six sterile syringe caps

Sealable bag

Beaker with ice bath

10-mL syringe without barrel (for temperature testing)

Temperature probe

Procedure

1. Place syringes in sterile beaker.
2. Fill beaker with iced water if iced injectate is used.
3. Determine position of pulmonary catheter on monitor, and ensure deflation of balloon.
4. Wash hands.
5. Place client in consistent position, either supine or 20° elevation. **Rationale:** Position change alters cardiac output reading (e.g., greater than 20° elevation results in lower cardiac output reading).
6. For iced injectate, place temperature probe in syringe without barrel and connect probe to computer.
7. Reassure client, and ensure that client is quiet. **Rationale:** Agitation increases cardiac output and thus causes an inaccurate reading.
8. Flush proximal lumen before injectate is infused. **Rationale:** If lumen is not fully patent, cardiac output measurement is inaccurate.
9. Check connection and proper function of cardiac output computer cable to thermister port of pulmonary artery catheter according to manufacturer's directions.
10. Turn on cardiac output computer according to manufacturer's directions.
11. Validate iced injectate temperature is 0–5°C.
12. Check and set computer constant to reflect volume and temperature of injectate being used. Table of computation constants are in computer manual.
13. Wait for light to indicate ready.
14. Obtain injectate-filled syringes from storage container.
15. Quickly connect syringe to stopcock, and open stopcock to syringe.
16. Push start button at end expiration, and rapidly inject solution into stopcock at proximal lumen of pulmonary artery catheter within 4 seconds. **Rationale:** Inaccurate cardiac output recording results with longer injectate times.

- Handling syringe barrel alters injectate temperature, thus altering cardiac output results. "Control syringes" with finger rings are preferred.

17. Observe for display of client's cardiac output.
18. Check cardiac rhythm and pulmonary artery pressure waveforms. **Rationale:** Bolus of cold injectate into right atrium can precipitate arrhythmias. Catheter can wedge or move into right ventricle.
19. Repeat procedure. **Rationale:** Three readings are taken to ensure accuracy.
20. Disconnect cable from catheter thermistry circuit, and replace protective cap on catheter.
21. Record client's cardiac output. The output is the average of the two most similar recordings. **Rationale:** By discarding the unusually high or low value, the average of remaining values yields a more accurate reading.
22. Calculate and record cardiac index, pulmonary vascular resistance, and systemic vascular resistance.
23. Fill four to six syringes with injectate, and place in cooler or ice bath if iced injectate procedure is used. **Rationale:** This ensures proper injectate temperature for next reading.

BALANCING THE TRANSDUCER

Procedure

1. Verbally reassure client.
2. Wash hands.
3. Position transducer at level of right atrium. **Rationale:** If level is not at right atrium, the pressure readings are inaccurate. Maintain transducer at proper level throughout monitoring.
4. Open stopcock. **Rationale:** This action opens transducer to air.

5. Close stopcock to client.
6. Push monitor button to zero, and check if monitor reading is zero. **Rationale:** When reading is at zero, transducer is balanced to atmospheric pressure.
7. Balance transducer by turning zero knob on monitor until reading is zero. Monitor does not have an automatic zero button.
8. Check that oscilloscope shows a flat wave at zero line. **Rationale:** This ensures accurate reading as it changes from zero point.
9. Close stopcock. The monitor and transducer are now ready to be calibrated.

■ CLINICAL ALERT

If the client moves, reposition and rebalance the transducer. For each inch away from the correct level, there is a 2 mm Hg error in the pressure reading.

CALIBRATING THE MONITOR AND TRANSDUCER

Procedure

1. Verbally reassure client.
2. Determine that transducer has been balanced.
3. Press zero button on monitor.
4. Press test–calibration button.
5. Turn sensitivity knob until reading is 100 mm Hg on the digital readout, or until reading is appropriate for the equipment being used. (Transducer and monitor are calibrated when reading is at 100 mm Hg.)

BALANCING AND CALIBRATING THE OSCILLOSCOPE

Procedure

1. Open transducer to air.
2. Press zero button on monitor.
3. Watch for baseline to register zero on oscilloscope, and then close port.
4. Select a pressure range for the modality you are monitoring, and press scale button. Choose a low pressure of 100 mm Hg for central venous pressure or left atrial pressure, or 200 mm Hg for arterial blood pressure.
5. Press test–calibration button, and observe oscilloscope for waveform. The waveform should be visible at pressure range selected (100 mm Hg or 200 mm Hg).
6. Adjust the sensitivity knob on the monitor so waveform reaches pressure range.

CHARTING for Pulmonary Artery Lines

- Size of pulmonary artery catheter inserted
- Placement and technique used to insert catheter (cutdown or percutaneous)
- Pressure readings obtained
- Expected outcomes and nursing interventions completed
- Client's response to and tolerance of procedure
- Cardiac output results

CRITICAL THINKING APPLICATION

CLINICAL PROBLEMS	CRITICAL THINKING OPTIONS
Catheter line not patent.	• Flush the line. • Attempt to aspirate clotted blood through line by pulling back on plunger of syringe. • Notify physician if unable to clear line.
Pulse waveforms abnormal.	• Deflate balloon on pulmonary artery catheter completely. Ask client to cough to help free catheter. • Test flush catheter line. • If condition persists, notify physician to reposition line. • Assess client for other signs and symptoms indicative of a change in clinical condition.
Infection occurs at site of insertion.	• Prepare to aid in removal of catheter and insertion of new catheter, if required. • Prepare to obtain tip of catheter as a specimen, and send to laboratory for culture. • Change dressing, and apply antiseptic ointment. • Observe for signs and symptoms of phlebitis. • Remind physician to change site every 72 hours. (This is ideal—many times it's 7–10 days.)
No pressure tracing.	• Determine that power is ON. • Check for loose connection. • Check for clotted blood in line (damping is an early sign). Try to aspirate; never flush. • Check stopcocks to make sure they are not turned the wrong way. • Check that dome on transducer is tight.
No pulmonary wedge pressure tracing.	• Suspect that catheter is not advanced far enough. Chest x-ray may be ordered to check placement of pulmonary artery catheter. • Reposition client. • Suspect possible balloon rupture. Notify physician. • Check and deflate balloon. Balloon may have caused catheter to wedge. If you cannot inflate balloon, it may be wedged. • For a brachial insertion of the catheter, reposition client's arm to float the balloon out of a smaller capillary.

unit 5 MECHANICAL VENTILATION

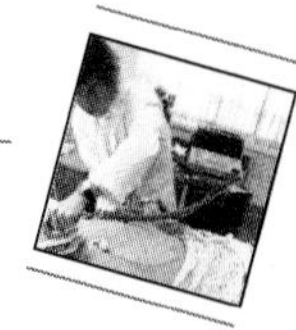

VENTILATION AND GAS EXCHANGE ALTERATIONS

Adequate gas exchange within the lung fields depends on the effective ventilation of air and perfusion of blood in both lungs. The thickness and permeability of the alveolar membrane, the amount of surface area available for diffusion, and the pressure gradient are also factors that affect gas exchange. The *pressure gradient* is the difference in partial pressures of PO_2 and PCO_2 and the alveolar air. The pressure gradients promote the transfer, or inward diffusion, of oxygen from alveolar air to the blood and the outward diffusion of carbon dioxide from the blood to the alveolar air.

Ventilation replenishes the supply of oxygen in the alveoli and removes the carbon dioxide released by the capillaries. If ventilation is not uniform throughout all the lung fields (due to a change in perfusion of one area of the lung), then the rate of oxygen replenishment is reduced, which can lead to hypoxemia.

Ventilation–perfusion problems are usually the result of chronic conditions, such as heart failure, asthma, and chronic obstructive pulmonary disease (COPD), as well as acute conditions such as pneumonia.

In the normal lung the capacity for diffusion of both oxygen and carbon dioxide is so great and the alveolar capillary membrane so thin that gas exchange occurs long before the blood reaches the end of the pulmonary capillary.

NURSING PROCESS DATA

ASSESSMENT Data Base

Assess client for presence of risk factors for acute respiratory distress syndrome: massive trauma, massive fat embolism, aspiration pneumonia, and other disorders characterized by abnormal gas distribution (due to airway or alveolar closure) and pulmonary interstitial edema.

Auscultate heart and lung sounds for baseline data.

Assess vital signs and measure arterial blood gases and hemodynamic pressures if CVP and Swan–Ganz lines are in place.

Identify if need for mechanical ventilation is present. Criteria for non-COPD clients.

- Vital capacity is less than 15 mL/kg of body weight.
- Inspiratory pressure is less than -25 cm H_2O.
- $PaCO_2$ is below 30 mm Hg or above 50 mm Hg.
- Alveolar–arterial oxygen difference (A–a Δ PO_2) is greater than 350 mm Hg on 100% oxygen.
- Pulmonary shunt is greater than 30%.
- Deadspace-tidal volume (V_D-V_T) ratio is greater than 60%.
- PaO_2 is less than 60 mm Hg on an FIO_2 of 1.0.

Observe for trend of respiratory values (trend is more important than isolated measurements).

Assess client for indications for PEEP:

- Inability to maintain arterial PO_2 of at least 70 mm Hg on 50% oxygen during continuous mechanical ventilation
- Failure of other methods to reduce pulmonary shunt (e.g., treatment of cardiac failure or pneumonia)
- Normovolemia (Normal blood volume)

Check physician's orders regarding amount and duration of PEEP. (Usual range is 5–15 cm H_2O although 20–35 cm H_2O have been used.)

Review physician's orders for amount of PEEP.

Assess client for indication for CPAP.

- Ability to breathe spontaneously.
- Inability to maintain Po_2 of 70 mm Hg.
- History of obstructive sleep apnea.
- Inability to reexpand atelectic lung tissue.

Assess client for indications for pressure support.

- Client is intubated and mechanically ventilated.
- Artificial airway imposes resistance to ventilation.

PLANNING Objectives

To provide or augment pulmonary functioning in respiratory center failure (brainstem injury or narcotic overdose), neuromuscular diseases (myasthenia gravis), musculoskeletal disorders (flail chest), and pulmonary disorders (adult respiratory distress syndrome)

To maintain acid–base balance of the body

For PEEP

To assist in keeping the alveoli open on expiration, thereby reducing shunt, increasing functional residual capacity (FRC), and improving compliance

To assist in surfactant stimulation

To improve oxygenation without prolonged use of high oxygenation concentrations

To maintain respiratory function in adult respiratory distress syndrome (ARDS)

For CPAP

To improve oxygenation for clients who are able to spontaneously ventilate without the use of mechanical ventilation.

To establish a resistance to expiration to enhance functional residual capacity.

To enable clients to avoid mechanical ventilation when pulmonary dysfunction is acute and reversible.

For PSV

To decrease the work of breathing for intubated clients.

IMPLEMENTATION Procedures

Caring for Clients on Ventilators

Providing Positive End-Expiratory Pressure (PEEP)

Providing Continuous Positive Airway Pressure (CPAP)

EVALUATION Expected Outcomes

Adequate respiratory function is maintained.

Acid–base balance is improved.

Oxygenation of tissue is improved and Po_2 is maintained at 80–100 mm Hg on low oxygen concentration with PEEP or CPAP.

Pulmonary pathology is reduced with PEEP or CPAP.

Functional residual capacity and compliance are increased with PEEP or CPAP.

Ventilator weaning is facilitated by CPAP or PSV.

Airway Pressure Modes

- Intermittent positive pressure breathing (IPPB)—inspiration by positive airway pressure; expiration is passive.
- Continuous mandatory ventilation (CMV)—total support ventilation with set ventilation rate (e.g., 12) and set tidal volume (e.g., 750 mL). Client-initiated breaths receive set volume and if client does not initiate breath, set rate and volume are guaranteed (sometimes referred to as assist control ventilation (ACV).
- Synchronous intermittent mandatory ventilation (SIMV)—spontaneous ventilation intermittently augmented by positive pressure ventilation.
- Positive end-expiratory pressure (PEEP)—an expiratory airway pressure modality in which the airway pressure is maintained above atmospheric at the end of expiration.
- Continuous positive airway pressure (CPAP)—spontaneous ventilation with maintenance of airway pressures above atmospheric throughout the respiratory cycle.
- Pressure support ventilation (PSV)—in addition to other ventilator settings, 6–10 cm H_20 pressure support is provided to compensate for the added resistance imposed by artificial airways, making breathing easier.

CARING FOR CLIENTS ON VENTILATORS

Equipment

Specific ventilator ordered (i.e., Bennett MA-1, Bennett 7200A, Servo 900C

Hand-held resuscitator connected to oxygen flowmeter (ambu or Laerdahl bag)

Sterile suction supplies

Ventilator flowsheet

Preparation

1. Double-check the ventilator settings against those ordered by the physician.
2. Plug the machine in, and turn it ON.
3. Familiarize yourself with location of alarm systems on the ventilator, and turn on all alarm systems.
4. Validate that tube cuff inflation is appropriate with minimal leak (squeak heard at end inspiration while auscultating over cuff at suprasternal notch).
5. Connect the ventilator tubing to client's endotracheal tube or tracheostomy tube.

Procedure

1. Monitor client's pulse and blood pressure until stable.
2. Obtain arterial blood gases 15 minutes after ventilation is established.
3. Monitor ventilator settings and delivered values: tidal volume, inspiratory pressure, peak pressure, rate, FIO_2, inspiratory–expiratory (I:E) ratio, ventilatory modes (e.g., SIMV). Modern ventilators monitor these parameters continuously.

Initial Ventilator Settings

- Tidal volume of 10–15 mL/kg (high tidal volumes help prevent atelectasis)
- Respiratory rate of 10–15 per minute
- Inspiratory–expiratory (I:E) ratio 1:2 (I:E ratio should be less than 1:1 to prevent air trapping in the lungs.)
- Pressure limit 20% above peak airway pressures delivered.
- FIO_2 of 40–100%.

4. Ensure adequate heat and 100% humidification of inspired gases.
5. Check humidifier fluid level every 8 hours, and refill as necessary.
6. Record intake, output, and daily weights.
7. Suspend ventilator tubing from an IV hook or support it on a pillow. **Rationale:** This reduces traction on the endotracheal or tracheostomy tube.
8. Change ventilator tubing weekly.
9. Check vital signs every hour, and auscultate lungs. **Rationale:** Positive pressure ventilation may decrease venous return and cardiac output. *Note: Continuous pulse oximetry facilitates constant assessment of clients receiving ventilatory assistance.*
10. Observe and listen for possible cuff leaks around tracheostomy or endotracheal tubes.
11. Discard accumulated water in the ventilator tubing. Disconnect the tubing, stretch it to release water trapped in the corrugated areas, and drain the water into a basin or trap in tubing. Do not drain water back into the humidifier. **Rationale:** Discarding the water decreases the risk of infection.
12. Provide client with a call bell and method of com-

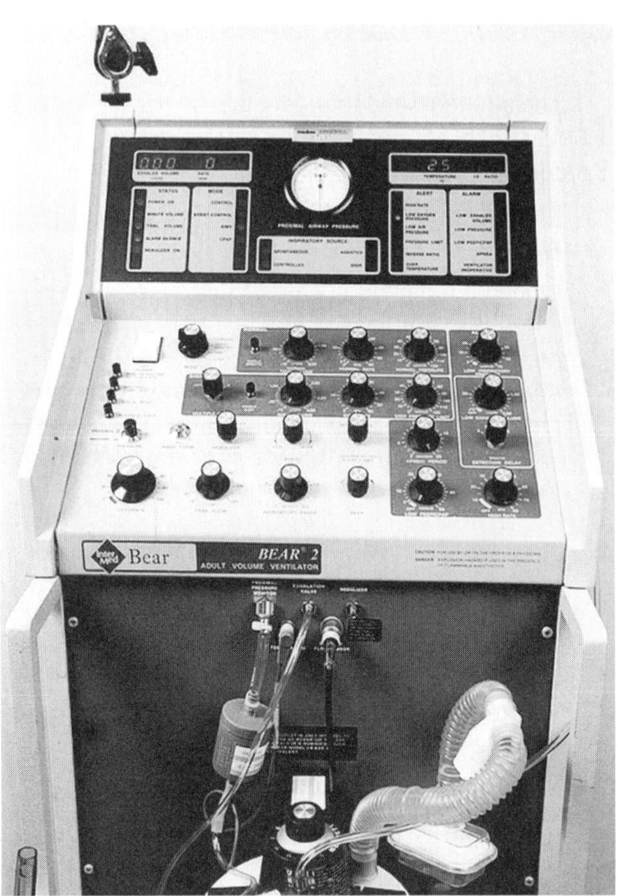

Double-check all ventilator settings against physician's orders.

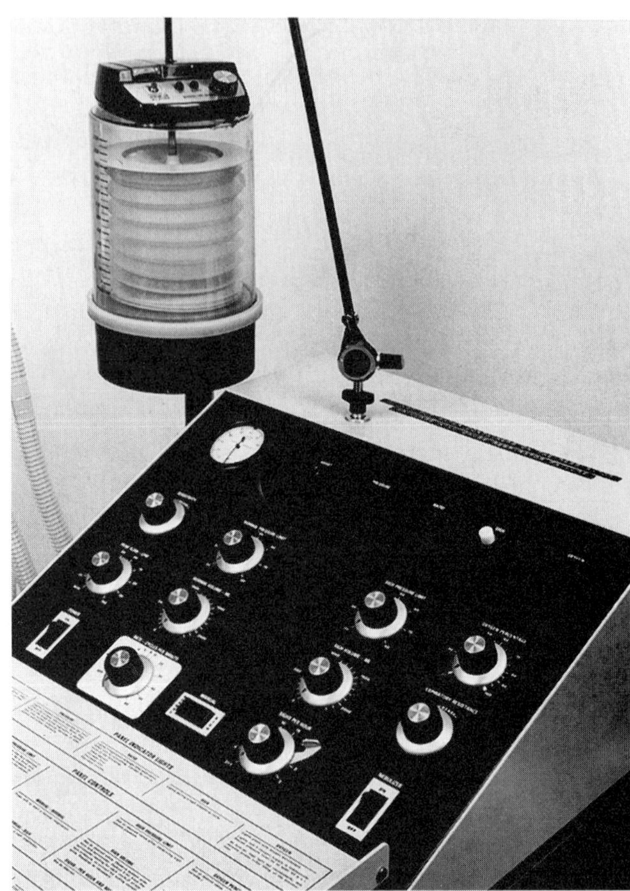
Identify location of alarm systems and what the alarm means when triggered.

munication, such as a "magic slate."

13. If ordered, test the nasogastric drainage pH every hour, and administer antacids as ordered. **Rationale:** Stress ulcers are frequently associated with mechanical ventilation, so pH should be maintained above 5.
14. Test the nasogastric drainage and stool daily for occult blood.
15. Assess lung compliance frequently. **Rationale:** Lung compliance falls before changes are evident in blood gas analysis or clinical manifestations.

Compliance is determined by

$$\frac{TV}{IPP - PEEP}$$

where TV = tidal volume; IPP = inspiratory plateau pressure; and PEEP = positive end-expiratory pressure.

16. Implement methods for stress reduction, such as careful explanation of procedures even if client appears comatose.
17. Keep ventilator alarms ON.

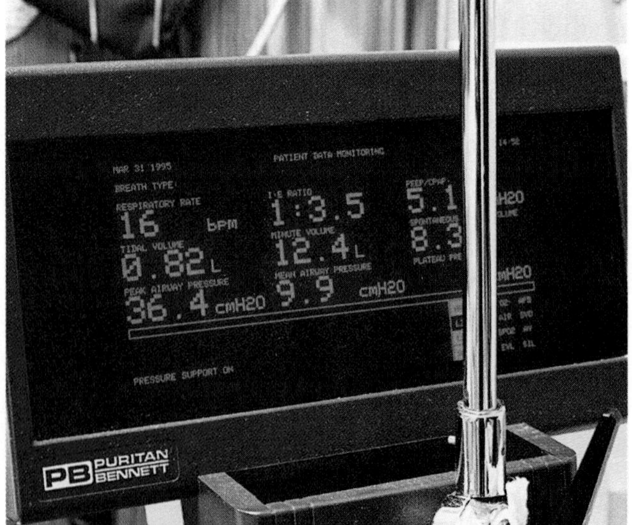

Continually monitor ventilator readings and delivered values.

18. Maintain appropriate "sigh" delivery. **Rationale:** This intervention assists in preventing atelectasis.

PROVIDING POSITIVE END-EXPIRATORY PRESSURE (PEEP)

Equipment

Mechanical ventilator with built-in PEEP device

Procedure

1. Notify respiratory therapist of order for PEEP.
2. Briefly explain procedure to client.
3. Gradually increase PEEP to specified level while monitoring respiratory and cardiovascular status.
4. Monitor vital signs every 15 minutes for 4 hours and hourly after that. **Rationale:** Transient hypotension is common with PEEP.
5. Check blood gases 15–30 minutes after stabilization, and adjust PEEP accordingly.
6. Check exhalation port tubing regularly. **Rationale:** Checking the tubing reveals kinks or other obstructions.
7. Monitor blood gases until the client is stable. Oximetry can also be used to monitor client. **Rationale:** Results determine oxygen requirements.
8. Inspect, palpate, and auscultate chest. **Rationale:** This action detects subcutaneous emphysema, or pneumothorax development.
9. Monitor cardiac output if Swan–Ganz catheter is in place and PEEP is more than 5 cm H_2O. **Rationale:** This information will identify a fall in cardiac output.
10. As condition improves, lower PEEP pressure.

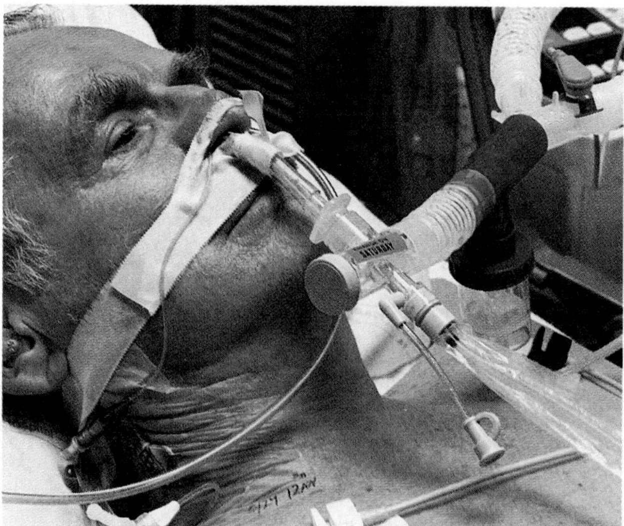

Ventilator with nebulizer for respiratory support.

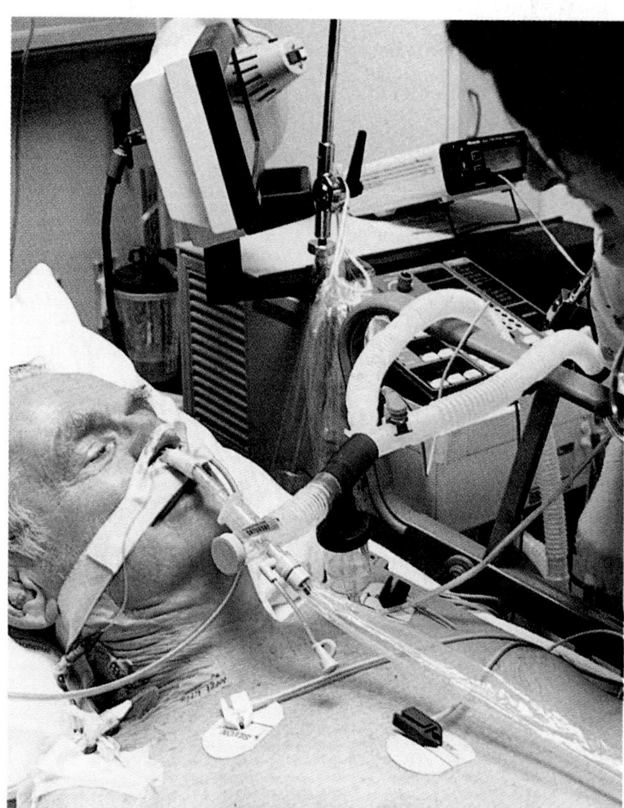

Appropriate positioning of ventilator reduces traction on ET tube.

PROVIDING CONTINUOUS POSITIVE AIRWAY PRESSURE (CPAP)

Equipment

Clear face mask with straps, nasal mask, or nasal pillows
Appropriate mechanical devices to achieve desired mode
Oxygen source with appropriate delivery device
Oxygen–air blender
Reservoir bag
Humidification warming device, if needed
CPAP devices with safety limit
Pressure gauge

CPAP is commonly used in the home setting to prevent obstructive sleep apnea.

Preparation

1. Notify respiratory therapist of physician's order.
2. Briefly explain procedure to client and family.
3. Start flow of warm, humidified oxygen through CPAP system.
4. Strap client to interface system to form tight seal.
5. Connect CPAP device.

Procedure

1. Slowly increase expiratory resistance to level specified by physician. CPAP is usually not delivered at more than 10 cm of H_2O.
2. Reassure client, especially if dyspneic, that CPAP helps to ease underlying condition.
3. Instruct client to breathe normally.
4. Monitor vital signs, blood gases, and respiratory and cardiovascular status. **Rationale:** CPAP may precipitate acute respiratory failure, due to CO_2 retention from fatigue, or cardiac failure due to increased intrathoracic pressure.
5. Observe frequently for air leaks in system, especially around mask.
6. Observe for abdominal distention. **Rationale:** This can be caused from air swallowing.
7. Clean and dry face as needed.
8. Supply another form of oxygen when client is off CPAP systems (e.g., nasal cannula) as needed.
9. Change the tubing as appropriate. **Rationale:** Frequent change of tubing minimizes infection.
10. Provide communication method such as a "magic slate" for client if mask is used.

CHARTING

- Type of device used
- Settings
- Time initiated
- Any problems and actions taken
- Results of suctioning (i.e., amount and character of secretions)
- Indicate if client is making spontaneous breathing efforts or is not triggering the machine
- Endotracheal tube location and minimal leak established
- Arterial blood gas values
- Hemodynamic monitoring values
- Findings on pulmonary and cardiac assessment

CRITICAL THINKING APPLICATION

CLINICAL PROBLEMS	CRITICAL THINKING OPTIONS
■ Adequate respiratory function is not maintained.	• Check for leaks in ventilator tubing and around humidifier. • Evaluate ventilator settings to see if they are correct. • Auscultate lungs to determine if air flow through the lungs is adequate. • Auscultate lungs to identify presence of adventitious lung sounds. • Suction airway frequently to increase pulmonary ventilation.
■ ABGs do not improve.	• Consult physician.
For Ventilator	
■ Client breathes out of synchronization with the ventilator.	• Check arterial blood gases—hypoxemia may cause anxiety. • Remove client from the ventilator, and hand ventilate at a rate faster than the machine (to blow off carbon dioxide and diminish client's ventilatory drive). Slowly decrease rate until it is the same as the ventilator setting. Place client back on the ventilator, while reassuring and coaching client to breathe in synchronization with ventilator. • If problem persists and arterial blood gas values and ventilator settings are adequate, consult with physician about the use of sedation or neuromuscular blocking agents to paralyze client.
■ Sudden respiratory distress, distended neck veins, or a possible tracheal shift occurs.	• Immediately remove client from ventilator and hand ventilate. • Immediately notify physician as these are signs of a tension pneumothorax. • Prepare equipment and client for chest tube insertion. • Assist the physician with chest tube insertion.
■ Client experiences decreased compliance, and diminished breath sounds.	• Check for signs of increased fluids in lungs (x-ray, increase in CVP or PAWP, crackles and wheezes on auscultation, decrease in urinary output). • Suction client more frequently. • Implement program of chest physical therapy. Provide percussion, vibration, and postural drainage. • Turn client frequently. • Sigh, cough, turn and deep breath client several times an hour to reopen atelectatic alveoli, hyperinflate lungs with a brief pause at the end of inspiration mimicking a normal sigh.

CLINICAL PROBLEMS	CRITICAL THINKING OPTIONS
Client experiences symptoms of dyspnea, burning chest pain on inspiration, decreasing Pa_{O_2}, and dry cough, indicating oxygen toxicity.	• Prevent oxygen toxicity by returning FI_{O_2} to specified setting after increasing it to 100% for oxygenation before and after suctioning, or for determination of A–a ΔP_{O_2} difference. • Obtain physician's order to reduce the FI_{O_2} as quickly as possible. (The danger of oxygen toxicity is increased with prolonged use of FI_{O_2} over 50%.) • Check FI_{O_2} settings.
Adventitious sounds, edema, weight gain, and pulmonary edema occur, indicating fluid overload.	• Slow IV rates and notify physician. • Administer diuretics and drugs to support cardiac output, as ordered by physician.
Pressure alarm is activated.	• Check for kinks or obstructions in tubing and take corrective measures. • Dispose of excess H_2O in ventilator tubing. • Suction client for possible mucous obstruction. • Obtain order for and administer bronchodilators. • Assess for pneumothorax. • Assess for decrease in lung compliance. If it has decreased, adjust alarm setting and consult physician. • If unable to find cause for alarm, discontinue ventilator treatment and hand ventilate while respirator is checked for malfunction.
Volume alarm is activated.	• Check if inspiratory phase is shortened due to pressure being reached earlier than normal. Tidal volume is decreased when this occurs. • Check for disconnected tubing. • Check for loose connections, and tighten them if present. • Check whether the plug has been pulled out of the wall socket. • Deflate and reinflate the airway cuff to adjust a cuff leak. • If unable to identify and relieve the cause immediately, disconnect the ventilator tubing, hand ventilate the client, and summon help.
Client has fever, elevated white blood cell count, or changed odor or color of respiratory secretions.	• Send sputum specimen for culture and sensitivity. • Administer antibiotics as ordered.

CLINICAL PROBLEMS	CRITICAL THINKING OPTIONS
For PEEP	
Mechanical ventilator fails or client needs to be transported.	• Start oxygen flow through hand-held ventilating device. • Attach expiratory resistance, for example PEEP valve. • Disconnect ventilator tubing from airway at end of inspiration. • Attach hand-held ventilator to airway during expiration. • Watch chest, and provide breaths in synchrony with client's inspirations (if any) or at rate of 10–12/minute. • Notify respiratory therapist to check machine.
Po_2 is not maintained at 80–100 mm Hg.	• Continue delivery of PEEP at ordered prescribed volume. If this is not effective, obtain an order for increased volume or more PEEP. • Do not attempt to wean client off PEEP until parameters are maintained or improved.
Pulmonary pathology is not reduced.	• Continue with PEEP. • Evaluate other treatment modalities for effectiveness. • Monitor drug therapy, such as antibiotic or diuretic and cardiotonic, for effectiveness. • Evaluate the results of respiratory toilet, and monitor amount, type, and consistency of secretions.
Cardiac output decreases significantly.	• Anticipate that clients with decreased sympathetic reserve may have difficulty adjusting to increased intrathoracic pressure. Examples are clients who are elderly, hypovolemic, or on sympatholytic medications. • If cardiac output falls abruptly, or severely decreases, terminate PEEP and notify physician.
Pneumothorax occurs.	• Discontinue PEEP, and take client off ventilator; hand ventilate with manual resuscitator and 100% oxygen. • Notify physician, and prepare to assist with chest tube insertion. • If tension pneumothorax occurs, assist with emergency chest decompression with large-bore needle, three-way stopcock, and large syringe.

CLINICAL PROBLEMS	CRITICAL THINKING OPTIONS
For CPAP	
■ Oxygenation is not improved.	• Monitor blood gases and pulmonary artery wedge pressures. If they remain abnormal even with treatment, notify physician for possible orders for mechanical ventilation and PEEP. • Continue to use CPAP and instruct client to breathe normally.
■ Pulmonary pathology is not decreased.	• Ensure adequate pulmonary toilet is being done in addition to CPAP with clients who have increased secretions. • Monitor effects of drug therapy for cardiac or pulmonary disorders. • Assess client's need for mechanical ventilation with PEEP.
■ Client complains of nausea.	• Immediately remove mask and supply oxygen via face tent while assessing cause of nausea. • Insert nasogastric tube to remove air and fluid from stomach. • If impending vomiting, turn client's head to side or place client on side to minimize risk of aspiration.
■ Client complains of fatigue; increasing dyspnea; coma, or apnea occurs.	• Assist physician with intubation and mechanical ventilation. • Discontinue CPAP, and bag ventilate the client with a manual resuscitator. Use 100% oxygen with bagging.
■ Pneumothorax occurs.	• Notify physician, and prepare to assist with chest tube insertion. • If tension pneumothorax occurs, assist with emergency chest decompression.

unit 6 VENTILATOR WEANING PROCESS

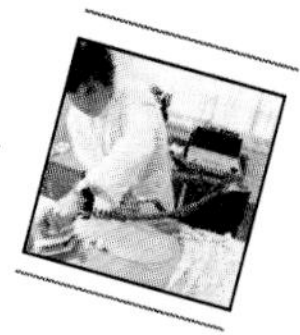

NURSING PROCESS DATA

ASSESSMENT Data Base

Measure vital signs, negative inspiratory pressure, vital capacity, and arterial blood gases.

Evaluate client parameters indicating readiness for weaning.

- PaO_2 of 70 mm Hg or better on an FIO_2 of 50% or less.
- PEEP 5 cm or less, if used.
- Vital capacity of 15 mL/kg or better.
- Inspiratory pressure of −25 cm H_2O or better.
- A–a ΔPO_2 difference less than 350 mm Hg on 100% oxygen.
- Shunt less than 30%.
- Respiratory rate between 12 and 20 breaths per minute.
- Blood pressure and pulse stable.

Note current ECG pattern as a baseline.

Review the physician's order regarding details of weaning.

PLANNING Objectives

To identify clients who are capable of maintaining breathing without the use of mechanical ventilators

To reestablish normal breathing patterns for clients on mechanical ventilators

IMPLEMENTATION Procedure

Weaning Long-Term Ventilated Client (T-Tube Trial)

EVALUATION Expected Outcomes

Laboratory parameters indicate client is ready for weaning.

Client is able to maintain respiratory status without mechanical ventilation.

Arterial blood gases maintained within normal range for client.

WEANING LONG-TERM VENTILATED CLIENT (T-TUBE TRIAL)

Equipment

Heated humidified oxygen source with wide-bore tubing

T-piece adaptor

Suctioning supplies

Arterial blood gas-sampling supplies

Continuous pulse oximetry unit

Procedure

1. Explain the discontinuation process to client. Reassure client that you will watch closely and, if necessary, discontinue weaning and attempt it again later.
2. Suction client. Hyperinflate client's lungs with 100% oxygen before and after suctioning.
3. Maintain endotracheal or tracheostomy cuff at minimal leak during weaning.
4. Elevate head of the bed to facilitate diaphragmatic excursion.

5. If physician orders cuff deflated during weaning, suction secretions that have accumulated above the cuff as follows:
   a. Provide positive pressure to end of tube with a hand-held resuscitation bag and 100% oxygen.
   b. Place tip of suction catheter in the posterior pharynx.
   c. Deflate cuff, and apply suction to catheter. **Rationale:** Positive pressure blows the secretions into the pharynx, where they can be suctioned out.
   d. Hyperinflate lungs with 100% oxygen for three to five breaths.
6. Connect T-piece to wide-bore oxygen tubing leading to the gas source.
7. Set oxygen concentration as ordered by physician, usually 10% higher than the ventilator FIO_2 the client has been receiving.

Note: Continuous pulse oximetry facilitates constant assessment of clients receiving ventilatory assistance

8. Remove ventilator tubing from airway, and connect airway to the T-piece.
9. Cover end of ventilator tubing with sterile gauze.
10. Observe for vital sign changes, apprehension, diaphoresis, and dysrhythmias. (A mild increase in blood pressure, pulse, and respiratory rate is normal. Mild-to-moderate anxiety is also normal.)
11. Monitor pulse oximetry continuously.
12. Measure arterial blood gases 15 minutes after initiating weaning.
13. Proceed with weaning procedure as ordered (e.g., time off ventilator). **Rationale:** Gradual weaning may be necessary.
14. Weaning the client on prolonged mechanical ventilation.
    a. Client is breathing spontaneously.
    b. Decrease SIMV rate to 2.
    c. Decrease FIO_2 to room air.
    d. Decrease PEEP to 0 cm H_2O.
    e. Decrease CPAP to 0 cm H_2O.
    f. Maintain PSV at 6 cm H_2O as long as mechanical ventilator in use.
    g. Monitor vital signs and oximetry.
15. If client tolerates no ventilator support (other than PSV), extubate client.
16. Following weaning, measure vital signs, vital capacity, inspiratory pressure, and blood gases.

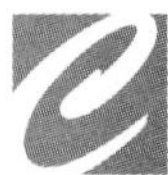

CHARTING for Ventilator Weaning

- Preweaning vital signs, vital capacity, inspiratory pressure, and blood gas values
- Method of weaning
- FIO_2
- Time weaning started and terminated
- Vital signs, blood gases, and physical signs and symptoms during weaning period

CRITICAL THINKING APPLICATION

CLINICAL PROBLEMS	CRITICAL THINKING OPTIONS
Laboratory parameters indicate client is not ready for weaning.	• Continue mechanical ventilation as ordered. • If ventilation settings do not improve client's respiratory status, notify physician for change in orders. • Ensure that client gets adequate periods of sleep. • Assess client for needed caloric intake and nutrition. • Assess client for possible respiratory complications that may be interfering with the weaning process.
Client is not able to maintain respiratory status without mechanical ventilation.	• Continue use of ventilator. • If client has been extubated, prepare equipment and client for intubation and placement on a ventilator. • If respiratory distress occurs with unintubated client, ventilate with ambu or Laerdahl bag, using a face mask.
Arterial blood gases (ABGs) are not maintained within normal range.	• Notify physician of abnormal ABGs, and obtain order for alteration in ventilation (i.e., increased percentage of oxygen, added dead space). • Maintain mechanical ventilation. Do not attempt to wean or extubate client. • Suction client frequently if secretions are thick or copious in amount. • If severe acidosis occurs, obtain order for increasing the respiratory rate to blow off carbon dioxide.
Decreased level of consciousness, dyspnea, severe anxiety, or severe fatigue occurs.	• Obtain arterial blood gases (anxiety may be due to hypoexemia). • Place client back on ventilator. • Provide thorough explanation, and increase reassurance. • Evaluate present use of sedatives or narcotics.
Client develops increased heart and respiratory rate, increased blood pressure, premature beats on ECG, or ST segment depression.	• Place client back on ventilator. • Monitor vital signs more frequently, and obtain blood gases to determine oxygen concentration. • Increase FIO_2.

34

Home Care Management

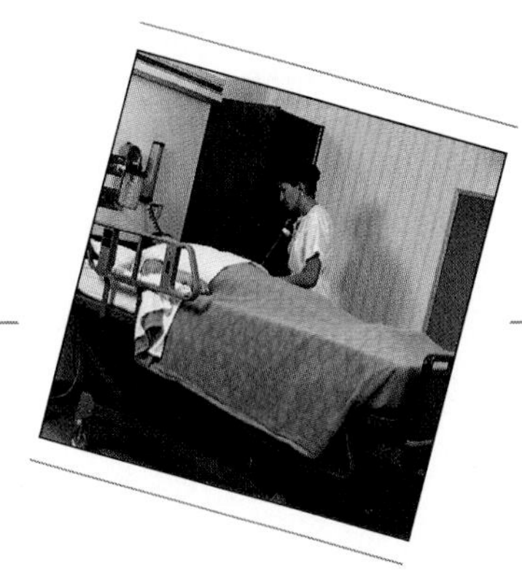

LEARNING OBJECTIVES

- Define the criteria for Medicare eligibility.
- Compare and contrast infection control practices in the home and hospital.
- Describe an alternative procedure for handwashing when soap and running water are not available.
- List the contents of the nursing bag carried by home care nurses.
- State at least three safety measures that should be carried out when placing a client into a tub or shower.
- List three areas in the home that should be evaluated for safety.
- Demonstrate at least three improvised nursing actions that promote good body mechanics when providing care in the home.
- Devise a method for assisting the client to remember to take medications.
- Compare and contrast the differences in administering parenteral nutrition in the home and hospital.
- Outline the steps in inserting a straight catheter for a home care client.
- Describe at least six safety measures for home care clients requiring oxygen therapy.
- List the steps for assessing pacemaker function using a pacemaker clinic.
- List two contraindications for using transtracheal oxygen.

INTRODUCTION

Home health care, a rapidly growing field of health care, has developed in response to recent changes in political and social forces in the United States. These changes have demanded that nurses expand their knowledge about home care and acquire skills needed to provide safe, competent care to clients in the home setting.

Several factors have contributed to the emergence of home health care as a primary delivery system. The fastest growing segment of the American population is 85 years of age or older. The elderly constitute the largest proportion of population currently using home health care services. Nine percent of those 65–74 years of age and 25% of those 75 years and older require some type of home care service. Many younger clients are receiving home care visits as a direct result of early discharge from hospitals. Home care visits are funded by private insurance companies and are a cost-effective measure for providing nursing care.

Another factor is the changing structure and role of the American family. Traditionally, women have provided health care for the family members at home. With more women working outside the home, the demand for home health services has increased.

Political factors have had an effect on health care delivery patterns. A cost-containment measure initiated by the federal government in 1983 to curb rising costs of hospitalized Medicare clients drastically altered the extent of care administered in the hospital setting. A prospective payment system (DRGs), rather than a retrospective payment system, was implemented. This resulted in shorter hospital stays for Medicare clients. With the shorter stays came a dramatic increase in the need for professional services to care for high acuity clients in the home. Additional types of services have also had to be added to the home care system to meet the needs of these clients. Even more changes are occurring with health care reform in the 1990s. Health maintenance organizations (HMOs) and reimbursement policies are directly affecting the home health care agencies.

The purpose of this chapter is to present clinical skills appropriate for the home setting. Many of the skills used in the home are exactly the same as those presented in other sections of this book; therefore, they are not repeated in this chapter. When a specific skill is not included in this unit, refer to a previous unit for that skill. Other skills require minor change for adaptation to the home environment, but, essentially, they are similar. Finally, a few skills are altered for the home setting.

The use of the nursing process is just as important in the home care setting as in the hospital setting. Actually, nursing care plans are required by Medicare regulations and are also used as a justification for skilled nursing services by private insurers. This chapter is presented in the nursing process format to assist in organizing nursing actions and evaluating health care.

Home Care Definition

The term "home health care" refers to all services that promote, maintain, or restore physical, social, or emotional health to clients in the home setting. Home care is provided in the individual's residence. For a smooth transition from hospital to home, the home care coordinator communicates with the family members and the home health nurse.

Home Health Team

A variety of health workers are needed to provide comprehensive home care services to clients and families. The following chart presents an overview of health care providers and their major responsibilities. The list and responsibilities are not inclusive; consult an additional home care reference for more detailed information.

Health Care Provider	Major Responsibilities
Registered Nurse	Performs as a case manager. Initiates physician-ordered plan of care, performs assessment, planning, and interventions for needed home care skills and teaching. Assists in evaluating treatment regimens for all services.
Home Care Aide	Performs hygienic care, skin care, exercise, ambulation, dressing, and elimination skills. Some may prepare and serve meals. They assist in maintaining a clean, safe, immediate client environment (e.g., client's bedroom).
Homemaker	Maintains the home environment, shops for and prepares meals, transports client, and runs errands.
Social Worker	Assists in planning for home care needs, instructs in use of social and community services and resources. Provides information relative to long-term planning and respite care in the home.
Physical Therapist	Evaluates environment in preparation for client's return home. Assists with safety adaptations for the home, instructs in exercise program, gait training, and use of special adaptive equipment.
Occupational Therapist	Instructs in activities of daily living, grooming, upper extremity strengthening, and function activities.
Speech Therapist	Evaluates swallowing and chewing ability; assists with increasing communication techniques for client, family, and health care provider; and provides speech reeducation program.
Nutritionist	Evaluates and provides for nutritional needs of client. Plans and instructs in appropriate diet.
Physician	Prescribes medical plan of treatment. Writes specific prescriptions for medications, diet, supplies, nursing interventions, and therapist parameters.

Referral to Home Care

It is necessary for nurses in all settings to be aware of the referral process and the type of client who should be referred for home care services. Although most home care clients have been hospitalized, it is not a prerequisite for service. Physicians, individual clients, families, and friends may refer a client by calling a home health agency and requesting service. A physician's approval is needed for reimbursement. An evaluation visit is made by the RN, PT, or ST to determine if service is needed, and if so, an appropriate plan of care is established.

Most hospitals have a designated protocol for making referrals, which is described in the hospital policy manual. In most hospitals it is the discharge planner or social worker who makes the referral. The nurse may alert the appropriate person to the client's need for home care. It is essential that the nurse provide complete and thorough information about the client's condition, including physical and psychosocial needs. This information is documented on a standard referral form or on an official form from the Department of Health and Human Services and sent to the home health agency. Accurate information and orders are needed to facilitate a smooth transition from hospital to home. Incomplete or inadequate communication could mean a lapse in service and inadequate care for the client.

All age groups use home health services. The criteria for referral depends on various factors, such as client need, agency protocol, and insurance criteria. Since the elderly on Medicare represent the largest segment of the population using home care services, it is important that all nurses know Medicare eligibility criteria for home visits. This ensures that accurate information is given to the client and family. In addition to eligibility criteria, many regulations govern the type and frequency of care. Since these regulations are subject to change and interpretation by the fiscal intermediaries who administer Medicare insurance, frequent review of Medicare regulations should be done. Eligibility for another funding agency, Medicaid, differs from state to state. It is the nurse's responsibility to be familiar with these policies. Each individual insurance company reimburses for services at different rates and for different levels of service. Each insurance plan needs to be reviewed to determine reimbursement.

Transition from Hospital to Home

A smooth transition from hospital to home depends on an appropriate discharge plan. The shorter duration in hospital stay requires a thorough, efficient discharge plan that must be initiated at the time of hospital admission. Identifying the client's needs and resources before planning for discharge results in a realistic plan. Since any illness causes additional stress in the family and necessitates an adaptive coping response, the needs of the family or significant other must be included in the teaching and discharge plan. In addition, accurate and comprehensive documentation must accompany the physician's plan of treatment to ensure a smooth transition. A description of the client at discharge should be provided; include physical assessment findings, ability to assist in ADL, adaptive devices needed for care, and a brief summary of hospitalization. These data greatly assist in the transition from hospital to home.

Client Teaching

Client teaching is an essential component of both hospital and home care. Since clients are discharged earlier and with a higher acuity level, the client and his or her family are expected to accept more responsibility for follow-up care. It is essential that client teaching begin in the hospital and provide a description of the disease or condition and the treatment regimen. The client and family should be instructed in skills and treatments necessary to restore health and prevent other illness or complications. The home health nurse builds on the teaching plan with the main emphasis on adapting care in the home environment. Continuity of care depends on comprehensive communication between the discharging and home care agencies.

Adapting Care to the Home Setting

The client is often a passive recipient of care in the hospital. In the home setting, on the other hand, the client is in control—it is his or her environment. That is, the environment is determined by the client and family according to their needs, desires, values, and resources. The nurse is a guest in this environment, which requires flexibility in adapting to a variety of situations.

In the hospital, equipment is readily available. Nurses perform procedures or treatments and provide 24-hour-a-day coverage of nursing care. In the home, equipment must be ordered or improvised and the emphasis is on teaching the client or caregiver self-care activities. The home care nurse must become very creative in adapting and improvising equipment and techniques.

unit 1 ADMISSION TO HOME CARE

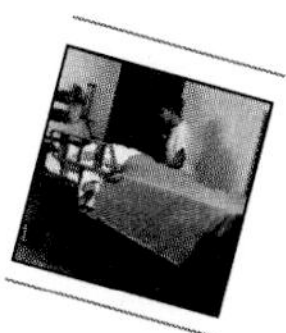

When a client referral is received by a home health agency, a nurse, physical therapist, or speech therapist makes an initial admission visit. This visit includes a thorough assessment of the client, family, and home environment. The home environment is evaluated for safety, and the client and family are assessed for knowledge of safety and emergency procedures. Assessment of the client includes physical, emotional, psychologic, and economic status. The home is assessed for any adaptations that must be made to enable the client to function optimally in his or her environment. Family members are assessed for understanding of the client's illness or needs; cultural, ethnic, and health beliefs and values; ability to cope with the current situation; the physical, emotional, and spiritual needs of family members; financial resources; and knowledge of how to use community resources. A complete list of assessment parameters for each of these areas is included on the initial assessment form.

Plan of Treatment

Based on admission findings, a plan of care is established. Since April, 1985, the Health Care Financing Administration (the federal office that administers the Medicare program) has required that all agencies certified to provide home health care to Medicare clients use the home health certification and plan of treatment form (form 485). This form must be completed on admission and signed by a physician. The plan of treatment is effective for 60 days, unless the client's condition changes. An updated plan must be signed and submitted to the Medicare office every 60 days.

In addition to form 485, the health care documentation includes admission worksheet, nursing care plan, medication profile, plan of treatment, and consent for admission and service.

Documentation

Accurate documentation of each visit is essential for both legal and fiscal purposes. The same legal considerations for charting apply to home care and the hospital. Legally, the documentation provides proof that care was given. Reimbursement of services is based on documentation. Documentation of visits can be done in a problem-oriented or narrative format, depending on agency policy. Charting must follow the nursing care plan.

Documentation takes a great deal of the nurse's time. Because of this, many agencies use standardized care plans and individualize them for each client. Flow sheets are used to expedite charting as much as possible.

The independent nature of home health nursing creates potential legal concerns for the nurse. Home care nurses must be adequately prepared and knowledgeable in current treatment procedures, protocols, and teaching modalities and be able to function independently.

Interventions are implemented by the client, family, and part-time caregivers; therefore, all are involved in the treatment plan. The nurse, as case manager, is responsible to coordinate and evaluate the care.

Currently, Medicare requires the nurse to make a home visit for the purpose of supervision at least every 14 days to reassess client and family needs and to revise the care plan.

Since home health aides provide care without direct daily supervision of a nurse, it is important that they have thorough training when they begin working for a home health agency and at periodic intervals receive continuing education. Most agencies hire only experienced nursing assistants (those who have worked in a hospital or nursing home), but it is still important to have a thorough orientation to the home setting. Training includes information about adapting skills to the home situation.

Currently, home health nurses must meet a national standard of care; no longer does the legal standard of care for nursing practice vary according to locale. Each practicing home health nurse must be aware of the national standards as published by the American Nurses' Association. The best preparation for home health nursing continues to be a sound base of nursing skills coupled with a broad knowledge of agency procedures and protocols.

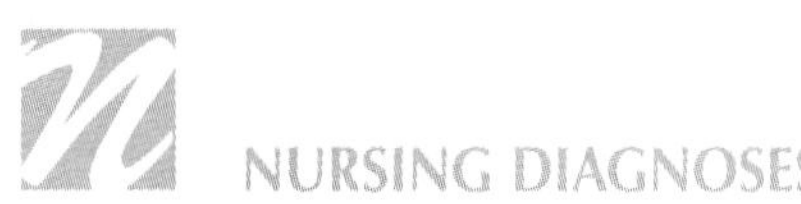

NURSING DIAGNOSES

The following nursing diagnoses may be appropriate to include in a client care plan when the components are related to admitting to the home care setting.

NURSING DIAGNOSIS	RELATED FACTORS
Anxiety	Fear of unknown outcome, actual or perceived threat to self-concept, threat to biologic integrity, change in socioeconomic status
Anticipatory Grieving	Loss of function, change in life style, lack of social support system, change in social role
Impaired Home Maintenance Management	Unavailable or inadequate support systems (spouse or children not available to provide care), insufficient finances, environmental barriers or physical facilities (lighting, condition of flooring, steps)
Risk for Injury	Impaired judgment, muscle weakness, disease process, safety factors in the home

NURSING PROCESS DATA

ASSESSMENT Data Base

Assess client's financial eligibility for home care service.

Assess client's care requirements.

Observe client's physical, emotional, and intellectual status.

Observe client's ability to adapt to the home setting.

Assess the client's level of comfort or discomfort.

Determine client's understanding of the disease and its limitations.

Assess home condition prior to client returning home.

Assess safety factors in the home.

Observe equipment for safety features.

PLANNING Objectives

To assist client to adapt to home care with minimal distress

To encourage client and family to participate in the plan of care

To provide a comfortable and safe environment for the client

To provide the necessary and appropriate home care treatment modalities

IMPLEMENTATION Procedures

Identifying Eligibility for Medicare Reimbursement

Assessing Home for Safe Environment

EVALUATION Expected Outcomes

Client adapts to home setting with minimal difficulties.

Safe environment is provided for client.

Client obtains necessary home care nursing modalities.

Client

No.

CLIENT HISTORY AND INITIAL ASSESSMENT

Code: + = Problem present Ø = No problem present

Name: ______ Age: ____ Date: ______
Address: ______ Tel: # ______
Information Obtained from Client: ______ Family Member: ______ Other: ______
Diagnosis: ______
History of Present Illness (include onset dates, operations, patient reactions, reason for home care): ______

Allergies:

SOCIAL & ENVIRONMENTAL HISTORY

Marital Status: ______ Religion: ______
Family Members in Home: ______
Name & Tel. # of Primary Care Giver: ______
Name & Tel. # of Person to Contact in case of emergency: ______
Are there steps in Client's Residence? Yes: ______ No: ______ Number: ______
Environmental Problems: None ____ Inadequate ____ Space ____ Utilities ____ Safety ____ Pests ____
Other Environmental Problems: ______
Is this Client known to other Community Agencies? if so, please list: ______

VITAL SIGNS

Temperature O ______ R ______ AX ______ RESP ______ BP Rt ______ Lt ______
Pulse AP ______ R ______ Sitting: ______
Height ______ Weight ______ Standing: ______
Recent Weight Loss/Gain: Yes ______ No ______ Lying: ______

REVIEW OF SYSTEMS

Vision: No Problem ____ Glasses ____ Last Checked ____ Blurring ____ Diplopia ____ Inflammation ____
Cataracts ____ Glaucoma ____ Pain ____ Contact Lenses ____
RN Observation/Physical Findings: ______
Hearing: No Problem ____ Limited ____ Aid ____ Pain ____ Tinnitus ____ Discharge ____
RN Observation/Physical Findings: ______

Speech: No Problem ____ Can Understand ____ Can Express ____ Language Barrier ____
Interpreter's Name and Telephone Number: ______

Skin: No Problem ____ Dryness ____ Color ____ Turgor ____ Nails ____ Toes ____
Rashes ______ Location ______
Lesions/Wounds ______ Location ______
RN Observation/Physical Findings: ______

Respiratory: No Problem ____ DOE ____ Pain ____ Cough ____ Sputum ____ Sinusitis ____
Tobacco ____ Expistaxis ____ Cold Freq. ____ D.A.R. ____ Orthopnea ____
Pillows: 1 ____ 2 ____ 3 ____ Tracheotomy Old ____ New ____ Rales ____ Rhonchi ____
IPPB ____ 02 ____ Vaporizer ____ Respirator ____ Other ______
RN Observation/Physical Findings: ______

Cardio-vascular: No Problem ____ Edema (location) ____ Numbness ____ Syncope ____
Dizziness ____ Cyanosis ____ Angina ____ Bruising ____ Pain ____ Palpitations ____
P.N.D. ____ Angina ____ Abnormal Heart Sounds ______
Pedal Pulse ______
RN Observation/Physical Findings: ______

G.I.: No Problem ____ Chewing Problems ____ Dysphagia ____ Dentures ____ Full ____ Partial ____
Mouth: Needs Care ____ Healthy ____ Lesions ____
RN Observation/Physical Findings: ______
Polydipsia ____ Polyphagia ____ Pain ____ Emesis ____ Hematemesis ____ Nausea ____
B.M.'s: No Problem ____ Loose ____ Constipated ____ Melena ____ Ostomy ____
Appliances Used: ______ Hemorrhoids ____ Incontinence ____
Abdomen: Soft ____ Tender ____ Distended ____ Bruits ____ Bowel Sounds ______
RN Observation/Physical Findings: ______

G.U.: No Problem ____ Dysuria ____ Frequency ____ Hesitancy ____ Urgency ____ Hematuria ____
Polyuria ____ Nocturia ____ Control ____ Pain ____ Ileostomy ____
Appliance Used: ______ Ureterostomy ____ Appliances Used ____
Catheter: Past ____ Present ____ Size ____ Type ____ Reason ____ Date ____
RN Observation/Physical Findings: ______

Musculoskeletal: No Problem ____ Deformities ____ Pain ____ Stiffness ____ Contractures ____
Arthritis ____ Exercises ____ Done by ______ Amputation ____
Prostheses: ______

No. ______

Neurological: No Problem ____ Seizures ____ Paralysis ____ Paresthesia ____ Weakness ____
Balance Problem ____ Gait Problem ____ Decreased Sensation ____ Dominant Hand ____ Pain ____
RN Observation/Physical Findings: ______
Present Mental Status: Alert ____ Confused ____ Forgetful ____ Orientation ______
Present Behavior: Cooperative ____ Anxious ____ Depressed ____ Isolated ____ Distrustful ____
Lethargic ____ Talkative ____ Withdrawn ____
RN Observation/Physical Findings: ______

Nutritional: Intake Route: Oral ____ Naso-Gastric Tube ____ Parenteral ____
Intake: Adequate ____ Excessive: ____ (Specify)
Dietary or Vitamin/Mineral Supplement Used: No ____ Yes ____ (Specify) ______
Special Diet ______ Appetite ______
Compliance ____ Copy of diet in Home: No ____ Yes ____ Instruction Needed ____ Person preparing food ____
RN Observation/Physical Findings: ______

ADL: No Problem ____ Needs Assistance with: Ambulation ____ Transfer ____ Hygiene ____ Bathing ____
Bed Bath ____ Shower ____ Tub Bath ____ Dressing ____ Feeding ____ Meal Prep. ____
Shopping ____ Housework ____ Laundry ____ Sleep: Hours ____ Naps ____ Aids ______
Insomnia ____ Due to: ______
Other Caregivers Assisting: ______ How Often ______
Housebound: Yes ____ No ____
RN Observation/Physical Findings: ______

Hobbies/Interest: Reading ____ T.V. ____ Games ____ Cards ____ Handwork ______
Other ______ Limitations Imposed by Illness: ______
RN Observation/Physical Findings: ______

Supplies/Equipment Needed: ______

Assessment of Client's Level of Understanding of Disease Process and Required Care: (Include learning abilities, present habits, etc.) ______

Additional information concerning this client which should be known to other staff members ______

Skilled needs to be included in Nursing Care Plan ______

Need Assessed for other disciplines
P.T. ____
O.T. ____
S.T. ____
MSW ____
HHA ____

ILLUSTRATE SKIN LESIONS, BRUISES, AMPUTATIONS, ETC.

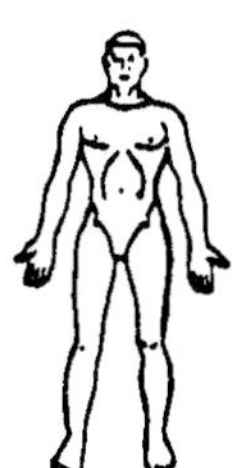
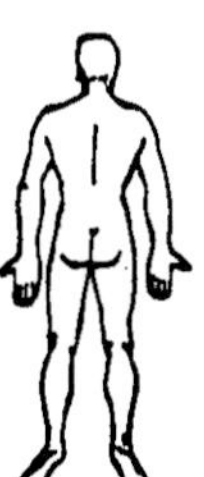

DEPARTMENT OF HEALTH AND HUMAN SERVICES
HEALTH CARE FINANCING ADMINISTRATION

FORM APPROVED
OMB No. 0938-0357

HOME HEALTH CERTIFICATION AND PLAN OF TREATMENT

1. Patient's HI Claim No.	2. SOC Date	3. Certification Period From: To:	4. Medical Record No.	5. Provider No.

6. Patient's Name and Address

7. Provider's Name and Address.

8. Date of Birth: 9. Sex ☐ M ☐ F

10. Medications: Dose/Frequency/Route (N)ew (C)hanged

11. ICD-9-CM	Principal Diagnosis	Date
12. ICD-9-CM	Surgical Procedure	Date
13. ICD-9-CM	Other Pertinent Diagnosis	Date

14. DME and Supplies

15. Safety Measures:

16. Nutritional Req.

17. Allergies:

18.A. Functional Limitations

1 ☐ Amputation
2 ☐ Bowel/Bladder (Incontinence)
3 ☐ Contracture
4 ☐ Hearing
5 ☐ Paralysis
6 ☐ Endurance
7 ☐ Ambulation
8 ☐ Speech
9 ☐ Legally Blind
A ☐ Dyspnea With Minimal Exertion
B ☐ Other (Specify)

18.B. Activities Permitted

1 ☐ Complete Bedrest
2 ☐ Bedrest BRP
3 ☐ Up As Tolerated
4 ☐ Transfer Bed/Chair
5 ☐ Exercises Prescribed
6 ☐ Partial Weight Bearing
7 ☐ Independent At Home
8 ☐ Crutches
9 ☐ Cane
A ☐ Wheelchair
B ☐ Walker
C ☐ No Restrictions
D ☐ Other (Specify)

19. Mental Status: 1 ☐ Oriented 2 ☐ Comatose 3 ☐ Forgetful 4 ☐ Depressed 5 ☐ Disoriented 6 ☐ Lethargic 7 ☐ Agitated 8 ☐ Other

20. Prognosis: 1 ☐ Poor 2 ☐ Guarded 3 ☐ Fair 4 ☐ Good 5 ☐ Excellent

21. Orders for Discipline and Treatments (Specify Amount/Frequency/Duration)

22. Goals/Rehabilitation Potential/Discharge Plans

23. Verbal Start of Care and Nurse's Signature and Date Where Applicable:

24. Physician's Name and Address

25. Date HHA Received Signed POT

26. I ☐ certify ☐ recertify that the above home health services are required and are authorized by me with a written plan for treatment which will be periodically reviewed by me. This patient is under my care, is confined to his home, and is in need of intermittent skilled nursing care and/or physical or speech therapy or has been furnished home health services based on such a need and no longer has a need for such care or therapy, but continues to need occupational therapy.

27. Attending Physician's Signature (Required on 485 Kept of File in Medical Records of HHA)

Date Signed

FORM HCFA-485 (C4) (4-87)

IDENTIFYING ELIGIBILITY FOR MEDICARE REIMBURSEMENT

Procedure

1. Check required criteria for Medicare coverage eligibility. **Rationale:** This prevents administering care for which reimbursement will not be received.
2. Identify client as homebound.
   a. Client's condition severely restricts leaving the home.
   b. Leaving the home requires considerable effort and assistance of another person.
   c. Special transportation is necessary.
   d. Absences from the home are infrequent and short.
3. Check that home service is considered skilled. To be skilled, service must be under the supervision of a registered nurse, a physical therapist, or a speech therapist.
   a. Registered nurse performs specific functions:
      Client teaching
      Dressings or irrigations
      Catheterization
      Parenteral therapies
      Medication administration and teaching
   b. Physical therapist performs certain functions:
      Gait training
      Therapeutic exercises
      Ultrasound, diathermy, TENS
      Restorative therapy
   c. Speech therapist performs certain functions:
      Therapy for clients with certain diagnoses (e.g., CVA, laryngectomies).
      Selected diagnostic and evaluative services.
4. Provide supplemental services from home health aide, social worker, or occupational therapist; care is reimbursed by Medicare only when one of the three skilled services is required.
   a. Supplemental services may be obtained even if one of the skilled services is not needed; however, Medicare does not reimburse, and client is responsible for payment.
   b. Home health aide services are reimbursable only if plan of care is established and supervised by registered nurse.
      Personal care (ADL)
      Light housekeeping (e.g., food preparation, client's laundry)
      Selected semiskilled care (e.g., PROM exercises)
   c. Social worker
      Interventions must contribute significantly to the improvement of the client's medical condition.
      Indication that social, environmental, or family conditions inhibit progress of recovery from medical condition.
   d. Occupational therapy
      Design maintenance program
      Design self-help devices to assist ADL
      Teach compensatory techniques
      Provide restorative therapy
5. Provide care that is part time and intermittent.
   a. Care must be episodic or acute and not chronic.
   b. Medically predictable recurring need for care must be present.
   c. Knowledge that condition will improve in a limited time frame.
   d. Frequency of service ranges from daily to every 90 days, depending on individual client's need.
6. Check that plan of treatment is authorized by physician and recertified every 60 days.
   a. Health Care Financing Administration form (485) is standardized for plan of treatment. This form is used by all home health agencies for Medicare clients.
   b. Form must include:
      Identifying data
      Diagnosis (ICD-9CM)
      Start of care
      Types of services required and frequency
      Functional limitations
      Activities permitted
      Safety measures
      Treatments
      Medications
      Mental status
      Nutritional status and diet orders
      Medical supplies and DME
      Goals and discharge plans
      Significant clinical findings

Prognosis
Physician's name, address, signature
Certification of homebound status

7. Assess that care is medically reasonable and necessary.
   a. Entire plan of care must correlate with client's medical problems and client's clinical status.
   b. Each service's goals (client outcomes) must be clearly stated and realistic for the client.

GUIDELINES FOR HOME CARE

- Take as little with you into the home as possible.
- Use appropriate nursing protocol in home setting.
- Wash your hands on entering and leaving home.
- Maintain clean technique in the home.
- Know the infection control guidelines (CDC).
- Review state and federal guidelines and protocol for reimbursement.

ASSESSING HOME FOR SAFE ENVIRONMENT

Equipment

Home Assessment Check List

Procedure

1. Identify type of dwelling.
2. Identify water source.
3. Identify sewer source.
4. Identify type of plumbing available.
5. Determine if any pollutants are present in the environment.
6. Assess exterior of the home for
   a. Condition of sidewalks and steps
   b. Presence of railings on steps
   c. Barriers that prevent easy access to the home
   d. Adequacy of lighting
7. Assess interior of the home for
   a. Presence of scatter rugs or worn carpeting
   b. Uncluttered pathways throughout the house
   c. Adequacy of lighting
   d. Doorways wide enough to permit assistive devices
   e. Cleanliness of house
   f. Presence of insects, rodents, or infective agents
   g. Presence of functioning smoke detectors
8. Determine if chemicals are safely stored.
9. Determine if medications can be adequately stored out of reach of children and impaired individuals.
10. Assess stairway and halls for
    a. Adequacy of light
    b. Handrails that are securely fastened to wall
    c. Flooring in good repair
    d. Rugs or carpeting in good repair
    e. Light switches in easy reach and accessible at both ends of stairs or hallway
11. Assess kitchen for
    a. Properly functioning stove
    b. Adequacy of light surrounding stove and sink
    c. Condition of small appliances
    d. Accessibility of appliances to clients in wheelchairs
12. Assess bathroom for
    a. Skidproof strips or mat in tub or shower
    b. Handrails around toilet and tub or shower
    c. Accessibility of medicine cabinet
    d. Adequate space if wheelchairs or walkers are used
    e. Temperature of hot water from faucets in sink, tub, or shower
13. Assess bedroom for
    a. Accessibility of closets and cabinets
    b. Ease in getting into and out of bed
    c. Adequate space, if commode or wheelchair is required
    d. Night light availability
    e. Accessibility of medications, water on a night stand
    f. Calling system to alert health care provider
    g. Flooring in good repair and nonslippery surface

unit 2 INFECTION CONTROL

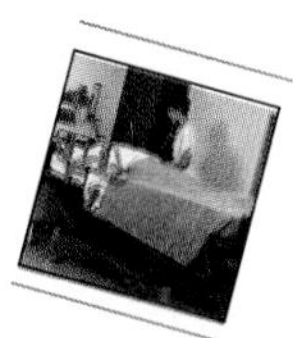

In the home setting, medical asepsis, or clean technique, is often used instead of sterile technique. The major reasons for this protocol change are the nature of the setting and the personnel providing care. The greatest infection control problem in hospitals is nosocomial infections due to the large numbers of antibiotic-resistant organisms present in a hospital setting. Although people are able to survive in what may be considered less than desirable environment without acquiring infections, they would not be protected or possess the acquired immunity to the bacteria in hospital setting. When clients are in their own environment, however, they tend to develop fewer infections because they are subjected to fewer organisms.

Nevertheless, sterile technique and equipment, such as prepackaged catheter and irrigation kits, parenteral fluid equipment, and dressings, are often purchased for home care. When sterile technique is required, it is the responsibility of the nurse to provide the instruction and evaluate the family's ability to perform the skill accurately. Hospital techniques may need to be modified for the home setting, and ideal environmental working conditions may not be present. Therefore, adaptations must be made, but the essential infection control measures must be maintained.

Just as in the hospital, effective handwashing is the *most* effective means of infection control in the home setting. There is one major difference between hospital and home. Equipment (soap, running water, and paper towels) that is readily available to the nurse in the hospital may not be available in the home. Even if running water is available, there may not be soap or clean towels. The nurse must carry handwashing supplies with her or him.

If the home care client is suspected of or diagnosed as having an infectious disease, the nurse should use the same protective equipment and protocol used in the hospital setting. The equipment includes gloves, disposable gown or apron, mask, cap, and goggles.

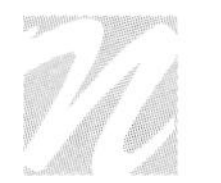

NURSING DIAGNOSES

The following nursing diagnoses may be appropriate to include in a client care plan when the components are related to clients requiring isolation protocol or sterile procedures.

NURSING DIAGNOSIS	RELATED FACTORS
Altered Health Maintenance	Diminished immune system function, steroid and antineoplastic drug therapy, substance abuse
Knowledge Deficit	Lack of access to health care facilities, lack of education, cognitive limitation, inadequate explanation or instruction
Noncompliance	Lack of understanding, lack of motivation, education or readiness, information misinterpretation, cultural or religious beliefs

NURSING PROCESS DATA

ASSESSMENT Data Base

Assess need for handwashing.
Identify clients at risk for infection.
Assess need for cleaning equipment and decontaminating equipment.
Identify type of waste material requiring special disposal.
Assess equipment needed to deliver care in the home.
Assess need for teaching preventive measures in the home of HIV or AIDS clients.

PLANNING Objectives

To deliver client care with pathogen-free hands
To clean equipment properly to prevent cross-contamination
To protect client from cross-contamination
To protect the nurse
To properly dispose of contaminated waste material
To protect client's significant others from contamination of infected material

IMPLEMENTATION Procedures

Preparing for Client Care
Disposing of Waste Material in the Home Setting
Cleansing Thermometer
Caring for an AIDS or HIV Client in the Home
Cleansing Equipment in the Home Setting
Teaching Preventive Measures in the Home
Teaching Safer Practices to IV Drug Users
(*For additional skills refer to Chapter 15*)

EVALUATION Expected Outcomes

Cross-contamination is prevented.
Nurse is protected from infection.
Equipment is cleaned appropriately.
Waste is disposed of in proper manner.
Thermometer is cleaned.

PREPARING FOR CLIENT CARE

Equipment

Community health nursing bag
Liquid soap
Paper towels
Germicide for handwashing
Disposable gloves
Disposable apron or gown
Goggles
Masks
Air-purifying mask
Thermometers (oral and rectal)
Thermometer sheaths

Vaseline or lubricant
Cotton balls
Alcohol, one small bottle
Cotton-tipped applicators
Tongue depressors
Sterile 4×4s
Band-Aids
Bandage scissors
Nonallergic tape
Plastic bags with ties
Ketodiastix and chemstrips
Sphygmomanometer
Stethoscope
Paper cups
Bleach, one small bottle

Procedure

1. Arrange equipment in bag prior to making home visit so that handwashing equipment is accessible. Bring only the supplies needed. **Rationale:** This procedure decreases the possibility of cross-contamination.
2. Place bag on flat, dry surface to establish a clean work area during visit. Place barrier such as newspaper under bag if necessary.
3. Wash hands.
    a. Use liquid soap and paper towels from bag and client's water supply; or
    b. Use client's soap and towels if you feel comfortable with this and client approves; *or*
    c. Use germicide as alternative for handwashing when soap and water are not available. Spray or squeeze small amount of germicide onto palm of hand and rub for 30 seconds along all surfaces of hands, fingers, and nails. Germicide evaporates into air, making towels unnecessary.
4. Don disposable gloves when appropriate for infection control, especially when handling blood and body fluids.
5. Take other equipment that will be needed during the visit out of the bag and place on clean work surface (use paper towel to make clean work area after washing hands).
6. Keep bag closed when not in use to promote cleanliness, safety, and security. Wash hands before entering the bag if additional equipment is needed during the visit. **Rationale:** This procedure keeps the inside of bag clean and prevents contamination.
7. Wear disposable apron or gown, goggles, or masks if necessary. **Rationale:** This protects the care giver from blood or body fluid exposure.
8. Cleanse thoroughly any equipment that left clean area and is to be returned to the bag on completing care.
    a. Rinse equipment (such as bandage scissors, forceps) under *cold* water, wash with soap and water, place in plastic bag, and take back to agency to sterilize.
    b. Return stethoscope and blood pressure cuff to plastic bag, and place in nursing bag.
9. Ensure nursing bag is monitored regularly for safety.
    a. Keep bag out of reach of children.
    b. Keep bag in trunk of car or keep in your home overnight. **Rationale:** Unattended bags in cars are more often stolen.
    c. Clean bag monthly and p.r.n.

DISPOSING OF WASTE MATERIAL IN THE HOME SETTING

Equipment

Plastic bags, heavy duty
Disposable gloves
Receptacle, rigid and puncture-proof
Bleach
Germicide

Procedure

1. Dispose of wastes contaminated with blood or body fluids.
    a. Place waste products in impenetrable, heavy-duty plastic bag.
    b. Remove plastic gloves by rolling inside out (so contaminated side is on inside) and drop into plastic bag.
    c. Seal plastic bag with tie.

d. Place plastic bag in second heavy-duty plastic bag and tie.
e. Discard in trash or bring to agency incinerator.
f. Wash hands with soap and water or germicide.

■ CLINICAL ALERT

All items contaminated with blood, exudates, or other body fluids should be considered to present a risk of transmission of HIV or hepatitis B. These items should be disposed of by incineration if possible. Use mechanisms for disposal of waste into normal trash only when incineration is not available.

2. Dispose of body wastes, such as urine, feces, respiratory secretions, vomitus, and blood, by flushing them down the toilet. (This is true whether the toilet empties into a septic tank or a sewage system.)
3. Dispose of needles and sharp objects.
   a. Do *not* remove needle from syringe or bend, break, clip, or recap after use.
   b. Drop entire disposable syringe and needle intact into rigid, puncture-proof receptacle provided by agency.
   c. Wash hands.
4. Discard other trash.
   a. Place in plastic bag.
   b. Discard in client's trash.

■ CLINICAL ALERT

Do not use glass bottles or plastic bottles that can be returned to store.
Bleach bottle with screw lid can be left in home for use as a sharp container. Tape closed before disposing of bottle. Small biohazard containers can be obtained from dry stores.

CLEANSING THERMOMETER

Equipment

Two alcohol wipes
Green soap or bar soap
Thermometer

Procedure

1. Prepare clean work area.
2. Tear one alcohol wipe in half, and apply soap to each half.
3. Cleanse thermometer with alcohol swab from distal end toward mercury tip using circular movements.
4. Repeat above using second swab.
5. Open remaining alcohol wipe, and wrap it around thermometer, letting it "soak" at least 10 minutes.
6. Discard swabs, and replace thermometer in case.
7. Wipe case with alcohol before replacing in nursing bag.

CARING FOR AN AIDS OR HIV CLIENT IN THE HOME

Equipment

Gloves
Disposable mask, gown, or apron
Protective eyewear
Specimen container if needed
Plastic bag for transport of specimen
Chlorine bleach solution (Clorox)

Procedure

1. Wash hands before and after client care and after disposing of soiled materials.
2. Don disposable gloves for any procedure.
   a. Don double gloves if tearing is likely during the procedure.
   b. If staff member has any type of open wounds or

weeping dermatitis, she or he should not administer care (even with gloves) until condition is resolved.

3. Don disposable gown or apron to protect clothing from soilage.
4. Put on mask and protective eyewear if splattering is anticipated during the procedure (e.g., suctioning, wound irrigations).
5. Collect specimens in appropriate containers labeled "Blood and Body Fluid Precautions."
6. Use extraordinary care to avoid puncture wounds with needles and other sharp objects.
   a. If puncture occurs, bleed wound, wash with soap and water.
   b. Notify supervisor immediately, and fill out unusual occurrence report.
7. Clean spills of blood and body fluids with 1:10 bleach solution (one part liquid chlorine bleach to nine parts water). Make solution fresh each time.
8. Wash eating utensils (dishes and silverware) in hot soapy water. Water should be hot enough to need gloves to tolerate the temperature. No other special precautions are required.
9. Store linens and laundry soiled with body fluids in a plastic bag and then wash separately with very hot water. Use a detergent and a 1:10 bleach solution. (Nonchlorine bleaches such as Clorox II are acceptable for colored clothing.)
10. Dispose of gown, apron, in plastic bag after completing care.
11. Take off gloves by peeling them down and turning them inside out so that contaminated side is on the inside. Place in plastic bag.
12. Wash hands.
13. Take off mask and goggles.
14. Wash hands.

CLEANSING EQUIPMENT IN THE HOME SETTING

Equipment

Article to be cleansed
Soap
Running water
Paper towels
Plastic bags
Disposable gloves

Procedure

1. Don gloves when working with equipment contaminated with any body fluid or blood.
2. Rinse article with cold running water. **Rationale:** Cold water releases organic material from the equipment and warm water may make it adhere to the surface.
3. Wash with hot, soapy water using friction.
4. Rinse well with clear water.
5. Dry thoroughly.
6. Disinfect equipment or article as indicated: one part chlorine bleach (Clorox) to nine parts water.
7. Dry thoroughly.
8. Remove disposable gloves.
9. Dispose of gloves (inside out) into plastic bag.
10. Wash hands.

■ CLINICAL ALERT

If durable medical equipment cannot be sterilized by ethyl oxide or autoclaved, it should be cleaned with 10% chlorine bleach solution after washing with hot soapy water.

TEACHING PREVENTIVE MEASURES IN THE HOME

Procedure

1. Discuss the inadvisability of allowing any person who is ill or who has depressed immune function to come in contact with the client.
2. Teach the client these appropriate hygiene principles:
   a. Wash hands after use of toilet or contact with any body fluids.
   b. Do not share thermometers, razors, razor

blades, toothbrushes, douche, or enema equipment.
   c. Do not cough without covering mouth.
   d. Be careful to dispose of nasal secretions in tissue, then in plastic bags.
3. Teach these guidelines for sharing kitchens and bathrooms:
   a. Good household cleaning practices prevent spread of infection.
   b. When eating utensils and dishes are shared, they must be cleaned with hot water (hot enough to necessitate use of gloves) and soap. Use of a dishwasher and soap is appropriate.
   c. Kitchen and bathroom surfaces should be cleaned every day with scouring powder or with chlorine bleach solution (1:10, one part bleach to nine parts water).
   d. Clean refrigerators regularly with soap and water; remove old food to prevent mold.
   e. Mop floors in bathroom and kitchen weekly. Pour dirty water down the toilet and disinfect with bleach solution.
   f. Clean toilet, tub, shower weekly or as often as necessary with bleach solution (1:10). If urine or diarrhea spills on toilet or floor, wipe immediately with the 1:10 bleach solution.
   g. Sponges used to clean floors or body fluid spills should be soaked for 5 minutes in a bleach solution (1:10).
4. Teach the following principles of food preparation:
   a. Discuss the fact that people infected with HIV may prepare food for others. They should follow usual practices for safe food preparation and be especially diligent about handwashing.
   b. Wash hands thoroughly before any food preparation.
   c. Do not lick fingers or taste from the mixing spoon while cooking.
   d. Avoid unpasteurized milk (danger of contact with *Salmonella*); do not eat old or moldy food (danger of food poisoning); and carefully wash and thoroughly cook chicken.
5. Teach how to care for linens and laundry.
   a. When clothing or linen is soiled with blood or body fluids, it should be stored separately in a plastic bag. Wash separately with very hot water, detergent, and bleach. Use Clorox II for colored clothing.
   b. Wear disposable gloves when touching soiled clothes or linen.
   c. Do not share used towels or washcloths, and wash separately. (Such towels and washcloths are, however, safe to use after washing.)
6. Inform client and family of measures for disposing of trash.
   a. Flush body wastes down the toilet.
   b. Discard dressings, diapers, Chux, or any materials soiled with secretions in a plastic bag. Then place into another plastic bag, seal, and discard into the regular trash.
   c. Sharp items (e.g., razors, needles) should be placed in a rigid, puncture-proof container with a solution of 1:10 bleach. Incinerate when container is full.
7. Discuss procedures for caring for pets.
   a. Clean bird cages wearing gloves. Birds can spread psittacosis (*Chlamydia psittaci*) or *Cryptococcus*.
   b. Clean cat litter boxes wearing gloves to prevent spread of toxoplasmosis.
   c. Tropical fish tanks should not be cleaned by the person with AIDS to prevent spread of *Mycobacterium*.
8. Teach general principles of preventing cross-infection.
   a. Wear gloves when handling body fluids, linens, or other objects contaminated with body fluids.
   b. Disposable gowns or aprons protect clothing from becoming soiled.
   c. Caregivers should not provide care when ill themselves. If this is not possible they should wear a mask when in close contact with the person with AIDS. AIDS clients are very susceptible to infections.
   d. Maintain adequate ventilation in the living quarters.

TEACHING SAFER PRACTICES TO IV DRUG USERS

Procedure

1. Inform persons of risk behaviors and factors associated with IV drug use.
   a. Direct transmission occurs with shared needles and syringes; permits blood-to-blood contact, the most direct method of transmitting the AIDS virus.
   b. Transmission to sexual partners; permits contact of body fluids
   c. Transmission to fetus during pregnancy
   d. Suppression of the immune system caused by alcohol or drug use
   e. Impaired judgment while under the influence of drugs
2. Teach IV drug users how to reduce the risk.
   a. Do not share needles or syringes with others.
   b. Clean needles and other equipment vigorously. Wash twice with full strength bleach or alcohol; rinse twice with water.
   c. Boil needles and other equipment for 15 minutes.
   d. Do not borrow or use needles or equipment from others, even if they appear healthy or say that they do not have AIDS.
3. Teach basic health maintenance measures.
   a. Decrease use of all immunosuppressive drugs (marijuana, speed, cocaine, alcohol).
   b. Maintain an adequate, nutritionally sound diet.
   c. Reduce stress on self through stress-reduction practices, or removing self from a stressful situation (living with others who routinely use drugs).
   d. Obtain regular medical and dental care.
   e. Follow life style that provides adequate rest and exercise.
   f. Obtain counseling to assist in living life without dependence on drugs.

unit 3 BODY MECHANICS

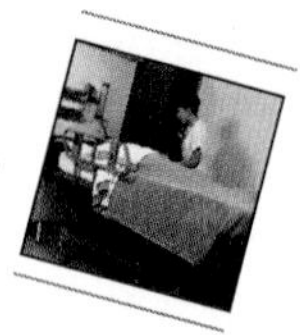

Knowledge of body mechanics and how to use these principles when giving care is important to both the health care provider and the client. Correct use of body mechanics decreases the caregiver's potential for injury and provides safety for the client. Recently, there has been an increase in the number of back injury accident claims among home health care providers. One reason for the increase is the improper use of body mechanics while performing skills in the home setting. Also, there may be no one to assist the care provider when lifting and turning clients in the home. The nurse may need to improvise, as the equipment may not be adequate or adjustable. The purpose of this unit is to consider adaptations necessary for providing safe care to the client while using proper body mechanics. In the home setting, much of the care is given by the family; therefore, it is essential that they are also taught good body mechanics.

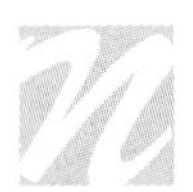

NURSING DIAGNOSES

The following nursing diagnoses are appropriate to use on client care plans when the components are related to body mechanics.

NURSING DIAGNOSIS	RELATED FACTORS
Activity Intolerance	Impaired motor function, pain
Risk for Disuse Syndrome	Debilitated state, immobility, muscle weakness, decreased motor agility, joint contractures
Injury, High Risk for	Altered mobility, impaired sensory function, prolonged bed rest
Impaired Physical Mobility	Trauma or musculoskeletal impairment, surgical procedure, muscle weakness, pain, decreased strength
Caregiver Role Strain	Insufficient resources, time, money, energy; family conflict regarding caregiver issue.

NURSING PROCESS DATA

ASSESSMENT Data Base

Assess family's knowledge of the principles of body mechanics.

Assess home care provider's knowledge of how to use correct muscle groups for specific activities.

Assess knowledge of how to improvise for a nonhospital bed.

Assess knowledge and correct any misinformation about body alignment and ability to move client up in bed without assistance.

PLANNING Objectives

To promote proper body mechanics while caring for clients

To move clients without assistance, preventing back injury

To provide knowledge of the musculoskeletal system, body alignment, and balance in order to prevent back injury when providing care for a client in the home

To provide methods of improvising for nonhospital bed

IMPLEMENTATION **Procedures**

Positioning Nonhospital Bed for Client Care

Moving a Helpless Client Up in Bed Without Assistance

EVALUATION **Expected Outcomes**

Correct body mechanics are used in caring for clients.

Injuries are prevented to both nurse and client.

Client care is facilitated by proper body mechanics.

Client is able to move without assistance.

Center of gravity is maintained when lifting objects.

Nonhospital bed is easily adapted for home care.

POSITIONING NONHOSPITAL BED FOR CLIENT CARE

Procedure

1. Position foam wedges to simulate change in position when head of bed does not move. High-Fowler's/90°;Fowler's/60°; semi-Fowler's/30°.
2. Use correct body mechanics to adjust height.
   a. Flex body at knees and keep back straight if bed is only slightly low.
   b. Kneel on pillow by bed or sit in chair alongside bed if bed is extremely low.
3. Lock each wheel or leg of bed in position by securing with bricks or blocks of wood.
4. Make footboard of lumber, or item such as a TV tray; position legs of tray under mattress so that tray becomes footboard.

CORRECT BODY MECHANICS

- Place both feet flat on the floor, and keep your back straight to prevent back injury.
- Hold objects close to the body to prevent muscle strain and possible back injury.
- Keep body in proper alignment by bending your knees and keeping back straight when lifting objects to prevent injury to back muscles.

MOVING A HELPLESS CLIENT UP IN BED WITHOUT ASSISTANCE

Procedure

1. Lower head of bed, and place pillow at head of bed.
2. Stand at side of client's bed.
   a. Face far corner at foot of bed.
   b. Place one foot behind the other, assume a broad stance, and flex knees.
3. Flex arms so forearms are level with bed. Place one arm under client's head and one under small of back.
4. Rock and shift weight from forward to rear foot; hips will move downward.
5. Guide the client as he or she slides diagonally across bed toward head.
6. Repeat for trunk and leg sections.
7. Move to other side of bed and repeat steps 2 through 5.
8. Repeat until client is satisfactorily positioned in bed.

unit 4 HYGIENIC CARE

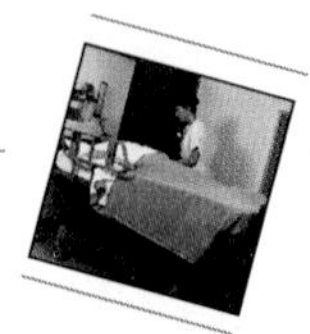

In the home care setting most hygienic care is provided by the home health aide (HHA) or the client and family members. The role of the nurse is to (1) assess the personal care needs of an individual client, (2) develop the care plan that is to be implemented by the home health aide, (3) supervise the home health aide, and (4) instruct the family members in how to provide safe, thorough, hygienic care when health care providers are not in the home.

The client care plan is developed by the nurse and implemented by the home health aide or caregiver. Skills include bathing, hair care, oral hygiene, shaving, TPR, toileting, dressing, ambulation, transfers, exercise, range of motion, assistance with assistive devices, feeding, and instructions for any specific observations to be made. The home health aide's responsibilities may include homemaking and supportive assistance activities, such as meal planning, marketing, linen change, light laundry, and light housekeeping. It is important to instruct the client and family that these activities are to be directed toward the client and not the entire household. A copy of the care plan is kept in the client's home for use by the home health aide. A second copy is placed in the permanent client record. The home health aide is responsible for documenting the care provided on each visit to the home. A sample is included in this unit. It is the nurse's responsibility to make sure the documentation is complete and accurate for legal and reimbursement purposes.

Bathing

The type and frequency of bathing depends on the client's condition, personal desires, and family and environmental situation. The client may be bathed in the bed, tub, or shower. The bathing may be done on a daily basis or once, twice, or three times a week. The home health aide may visit two to three times per week for personal care, and the family may perform the care between visits. The nurse's role is to instruct all persons involved in the client's care to perform procedures correctly and safely.

Skin Care

Just as in the hospital, skin care is an important component of personal care. The home health nurse must assess the condition of the client's skin and teach skin care techniques to all caregivers. The instructions should include keeping the skin clean and dry, providing special care to buttocks and perineal area, and obtaining available products such as Chux for incontinent clients to protect the skin. A skin care program should be initiated by the nurse. All care givers should follow the plan of action. The program addresses ways to prevent friction, shearing, and pressure.

Pressure Ulcer Care

If skin breakdown is present, special treatment is necessary. The stage of pressure ulcer dictates the specific protocol needed. Pressure ulcer treatments for the homebound client are the same as for the hospitalized client. Refer to Chapter 24 for specific protocols.

Hair Care

Shampooing the hair of a client on bed rest is similar to the skill in a hospital setting. Rather than using a basin to catch the water, a bucket or pail may be substituted. For long-term bedridden clients, commercial shampoo boards are available.

"Dry shampoo" is available at local pharmacies. This is often used for a client on bed rest for a short time or between regular shampoos. Regular shampooing is necessary to maintain scalp integrity.

Pediculosis is an infestation of lice on the body. It is very contagious by either direct contact with the infected person or by indirect contact with contaminated articles, such as combs, clothing, and bed linen. Although lice can infest the head, body, or pubic area, the head is the most common area of infestation.

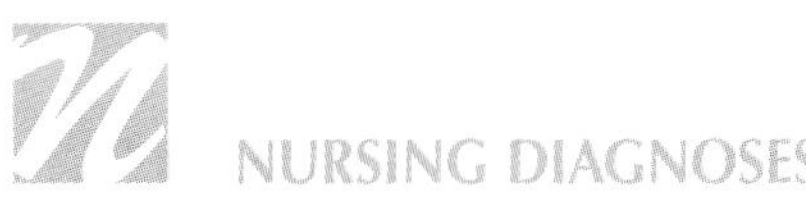

NURSING DIAGNOSES

The following nursing diagnoses may be appropriate to include in a client care plan when the components are related to hygienic care.

NURSING DIAGNOSIS	RELATED FACTORS
Activity Intolerance	Prolonged bed rest, surgery, pain, treatment schedule, weakness, fatigue
Health Maintenance, Altered	Ineffective coping, lack of motivation, motor impairment, lack of financial resources
Self-Care Deficit: Bathing/Hygiene	Dependence on others for assistance, motor impairment, visual disorders, surgery, muscle weakness, pain
Skin Integrity, Impaired	Surgery, immobility, prolonged bed rest, mechanical factors (shearing force, pressure), lack of adherence to diet, inadequately prepared caregiver

NURSING PROCESS DATA

ASSESSMENT Data Base

Assess for signs of skin breakdown or stage of pressure ulcer.

Assess color of skin.

Check for alterations in skin turgor.

Assess ability to assist with transfer to tub or shower.

Check general hygienic state.

Assess for presence of lice.

PLANNING Objectives

To maintain intact skin without signs of ischemia, hyperemia, or necrosis

To recognize a break in skin integrity

To avoid introduction of pathogens through a break in skin integrity

To prepare sterilized normal saline solution for home care

To promote wound closure for Pressure ulcer

To shampoo hair for client on bed rest

To transfer client safely to tub or shower

To eradicate lice from client and belongings

IMPLEMENTATION Procedures

Bathing Client in the Home

Transferring Client to Tub or Shower

Adapting Bedmaking to the Home

Providing Pressure Ulcer Care

Preparing Normal Saline

Removing Lice

(*For additional skills see Chapters 9 and 10*)

EVALUATION Expected Outcomes

Client's skin remains intact without signs of ischemia, hyperemia, or necrosis.

Client is free of lice infestation.

Pressure ulcer heals.

Bathing and bedmaking are accomplished for client on bed rest.

Client is transferred safely to tub or shower.

BATHING CLIENT IN THE HOME

Equipment

Personal care items (i.e., soap, deodorant, toothbrush)
Tray for personal items
Beach towel
Large piece of plastic
Call bell, dinner bell, or smoke alarm
Nonskid strips for tub
Shower chair or suction tips for chair legs

Procedure

1. Keep all personal care items (soap, deodorant, lotion, powder, cosmetics, cologne, hair products, oral hygiene supplies, and other personal items) on a tray or in a handy carry tote (e.g., the type of rubber or plastic tote that can be purchased to carry household cleaning supplies).
2. Use old beach towel for bath blanket.
3. Place plastic under towel to protect mattress prior to beginning the bath.
4. Ensure that nonskid strips or mats are on the floor of tub or shower.
   a. Ask family to purchase strips.
   b. Place wet terrycloth towel on floor of tub or shower if strips or mat not available. **Rationale:** A wet towel provides a temporary nonskid surface during bath or shower.
5. Provide tub or shower stool or chair.
   a. Order from supply company, if family desires and can afford.
   b. Improvise shower chair by using straight-backed chair and attaching suction cups to legs to prevent sliding. (Suction cups are available at hardware stores.)
6. Simulate a client call bell by placing dinner bell or battery-powered smoke detector that emits a loud alarm within easy reach of client.

TRANSFERRING CLIENT TO TUB OR SHOWER

Equipment

Towels
Shower or tub chair
Grips in bathtub or bath mat
Safety bars on tub or wall
Assistive devices (e.g., walker, wheelchair, cane, to assist to shower or tub if needed)

Procedure

1. Gather equipment.
2. Place wet bath towel on the floor of tub or shower if safety grips or mats are not available.
3. Position chair or shower stool securely in the tub or shower. Place second chair or wheelchair outside tub.
4. Assist client to bathroom.
5. Transfer client to tub or shower chair before putting water in tub.
   a. Stand in front of client.
   b. Lower client into chair, bending your knees and keeping your back straight. **Rationale:** This provides most secure balance and aids in preventing back injuries.
   c. Flex your knees, move to kneeling position, and keep your back straight while assisting client to swing legs over side of tub.

ADAPTING BEDMAKING TO THE HOME

Equipment

Sheets
Pillowcases
Plastic trash bag
Cotton flannel
Plastic shower curtain

Procedure

1. Follow directions for making an occupied or unoccupied bed outlined in Chapter 9.
2. Turn pillowcase inside out and use as laundry bag, or use plastic trash bag.
3. Place one knee on bed if bed cannot be moved away from wall. This is especially useful when making water beds.
4. Making incontinent pads with cotton flannel if commercial pads are not available. **Rationale:** This material is soft and easily laundered.
5. Make bed protectors by cutting a piece of plastic shower curtain or heavy trash bag. Cover with draw sheet or cotton flannel. **Rationale:** This protects skin from direct contact with plastic.

PROVIDING PRESSURE ULCER CARE

Equipment

Normal saline solution
Medicated ointment (if prescribed)
Irrigation set (if needed)
Asepto syringe
Dressings—hydrocolloid or transparent adhesive film
Nonallergic tape
Clean gloves
Plastic bags

Procedure

1. Wash hands.
2. Don clean gloves.
3. Remove dressings. Discard in plastic bag.
4. Cleanse with solution such as normal saline. Irrigate the wound if excessive drainage is present.
5. Allow to dry or apply medicated ointment, as ordered.
6. Apply dressing as ordered.
7. Dispose of waste according to protocol.
8. Remove gloves, and wash hands.

PREPARING NORMAL SALINE

Equipment

Large pan
Jar with lid
Cold water to cover jar and lid
1 teaspoon salt
500 mL (1 pint) water

Procedure

1. Sterilize jar for storage.
   a. Place cover and jar in large pan of cold water, completely immersing jar and lid in water.
   b. Bring to a boil.
   c. Boil 20 minutes.
   d. Pour off water.
   e. Handle only outside of jar and lid.
2. Add 1 teaspoon salt to 500 mL (1 pint) water.
3. Boil salted water for 20 minutes to sterilize.
4. Pour water into sterilized jar for storage.

REMOVING LICE

Equipment

Isolation bag or plastic bag

Treatment solution as ordered (i.e., gamma benzene hexachloride (Kwell) or nonprescription drug)

Clean linen

Fine-toothed comb

Disinfectant for comb

Clean towel

Spray for fomites

Procedure

1. Obtain order for treatment and notify family members and health care giver. **Rationale:** All household members and caregivers must be treated to prevent the spread of lice to others.
2. Remove and bag client's clothing and linens, and place in plastic bag. Launder these articles separately. Use hot water at 125°F and detergent. **Rationale:** This prevents cross-contamination of lice to other family members.
3. Items that cannot be washed should be dry cleaned. Place in plastic bag, seal, and bring to dry cleaner.
4. Begin treatment as ordered by physician. Common treatment is gamma benzene hexachloride applied as a cream, lotion, or shampoo. **Rationale:** Head lice infestation requires shampoo. Body and pubic lice require shower with soap followed by lotion application for 24 hours.
5. Apply shampoo, and leave in place several minutes. **Rationale:** Prolonged use of shampoo can burn scalp.
6. Rinse thoroughly.
7. Comb through hair with fine-toothed comb.
8. Disinfect comb and brushes with Kwell shampoo.
9. Wash your hands.
10. Instruct client to vacuum rugs, upholstery, and furniture. Then, spray with a commercial spray. Empty vacuum cleaner bag into trash bag, and seal.
11. Discuss with client and family the cause, treatment, and preventive measures regarding lice infestation.
12. Instruct client or family to repeat treatment in 7–10 days. **Rationale:** Initial application only rids the client of lice. Eggs hatch after this and thus a repeat treatment is needed to rid the body of new lice.

unit 5 MEDICATIONS

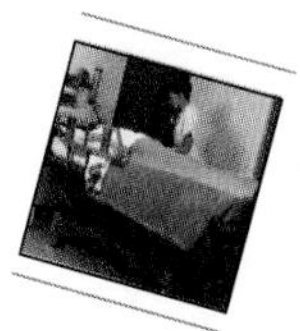

In the hospital, medications are given at designated time. The time that the client takes the medication is determined by physician's orders and the hospital, not the client. In the home setting, however, the nurse works with the client and family to establish a medication schedule. This regimen fits their life style, yet comes within the prescribed medication parameters (e.g., number of dosages, blood levels). Since the nurse is not present in the home at all times, the client and family must take responsibility for the routine administration of medications.

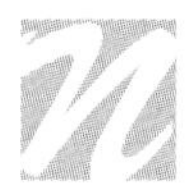

NURSING DIAGNOSES

The following nursing diagnoses may be appropriate to include in a client care plan when the components relate to a client who requires medication.

NURSING DIAGNOSIS	RELATED FACTORS
Altered Health Maintenance	Lack of education or readiness to learn, cognitive impairment, lack of equipment, inadequate support systems, inadequate financial resources, religious beliefs, cultural beliefs.
Risk for Infection	Contamination of equipment, improper storage, improper technique, traumatized tissue, malnutrition.
Knowledge Deficit	Inadequate understanding of condition, misinformation, cognitive impairment.
Noncompliance	Impaired ability to perform tasks, side effects of therapy, nontherapeutic environment, denial of condition, lack of information, poor self-esteem, nonsupportive family.

NURSING PROCESS DATA

ASSESSMENT Data Base

Assess that client and family understand time and dosage for medication administration.

Assess most appropriate methods for aiding a client to remember to take medications.

Assess client and family's knowledge and skill in sterilizing medication equipment.

Determine client's physical ability to take medication as ordered.

- Swallow reflex present
- State of consciousness
- Signs of nausea and vomiting
- Uncooperative behavior

PLANNING Objectives

To ensure that medications are taken according to physician's orders

To provide an easy method to sterilize nondisposable medication equipment

To provide client and family education about medications

To determine appropriate aids to assist the client to take medications as ordered

IMPLEMENTATION Procedures

Administering Medications

Sterilizing Nondisposable Medication Equipment

(*For additional skills refer to Chapter 16*)

EVALUATION Expected Outcomes

Equipment is sterilized and infection prevented.

Medications are taken at appropriate times.

Creative device for remembering to take medications is identified.

ADMINISTERING MEDICATIONS

Procedure

1. Examine all medications taken by the client during your admission visit and subsequent visits. Include all over-the-counter (OTC), as well as prescription drugs.
2. Discuss life style with client and family as it relates to medication schedule and their beliefs about medications.
3. Establish the medication regimen based on physician's orders or prescribed drugs and client's schedule.
4. Teach client and family the medication regimen.
5. Teach client and family how to monitor for effects and side effects of drugs.
6. Design medication aids, such as a calendar of drugs or daily/weekly pill reminder boxes, to help client and family remember to take medications.
   a. Investigate and share with the client and family those aids that are commercially available.
   b. Improvise using household items, such as egg cartons, tiny paper cups attached together or stacked, or empty match boxes glued together to make a row of pill containers that can be labeled with time and day.
7. Design creative methods to assist client and family to administer medication.
   a. If client has trouble seeing the markings on a syringe or on medication bottles, the nurse may recommend a magnifying glass, magnifying syringe, or marking the bottles or syringes with tape at the appropriate dosage.
   b. If a client lives alone, needs daily insulin, and knows the procedures but cannot see well enough to fill the syringes accurately, the nurse may prefill the syringes and leave them in the refrigerator for use between visits. Mixed insulin can be prefilled but must be used within 24 hours.
   c. Take syringe out of refrigerator 1 hour before administration.
8. Discard uncapped needles and syringes in sharps container.
9. Document all teaching and learning outcomes, administration of medication, and client response to medications.

■ CLINICAL ALERT

Home health aides and homemakers are not allowed to administer medications to clients in the home setting. Families should be instructed not to ask home health aides or homemakers to give medication.

STERILIZING NONDISPOSABLE MEDICATION EQUIPMENT

Equipment

Large pan or kettle
Jar or container with lid for storage
Equipment to be sterilized
Tongs or forceps for handling sterile equipment

Procedure

1. Place jar, lid, tongs, and equipment in large clean pan.
2. Fill pan with cold water until all equipment is covered.
3. Place pan on stove.
4. Boil water for 20 minutes.
5. Pour off water.
6. Lift equipment out of pan, using tongs. Remove jar from pan by touching only the outside.
7. Position jar so sterile equipment can easily be inserted without touching edges of the jar.
8. Place lid on jar by grasping outside edge and twisting tightly.

unit 6 TOTAL PARENTERAL NUTRITION

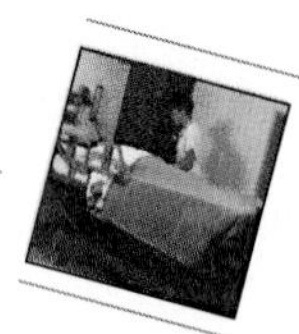

NUTRITION

Nutritional support in the home is not significantly different from that in a hospital setting. Gastrostomy and nasogastric tube feedings are frequently performed in the home setting using small feeding tubes and maintained via continuous feeding pumps. The only difference in the procedure at home is that the family is taught how to provide the feeding. The nurse's role is to change the nasogastric tube and to teach and monitor the family's ability to administer the feeding. Intake and output records are maintained by the family and monitored by the nurse when the client's condition warrants it.

Nutritional teaching principles and information that should be provided to client and family include

- Instruction in positioning client and providing assistance for eating
- Special eating utensils that can be purchased or made for self-feeding
- Instruction in Heimlich maneuver in case of choking
- Method of gently stroking throat if client doesn't remember to swallow
- Resources available in the community to assist with nutritional support:
  Meals on wheels: Meals can be ordered for cardiac and diabetic clients as well
  Food stamps
  Senior nutrition sites that usually serve a hot meal at noon
- Dietary supplements readily available
  Instant breakfast (*not* the diet type) when added to milk provides a less expensive nutritional supplement than some commercially canned ones
  Nutritional supplements frozen into cubes for clients to suck on if they don't like to drink
- Gatorade, a 5% glucose solution, may be used as a supplement if body fluids need replacing

Total Parenteral Nutrition (TPN)

Total parenteral nutrition is now being used in the home. The procedure and equipment are similar to that used in the hospital, including the use of sterile technique when preparing and discontinuing the infusion.

Home health agencies have specified policies and procedures for TPN that the nurse must follow to practice within legal parameters. The first dosage of any TPN solution or any IV medication must be given in the hospital or emergency room (where emergency intervention is available if an adverse reaction occurs).

In the home care setting, the client or family is taught how to administer TPN after the first dose. Many clients prefer to infuse TPN at night while they sleep, since the procedure takes about 12 hours. The client or family must be taught proper storage, fluid administration, volumetric pump use, and site care. Most people use preprepared TPN solutions that are available at the hospital pharmacy. Clients and families must be given careful instruction on sterile technique used in preparing TPN solutions. Catheter site care is performed the same as in the hospital.

NURSING DIAGNOSES

The following nursing diagnoses may be appropriate to include in a client care plan when the components of the plan are related to nutritional problems or nutritional health maintenance.

NURSING DIAGNOSIS	RELATED FACTORS
Impaired Home Maintenance Management	Chronic debilitating disease (cancer, neuromuscular diseases), surgery, injury
Knowledge Deficit	Lack of client and family education, poor understanding of equipment or procedure

NURSING DIAGNOSIS	RELATED FACTORS
Noncompliance	Improper nutritional intake or balance of nutrients, inadequate knowledge base, denial of disease process, chronic illness
Altered Nutrition: Less than Body Requirements	Impaired swallowing, faulty metabolism, dysphagia, altered level of consciousness, inadequate absorption

NURSING PROCESS DATA

ASSESSMENT Data Base

Observe for correct additives in each hyperalimentation bag.
Check label on solution bag.
Check rate of infusion on volumetric pump.
Assess ability of client to understand instructions during procedure.
Ensure patency of central venous line.
Observe catheter insertion site for signs of infection, thrombophlebitis, or possible infiltration.
Inspect dressing over central line to ensure a dry, noncontaminated dressing.
Identify client and family's ability to provide TPN in the home.

PLANNING Objectives

To provide adequate calories and nutrition for clients unable to tolerate oral feedings
To provide increased calories when oral route is not accessible
To provide a contamination-free mode of delivering the hyperalimentation solution
To heparinize TPN catheter between infusions
To discontinue TPN infusions maintaining sterile technique

IMPLEMENTATION Procedures

Administering Total Parenteral Nutrition in the Home
Discontinuing TPN Infusion
(*For additional skills refer to Chapter 28*)

EVALUATION Expected Outcomes

Solution is infused at prescribed flow rate and tolerated by client.
Dressing remains dry and intact during interval between changes.
Insertion site remains free of infection and inflammation.
Client receives nutrients necessary for tissue repair and sustenance.
Client and family understand procedure and infuse TPN correctly.
Heparinization of TPN catheter accomplished.

ADMINISTERING TOTAL PARENTERAL NUTRITION IN THE HOME

Equipment

TPN solution bag
IV tubing with in-line filter
Volutrol
Controller or pump
Povidone-iodine swab
Padded Kelly forceps, tape
Sugar and acetone test equipment
Intake and output and TPN record
Clean gloves

Procedure

1. Remove TPN solution from refrigerator at least 1 hour before using. **Rationale:** Warming the solution prevents venospasm and hypothermia.
2. Gather equipment.
3. Wash hands, and don gloves.
4. Inspect TPN solution for cloudiness, clarity, and intact bag. **Rationale:** Contamination of the solution causes a cloudy or milky precipitate.
5. Prepare to administer TPN solution by spiking bag with tubing, then flush tubing of all air.
6. Prepare catheter when solution is ready for infusion by clamping catheter with a padded Kelly forceps and removing injection cap.
7. Cleanse end of catheter with povidone-iodine swab.
8. Remove protective cap from IV tubing and insert tubing into catheter.
9. Tape connection site. **Rationale:** Taping prevents accidental dislodging of the tubing from catheter and lessens chance of contamination.
10. Remove gloves.
11. Thread IV tubing through volumetric pump according to manufacturer's directions, and set machine to deliver appropriate rate.
12. Monitor infusion rate, and assess IV site throughout procedure. Procedure takes about 12 hours; therefore, many clients prefer to infuse the solution during their sleeping hours. **Rationale:** If flow rate is too rapid, excess sugar may cause seizures.
13. Monitor blood glucose daily using Accu-chek or autolet and chemstrips. Report 3+ or 4+ or positive urine acetone findings to physician. **Rationale:** Insulin may need to be ordered.
14. Maintain accurate intake and output and TPN sheet.

DISCONTINUING TPN INFUSION

Equipment

Tape
Sterile injection cap
4×4 gauze pad
Normal saline 2 mL
20-gauge needle
25-gauge needle
2-mL syringe
Alcohol swab
Povidone-iodine swab
Padded Kelly clamp
Clean gloves

Procedure

1. Gather equipment.
2. Wash hands, and don clean gloves.
3. Withdraw 2 mL normal saline into syringe.
4. Turn IV solution off by closing roller clamp and turning off controller or pump.
5. Clamp catheter with padded Kelly forceps.
6. Disconnect IV tubing from catheter.
7. Cleanse catheter site with a povidone-iodine swab.
8. Place sterile injection cap on catheter.
9. Wipe injection cap with alcohol swab.
10. Inject 2 mL of normal saline solution through cap.
11. Withdraw needle.
12. Coil catheter and place 4×4 gauze pad over catheter and tape catheter to chest or abdomen. Site care is performed every 48 hours using same sterile technique as in hospital. See Chapter 28.
13. Discard used equipment.
14. Wash your hands, and remove gloves.

unit 7 URINARY ELIMINATION

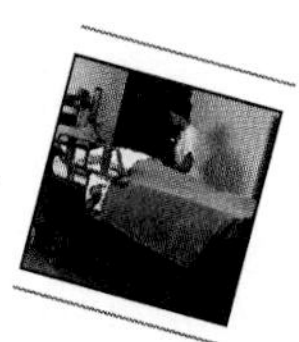

Home care clients who require assistance with emptying their bladders are usually placed on intermittent clean catheterization protocols rather than having an indwelling catheter. This procedure assists in preventing penoscrotal abscess formation, overwhelming infection, and altered body image. Fluid intake needs to be monitored and restricted to 1500 mL per day to avoid bladder distention. If spontaneous voiding returns, frequency of catheterizations can be extended to every 12 hours and discontinued when the residual urine is consistently less than 100 mL in 24 hours.

When an indwelling catheter is used, it is important to be aware that it may lead to urinary tract infection. The nurse must teach the client and family to observe for signs and symptoms of urinary tract infections and sepsis. They should note odor, color, and consistency of the urine. Catheter changes are the responsibility of the nurse and are usually performed once a month. Encouraging fluids becomes a major role assumed by family members and monitored by the nurse. Urinary antiseptics are adjunctive measures when catheterizations are required.

Home care dialysis is common in many areas of the country. The principles and procedures are similar to those in a hospital or free-standing dialysis unit. The major change is the advent of portable dialysis methods such as chronic ambulatory peritoneal dialysis (CAPD) and chronic continuous peritoneal dialysis (CCPD). These procedures allow individuals to participate in a normal life style. However, use of these methods requires monitoring by the nurse and specific teaching of the essential components to prevent complications and promote health.

NURSING DIAGNOSES

The following nursing diagnoses may be appropriate to include in a client care plan when the components are related to promoting urine elimination.

NURSING DIAGNOSIS	RELATED FACTORS
Body Image Disturbance	Alteration in body appearance, urinary diversion stoma
Fluid Volume Excess	Decreased urine output, renal system dysfunction, decreased cardiac output
Ineffective Individual Coping	Poor adjustment to illness or treatment, chronic disease state
Noncompliance	Inadequate knowledge base, denial of health status, cultural or spiritual beliefs
Altered Urinary Elimination	Incontinence, lack of muscle tone, urinary tract infection, motor or sensory impairment, abdominal surgery
Urinary Retention	Inability to void, bladder distention or atony, surgical repair

NURSING PROCESS DATA

ASSESSMENT Data Base

Assess the client's bladder for distention.

Assess the client's physical ability to cooperate with positioning.

Assess urinary meatus and catheter for exudate, edema, inflammation, and general cleanliness.
Assess need for perineal care before catheterization procedure.
Assess condition of skin surrounding catheter.
Assess dialysate solution for clarity.
Assess dialysis returns for cloudiness.
Assess family's ability to use gloving technique and maintain asepsis.
Assess need for catheterization procedure.
Assess for proper function of dialysis machine.

PLANNING Objectives

To prevent or relieve discomfort due to bladder distention
To promote urinary elimination
To identify family's knowledge related to signs and symptoms of dialysis-related infections
To prevent urinary tract infections through aseptic catheter care
To prevent infection at peritoneal catheter site
To use aseptic technique when instituting CAPD
To identify client's and family's knowledge base regarding CAPD or CCPD

IMPLEMENTATION Procedures

Using Clean Technique for Intermittent Self-Catheterization
For Female Client
For Male Patient
Administering Chronic Ambulatory Peritoneal Dialysis (CAPD)
Changing Dressing for CAPD Client
(*For additional skills refer to Chapter 21*)

EVALUATION Expected Outcomes

Catheterization performed using aseptic technique.
Bladder emptied when client is unable to void.
Urinary tract infection prevented through aseptic catheter care.
Aseptic peritoneal dialysis procedure used.
Catheter site remains free of infection.

USING CLEAN TECHNIQUE FOR INTERMITTENT SELF-CATHETERIZATION

Equipment

Straight catheters in clean container, plastic bag, or wrapped in aluminum foil
Washcloth, soap, water
Water-soluble lubricant (K-Y; Surgilube)
Plastic bags
Basin or container
Mirror

Procedure

for Female Client

1. Attempt to urinate. If unable to do so, continue to follow these steps.
2. Wash hands, and gather equipment. (Keep equipment in one large container.)
3. Assume sitting position on the bed or commode. (Place plastic under towel if bed is used.)
4. Separate labia with one hand while cleaning with soap and water front to back with other hand.
5. Position mirror to visualize urinary meatus.

6. Remove catheter from container (plastic bag or aluminum foil).
7. Lubricate end of catheter with water-soluble lubricant and place other end in container to catch urine.
8. While holding labia apart with one hand, insert catheter about 3 inches or until urine flows.
9. Press down with abdominal muscles to promote bladder's emptying.
10. Pinch off catheter after all urine has drained and withdraw gently, holding tip of catheter upright.
11. Wash and dry perineal area.
12. Wash catheter in warm, soapy water.
13. Rinse with clear water and dry outside with paper towel.
14. Place in plastic bag for storage.
15. Use catheters for 2–4 weeks and then discard.
16. Wash hands.

for Male Client

1. Attempt to urinate. If unable to do so, continue to follow these steps.
2. Wash hands, and gather equipment. (Keep equipment in one large container.)
3. Assume sitting position on the bed or commode. (Place plastic under towel if bed is used.)
4. Retract the foreskin, if present, and wash tip of penis with soap and water.
5. Remove catheter from container (plastic bag or aluminum foil).
6. Lubricate the first 7–10 inches of catheter with water-soluble lubricant. Place other end in container to catch urine.
7. Hold penis at right angle to body, keeping foreskin retracted. Insert catheter 7–10 inches into penis or until urine begins to flow. Then insert catheter 1 inch further.
8. Press down with abdominal muscles to promote bladder's emptying.
9. Pinch off catheter after all urine has drained and gently withdraw, holding tip of catheter upright.
10. Wash and dry area.
11. Wash catheter in warm, soapy water.
12. Rinse with clear water and dry outside with paper towel.
13. Place in plastic bag for storage.
14. Use catheters for 2–4 weeks and then discard.
15. Wash hands.

ADMINISTERING CHRONIC AMBULATORY PERITONEAL DIALYSIS (CAPD)

Equipment

Sterile dialysate solution
Sterile dialysate inflow tubing set
IV pole or permanent hook on wall of room used for dialysis
Low stool or table
Intake and output record
Clean gloves

Preparation

1. Wash hands thoroughly.
2. Obtain container of sterile dialysate.
3. Check that strength and amount of solution are accurate as ordered.

Procedure

1. Use clean gloves when working with dialysis equipment. **Rationale:** Infection control precaution for caregiver when there is potential contact with blood or body fluids.
2. Remove empty, folded solution bag from client's waist pouch.
3. Place pouch on low stool or table below level of client's abdomen. **Rationale:** This position allows fluid to drain by gravity from client's peritoneal cavity.
4. Unclamp tubing.
5. Allow fluid to drain into bag from abdomen until flow ceases, approximately 20 minutes.
6. Reclamp tubing.
7. Examine drainage for discoloration or cloudiness. **Rationale:** Change in color may indicate presence of infection.
8. Check blood pressure and pulse. **Rationale:** Rapid fluid shift may cause hypotension.
9. Add medications to dialysate, if ordered.
10. Disconnect tubing from drainage bag while maintaining strict aseptic technique. **Rationale:** The glu-

cose in the dialysate solution predisposes the client to infection.

11. Attach tubing to new sterile dialysate bag by spiking port, continuing to maintain strict aseptic technique.
12. Hang new dialysate bag on IV pole or hook, which is positioned above client at shoulder height.
13. Open clamp and adjust height to ensure inflow of solution by gravity over a 10- to 20-minute period.
14. Clamp tubing.
15. Fold empty dialysate bag and place in carrying–holding pouch at client's waist.
16. Allow fluid to remain in peritoneal cavity approximately 4 hours.
17. Repeat procedure four times daily, the last time at bedtime, allowing fluid to remain in peritoneal cavity overnight.
18. Change tubing every 24 hours, using strict aseptic technique.
19. Ensure that client and caregiver are knowledgeable in strict aseptic technique.
20. Instruct client to notify physician if there is evidence of infection.

CHANGING DRESSING FOR CAPD CLIENT

Equipment

4 × 4 gauze pads
ABD pad
Tape
Povidone-iodine swab or solution
Applicator sticks
Hydrogen peroxide
Sterile saline
Sterile gloves (two pair)
Forceps (optional)

Procedure

1. Wash hands.
2. Don gloves.
3. Remove old dressing with forceps or sterile gloves.
4. Inspect site for infection (erythema, edema, warmth, exudate).
5. Remove any dried blood or drainage using hydrogen peroxide or normal saline solution.
6. Rinse area with normal saline.
7. Dry area thoroughly.
8. Change gloves.
9. Cleanse area surrounding catheter with povidone-iodine swab or applicator sticks.
10. Apply sterile 4 × 4 gauze pads around catheter at exit site and on top of catheter.
11. Place ABD pad over area.
12. Remove gloves.
13. Tape dressing using occlusive technique.

unit 8 RESPIRATORY CARE

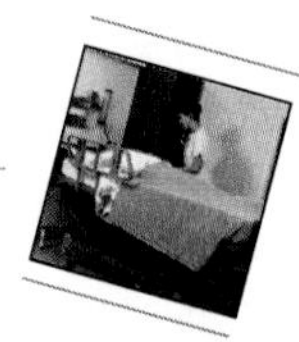

Oxygen therapy is most commonly used in the home situation for clients who have chronic obstructive pulmonary disease (COPD). The type of oxygen equipment used is different from that used in the hospital because there is no "wall oxygen." The systems most frequently used include cylinder tanks, portable walking cylinders, or oxygen concentrators or compressors. If the compressor or concentrator is used, it is plugged into the electrical system. However, it is necessary to have a portable tank or cylinder available in case of power failure. Most people use a portable tank when going outside the home.

Low-flow (2 L) oxygen is usually administered by nasal cannula or Venturi mask. Short and long oxygen tubing is needed to connect the oxygen source to the client. Long tubing is used during the day to allow more flexibility for moving about the house. COPD clients and their families need to be alerted to the signs and symptoms of carbon dioxide narcosis to prevent respiratory distress.

Clients on respirators are now cared for in the home. Since the hospital-type positive pressure machines are too complicated for home use, a more simplified respirator is selected. Positive pressure home respirators have alarms that signal power loss or indicate when pressures are too high or too low. Most respirators function with either electricity or battery power. Each machine has specific operating procedures that must be followed. Before caring for a home care client on a respirator, the nurse must be familiar with the specific equipment.

Clients with neuromuscular diseases can use an external negative pressure ventilator when they do not have an artificial airway and there is no problem with decreased lung compliance. In addition, clients must be able to handle their own secretions to be able to use this type of ventilator. These machines cause the intraairway pressure to become negative as a result of the pressure surrounding the chest wall. The negative pressure ventilators, (Poncho or Pulmo-wrap) are designed to model the old iron lung.

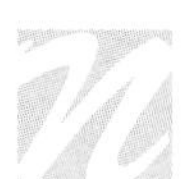

NURSING DIAGNOSES

The following nursing diagnoses are appropriate to use on client care plans when the components are related to respiratory conditions.

NURSING DIAGNOSIS	RELATED FACTORS
Activity Intolerance	Fatigue, pain, inadequate oxygenation
Anxiety	Pulmonary congestion, chronic respiratory disorders (COPD), pain
Impaired Gas Exchange	Ventilation–perfusion imbalance, diminished functional lung tissue, changes in arterial blood gases
Ineffective Airway Clearance	Inability to clear secretions, excessive secretions, obstructed respiratory tract, chest trauma, surgical interventions, pain, edema
Ineffective Breathing Pattern	Inability to maintain sufficient oxygen supply to cells, neuromuscular impairment, chronic respiratory disease states
Altered Oral Mucous Membrane	Prolonged mouth breathing, bypassed airway, disease state, intubation, comatose state
Bathing/Hygiene Self-Care Deficit	Fatigue, hypoxic states (confusion), chronic respiratory disorders, impaired gas exchange

NURSING PROCESS DATA

ASSESSMENT Data Base

Check if client has patent airway.

Assess need for oxygen therapy.

Assess family's ability to suction using aseptic technique.

Observe for cleanliness of equipment (tubing or reservoir).

Assess family's knowledge about safety factors when oxygen is in use.

Assess family's knowledge base related to set-up and monitoring of ventilator.

Determine if client has contraindications to using transtracheal oxygenation.

Determine client's willingness to comply with daily routine.

PLANNING Objectives

To return or maintain client's arterial Po_2 to normal range

To provide ventilatory assistance for clients with COPD or neuromuscular disorders

To teach safety measures when oxygen is used in the home setting

To promote accurate management of ventilator equipment

To increase client's comfort level when continuous oxygen is required

To prevent nasal irritation or facial skin pressure from continuous nasal cannula use

To promote independence and increase self-esteem in clients requiring continuous oxygenation

IMPLEMENTATION Procedures

Caring for Oxygen Equipment

Teaching Safety Measures for Oxygen Use

Managing Ventilator Equipment

(For additional skills refer to Chapter 25)

Providing Catheter Care for Transtracheal Catheter

for Heimlich Micro-Trach

for SCOOP 1

for SCOOP 2

Teaching the Client Catheter Care

EVALUATION Expected Outcomes

Safety measures are instituted when oxygen is in use.

Clients are safely maintained on ventilator.

Ventilators are cleaned appropriately.

Arterial Pao_2 is maintained at specified level (usually 65–80 mm Hg).

Client comfort is attained.

Catheter remains patent.

Client is able to provide self-care.

CARING FOR OXYGEN EQUIPMENT

Equipment

Soap
Water
Paper towel
Plastic bag
Distilled water for humidifier

Procedure

1. Obtain order for oxygen therapy.
2. Determine type of oxygen system to be used.
3. Contact inhalation therapy company and ensure company offers 24-hour emergency service. (Usually the company sends a representative to set up the equipment and instruct the client or family on its use and care.)
4. Rinse cannula or mask clean with water and dry with paper towel daily.
5. Wash tubing daily. Hang in bathroom to dry. Store in clean plastic bag when not in use.
6. Wash long tubing weekly. Replace monthly.
7. Clean compressor filter daily with water or according to company instructions.
8. Use distilled water in humidifier. (Store distilled water in refrigerator.) Wash humidifier with soap and water every few days.

SAFETY PRECAUTIONS

- Set up "No Smoking" and "Oxygen in use" signs at the site of administration and at the door.
- Remove matches and lighters from bedside.
- Disconnect grounded electric equipment.
- Remove all volatile materials except solutions and equipment to be used during intervention.
- Place fire extinguishers near room where oxygen is in use.

TEACHING SAFETY MEASURES FOR OXYGEN USE

Equipment

No smoking sign
Emergency number of oxygen company
Alternate oxygen supply
Cotton dust cloth

Procedure

1. Post "No Smoking" signs.
2. Keep room temperature at 65–70°F.
3. Keep an alternative supply of oxygen (e.g., tank), which is not dependent on electrical system.
4. Post emergency number of oxygen company by the phone.
5. Avoid clothing with nylon or wool, which produces static electricity and sparks.
6. Store oxygen away from heat, open flames, or flammable materials.
7. Do not use electric equipment, such as hair dryers and shavers, when oxygen is in use.
8. Keep environment dust free. Damp dust three and four times per week with cotton cloth. Use oxygen equipment in noncarpeted room if possible.

MANAGING VENTILATOR EQUIPMENT

Equipment

Ventilator and accessory equipment (positive or negative pressure ventilator)
Two humidifiers
Distilled water
Sterile tracheostomy tube replacement set as needed
Suctioning equipment
Oxygen or compressed air administration equipment
Tubing
Compressor filter
Bucket or bowl
Weak bleach solution
Plastic bag

Preparation

1. Evaluate home for best room in which to place client and equipment.
2. Order necessary equipment from vendor, based on type of ventilator being used (positive pressure or negative pressure ventilator).
3. Evaluate client and family's understanding of principles of ventilator care before client begins treatment.
4. Ensure that fire department, electric company, and telephone company are aware that ventilator-dependent client is in the home. Have electric company place home on high-risk list.
5. Check home environment for cleanliness and safety prevention, such as condition of floors.

Procedure

1. Read manufacturer's directions for setting up ventilator.
2. Attach ventilator to oxygen or compressed air source.
3. Fill humidifier with distilled water.
4. Set ventilator parameters for tidal volume and rate.
5. Set alarm parameters.
6. Analyze oxygen concentration at least every 8 hours or as ordered.
7. Measure tidal volume at least every 8 hours or as ordered.
8. Suction airway as needed.
9. Provide a communication with the client if tracheostomy tube is in place.
10. Provide oral hygiene for clients with tracheostomy tubes.
11. Force fluids if tolerated. **Rationale:** Fluids aid in liquifying secretions for easy removal.
12. Observe for signs and symptoms of respiratory infection.
13. Drain condensation from tubing by draining fluid into bucket or large bowl. **Rationale:** Draining fluid back into humidifier can lead to bacterial contamination.
14. Change ventilator tubing, compressor filter, and humidifier every 24 hours. **Rationale:** This prevents contamination.
15. Clean tubing and humidifier reservoir using a weak bleach solution (nine parts water to one part bleach).
16. Rinse thoroughly and allow tubing to hang dry.
17. Store clean equipment in plastic bag.

PROVIDING CATHETER CARE FOR TRANSTRACHEAL CATHETER

Equipment

Cotton swab
Mild bar soap
Vial of sterile normal saline
Cleaning rod for SCOOP 1 catheter

Preparation

1. Cleanse catheter site with cotton swab and tap water twice a day. Use mild bar soap if secretions are thick.
2. Rinse well following use of soap.

Procedure

for Heimlich Micro-Trach

1. Apply nasal cannula oxygen during cleaning procedure.

CONTRAINDICATIONS FOR USE OF TRANSTRACHEAL OXYGEN

- Tracheal deformities
- Disabling anxiety
- Acute respiratory failure
- Pleural herniation
- Arrhythmias
- Bleeding disorders
- Severe bronchospasm
- High steroid dosage

2. Disconnect oxygen tubing from catheter and connect to nasal catheter.
3. Observe for edema, erythema, or excess drainage around catheter site.
4. Instill 0.5–1.0 mL sterile normal saline into catheter. **Rationale:** Saline stimulates coughing and

clearing of accumulated secretions in the lungs. Repeat instillation two to three times each day.

5. Reconnect oxygen tubing to catheter.
6. Reestablish oxygen flow at ordered amount, usually 1–2 L/minute.
7. Replace catheter if dislodged during coughing. Swab catheter with alcohol, and reinsert.

for Spofford Christopher Oxygen Optimizing Prosthesis (SCOOP) 1 Catheter

1. Apply nasal cannula oxygen during cleaning procedure.
2. Disconnect oxygen tubing from catheter, and connect to nasal catheter.
3. Observe for edema, erythema, or excess drainage.
4. Instill 1.5 mL sterile saline solution into catheter.
5. Insert cleaning rod into catheter. Pull back and forth three times. **Rationale:** This action removes mucus attached to the catheter.
6. Instill additional 1.5 mL normal saline into catheter.
7. Reconnect catheter to oxygen tubing.
8. Catheter remains in place for 6–8 weeks. **Rationale:** This allows time for tract to mature.

for SCOOP 2 Catheter

1. Apply nasal cannula oxygen during cleaning procedure.
2. Disconnect oxygen tubing from catheter and connect to nasal catheter.
3. Observe for edema, erythema, or excess drainage.
4. Clean around catheter site with warm water and mild bar soap if necessary.
5. Remove SCOOP 2 catheter. Never remove catheter when oxygen is flowing into catheter.
6. Lubricate a second SCOOP 2 catheter with water-soluble jelly, and insert immediately into tract. **Rationale:** If catheter remains out of place for more than 30 minutes, the insertion procedure may have to be repeated.
7. Reconnect oxygen tubing to catheter. Oxygen source may be portable.
8. Secure catheter in place. (Clients may secure catheter to a metal necklace that goes around the neck.)
9. Clean soiled catheter by using antimicrobial soap and cleaning rod. Rinse under tepid tap water. **Rationale:** Hot water may damage the plastic catheter.
10. Allow catheter to dry and store in clean, dry area away from direct sunlight. **Rationale:** Catheter becomes brittle when stored in hot, sunny area.
11. Repeat cleaning procedure twice each day. **Rationale:** More frequent catheter changes can traumatize tract and lead to scar tissue formation.

TEACHING THE CLIENT CATHETER CARE

Equipment

Catheter kit
Pulse oximeter
Written information for catheter care

Preparation

1. Ensure client's readiness to learn catheter care.
2. Evaluate client's level of understanding.
3. Determine appropriate time and place for teaching.
4. Arrange for family members to attend teaching session.

Procedure

1. Review verbally and in writing signs and symptoms of infection, bronchospasm, bleeding, respiratory failure, subcutaneous emphysema, and pneumothorax with client and family prior to discharge from hospital. **Rationale:** Understanding catheter insertion complications alert client to notify physician before complications become critical.
2. Instruct client to take oral temperature twice a day for 1 week and to report fever greater than 99.5°F. **Rationale:** Increased temperature indicates possible infection.
3. Review instructions for ordered medications. **Rationale:** Antibiotics are usually prescribed for 1 week to prevent infection. These drugs need to be taken on schedule and for length of time ordered.
4. Instruct client about follow-up hospital and physician visits. Clients with SCOOP catheters have at least two physician visits for catheter change.
5. Instruct in use of pulse oximeter as needed.

Rationale: Transtracheal oxygen flow rates are adjusted according to these readings.

6. Instruct to return to physician for catheter change every 6 months for Micro-Trach or every 3 months for SCOOP catheter.

CHARTING for Transtracheal Oxygen Delivery

- Respiratory assessment before and after cleaning
- Client instructions provided for catheter care
- Results of return demonstration of cleaning procedure.
- Catheter site assessment.
- Irrigation solution type and amount instilled each time
- Catheter cleaning procedure

unit 9

CIRCULATORY CARE

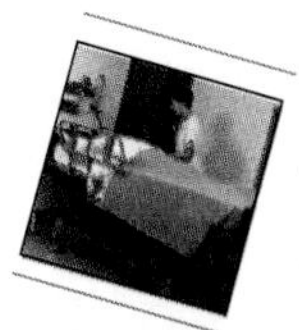

Circulatory skills performed in the home setting are similar to those in the hospital. Vital signs are taken using the same equipment and procedures. CPR and the Heimlich maneuver are performed exactly the same way. Care of the pacemaker client, however, is somewhat different.

Clients with permanent pacemakers are expected to monitor pacemaker function on a daily basis. While in the hospital, the client is taught how to monitor pulse, vital signs, symptoms of pacemaker failure, and indications of infection at the pacemaker insertion site. When the client returns home, the home health nurse needs to reinforce the teaching that was initiated in the hospital.

The client should be taught to monitor the pulse daily on awakening to identify altered pacemaker function. This may indicate a need for a battery change earlier than scheduled. Normally, lithium batteries last 6 years or more, whereas mercury-zinc batteries last 5 years. Nuclear-powered pacemakers (plutonium-238) can last 20 years or more. Some batteries can be recharged externally.

The generator is usually placed in the abdominal subcutaneous tissue or under the clavicle on the left side where the outline of the generator can be easily observed. The client must be taught to assess the site during the postoperative period for erythema, edema and warmth, which may indicate the presence of infection.

A periodic telephone pacemaker check can be used for clients living in rural settings or in areas where a cardiologist is not easily available. Heart sounds are transmitted via telephone signals and recorded on an ECG strip. The technician at the clinic compares a baseline ECG strip that is on file to that of the newly recorded ECG. If there are any alterations from normal, the client is asked to call his physician and the technician also notifies the physician. This procedure identifies early pacemaker dysfunction and aids in preventing complications.

For client safety, it is imperative to stress the importance of having someone present while checking for pacemaker malfunction when a magnet is used. The telephone number of the pacemaker clinic should be kept readily accessible in case of an emergency situation, particularly when testing with the magnet.

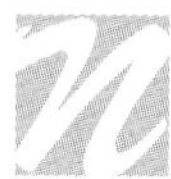

NURSING DIAGNOSES

The following nursing diagnoses are appropriate to use on client care plans when the components are related to pacemaker function.

NURSING DIAGNOSIS	RELATED FACTORS
Decreased Cardiac Output	Cardiac disease states, altered electrical conduction, drug side effects, hypovolemia.
Fluid Volume Excess	Decompensated cardiovascular system, disease states, increased fluid intake secondary to excess sodium, drugs
Risk for Infection	Pacemaker implantation site, altered circulation.
Knowledge Deficit	Incomplete understanding or instruction regarding pacemaker function or monitor management

NURSING PROCESS DATA

ASSESSMENT Data Base

Assess client's ability to monitor pulse accurately.

Identify client's and/or family's knowledge of pacemaker function and safety measures.

Assess pacemaker site for signs and symptoms of infection.

Assess for signs and symptoms related to pacemaker dysfunction, including dizziness, weakness, altered level of consciousness, irregular pulse, low blood pressure, decreased urine output, fatigue.

Assess client's ability and knowledge related to contacting the pacemaker clinic.

PLANNING Objectives

To provide client teaching related to monitoring pulse and use of magnet

To evaluate client's knowledge-base about pacemaker clinic

To increase client's knowledge-base about pacemaker function

INTERVENTIONS Procedures

Monitoring Pacemaker at Home

Checking with Pacemaker Clinic via Telephone

Instructing in Use of Holter Monitor

(*For additional skills refer to Chapter 26*)

EVALUATION Expected Outcomes

Client is able to accurately monitor pulse.

Client's cardiac rate and rhythm are maintained through use of a pacemaker.

Battery failure is identified early and major complications prevented.

Client is knowledgeable about pacemaker function.

Client is able to contact pacemaker clinic easily and comply with directions for pacemaker check.

MONITORING PACEMAKER AT HOME

Equipment

Clock or watch with second hand

Daily record

Pacemaker magnet

Procedure

1. Establish a daily routine check. **Rationale:** Battery failure can be identified in early stages by routine monitoring of pulse.
   a. Sit on side of bed.
   b. Check pulse for 1 full minute before arising.
   c. Record on daily record.
2. Contact physician if any of these symptoms occur:
   a. Sudden slowing or increasing in pulse rate
   b. Irregular pulse
   c. Pain or erythema over incision site
3. Check with pacemaker magnet if ordered by physician.
   a. Sit on side of bed.
   b. Place magnet over pacemaker generator.
   c. Take pulse for 1 full minute.
   d. Record.

■ CLINICAL ALERT

Pacemaker check with magnet should be done only if someone else is present, never if client is alone, because of possible magnet-induced ventricular arrhythmias.

4. Observe for signs and symptoms of infection at pacemaker insertion site when pacemaker is newly implanted.
5. Teach safety factors to client and family.
   a. Wear Medic-Alert identification band, and carry pacemaker identification card at all times. **Rationale:** This alerts health care providers to the fact that pacemaker is in place and identifies manufacturer's name.
   b. Avoid sources of electromagnetic interference (i.e., large engines, telephone transmitters, airport screening devices, alarm systems). **Rationale:** These devices emit intense magnetic fields that cause temporary pacemaker dysfunction.
   c. If dizziness occurs, then check pulse. Pulse should return to normal within 5 minutes; otherwise, seek medical attention.

CHECKING WITH PACEMAKER CLINIC VIA TELEPHONE

Equipment

Electrodes (e.g., finger, wrist, underarm)
Telephone
ECG transmitter
Magnet

Procedure

1. Arrange schedule of calls with nurse at pacemaker clinic.
2. Follow these steps when clinic calls.
   a. Place electrodes on the skin.
   b. Turn on ECG transmitter.
   c. Place telephone mouthpiece over transmitter's audio output. **Rationale:** This transmits a single-lead ECG pattern to a monitor in the clinic.
   d. Place the magnet over generator if requested by clinic technician to check pacemaker functioning. **Rationale:** This places the pacemaker in the fixed-rate mode to allow for reflection of pacemaker function.
3. Instruct client to contact physician if
   a. Pulse is 5 beats or more per minute less than before magnet use.
   b. ECG pattern is altered from baseline ECG on file in clinic.

INSTRUCTING IN USE OF HOLTER MONITOR

Equipment

Electrodes
Magnetic recorder
Shoulder strap or belt clip
Paper and pencil

Procedure

1. Explain that heart rate and rhythm is monitored during entire time monitor in place.The Holter monitor is used to obtain a continuous graphic tracing of a client's pulse while ADLs are performed.
2. Explain that Holter monitor will be in place 12–24 hours.
3. Place electrodes at both negative and positive poles, as directed by laboratory staff.
4. Assist client in strapping monitor in place.
5. Connect electrodes to recorder.
6. Instruct client to record any unusual pain, abnormal sign or symptom or activity, stating exact time. **Rationale:** All unusual pain, signs or symptoms or activity are evaluated with findings from ECG tape.
7. Explain to client that he or she can call the laboratory or clinic any time during the period the Holter monitor is in place if they have questions. Provide client with phone number of appropriate facility.
8. Instruct client to take recorder, strap, and paper documentation to laboratory as directed.

Bibliography

Abrams AC. *Clinical Drug Therapy: Rationales for Nursing Practice.* 3rd ed. Philadelphia: J. B. Lippincott; 1991.

Abrams WB, Berkow, R (eds). *The Merck Manual of Geriatrics.* Rahway, NJ: Merck Sharp & Dohme Research Laboratories; 1990.

Adelman E. When the patient's blood pressure falls. *Nursing87.* October 1987; 17(10):66–73.

Agee BL, Herman C. Cervical logrolling on a standard bed. *Am J Nurs.* March 1984; 84(3):318–320.

Aguilera D. *Crisis Intervention: Theory and Methodology.* 7th ed. St. Louis: C. V. Mosby; 1994.

Alfaro R. *Applying Nursing Diagnosis and Nursing Process.* 3rd ed. Philadelphia: J. B. Lippincott; 1994.

Alfaro-LeFevre, R. *Critical Thinking in Nursing: A Practical Approach.* Philadelphia: W.B. Saunders; 1995.

Alspach J, Williams S. *Core Curriculum for Critical Care Nursing.* 4th ed. Philadelphia: W. B. Saunders; 1991.

Alternative Medicine: Expanding Medical Horizons. A Report to the National Institute of Health, Workshop on Alternative Medicine. Chantilly, OR: US Government Printing Office; 1992.

Amas G. *The Rights of the Hospital Patients.* ACLU Handbook. New York: Avon Books, 1975.

American College of Chest Physicians and American Thoracic Society Joint Committee on Pulmonary Nomenclature. Pulmonary terms and symbols. *Chest.* 1975; 67:583–593.

American Nurses' Association. *The Nursing Practice Act: Suggested State Legislation.* 1981.

Anderson F, Maloney J. Taking blood pressure correctly: It's no off-the-cuff matter. *Nursing94.* November 1994; 24(11):34–39.

Anderson K, Anderson L. *Mosby's Medicine, Nursing, and Allied Health Dictionary.* 4th ed. St. Louis: C. V. Mosby; 1994.

Anderson M, Braun JV. *Caring for the Elderly Client.* Philadelphia; F.A. Davis Company; 1995.

Anderson RD. *Legal Boundaries of California Nursing Practice.* 4th ed. Sacramento: R. D. Anderson; 1988.

Arbour R. Weaning a patient from a ventilator. *Nursing93.* 23(2):52.

Ashworth L. Pressure support ventilation. *Crit Care Nurs.* July/August 1990; 10(7):20–25.

Babcock D. *Client Education: Theory & Practice.* St. Louis: C. V. Mosby; 1994.

Ball J, Bindler R. *Pediatric Nursing.* Norwalk, CT: Appleton & Lange; 1995.

Bandman E, Bandman B. *Critical Thinking in Nursing.* 2nd ed. Norwalk CT: Appleton and Lange; 1995.

Baranowski I. Central venous access devices: Current technologies, uses and management strategies. *J Intravenous Nurs.* May–June 1993; 16:167–194.

Barnard MU, et al. *Human Sexuality for Health Professionals.* Philadelphia: W. B. Saunders; 1978.

Barnes H. Alternating transparent and hydrocolloid dressings. *Nursing93.* March 1993; 23(3):59–61.

Barkauskas VH, Stoltenberg-Allen K, Baumann LC, Darling-Fisher C. *Health and Physical Assessment.* St. Louis: C. V. Mosby; 1994.

Barrick B. Light at the end of a decade. *Am J Nurs.* November 1990; 90(11):37–40.

Basmajian JV (ed). *Biofeedback: Principles and Practice for Clinicians.* 3rd ed. Baltimore: Williams & Wilkins; 1989.

Bates B. *A Guide to Physical Examination.* 5th ed. Philadelphia: J. B. Lippincott; 1991.

Beare P, Myers J. *Principles and Practices of Adult Health Nursing,* 2nd ed. St. Louis: C. V. Mosby; 1994.

Behrman R, Vaughn V. *Nelson Textbook of Pediatrics.* 13th ed. Philadelphia: W. B. Saunders; 1987.

Beiderman RP. Seeking the Rational Alternative: The National College of Chiropractic 1906 to 1982. Chiropractic History, 1983; 3:17.

Bellack JP, Bamford PA. *Nursing Assessment and Diagnosis.* 2nd ed. Boston: Jones & Barlett; 1992.

Benson H. *The Relaxation Response.* New York: Times Books, 1984.

Benson H. *Beyond the Relaxation Response.* New York: Times Books, 1984.

Bergmann TF, Peterson PH, Lawrence DJ. *Chiropractic Techniques.* Vol. 5. Livingstone, NY: Churchill; 1993.

Bernstein L, et al. *Primary Care in the Home.* Philadelphia: J. B. Lippincott; 1987.

Black J, Matassarin-Jacobs E. *Luckmann and Sorensen's Medical–Surgical Nursing.* 4th ed. Philadelphia: Saunders; 1993.

Bloom BS, ed. *Taxonomy of Educational Objectives, Handbook I: Cognitive Domain.* New York: David McKay; 1956.

Bobak I. *Maternity and Gynecologic Care: The Nurse and the Family.* 5th ed. St. Louis: C. V. Mosby; 1993.

Bockus S. Troubleshooting your tube feedings. *Am J Nurs.* May 1991; 91(5):24–28.

Bodinski L. *The Nurses' Guide to Diet Therapy.* 2nd ed. Albany: Delmar; 1987.

Boggs R, Wooldridge-King M (eds). *Critical Care Procedures Performance Evaluation.* Philadelphia: W. B. Saunders; 1993.

Bolander V. *Sorenson and Luckmann's Basic Nursing: A Psychophysiologic Approach.* 3rd ed. Philadelphia: W. B. Saunders; 1994.

Bolgiano CS, Bunting K, Shoenberger MM. Administering oxygen therapy: What you need to know. *Nursing90.* June 1990; 20(6):47–51.

Bolton P. Understanding modes of mechanical ventilation. *Am J Nurs.* June 1994; 94(6):36–43.

Boltz M. Identifying cardiac rhythms. *Nursing94.* April 1994; 24(4):54–58.

Bordick K. *Patterns of Shock: Implications for Nursing Care.* New York: Macmillan; 1980.

Boyer MJ. *Math for Nurses: A Pocket Guide to Dosage Calculations and Drug Preparations.* 3rd ed. Philadelphia: J. B. Lippincott; 1994.

Brallier L. *Successfully Managing Stress.* Los Altos, CA: National Nursing Review; 1982.

Braun A. Defibrillation or cardioversion. *Nursing91.* July 1991; 21(7):50–54.

Brennan B. *Hands of Light.* New York: Bantam Books; 1987.

Brighton CT, Pollack SR (eds). *Electromagnetics in Medicine and Biology.* San Francisco: San Francisco Press, Inc; 1991.

Brooten DN, et al. *Leadership for Change: An Action Guide for Nurses.* 2nd ed. Philadelphia: J. B. Lippincott; 1988.

Brower R. The alternatives to restraints. *J Gerontol Nurs:* 1991; 17(2):18–22.

Brown B. *New Mind, New Body.* New York: Harper & Row, 1982.

Brown B. *Stress and the Art of Biofeedback.* New York: Harper & Row, 1977.

Brown KR, Jacobson S. Interpreting ECG tracings. *Nursing90.* September 1990; 20(9).

Brungardt G. Patient restraints: New guidelines for a less restrictive approach. *Geriatrics.* 1994; 49(6):43–50.

Bryant R. *Acute and Chronic Wounds.* St. Louis: C. V. Mosby Co; 1992.

Burgess AW, Lazare A. *Psychiatric Nursing in the Hospital and the Community.* 5th ed. Norwalk: Appleton & Lange; 1990.

Buttaro M. Staying on top of transdermal drug patches. *Nursing94.* November 1994; 24(11):41–44.

Cahill M, McVan B. *Patient Teaching.* Springhouse: Springhouse, PA; 1987.

Camp D, Otten N. How to insert and remove nasogastric tubes quickly and easily. *Nursing90.* September 1990; 20(9):59–64.

Campbell CD, Newsome JA. Detecting life-threatening arrhythmias. *Nursing90.* December 1990; 20(12):34–39.

Cannon WB. *Bodily Changes in Pain, Hunger, Fear, and Rage: An Account of Recent Researches into the Function of Emotional Excitement.* New York: D. Appleton and Co; 1929.

Cannon WB. *The Wisdom of the Body.* New York: Norton; 1942.

Carnevali D, Patrick M. *Nursing Management for the Elderly.* 3rd ed. Philadelphia: J. B. Lippincott; 1993.

Carpenito LJ. *Nursing Care Plans and Documentation.* 2nd ed. Philadelphia: J. B. Lippincott; 1995.

Carpenito L. *Nursing Diagnosis: Application to Clinical Practice.* 6th ed. Philadelphia: J.B. Lippincott; 1995.

Carroll P. A med/surg nurse's guide to mechanical ventilation. *RN Magazine.* February 1995; 58(2):26–31.

Carroll P. Lowering the risks of endotracheal suctioning. *Nursing88.* 1988; 18(5):46–50.

Carroll P. Safe suctioning. *RN Magazine.* May 1994; 57(5):32–36.

Carroll P. The right way to do chest physiotherapy. *RN Magazine.* May 1987; 50(5):26–29.

Chernecky C. *Laboratory Tests and Diagnostic Procedures.* W. B. Saunders; 1993.

Christianson D. Caring for a patient who has an implanted venous port. *Am J Nurs.* November 1994; 94(11):40–44.

Cobb MD. Dealing fairly with medication errors. *Nursing90.* March 1990; 20(3):42–43.

Conway B. *Carini and Owens' Neurological and Neurosurgical Nursing.* 8th ed. St. Louis: C. V. Mosby; 1982.

Corbett J. *Laboratory Tests and Diagnostic Procedures with Nursing Diagnoses.* 3rd ed. Norwalk, CT: Appleton & Lange; 1992.

Creighton H. *Law Every Nurse Should Know.* 5th ed. Philadelphia: W. B. Saunders; 1986.

Cuzzell J. Back to basics: Test your wound assessment skills. *Am J Nurs.* June 1994; 94(6):34–35.

Dabbs A, Kline L. The new modes of mechanical ventilation. *Am J Nurs.* 1994; 94(8):42–45.

Daily EK, Schroeder JS. *Techniques in Bedside Hemodynamic Monitoring.* 5th ed. St. Louis: C. V. Mosby; 1994.

Darovic G. *Hemodynamic Monitoring: Invasive and Non-Invasive Clinical Application.* Philadelphia: W. B. Saunders; 1987.

Dennison R. Making sense of hemodynamic monitoring. *Am J Nurs.* 1994; 94(8):24–31.

Doenges M, Moorhouse M. *Nurse's Pocket Guide: Nursing Diagnosis with Interventions.* 4th ed. Philadelphia: F. A. Davis; 1993.

Doenges M, et al. *Nursing Care Plans: Guidelines for Planning Patient Care.* 3rd ed. Philadelphia: F. A. Davis; 1993.

Dolan JT. *Critical Care Nursing: Clinical Management through the Nursing Process.* Philadelphia: F. A. Davis; 1991.

Dossey B. A wonderful prerequisite—Relaxation. *Nursing84.* January 1984; 14(1):97–99.

Duke University Hospital Nursing Services. *Guidelines for Nursing Care: Process and Outcome.* Philadelphia: J. B. Lippincott; 1983.

Dunston J. How managed care can work for you. *Nursing90.* October 1990; 20(10):56–59.

Ebersole P, Hess P. *Toward Healthy Aging.* 4th ed. St. Louis: C. V. Mosby Co; 1994.

Eggland E. *Nursing Documentation: Charting, Recording, and Reporting.* Philadelphia: Lippincott; 1994.

Ehrhardt BS, Graham M. Pulse oximetry: An easy way to check oxygen saturation. *Nursing90.* March 1990; 20(3):50–54.

Eisenberg P. Gastronomy and jejunostomy tubes. *RN Magazine.* November 1994; 57(11):54–59.

Eisenberg P. Nasoenteral tubes. *RN Magazine.* October 1994; 57(10):62–69.

Elder AN. Setting up and using a cardiac monitor. *Nursing91.* March 1991; 21(3):58–63.

Eliopoulos C. *Caring for the Elderly in Diverse Care Settings.* Philadelphia: J. B. Lippincott; 1990.

Eliopoulos C. *Gerontological Nursing.* 3rd ed. Philadelphia: J. B. Lippincott; 1993.

Ellstrom K, DellaBella L. Understanding your role during a code. *Nursing90.* May 1990; 20(5):37–43.

Erickson EH. *Childhood and Society.* New York: W. W. Norton; 1963.

Erickson R. Accuracy of infrared ear thermometry and traditional temperature methods in young children. *Heart Lung.* May–June 1994; 23(3):181–195.

Erwin-Toth P. Wound care: Selecting the right dressing. *Am J Nurs.* February 1995; 95(2):46–51.

Evaluation and Management of Early HIV Infection. US Department of Health and Human Services. January 1994; Number 7. AHCPR Publication No. 94-0572.

Fagerhough SY, Strauss A. How to manage your patient's pain . . . and how not to. *Nursing80.* February 1980. From *Politics of Pain Management: Staff-Patient Interaction.* Fagerhough SY, Strauss A. Menlo Park: Addison-Wesley; 1977.

Farrell J. *Illustrated Guide to Orthopedic Nursing.* 3rd ed. Philadelphia: J. B. Lippincott; 1988.

Ferland P. Are you ready for ventilator patients? *Nursing91.* January 1991; 21(1):42–47.

Fischbach F. *A Manual of Laboratory Diagnostic Tests.* 4th ed. Philadelphia: J. B. Lippincott; 1994.

Fisher J. What you need to know about neurological testing. *RN Magazine.* January 1987; 50(1).

Flynn J, Bruce N. *Introduction to Critical Care Skills.* St. Louis: C. V. Mosby Co; 1993.

Food and Nutrition Board, National Research Council—National Academy of Sciences. *Recommended Dietary Allowances.* Washington, DC; 1990.

Fowler E, et al. Healing with hydrocolloid. *Am J Nurs.* February 1991; 21(2).

Frohmagen J. *Current Management of Wounds.* Cabrillo College Syllabus, Level I. 1992.

Gahart B. *Intravenous Medications: A Handbook for Nurses and Allied Health Professionals.* 11th ed. St. Louis: C. V. Mosby; 1995.

Gallagher M, Kahn C. Lasers: Scalpels of light. *RN Magazine.* May 1990; 53(5):46–52.

Gerber R. *Vibrational Medicine—New Choices for Healing Ourselves.* Claremont, CA: Bear & Co. Publishing; 1988.

Goleman D, Gurin J. *Mind-Body Medicine.* Yonkers, NY: Consumers Union of United States, Inc; 1993.

Gordon M. *Manual of Nursing Diagnosis 1995–1996.* St. Louis: C. V. Mosby; 1995.

Green E, Green A. *Beyond Biofeedback.* New York: Dell Publishing Co., Inc; 1978.

Green L, Gerlach CJ. Central lines have moved out. *RN Magazine.* May 1994; 57(5):26–30.

Guidelines for Isolation Precautions in Hospitals: Part I: Evolution of Isolation Practices and Part II: Recommendations for Isolation Precautions in Hospital (draft). Centers for Disease Control and Prevention. Federal Register. 59(214) Nov 7, 1994: 55552-55568.

Guido G. *Legal Issues in Nursing: A Source Book for Practice.* Norwalk, CT: Appleton & Lange; 1988.

Guthrie HA. *Introductory Nutrition.* 7th ed. St. Louis: C. V. Mosby; 1988.

Guyton AC. *Textbook of Medical Physiology.* 8th ed. Philadelphia: W. B. Saunders; 1990.

Guyton-Simmons J, Ehrmin J. Problem solving pain management by expert intensive care nurses. *Crit Care Nurs.* October 1994; 14(5):37–44.

Haber J, et al. *Comprehensive Psychiatric Nursing.* 4th ed. New York: McGraw-Hill; 1992.

Hagle M, McDonagh L, Rapp C. Patients with long-term vascular access devices: Care and complications. *Orthoped Nurs.* September/October 1994; 13(5):41–51.

Hahn K. Teaching patients to administer insulin. *Nursing90.* April 1990; 20(4):70.

Hall L. Cardiovascular lasers: A look into the future. *Am J Nurs.* July 1990; 90(7):27–30.

Hambleton N. Dealing with complication of epidural analgesia. *Nursing94.* October 1994; 24(10):55–57.

Harovas J, Anthony H. Your guide to trouble-free transfusions. *RN Magazine.* November 1993; 56(11):27–34.

Hays JS, Larson K. *Interacting with Patients.* New York: Macmillan; 1965.

Henrickson M. How to access an implanted port. *Nursing93.* January 1993; 23(1):50–53.

Hersen M, ed. *The Clinical Psychology Handbook.* New York: Pergamon Press; 1983.

Hill MN, Grim CM. How to take a precise blood pressure. *Am J Nurs.* February 1991; 91(2):38–42.

Hoffmann K, et al. Transparent polyurethane film as an intravenous catheter dressing. *JAMA.* April 1992; 267(15):2072–2076.

Holloway NM. *Nursing the Critically Ill Adult.* 4th ed. Menlo Park: Addison-Wesley; 1993.

Holmes TH, Rahe RH. Social readjustment rating scale. *J Psychosom Res.* 1967; 11:213.

Hudak, CM, et al. *Critical Care Nursing: A Holistic Approach.* 6th ed. Philadelphia: J. B. Lippincott; 1994.

Humphrey C. *Home Care Nursing Handbook.* 2nd ed. Aspen; 1994.

Ignatavicius D, Bayne M. *Medical-Surgical Nursing: A Nursing Process Approach.* 2nd ed. Philadelphia: W. B. Saunders; 1995.

Illustrated Manual of Nursing Practice. 2nd ed. Springhouse: Springhouse; 1994.

Ilyer P, Camp N. *Nursing Documentation: A Nursing Process Approach.* St. Louis: C. V. Mosby; 1991.

Iyer P, et al. *Nursing Process and Nursing Diagnoses.* 2nd ed. Philadelphia: W. B. Saunders; 1991.

Jacobs B. Working on the right move. *Nursing94.* October 1994; 24(10):58–62.

Jarvis C. *Physical Examination and Health Assessment.* Philadelphia: W. B. Saunders Co; 1992.

Jones L, Brooks J. The ABCs of PCA. *RN Magazine.* 1990; 53(5):54–60.

Jubeck M. Teaching the elderly: A commonsense approach. *Nursing94.* May 1994; 24(5):70–71.

Kaufman J. Assessing the 12 cranial nerves. *Nursing90.* June 1990; 20(6):56–58.

Katzung BG. *Basic and Clinical Pharmacology.* 3rd ed. Norwalk, CT: Appleton & Lange; 1987.

Keddington R. Emergency cardiac care: New pediatric guidelines. *RN Magazine.* May 1994; 57(5):44–51.

Kee J. *Laboratory and Diagnostic Tests with Nursing Implications.* 4th ed. Norwalk, CT: Appleton & Lange; 1995.

Kee J. *Pharmacology: Nursing Process Approach.* Philadelphia: W. B. Saunders; 1993.

Keen MF. Get on the right track with Z-track injections. *Nursing90.* August 1990; 20(8):59.

Kelly A. Human immunodeficiency virus: Current trends in assessment, diagnosis, and treatment. *J Intravenous Ther.* March/April 1994; 17(2):83–92.

Kemp MG. Troubleshooting ostomy problems. *Geriatr Nurs.* September/October 1990; 11(5):233–236.

Kestel F. Using blood glucose meters: What you and your patient need to know. *Nursing93.* March 1993; 23(3):34–41.

Kim MJ, et al, eds. *Pocket Guide to Nursing Diagnosis.* 6th ed. St. Louis: C. V. Mosby; 1995.

Kinkade S, Lehrman J. *Critical Care Nursing Procedures: A Team Approach.* St. Louis: C. V. Mosby; 1990.

Kinney MR, et al. AACN's *Clinical Reference for Critical-Care Nursing.* 3rd ed. St. Louis: C. V. Mosby; 1993.

Kohr J. Measuring your patient's pain. *RN Magazine.* April, 1995; 58(4):39–40.

Konstantinides N. The impact of nutrition on wound healing. *Crit Care Nurs.* October 1993; 13(5):25–33.

Kozier B, Erb G, Olivieri R. *Fundamentals of Nursing: Concepts, Process and Practice.* 4th ed. Redwood City, CA: Addison-Wesley; 1991.

Kozier B, et al. *Techniques in Clinical Nursing.* 4th ed. Redwood City, CA: Addison-Wesley; 1993.

Krasner D. *Chronic Wound Care.* King of Prussia, PA: Health Management Publications; 1990.

Krasner D. The 12 commandments of wound care. *Nursing92.* December 1992; 22(12):34–41.

Krasner D. What's wrong with this stoma? *Am J Nurs.* 1990; 90(4):46–47.

Krasner D. Wound care: How to use the red-yellow-black system. *Am J Nurs.* May 1995; 95(5):44–47.

Krupp MA, et al. *Physician's Handbook.* 21st ed. Norwalk, CT: Appleton & Lange; 1985.

Kubler-Ross E. *On Death and Dying.* New York: Macmillan Publishing Company, Inc.; 1993.

Lammon C, et al. *Clinical Nursing Skills.* Philadelphia: Saunders; 1995.

Kuhar PA, Hill KM. White clot syndrome: When heparin goes haywire. *Am J Nurs.* March 1991; 91(3):59–60.

Leckrone L. Preparing your patient for surgery. *Nursing91.* July 1991; 21(7):46–49.

Lederer J, et al. *Care Planning Pocket Guide: A Nursing Diagnosis Approach.* 3rd ed. Menlo Park: Addison-Wesley; 1991.

Lenox AC. IV therapy: Reducing the risk of infection. *Nursing90.* March 1990; 20(3):60–61.

Lepler M. HIV guidelines inform nonspecialists. *Nurseweek.* March 1994; 7(5):7–20.

Lewis L, Timby B. Fundamental Skills and Concepts in Patient Care. 4th ed. Philadelphia: J. B. Lippincott Company; 1988.

Lewis SM, Collier IC. *Medical-Surgical Nursing: Assessment and Management of Critical Problems.* 3rd ed. New York: McGraw-Hill; 1992.

Liberman J. *Light—Medicine of the Future.* Claremont, CA: Bear & Co. Publishing; 1988.

Lorenz BL. Are you using the right IV pump? *RN Magazine.* May 1990; 53(5):31–36.

Lorenzo L. Making codes as easy as ABC . . . CD. *Nursing91.* 1991; 21(2).

Lovell H, Anderson C. Put your patient on the right bed. *RN Magazine.* May 1990; 53(5):66–72.

Lueckenotte AG. *Pocket Guide to Gerontologic Assessment.* 2nd ed. St. Louis: C. V. Mosby; 1994.

Luckmann J, Black J, Sorensen KC. *Medical-Surgical Nursing: A Psychophysiologic Approach.* 4th ed. Philadelphia: W. B. Saunders; 1993.

Maier P. Taking the work out of range-of-motion exercises. *RN Magazine.* September 1986; 49(9).

Malasanos L, et al. *Health Assessment.* 4th ed. St. Louis: C. V. Mosby; 1989.

Managing Early HIV Infection. U.S. Department of Health and Human Services. January 1994. Number 7. AHCPR Publication No. 94-0573.

Maran J, Monroe M. Pulmonary laser therapy. *Am J Nurs.* 1988; 88(6):828–831.

Marlow DR, Redding B. *Textbook of Pediatric Nursing.* 6th ed. Philadelphia: W. B. Saunders; 1988.

Masoorli S, Angeles T. PICC lines: The latest home care challenge. *RN Magazine.* January 1990; 53(1):44–51.

Mathews J. How to use an automated vital signs monitor. *Nursing91.* February 1991; 21(2).

McAfee T, Garland LR, McNabb TS. How to safely draw blood from a vascular access device. *Nursing90.* November 1990; 20(11):42–44.

McCaffery M, Beebe A. *Pain: Clinical Manual for Nursing Practice.* St. Louis: C. V. Mosby Co; 1989.

McCance K, Huether S. *Pathophysiology: The Biologic Basis for Disease in Adults and Children.* 2nd ed. St. Louis: C. V. Mosby; 1994.

McConnell E. Clinical do's and don'ts: Assessing an arteriovenous fistula. *Nursing95.* February 1995; 25(2):22.

McDonagh A. Getting your patient ready for a nuclear medicine scan. *Nursing91.* February 1991; 21(2).

McFarland G, et al. *Nursing Leadership and Management: Contemporary Strategies.* Albany: Delmar; 1984.

McFarland MB, Grant MM. *Nursing Implications of Laboratory Tests.* 2nd ed. New York: John Wiley; 1988.

McFarland MB. *Nursing Diagnosis Theory and Practice.* 2nd ed. St. Louis: C. V. Mosby; 1993.

McKenry F. *Mosby's Pharmacology in Nursing.* 17th ed. St. Louis: C. V. Mosby; 1989.

Meares C. P.I.C.C. and M.L.C. lines: Options worth exploring. *Nursing92.* 1992; 22(10):52–55.

Mehler E. Preparing your patient to use a fecal occult blood test. *Nursing94.* May 1994; 24(5):XX–XX.

Meissner J. Measuring patient stress with the hospital stress rating scale. *Nursing80.* August 1980; 43(8).

Metheny N. *Fluid and Electrolyte Balance: Nursing Considerations.* 2nd ed. Philadelphia: J.B. Lippincott Co.; 1992.

Mezzanotte J. A checklist for better discharge planning. *Nursing87.* October 1987; 17(10):82–83.

Millam DA. Controlling the flow: electronic infusion devices. *Nursing90.* August 1990; 20(8):65–68.

Millam D. Tips on improving your venipuncture techniques. *Nursing87.* June 1987; 17(6).

Millar S. *Procedure Manual for Critical Care: The AACN Manual.* 2nd ed. Philadelphia: W. B. Saunders; 1985.

Miller D, Miller H. A nurse's guide to tube feeding. *RN Magazine.* January 1995; 58(1):49–51.

Miller LA. At-home help for the CAPD patient. *RN Magazine.* August 1990; 53(8):77–80.

Miracle V, Allnutt D. Using a manual resuscitator correctly. *Nursing90.* May 1990; 20(5):49–51.

Monroe D. Patient teaching for x-ray and other diagnostics. *RN Magazine.* April 1990; 53(4):52–56.

Morrissey BG. *Quick Reference to Therapeutic Nutrition.* Philadelphia: J. B. Lippincott; 1984.

Morton P. Health Assessment. In: *Nursing.* 2nd ed. Springhouse, PA: Springhouse; 1993.

Motta G. Dressed for success: How moisture-retentive dressings promote healing. *Nursing93.* December 1993; 23(12):26–33.

Muma R, et al. *HIV Manual for Health Care Professionals.* Norwalk, CT: Appleton & Lange; 1994.

Murphy J, Burke LJ. Charting by exception: a more efficient way to document. *Nursing90.* May 1990; 20(5):65–69.

Murray SM, Thompson R. We've organized our approach to pressure sores. *RN Magazine.* January 1991; 54(1):42–44.

NANDA Classification of Nursing. 10th Conference. Philadelphia: J. B. Lippincott; 1994.

Narrow BW. *Patient Teaching in Nursing Practice, a Patient and Family-Centered Approach.* New York: John Wiley; 1979.

National Research Council. *Diet and Health: Implications for Reducing Chronic Disease Risk.* Washington: National Academy Press, 1989.

Newton M, Newton D, Fudin J. Reviewing the "Big Three" injection routes. *Nursing92.* February 1992; 22(2):34–41.

Noah V. Preop teaching is the key to PCA success. *RN Magazine.* May 1990; 53(5):60–63.

North American Nursing Diagnosis Association. *Classification of Nursing Diagnoses.* 1995.

O'Connor ME, Bentall RHC, Monahan JC (eds). *Emerging Electromagnetic Medicine.* Conference Proceedings. New York: Springer Verlag; 1990.

Olsson GL, Leddo CC, Wild L. Nursing management of patients receiving epidural narcotics. *Heart Lung.* March 1989; 18(2):130–136.

Orque M, et al. *Ethnic Nursing Care: A Multi Cultural Approach.* St. Louis: C. V. Mosby; 1983.

Pagana K, Pagana T. *Diagnostic Testing and Nursing Implications.* 4th ed. St. Louis: C. V. Mosby; 1994.

Peplau H. Talking with patients. *Am J Nurs.* 1960.

Phipps W, Cassmeyer V, Sands J, Lehman M (eds). *Medical-Surgical Nursing. Concepts and Clinical Practice.* 5th ed. St. Louis: C. V. Mosby Co; 1995.

Physician's Desk Reference to Pharmaceutical Specialties and Biologicals. Oradell: Medical Economics; 1995.

Pinderman M. Indwelling urinary catheters: Reducing infection risks. *Nursing94.* September 1994; 24(9):66–68.

Plankey ED, Knauf J. What patients need to know about magnetic resonance imaging. *Am J Nurs.* January 1991; 91(1):27–28.

Plumer A. *Principles and Practice of Intravenous Therapy.* 4th ed. Boston: Little, Brown and Company; 1987.

Poleman C, Peckenpough N. *Nutrition: Essentials and Diet Therapy.* 6th ed. Philadelphia: W. B. Saunders; 1991.

Potter P. *Basic Nursing: Theory and Practice.* 3rd ed. St. Louis: C. V. Mosby; 1995.

Potter P, *Pocket Nurse Guide to Physical Assessment.* 3rd ed. St. Louis: C. V. Mosby; 1994.

Pressure Ulcers in Adults: Prediction and Prevention. U.S Department of Health and Human Services. May 1992. AHCPR Publication No. 92-0047.

Price S, Wilson L. *Pathophysiology: Clinical Concepts of Disease Processes.* 3rd ed. New York: McGraw-Hill; 1986.

Querin J, Stahl L. 12 simple sensible steps for successful blood transfusions. *Nursing90.* October 1990; 20(10):68–81.

Questions and answers about blood transfusions. *Nursing95.* February 1995; 25(2):32c–32d.

Radcliff R. *Calculations of Drug Dosages.* 4th ed. St. Louis: C. V. Mosby; 1990.

Raimer F. How to identify electrolyte imbalances on your patient's ECG. *Nursing94.* June 1994; 24(6):54–58.

Raffensperger EB, et al. *Clinical Nursing Handbook.* Philadelphia: J. B. Lippincott; 1986.

Rankin S, Stallings KD. *Patient Education.* 2nd ed. Philadelphia: J. B. Lippincott; 1990.

Ratto T. The Truth About Protein. *Med SelfCare.* Nov–Dec 1986.

Redman BK. *The Process of Patient Education.* 7th ed. St. Louis: C. V. Mosby; 1993.

Reeder S, et al. *Maternity Nursing.* 17th ed. Philadelphia: J. B. Lippincott; 1992.

Reilly N, Torosian L. The new wave in lithotripsy: Implications for nursing. *RN Magazine.* March 1988; 51(3):44–49.

Renkes J. GI: endoscopy: Managing the full scope of care. *Nursing93.* June 1993; 23(6):50–55.

Reusch J. *Therapeutic Communication.* New York: W. W. Norton; 1961.

Rice R. *Home Health Nursing Practice: Concepts and Applications.* St. Louis: C. V. Mosby; 1992.

Rice R. *Manual of Home Health Nursing Procedures.* St. Louis: C. V. Mosby; 1995.

Rodts B, Meister S. Infection control takes top priority. *RN Magazine.* December 1990; 53(12):59–62.

Rovinski C, Zastocki D. *Home Care: A Technical Manual for the Professional Nurse.* Philadelphia: W. B. Saunders; 1989.

Rubenfeld MG, Scheffer BK. *Critical Thinking in Nursing: An Interactive Approach.* Philadelphia, PA: J. B. Lippincott Co.; 1995.

Saltman P, Gurin J, Mothner I. *The California Nutrition Book: A Food Guide for the '90s From Faculty at the University of California and the Editors of American Health.* Boston: Little, Brown and Company; 1987.

Samuels M. *Healing With the Mind's Eye.* New York: Random House; 1992.

Sanderson R, Kurth C. *The Cardiac Patient, a Comprehensive Approach.* 3rd ed. Philadelphia: W. B. Saunders; 1983.

Satir V. *Conjoint Family Theory.* Palo Alto: Science & Behavior Books; 1967.

Saul L. Arrhythmia mimics. *Am J Nurs.* March 1991; 91(3):40–43.

Scherer JC. *Introductory Clinical Pharmacology.* 4th ed. Philadelphia: J. B. Lippincott; 1992.

Scherer P. How HIV attacks the peripheral nervous system. *Am J Nurs.* May 1990; 90(5):66–70.

Schlafer M. *The Nurse, Pharmacology, and Drug Therapy.* 2nd ed. Redwood City, CA: Addison-Wesley; 1993.

Schroeder J, Daily E. *Techniques in Bedside Hemodynamic Monitoring.* St. Louis: C. V. Mosby; 1985.

Schroeder SA, et al. *Current Medical Diagnosis and Treatment 1991.* 30th ed. Norwalk: Appleton & Lange; 1990.

Schultheis A. When and how to extubate in the recovery room. *Am J Nurs.* 1989; 89(8):1040–1045.

Schweisguth D. Setting up a cardiac monitor without missing a beat. *Nursing88.* 1988; 18(11):43–49.

Scipien G, et al. *Comprehensive Pediatric Nursing.* 4th ed. New York: McGraw-Hill; 1989.

Seidel H, et al. *Mosby's Guide to Physical Examination.* 2nd ed. St. Louis: C. V. Mosby; 1990.

Selye H. *Stress Without Distress.* New York: Signet; 1974.

Selye H. *The Stress of Life.* New York: McGraw-Hill; 1965.

Sergeant L. Tracking your outpatient's EKG with a Holter monitor. *Nursing86.* October 1986; 49(10).

Sheehy SB. *Emergency Nursing: Principles and Practices.* 3rd ed. St. Louis: C. V. Mosby; 1992.

Shils ME, Coiro D. *Nutrition Assessment of the Cancer Patient: Report of a Pilot Study.* New York: Memorial Sloan Kettering Cancer Center; 1990.

Silver HK, et al. *Handbook of Pediatrics.* 15th ed. Norwalk: Appleton & Lange; 1987.

Simonton OC, Matthews-Simonton S, Creighton J. *Getting Well Again.* Los Angeles: J.P. Tareher, Inc.; 1978.

Smeltzer S. *Brunner and Suddarth's Textbook of Medical–Surgical Nursing.* 7th ed. Philadelphia: Lippincott; 1992.

Sloane P. Alternatives to physical and pharmacologic restraints in long-term care. *Am Fam Physician.* February 1992; p. 763–769.

Smith D, et al. *Comprehensive Child and Family Nursing Skills.* St. Louis. Mosby Year-Book; 1991.

Smith RN, et al. Underwater chest drainage: Bringing the facts to surface. *Nursing95.* February 1995; 25(2):60–63.

Smith R. A nurse's guide to implanted ports. *RN Magazine.* April 1993; 56(4):48–52.

Smith S, Smith C. *Personal Health Choices.* Boston: Jones and Bartlett; 1990.

Smith S. *Sandra Smith's Review of Nursing for NCLEX-RN.* 8th ed. Los Altos, CA: National Nursing Review; 1994.

Smith-Temple I. *Nurses' Guide to Clinical Procedures.* 2nd ed. Philadelphia: Lippincott; 1994.

Snowberger P. Premature ventricular contractions. *RN Magazine.* October 1994; 57(10):59–61.

Sorenson KC, Luckmann J. *Basic Nursing: A Psychophysiologic Approach.* 2nd ed. Philadelphia: W. B. Saunders; 1986.

Sparks S, Taylor C. *Nursing Diagnosis Reference Manual.* 3rd ed. Springhouse, PA: Springhouse Corp; 1995.

Spradley B. *Community Health Nursing: Concepts and Practice.* 3rd ed. Boston: Little, Brown; 1989.

Springhouse Corporation. *Normal & Abnormal Heart Sounds.* Springhouse, PA: Springhouse Corp; 1990.

Spyr J, Preac MA. Pulse oximetry: Understanding the concept, knowing the limits. *RN Magazine.* May 1990; 53(5):38–43.

Stanford University Medical Center, Department of Anesthesia. Epidural narcotic analgesia protocol. May 1988.

Stillman R. *A Lange Chemical Manual: Surgery Diagnosis and Therapy.* Norwalk, CT: Appleton & Lange; 1989/90.

Stotts N. Seeing red and yellow and black: The three color concepts of wound care. *Nursing90.* February 1990; 20(2):59–61.

Strowig S. Insulin therapy. *RN Magazine.* June, 1995; 58(6):30–36.

Stuart G, Sundeen S. *Principles and Practice of Psychiatric Nursing.* 5th ed. St. Louis: C. V. Mosby; 1995.

Suddarth D, Brunner LS. *Lippincott Manual of Nursing Practice.* 5th ed. Philadelphia: J. B. Lippincott; 1991.

Suitor CW, Hunter MF. *Nutrition: Principles and Application in Health Promotion.* 2nd ed. Philadelphia: J. B. Lippincott; 1984.

Sullivan-Marx E. Delirium and physical restraints in the hospitalized elderly. *Image Nurs Scholarship.* Winter 1994; 26(4):295–300.

Swackhamer A. Alternatives-complementary therapies. *RN Magazine.* January 1995; 58(1):49–51.

Swearington PL, ed. *Photo-Atlas of Nursing Procedures.* 2nd ed. Menlo Park: Addison-Wesley; 1991.

Swearington PL, et al. *Manual of Critical Care.* St. Louis: C. V. Mosby; 1988.

Tasota F, Wesmiller S. Assessing ABGs: Maintaining the delicate balance. *Nursing94.* May 1994; 24(5):34–45.

Thieh NH. *The Miracle of Mindfulness: A Manual on Meditation.* 2nd ed. Boston: Beacon; 1988.

Thompson J, et al. *Mosby's Manual of Clinical Nursing.* 3rd ed. St. Louis: C. V. Mosby; 1995.

Tiernan PJ. Independent nursing interventions: Relaxation and guided imagery in critical care. *Crit Care Nurs.* October 1994; 14(5):47–51.

Tomky D. Advances in monitoring. *RN Magazine.* March 1995; 58(3):38–44.

Transtracheal oxygen: The nose knows the difference. *Am J Nurs.* April 1987; 87(4):421–424.

Travelbee J. *Intervention in Psychiatric Nursing. Process in the One-to-One Relationship.* 2nd ed. Philadelphia: F. A. Davis; 1985.

Tucker SM, et al. *Patient Care Standards.* 5th ed. St. Louis: C. V. Mosby; 1992.

U.S. Department of Agriculture. *A Daily Food Guide: The Basic Four.* Rev. ed. Washington, DC: Government Printing Office; 1979.

US Department of Agriculture and US Department of Health and Human Services. *Food Guide Pyramid—A Guide to Daily Food Choices.* Washington, DC; 1992 USDA/HNIS.

US Department of Health and Human Services, Public Health Service. *Acute Pain Management: Operative or Medical Procedures and Trauma.* February 1992 Pub. no. 92-0032.

Urdang L, ed. *Mosby's Medical and Nursing and Allied Health Dictionary and Data Base.* St. Louis: C. V. Mosby; 1995.

Viall C. Taking the mystery out of TPN, Part I. *Nursing95.* April 1995; 25(4):34–41.

Viall C. Taking the mystery out of TPN, Part II. *Nursing95.* May 1995; 25(5):57–59.

Viall CD. Your complete guide to central venous catheters. *Nursing90.* February 1990; 20(2):34–41.

Wade J. *Respiratory Nursing Care: Physiology and Techniques.* 3rd ed. St. Louis: C. V. Mosby; 1982.

Walker J. *Psychiatric Emergencies: Intervention and Resolution.* Philadelphia: J. B. Lippincott; 1983.

Walsh J, et al. *Manual of Home Health Care Nursing.* Philadelphia: J. B. Lippincott; 1987.

Walsh SM, Banks LA. How to insert a small-bore feeding tube safely. *Nursing90.* March 1990; 20(3):55–59.

Way L. *Current Surgical Diagnosis and Treatment.* 9th ed. Menlo Park: Appleton & Lange; 1991.

Weber J. *Nurses' Handbook of Health Assessment.* 2nd ed. Philadelphia: J. B. Lippincott; 1993.

Wesmiller SW, Hoffman LA, Wiseman M. Understanding transtracheal oxygen delivery. *Nursing89.* December 1989; 19(12):43–47.

West BA. Understanding endorphins: Our natural pain relief system. *Nursing81.* February 1981; 11(2).

Wong D. *Whaley and Wong's Essentials of Pediatric Nursing.* 4th ed. St. Louis: C. V. Mosby; 1993.

Widmann F. *Clinical Interpretation of Laboratory Tests.* 10th ed. Philadelphia: F. A. Davis; 1989.

Wiggins MS, Sesin P. Guidelines for administering IV drugs. *Nursing90.* April 1990; 20(4):145–152.

Wilkinson J. *Nursing Process in Action: A Clinical Thinking Approach.* Redwood City, CA: Addison-Wesley; 1992.

Williams SR. *Nutrition and Diet Therapy.* 7th ed. St. Louis: C. V. Mosby; 1993.

Wills SL, Tremblay SF. *Critical Care Review for Nurses.* Monterey: Wadsworth Health Sciences Division; 1984.

Wilson HS, Kneisl CR. *Psychiatric Nursing.* 3rd ed. Menlo Park: Addison-Wesley; 1988.

Woods NF. *Human Sexuality in Health and Illness.* St. Louis: C. V. Mosby; 1983.

Yura H, Walsh MB. *The Nursing Process: Assessing, Planning, Implementing, Evaluating.* 5th ed. Norwalk, CT: Appleton & Lange, 1988.

Index

A

Page numbers followed by t refer to tables. Page numbers followed by f refer to figures.

C

E

F

G

H

M

N

O

P

Q

R

S

U

V

W

X

Y

Z